3. EYE

A. Gently wash eye immediately, using plenty of water (or milk in an emergency), for five minutes with eyelids held open.
B. Remove contact lenses if worn; never permit the eye to be rubbed.
C. Call physician, hospital, poison control center, or rescue unit, and transport victim to a medical facility promptly.

4. SKIN (acids, lye, other caustics, pesticides, etc.)

A. Wash off skin immediately with a large amount of water; use soap if available.
B. Remove any contaminated clothing.
C. Call physician, hospital, poison control center, or rescue unit, and transport victim to a medical facility if necessary.

5. POISONOUS BITES

A. SNAKES
   1. Don't let victim walk; keep him as quiet as possible.
   2. Do not give alcohol.
   3. Call physician, hospital, poison control center, or rescue unit, and transport victim promptly to a medical facility.

Enroute, or while awaiting transportation
   4. Apply suction to bite wound with mouth or suction cup.
   5. If victim stops breathing use artificial respiration.

B. INSECTS (Spiders, scorpions, or unusual reaction to other stinging insects such as bees, wasps, hornets, etc.)
   1. Do not let victim walk or exercise.
   2. Place any available cold substance on bite area to relieve pain.
   3. A paste of Adolph's® Meat Tenderizer applied to the bite will often reduce the swelling and itching by its enzymatic action.
   4. If victim stops breathing, use artificial respiration.
   5. Call physician, hospital, poison control center, or rescue unit, and transport victim promptly to a medical facility. (Persons with known unusual reactions to insect stings should carry emergency treatment kits and an emergency identity card).

C. ANIMAL BITES
Bat and skunk bites, and other unprovoked animal bites, may be from a rabid animal. Call physician or medical facility; wash wound gently but thoroughly with soap and water. Human bites, because of the infection which so often develops, can also be serious and should be treated in a similar fashion as the animal bite.

D. POISONOUS MARINE ANIMALS
Apply any cold substance to relieve pain. (For "sting ray," heat is better).
Call physician or medical facility if severe reaction.

Permission and courtesy of the American Academy of Pediatrics, Inc., Evanston, Illinois, U.S.A. (with modifications)

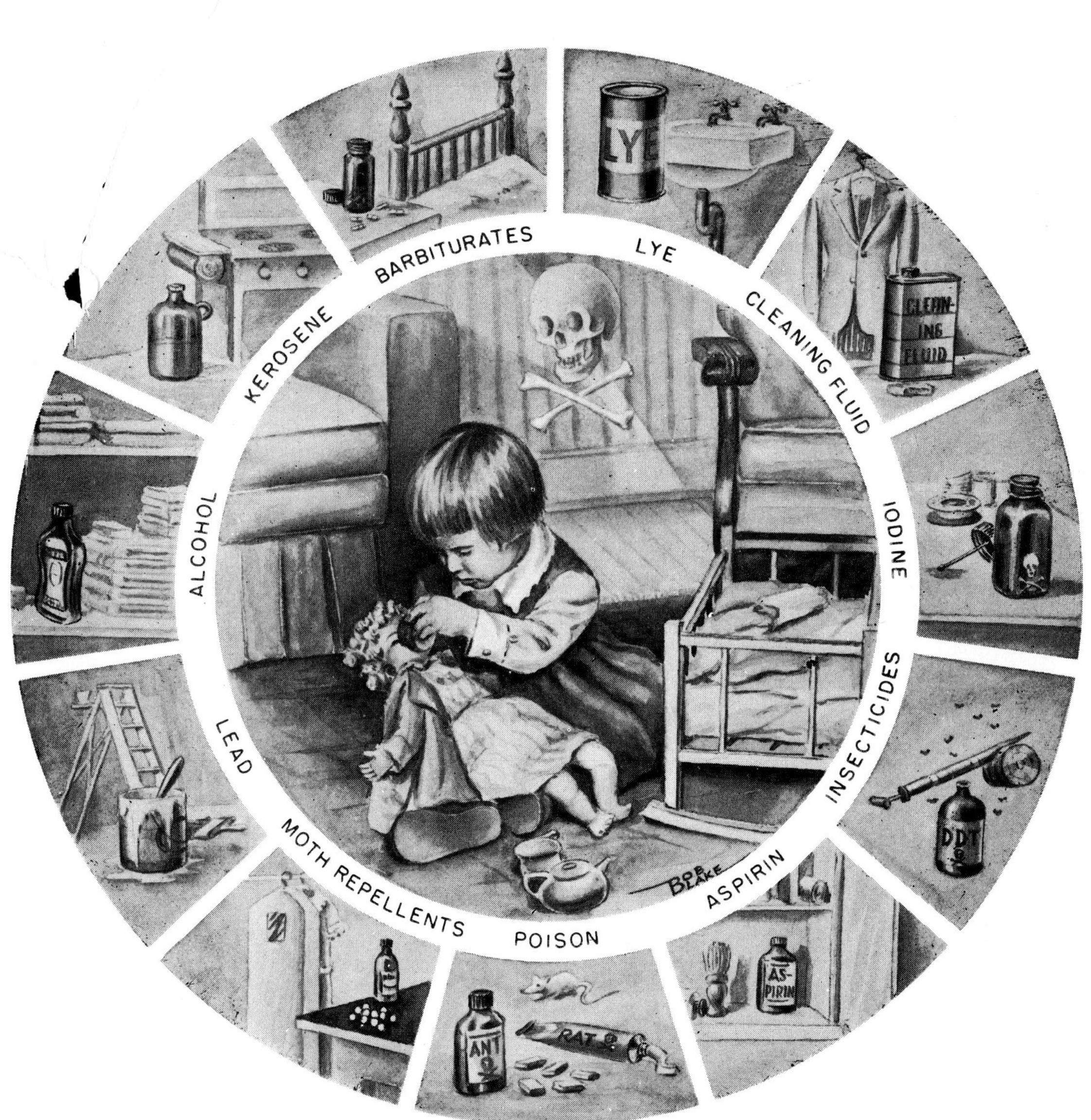
BARBITURATES
LYE
CLEANING FLUID
IODINE
INSECTICIDES
ASPIRIN
POISON
MOTH REPELLENTS
LEAD
ALCOHOL
KEROSENE
LYE
CLEANING FLUID
DDT
AS-PIRIN
ANT
RAT
BOB BLAKE

# POISONING

*Publication Number 1019*
AMERICAN LECTURE SERIES®

*A Monograph in*
*The* BANNERSTONE DIVISION *of*
AMERICAN LECTURES IN LIVING CHEMISTRY

*Edited by*
I. NEWTON KUGELMASS, M.D., Ph.D., Sc.D.

*Consultant to the Department of Health and Hospitals*
*New York, New York*

FOURTH EDITION

# POISONING

## TOXICOLOGY • SYMPTOMS • TREATMENTS

*By*

**JAY M. ARENA, M.D.**

*Professor of Pediatrics and Community Health Services*
*Director, Poison Control Unit*
*Duke University Medical Center*
*Durham, North Carolina*
*Member, Executive Committee and Past President*
*American Association of Poison Control Centers*
*Past President, American Academy of Pediatrics*
*Member, National Advisory Committee on Consumer and Product Safety*
*Food and Drug Administration*

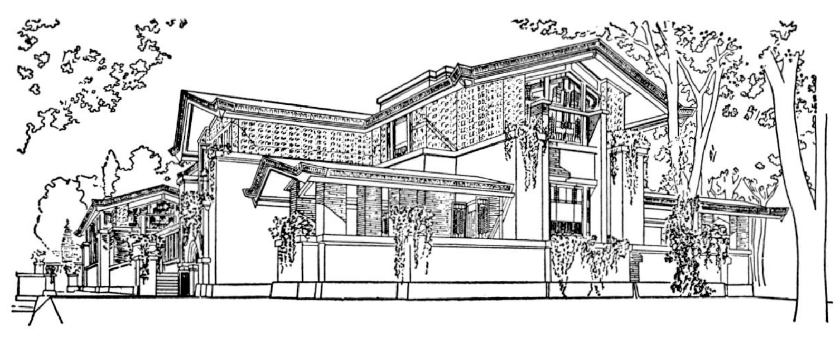

**CHARLES C THOMAS • PUBLISHER**

***Springfield · Illinois · U.S.A.***

*Published and Distributed Throughout the World by*

CHARLES C THOMAS • PUBLISHER
Bannerstone House
301-327 East Lawrence Avenue, Springfield, Illinois, U.S.A.



ISBN 0-398-03767-1

Library of Congress Catalog Card Number: 78-5382

*With THOMAS BOOKS careful attention is given to all details of manufacturing and design. It is the Publisher's desire to present books that are satisfactory as to their physical qualities and artistic possibilities and appropriate for their particular use. THOMAS BOOKS will be true to those laws of quality that assure a good name and good will.*

*Printed in the United States of America*
M-3

**Library of Congress Cataloging in Publication Data**
Arena, Jay M.
Poisoning.

(American lecture series; publication no. 1019)
Bibliography: p.
Includes index.
1. Toxicology. I. Title.
RA1216.A69 1978 615.9 78-5382
ISBN 0-398-03767-1

To my seven children and their children
who by their escapades over the years
compounded my interest in poisoning

*And*

To Polly who withstood it all

# PREFACE TO THE FOURTH EDITION

Albert Schweitzer once said "Man can hardly even recognize the devils of his own creation." The most alarming of these creations is man's assault upon his own environment in the contamination of air, earth, water and himself. An incredible series of recent disasters implicating new chemicals in the marketplace is sending growing numbers of patients exposed to these agents to physicians who are often unaware of either the magnitude or the precise nature of the chemical hazard.

Among the bewildering array of life-threatening substances headlined in the news media are PCB (polychlorinated biphenyl) from industrial waste discharged into many waterways, linked to cancer and birth defects and detected in the milk of nursing mothers; PBB (polybrominated biphenyl), a fire retardant accidentally mixed with animal feed, which found its way into the food chain and mother's milk; mirex, the carcinogenic persistent pesticide used against fire ants in the South, which has leached into soil and water; kepone, another pesticide contaminating Virginia's James River and Chesapeake Bay, causing tremors and liver disorders, as well as decreased sperm production in men; VC (vinyl chloride), which is used to manufacture polyvinyl chloride plastic, carrying a threat of angiosarcoma of the liver; dioxin, the teratogenic skin-burning compound used to make a bactericide and herbicide, which spread a poisonous cloud over the Italian town of Seveso; mercury, cause of the devastating Minamata disease affecting the nervous system and named for Minamata Bay, Japan, into which mercury-laden industrial waste was discharged, poisoning fish and those who ate them.

The wide publicity given these plagues of modern technology, plus steadily increasing pressure from environmentalists and their physician-supporters, culminated in passage of the Toxic Substances Control Act in October of 1976. This important legislation now places a challenge before physicians and scientists, because the science needed to accomplish the law's purposes is not yet available.

Numerous additions, changes in many sections and a number of new topics and items have been added to this fourth edition. Hopefully, this edition, revised and updated from current literature on poisoning and toxicological and environmental hazards from here and abroad, which I diligently extract almost daily, will help physicians meet the challenge that the Toxic Substances Control Act presents. Few epidemiologic studies are mounted unless there is a guess, hint or suspicion from the practicing physician, who is the front line of defense.

In the completion of this fourth edition, again I am indebted to many: to my toxicology and pediatric colleagues who have permitted me the use of their material, particularly to Jane H. Speaker, Ph.D., Chief Toxicologist, Office of the Medical Examiner, Philadelphia, Pennsylvania, for her section on Routine Toxicology Screening Tests; to the Duke Pediatrics Department and House Staff whose interest and concern for poisoned children is a constant satisfaction and rewarding experience; to Charles C Thomas, Publisher, for their careful attention to all the details needed to produce a quality book; and finally to my secretary Cathy Cotten and substitute Donna Cain, for their good humor and efficiency in putting all the pieces together, and to Barbara Wengert for her thorough index.

J.M.A.

# PREFACE TO THE THIRD EDITION

The second edition of *Poisoning* has sold out sooner than anticipated. Because of a number of important additions as well as numerous changes in the present material, in order to keep it current, it was decided to go to a new third edition instead of reprinting. Substantial changes have been made in all sections, and many new items are included for the first time, e.g. tricyclic drugs, methadone, Narcan® (naloxone hydrochloride), drugs and chemicals in breast milk, methyl mercury in fish and humans, polychlorinated biphenyl (PCB), pentachlorophenol (PCP), isoniazid, animal poisons, a table of signs and symptoms of poisoning, and many other additional tables and materials.

Poisoning has an interface with many specialties and disciplines: the Internist and Family Practitioner with the more than 6000 annual deliberate poisonings and suicides from drugs and chemicals; the Obstetrician and his involvement in preventing teratogenic effects in the fetus and toxic excretions in breast milk; the Medical Examiner and Pathologist, the Toxicologist, the Environmentalist and, of course, the Pediatrician, who bears the brunt of most acute poisoning in this country.

Mothers have never deliberately gone shopping for poisons, but the fact is that they buy several every time they go to the grocery store or market. They use them whenever they clean house, polish the furniture, wash the dishes, paint the kitchen or clean a spot off their husband's tie. Most of the time they are not aware of the danger or the toxic potential of these household products for *all too often they do not read or heed the labels,* and their children can't!

The natural curiosity of children to learn by exploration, questioning, sampling and trial and error leads them to investigate the more than a quarter million products and the myriad of drugs which are now available and many of which are often present in the home.

Few practicing physicians escape the anxiety in treating incidents of acute poisoning, accidental or willful, in children or adults, as an emergency event. When encountered, it is imperative for them to have some firsthand information on the basic principles of the diagnosis and treatment of these tragic occasions. Therefore I am pleased to hear and to find that this publication has been useful to many physicians and nonphysicians, not only in Poison Control Centers, in libraries and emergency rooms of medical centers and community hospitals, and in Public Health Departments, but also in the offices of the generalists and specialists. The practitioner is often the physician who is first involved, and what he does or does not do can be critical and affect the ultimate outcome of a serious poisoning.

As usual, I am indebted to many individuals in the process of completing this third edition, many of whom have already been acknowledged and thanked in previous prefaces. This time I particularly owe a debt of gratitude to my present secretary, Mrs. Glenn Newman, who has done yeoman work in all aspects of this revision.

J.M.A.

# PREFACE TO THE SECOND EDITION

The second edition has been entirely revised and updated with most of the current literature on poisoning here and abroad, which I have been trying diligently to extract for years. Over one hundred new items and tables (solvents, pneumoconioses, food poisoning, detergents, zoonoses, veterinary toxicology, hypoglycemic agents, various drug charts, etc.) have been added to make this book more complete and useful.

Continual advances in organic and inorganic chemistry, in manufacturing processes, pesticide control, advertising, marketing and distribution have put a huge variety of synthetic and natural compounds of a potentially toxic nature in almost every household and its environs. It is not surprising, then, that the problem of poisoning, both acute and chronic, remains critical and urgent, often requiring immediate attention and heroic measures from the busy practitioner.

To quote from J.C. Furnas in *Goodbye to Uncle Tom:* "Thanking individuals in print for help in such books as this is risky. Somebody always gets left out. Will all who gave me advice or information—and there are hundreds of them—take this please, as a personal and hearty thanks." I would be amiss, however, not to specifically mention the Mary Duke Biddle Foundation for its support in the preparation of the index; Mrs. Edna R. Fortner, Mrs. Pamela Leight, and Mrs. Clarice Harton, capable and industrious pediatric secretaries; Doctor Roscoe R. Robinson, Professor of Medicine, Duke University Medical Center, for his splendid contribution on barbiturates; and Doctor Shirley Osterhout, Associate Director of the Duke Poison Control Center, without whose interest, dedication and assistance, this endeavor might never have been completed. I am particularly indebted to our House officers and the Duke telephone operators, who unselfishly man our Poison Control Center facilities, twenty-four hours daily, every day, and who are largely responsible for the successful emergency service that is offered to physicians and the public alike. This source of action is invaluable in collecting data on trends in poisoning and developing current therapy. I trust that this second edition will serve effectively for those who are interested in and concerned about the prevention and treatment of poisoning in the unstable or careless adult as well as in the inquisitive, sampling and exploring child. Somehow, parents must be made to realize that, in the final analysis, it is their responsibility to prevent these tragic accidents.

> To guard is better than to heal
> The shield is nobler than the spear!
> HOLMES

J.M.A.

# PREFACE TO THE FIRST EDITION

This book, like a newborn babe, was easy to conceive but difficult to deliver. It had its inception many years ago, when as a student and later a house officer in the spanking new Duke University Medical Center, it was my unfortunate lot to see and to care for many children with acute caustic alkali ("lye") poisoning. The sad and unforgettable part of this experience was that toddlers and infants were mainly involved. Deaths were few; however, the heartaches of months and sometimes years of painful dilatations to keep a patent esophagus, followed later by definitive surgery for those whose esophagi finally closed off, left an indelible imprint. It aroused an interest in poisoning in general and in the prevention of these tragic accidents in particular. My seven inquisitive and exploring children at home compounded this interest and kept it at a fever pitch. Then came the busy years of a part-time practice and the increasing number of frantic calls from parents. The ingestion of drugs, household agents and insecticides was becoming my most prevalent medical emergency. Although the facts of these ever-increasing incidents were not being publicized or even mentioned in the medical literature, in discussions at medical meetings and through personal communications, I found that the problem of poisoning existed and was frequently encountered by pediatricians and general practitioners everywhere. Many cases were being treated each day with the meager knowledge available. Unfortunately, many of the larger medical centers were unaware of this particular trend; and therefore, few of their house officers—the future pediatricians—were given adequate information and the necessary training in this particular field. In 1951, the Academy of Pediatrics, through a survey of its Committee on Accident Prevention, found that a majority of the accidents encountered in pediatric practice was due to poisoning. The study brought forth many requests for up-to-date information on toxic ingredients in common household products as well as for improved therapeutic measures. In 1953, the first Poison Control Center was established in Chicago, and a few months later the Duke organization was activated. This unit was actually a continuation and broadening of a program that the Department of Pediatrics at Duke, because of its interest, had been carrying out for years. As of July, 1961, there were 460 Poison Control Centers in the United States. One or more are in each of forty-seven states and four territories.

This book could never have been written without the assistance of many dedicated people, friends, and the Pediatric Staff (Upper and House) of the Duke University Medical Center, whose Department Chairman, Doctor Jerome S. Harris, has been particularly helpful with his support and enthusiasm. To the former Dean of Duke University Medical School and Chairman of its Pediatric Department, Doctor Wilburt C. Davison, I owe a special debt of gratitude. In a thirty-year association as his student, house officer and staff member, he was instrumental not only in arousing my interest in poisoning but also in encouraging continued interest throughout the years. More than that, he taught me much by his own sense of values and by his integrity and loyalty. To Mrs. Carl H. Weber, my faithful and efficient secretary, without whose collaboration this book may never have been completed, I am indeed thankful. To my associate, Doctor Charles B. Neal III, who assumed the heavy burden of co-reading the proof, I am particularly indebted. Finally to my wife, Polly, for her inspirations, help and for sharing my interest, I am eternally grateful.

Encouragement and financial assistance from the Hanes Committee, the United Medical Research Foundation and the Mary Duke Biddle Foundation have greatly facilitated the completion and publication of this book.

As I said at the outset, this book was easy to conceive, and now the time that it should be delivered is at hand, for the manuscript is completed. This does not mean the end however—as there is no ending to this problem. As long as we have thousands of household agents with toxic compounds and miniature drugstores in the home, disturbed adults and inquisitive children will be poisoned. Regardless of what precautions are taken, some will circumvent them. Therefore, in addition to taking all the precautions and preventive measures now available and yet to be found, every physician (no one is immune to an emergency call when poisoning has occurred regardless of his specialty) should be alert at least to first aid measures and the basic principles of diagnosis and treatment.

J.M.A.

# CONTENTS

*Page*

*Preface to the Fourth Edition* vii
*Preface to the Third Edition* ix
*Preface to the Second Edition* xi
*Preface to the First Edition* xiii

*Chapter*

1. GENERAL CONSIDERATIONS OF POISONING .......... 3
   - Prevention .......... 3
   - General Diagnostic Considerations .......... 6
   - Methemoglobinemia .......... 17
   - Emergency Drugs and Equipment .......... 19
   - Gastric Lavage .......... 28
   - Treatment .......... 31
   - Antidotes .......... 47
   - Supportive Measures .......... 47
   - Artificial Respiration .......... 59
   - Cardiac Therapy .......... 61
   - Blood Transfusions (Exchange Transfusions and Plasmapheresis) .......... 63
   - Extracorporeal Dialyzer (Artificial Kidney) .......... 64
   - Lipid Dialysis .......... 66
   - Peritoneal Dialysis .......... 67
   - Shock Therapy .......... 69
   - Disseminated Intravascular Coagulation (DIC) .......... 70
   - Cranial Hypertension .......... 70
   - Treatment of Convulsions .......... 71
   - Coma .......... 71
   - Respiratory Insufficiency .......... 73
   - Toxic Hepatitis (Drug-induced and Chemical) .......... 75
   - Renal Failure .......... 82
   - Antibiotics and General Therapeutic Agents .......... 82
   - Toxicology (Selection of Specimens in Poisoning Cases) .......... 84
   - Toxicological Screening Tests .......... 89
   - Lethal Doses .......... 91
   - Poisons and Mental Function (Psychosis-Hallucinogens) .......... 93

Page

Toxic Episodes in the Fetus and Infant (Maternal Medication and Drug Dangers) 102
Fetal Alcohol Syndrome 103
Environmental Fetal and Infant Pollutants 109
Drugs and Chemicals In Breast Milk 115

2. INSECTICIDES 126
Synthetic Organic Insecticides 127
Inorganic Chemical-Type Insecticides 138
Insecticides from Botanical Sources 156
Biological Pesticides 158

3. RODENTICIDES, FUNGICIDES, HERBICIDES, FUMIGANTS AND REPELLENTS 173
Rodenticides 173
Fungicides 179
Herbicides 182
Fumigants and Repellents 186

4. INDUSTRIAL HAZARDS 202
Nitrogen Compounds 203
Halogenated Hydrocarbons 205
Alcohols and Glycols 209
Aldehydes, Ketones, Ethers and Esters 219
Hydrocarbons 222
Corrosives 226
Metallic Poisons 252

5. OCCUPATIONAL HAZARDS 273
The Forgotten Casualty 311
Occupational Hazards of Painters and Sculptors 313
Pneumoconioses 314
Environmental Hazards 322

6. DRUGS 332
Food-Drug Interactions 333
Role of Drugs in Suicide 334
Drug-induced Hemolytic Anemia and Altered Therapeutic Responses (Inborn Errors of Metabolism) 336
Known Retinotoxic Drugs 344
Acetaminophen (Paracetamol) 346
Aconitine (Aconite) 350

*Page*

Aluminum Compounds.................................................... 350
Amphetamines (*See* Sympathomimetic Amines).............................. 351
Anesthetic, General.................................................... 351
Anesthetics, Local..................................................... 351
Anthelmintics.......................................................... 353
Antibiotics and Chemotherapeutics...................................... 354
Anticholinergic Compounds.............................................. 358
Anticonvulsants for Epileptic Therapy.................................. 359
Antihistamines (Diphenhydramine, Tripelennamine,
Chlorpheniramine, etc.)................................................ 364
Arsphenamine and Neoarsphenamine....................................... 367
Ataractics, Tranquilizing (Psychotropic) Drugs......................... 370
Atropine (Belladonna, Stramonium)...................................... 376
Barbiturates........................................................... 378
Bismuth Compounds...................................................... 391
Bromide................................................................ 392
Caffeine............................................................... 394
Calcium................................................................ 394
Cancer Chemotherapeutic Agents......................................... 395
Camphor and Camphorated Oil............................................ 404
Cantharidin (Spanish Fly).............................................. 405
Cathartics............................................................. 405
Chloral Hydrate........................................................ 408
Cinchophen (Neocinchophen)............................................. 409
Citric Acid............................................................ 409
Cobalt................................................................. 410
Cocaine................................................................ 410
Codeine................................................................ 412
Colchicine (Colchicum)................................................. 412
Contraceptives, Oral................................................... 413
Corticosteroids........................................................ 413
Curare (Chondodendron Tomentosum Extract, Dimethyl
Tubocurarine Chloride, Iodide, etc.)................................... 415
Dextromethorphan Hydrobromide.......................................... 416
Dextropropoxyphene Hydrochloride (Darvon)............................... 416
Diamethazole (Asterol).................................................. 417
Digitalis............................................................... 417
Diphenoxylate Hydrochloride (Lomotil).................................. 422
Ergot and Ergot Alkaloids.............................................. 423
Estrogens, Conjugated U.S.P............................................ 426
Ether and Other Anesthetic Agents...................................... 426

*Page*

Glutethimide (Doriden) .......... 427
Gold .......... 428
Hydralazine .......... 428
Hypoglycemic Agents (Oral) .......... 429
Iodine and Its Compounds .......... 429
Iproniazid Phosphate-Marsilid (Isonicotinoyl-2-Isopropylhydrazine) .......... 431
Iron Compounds .......... 431
Isoniazid (Isonicotinic Acid Hydrazide, I.N.H. Nydrazid, Niconyl) .......... 437
Magnesium .......... 438
Marihuana (Cannabis) .......... 439
Methadone (Dolophine) .......... 440
Monoamine Oxidase Inhibitors (Marplan, Nardil, Niamid, Parnate, etc.) .......... 442
Morphine (Narcotics) .......... 444
Morphine (Narcotic) Addiction .......... 447
Myristicin (Nutmeg, Mace) .......... 449
Nitrites, Nitrates, Glyceryl Trinitrate .......... 449
Para-Aminophenol Analgesic Compounds (Acetanilid, Phenacetin [Acetophenetidin], etc.) .......... 451
Parasympathomimetic (Cholinergic) Agents .......... 452
Paregoric (Camphorated Tincture of Opium) .......... 453
Phenol and Derivatives (Cresol, Naphthol, Menthol, Thymol, Guaiacol, Resorcinol, etc.) .......... 453
Phenolphthalein .......... 454
Phosphate Compounds .......... 455
Photosensitizing Compounds .......... 455
Picric Acid .......... 456
Procaine (Tetracaine, Dibucaine, Piperocaine, Dimethisoquin [Quotane], etc.) .......... 457
Pyrazolon Analgesics (Aminopyrine, Dipyrone, Antipyrine, Phenylbutazone, etc.) .......... 457
Quinine and Cinchona Compounds .......... 457
Salicylamide .......... 461
Salicylate .......... 461
Silver Salts .......... 467
Sulfones, Ethyl (Sulfonal, Trional, Tetronal) .......... 468
Sulfonamides .......... 468
Sulfonamide (Thiazide) Diuretics .......... 469
Sympathomimetic Amines .......... 470

*Page*

Tricyclic Compounds.......... 472
Vanadium.......... 474
Veratrum (Veratramine, Veratrine, etc.).......... 474
Vitamins.......... 475
Volatile Oils.......... 479
Xanthines (Aminophylline, Theophylline, Theobromine, Caffeine, etc.).......... 480
Oral Anticoagulants vs. Other Drugs.......... 503
Drug Information Centers.......... 504

7. Soap, Detergent, Polishing and Sanitizing Agents.......... 517
Detergents.......... 517

8. Cosmetics and Toilet Articles.......... 532
Shampoos.......... 532
Hair-Waving Preparations.......... 533
Hair-Straightening Solutions.......... 533
Hair Tints and Dyes.......... 533
Hairsprays.......... 535
Depilatories.......... 535
Deodorants.......... 536
Royal Jelly.......... 536
Suntan Preparations.......... 536
"Suntan Pills" (Psoralens).......... 537
Miscellaneous Cosmetic Products.......... 537

9. Poisonous Plants, Reptiles, Arthropods, Insects and Fish.......... 538
Poisonous Plants.......... 538
Poisonous Snakes (Ophidism).......... 558
Arthropods and Insects.......... 570
Poisonous Fish.......... 581
Zoonoses.......... 591
Veterinary Toxicology.......... 604

10. Miscellaneous Compounds.......... 608
Acrodynia (Mercury, Copper).......... 608
Aerosols.......... 608
Alphazurine 2 G.......... 609
Aqua Fortis.......... 609
Aquarium Products.......... 609
Aromatics.......... 610
Balsam of Peru (Peruvian, Indian Balsam).......... 610
Batteries.......... 610
Benzene (Benzol).......... 611

*Page*
Benzoic Acid U.S.P. .... 611
Blue Velvet .... 611
Borax (Sodium Tetraborate) .... 612
Bordeaux Mixture .... 612
Boroglycerin .... 612
Brown Mixture .... 612
Burow's Solution .... 612
Calamine U.S.P. .... 612
Cataria (Catnep, Catnip, Catmint) .... 613
Cellosolves (Methyl, Ethyl, Butyl, Diethyl) .... 613
Chalk .... 613
Chemistry Sets .... 613
Chloracetophenone .... 616
Chlorothen (Chloromethapyrilene) .... 617
Citronella Oil (Lemon Grass Oil) .... 617
Clove Oil U.S.P. .... 617
Cocillana .... 617
Collodion U.S.P. .... 617
Crayons (Art Material) .... 618
Creosote (Creosote Oil) .... 618
Dichloroisocyanurates, Sodium or Potassium .... 618
Dimethyl Sulfoxide (DMSO) .... 618
Dioctyl Sodium Sulfosuccinate .... 619
Donovan's Solution .... 619
Electric Shock .... 620
Epoxy Resin Glues .... 620
Ferbam (Fermate) .... 621
Fertilizers and Plant Foods .... 621
Fiberglass and Resin Plastics .... 623
Freon (Dichlorodifluoromethane) .... 624
Gas (Natural, Manufactured, Propane) .... 625
Gibberellic Acid .... 626
Glycerin (Glycerol) .... 626
Glycyrrhizin (Licorice) .... 626
Golf Balls .... 626
Graphite (Plumbago) .... 626
Hexachlorophene .... 626
Hexachlorophene and Skin Care of Newborn Infants .... 627
Javelle Water .... 629
Labarraque's Solution .... 629
Lanolin .... 629

| | Page |
|---|---|
| Lime | 629 |
| Linseed Oil (Flaxseed Oil) | 630 |
| Lithium Salts | 630 |
| Mace | 631 |
| Maté | 631 |
| Mescal (Peyote) | 632 |
| Methylbenzethonium Chloride (Diaparene) | 632 |
| Methylparaben U.S.P. (Methyl-*p*-Hydroxybenzoate, Methyl Parasept) | 632 |
| Mirbane, Essence or Oil (Nitrobenzene) | 632 |
| Monsel's Solution | 632 |
| Muriatic (Hydrochloric) Acid | 633 |
| Neatsfoot Oil | 633 |
| Oil of Sassafras | 633 |
| Paris Green (Schweinfurth Green) | 633 |
| Pencils | 633 |
| Permanganate, Potassium | 633 |
| Phenyl Salicylate (Salol) | 634 |
| Photographic (Polaroid) Material | 634 |
| Pine Oil | 636 |
| Plaster of Paris (Gypsum) | 636 |
| Plastic Cement | 636 |
| Pomegranate | 636 |
| Polymer Fume Fever | 637 |
| Propane, Liquid | 637 |
| Prussic Acid | 637 |
| Pumice | 637 |
| Quince Seed | 637 |
| Radiation Syndrome | 638 |
| Radioactive Isotope Poisoning | 642 |
| Rocket Fuels (Boron Hydride) | 644 |
| Rosin (Abietic Anhydride, Yellow Resin, Colophony) | 645 |
| Saffron | 645 |
| Salt (Sodium Chloride) | 645 |
| Selenium Derivatives | 646 |
| Sesame Oil | 647 |
| Shellac | 647 |
| Silica (Silicone Dioxide) | 647 |
| Silicones (Methyl Polysiloxane) | 647 |
| Smoke Poisoning | 647 |
| Smoking Deterrents | 649 |

*Page*

Sodium Alginate (Algin) ... 649
Solox ... 649
Spermaceti ... 650
Starch ... 650
Stearic Acid (Octadecanoic Acid) ... 650
Stoddard Solvent (Varsol) ... 650
Sulfosalicylic Acid ... 650
Sulfur ... 651
Sweetening Agents ... 651
Swimming Pool Disinfectants (Purifiers) ... 652
Talc (Talcum) U.S.P. ... 653
Tannic Acid NF ... 653
Tear Gases ... 654
Teflon, Kel-F ... 654
Thiocyanates ... 654
Thioglycolate Salts ... 655
Thuja (Yellow Cedar, Arbor Vitae) ... 655
Tobacco ... 655
Tricalcium Phosphate ... 655
Trichloroacetic Acid ... 655
Tris-BP ... 656
Turkey Red Oil ... 656
Uva Ursi ... 656
Vitriolic Acid ... 656
Water Glass ... 656
Welding Hazards ... 656
Witch Hazel (Hamamelis Winter Bloom, Snapping Hazel, Striped or Spotted Alder, Tobacco Wood) ... 657
Xylene (Benzene, Toluene, Cumene, Mesitylene) ... 658

11. Public Safety Education ... 660
Poison Control Centers ... 661
Status of Household Articles Under Federal Laws as to Identity of Contents and Precautions in Labeling ... 701
Federal Hazardous Substances Labeling Act ... 702
Food Additives ... 703
Food Poisoning ... 710
Recommendations to the Public on First Aid Measures for Poisoning ... 720
Carbon Monoxide Poisoning ... 722
Hazards of Solvents at Home and On the Job ... 724

Page

Pests About the Home ........ 730
Matches ........ 736
Fireworks Hazards ........ 738
Toxic Christmas Decorations ........ 739
Insects and Man ........ 741

*Appendix*

A. Pamphlets and Other Media ........ 744
B. Normal Laboratory Values in the Diagnosis and Treatment of Poisoning (Alteration by Drugs) ........ 752

*Index* ........ 773

# LIST OF ILLUSTRATIONS


*Figure* *Page*

1. 85% of all poisoning cases involve children .......... 4
2. Body surface area .......... 27
3. Gastric lavage tube .......... 29
4. Efficient lavage technique .......... 30
5. Artificial respiration, standard technique .......... 60
6. Artificial respiration, mouth-to-mouth technique .......... 61
7. Closed-chest cardiac massage .......... 63
8. Conway dish for routine toxicology screening tests .......... 89
9. Proposed mechanism of action of phosgene .......... 251
10. Air pollution .......... 328
11. Public drug spending in 1971 and 1976 .......... 332
12. Methods of suicide used by Americans in 1964 and 1972 .......... 337
13. Drug reactions .......... 339-340
14. Forrest rapid urine color tests for phenothiazine .......... 372
15. Chemical structure for derivatives of barbituric acid .......... 379
16. Titration curve for a weak organic acid against a base .......... 380
17. Proposed pathogenesis of the acid-base disturbances of salicylate intoxication in children .......... 463
18. Serum salicylate concentration and severity of intoxication .......... 465
19. Poisonous flowering plants .......... 541
20. Poisonous fruit-bearing plants .......... 542
21. Mushrooms, edible .......... 556
22. Mushrooms, edible and poisonous .......... 557
23. Some identifying features of poisonous and harmless snakes .......... 563
24. Identifying features of the moccasin, copperhead and rattlesnake... 564
25. Coral snake .......... 564
26. Brown recluse spider .......... 572
27. Habits and effects of various arthropods .......... 576

# LIST OF TABLES


*Tables* *Page*

1. General signs and symptoms of poisoning ........ 6
2. Urine color ........ 10
3. Discoloration of the urine by drugs ........ 11
4. Discoloration of the feces by drugs ........ 12
5. Known compounds producing methemoglobin ........ 12
6. Anemias ........ 13
7. Drugs associated with eosinophilia ........ 15
8. Drugs associated with thrombocytopenia ........ 16
9. Emergency drugs (general) ........ 19
10. Emergency drugs (specific) ........ 21
11. Factors useful in calculating children's doses ........ 23
12. Determination of children's doses from adult doses on basis of body surface area ........ 23
13. Approximate dosage equivalents for grains and grams ........ 23
14. Approximate household measures ........ 24
15. Numerical equivalents ........ 25
16. Approximate amount of solution ........ 26
17. Some relations of drug toxicity in experimental animals compared with man ........ 26
18. Approximate amount of substance adsorbed by 1 gm charcoal ........ 35
19. Dosage of some antiarrhythmic drugs ........ 48
20. Adverse effects of some antiarrhythmic drugs ........ 49
21. Some specific antidotes ........ 50
22. Broad-spectrum and household antidotes ........ 56
23. Effects of water and certain solutes ........ 57
24. Rough guide to maintaining body water needs and correcting fluid deficits ........ 57
25. Electrolyte concentrations of several commonly used parenteral fluids ........ 58
26. Factors for converting blood chemistry values to milliequivalents per liter ........ 59
27. Myocardiopathy ........ 62
28. Known dialyzable poisons ........ 65
29. Composition of dialysis fluids ........ 68
30. Treatment of convulsions ........ 72

*Tables* *Page*


31. Coma ........ 74
32. Conditions causing coma ........ 75
33. Drug-induced hepatotoxicity ........ 79
34. Nephrotoxic chemical compounds ........ 82
35. Infrared analysis of gases and vapors in expired air ........ 87
36. Screening tests for general drug category ........ 92
37. Poisonous substances found in the household ........ 94
38. Lethal doses ........ 97
39. Source and comparative strengths of LSD and other hallucinogens (approximate) ........ 102
40. Psychotic states associated with misuse or abuse of ordinarily useful drugs and other substances: differentiation and treatment ........ 104
41. Medication and therapy which may affect the fetus and newborn ... 110
42. Categorical effects of maternal drug therapy on the fetus and newborn ........ 112
43. Drugs excreted in human milk ........ 117
44. Antimicrobials in breast milk (milk-plasma ratio) ........ 118
45. Adverse reactions and antibiotic dosage in the premature and newborn infant ........ 121
46. Drugs capable of in vitro displacement of bilirubin from albumin in the newborn ........ 124
47. Estimated lethal doses of chlorinated hydrocarbon insecticides ........ 130
48. Organic phosphate ester poisoning symptoms ........ 131
49. Acute toxicity of organic phosphorus-containing insecticides ........ 132
50. Insecticides ........ 137
51. Chemicals and drugs producing alopecia ........ 143
52. Acute toxicity to man of some inorganic insecticides ........ 155
53. Toxicity of insecticides of botanic origin to man ........ 158
54. Insecticides ........ 159
55. Miscellaneous insecticides (combination sprays and powders) ........ 171
56. Estimated fatal doses of rodenticides to man ........ 179
57. Relative toxicity of herbicides to mammals ........ 187
58. Rodenticides, herbicides, fungicides ........ 194
59. Chart of approximate blood alcohol percentage ........ 211
60. Some drug interactions with alcohol ........ 214
61. Alcohol and toxic substitutes ........ 220
62. Contents of common household bleaches ........ 233
63. Effects of bleach and household product mixtures ........ 234
64. Variation of child's sodium nitrite dose with hemoglobin concentration ........ 237
65. Carbon monoxide poisoning ........ 242

*Tables* *Page*

66. Maximum allowable concentrations for gases and vapors ........ 247
67. Function of metals in man ........ 252
68. Calculation of tolerable levels of lead intake to reflect body size of young children ........ 256
69. Average levels of trace metals (gm/70-kg man) ........ 270
70. Maximum biological allowable concentrations ........ 271
71. Blood, urine and tissue levels of metals (micrograms per 100 ml or 100 gm) ........ 272
72. Occupational hazards ........ 274
73. Maximum allowable concentrations for toxic fumes and dusts ........ 311
74. Maximum allowable concentrations for mineral and inert dusts ........ 311
75. A. Materials and industrial exposures associated with occupational dermatitis and/or asthma ........ 313
B. Materials and industrial exposures associated with urticaria ........ 313
76. Antigens causing hypersensitivity pneumonitis ........ 322
77. Occupations potentially associated with pneumoconioses ........ 323
78. Pollutants ........ 324
79. Air pollutants ........ 329
80. Water pollutants ........ 330
81. Some leading occupational carcinogens ........ 331
82. A sampling of possible food-drug reactions ........ 334
83. United States suicide rates ........ 335
84. International suicide rates ........ 335
85. Number of suicidal deaths by specific causes according to international classification ........ 335
86. Number of suicidal deaths by specific cause in international classification E 970 (suicide and self-inflicted poisoning by analgesic and soporific substances) ........ 336
87. Number of suicides due to barbiturates (class E970 B), other analgesic and soporific substances (class E970 H), and meprobamate during 1954-1963 ........ 336
88. Genetic polymorphisms producing drug-induced hemolytic anemia or altered therapeutic response ........ 338
89. Some oxidants and drugs that may cause hemolysis in G-6-PD deficiency ........ 343
90. Gastroduodenal ulcers—role of drugs ........ 345
91. Drug-induced systemic lupus erythematosus ........ 345
92. Drug reactions in the aged ........ 345
93. Drugs capable of causing fixed eruptions ........ 346
94. Drugs and Stevens-Johnson syndrome (erythema multiforme) ........ 347
95. Drugs and exfoliative dermatitis ........ 347

*Tables* *Page*

96. Drugs and toxic epidermal necrolysis .......... 347
97. Drug-induced malabsorption .......... 347
98. Drugs producing hyperglycemia .......... 347
99. Drugs producing gynecomastia .......... 348
100. Local anesthetics .......... 352
101. Anthelmintics .......... 353
102. Antibiotic and chemotherapeutic agents .......... 355
103. Drugs and chemicals capable of producing the anticholinergic syndrome .......... 358
104. Common untoward reactions of anticonvulsant (epileptic) drugs .......... 362
105. Guide to antihistamine agents .......... 365
106. Common antihistamine-drug interactions .......... 366
107. Psychotropic agents .......... 368
108. Ocular phenothiazine effects .......... 371
109. Adverse reactions to phenothiazines .......... 374
110. Physicochemical properties of common barbiturates .......... 379
111. Barbiturate blood levels at conscious return .......... 383
112. Treatment of barbiturate intoxication .......... 388
113. Manifestations of chronic bromide intoxication .......... 393
114. Toxicity of cancer chemotherapeutic agents .......... 396
115. Cathartics .......... 406
116. The "caine" phases .......... 411
117. Complications due to infection-promoting and anti-inflammatory effect in steroid treatment .......... 414
118. Complications due to hormone excess encountered in treatment with steroids .......... 414
119. Available corticosteroids and their relative potencies .......... 415
120. Drug therapy for digitalis toxicity .......... 421
121. Ergot derivatives maximum dosage in use for migraine .......... 424
122. Recommended dosage regimens for deferoxamine .......... 436
123. First-line antituberculosis drugs .......... 437
124. Adverse effects with concurrent administration of other agents and MAO inhibitors .......... 443
125. Tyramine in foods and beverages (μg/gm or μg/ml) .......... 444
126. Vitamins—physiologic requirements .......... 476
127. Vitamins .......... 477
128. Miscellaneous drug compounds .......... 481
129. Oral anticoagulants vs. other drugs .......... 503
130. Drug information centers .......... 504
131. Blood levels .......... 513
132. Chemical classification of detergents .......... 518

*Tables* *Page*

133. Toxicity of soaps and detergents ........ 521
134. Composition of soap and detergent products ........ 522
135. Cleaning, polishing, and sanitizing agents ........ 526
136. Herbal preparations with psychoactive effects ........ 546
137. Mushroom poisoning ........ 559
138. Plants producing photosensitization ........ 548
139. Poisonous plants ........ 548
140. Ophidism: a guide to therapy ........ 569
141. North American spiders and insects potentially harmful to man ..... 573
142. Reactions to Hymenoptera stings ........ 577
143. Poisonous fish ........ 586
144. Guide for specific antirabies prophylaxis ........ 593
145. Epidemiological aspects of some zoonoses ........ 594
146. Common animal poisons ........ 605
147. Chemistry sets:
   A. Very low toxicity ........ 614
   B. Low toxicity ........ 614
   C. Potentially toxic ........ 615
148. Toxicity of epoxy resin elements ........ 622
149. Side-effects associated with lithium therapy ........ 631
150. Radiation effects at various doses ........ 640
151. Representative radioisotope diagnostic procedures ........ 641
152. Important radioisotopes used in medicine and biology ........ 643
153. Radioisotopes and organs currently subject to scanning ........ 644
154. Principal toxic combustion products of common substances ........ 648
155. United States directory of poison control centers, 1977 ........ 662
156. State drug laws (enforcement agencies and principal provisions) ..... 704
157. Functions of some commonly used additives ........ 708
158. Symptoms which may indicate that an individual is taking drugs .... 722
159. Comparison of carbon disulfide and acetone ........ 725
160. Solvent effects ........ 729
161. Potential toxicity of pesticides ........ 734

# POISONING

## Chapter 1

# GENERAL CONSIDERATIONS OF POISONING

The causes of poisoning are many—civilian and industrial, accidental and deliberate. An eight-year study in San Francisco indicates that poisoning is possibly the major means of suicide in the nation. Some form of poison accounts for more than 1 million illnesses* (It has been estimated that there are over 200 incidents of poisoning for each fatality.) About one half the deaths are accidental with one third occurring in children. The last vital statistics report listed 2742 accidental deaths from solids and liquids and 1274 accidental deaths from gases and vapors.

* This figure could be just the tip of the iceberg since poisoning is not a reportable condition. Not even all the poison control centers (less than 75%) report their incidences to the National Clearing House for Poison Control Centers in Washington, D.C.

These are rather somber statistics for a cause of injury and death which is known to be largely preventable. Poisoning is now the most common *medical* emergency among young children: child deaths from poisoning exceed those from poliomyelitis, measles, scarlet fever and diphtheria combined. Children, who learn by exploration, questioning, sampling and trial and error, are constantly exposed to more than one quarter million products and to myriads of drugs now available and often present in the home. It is not surprising then that not many days pass without the busy practitioner or pediatrician getting one or more frantic calls from a distraught parent saying, "Johnny has just taken . . . what shall I do?"

## PREVENTION

The prevention of poisoning requires protection as well as education. Although protection is paramount in the age-group most frequently involved, children under five, effective educational experiences adapted to the child's level of development may further decrease the risk. Parents can profit even more from education. They should be told the facts in a positive manner and reminded by all available media that 75 per cent of all poisoning in children occurs from the ingestion of "in sight" compounds or drugs and only 25 per cent from the "out of sight" agents. Related, with better and more telling effect, is to emphasize that three out of every four children's poisonings could be prevented simply by putting all drugs and household products "out of sight" and "out of reach."

The physician has an unparalleled opportunity during home visits, for whatever purpose, to observe existing hazards, to pinpoint them and to advise and motivate the family to eliminate them. Unlike other factors, the physical environment can easily be altered and made safer for children. Parents need advice and counsel from a physician whom they know and respect concerning the maintenance of safety precautions in and about the home. The physician's waiting room should include information and reliable health edu-

# 85% Of All Poisoning Cases

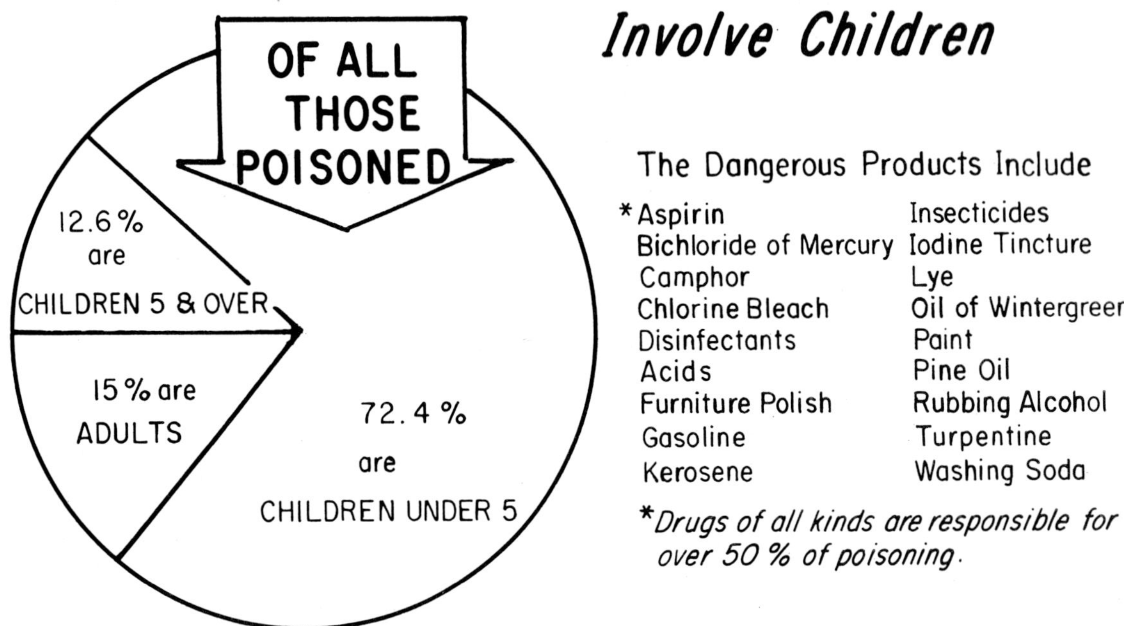


## ☆ *Chief Reasons Why these Products have Proved Dangerous*

1. They are kept in old bottles or cans instead of the original containers.
2. They are removed from their usual storage places.
3. The storage place is unlocked ··· and easily accessible to children
4. 75 % are "in sight" and therefore sought.
5. Failure to properly reapply safety closures or the purchasing of household products, for homes in which small children reside, that are not in safety packaging.

## ☆ *Here is where the Accidents Occur*

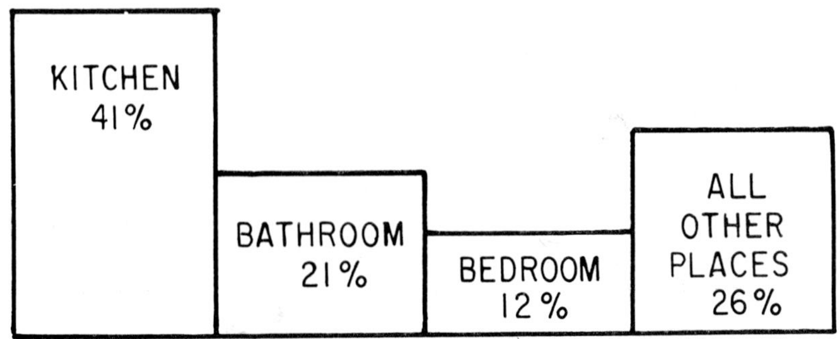


Figure 1.

cation literature and visual aids on the occurrence and prevention of accidental household and drug poisoning. The educational use of a home checklist of poison hazards may succeed with those deaf to other warnings. All medicines should be kept in a locked medicine cabinet or closet. No inflammable liquids and no cleaning or polishing materials should be placed on lower shelves or floors, and there should be no pennypinching saving of solvents and insecticides in pop bottles. Unfortunately, physicians are often guilty of bringing home samples of new and unfamiliar drugs and are also culpable for their tacit approval of many home remedies of dubious worth. The prevention of poisoning usually requires a somewhat different approach than is generally used in the prevention of other types of accidents. Here the age-group of children most frequently involved is under five years, and it is easier to alter their physical environment and make it safe for them. The solution is manifold and complex. The following preventive measures, among others, are needed and worth striving for.

1. Physicians, as well as the public, should be educated as to the intention and significance of the Federal Uniform Hazardous Substance Act, enacted July 12, 1960. An amendment to this act providing for safe packaging of toxic household substances has also been implemented. In addition, new labeling requirements under the Fair Packaging and Labeling Act dealing with nonprescription drugs, medical devices and cosmetics went into effect July 1, 1968. It requires that hazardous household products bear information to protect and warn users against accidental ingestion by children. The law compels labeling to include the common, usual or chemical name of the hazardous substance and the single word "Poison," "Danger," "Warning" or "Caution," depending on the chemical's potential and degree of toxicity. Also required is an affirmative statement of the principal hazard or hazards, such as "Flammable," "Vapor Harmful," "Causes Burns," etc.; precautionary measures describing the action to be taken or avoided; instructions, when necessary or appropriate, for first aid treatment; and finally the statement, "Keep out of reach of children," or its practical equivalent.
2. Use of effective safety containers and closures for drugs and poisonous household agents by the drug and chemical industries. Some children can at times circumvent any and all precautionary measures; yet, for each child successful in removing a grip-tight cap or similar safety device, there are many who are not able to do so.
3. Education of laymen, children, parents, physicians and particularly manufacturers of their responsibility to the public health and safety of all products.
4. Drugs should be administered to children seriously, with a matter-of-fact attitude, and should not be made a game. Drugs should never be referred to as *candy,* and children should never be bribed by such inducements. Parents, especially those taking medications or vitamins regularly, should take their pills and elixirs in privacy and not in the presence of small children. They are great imitators.
5. Preventive and educational efforts by physicians, nurses and community organizations at the local level often accomplish more than well-published advisory measures on a national scale.
6. Training of toxicologists in a scientific discipline on the positive approach to the problems of producing, handling, storing, using or discarding safely the innumerable dangerous substances with which we are learning to live. The negative attitude of the past, "What will kill?" must be replaced by the positive position for the future, "What is safe?"
7. Establishment of properly functioning poison control centers. These centers perform a vital public health service. However, this problem shall never be eliminated unless parents and those responsible for the care of small children create their own

poison control center at home. To prevent tragic poisoning accidents, children must be protected. This can only be done by a responsible parent or an individual educated and personally aware of the potential dangers that the poorly supervised child can encounter in each and every room of his home and outdoor environment.

8. A perpetual slogan should be—
   Poisoning and Children
   Store one—Save the other

## GENERAL DIAGNOSTIC CONSIDERATIONS

In the absence of a definite history of the ingestion of, or contact with, a known poisonous substance, the symptoms and signs presented by a case seen as an emergency may not suggest a diagnosis of poisoning. However, the possibility of poisoning should always be considered in a puzzling situation when differential diagnosis presents a difficult problem. This is especially true if children are involved.

The ingestion as well as (though less frequently) the inhalation or skin absorption of poisons generally causes gastrointestinal disturbances, including anorexia, abdominal pain, nausea, vomiting and diarrhea. However, such symptoms are not diagnostic since they occur in many disorders of childhood. Respiratory and circulatory symptoms are also prominent in most cases of acute poisoning. The diagnosis should be considered whenever one is confronted with unexplained cyanosis, shock, collapse, sudden loss of consciousness or convulsions. Again, these symptoms are not pathognomonic since they may occur as a result of many severe overwhelming infections.

TABLE 1
GENERAL SIGNS AND SYMPTOMS OF POISONING

| SIGN OR SYMPTOM | POISON |
|---|---|
| | *Eye* |
| Dilation of pupil (mydriasis) | Belladonna group, meperidine, alcohols, ether, chloroform, papaverine, sympathomimetics, parasympatholytics, antihistamines, gelsemium, cocaine, camphor, aconitine, benzene, barium, thallium, botulinus toxin, cyanide, carbon monoxide, carbon dioxide |
| Constriction of pupil (miosis) | Opium, morphine group, sympatholytics (ergot), parasympathomimetics, dibenamine, barbiturates, cholinesterase inhibitors, chloral hydrate, picrotoxin, nicotine, caffeine, phenothiazines, ethanol |
| Purple-yellow vision | Marihuana, digitalis, carbon monoxide, santonin |
| Blurred vision | Belladonna group (atropine), methyl alcohol, ethyl alcohol, ergot, carbon tetrachloride, irreversible cholinesterase inhibitors (DFP, TEPP, HETP), vesicant war gases (mustard gas), camphor |
| Partial or total blindness | Methyl alcohol |
| Photophobia, lacrimation, pain | Vesicant war gases (mustard gas), Mace, tear gases (bromacetone, etc.) |
| | *Face and Scalp* |
| Dull and mask-like expression | Barbiturates, bromides, gelsemine, manganese, thallium |
| Facial twitchings | Lead, mercury |
| Alopecia | Thallium, arsenic, ergot, hypervitaminosis A, gold, lead, boric acid, thiocyanates, drugs containing heparin and coumarin |

TABLE 1—*Continued*
GENERAL SIGNS AND SYMPTOMS OF POISONING

| SIGN OR SYMPTOM | POISON |
|---|---|
| | *Skin and Mucous Membranes* |
| Pale | Aniline derivatives, colchicine, sympathomimetics (epinephrine), insulin, pilocarpine |
| Livid, ashy pale | Dinitrocresol, dinitrophenol, ergot, lead, phenacetin |
| Cyanotic, brown-bluish (in absence of respiratory depression and shock) | Nitrobenzene, chlorates, acetanilids, carbon dioxide, methane, nitrous oxide, aniline derivatives, nitrites, morphine, sulfides, ergot, amyl nitrite, and well over 100 other drugs and chemicals |
| Pink | Carbon monoxide, cyanides |
| Yellow | Atabrine; jaundice from hepatic injury (chlorinated compounds, arsenic and other heavy metals, chromates, mushrooms, and many drugs); jaundice from hemolytic anemias (aniline, nitrobenzene, quinine derivatives, arsine, fava beans, and many drugs) |
| Sweating | Pilocarpine, nicotine, physostigmine, picrotoxin |
| Dry, hot skin | Belladonna group (atropine), botulinus toxin |
| Blue-gray | Silver salts |
| | *Local Coloring of the Skin* |
| Brown, black | Iodine, silver nitrate |
| Deep brown | Bromine |
| Yellow | Nitric acid, picric acid |
| White | Phenol derivatives |
| Gray | Mercuric chloride |
| | *Nervous System* |
| Coma | Morphine derivatives and analogues, all hypnotics, sedatives and general anesthetics, barbiturates, chloral hydrate, sulfonal, trional, paraldehyde, chloroform, ethers, bromides, alcohols, lead, cyanide, carbon monoxide, carbon dioxide, nicotine, benzene, atropine, phenols, scopolamine, xylene, irreversible cholinesterase inhibitors (DFP, TEPP, HETP, parathion), insulin, aniline derivatives, mushrooms, salicylates, copper salts |
| Delirium, mental disturbances | Belladonna group (atropine, hyoscine), cocaine, alcohol, lead, marihuana, arsenic, ergot, amphetamine and derivatives, antihistamines, camphor, benzene, barbiturates, DDT, aniline derivatives, physostigmine, veratrine, nerve gases (DFP, TEPP) |
| Convulsions | Strychnine, picrotoxin, camphor, santonin, cocaine, belladonna group (atropine), veratrine, aconite, irreversible cholinesterase inhibitors (DFP, TEPP, HETP, parathion), pentylenetetrazol, amphetamine and derivatives, ergot, nicotine, lead, antipyrine, barium, sodium fluoroacetate, mushrooms, caffeine, carbon monoxide, cyanides, salicylates, copper salts |
| Headache | Carbon monoxide, phenol, benzene, nitrobenzene, nitrates, nitrites, aniline, lead, indomethacin (Indocin) |
| Muscle spasms | Atropine, cadmium, strychnine, copper salts, bites of black widow spider, scorpion, and sting ray |
| General or partial paralysis | Carbon monoxide, carbon dioxide, botulinus toxin, alcohols, physostigmine, curare group, DDT, aconite, nicotine, barium, cyanide, mercury, arsenics, lead |
| | *Gastrointestinal Tract* |
| Nausea, vomiting, diarrhea, dehydration, abdominal pain | Heavy metal salts, corrosive acids and alkalis, halogens, cathartics (croton oil, castor oil), ergot, nicotine, aconitine, cantharides, solanine, acetanilid and derivatives, phosphorus, phenols, cresol, methyl alcohol, muscarine, cardioactive glycosides (digitalis), fluorides, morphine and analogues, DDT, irreversible cholinesterase inhibitors (DFP, TEPP, HETP, OMPA, parathion), pilocarpine, veratrine, colchicine, botulinus toxin, mushrooms, boric acid and sodium borate, cocaine, procaine and local anesthetics, salicylates |
| "Burning" throat and stomach | Camphor, picrotoxin, iodine, arsenicals, antimony compounds |

TABLE 1—*Continued*
GENERAL SIGNS AND SYMPTOMS OF POISONING

| SIGN OR SYMPTOM | POISON |
|---|---|
| | *Odor of Vomitus, Breath, or Body Fluids* |
| Phenolic | Phenols, cresol |
| Etheric, ethereal sweet | Ether |
| Sweet | Chloroform, acetone |
| Bitter almond-like | Cyanides |
| Stale tobacco-like | Nicotine |
| Pear-like | Chloral hydrate |
| Alcoholic | Alcohols |
| Garlic-like | Phosphorus, tellurium, arsenic |
| Shoe polish-like | Nitrobenzene |
| Violets | Turpentine |
| | *Colored Material in Gastric Lavage or Vomitus* |
| Pink or purple | Potassium permanganate |
| Blue, green | Copper salts, chemical dyes added to fluorides or mercury bichloride |
| Green | Nickel salts |
| Pink | Cobalt salts |
| Yellow | Picric acid, nitric acid |
| Bright red | Mercurochrome, nitric acid |
| Black, coffee-like grounds | Sulfuric acid, oxalic acid, nitric acid |
| Brown | Hydrochloric acid |
| Luminescent in dark | Yellow phosphorus |
| Discolored, bloody (hematemesis) | Alkalis, acids, fluoride, phosphorus, salicylates, iron |
| | *Mouth* |
| Excess salivation | Ammonia, cantharides, pilocarpine, arecoline, physostigmine, muscarine, nicotine, mercury, irreversible cholinesterase inhibitors (DFP, HETP, TEPP), salicylates |
| Dry mouth | Belladonna group (atropine), botulinus toxin, barium, diphenhydramine, ephedrine |
| | *Ears* |
| Impaired hearing ("roaring") | Salicylates, quinine, streptomycin |
| "Buzzing" | Camphor, tobacco, ergot, methyl alcohol, quinidine |
| | *Genitourinary System* |
| Uterine cramps, uterine bleeding, abortion | Phosphorus, lead, pilocarpine, physostigmine, nicotine, ergot, quinine, mustard, cantharides, apiol, cathartics (croton oil, castor oil) |
| Porphyria | Barbiturates, sodium phenobarbital, sulfonethylmethane (Trional), glutethimide (Doriden), diphenylhydantoin (Dilantin), bemegride (Megimide), phensuximide (Milontin), hexachlorobenzene, diallyl-barbituric acid (Dial), sulfonmethane (Sulfonal), methyprylon (Noludar), mephenytoin (Mesantoin), meprobamate (Miltown), methsuximide (Celontin), griseofulvin<br>*Note:* These compounds have demonstrated a definite potential for inducing porphyria in vitro. Therefore they should be considered to be contraindicated in patients with known hepatic porphyria and in their near relatives. |
| | *Respiratory System* |
| Slow respiration | Opium, morphine derivatives and analogues, hydrate alcohols, picrotoxin, fluorides, cyanides |

TABLE 1—*Continued*
GENERAL SIGNS AND SYMPTOMS OF POISONING

| SIGN OR SYMPTOM | POISON |
|---|---|
| Rapid or deep respiration, or both | Belladonna group (atropine), cocaine, amphetamine and derivatives, strychnine, carbon dioxide, lobeline, salicylates, nikethamide, camphor |
| Dyspnea | Cyanides, carbon monoxide, volatile organic solvents (benzene), snake venoms, suffocating war gases (phosgene), carbon dioxide |
| Respiratory paralysis | Morphine derivatives and analogues, general anesthesia, hypnotics and sedatives (barbiturates), alcohols, snake venoms, carbon monoxide |
| Edema | Chlorine, bromine, phosgene, methyl perchloroformate |
| Burning pain in chest and throat | Tear gases |
| Sneezing | Adamsite, Clarc I, Clarc II |
| Restlessness | Caffeine |
| Laryngitis, coughing | Vesicant war gases (mustard gas, Lewisite, etc.), nerve gases (DFP, TEPP) |
| Difficult breathing | Alkalis |
| | *Cardiovascular System* |
| Slow pulse (bradycardia) | Barium, aconite, cardioactive glycosides (digitalis), muscarine, physostigmine, pilocarpine, quinine, quinidine, veratrine, picrotoxin, lead, phenylephrine |
| Fast pulse (tachycardia) | Amphetamine and derivatives, atropine, cocaine, sympathomimetics (ephedrine), epinephrine, caffeine, alkalis |
| Angina pectoris-type pain | Nicotine |
| Pain in heart area | Sternutators (Adamsite, Clarc I, Clarc II) |
| Hypotension | Chloral hydrate, alkalis, nitrites, nitrates, quinine, volatile oils, iron salts, chlorpromazine (Thorazine), veratrum |
| Hypertension | Epinephrine or substitutes, ergot, cortisone, vanadium, lead, nicotine |
| Vascular collapse | Lead, acids, alkalis |

Despite the obstacles imposed by the lack of distinguishing symptoms and by the difficulty or impossibility of obtaining a history from patients who are too young, too ill or too frightened to be of assistance, a high index of suspicion and a little ingenious investigation can often establish the correct diagnosis and lead to identification of the poison. Knowledge of the sources, actions and therapy of every known poison is an impossibility. However, command of the basic and general principles of management is even more desirable, for too often the next case of poisoning encountered will be due to a new or not readily identifiable substance. Clues can sometimes be obtained from relatives, friends or bystanders. The characteristic odors of many poisons may be detected on the patient's breath. In addition, the vomitus, the material obtained by gastric lavage, and the first urine specimen (*see* Tables 2 and 3) may yield decisive evidence.

A number of drugs are detected in the urine by impregnated paper-reagent strips (Phenistix®). The test is especially useful for determining failure of hospitalized patients to take prescribed drugs, in addition to overdosing and poisoning.

A gray to blue-purple color is produced on the test strip for as long as thirty-six hours after chlorpromazine is withdrawn. Other distinct color changes produced by drugs are purple for aspirin and related drugs, gray-purple for promazine, brown for sulfonamide, green for tetracycline and gray-blue for promethazine. All are distinct from the gray-green color change caused by phenylpyruvic acid.

The test is best performed on the first specimen of urine passed by the patient on arising. The chemically impregnated end of the paper-reagent strip is dipped into the urine, placed flat on a white porcelain tray and examined under daylight-type fluorescent

TABLE 2
URINE COLOR

| *Dark* | *Red to Red Brown* | *Greenish or Bluish* |
|---|---|---|
| Aniline dyes | Aminopyrine | Amitriptylin (Elavil®) |
| Cadmium | Anticoagulants | Anthraquinone |
| Cascara | Beets* | Arbutin |
| Chlorobenzenes | Blood | Bile pigments |
| Chloronaphthalene | Cascara | Indomethacin (Indocin) |
| Hydroquinone | Chrysarobin (alk.sol.) | Methylene blue |
| Iron salts | Cinchophen | Resorcinol |
| Naphthol | Deferoxamine (Desferal®) | Tetrahydronaphthalene |
| Nitrites | Diphenylhydantoin | Thymol |
| Nitrobenzene | Dorbane® | Triamterene (Dyrenium®) |
| Metronidazole (Flagyl®) | Emodin (alk.sol.) | |
| Phenol | Fava beans | |
| Phenylsalicylate | Hemoglobin | |
| Pyrogallol | Phenindione | |
| Quinine | Phenolphthalein (alk.sol.) | |
| Resorcinol | Phenazopyridine (Pyridium®) | |
| Rhubarb | Phensuximide | |
| Santonin | Porphyrins | |
| Senna | Pyrazolon | |
| Thymol | Rifampin | |
| Trinitrotoluene | Santonin (alk.sol.) | |
| | Senna | |
| | Urates | |

*The dye authocyanin is responsible for the occasional red urine from eating beets.

tubes. The color change appears immediately and fades within a few seconds. The change may be more apparent if the test strip is examined together with one from a person who is not suspected of toxicity or receiving the drug.

In some acute and in many chronic types of poisoning, the blood picture can show various changes that may be of considerable assistance in making the diagnosis as well as in determining the prognosis (*see* Tables 5 and 6). However, definitive laboratory studies of the blood unfortunately require time, even if facilities for them are available. When it is possible, spectroscopic examination of the blood establishes the presence or absence of methemoglobin, sulfhemoglobin and carboxyhemoglobin. Also, lead, bromine, thymol and many other toxic substances can be detected by use of a photoelectric colorimeter. X-ray studies of the bone are, of course, valuable in lead, bismuth and other heavy metal poisoning.

## Drug-induced Eosinophilia

Eosinophilia is an increase in eosinophilic granulocytes above 500/cu. mm. It is associated with parasitic infections, acute allergic attacks, certain extensive chronic skin diseases and some rheumatic and neoplastic diseases. Drug-induced eosinophilia may complicate the diagnosis of these conditions in addition to causing confusion in the management of other diseases for which the drugs in Table 7 are used.

## Drug-induced Thrombocytopenia

Drug-induced thrombocytopenia is a dose-related phenomenon that results either from

TABLE 3
DISCOLORATION OF THE URINE BY DRUGS

| *Therapeutic Use* | *Color* | *Drug(s)* |
|---|---|---|
| Analgesics (urinary) | Orange to orange-red | Ethoxazene (Serenium®); phenazopyridine * (Pyridium®) |
| Antibacterial agents | Orange-yellow (in alkaline urine) | Salicylazosulfapyridine (Azulfidine®) |
| | Discoloration (no specific effect) | p-aminosalicylic acid and derivatives |
| | Rust yellow or brownish | Sulfonamides, nitrofurantoin and derivatives, e.g. furazolidone (Furoxone®) |
| | Red-orange | Rifampin |
| Anticoagulants | Orange (in alkaline urine); pink or red to red-brown | Indandione derivatives, e.g., anisindione (Miradon®), phenindione (Hedulin®) |
| Anticonvulsants | Pink or red to red-brown | Diphenylhydantoin (Dilantin®)<br>Phensuximide (Milontin®) |
| Antidepressants | Blue-green | Amitriptyline (Elavil®) |
| Antidote to cyanide poisoning | Blue or green | Methylene blue |
| Antiprotozoal agents | Brown to black | Quinine and derivatives |
| | Rust yellow or brown | Pamaquine naphthoate (Plasmochin®)<br>Primaquine<br>Chloroquine (Aralen®) |
| | Yellow | Quinacrine (Atabrine®) |
| | Dark | Metronidazole (Flagyl®) |
| Diuretics | Pale blue fluorescence | Triamterene (Dyrenium®) |
| Hemostatic agents | Blue-green | Tolonium (Blutene®) |
| Hematinic agents | Black | Iron-sorbitol-citric acid complex (Jectofer®) |
| Laxatives, cathartics | Brown to black | Cascara; rhubarb |
| | Pink to red or red-brown | 1,8-dihydroxyanthraquinone **<br>Emodin (in alkaline urine)<br>Phenolphthalein † |
| Skeletal muscle relaxants | Orange or purplish-red | Chlorzoxazone (Paraflex®) |
| | Dark brown to black or green on standing | Methocarbamol (Robaxin®) |
| Tranquilizers | Pink to red or red-brown | Phenothiazines |
| Vitamins | Yellow | Riboflavin |

From *Resident Physician*, Feb., 1969.

* *Often used in combination with other antibacterials, e.g., Azotrex, Azo-Gantrisin.*

** *Often present in combination with dioctyl sodium sulfosuccinate, e.g., Dorbantyl, Doxidan. Also used in combination with calcium pantothenate (Modane).*

† *May even produce a magenta coloration in alkaline urine.*

drug-induced suppression of the platelet production in the marrow or from destruction of formed platelets in the blood. Toxic mechanisms are common; allergic mechanisms appear to be relatively rare. Most such toxicities are reversible upon discontinuation of the offending drug. The drugs that have been associated with drug-induced thrombocytopenia are indicated in Table 8.

TABLE 4
DISCOLORATION OF THE FECES BY DRUGS

| *Therapeutic Use* | *Color* | *Drug(s)* |
|---|---|---|
| Analgesics (CNS) (anti-inflammatory) | Pink to red to black (resulting from internal bleeding) | Salicylates<br>Phenylbutazone-oxyphenbutazone<br>Indomethacin |
| Analgesics (urinary) | Orange-red | Phenazopyridine (Pyridium®)<br>Azo Gantanol® (Azo Gantrisin®) |
| Antacids | Whitish discoloration or speckling of feces<br>Gray-white | Aluminum hydroxide preparations |
| Anthelmintics | Blue<br>Red | Dithiazanine (Delvex®)<br>Pyrvinium pamoate (Povan®) |
| Antibacterial agents | Black<br><br>Orange-red | Bismuth sodium triglycollamate (Bistrimate®)<br>Rifampin |
| Anticoagulants | Pink to red to black (resulting from internal bleeding) | All anticoagulants |
| Antiprotozoal agents | Black | Bismuth glycolylarsanilate (Milibis®) |
| Hematinic agents | Black | Iron preparations (e.g., ferrous sulfate) |
| Laxatives, cathartics | Can lead to a brownish staining of the rectal mucosa<br>Yellow-green | 1,8-dihydroxyanthraquinone (Dorbane®; Doxan®)<br>Senna |

TABLE 5
KNOWN COMPOUNDS PRODUCING METHEMOGLOBIN

| | | |
|---|---|---|
| Acetanilid | Erythrityl tetranitrate | Pentaerythritol tetranitrate |
| Acetophenetidin (phenacetin) | Ethylene glycol dinitrate | Phenetidin |
| Alloxans | Ethyl nitrite | Phenols |
| Aminophenols | Ethyl *p*-aminobenzoate (idiosyncracy) | Phenylazopyridine |
| Amyl nitrite | Hydroquinone (oral) | Phenylenediamine |
| Aniline derivatives | Hydroxylamine | Phenylhydroxylamine |
| Anilinoethanol | Inks, marking | Piperazine (also EEG changes) |
| Antipyrine | Kiszka | Plasmoquine |
| Benzocaine* | Lidocaine* | Prilocaine |
| Bismuth subnitrate* | Menthol* | Primaquine |
| Bitter almond oil, false | Metachloroaniline | Pyridium |
| Chloranilines | Methylene blue (IV) | Quinones |
| Chlorates | Naphthylamines* | Resorcinol |
| Cholorbenzene (oral) | Nitrates (if reduced)* | Shoe dye or polish |
| Chloronitrobenzene (oral) | Nitrites | Spinach* |
| Cobalt preparations | Nitrobenzene (Dinitrobenzene) | Sulfanilamide |
| Corning extract | Nitrochlorobenzene | Sulfonamides |
| Crayons, wax (red or orange)* | Nitrofurans | Sulfones |
| Dapsone (Avlosulfon) | Nitrogen oxide | Tetralin |
| Diaminodiphenyl sulfone | Nitroglycerol | Tetranitromethane |
| Diesel fuel additives | Nitrosobenzene | Tetronal |
| Dimethylaniline | Para-bromoaniline | Trional |
| Dinitrobenzene | Para-chloroaniline | Toluidine |
| Dinitrophenol | Para-nitroaniline | Trichlorocarbanilide (TCC degradation) |
| Dinitrotoluene | Para-toluidine | Trinitrotoluene |
| Diphenylhydantoin* | | |

*Likely to cause significant methemoglobinemia only in infants or young children.

TABLE 6
ANEMIAS

| | *Pancytopenia* | Thrombocytopenia* | *Unspecified* | *Hemolytic* | *Aplastic* | *Leukopenia* | *Agranulocytosis* | *Miscellaneous* |
|---|---|---|---|---|---|---|---|---|
| Acetarsone | x | | | | x | | | Heinz bodies |
| Acetaminophen | x | | x | | | | | |
| Acetazolamide | x | x | | x | | x | | |
| Acetophenetidin | x | | | | | | x | |
| *Amanita phalloides* | | | | x | | | | |
| Aminopyrine | x | x | | | | x | | |
| Amobarbital | x | | x | | | x | | Eosin (Eosinophilia) |
| Amodiaquin | | | | | | x | | |
| Aniline | | | | x | | | | Heinz bodies |
| Arsenic trioxide | x | | | x | | | x | Stippled cells |
| Arsine | | | | x | | | | Nucleated RBC's, stippled cells |
| Aspirin | x | x | x | | | x | | Eosin (C. D. Coagulation defect) |
| Benzene | x | | | x | | | x | Nucleated RBC's |
| Benzol | x | | x | | | | | |
| Carbon monoxide | | | | x | | | | Polycythemia |
| Carbon tetrachloride | x | | | | x | | | |
| Chloramphenicol | x | x | x | | | x | | Heinz bodies |
| Chlorates | | | | x | | | | Heinz bodies |
| Chlordane | x | | | | | x | | |
| Chlorobenzene | | | | x | | | | Heinz bodies |
| Chlorophenothane (DDT) | x | x | | | | x | | |
| Chlorothiazide | x | x | x | | | x | | |
| Chlorpheniramine maleate | x | x | | x | | | x | Eosin |
| Chlorpromazine | x | x | x | | | x | | |
| Chlortetracycline | x | | | | | x | | |
| Codeine | x | x | x | | | x | | |
| Colchicine | x | x | | | | x | | |
| Corticotropin | x | | x | | | x | | |
| Dextroamphetamine sulfate | x | x | | | | x | | Eosin |
| Diethylstilbestrol | | | | | | x | | |
| Digitalis | x | x | | | | | | Allergic purpura |
| Digitoxin | x | x | x | | | x | | |
| Digoxin | x | x | x | | | x | | |
| Dihydrocodeinone bitartrate | x | | | | | | | |
| Dihydrostreptomycin | x | | | | | x | | |
| Diphenylhydantoin sodium | x | x | x | | | x | | Eosin |
| Dipyrone (analgesic) | | | | | | x | | |
| Ephedrine | x | | | | | x | | |
| Erythromycin | x | x | x | | | x | | |
| Fava bean | | | | x | | | | |
| Gamma benzene hexachloride | x | | | | | x | | |

TABLE 6—*Continued*
ANEMIAS

| | *Pancytopenia* | *Thrombocytopenia* * | *Unspecified* | *Hemolytic* | *Aplastic* | *Leukopenia* | *Agranulocytosis* | *Miscellaneous* |
|---|---|---|---|---|---|---|---|---|
| Glutethimide (Doriden) | x | x | | | | x | | |
| Guaiacol | | | | x | | | | Heinz bodies |
| Hydrocortisone | x | x | | | | x | | |
| Hyoscyamine sulfate | x | | x | | | x | | |
| Imipramine (Tofrãnil®) | | | | | | | x | |
| Isoniazid | x | | x | | | x | | Stippled RBC's. Red fluorescence under ultraviolet light |
| Lead | x | | | | | | | |
| Manganese | x | | | | | | | |
| Mepazine | x | x | | | | | | |
| Meprobamate | x | x | | | | x | | (C.D.) |
| Methanol | x | | | | | | | |
| Methimazole | | | | | | x | | |
| Methylphenidate HCL | | x | | | | x | | |
| Methylphenylethyl hydantoin (Mesantoin®) | x | | x | | | x | | Eosin |
| Naphthol | | | | | x | | | Heinz bodies |
| Nitrites | | | | | x | | | |
| Nitrobenzene | | | | | x | | | Heinz bodies |
| Nitrofurantoin | x | | x | | | x | | |
| Novobiocin | x | x | x | | | x | | |
| Oleandomycin (in association with other drugs) | x | x | | | | x | | |
| Oxytetracycline | x | x | x | | | x | | |
| Paints | x | | x | | | x | | |
| Paint thinners | x | | | | | x | | |
| Para-aminosalicylic acid | | | x | | | x | | |
| Penicillin | x | x | x | | | x | | (C.D.) |
| Pentobarbital sodium | x | x | | | | x | | |
| Perphenazine | | | x | | | x | | |
| Petroleum distillates | x | x | | | | x | | |
| Pheniramine maleate | x | | | | | | | |
| Phenobarbital | x | x | x | | | x | | Eosin |
| Phenol | x | | | x | | | | |
| Phenolphthalein | x | x | | | | x | | |
| Phenylbutazone | x | x | x | | | x | | |
| Phenylephrine HCL | x | | | | | | | |
| Phosgene | x | | | | | | | Polycythemia |
| Piperonyl butoxide | x | x | x | | | x | | |
| Prednisone | x | x | | | | x | | |
| Primidone | x | | x | | | x | | |
| Prochlorperazine | | x | x | | | x | | |
| Promazine HCL | | x | | | x | | | |
| Promethazine | x | | | | | x | | |
| Pyrogallol | | | | x | | | | |
| Quinidine | x | x | x | | | x | | |

TABLE 6—*Continued*
ANEMIAS

| | *Pancytopenia* | *Thrombocytopenia* * | *Unspecified* | *Hemolytic* | *Aplastic* | *Leukopenia* | *Agranulocytosis* | *Miscellaneous* |
|---|---|---|---|---|---|---|---|---|
| Quinine | | x | | x | | x | | |
| Reserpine | x | x | | | | x | | |
| Resorcinol | | | | x | | | | |
| Ristocetin | x | x | x | | | | x | |
| Salicylazosulfapyridine | | | x | | | | x | |
| Secobarbital sodium | x | x | x | | | | x | Eosin |
| Snake venoms | | | | x | | | | |
| Solvents | x | x | | | | | | (C.D.) |
| Streptomycin | x | x | x | | | | x | |
| Sulfadiazine | x | x | x | | | | x | |
| Sulfamethazine | x | | | | | | x | |
| Sulfamethoxypyridazine | x | x | x | | | | x | |
| Sulfisoxazole | x | x | x | | | | x | |
| Sulfonamides (general) | x | x | | x | x | x | x | Heinz bodies |
| Sulfur dioxide | | | | | | | | Polycythemia |
| Tetracycline | x | x | x | | | | x | |
| Thenalidine tartrate | | | | | | | x | |
| Thiopental | | | | | | | x | |
| Thiouracil | | x | | | | | x | (C.D.) |
| Thorium dioxide | | | | | x | | | |
| Tolbutamide (Orinase®) | x | | | | | | x | |
| Toluene | x | | | x | | | | |
| Triamcinolone | | | | | | | x | |
| Triflupromazine (Vesprin®) | | | | | | | | |
| Trimethadione | | | | | | | x | |
| Trinitrotoluene | | | | | | | | Nucleated RBC's, Heinz bodies |
| Tripelennamine HCL | x | | | | | | x | |

* IgM antibody (macroglobulin) has been found responsible for several thrombocytopenic drug purpuras (chlorothiazide, sulfonamides, digitoxin, and others).

TABLE 7
DRUGS ASSOCIATED WITH EOSINOPHILIA

| *Drug* | *Comments* |
|---|---|
| Aldomet® (methyldopa) | Uncommon occurrence |
| Antidepressants, tricyclic | Imipramine and desipramine reported; other drugs in this class also may be associated with eosinophilia |
| Aminosalicylic acid (PAS) | Often accompanied by fever |
| Apresoline® (hydralazine) | May be dose-related |
| Atarax®, Vistaril® (hydroxyzine) | Seen with or without rash |
| Capastat® (capreomycin) | Frequent occurrence |
| Cephalosporin antibiotics | Often accompanied by rash or fever or both |
| Digitalis glycosides | Rare occurrence |
| Dyrenium® (triamterene) | Rare occurrence usually seen with syndrome of GI upset, headache, rash |
| Fluothane® (halothane) | Seen with hepatotoxic syndrome |

TABLE 7—*Continued*
DRUGS ASSOCIATED WITH EOSINOPHILIA

| *Drug* | *Comments* |
|---|---|
| Indandione oral anticoagulants | Uncommon occurrence |
| Ilosone® (erythromycin estolate) | Very rare with base and other erythromycin salts |
| Iodine radiologic contrast media | Especially diatrizoates |
| Isoniazid (INH) | Associated with hypersensitivity reaction |
| Kantrex® (kanamycin) | Often accompanied by rash and fever |
| Macrodantin®, Furadantin®, etc. (nitrofurantoin) | Often accompanied by headache, rash, and fever |
| Penicillins | Often accompanied by rash or fever or both; may be seen with all penicillins, but most often with ampicillin |
| Pronestyl® (procainamide) | Rare occurrence usually accompanied by fever |
| Pyrazinamide (PZA) | Often accompanied by chills and fever |
| Sulfonamides | Often accompanied by rash or fever or both |
| Tegretol® (carbamazepine) | Frequent occurrence |
| Vancocin® (vancomycin) | Common occurrence |
| Zyloprim® (allopurinol) | Uncommon occurrence |

From Arthur G. Lipman, reprinted from *Modern Medicine* © 1976 by Harcourt Brace Jovanovich.

TABLE 8
DRUGS ASSOCIATED WITH THROMBOCYTOPENIA

| *Drug* | *Effect* |
|---|---|
| Aldomet® (methyldopa) | Uncommon occurrence |
| Antidepressants, tricyclic | Several tricyclic antidepressants implicated, but interdrug sensitivity does not necessarily occur; allergic mechanism |
| Antineoplastic agents | Direct marrow toxicity from many cancer chemotherapeutic agents |
| Butazolidin®, Azolid® (phenylbutazone) Tandearil®, Oxalid® (oxyphenbutazone) | Occurs with normal doses; allergic mechanism |
| Cephalosporins | Thrombocytopenia reported with Keflin® (cephalothin) in a patient allergic to penicillin; allergic mechanism |
| Chloromycetin® (chloramphenicol) | Rapid onset, reversible reaction; toxic mechanism |
| Cuprimine® (penicillamine) | Mechanism not known |
| Daraprim® (pyrimethamine) | One case of thrombocytopenic purpura reported |
| Diamox®, Hydrazol® (acetazolamide) | Thrombocytopenia has occurred with normal doses within a few weeks of initiation of therapy |
| Diethylstilbestrol | Two case reports resulting from high doses used in prostatic carcinoma |
| Digitalis glycosides | Patients who react to digoxin may not react to digitoxin and vice versa |
| Diuretics: thiazide diuretics; Hygroton® (chlorthalidone) Lasix® (furosemide) mercurial diuretics | Occurs with normal doses; toxic mechanism |
| Gold salts | Due to slow excretion, chelating agents indicated in gold-induced thrombocytopenia |
| Heparin | Mild platelet depression is common; serious thrombocytopenia has been reported |
| Histadyl® (methapyrilene) | A common component of nonprescription sleep and cold medications; toxic mechanism |

TABLE 8—*Continued*
DRUGS ASSOCIATED WITH THROMBOCYTOPENIA

| *Drug* | *Effect* |
|---|---|
| Indanedione anticoagulants: Dipaxin® (diphenadine), Hedulin® (phenindione), Miradon® (anisindione) | Thrombocytopenia is a common part of the hypersensitivity reaction that occurs in about 0.2 per cent of patients receiving these drugs |
| Inderal® (propranolol) | One case report of thrombocytopenic purpura |
| Indocin® (indomethacin) | Rare occurrence |
| Naprosyn® (naproxen) | Collagen-induced platelet aggregation may be inhibited |
| Nitroglycerin | One case report; effect recurred on rechallenge |
| Penicillin, Ampicillin | Rare occurrence; allergic mechanism |
| Placidyl® (ethchlorvynol) | One case report; effect recurred with multiple rechallenges; final exposure fatal |
| Proglycem® (oral diazoxide) | Reported in a hypoglycemic infant receiving the drug in experimental trials |
| Quinine, Quinidine | Patients experiencing thrombocytopenia with one drug may not have it with the other and vice versa |
| Rifadin®, Rimactane® (rifampin) | Allergic mechanism |
| Salicylates | Allergic mechanism |
| Sulfonamides | Occurs with normal doses; greater risk with Bactrim® and Septra® (sulfamethoxazole-trimethoprim) combination than with sulfonamides alone |
| Tegretol® (carbamazepine) | Reported after many months of therapy |
| Vaccines: measles, mumps, rubella | May be due to virus from live vaccines disrupting megakaryocytes |
| Vitamin A | Hypervitaminosis A has produced thrombocytopenia |

From Arthur G. Lipman, reprinted from *Modern Medicine* © 1976 by Harcourt Brace Jovanovich.

## METHEMOGLOBINEMIA

Under normal circumstances, 99 per cent of the hemoglobin in the blood exists in the reduced ferrous state. Methemoglobinemia is produced by the oxidation of the ferrous ($Fe^{++}$) iron of hemoglobin to the ferric ($Fe^{+++}$) form by the action of a number of chemicals and drugs. These include nitrites, aniline derivatives, acetanilid, pyridium, dinitrophenol, chlorates, methylene blue and many others. Sodium nitrite used in meat curing may be present in excess in home-cured meats, or the salt may be used accidentally as table salt. The agricultural use of fertilizers in the soil can frequently cause the nitrate contamination of well water. The drinking of such contaminated water by children or its use in formulas for infants can produce methemoglobinemia. The oral use of bismuth subnitrate can also cause this to occur. The nitrates are reduced by the bacterial flora of the intestinal tract to nitrites, which are responsible for the formation of methemoglobin. Organic nitrates and nitrites as well as nitro and amino organic compounds are also capable of forming methemoglobin.

The ferric iron of methemoglobin can be reduced to ferrous iron (hemoglobin) most promptly by the administration of methylene blue. Although methylene blue in large doses is itself capable of causing methemoglobinemia, a point of equilibrium is reached when not more than 5 to 10 per cent of the hemoglobin has been changed to methemoglobin. After administration, the colored methylene blue is rapidly converted to a leuko base by the coenzyme diphosphopyridine nucleotide (DPN). This leuko base rapidly reduces ferric iron ($Fe^{+++}$). The reactions are as follows:

$$\text{Reduced DPN} + \text{Methylene blue} \longrightarrow \text{DPN} + \text{Leuko methylene blue}$$

$$\text{Leuko methylene blue} + \underset{(Fe^{+++})}{\text{Methemoglobin}} \longrightarrow \underset{(Fe^{++})}{\text{Hemoglobin}} + \text{Methylene blue}$$

The reaction continues in the presence of reduced DPN.

Ascorbic acid is also capable of reducing the ferric iron of methemoglobin to the ferrous iron of hemoglobin, but the action is slower than that of methylene blue. When the blood is examined on a slide beside normal blood or is agitated, it does not change from its characteristic chocolate color. Only sulfhemoglobin and methemoglobin have this property, owing to the fact that the iron is permanently in the ferric state, in which it is incapable of transporting oxygen. The distinction between methemoglobin and sulfhemoglobin can be made by a hand spectroscope. The blood is diluted with water (10 to 100 times), and a characteristic band can be seen at 630 mμ. The addition of 2 or 3 drops of 5% potassium cyanide causes the disappearance of this band if it is due to methemoglobin. The sulfhemoglobin band, which has an absorption of 618 mμ, may be difficult to distinguish from methemoglobin, but the band is not abolished by potassium cyanide.

Cyanosis occurs when 15 per cent of hemoblobin has been converted to methemoglobin, but symptoms of headache, dizziness, weakness and dyspnea are not likely to develop until the concentration reaches 30 to 40 per cent. At levels of 60 per cent, stupor and respiratory depression occur.

Without treatment, methemoglobin levels of 20 to 30 per cent revert to normal in one to three days, but a concentration above 40 per cent necessitates the use of methylene blue. Spectrophotometric analysis gives the concentration of methemoglobin in the blood.

Treatment consists of giving 100% oxygen to increase the saturation of unchanged hemoglobin. If the poison has been ingested, it should be removed by gastric lavage or emesis followed by a saline cathartic. For skin contamination, the skin should be washed thoroughly with soap and water for fifteen minutes. The specific antidote is methylene blue, which should be used for concentrations of methemoglobin above 40 per cent or, if analysis is not immediately available, when the symptoms are serious enough to warrant therapy.

This should be administered slowly over five to ten minutes in a 1% solution, using 1 mg (0.1 ml) lb. of body weight. Perivenous infiltration should be avoided since rather severe necrosis of soft tissue may occur. If there is no great improvement within one to two hours, methylene blue can be repeated. In young infants hemolysis may readily occur and partial blood exchange may be indicated. Ascorbic acid 1 gm intravenously can be given in addition to or in place of methylene blue if it is not available. However, the rate of conversion of methemoglobinemia is so slow that ascorbic acid is not often used now in treatment. General measures should include absolute bedrest and the continuation of oxygen (hyperbaric oxygen has been used successfully) for at least two hours after methylene blue has been given. (For Drug-induced Hemolytic Anemias and G-6-PD Deficiency, *see* pages 336 through 344.) An associated G-6-PD deficiency may interfere with or completely negate methylene blue therapy.

## EMERGENCY DRUGS AND EQUIPMENT

Hospitals and clinics wishing to provide for emergency treatment of common forms of poisoning should have all supplies and drugs indexed as listed in Table 9 and available for immediate use. A less comprehensive but current list is found in Table 10. Other drugs should be added to this list as local medical practice dictates.

TABLE 9

EMERGENCY DRUGS (GENERAL)

| *Drug list A (For injection)* | *Unit* | *Amt./unit* | *Amt./ml* | *No.* |
|---|---|---|---|---|
| ACTH (corticotropin) | Vial 5 ml | 200 units | 40 u/ml | 1 |
| Aminophylline | Amp. 10 ml | 250 mg | 25 mg/ml | 4 |
| Amytal® Sodium | Amp. Dry | 250 mg | | 6 |
| Apomorphine HCl | Hypo. Tab | 6 mg | | 10 |
| Ascorbic acid (ascorbate sodium) | Amp. 1 ml | | 250 mg/ml | 6 |
| Atropine sulfate | Amp. 4.5 ml | 450 mg | 100 mg/ml | 5 |
| BAL in oil (dimercaprol) 10% | Hypo. Tab. | 0.4 mg | | 10 |
| Benadryl® | Vial 10 ml | 100 mg | 10 mg/ml | 1 |
| Caffeine & sodium benzoate | Amp. 2 ml | 500 mg | 250 mg/ml | 6 |
| Calcium disodium versenate | Amp. 5 ml | 1.0 gm | 0.2 gm/ml | 3 |
| Calcium gluconate 10% | Amp. 10 ml | 1.0 gm | 0.1 gm/ml | 4 |
| Camphor in oil | Amp. 1 ml | 0.2 gm | | 1 |
| Cedilanid® (lanatoside C) | Amp. 4 ml | 0.8 mg | 0.2 mg/ml | 4 |
| Codeine phosphate | Hypo. Tab. | 30 mg | | 6 |
| Coramine® (nikethamide 25%) | Amp. 1.5 ml | | 250 mg/ml | 4 |
| Dexedrine® (d-amphetamine $SO_4$) | Amp. 1 ml | 20 mg | | 4 |
| Dextrose (50%) | Amp. 50 ml | | | 2 |
| Digitoxin | Amp. 1 ml | 0.2 mg | | 4 |
| Dramamine® | Vial 5 ml | 250 mg | 50 mg/ml | 1 |
| Ephedrine sulfate | Amp. 1 ml | 50 mg | | 6 |
| Epinephrine (adrenalin) aq. 1:1000 | Amp. 1 ml | 1 mg | | 10 |
| Epinephrine in oil 1:500 | Amp. 1 ml | 2 mg | | 4 |
| Hydrocortisone (Solu-Cortef®) | Vial 2 ml | 100 mg | 50 mg/ml | 1 |
| Levallorphan (Lorfan®) | Amp. 1 ml | 1 mg | 1 mg/ml | 4 |
| Levophed® bitartrate (norepinephrine) | Amp. 4 ml | 8 mg | 2 mg/ml | 4 |
| Magnesium sulfate (25%) | Amp. 10 ml | 2.5 gm | 250 mg/ml | 4 |
| Mephyton® (vitamin $K_1$ emulsion) | Amp. 1 ml | 50 mg | | 2 |
| Methylene blue (1%) | Amp. 10 ml | 100 mg | 10 mg/ml | 2 |
| Metrazol® | Amp 1 ml | 100 mg | | 4 |
| Morphine sulfate | Hypo. Tab. | 15 mg | | 6 |
| N-allylnormorphine HCl (Nalline®) | Amp. 1 ml | 5 mg | | 4 |
| Naloxone HCl (Narcan®) | Amp. 10 ml | 4 mg | 0.4 mg/ml | 5 |
| Neostigmine bromide (Prostigmin®) 1:2000 | Vial 10 ml | 5 mg | 0.5 mg/ml | 1 |
| Paraldehyde | Amp. 5 ml | | | 4 |
| Phenobarbital sodium (Luminal®) | Amp. Dry | 120–300 mg | | 6 |
| Picrotoxin | Vial 20 ml | 60 mg | 3 mg/ml | 1 |
| Procainamide HCl (Pronestyl®) | Vial 10 ml | 1.0 gm | 100 mg/ml | 1 |
| Pyribenzamine® HCl | Amp 1 ml | 25 mg | | 6 |
| Quinidine HCl | Amp. 5 ml | 0.6 gm | .12 gm/ml | 1 |
| Sodium bicarbonate (6%) | Amp. 50 ml | 3.0 gm | | 4 |
| Sodium formaldehyde sulfoxylate | Amp. Dry | 20 gm | as 5% sol. | 1 |
| Sodium lactate (IV) | Amp. 40 ml | | | 4 |

TABLE 9—*Continued*

EMERGENCY DRUGS

| *Drug list A (For injection)* | *Unit* | *Amt./unit* | *Amt./ml* | *No.* |
|---|---|---|---|---|
| Sodium nitrite } | Amp. 10 ml | 0.3 gm | (2 amps. each of these | |
| Sodium thiosulfate } | Amp. 50 ml | 12.5 gm | in cyanide kit) | 1 |
| Sodium thiosulfate | Amp. 10 ml | 1.0 gm | 100 mg/ml | 2 |
| Synkayvite® (vitamin $K_1$) | Amp. 1 ml | 10 mg | | 6 |
| Thiamine HCl (vitamin $B_1$) | Vial 25 ml | 2.5 gm | 100 mg/ml | 1 |
| *Drug List B (For oral use)* | *Preparation* | *Amount* | *Strength* | *No.* |
| Acetic acid (5%) | Liquid * | 500 ml | | 1 |
| Aluminum hydroxide gel | Liquid | 240 ml | | 1 |
| Aminophylline | Tablet | | 100 mg | 12 |
| Ammonium hydroxide (0.2%) | Liquid | 1000 ml | | 1 |
| Ascorbic acid | Tablet | | 100 mg | 12 |
| Benadryl HCl | Capsule | | 25 mg | 12 |
| Brewer's yeast | Tablet | | 400 mg | 12 |
| Calcium hydroxide | Liquid | 500 ml | | 1 |
| Calcium lactate | Powder * | | 100 gm | 1 |
| Charcoal, activated | Powder or Tablet 500 gm (1 can) | | 1 gm | 1 |
| Codeine phosphate | Tablet | | 30 mg | 12 |
| Dexedrine sulfate | Tablet | | 5 mg | 12 |
| Ephedrine sulfate | Tablet | | 25 mg | 12 |
| Glycerin | Liquid | 240 ml | | 6 |
| Ipecac, syrup | Liquid | 120 ml | | 1 |
| Magnesium oxide | Powder * | | 25 gm | 6 |
| Magnesium sulfate (50%) | Liquid | 240 ml | | 4 |
| Milk, evaporated | Liquid | 500 ml (1 can) | | 1 |
| Mineral oil | Liquid | 500 ml | | 1 |
| Nitroglycerin, sublingual | Tablet | | .32 mg | 6 |
| Paraldehyde | Liquid | 120 ml | | 1 |
| Paregoric | Liquid | 120 ml | | 1 |
| Phenobarbital | Tablet | | 30–100 mg | 12 |
| Phenobarbital, elixir | Liquid | 240 ml | 4 mg | 1 |
| Potassium permanganate | Tablet * | | 0.1 gm | 12 |
| Procainamide (Pronestyl) | Tablet | | .25 gm | 6 |
| Pyribenzamine® HCl | Tablet | | 50 mg | 12 |
| Quinidine sulfate | Tablet | | 0.2 gm | 6 |
| Sodium bicarbonate | Powder * | | 50 gm | 4 |
| Sodium sulfate (40%) | Liquid | 240 ml | | 1 |
| Starch | Powder * | | 80 gm | 1 |
| Tannic acid | Powder * | | 40 gm | 1 |
| *Drug List C (Miscellaneous)* | *Amount* | *No.* | | |
| Alcohol, ethyl 95% | 120 ml | 1 | | |
| Aminophylline suppositories | 250 mg | 6 | | |
| Ammonia, arom. spirits | 120 ml | 1 | | |
| Amyl nitrite pearls | 0.3 ml | 12 | | |
| Antivenin (*Crotalus, Micrurus fulvius*) | Unit | 4 | | |
| Botulism antitoxin (trivalent A,B,E) | Amp. | 2 | | |
| Chloroform | 120 ml | 1 | | |
| Iodine, tincture | 120 ml | 1 | | |
| Tribromoethanol (Avertin®) | 25 ml | 1 | | |

Several rules should be followed to decrease chance of error:

1. All containers labeled clearly with name and amount of material.
2. Index file should always be consulted regarding indication and dosage.
3. Only one size of unit for injection of any particular drug should be kept on hand.
4. Volume should be stated in *cc* and *ml* to avoid misreading as mg (for index file only).
5. For labeling gram should be abbreviated with capital, Gm., again to avoid error or misreading.

TABLE 9—*Continued*

EMERGENCY DRUGS

6. Particularly dangerous drugs should bear red label.
7. Emphasis (in training, in wording of materials) should be on the hazards of overtreatment.

* *Special units:* Dry powder is placed in 1000 ml bottle and stored on shelf in this fashion. When necessary to use for lavage, material is dissolved in water by filling bottle. Weights calculated to given amount for strength of solution to be used. Directions on label.

*Example:* *Tannic Acid* 40 Gm
4% Solution
(When dissolved in container full of water)

TABLE 10
EMERGENCY DRUGS (SPECIFIC)

| *Drug* | *Concentration, unit size, No. of Units* | *Route* | *Pharmacologic Use* |
|---|---|---|---|
| Aminophylline | 25 mg/ml; 20ml ampul; 2 | IV push | Spasmolytic |
| Atropine | 100 μg/ml; 10 ml syringe*; 2 | IV push | Anticholinergic |
| Calcium chloride | 100 mg/ml; 10 ml syringe*; 5 | IV | Electrolyte |
| Dexamethasone (Decadron®) | 4 mg/ml; 1 ml syringe†; 2 | IV | Adrenocorticosteroid |
| Diazepam‡ (Valium®) | 5 mg/ml; 2 ml syringe†; 2 | IV push | Anticonvulsant, sedative |
| Digoxin (Lanoxin®) | 250 μg/ml; 2 ml ampul; 2 | IV | Cardiac glycoside |
| Diphenhydramine (Benadryl®) | 50 mg/ml; 1 ml syringe†; 2 | IM | Antihistamine |
| Dopamine (Intropin®) | 40 mg/ml; 5 ml ampul; 2 | IV infusion | Catecholamine precursor |
| Edrophonium (Tensilon®) | 10 mg/ml; 1 ml ampul; 2 | IV | Curariform drug antidote |
| Epinephrine (Adrenalin®) | 1 mg/ml (1:100); 1 ml ampul; 2<br>100 μg/ml (1:10,000); 10 ml syringe; 2 | IV<br>IC | Sympathomimetic (alpha-beta) |
| Furosemide (Lasix®) | 10 mg/ml; 2 ml ampul; 2 | IV push | Diuretic |
| Hydrocortisone sodium succinate (Solu-Cortef®) | 1 gm/vial; 2 | IV | Adrenocorticosteroid |
| Isoproterenol (Isuprel®) | 200 μg/ml; 5 ml ampul; 4 | IV | Sympathomimetic (beta) |
| Levarterenol (Levophed®) | 2 mg/ml; 4 ml ampul; 8 | IV | Sympathomimetic (alpha, 90%; beta, 10%) |

TABLE 10—*Continued*
EMERGENCY DRUGS

| *Drug* | *Concentration, unit size, No. of Units* | *Route* | *Pharmacologic Use* |
|---|---|---|---|
| Lidocaine (Xylocaine®) | 20 mg/ml; 5 ml syringe; 4<br>40 mg/ml; 50 ml vial; 2 | IV push<br>IV infusion | Antiarrhythmic |
| Mannitol | 250 mg/ml; 50 ml vial; 2 | IV infusion | Osmotic diuretic |
| Mephentermine (Wyamine®) | 15 mg/ml; 1 ml ampul; 2 | IM<br>IV infusion | Sympathomimetic (primarily alpha) |
| Metaraminol (Aramine®) | 10 mg/ml; 10 ml vial; 1 | IM<br>IV infusion | Sympathomimetic (primarily alpha) |
| Methylprednisolone sodium succinate (Solu-Medrol®) | 500 mg/vial; 2 | IV | Adrenocorticosteroid |
| Naloxone (Narcan®) | 400 μg/ml; 1 ml ampul; 2 | IV | Narcotic antagonist |
| Nitroprusside sodium (Nipride®) | 50 mg/vial; 2 | IV infusion | Antihypertensive |
| Phentolamine mesylate (Regitine®) | 5 mg/ampul; 2 | IV | Antihypertensive (alpha sympatholytic) |
| Phenytoin (Dilantin®) | 250 mg/syringe†; 2 | IV push | Antiarrhythmic, anticonvulsant |
| Phenylephrine (Neosynephrine®) | 10 mg/ml; 10 ml ampul; 3 | IV | Sympathomimetic (alpha) |
| Phytonadione (vitamin $K_1$) (Aquamephyton®) | 10 mg/ml; 1 ml ampul; 2 | IV | Coagulant in coumarin overdose |
| Potassium chloride | 20 mEq/10 ml vial; 3 | IV infusion | Electrolyte |
| Procainamide (Pronestyl®) | 100 mg/ml; 10 ml vial; 1 | IV infusion | Antiarrhythmic |
| Quinidine gluconate | 80 mg/ml; 10 ml vial; 1 | IV infusion | Antiarrhythmic |
| Sodium bicarbonate | 1 mEq/ml; 50 ml syringe*; 2 | IV | Alkalinizer |
| Sterile water for injection | 20 ml ampul; 2 | | Diluent |

*Available in prefilled syringe as generic drug from Abbott Laboratories, Bristol Laboratories, International Medication Systems, Ltd.
†Available in prefilled syringe from manufacturer of drug.
‡Controlled substance (federal law).
From Arthur G. Lipman, reprinted from *Modern Medicine* © 1975 by Harcourt Brace Jovanovich.

## Drug Dosage

### *For Infants and Children*

For almost all drugs, immaturity of renal and hepatic functions and of enzyme activity in early infancy presents challenging problems in dose estimation. These functions improve during and after the neonatal period, and differences may be insignificant in three to six months, but variations in response to drugs among infants, and even in the same infant, are often so great as to make it difficult to predict either therapeutic or toxic effects. The following charts of children's dosages can be helpful in this regard.

## Drug Dosage Equivalents

In order to determine the correct drug dosage, it is essential to determine the various dosage equivalents. Table 13 charts the approximate equivalents for grains, grams and milligrams, while Tables 14 and 15 show the various equivalent measures.

## Making Weight in Weight Percentage Solution

Table 16 gives the proportions of material and solvent weight in weight to be used for making solutions in quantities of 1 fl. oz., 1 pt., 100 ml and 500 ml. Multiples or fractions of these values may be calculated from these figures. Where exactness is desired, use the amount of water shown. If slight variations are not objectionable, the material may be dissolved in water sufficient to make the volume given at the top of the column.

TABLE 11
FACTORS USEFUL IN CALCULATING CHILDREN'S DOSES

In general, Young's rule is applicable:

$$\text{Children's doses} = \frac{\text{Age x Adult dose}}{\text{Age} + 12}$$

FRACTION OF ADULT DOSES

| | New-born | 6 mo. | 1 yr. | 2 yr. | 5 yr. | 10 yr. | Adult |
|---|---|---|---|---|---|---|---|
| By age | ...... | 0.04 | 0.08 | 0.15 | 0.29 | 0.45 | 1 |
| By weight | 0.05 | 0.11 | 0.14 | 0.18 | 0.26 | 0.45 | 1 |
| By surface area | 0.12 | 0.21 | 0.26 | 0.31 | 0.42 | 0.64 | 1 |

TABLE 12
DETERMINATION OF CHILDREN'S DOSES FROM ADULT DOSES ON BASIS OF BODY SURFACE AREA

| Weight (kg) | Weight (lb.) | BSA (sq. m.) | Approximate Percentage of Adult Dose |
|---|---|---|---|
| 2 | 4.4 | 0.15 | 9 |
| 4 | 8.8 | 0.25 | 14 |
| 6 | 13.2 | 0.33 | 19 |
| 8 | 17.6 | 0.40 | 23 |
| 10 | 22.0 | 0.46 | 27 |
| 15 | 33.0 | 0.63 | 36 |
| 20 | 44.0 | 0.83 | 48 |
| 25 | 55.0 | 0.95 | 55 |
| 30 | 66.0 | 1.08 | 62 |
| 35 | 77.0 | 1.20 | 69 |
| 40 | 88.0 | 1.30 | 75 |
| 45 | 99.0 | 1.40 | 81 |
| 50 | 110.0 | 1.51 | 87 |
| 55 | 121.0 | 1.58 | 91 |

TABLE 13
APPROXIMATE DOSAGE EQUIVALENTS FOR GRAINS AND GRAMS

| gr | gm | mg | gr | gm | mg | gr | gm | mg |
|---|---|---|---|---|---|---|---|---|
| 1/600 | .0001 | 0.1 | 1/20 | .003 | 3 | 1½ | .100 | |
| 1/500 | .00012 | 0.12 | 1/15 | .004 | 4 | 2 | .130 | |
| 1/400 | .00015 | 0.15 | 1/12 | .005 | 5 | 2½ | .150 | |
| 1/300 | .0002 | 0.2 | 1/10 | .006 | 6 | 3 | .200 | |
| 1/250 | .00025 | 0.25 | 1/8 | .008 | 8 | 4 | .250 | |
| 1/200 | .0003 | 0.3 | 1/6 | .010 | 10 | 5 | .325 | |
| 1/150 | .0004 | 0.4 | 1/4 | .015 | 15 | 7½ | .500 | |
| 1/120 | .0005 | 0.5 | 1/3 | .020 | 20 | 10 | .650 | |
| 1/100 | .0006 | 0.6 | 3/8 | .025 | 25 | 15 | 1 | |
| 1/80 | .0008 | 0.8 | 1/2 | .032 | 32 | 30 | 2 | |
| 1/60 | .001 | 1 | 3/4 | .050 | 50 | 45 | 3 | |
| 1/30 | .002 | 2 | 1 | .065 | 65 | 60 | 4 | |

gr = grains; gm = grams; mg = milligrams.

TABLE 14
APPROXIMATE HOUSEHOLD MEASURES

| | | |
|---|---|---|
| 1 Teaspoonful | 1 fl dram | 4–5 ml |
| 1 Dessertspoonful | 2 fl drams | 8 ml |
| 1 Tablespoonful | ½ fl oz. | 15 ml |
| 1 Jigger | 1 fl oz. | 30 ml |
| 1 Wineglass | 2 fl oz. | 60 ml |
| 1 Teacup | 4 fl oz. | 120 ml |
| 1 Drinking Glass | 8 fl oz. | 240 ml |

TABLE 15
NUMERICAL EQUIVALENTS

**Length**

1 cm = 0.3937 inch
1 meter = 39.37 inches
= 3.28 feet
1 km = 0.6214 mile

1 inch = 2.54 cm
1 foot = 30.48 cm
= 0.3048 meter
1 miles = 1.609 km

**Area**

1 sq. mm = 0.0015 sq. in.
1 sq. cm = 0.1549 sq. in.
1 sq. m = 1549.99 sq. in.
= 10.75 sq. ft.
1 sq. km = 0.3861 sq. mile

1 sq. in. = 6.45 sq. cm
1 sq. ft. = 929.03 sq. cm
= .0929 sq. m
1 sq. mile = 2.58 sq. km

**Volume**

1 liter = 1.057 qt.
= 61 cu. in.
1 cu. m = 35.26 cu. ft.
1 ml = 0.0338 oz.
= 0.068 tablespoon
= 0.203 teaspoon
= 16.231 minims

1 cu. ft. = 0.028 cu. m
1 qt. = 0.946 liter
= 946 ml
1 cup = 2.36 × $10^{-4}$cu. m
1 US fluid oz = 29.57 ml
1 tablespoon = 14.7 ml
1 teaspoon = 4.92 ml
1 minim 0.0616 ml

**Mass or Weight**

1 kg = 2.205 lb.
1 gm = 0.035 oz.
= 15.45 grains
1 mg = 0.015 grain

1 lb. (avoirdupois) = 0.453 kg
1 oz. (avoirdupois) = 28 gm
1 grain = 0.0647 gm
= 64.7 mg

**Force**

1 dyne = 2.24 × $10^{-6}$ pound weight*
= 1.01 × $10^{-3}$ gram weight
= 0.015 grain weight
1 newton = $10^{5}$ dynes = 0.224 lb. weight
= 101 gm weight
= 1573 grain weight
1 gram weight = 980.665 dynes
1 kilogram weight = 9.80 × $10^{5}$ dynes
= 9.8 newtons

1 lb. weight = 453.59 gm weight
= 4.44 × $10^{5}$ dynes
= 4.44 newtons

*All weights based on acceleration due to gravity of 9.8 meters/sq. sec.

**Pressure**

1 mm Hg = 0.019 lb./sq. in.
= 1.35 gm/sq. cm

TABLE 15—*Continued*
NUMERICAL EQUIVALENTS

= 13.5 kg/sq. m
= 1333.22 dynes/sq. cm
= 133.32 newtons/sq. m

1 lb./sq. in.(psi) = 51.715 mm Hg
= 70.307 gm/sq. cm
= 6.8 × $10^4$ dynes/sq. cm
= 6.8 × $10^3$ newtons/sq. m
= 703.07 kg/sq. m

**Work or Energy**

1 joule = 0.239 calorie (gram)
= 2.39 × $10^{-4}$ calories (kilogram)
= 9.48 × $10^{-4}$ BTU
= 2.77 × $10^{-7}$ kw-hr
= 1 watt-sec
= 0.62 × $10^{19}$ electron volts

1 curie = 3.7 × $10^{10}$ disintegration/ sec
1 rad (radiation absorbed dose) = 1 × $10^{-2}$ joule/kg
1 roentgen = 2.57 × $10^{-4}$ coulomb/kg

1 calorie = 4.18 joules
1 BTU = 1054.8 joule

1 kw-hr = 3.6 × $10^6$ joules
1 watt-sec = 1 joule
1 electron volt = 1.6 × $10^{-19}$ joule

**Power**

1 watt = 0.056 BTU/minute
= 0.00131 horse power
= 0.00134 horse power (electrical)
= 0.737 ft.-lb./sec.
= 1 × $10^7$ erg/sec.
= 0.239 calories/sec.

1 BTU/minute = 17.58 watts
1 horse power = 745.7 watts
1 horse power (electrical) = 746 watts
1 ft.-lb./second = 1.35 watts
1 gm-cm/sec. = 9.8 × $1^{-5}$ watts
1 erg/sec. = 1 × $10^{-7}$ watts
1 calorie/sec. = 4.18 watts

**Temperature**

Temperature Fahrenheit = 9/5 × C + 32
Temperature centigrade = 5/9 (F − 32)
Temperature Kelvin = 273.15 + C

To convert:
A Fahrenheit reading to Celsius, subtract 32 from —°F, multiply by five, and divide by nine; A Celsius reading to Fahrenheit, divide—°C by five, multiply by nine, and add 32.

## *Parts Per Thousand Solutions*

The term "parts per thousand" is used to express parts of solids per thousand parts of solution. It is a convenient method of expressing the strength of very dilute solutions and is written 1/1000 or 1:1000. The following method applies also to "parts per 100," "parts per 10,000," etc.

In all these solutions, regardless of strength, in order to find the amount of solid required, divide the amount of the solution desired by the second figure of the strength necessary. If for example, 500 ml of a 1:1000 solution of $KMNO_4$ is needed, divide 500 by 1000, i.e. 500 ÷ 1000 = 0.5 gm. Thus, 0.5 gm (½ gm) of $KMNO_4$ must be dissolved in 500 ml of water.

*Example:* 2000 ml of a 1:8000 solution of $KMNO_4$
2000 ÷ 8000 = 0.25 gm

*Example:* 500 ml of a 1:500 solution of $KMNO_4$
500 ÷ 500 = 1 gm

TABLE 16
APPROXIMATE AMOUNT OF SOLUTION

| *Strength of Solution* | *100 ml* | | *500 ml* | | *1 fl. oz.* | | *1 pt.* | |
|---|---|---|---|---|---|---|---|---|
| | *Material* | *Distilled Water* | *Material* | *Distilled Water* | *Material* | *Distilled Water* | *Material* | *Distilled Water* |
| 1:5000 | 0.02 gm | 100.0 ml | 0.1 gm | 500.0 ml | 1/10 gr | 500 gr | 1 1/2 gr | 7498 gr |
| 1:2000 | 0.05 gm | 100.0 ml | 0.25 gm | 500.0 ml | 1/4 gr | 500 gr | 3 3/4 gr | 7496 gr |
| 1:1000 | 0.1 gm | 100.0 ml | 0.5 gm | 500.0 ml | 1/2 gr | 500 gr | 7 1/2 gr | 7492 gr |
| 1:500 | 0.2 gm | 100.0 ml | 1 gm | 499.0 ml | 1 gr | 499 gr | 15 gr | 7485 gr |
| 1:200 | 0.5 gm | 100.0 ml | 2.5 gm | 497.5 ml | 2 3/10 gr | 458 gr | 37 gr | 7363 gr |
| 1 % | 1 gm | 99.0 ml | 5 gm | 495.0 ml | 4 3/5 gr | 455 gr | 74 gr | 7326 gr |
| 2 % | 2.02 gm | 99.1 ml | 10.1 gm | 495.5 ml | 9 1/4 gr | 452 gr | 148 gr | 7252 gr |
| 3 % | 3.05 gm | 98.5 ml | 15.25 gm | 492.5 ml | 14 gr | 453 gr | 224 gr | 7243 gr |
| 4 % | 4.08 gm | 98.0 ml | 20.4 gm | 490.0 ml | 19 gr | 456 gr | 300 gr | 7200 gr |
| 5 % | 5.13 gm | 97.5 ml | 25.6 gm | 487.5 ml | 24 gr | 456 gr | 380 gr | 7220 gr |
| 6 % | 6.2 gm | 96.9 ml | 31 gm | 484.5 ml | 29 gr | 454 gr | 455 gr | 7136 gr |
| 8 % | 8.33 gm | 95.8 ml | 41.7 gm | 479.0 ml | 39 gr | 448 gr | 612 gr | 7044 gr |
| 10 % | 10.5 gm | 94.8 ml | 52.6 gm | 474.0 ml | 48 gr | 432 gr | 772 gr | 6952 gr |
| 12 1/2% | 13.3 gm | 93.1 ml | 66.5 gm | 465.5 ml | 62 gr | 427 gr | 976 gr | 6832 gr |
| 15 % | 16.13 gm | 91.4 ml | 80.6 gm | 457 ml | 75 gr | 425 gr | 1188 gr | 6732 gr |
| 16 2/3% | 18.11 gm | 90.6 ml | 90.6 gm | 453.0 ml | 84 gr | 420 gr | 1336 gr | 6682 gr |
| 20 % | 22.12 gm | 88.5 ml | 110.6 gm | 442.5 ml | 102 gr | 408 gr | 1634 gr | 6538 gr |
| 25 % | 28.4 gm | 85.2 ml | 142 gm | 426 ml | 132 gr | 396 gr | 2104 gr | 6312 gr |
| 30 % | 35.04 gm | 81.8 ml | 175.2 gm | 409 ml | 165 gr | 385 gr | 2625 gr | 6125 gr |
| 33 1/3% | 39.5 gm | 79.0 ml | 197.6 gm | 395 ml | 185 gr | 370 gr | 2954 gr | 5908 gr |
| 50 % | 64.5 gm | 64.5 ml | 322.5 gm | 322.5 ml | 295 gr | 295 gr | 4720 gr | 4720 gr |

437.5 gr = 1 avoirdupois ounce; 480 gr = 1 apothecaries ounce.

TABLE 17
SOME RELATIONS OF DRUG TOXICITY IN EXPERIMENTAL ANIMALS COMPARED WITH MAN

| *Animal* | *Weight in kg* | *Wt. Ratio (An./Man)* | *Drug Dose Ratio (An./Man)* | *Sensitivity (Drug Dose Ratio/Wt. Ratio)* |
|---|---|---|---|---|
| Man | 60 | 1 | 1 | 1 |
| Cow | 500 | 8 | 24 | Man is 3 times as sensitive. |
| Horse | 500 | 8 | 16 | Man is 2 times as sensitive. |
| Sheep | 60 | 1 | 3 | Man is 3 times as sensitive. |
| Goat | 60 | 1 | 3 | Man is 3 times as sensitive. |
| Swine | 60 | 1 | 2 | Man is 2 times as sensitive. |
| Dog | 10 | 1/6 | 1 | Man is 6 times as sensitive. |
| Cat | 3 | 1/20 | 1/2 | Man is 10 times as sensitive. |
| Rat | 0.4 | 1/150 | 1/15 | Man is 10 times as sensitive. |

## Emergency Equipment

1. Stomach tubes of different calibers suitable for use in infants, children and adults. Davol plastic duodenal tubes, sizes 8, 12, 14 and 16 and varying from 15 to 50 in. in length, are more practical than rubber lavage tubes which deteriorate with constant sterilization and use. The plastic variety can be chilled for further rigidity or warmed for greater flexibility. They also have the great advantage of being able to be passed after immersion in water, obviating the use of oil for this purpose.

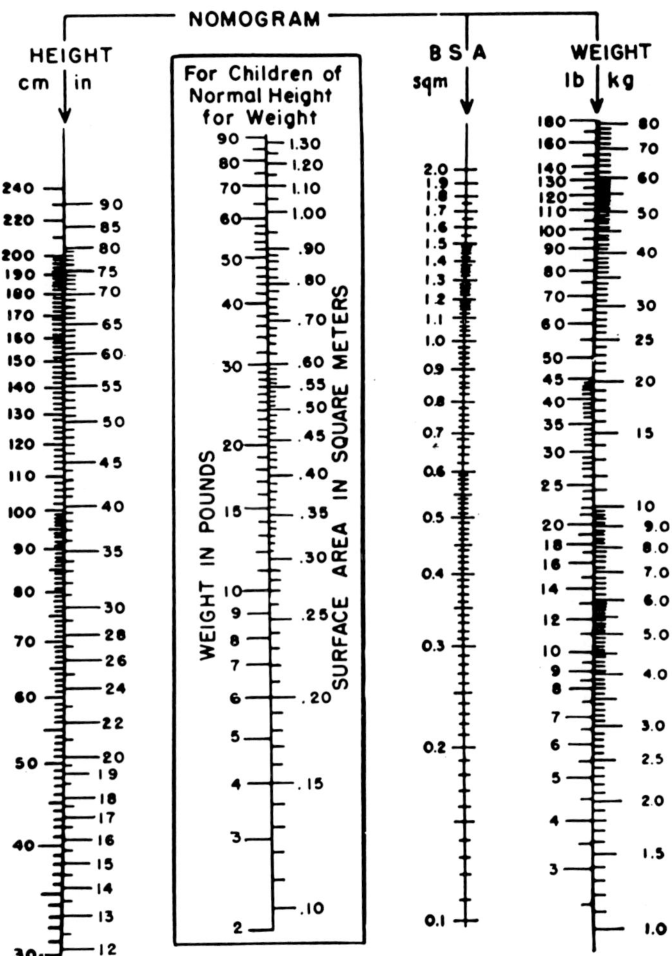


Figure 2. Body surface area (BSA) is indicated where straight line that connects height and weight levels intersects BSA column or, if patient is about average size, from weight alone (enclosed area). (Modified from data of E. Boyd by C.D. West, from Shirkey and Barba.)

2. Three 4 oz. Asepto® irrigating syringes.
3. 1, 2, 5, 10, 20 and 50 ml syringes and needles.
4. A rubber bulb and an ear syringe for suction on the stomach tube.
5. Airways for infants, children and adults.
6. Oxygen inhalation apparatus.

## Management (General)

Acute poisoning, unfortunately, is often mismanaged. It is impossible at times to determine whether recovery occurred because of or in spite of the treatment used. Although poisoning is a common pediatric problem, many other specialists are involved (obstetrician, neonatologist, internist, family physician, surgeon, etc.), and it has an interface with many disciplines.

The basic treatment for acute poisoning, whether drug or chemical, is mainly symptomatic and supportive. Overtreatment of the poisoned patient with large doses of nonspecific and questionably effective antidotes, stimulants, sedatives and other therapeutic agents often does far more harm and damage than the poison itself. A calm attitude, with the judicious use of drugs, parenteral fluids, electrolytes for homeostasis and the maintenance of an adequate airway are far more effective than heroic measures, which usually are unnecessary. Remember, *"Treat the patient, not the poison."*

The four cardinal principles of good management are (1) identification of the drug or chemical as quickly as possible, (2) evacuation of the poison from the stomach, except when contraindicated (discussed under gastric lavage), (3) administration of an antidote if available, and (4) symptomatic and supportive therapy as indicated.

## GASTRIC LAVAGE

Gastric lavage may be lifesaving and is clearly indicated within three hours after ingestion of a poison and even later if large amounts of milk or food were given beforehand or if enteric-coated drugs had been taken. However, the contraindications to this procedure should be kept in mind. Following the ingestion of strong corrosive agents like alkali (concentrated ammonia water, lye, etc.) or mineral acids (considered safe here if done within an hour), intubation is impractical and dangerous in that it may lead to perforation. In those who have ingested strychnine, a convulsion may be induced by this manipulation if much time has elapsed. Lavage is also contraindicated in petroleum distillate poisoning (kerosene, mineral seal oil, etc.) or in the presence of coma, since pneumonia may follow depression of the cough reflex and aspiration of stomach contents into the lungs.

The only equipment needed for gastric lavage in children is a common urethral catheter (No. 8 to 12 F.) and a 4 oz. size Asepto irrigating or glass syringe (20 or 50 ml, preferably the latter). Davol plastic duodenal tubes are preferable, however, because of their durability, flexibility and ease in passage without lubrication. For adults, a tube with a diameter between 5/16 and ½ in. (No. 24 F. or greater) is usually satisfactory. At any rate, use as large a tube as accessible so that the wash solution flows freely and the lavage is carried out as quickly as possible. In older children and adults, the nasal route is preferred, whereas the oral passage is easier and less traumatic for infants and young children. The tube should be inserted the length of the distance measured from the bridge of the nose to the tip of the xiphoid process. Marking the distance on the lavage tube with adhesive tape and immersing in cold water or a water-miscible jelly (avoid oils) greatly facilitates this procedure. Dentures and other foreign objects should be removed from the mouth. Restraints are required for most children. In centers where anesthesiologists are readily available, patients can be lightly anesthetized, given succinylcholine and lavaged, after inserting into the trachea an endotracheal tube with an inflatable cuff. In most community hospitals and in physicians' offices, this method, although ideal, would be impractical.

During gastric lavage the patient should be placed on his left side with the head hanging over the edge of the examining table and with the face down. If possible, the foot of the bed or table should be elevated. This technique is particularly important if the patient is drowsy or comatose so that the chances of aspiration from reflex vomiting are minimized. Pass the tube gently; no great force is necessary. If the patient cooperates, have him swallow frequently; this permits the tube to move easily and rapidly. If the catheter enters the larynx instead of the esophagus, dyspnea and severe coughing are produced (but may be absent if patient is deeply narcotized). If this occurs, the tube should be partially withdrawn before proceeding and if in doubt, test the free end of the tube in a glass of water. Continuous bubbling on expiration implies placement in the trachea, whereas gas from the stomach is usually expelled in two or three exhalations. In every instance, however, before instilling lavage solution or an antidote, always aspirate first. When the tube has reached the stomach, the glass syringe is then attached and the stomach contents aspirated.

Although tap water, containing an antidote if one is available, is the type of fluid ordinarily used by most physicians for this purpose, the substitution of isotonic or half isotonic (never hypertonic) saline solution is far safer, particularly for children, since there is a limited tolerance of the organism to electrolyte-free solutions. An increase of the body fluid volume with electrolyte-free water of 5 per cent is sufficient to initiate the cardinal symptoms of water intoxication, which are tonic and clonic seizures with coma. These may start without any prodromes. Only small amounts of fluid should be injected at one time so that the passage of the poison into the upper intestinal tract is not promoted. Repeat lavage ten or twelve times or until the returns are clear. Save all washings, separating the first from the others, for any analysis that might be indicated. At the completion of lavage, the antidote if indicated should be instilled through the tube and allowed to remain in the stomach. Before the catheter is withdrawn, it should be either pinched off or suction maintained in order to prevent aspiration of material into the lungs.

A new technique of using a device consisting of a double lumen tube both to deliver fluid and to aspirate simultaneously or separately allows the entire procedure of thorough gastric lavage to be done in as little as five minutes (*see* Fig. 3.)

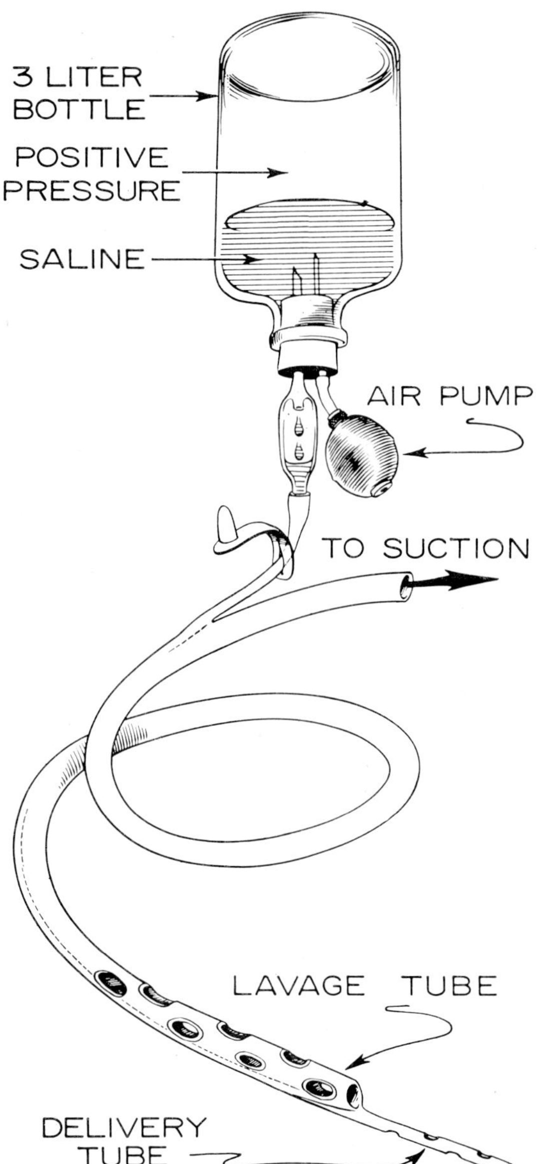


Figure 3. Gastric lavage tube. (Reprinted with permission of United States Catheter and Instrument Corporation, Glen Falls, New York.)

In adults the combined tube contains a No. 12 F. delivery tube and a No. 30 F. suction tube. The delivery tube is connected to a pressurized 3 liter bottle of lavaging fluid; the distal end protrudes past the suction tube. The large bore of the suction tube allows ready removal of matter.

In children, a smaller No. 18 F. unit is utilized. In children (not infants) and adults, these large tubes are passed nasally without undue difficulty (Moss, G.: *Surg Gynecol Obstet, 119*:1325, 1964).

Of fundamental importance is the recent recognition that absolute solubility characteristics of individual drugs are misleading in the oral clinical overdosage context. Stated solubilities for any chemical or drug are derived from use of crystalline or powdered material *in vitro,* with additional data as to tablet or capsule dissolution *in vitro* under U.S.P.

conditions. Only rarely are there data available as to dissolution in the GI tract of higher species of laboratory animals or in man, and such data are based upon ingestion of therapeutic dosages as a rule.

In gross overdosage, with large numbers of tablets or capsules ingested over a short period of time, gastric or bowel "concretions" commonly occur, even with substances that in normal usage are readily dissolved in the GI tract. Undissolved or partially dissolved tablets of glutethimide may be found at postmortem or removed by adequate lavage long after ingestion, as is true for barbiturates and many other drugs (even noted with massive overdosage of aspirin). One of the most dramatic examples has been the documentation and reporting of a case of gross overdosage of meprobamate (Jenis, E.H., et al.: *JAMA, 207*:361-362, 1969).

Among others, Schreiner et al. (as long ago as 1958) recommended and practiced gastric lavage even many hours after overdosage ingestion of various CNS-depressant drugs. In recent years, more use has been made of castor-oil-emulsion lavage, both because of relative water insolubility of certain drugs and because a large tablet or capsule bolus may be refractory to aqueous lavage even for ordinarily water-soluble substances. Some clinicians routinely use copious water lavage followed by castor oil lavage per wide-bore tube, with a cuffed endotracheal tube in place to protect against aspiration of gastric contents or lavage material. They have been able to wash out from 5 to 15 gm of Doriden® in this way a good many hours after known or estimated ingestion time. This procedure, followed by an activated charcoal slurry, as part of intensive conservative treatment, appears very important in the successful management not requiring hemodialysis and probably should be used for overdosage of CNS-depressant drugs in general, regardless of absolute solubilities in nonclinical situations.

A simple and efficient lavage technique illustrated below uses a 1000 or 2000 ml enema bag hung from an IV pole and a wall-mounted suction bottle, both connected via a **Y**-tube to a large-bore nasogastric tube (either Levin or Ewald). By simply moving a Kelly clamp from one arm of the set-up to the other, it is possible to rapidly and effortlessly irrigate the stomach with 100 to 200 ml of solution at a time and then withdraw the solution by vacuum from the stomach.

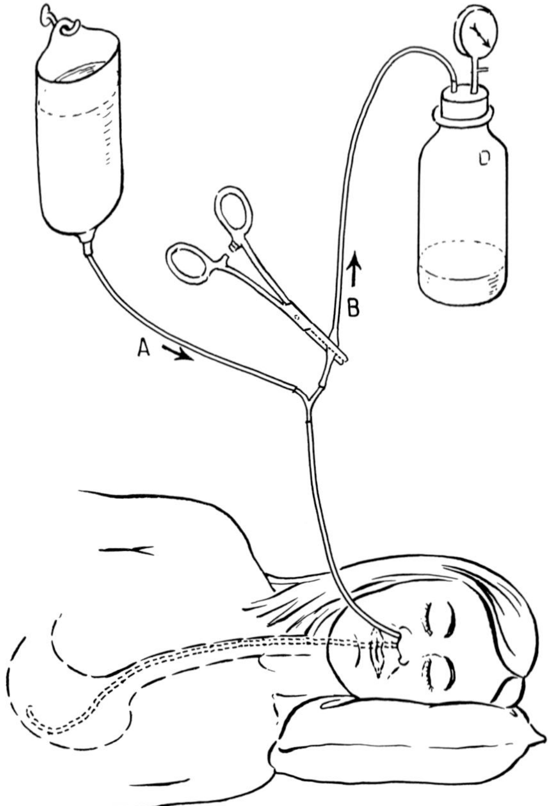


Figure 4. Efficient lavage technique.

1. Place the patient on his left side to minimize the amount of irrigating solution lost through the pylorus.
2. Position the nasogastric tube in the stomach.
3. Clamp the suction arm (B) with a Kelly clamp and run in 100 to 200 ml of fluid from the enema bag. (Use iced saline for GI bleeders and room-temperature saline for overdose victims.)
4. Switch the clamp to the irrigation arm (A). With the pressure gauge on the suction apparatus set between 40 and 60 mm Hg, suction continuously until most of the instilled solution is recovered.
5. Switch the Kelly clamp back to the suction arm and repeat the cycle as often as necessary.

Modified from *Hospital Physician,* July 1975.

## TREATMENT

*Acetic Acid (1%)*

*Oral:* Dilute 1:1 with water in instances of alkali ingestion.

*Topically:* Following alkali burns, wash copiously with 1% solution.

*Note:* Vinegar is 5% acetic acid and may be used diluted 1:4 for 1% solution.

*Aluminum Hydroxide Gel*

Supplement to treatment of gastritis and chemical inflammation of the gastric mucosa.

*Aminophylline (250 mg ampules, tablets or suppositories)*

Coronary, bronchial and smooth muscle dilator. Also, reduces clotting time by increasing prothrombin and fibrinogen levels.

Avoid oral route if gastric mucosa is not intact.

*Dose:* 3 to 6 mg/kg via all routes. Toxic manifestations and deaths, particularly in small children, have been reported from rectal suppositories. Overdosage must be avoided via all routes.

*Ammonium Acetate*

Ammonium acetate or dilute ammonia water approximately 4 ml to 500 ml of water. Combines with formaldehyde to form relatively harmless methenamine.

*Ammonium Hydroxide (0.2%)*

Use as lavage solution in formalin (formaldehyde) ingestion.

*Amphetamine (5 mg tablets)*

Brain stem and cortical stimulant with hypertensive effects.

*Amyl Nitrite® Pearls (0.3 ml)*

First step in the treatment of acute cyanide poisoning. Have patient inhale fumes until such time sodium nitrite can be given intravenously (*see* Cyanide Poisoning).

*Apomorphine Hypodermic Tabs (6 mg, Lilly & Co.)*

Powerful emetic, but also strong respiratory depressant. Thus, do not use in any patient with central depression. *Do not repeat if first dose ineffectual.*

A 6 mg tablet is placed in a 10 ml syringe and crushed. Then 6 ml of sterile water is drawn and agitated, which readily dissolves the crushed tablet. Light and air gradually decompose apomorphine tablets; therefore, they should be kept in a dark, tightly stoppered bottle.

*Dose:* one– to two-year-old child, 1 to 2 mg, or 0.03 mg/lb. SC or IM; adult, 6 mg (*also see* pages 43 through 44).

*Aromatic Spirits of Ammonia*

To be swallowed following ingestion of formalin.

*Ascorbic Acid-Ascorbate Sodium (injectable 250 mg/ml)*

Powerful reducing agent. Useful in methemoglobinemia in conjunction with methylene blue and as an accessory agent in benzene, lead and arsenic poisoning; nicotine intoxication; bacterial toxins and anaphylactoid reactions.

*Dose:* 250 to 1000 mg, IV, well diluted (can cause hemolysis in strong concentrations) in normal saline or 5% glucose solution.

*Atropine Sulfate Hypodermic Tab (0.4 mg)*

Antagonist of muscarine effects of acetylcholine and methacholine (from poisonous mushrooms and certain insecticides). Useful in overdosage effects from arecoline and pilocarpine. Should be used until desired effect is produced or toxicity is present (dilated pupils, flushed skin, elevated temperature, tachycardia and excitement).

In organic phosphate poisoning, fasciculations or convulsions may occur which require, in addition to atropine, anticonvulsive therapy (*see* Table 30).

*Dose:* Subcutaneous or oral, may be repeated every thirty minutes until desired effect is achieved, then every four to eight hours.

| | |
|---|---|
| 6 mo. | 0.12 mg |
| 1 yr. | 0.16 mg |
| 2 yr. | 0.2 mg |
| 5 yr. | 0.3 mg |
| 10 yr. | 0.5 mg |
| Adult | 0.6 mg |

### *Avertin (Tribromoethanol)*

Rectally 50 to 60 mg/kg. Preferably should be given by an anesthetist. Useful for anesthesia in child who is convulsing from ingested poison.

### *BAL (2,3-Dimercaptopropanol, Dimercaprol, British Anti-Lewisite) 10% Solution in Oil (4.5 ml: 100 mg/ml)*

BAL is a good antidote for mercury, copper, arsenic, gold, nickel, lead and antimony. It is less effective for silver and practically ineffective if tissue damage is extensive. It may aggravate cadmium poisoning since the BAL-cadmium complex has a nephrotoxic action. BAL should be given as soon as possible for best results, and its administration should be continued until the urinary excretion of the metal is negligible. The usual recommended dosage is 3 to 4 mg/kg IM every four to six hours first day, every six to eight hours the second day and then tapered according to symptoms. However, in mercury poisoning larger doses are indicated: 5 mg/kg immediately and repeated in two hours. Then 2.5 mg/kg every six hours for three doses, followed by two doses the second day and one dose the third and subsequent days. Since the amounts listed are approximately half the toxic dose, undesirable side-effects are often encountered (hemolysis has been reported in two G-6-PD deficient children). These include lacrimation; salivation; rhinorrhea; sense of constriction in the throat and chest; burning sensation in the mouth, throat, eyes, extremities, and penis; sweating of forehead and hands; flushing of the face; muscular cramps; nausea; vomiting; fall in blood pressure and pulmonary edema. In children fever develops rather frequently after the first few injections of BAL and may persist until treatment is completed or discontinued. Prophylactic administration of 25 mg of ephedrine by mouth half an hour before injection of BAL may prevent or modify these symptoms. If symptoms develop later, 0.6 ml of 1:1000 epinephrine solution can be administered intramuscularly to adults. Correspondingly smaller doses should be given to infants. The chart below is useful as a basis for all treatment when BAL is indicated.

BAL Disposable Unit (in packages of five) contains a 3 ml size ampule of BAL, a sterile syringe calibrated with the 2.5 mg/kg dosage, sterile needle and alcohol swab. The prefigured dosage schedule imprinted on the syringe facilitates the administration of this heavy metal antidote in cases of emergency where too often time is of critical essence.

BAL (IM)

| | *Severe Intoxication* | *Mild Intoxication* |
|---|---|---|
| 1st day | 3.0 mg/kg q.4h. (6 inj.) | 2.5 mg/kg q.4h. (6 inj.) |
| 2nd day | Same | Same |
| 3rd day | 3.0 mg/kg q.6h. (4 inj.) | 2.5 mg/kg q.12h. (2 inj.) |
| 10 subsequent days (or until recovery) | 3.0 mg/kg q.12h. (2 inj.) | 2.5 mg/kg q.d. (1 inj.) |

*Brewer's Yeast®, Tablets (0.4 gm)*

*Indications:* Thallium ingestion (depilatories and rat bait).

*Dose:* Children of two to three years, 3 to 4 gm/day.

*Bromobenzene (1 gm units)*

For selenium intoxication.

*Dose:* Adults, 1 gm; one year, 0.25 gm.

Use 1 gm in lavage solution and administer appropriate dose every twelve hours.

*Caffeine and Sodium Benzoate (250 mg/ml)*

Mild cerebral and respiratory stimulant. Useful in alcohol, morphine, chloral hydrate and some organic alkaloid intoxications. Avoid use in chlorinated hydrocarbon and barbiturate poisoning.

*Dose:* IV or IM, may be repeated every thirty minutes.

| | | |
|---|---|---|
| 1-2 yr. | 60-180 mg | 0.2-0.7 ml |
| 5 yr. | 200 mg | 0.8 ml |
| 10 yr. | 300 mg | 1.2 ml |
| Adult | 500 mg | 2.0 ml |

*Calcium Disodium Edetate or Versenate® (EDTA—Ethylenediaminetetra-acetate) 0.2 gm/ml (*Also see *Lead, for use and adverse effects)*

Combines with metallic ions to form water-soluble complexes or chelates, which are non-ionizable, nonmetabolized and excreted intact.

The word "chelate" is derived from the Greek *chele,* which refers to the claw of a lobster. The term describes the firm, pincer-like binding of metal ions by complexing substances called ligands. This binding is accomplished through the sharing of pairs of electrons by the metal ion and the ligand molecule. Both electrons of the shared pair usually come from the ligand molecule. Nitrogen, sulfur and oxygen are the most common "donor atoms" supplying these electrons. A chelate has behavioral properties not possessed by either the metal or the ligand alone. Solubility, color, chemical reactivity, catalytic properties, stability and optical activity of the new complex are altered from those of either the metal or the free ligand.

*Indications:* Lead, nickel, copper, manganese, iron and radioelements (except strontium). To be effective, chelates must be used before skeletal growth transforms the particles into an inaccessible form.

*Method:* (IV) Use a 3% solution maximum. Safest for children is a 2% solution of a slow intravenous drip of one to two hours for total dose of 0.5 gm/30 lb. of weight (36 mg/kg) twice daily up to five days. Intermittent intramuscular injections of a 20% solution (0.5% procaine) of a total dosage range of 50 to 75 mg/kg body weight for five to seven days may be substituted for intravenous therapy, although not recommended by the AMA Council on Drugs.

If repeat therapy is necessary, wait two days then give for an additional five days. Or 75 mg/kg can be given orally in divided doses four times a day for nine days as an addition to parenteral therapy. It has also been taken orally daily, though not recommended, by exposed industrial lead workers as a prophylactic measure in prevention.

Dipotassium or disodium edetate (sodium versenate) 50 mg/kg IV chelates calcium ion, producing a hypocalcemia which reduces the synergistic action of calcium with digitalis. This effect made them valuable agents as antidotes for digitalis intoxication, but they are not used for this purpose in present day therapy.

*Calcium Gluconate 10%*

*Indications:* Poisoning from chlorinated hydrocarbons, fluorides and oxalates. Circulating calcium has great affinity for these compounds and tetany may result. Also useful in black widow spider and other insect bites for relief of muscle spasm.

### *Calcium Lactate 10% Solution and Powder*

*Indications:* For lavage in instances of ingestion of fluorides, oxalates and chlorinated hydrocarbons.

*Administration:* Intravenous or oral solution, calcium lactate or gluconate 1.5% to 3.0%, calcium chloride 0.4%.

*Dose:* Oral; lactate; 0.48 gm/kg three times daily; gluconate, 0.73 gm/kg three times daily.

### *Codeine Phosphate Hypodermic Tablets (30 mg)*

| *Dosage* | *PO* | *SC* |
|---|---|---|
| 1 yr. | 8-15 mg | 8 mg |
| 2 yr. | 10-20 mg | 10 mg |
| 5 yr. | 15-25 mg | 15 mg |
| 10 yr. | 15-35 mg | 20 mg |
| Adult | 15-60 mg | 30 mg |

### *Charcoal, Activated (finely powdered) (1 gm units)*

Charcoal, activated (residue from the destructive distillation of various organic materials, treated to increase its absorptive powers; source materials now largely are coal, lignite or waste from paper manufacture, rather than the original carbonized wood [charcoal]; vegetable charcoals made from wood pulp, which are porous, have a low ash content and very high surface areas, usually in the range of 1000 sq. m/gm, and are of particular value) is a potent adsorbent that rapidly inactivates many poisons, if it is given *early* before much adsorption takes place. It is effective for most chemicals (with few exceptions) whether they be organic, inorganic, large– or small-moleculed compounds (Table 18). Potency of adsorption is not reduced by acidity or alkalinity of the poison or by wide range of pH in the gastrointestinal tract. Adsorbed material is retained tenaciously throughout passage in the gut. The concern that part of the intoxicant in the intestine may be later released because of a less favorable pH has been investigated by Doctors L. Chin and Picchioni at the University of Arizona, College of Pharmacy. They found that the marked reduction of available poison in the gastrointestinal tract eclipses the insignificant elution of the poison in the intestines. Activated charcoal was restored to the *United States Pharmacopeia,* Seventeenth Edition (1965) and Eighteenth Edition (1970), not as a remedy for flatulence or intestinal intoxication, but as one of the best, least expensive and most practical emergency antidotes available. An effective concentration for oral use or lavaging is 1 to 2 tbsp. (50 gm for adults, 20 gm for children) to a 6 to 8 oz. glass of water or a mixture of soupy consistency. The adsorptive capacity of activated charcoal has been shown to be significantly decreased when ice cream (or sherbert) is mixed with the charcoal in a 2.5:1 ratio by weight. There is no great alteration, however, when concentrated fruit juice or chocolate powder is used or when suspended in water for immediate use for as long as one year. Tablets or granules of activated charcoal are less effective than the powder form and should not be used unless they are the only forms available. Bone chars are not suitable because of their high mineral content, and the mineral charcoals are relatively little used. Favorable experience with five products on the American market are (1) Activated Charcoal (Merck) *in vivo* comparison is one of the most effective brands; (2) Norit A. (American Norit Company, Jacksonville, Florida); (3) Darco G. 60 (Atlas Powder Company, Wilmington, Delaware); (4) Nuchar C. (West Virginia Pulp and Paper Company, 230 Park Avenue, New York, New York); (5) Requa's (Requa Manufacturing Company, Inc., 4510 Bullard Avenue, Bronx, New York). There are doubtless many good ones other than these also available.

A minor drawback to this agent is that it is *black.* Many children refuse to drink it; it is gritty and the carbon sticks in the back of the throat, producing gagging, and if spewed, it spots uniforms, clothes, walls and personnel. However, a firm but kindly positive approach, assuring the child of the innocuousness and benefit of the activated charcoal suspension, should result in successful administration in most cases.

An effective suspension or liquid preparation of charcoal may soon be on the market. This would have many advantages in being more palatable, easier to administer and more readily available for immediate use.

Activated charcoal should not be used simultaneously with syrup of ipecac, since it is capable of adsorbing the emetic principle and inactivating it. It should be administered only after emesis has been successfully induced. Of course, it can be administered before (preferable), at the same time or later with parenteral apomorphine.

*Cystine*

*Indications:* Used rarely with brewer's yeast in thallium ingestion (rat bait or depilatories).

*Dexedrine® or d-Amphetamine Sulfate (5 mg tablets and 20 mg ampules)*

Very effective cerebral and medullary respiratory center stimulant; minimal vascular effect.

*Indications:* Central depression by anesthetic, narcotic or hypnotic drugs.

TABLE 18
APPROXIMATE AMOUNT OF SUBSTANCE ADSORBED BY 1 GM CHARCOAL

| *Adsorbendum* | *Maximal adsorption in mg* |
|---|---|
| Mercuric chloride | 1800 |
| Sulfanilamide | 1000 |
| Strychnine nitrate | 950 |
| Morphine hydrochloride | 800 |
| Atropine sulfate | 700 |
| Nicotine | 700 |
| Barbital (Veronal®) | 700 |
| Barbital sodium (Medinal®) | 150 |
| Phenobarbital sodium (Luminal®)<br>Alurate® sodium<br>Dial® sodium<br>Evipal® sodium<br>Phanodorn® calcium | 300–350 |
| Salicylic acid | 550 |
| Phenol | 400 |
| Alcohol | 300 |
| Potassium cyanide | 35 |

SOME SUBSTANCES EFFECTIVELY ADSORBED BY ACTIVATED CHARCOAL

| *Organic Compounds* | | *Inorganic Substances* |
|---|---|---|
| Aconite | Muscarine | As (Arsenic) |
| Alcohol | Nicotine | Ag (Silver) |
| Antipyrine | Opium | $HgCl_2$ (Mecuric chloride) |
| Atropine | Oxalates | I (Iodine) |
| Barbiturates | Parathion | $KMN0_4$ (Potassium parmanganate) |
| Cantharides | Penicillin | P (Phosphorus) |
| Camphor | Phenolphthalein | Pb (to limited extent) (Lead) |
| Cocaine | Phenol | Sb (Antimony) |
| Delphinium | Quinine | Sn (Tin) |
| Digitalis | Salicylates | Ti (Titanium) |
| Elaterin | Stramonium | |
| Hemlock | Strychnine | |
| Ipecac | Sulfonamides | |
| Methylene blue | Veratrum | |
| Morphine | | |

Cyanide, alcohols, boric acid, corrosives and ferrous sulfate are known exceptions. Courtesy of L.E. Holt, Jr. M.D.

*Antidote:* Sedatives or chlorpromazine.

*Dose:* (Severe depression only). Thirty-pound child, 5 to 25 mg orally or 2 to 6 mg IV; adult, 15 to 50 mg orally or 5 to 15 mg IV.

### *Ephedrine Sulfate (25 mg capsules and tablets, 50 mg ampules)*

Useful in preventing hypotension in conditions other than shock, in relieving bronchiolar spasm, and in morphine and barbiturate intoxication to combat respiratory depression.

Prevents side-reactions from administration of BAL if given one-half hour beforehand.

*Oral dose:* Children, 3 mg/kg/24 hr.; adult, 15 to 60 mg.

### *Epinephrine 1:1000 (1 ml ampule)*

*Indications:* Anaphylactoid reactions. For relief of symptoms due to BAL administration.

| *Administration* | *Subcutaneously* |
|---|---|
| 1 yr. | 0.2 ml |
| 2 yr. | 0.3 ml |
| 5 yr. | 0.5 ml |
| 10 yr. | 0.5-0.8 ml |
| Adult | 0.5-1.0 ml |

Every fifteen minutes for four doses. Use caution if heart rate exceeds 140.

### *Ethyl Alcohol (95%)*

Use as 10% solution for lavage.

*Indications:* Ingestion of any soluble derivative (*also see* IV use for methyl alcohol and glycol poisoning).

### *Iodine (Tincture)*

An iodine solution of about 15 drops of the tincture in 4 oz. of water precipitates lead, mercury, silver, quinine and strychnine. Precipitants must be thoroughly removed by gastric lavage.

### *Kwik-Kold ® (International Latex)*

This product is a 6 × 9 in. plastic bag which, when squeezed, turns colder than ice. It contains water and, in an inner film pouch, crystalline ammonium nitrate mix, immediately producing 20° F cold. Kwik-Kold is ideal for first aid treatment and injuries that require cold therapy.

### *Levophed ® Bitartrate (Norepinephrine) (4 ml ampule of 0.2% solution)*

To combat circulatory collapse.

*Dose:* 0.1 to 0.4 μg/kg/min.

*Method:* Dilute ampule contents to 1 liter with 5% dextrose water or saline. Levarterenol base equals 4 μg/ml. Care should be taken that extravasation does not occur, since tissue sloughs and ischemic necrosis of the skin may result.

### *Limewater (Calcium Hydroxide solution, U.S.P.)*

Limewater is a widely recommended antacid antidote. It is a clear, colorless liquid with an alkaline taste containing 0.14% calcium hydroxide. Since it is often not readily available in the home, other antacid agents (magnesium hydroxide [milk of magnesia] etc.) are used more frequently.

### *Magnesium Oxide (25 gm units)*

This is used primarily as a neutralizing agent for acidic substances, including aspirin, sulfuric and other mineral acids, oxalic acid, etc. It does not release $CO_2$ to distend the stomach, and if not too much is allowed to remain in the stomach, the depressant effect of magnesium on the central nervous system is negligible. Approximately 25 gm of magnesium oxide per 1000 ml of water is the concentration used.

### *Magnesium Sulfate (Epsom Salts) (50% solution)*

*Indications:* (1) Lead or soluble barium salt (carbonate or sulfate) ingestion. May precipitate out the harmful complex. (2) Any toxic agent for which rapid elimination from the GI tract is desired.

*Caution:* Avoid if kidneys damaged.

*Dose:* Oral.

| | | | |
|---|---|---|---|
| 1 yr. | 2.0 gm | 4 | ml of 50% solution |
| 2 yr. | 2.5 gm | 5 | ml of 50% solution |
| 5 yr. | 3.7 gm | 7.5 | ml of 50% solution |
| 10 yr. | 5.0 gm | 10 | ml of 50% solution |
| Adult | 10-15 gm | 20-30 | ml of 50% solution |

### *Methylene Blue (1%, 10 ml ampule)*

Methylene blue is an aniline dye which produces methemoglobin and the potential for hemolysis in those individuals with glucose-6-phosphate dehydrogenase (G-6-PD) enzymic deficiency. Since the methemoglobin binds the cyanide ion and prevents damage of the respiratory enzyme by cyanide, this action is utilized in the treatment of cyanide poisoning. However, amyl nitrite and sodium nitrite are much more effective in forming methemoglobin and have, therefore, largely supplanted methylene blue. Strangely enough, methylene blue can also reduce methemoglobin to normal hemoglobin so that it is used for treatment of methemoglobinemia caused by nitrites, aniline dyes, and other drugs.

The recommended dose is 2.2 mg of methylene blue per kg of body weight (1 mg/lb.). This is given as an intravenous injection of a 1.0% solution. The injection should be made slowly; at least five minutes should be required to give the total dosage. Hypertension, sweating, chest pain, confusion, nausea and vomiting, dizziness and cyanosis are self-limited reactions. Care should be taken to avoid perivenous infiltration, which can cause tissue necrosis. This dose may be repeated in an hour if needed. Its effectiveness in reducing the methemoglobin to normal hemoglobin is only moderate but is enhanced by large parenteral doses (100 to 500 mg/24 hr.) of ascorbic acid. A dose of 3 to 5 mg/kg can also be given orally. The action however is much slower by this route and is not practical for true emergency use.

### *Methyl-Ethyl Glutarimide (Megimide ®)*

This agent has been used with considerable enthusiasm as a barbiturate antagonist in Australia and England under the trade name of Megimide. It is also available here as Megimide (bemegride). Results in this country have been equivocal. The general opinion now is that its original promise has not been fulfilled, but that it probably has a place when respiratory depression is marked.

### *Milk or Evaporated Milk*

Canned evaporated milk keeps well and is inexpensive. It may be diluted with an equal part of water or used without dilution, the latter particularly when the demulcent action is desired, e.g. with copper sulfate, croton oil, chlorates and thioglycolic acid ingestion.

### *Mineral Oil (U.S.P.)*

May be given with caution following kerosene ingestion, although vegetable oils are preferable, to prevent possible (equivocal) gastric absorption as well as hurry it through the intestinal tract. However, care must be taken to prevent gagging, vomiting and aspiration.

### *Nalorphine (Nalline ®) (1 ml 5 mg ampule), Levallorphan (Lorfan®) (1 ml 1 mg ampule) and Naloxone (Narcan®) (1 ml 0.4 mg ampule)*

Nalorphine is effective in combating the respiratory depression of morphine and pharmacologically related drugs such as heroin, Dilaudid®, dextropropoxyphene, methadone, Pantopon® and even meperidine

(Demerol®). It is not effective in respiratory depression due to barbiturates. The adult dose of nalorphine is 15 mg subcutaneously or 10 mg intravenously. Infants and children should receive proportionately smaller doses (0.1 mg has been given to the newborn infant intravenously through the umbilical vein). For children one to two years old, 1 to 2 mg subcutaneously can be given, and if the response is inadequate, this may be cautiously repeated in fifteen minutes. The use of nalorphine in addicts presents the hazard of inducing withdrawal symptoms. Levallorphan (Lorfan) is a drug with actions and uses similar to, if not identical with, those of nalorphine. Nalline and Lorfan can now be purchased by all classes of registrants without filling out the federal narcotic order forms or maintaining inventory records (*see* page 441 for discussion of the preferable narcotic antagonist naloxone [Narcan]).

### *Nikethamide (Coramine ®) (25% solution) (1.5 to 5 ml ampules)*

Respiratory stimulant in opiate poisoning, central depression from general anesthesia, and some hypnotics. Questionable effectiveness in severe barbiturate poisoning. Is more prone to produce convulsion than picrotoxin or Metrazol®.

*Dose:* Adult, 1 to 4 ml of 25% solution. Can be used in dose of 5 ml IV every fifteen to thirty minutes in severe opium poisoning.

| | |
|---|---|
| 6 mo. | 0.3 ml |
| 1 yr. | 0.4 ml |
| 2 yr. | 0.5 ml |
| 5 yr. | 0.7 ml |
| 10 yr. | 1.0 ml |

### *Nitroglycerin Tablets, Sublingual (0.3 mg)**

Useful in barium poisoning, which causes marked ateriolar spasm (plus marked GI activity, myocardial stimulation, muscle tremors).

*Use:* Sublingually only.

**Note:* Must be fresh and kept in glass container to prevent potency loss.

### *Paraldehyde (U.S.P.) (5 ml ampule)*

Analgesic and hypnotic. Useful in any poisoning causing delerium tremens, pain and/or excitement, but it has its drawbacks in taste and odor. Though no longer employed to any great extent except in the management of alcoholics, it is still a very useful and practical preparation. This drug is rarely used intravenously now in present therapy.

Paraldehyde should be kept in a well-filled, light-resistant, tightly closed container which holds not more than 120 gm, preferably at a temperature not above 30° C. When stored for a long time in a partially filled and loosely stoppered bottle, paraldehyde can break down to acetaldehyde and acetic acid. At least one death reportedly caused by paraldehyde was later discovered to be due to the breakdown chemical acetic acid.

*Dose:*

| | *Oral* | *Rectal* | *IM* | *IV (5%)* |
|---|---|---|---|---|
| 6 mo. | 0.8 ml | 1.6 ml | | 1.5 ml |
| 1 yr. | 1.0 ml | 2.0 ml | | 2.0 ml |
| 2 yr. | 1.2 ml | 2.4 ml | | 2.5 ml |
| 5 yr. | 2.0 ml | 4.0 ml | | 4.0 ml |
| 10 yr. | 3.0 ml | 6.0 ml | | 6.0 ml |
| Adult | 5.0 ml | 15-30 ml | 5-8 ml | 10.0 ml |

### *Pentylenetetrazol (Metrazol®) (1 ml 100 mg ampule)*

Metrazol is used in much the same way as picrotoxin as a medullary stimulant in poisoning with depression of vital centers. Its effectiveness in the treatment of barbiturate poisoning is controversial.

### *Phenobarbital (tablets 30 mg; ampules 0.12 to 0.3 gm, elixir 4 mg/ml)*

Slow-acting with prolonged effect.

| | *Oral* | *IM* | *IV* |
|---|---|---|---|
| Newborn | 4-12 mg | 8-16 mg | 4 mg |
| 1 yr. | 8-24 mg | 24-50 mg | 8 mg |
| 2 yr. | 10-30 mg | 30-65 mg | 15 mg |
| 5 yr. | 12-45 mg | 40-90 mg | 30 mg |
| 10 yr. | 20-65 mg | 45-120 mg | 30 mg |
| Adult | 30-100 mg | 100-320 mg | 65 mg |

Subcutaneous, intramuscular and intravenous doses are for controlling convulsions only. Oral doses are for sedation or hypnosis.

### *Physostigmine Salicylate (Antilirium®) (ampule 2 ml, 1 mg/ml)*

Physostigmine has been used as an antidote for delirium and prolonged somnolence caused by atropine and scopolamine. It is particularly effective in relieving the cardiac (arrhythmias) and central nervous system toxic effects of the tricyclic antidepressant drugs as well as the many other anticholinergic compounds (antidepressants, antihistamines, antispasmodics, antiparkinsonians, and antipsychotics).

*Dose:* Adult, 1 to 2 mg IM or IV (slow). Repeat in thirty minutes if necessary. Child or elderly adult, 0.5 to 1 mg IM or IV (slow).

An excess of physostigmine can produce bradycardia, diarrhea, hypersalivation and rhinorrhea all the way to cholinergic crisis. These symptoms can be quickly reversed with a peripherally acting anticholinergic agent such as propantheline bromide (Pro-Banthine®). Atropine is a second choice drug for this purpose since its central action could potentiate the CNS effect of the original intoxicant.

### *Picrotoxin (1 and 20 ml, 3 mg/ml, ampules)*

This drug has a selective stimulant action on the cortical and subcortical areas of the brain. In toxic doses, however, it causes delirium and generalized convulsions and is often followed by vomiting, bradycardia and tachypnea.

Picrotoxin may be useful for its antagonism of the central depression caused by barbiturates. It can be given for such depression in initial doses of 3 to 20 mg and then repeated once or twice at thirty-minute intervals, until there are signs of returning consciousness, swallowing movements, stirring, returning corneal and other reflexes.

Picrotoxin's full effects develop slowly, even after intravenous injection. An additional dose should not be given, therefore, until after a thirty-minute waiting period. Failure to observe this precaution has resulted in severe picrotoxin intoxication.

A slow intravenous drip, 1.0 mg/min. for adults and about one-sixth to one-third this rate (5 mg total) for small children, is safe, but here, too, the injection is temporarily discontinued as soon as signs of activity appear. The objective of treatment is to reactivate the respiratory and cardiac centers without causing convulsions. When the respiration and cardiodynamics are adequate, there seems to be no further indication for its use.

In any event, attention to vital signs, clear airway, artificial respiration when necessary, plasma or plasma expanders for shock, and penicillin or other antibiotics to prevent pneumonia is of first importance in the treatment of poisoning which causes severe central depression.

### *Pilocarpine*

Pilocarpine is used to antagonize the toxic effects of atropine and related alkaloids. This action is exerted chiefly against the peripheral effects of atropine rather than the more important central effects. Tablets formerly marketed by Wyeth Laboratories have been discontinued, but the drug is still available in powder form. Doses of 2 or 3 mg of pilocarpine nitrate orally for a four-year-old child may be used. Adult doses are correspondingly larger. Most authorities feel that physostigmine is more effective than pilocarpine in treating atropine poisoning.

### *Potassium Permanganate (0.1 gm tablets)*

Oxidizing agent that reacts well with organic substances. It is effective in neutralizing such compounds as strychnine, nicotine, physostigmine and quinine. Because potassium permanganate is itself a strong irritant, care must be taken to use it well diluted (1:10,000 approximately, and not stronger than 1:5000) and to be sure that no undissolved particles come in contact with the stomach or other tissues. It is recommended that a thoroughly dissolved 5% solution be kept on hand to be diluted to the needed strength. A 1:10,000 solution may be prepared by dissolving 0.1 gm in 1 liter of water, or 1 gm may be dissolved in 100 ml of water and 10 ml of this added to 1000 ml of water to make a 1:10,000 solution.

### *Procainamide HCl (Pronestyl ®)*

This compound depresses the excitability of cardiac muscle to electrical stimulation and slows conduction in the atrium, bundle of His and the ventricle. The effects of procainamide hydrochloride are more beneficial in ventricular than in auricular arrhythmias. It is an excellent substitute for those who cannot tolerate quinidine. Ventricular extrasystoles and ventricular tachycardia are controlled within an hour after oral or intramuscular administration or in just a few minutes after intravenous infusion.

*Dose:*

*Oral:* Adult, 0.5 to 1.0 gm every four to six hours; child, 25 to 50 mg/kg/24 hr.

*IM:* Adult, 0.5 to 1.0 gm every six hours until oral dose is feasible; child, 50 to 150 mg in a 10% solution every six hours.

*IV:* 0.2 to 1.0 gm. Should not be given at a rate exceeding 25 to 50 mg/min. since precipitous hypotensive response sometimes occurs.

The principal side-effects arising from drug abuse are ventricular tachycardia and severe hypotension. Excess oral doses may sometimes produce anorexia, nausea, urticaria with pruritus and agranulocytosis. Rare adverse effects are fever, chills and profuse sweating. A lupus-erythematosus-syndrome-like condition has also been reported with arthralgia, pleuritic pain with roentgenologic evidence of pleuropulmonary disease and cutaneous lesions. Positive lupus erythematosus phenomenon and antinuclear antibodies are usually found. Less commonly, splenomegaly, anemia, positive direct Coombs' reaction, leukopenia, granulocytopenia and hypergammaglobulinemia occur. Interval from initiation of therapy to lupus-like symptoms is one to nine months. Other drugs incriminated in precipitating overt systemic lupus erythematosus (SLE) are isoniazid, oral contraceptives, sulfonamides, thiouracils, alpha-methyldopa, phenothiazines (chlorpromazine, etc.), hydralazine (Apresoline®) and several anticonvulsant agents. The relationship between drug and disease is unclear, but certain persons may have an inherent SLE diathesis which is unmasked by the drug. A simple drug allergy might cause the disease, or its occurrence during drug administration might be coincidental.

### *Quinidine Sulfate (0.12, 0.2, 0.3 gm tablets)*

In instances of cardiac arrhythmias, effect produced.

| | |
|---|---|
| Orally | 1-3 hr. |
| IM | 30-90 min. |
| IV | 10-20 min. |

*Dose:* Oral (adult), 0.2 gm, repeated in two hours and twelve hours if no untoward symptoms develop; then 0.4 gm every three to eight hours.

*Quinidine HCl* is an intramuscular preparation of 0.6 gm in a 5 ml ampule. Its action is no more rapid than with the oral salts.

For critical patients, intravenous *quinidine gluconate* (0.8 gm in 10 ml ampule) diluted in 250 ml of 5% glucose in water should be given slowly until normal sinus rhythm occurs, otherwise it can be given in a dosage of 0.4 gm IM every two hours. Overdosage or prolonged use can produce deafness (cinchonism), skin rash or gastrointestinal symptoms. Cardiotoxicity may be reversed by IV M solution of sodium lactate at a rate of 5 to 10 ml/min.

*Sodium Amytal (barbiturate with relatively fast onset of action) (0.25 to 0.5 gm ampules)*

| | mg PO | mg IM | 10% | (IM) ml |
|---|---|---|---|---|
| 1 yr. | 15 | 50 | | 0.5 ml |
| 2 yr. | 18 | 65 | | 0.6 ml |
| 5 yr. | 25 | 90 | | 0.9 ml |
| 10 yr. | 65 | 120 | | 1.2 ml |
| Adult | 100 | 200 | | 2.0 ml |

Use intravenously as 10% aqueous solution. Do not exceed the rate of 1 ml/min.

*Sodium Bicarbonate (50 gm units)*

A 5% solution (empty one 50 gm unit into a liter of water) is advised for gastric lavage in cases of ferrous sulfate poisoning, since it forms the less corrosive and more insoluble ferrous carbonate. Bicarbonate, although an effective alkaline solution, is usually not recommended for neutralizing acids because of the possibility that the liberated $CO_2$ might cause increased gastric distention and thus predispose to perforation if the stomach wall has been partly corroded by the acid.

*Sodium Chloride*

A normal saline solution (0.8%), approximately 1 tsp./1 pt. of water, is an effective gastric lavage solution for silver nitrate. A relatively insoluble and noncorrosive silver chloride is formed in this reaction.

*Sodium Formaldehyde Sulfoxalate (20 gm ampule)*

A chemical antidote for mercury poisoning, it reduces mercuric chloride and other mercury salts to metallic mercury, which is much less soluble. This action is enhanced by a 5% solution of sodium bicarbonate. The sodium formaldehyde sulfoxalate should be made as a fresh solution in water; a concentration of 5% is recommended. Prior to the advent of BAL, a sterile solution of the same concentration was injected intravenously, but BAL is much more effective and the sulfoxalate is now limited to use as a lavage fluid.

*Sodium Lactate (40 ml ampules of molar solution)*

*Indications:* Acidosis due to methyl alcohol ingestion and other poisonous compounds.

Use as M/6 solution, 4.2 ml of sodium lactate per kg of body weight raises serum bicarbonate concentration 1.0 mEq/liter (2.2 vol%).

*Calculation:* For mEq $CO_2$ desired, mEq $CO_2$ actual × 4.2 ml × body weight in kg = ml required.

*Sodium Nitrite (0.3 gm in 10 ml vial) (found in cyanide poisoning kit)*

*Indications:* Cyanide poisoning. Converts hemoglobin to methemoglobin.

*Dose:* Adult, 10 ml of 3% solution IV; two- or three-year-old child, 1.5 ml of 3% solution IV. Follow by sodium thiosulfate (same needle, different syringe).

*Sodium Sulfate (40% solution)*

Same indications as for magnesium sulfate. If any kidney damage is present, it is safer and preferable.

For *dose, see* schedule for Magnesium Sulfate.

*Sodium Thiosulfate (12.5 gm in 50 ml)*

In addition to its use in the treatment of cyanide poisoning, sodium thiosulfate is recommended for iodine poisoning. It combines with iodine to form relatively harmless sodium iodide. It may be given orally three times a day in doses of approximately 2 to 3 gm well diluted, or intravenously in a 10% or 25% solution in similar doses for a thirty-pound child. Adult dosage is correspondingly larger. This may be repeated if necessary in three to four hours.

*Starch (80 gm units)*

A starch solution is considered particularly efficacious in neutralizing iodine. About 80 gm of starch per 1000 ml of water is used, and the lavage is continued until the returning fluid is no longer blue.

*Tannic Acid (40 gm units)*

Use a 4% solution for lavage.

Tannic acid is mildly acidic and precipitates a large number of organic and inorganic compounds (apomorphine, hydrastine, strychnine, veratrine, aluminum, lead and silver salts), including alkaloids, metals and some glucosides. The tannates formed often redissolve and hydrolyze later and therefore should not be allowed to remain in the stomach. (For neutralizing strong alkalis, diluted acetic acid is more effective.) Approximately 40 gm/1000 ml of water is an effective concentration of tannic acid.

*Vitamin K (Menadione) Synkayvite® (10 mg/ml) Mephyton® (Vitamin $K_1$ U.S.P.) (10 and 37.5 mg/ml)*

Useful for hemorrhagic manifestations associated with prolonged prothrombin time. It is an especially effective antidote for Dicumarol® and related drugs. A dose of 10 to 20 mg can be given intramuscularly or intravenously to a thirty-pound child and repeated only when necessary to obtain a normal prothrombin time. Prolonged and unnecessary therapy can be injurious. The adult requires about five times as much. The naturally occurring form of vitamin K is superior and safer in combating the anticoagulant effect of prothrombin-depressing agents and hypoprothrombinemia due to other causes than are synthetic vitamin-K-like substances.

## General Principles of Treatment

The management of acute poisoning is often mis-managed. Overtreatment of the poisoned patient with large doses of antidote, sedatives or stimulants often does far more damage than the poison itself. The judicious use of drugs and therapeutic measures with a calm and collected attitude is far more effective than heroic measures, which usually are unnecessary. In the handling of cases of acute poisoning, the following principles should be kept in mind.

*Oral Poisons*

When poisons have been taken by mouth, obviously it is important to remove the unabsorbed poison. Most poisons are themselves emetics, but if vomiting does not occur spontaneously, the simplest procedure then is to induce vomiting. As far as children are concerned, this is best done by having them drink a glass of water or milk, after which they should be gagged with the finger (with precautions being taken to prevent biting) or have the posterior pharynx stroked with a blunt object. To prevent aspiration in small children, the body should be inverted with the head down, but supported, and the feet elevated. Unfortunately, mechanically induced evacuation is often unsuccessful and incomplete, with mean volume of vomitus about one-third that obtained by other methods. The use of warm saline (or mustard) water as an emetic is not only dangerous (severe and occasionally fatal hypernatremia) but impractical in most instances, since children refuse (fortunately) to drink this type of concoction and much valuable time is lost coaxing them to do so. One tablespoon of salt contains at least 250 mEq of sodium and, if retained and absorbed, would be expected to raise the serum sodium level by 25 mEq/liter (based on a total body water of about 10 liters in a three-year-old child). Salt may be an occasionally successful emetic; certainly it is a reliable poison. It is high time that the use of salt as an emetic be deleted from first aid charts and other informational material. There have been enough documented deaths from salt poisoning (hypernatremia) even in adults, especially those who have taken anti-emetic compounds, to warrant discontinuing this dangerous, unnecessary and often ineffective method of producing vomiting. However, syrup of ipecac (not the fluidextract), if available, can be given in doses of 10 to 15 ml and repeated in fifteen to thirty minutes if emesis does not occur. Activated charcoal negates the ipecac effects by adsorption; therefore, they should not be used simultaneously. To obtain maximum results, one or two glasses of water (not carbonated fluids) should be given after the administration of syrup of ipecac, since emesis may not occur if the stomach is empty. Milk should not be substituted for water since it has been demonstrated in human volunteers that emesis is delayed on the average of eleven minutes (thirty-five versus twenty-four minutes). In addition to being more accessible than milk, water enables the physician to more rapidly and accurately evaluate the color, odor and pill or particle content of the emesis. Contraindications are the same as for gastric lavage. In addition, if vomiting does not occur after antiemetic drug ingestion, gastric lavage should be done. Recent studies indicating that ipecac-induced vomiting empties the stomach of ingested poisons more effectively than does gastric lavage have produced an increased enthusiasm for its use. However, x-ray investigations with radiopaque contrast material show that neither method has any superiority and that both appear far less than ideal in accomplishing evacuation. Nevertheless, the ipecac that fails to effect vomiting either remains in the gastrointestinal tract as an irritant or is absorbed and exerts systemic actions concomitantly with the toxins already present.

Ipecac is a specific cardiotoxin producing reversible progressive depression or inversion of T waves, disturbances in intraventricular conduction, bradycardia, prolonged atrioventricular conduction time, atrial fibrillation, myocardial infarction or fatal myocarditis. If emesis does not occur, these effects should always be kept in mind, although ordinarily it would require more than 30 ml of syrup of ipecac to produce toxic effects.

Until clearer data are forthcoming on the method of choice of inducing vomiting, syrup of ipecac is the safest and the most available form of treatment in the home and should be tried first.

If vomiting has not occurred or cannot be induced, institute gastric lavage at once. *The importance of emptying the stomach quickly cannot be overemphasized, for this is the essence of treatment of any poison and is often a lifesaving procedure. This is not the time for procrastination. Except when the patient is comatose, or if the poison was a petroleum distillate or corrosive, or if too much time has elapsed, gastric lavage should be carried out in every instance.*

Apomorphine. Given subcutaneously, this drug (acting on the chemoreceptor trigger zone) usually causes prompt vomiting (within three to five minutes). Since it is a respiratory depressant, it should not be given if the patient is comatose, if the respiration is slow and labored or if the poisoning is by a respiratory depressant. Because of its narcotizing action, some authorities prefer other emetics or gastric lavage if it can be performed safely. The recommended subcutaneous dose is 6 mg for adults and 1 or 2 mg for children one to two years old (0.03 mg/lb.).

It should be understood that emesis does not occur readily if the stomach is empty, and so fluids should be given beforehand, orally or by nasogastric tube, if this be necessary (also true for best results in syrup of ipecac therapy).

Naloxone hydrochloride (Narcan), a narcotic antagonist, rapidly terminates the emetic effects of apomorphine and helps to diminish the subsequent depression, which is usually mild with the recommended dosage. The combined use of these compounds for emptying the stomach in acute poisonings has clearly been shown to be effective and reasonably safe, both experimentally and clinically, and has gained wide use in many medical and poison control centers in an emergency room setting. In children the dosages used are 0.03 mg/lb. SC or IM for apomorphine, followed soon after vomiting has been initiated with 0.01 mg/kg of naloxone hydrochloride. Narcan Neonatal in a 2 ml ampule at a concentration of 0.02 mg/ml is available for the neonate and infant. It is not necessary, however, to use Narcan routinely, since the apomorphine side-effects may be such as not to require an antagonist.

*Advantages*

1. Rapid emesis with removal of all gastric contents (large particles of food, enteric-coated tablets, etc.) within three to five minutes.
2. No obstruction of lavage tubes, producing delays and incomplete emptying.
3. Reflux of contents (enteric-coated tablets, etc.) from the upper intestinal tract into the stomach.

*Disadvantages*

1. Treatment should not be used if patient is greatly depressed.
2. Stomach does not evacuate well if empty. (Fluids should be given beforehand. This also applies in the use of syrup of ipecac.)
3. Used only in conscious patients. (One half to one hour of sleep usually follows.)
4. Treatment should be under the supervision of a physician.
5. Should not be used if the solution is green, which indicates decomposition.

To prepare apomorphine for use, a 6 mg tablet (Lilly) is placed in a 10 ml syringe and crushed with the plunger. Sterile water, 6 ml, is drawn into the syringe and agitated until the tablet is dissolved. This usually requires about 30 seconds. The appropriate dose can then be found in the dosage schedule below. For accuracy in administering the dose to a small child, a 2.5 ml syringe and needle can be used to withdraw the solution from the hub of the larger syringe.

DOSE SCHEDULE FOR APOMORPHINE-NALOXONE INDUCED EMESIS

| APOMORPHINE HYDROCHLORIDE[1] 0.03 mg/lb. = 0.066 mg/kg | BODY WEIGHT | | NALOXONE HYDROCHLORIDE[2] 0.01 mg/kg 0.4 mg/ml | |
|---|---|---|---|---|
| mg = ml[3] | lb. | kg | mg | ml |
| 0.39 | 13 | 6 | 0.06 | 0.15 |
| 0.81 | 27 | 12 | 0.12 | 0.30 |
| 1.2 | 40 | 19 | 0.19 | 0.48 |
| 1.6 | 55 | 25 | 0.25 | 0.62 |
| 2.0 | 68 | 31 | 0.31 | 0.78 |
| 2.5 | 82 | 37 | 0.37 | 0.92 |
| 2.8 | 95 | 43 | 0.40 | 1.0 |
| 3.3 | 110 | 50 | 0.50 | 1.2 |
| 3.7 | 123 | 56 | 0.56 | 1.4 |
| 4.1 | 137 | 62 | 0.62 | 1.6 |
| 4.5 | 150 | 68 | 0.68 | 1.7 |
| 4.6 | 155 | 70 | 0.70 | 1.8 |
| 5.0 | 165 | 75 | 0.75 | 1.9 |

1. Do not repeat the apomorphine dose.
2. It is safe to double the dose of naloxone or it may be repeated.
3. Based on the dissolution of a 6 mg tablet in 6 ml of water.

Copper and Zinc Sulfate. Copper sulfate induced emesis in a significantly higher number of cases, more rapidly, with fewer episodes of vomiting and a shorter period of nausea than did ipecacuanha (ipecac) in a study comparing single doses of each. Copper sulfate was given to 132 children and ipecac given to 125 children, of similar age distribution, to combat intoxication or suspected intoxication caused by ingested agents. Of the patients who received copper sulfate, 85 per cent vomited, 65 per cent within four minutes and 98 per cent within fourteen minutes. Only 55 per cent of the ipecac patients vomited, 50 per cent of them after a latent period of fifteen minutes or more.

For the most rapid effect with the highest incidence of positive results, the following method to induce vomiting was suggested: (1)

administer 100 to 200 ml of juice or other appropriate fluid; (2) then give 0.25 gm copper sulfate in 1% solution; (3) if vomiting has not occurred within fifteen minutes, administer 0.15 gm potassium ferrocyanide in 1% solution. Stomach contents are then aspirated and gastric lavage performed (Karlsson, B. and Noren, L: *Acta Paediat, 54*:331, 1965). In another study (*Pediatrics, 42*:189-193, 1968), elevated serum copper levels were found in a group of children thus treated, but more disconcerting was the inability to account for 30 per cent of the administered copper sulfate in the vomitus. The fact that significant elevations of serum copper (nephrotoxic, hepatotoxic and hemolytic properties) can occur makes this procedure hazardous and a poor substitute for other emetics. Since this agent is corrosive to the gastrointestinal tract, its use following ingestion of corrosive compounds (caustics, ferrous sulfate, salicylates, etc.) also appears to be dangerous.

The emetic dose of zinc sulfate is 0.6 to 2.0 gm dissolved in 200 ml of water and repeated at fifteen-minute intervals until vomiting occurs. However, the lethal dose of zinc sulfate is 15 gm and the symptoms of poisoning are similar to those of copper sulfate. Removal of the zinc sulfate by stomach tube is necessary when emesis does not occur.

### *Five Important Actions*

1. Identify the poison as soon as possible, so that specific measures may be promptly instituted. The label on the container, if still present and legible, often gives the ingredients and may also list specific antidotes. A telegram or telephone call to the manufacturer or to a Poison Control Center for identification may be necessary.
2. Administer an antidote, when indicated, for the residual poison not removed by emetics or gastric lavage. When a stomach tube is used, leave the antidote and other remedies in the stomach before removing the tube.
3. Give an antagonist when available.
4. Administer symptomatic and supportive treatment as indicated.
5. When the nature of the poison is unknown, one should not give the "universal antidote." Its effectiveness is questionable, as noted below. Activated charcoal is capable of absorbing large amounts of alkaloids like strychnine, morphine and atropine, as well as inorganic substances such as mercuric and arsenic compounds. One gram of charcoal absorbs 400 mg of phenol and more than 950 mg of strychnine. The tannic acid precipitates alkaloids, certain glucosides and many metals. The magnesium hydroxide neutralizes acids. Burnt toast is probably useless and if activated charcoal is not available, no time should be wasted in preparing it.

Universal Antidote

Activated charcoal..................... burned toast (nonactivated charcoal)

Two Parts

Magnesium hydroxide...... milk of magnesia

One Part

Tannic acid........................ strong tea solution

One Part

This "universal antidote" is ineffective and may even be harmful in that it can give a false sense of security to those who use it. It is only included here to deemphasize its popularity in lay journals and other media. The use of activated charcoal alone would be far more effective therapy, with magnesium hydroxide and tannic acid being administered only when specifically indicated. Actually there is some evidence to prove that these two agents interfere with the absorptive activity of activated charcoal when used conjointly.

Antidotes are given after ingestion of a poison only to render it inert or prevent its absorption by changing its physical nature. In general, soap or milk of magnesia may be used in poisoning due to acids; diluted vinegar, orange or lemon juice after ingestion of alkalis. Sodium thiosulfate, 15 gm in 2 liters of water, is recommended for heavy metals.

Intoxication due to alkaloids such as atropine or morphine is combated with solutions of potassium permanganate 1:5000 or tannic acid 4.0%. Milk, raw egg whites and flour or starches are generally useful household antidotal substances. Starch is an especially effective precipitant for iodine, while milk and raw egg whites may act as precipitants for mercury, arsenic and other heavy metals due to their protein content. All have demulcent properties also.

### *Inhaled Poisons*

In cases of gas poisoning, the first act should be to remove the victim from the presence of the gas and apply artificial respiration and give oxygen if necessary.

### *Injected Poisons*

If an injection of a poison has occurred, application of tourniquets central to the point of injection may slow absorption. Quantities of unabsorbed poison may be removed by means of incision and suction similar to that commonly advised for the treatment of snakebite. Cryotherapy is also beneficial in delaying absorption.

### *Adsorbed Dermal Poisons*

There are any number of poisonous compounds that are capable of producing intoxication of various degrees through transcutaneous adsorption, as well as local dermatitis of many kinds. These compounds include the chlorinated and organic phosphate insecticides, the halogenated hydrocarbons, the caustics and corrosives and many others. In the treatment, the contaminated skin should be thoroughly washed with water from a hose, shower or even poured from a bucket. Clothing should be removed while a continuous stream of water is played on the skin. A twenty-four-hour continuous shower has been found effective for chemical burns. Concentrated chemical antidotes should not be used as the heat liberated from the chemical reaction may increase the extent of injury. Corroded and burnt areas should be treated as for any burn.

### *Chemical Burns (Eye)*

A chemical burn of the eye results from local contact with a chemical—solid, liquid, dust, mist or vapor—of such degree as to alter the structure of the cornea and conjunctiva. Some alterations not visualized readily may be demonstrated by staining with a 2% solution of fluorescein after a local anesthetic.

Industries where this type of injury is particularly prevalent have adopted measures for prevention and have established facilities for first aid treatment. Any attempt to treat a chemical eye injury with a specific neutralizing material is now considered detrimental. The two exceptions to this rule are the treatment of lewisite burns with dimercaptopropanol (BAL) and the commonly used cocaine hydrochloride for neutralizing the iodine used as a cauterizing agent in the treatment of dendritic (herpes simplex) ulcers of the corneal epithelium.

The basic treatment of all types of chemical eye injuries is the quick, thorough irrigation of the eye with water at the nearest source of supply for five minutes. After instillation of a local anesthetic, irrigation with water or normal saline is continued for half an hour (neutralizing solutions should not be used). During this period the eye is carefully inspected, under loupe or slit-lamp magnification, and any insoluble particles on the ocular surfaces are removed using applicators or forceps. Gentle mechanical removal of injured or possibly contaminated tissue may be required. An antibiotic ointment is used to prevent adhesions. Use of local anesthetics is not continuous because of their detrimental effect on epithelial regeneration. A cycloplegic is indicated for any associated iritis. Atropine is used for the more severe cases. Firm eye dressings give comfort, promote healing and prevent mechanical disturbance of the regenerating epithelium. Use of cortisone reduces the inflammation and scarring and corneal vascularization, but it should not be used in the presence of uncontrollable infection nor for any great length of time. A recent approach in medication is use of a collagenase inhibitor such as cysteine. The destruction of the cornea in these cases is not due to the foreign alkali or acid; the cornea eats itself up with collagenase and perforates. This perforation can be prevented by the use of cysteine.

It is important to know the chemical nature of the substance causing the injury for predicting the probable course, prognosis and extent of treatment necessary. The action of acids of considerable strength is one of coagulation of all protein with which contact is made, forming insoluble acid proteinates—an instantaneous irreversible reaction. Penetration of the acid is limited by the barrier made by the dense layer of precipitated protein. A whole layer such as the cornea may be lost only when the injuring acid is great in concentration and amount.

Alkalis produce some of the most severe chemical eye injuries. The increase in hydroxyl ion concentration beyond the limits of tissue protein stability results in the formation of gel-like alkaline proteinates. In addition, alkalis combine with fats to form soaps and in this way they destroy the structure of the cell membranes and thus penetrate rapidly into the tissues. This speed of penetration is responsible for the capacity of alkalis to cause great ocular damage.

Some other chemicals produce changes in the tissue proteins, without altering the hydrogen ion concentration, which disable performance of their function and result in inflammatory and degenerative reactions. The injury to the eye from such a chemical may be just as severe as from alkalis and acids. Examples of these are the war gases, lewisite and mustard gas.

Study of the chemical properties of the involved agent is particularly important now that such a variety of products is being used in industry and the home, with new chemicals being added daily.

The amount of light energy reaching the retina from flashlight photographs in a young infant is insignificant and much less than that required to cause a retinal burn.

## ANTIDOTES

Effective and useful specific antidotes for poisoning are limited in number and by their overuse often complicate the initial injury by producing other forms of poisoning. The sensible selection and use of drugs and therapeutic measures for the general and supportive treatment of poisoning are more likely to save lives than ill-considered and heroically applied specific antidotes. Table 21 outlines alphabetically most of the useful and practical antidotes which are now available to the physician for emergency use, and these combined with the symptomatic and supportive drugs and measures on hand are all that are usually necessary.

## SUPPORTIVE MEASURES

### *Fluid Therapy*

Administration of adequate amounts of fluid is important in all cases and especially if the poison is excreted in the urine. If the patient is conscious and able to swallow, copious amounts of water are usually indicated. If the patient is unconscious or unable to swallow, fluids must be given by vein.

TABLE 19
DOSAGE* OF SOME ANTIARRHYTHMIC AGENTS

| | *Quinidine* | *Procain-amide* | *Lidocaine* | *Diphenyl-hydantoin* | *Propranolol* | *Bretylium* | *Potassium* |
|---|---|---|---|---|---|---|---|
| *Parenteral* | (Gluconate) *Intramuscular:* 0.2–0.4 Gm<br><br>*Intravenous:* 25 mg/min (total less than 800 mg) | *Intramuscular:* 250–500 mg<br><br>*Intravenous:* 100 mg every 5 min (total less than 1000 mg) | *Intravenous:* 50–100 mg every 5 min (total less than 350 mg)<br><br>Maintenance: 1–4 mg/min | *Intravenous:* 100 mg every 5 min (total less than 1000 mg) | *Intravenous:* 1–3 mg initially (total less than 0.1 mg/kg) | *Intramuscular* or *Intravenous:* 3–5 mg/kg<br><br>Maintenance: 2–5 mg/kg every 8 to 12 hours | (Chloride) *Intravenous:* 3 Gm (40 mEq) in more than 2 hours |
| *Oral* | (Sulfate) 0.2–0.4 Gm every 6 hours | 250–500 mg every 6 hours | | 100 mg every 6 hours | 10–30 mg every 6 to 8 hours | 300–600 mg every 8 to 12 hours | (Chloride) 1–3 Gm every 6 to 8 hours |

*Adult doses

TABLE 20
ADVERSE EFFECTS OF SOME ANTIARRHYTHMIC DRUGS

| *Drug* | *Adverse Effect* |
|---|---|
| Digitalis | Ventricular premature beats, ventricular tachycardia and fibrillation, atrial tachycardia with A-V block, Wenckebach phenomenon, complete A-V block, and complex arrhythmias. |
| Procainamide (Pronestyl) | Lupus-like picture with arthralgia, cutaneous lesions and pleuropulmonary disease; hypotension, GI symptoms, urticaria, lymphadenopathy, eosinophilia, serious arrhythmias, agranulocytosis. |
| Quinidine sulfate | GI symptoms, photophobia and diplopia, urticarial, or macular or papular rashes, fever, thrombocytopenia, hemolytic anemia, hypotension, serious arrhythmias and block. |
| Propranolol hydrochloride (Inderal) | Congestive heart failure, asthma, bradycardia, hypotension, shock. |
| Diphenylhydantoin (Dilantin®) | Hypotension, S-A node or A-V node depression, hematological effects, ataxia; cardiac arrest has been reported after IV therapy. |
| Lidocaine (Xylocaine®) | Drowsiness, euphoria, muscle twitching, disorientation, medullary depression, convulsions, cardiovascular depression. |
| Edrophonium (Tensilon®) | Salivation, perspiration (profuse), tachypnea. |
| Epinephrine and Isoproterenol | Ventricular arrhythmias, tachycardia. |

The three principles of fluid therapy which must be considered include the following:

1. Deficit therapy
2. Maintenance therapy
3. Concomitant replacement of abnormal losses

The first involves the replacement of any deficits of water and electrolytes that are present at the beginning of fluid therapy. The amount and kind of deficit must be estimated as accurately as possible from the patient's history, physical findings and laboratory data. The second general principle of fluid therapy is the supply of water, electrolytes, protein, calories and vitamins at a rate that approximates the rate of turnover of these substances under ordinary circumstances—so-called maintenance therapy. This turnover is a function not simply of weight or surface area but rather of total heat production—in other words, of energy expenditure. Actually, determining parenteral fluid needs by body surface area is not necessarily valid. Surface area is not an accurate indicator of body needs because (1) it cannot be accurately estimated by ordinary methods; (2) physiologic functions do not correlate with body surface; and (3) total metabolism increases with size but not consistently with area or any other unit yet ascertained.

A simple rule of thumb based on weight alone is sufficiently accurate and less misleading. The rule for infants less than one year of age is 60 ml ± 15 ml of fluid per pound of body weight for twenty-four hours; for children from one to five years, 50 ml ± 15 ml; and for children over five years, 40 ml ± 15 ml. Fluid maintenance in adults can also be based on weight; 30 ml or 1 ounce of fluid per pound for twenty-four hours is usually adequate to begin with. Such conditions as fever and polyuria may necessitate larger amounts. Skin turgor, daily weight, volume of urine output and appearance of the patient should all be considered.

### *Acidosis*

The acidosis that occurs in poisoning may be due to either of two mechanisms: (1) loss of base with reduction in pH and $CO_2$ combining

TABLE 21
SOME SPECIFIC ANTIDOTES

| *Poison* | *Antidote* | *Poison* | *Antidote* |
|---|---|---|---|
| acid, corrosive | alkali, weak | lead | iodine |
| alkali, caustic | acids, weak | lead | magnesium sulfate |
| alkaloids | potassium permanganate | malathion | atropine sulfate |
| amphetamine | chlorpromazine | meperidine | narcotic antagonist |
| anticoagulants, oral | phytonadione | mercury | dimercaprol |
| antimony | dimercaprol | mercury | iodine |
| arsenic | dimercaprol | mercury | penicillamine |
| atropine | physostigmine | mercury salts | formaldehyde sodium sulfoxylate |
| atropine | pilocarpine | | |
| barbiturates* | ——— | metals | edetate disodium calcium |
| barium | magnesium sulfate | metals, heavy | penicillamine |
| bismuth | dimercaprol | methadone | narcotic antagonist |
| bromides | sodium chloride | methyl alcohol | alcohol, ethyl |
| cadmium | edetate disodium calcium | morphine | narcotic antagonist |
| chlorinated hydrocarbons | calcium lactate | mushrooms | atropine sulfate |
| cholinesterase inhibitors | atropine sulfate | nickel | dimercaprol |
| cholinesterase inhibitors | pralidoxime | nickel | edetate disodium calcium |
| cobalt | edetate disodium calcium | nicotine | potassium permanganate |
| codeine | narcotic antagonist | opium alkaloids | narcotic antagonist |
| copper | edetate disodium calcium | organic compounds | potassium permanganate |
| coumarin derivatives | phytonadione | organic phosphate esters | atropine sulfate |
| cyanide | cyanide poison kit | organic phosphate esters | pralidoxime |
| cyanide | sodium thiosulfate | oxalates | calcium lactate |
| diazepam | physostigmine | parathion | atropine sulfate |
| digitalis | antiarrhythmic agents | phenothiazine tranquilizers | diphenhydramine |
| ethylene glycol | alcohol, ethyl | phosphorus | copper sulfate |
| ethylmorphine HCI | narcotic antagonist | physostigmine | potassium permanganate |
| fluoride | calcium lactate | potassium permanganate | hydrogen peroxide |
| formaldehyde | ammonium acetate | quinine | iodine |
| gluthion | atropine sulfate | quinine | potassium permanganate |
| glycols | alcohol, ethyl | scopolamine | physostigmine |
| gold | dimercaprol | selenium | bromobenzene |
| hemochromatosis | deferoxamine | silver | iodine |
| heparin | protamine sulfate | silver nitrate | sodium chloride |
| heroin | narcotic antagonist | snake venoms | antivenins |
| hypercalcemia | sodium sulfate | sodium fluroacetate | monoacetin |
| hypervitaminois D | sodium sulfate | sodium hypochlorite | alkali, weak |
| insect bites | calcium gluconate | spider venoms | antivenins |
| iodine | cyanide poison kit | spider venoms | calcium gluconate |
| iodine | sodium thiosulfate | strychnine | iodine |
| iodine | starch | strychnine | potassium permanganate |
| iron | edetate disodium calcium | tetraethyl pyrophosphate | atropine sulfate |

| | | | |
|---|---|---|---|
| iron | deferoxamine | thallium | dithizone |
| lead | dimercaprol | tricyclic antidepressants | physostigmine |
| lead | edetate disodium calcium | trithion | atropine sulfate |

*There is no specific antidote for the barbiturates. In acute poisoning, current practices in most centers with much experience consider the immediate establishment of adequate pulmonary ventilation as well as control of shock of prime importance while analeptics are considered subsidiary, if not actually contraindicated. The evidence indicates that the most favorable results are obtained by careful attention to respiratory and circulatory functions. Forced diuresis by giving large amounts of fluids IV and also giving diuretics (acetazolamide [Diamox] or mercurials) reduces the need for vasopressor drugs, prevents renal complications and hyperthermia, and lessens crust formation in the respiratory tract. Contraindications are cardiac and renal disease. Pulmonary edema does not seem to be a serious hazard. Hemodialysis should be resorted to when indicated. See Barbiturates pages 378-391.

| *Antidote* | *Dose* | *Poison* | *Reaction (to antidote) and Comments* |
|---|---|---|---|
| Acids, weak<br>Acetic acid, 1%<br>Vinegar, 5% acetic acid (diluted 1:4 with water)<br>Hydrochloric acid, 0.5% | 100 to 200 ml | Alkali, caustic | |
| Alcohol, ethyl | IV as 5% solution in bicarbonate or saline solution, orally as 3 to 4 oz. of whiskey (45%) every 4 hr. for 1 to 3 days | Methyl alcohol; Ethylene glycol (and other glycols) | Competes effectively for hepatic enzyme (alcohol dehydrogenase) with methyl alcohol and prevents formation of toxic formic acid and formates; prevents breakdown of glycols into toxic oxalic acid and oxalates |
| Alkali, weak<br>Magnesium oxide (preferred)*<br>Sodium bicarbonate | 2.5% solution (25 gm/liter)<br>5% solution (50 gm/liter) | Acid, corrosive<br>sodium hypochlorite | Gastric distention from liberated $CO_2$ (from use of $NaHCO_3$) |
| Ammonium acetate | 5 ml in 500 ml water, for gastric lavage | Formaldehyde (formalin) | Forms relatively harmless methenamine |
| Ammonium hydroxide | 0.2% solution, for gastric lavage | | |

*Paradoxical as it may seem, magnesium oxide or hydroxide should be used for hypochlorite (bleaches) ingestion to prevent the formation of irritating hypochlorcous acid.

TABLE 21—*Continued*
SOME SPECIFIC ANTIDOTES

| *Antidote* | *Dose* | *Poison* | *Reaction (to antidote) and Comments* |
|---|---|---|---|
| Atropine sulfate | 1 to 2 mg IM and repeat in 30 min. | Organic phosphate esters: gluthion, malathion, parathion, mushroom, tetraethyl pyrophosphate, trithion, etc.; other cholinesterases inhibitors | Atropinization |
| Antivenins | See circular for dosage instruction | | |
| *specific* Crotalidae polyvalent (Wyeth) | | North and South American snakebite venoms | |
| Latrodectus, Mactans and Curacaviensis (Merck) | | Black widow spider venom | |
| Micrurus (Wyeth Laboratories and C. Amaral and Cia L.T.D.A. Cloria 34, P.O. Box 2123, São Paulo, Brazil) | | Coral snake venom | |
| *nonspecific* Adult (may be used without antivenin, for adult only) | | Black widow spider venon | |
| Methocarbamol (Robaxin®) | On diagnosis, 1 amp. (1 gm, 10 ml) IV in 15 ml isotonic saline over 5 min. period or in IV drip; follow in 12 hr. with 2 tablets (1500 mg) 3 times a day for 2 days | | Muscle relaxant |
| Orphenadrine citrate (Norflex®) | On diagnosis, 1 amp. (2 ml, 60 mg) IV in 5 ml isotonic saline followed in 12 hr. by 1 tablet (100 mg) 2 times a day for 2 days | | Muscle relaxant |
| Antivenin child | Antivenin IV followed in 1 hr. by methocarbamol 1 tablet (500 mg) and 1 every 12 hr. for 2 days | | In children the antivenin should be used; this may be supplemented with the muscle relaxant when necessary. |
| Bromobenzene | Adult: 1 gm<br>Child: 0.25 gm (in lavage solution) | Selenium | |
| Calcium gluconate | 10% solution, 5 to 10 ml IM or IV, may be repeated in 8 to 12 hr. | Black widow spider and other insect bites | Muscle relaxant; bradycardia; flushing; local necrosis from perivenous infiltration (methocarbamol, etc., also effective) |

| | | | |
|---|---|---|---|
| Calcium lactate | 10% solution (in lavage solution) | Chlorinated hydrocarbons, fluoride, oxalates | |
| Chlorpromazine | 1 to 2 mg/kg IM | Amphetamine | Drowsiness; hypotension; neuromuscular (parkinsonian) |
| Copper sulfate | 0.25 to 3 gm in glass of water | Phosphorus | Forms insoluble copper phosphide |
| Cyanide poison kit (Eli Lilly stock M76) | | Cyanide | Hypotension; pearls, should be replaced annually for freshness |
| Amyl nitrite pearls, sodium nitrite | 0.2 ml (inhaled) follow with 3% solution (10 ml) in 2 to 4 min., and | | |
| Sodium thiosulfate | 25% solution (50 ml) in 10 min. through same needle and vein (Repeat with ½ doses if necessary.) | Iodine | Sodium thiosulfate used alone for iodine; forms harmless sodium iodide |
| Deferoxamine mesylate (Desferal®), Desferal isolated from *Streptomyces pilosus* | 1 to 2 gm IM or IV (adults), repeat if necessary every 4 to 12 hr.; also 5 to 10 gm via nasogastric tube after gastric lavage *(see comment)* | Iron, hemochromatosis | Diarrhea; hypotension; large oral doses can be absorbed and may result in systemic toxicity and its use is now being questioned |
| Dimercaprol | *Severe intoxication;* day 1: 3 mg/kg every 4 hr. (6 injections); day 2: same; day 3: 3 mg/kg every 6 hr. (4 injections); days 4 to 13 (or until recovery): 3 mg/kg every 12 hr. (2 injections)<br><br>*Mild intoxication;* day 1: 2.5 mg/kg every 4 hr. (6 injections); day 2: same; day 3: 2.5 mg/kg every 12 hr.; days 4 to 13 (or until recovery): 2.5 mg/kg daily (1 injection) | Antimony, arsenic, bismuth, gold, mercury (acrodynia), nickel, lead (combined therapy with edetic acid for encephalitis); contraindicated for iron | Flushing; myalgia; nausea and vomiting; nephrotoxic; hypotension; pulmonary edema; salivaton and lacrimation; fever (children) |
| Diphenhydramine hydrochloride | 10 to 50 mg IV or IM | Phenothiazine tranquilizers (for extrapyramidal neuromuscular manifestations) | Atropinelike effect; drowsiness |
| Dithizone | 10 mg/kg twice a day orally with 10 ml 10% glucose solution for 5 days | Thallium | Diabetogenic; not available for therapeutic use; may be obtained through a chemical supply company |
| Edetate disodium calcium or edetic acid (versene) (ethylenediamine tetra-acetic acid); pentetic acid ([diethylenetriamine pentaacetic acid], more promising analog) | 25 to 50 mg/kg, 20% solution 2 times a day for 5 days<br>50 mg/kg 20% solution (0.5% procaine) IM daily for 5 to 7 days<br>Repeat these courses after 2-day rest period. | Cadmium, cobalt, copper, digitalis, iron, lead (combined therapy with dimercaprol for encephalitis), nickel, and other metals | Nephrotoxic; increases urinary potassium excretion; use sodium salt for digitalis in place of edetate disodium calcium, which chelates Ca ion, producing hypocalcemia and reducing synergistic action of the Ca and digital- |

TABLE 21—*Continued*
SOME SPECIFIC ANTIDOTES

| *Antidote* | *Dose* | *Poison* | *Reaction (to antidote) and Comments* |
|---|---|---|---|
| | | | is, converting dangerous arrhythmias to sinus arrhythmias (other digitalis therapy preferable); orally given edetic acid should not be used until all lead has been removed or absorbed from the gastrointestinal tract. |
| Hydrogen peroxide | 3% solution (10 ml in 100 ml water as lavage solution) | Potassium permanganate; oxidizing agent for many other compounds | Irritation of mucous membranes; distention of abdomen from release of gas |
| Iodine, tincture | 15 drops in 120 ml water | Precipitant for lead, mercury, quinine, silver, strychnine | Precipitants must be thoroughly removed by gastric lavage. |
| Magnesium sulfate | 2 to 5% solution for lavage | Precipitant for barium, lead | |
| Monoacetin (glyceryl monoacetate) | 0.5 ml/kg IM or in saline solution IV; repeat as necessary | Sodium fluoroacetate 1080 | Not available commercially; if parenteral therapy not feasible, can give 100 ml. of monoacetin in water |
| Narcotic antagonists | | | |
| Nalorphine (Nalline®) hydrochloride | Adult: 5 to 10 mg IM or IV and repeat in ½ hr.<br>Child: 0.1 to 0.2 mg/kg IM or IV and repeat in ½ hr. | Codeine, meperidine hydrochloride (Demerol), ethylmorphine hydrochloride (Dionin), heroin, methadone, morphine, opium alkaloids (Pantopon) (For respiratory and cardiovascular depression) | Withdrawal symptoms; depressant effects in other than narcotic compounds |
| Levallorphan tartrate (Lorlan®) | Adult: 0.5 to 1 mg IM or IV<br>Child: 0.01 to 0.02 mg/kg IM or IV | | |
| Naloxone hydrochloride (Narcan®) | 0.01 mg/kg IV, IM, or SC | | |
| Penicillamine and its derivatives (Cuprimine®) | 1 to 5 gm orally | Mercury and other heavy metals | Fever; stupor; nausea and vomiting; taste dysfunction; myalgia; leukopenia, thrombocytopenia; nephrosis, reversible; optic axial neuritis, reversible; ineffective when severe vomiting is prominent |
| Physostigmine salicylate (Antilirium®) | 1 to 2 mg IM or IV* | Atropine, scopolamine, are particularly effective for cardiac arrhythmias and CNS toxic effects of the tricyclic antidepressant drugs and diazepam (*Valium)* intoxication | Anticholinesterase agent that reverses the action of anticholinergic drugs; the only cholinergic drug that crosses blood-brain barrier. Excess physostigmine can produce diarrhea, bradycardia, hypersalivation, rhinorrhea, and |

| | | | |
|---|---|---|---|
| | | | cholinergic crises, which would require treatment with propantheline (*Pro-Banthine*) parenterally (atropine second choice) |
| Phytonadione (vitamin $K_1$) | 25 to 150 mg IV; rate not to exceed 10 mg/min. or 2.5 to 10 mg orally | Coumarin derivatives; coumarin, phenprocoumon, warfarin, and other oral anticoagulants | Bleeding; focal hemorrhages; whole blood transfusion may be needed |
| Pilocarpine | 2 to 4 mg orally | Atropine and related alkaloids | Antagonizes the parasympathetic (mydriasis and dry mouth), not central, effects of atropine |
| Potassium permanganate | 1:5000 and 1:10,000 solution for gastric lavage | Nicotine, physostigmine, quinine, strychnine; oxidizing agent for many alkaloids and organic poisons | Severe irritant and should not be used in strong dilutions or with any residual particles |
| Pralidoxime iodide<br>Pralidoxime chloride | adult: 1 to 2 gm<br>child: 25 to 50 mg/kg IM or IV as 5% solution | Organic phosphate esters; cholinesterase inhibition by any agent: chemical, drug, etc. | Diplopia; dizziness; headache |
| Protamine sulfate | 1% solution IV slowly mg/mg to that of heparin | Heparin | Sensitivity effects; whole blood transfusions may be needed |
| Sodium chloride | 1 tsp. salt to 1 pt. water (approximately normal saline solution) | Silver nitrate | Forms noncorrosive silver chloride; hypernatremia |
| | 6 to 12 gm orally in divided doses or in isotonic saline IV | Bromides | |
| Sodium sulfate | 10% solution IM and repeat in 30 min.; also as catharsis for rapid elimination of toxic agent from gastrointestinal tract | Hypervitaminosis D; hypercalcemia | Glucocorticoids are more rapid and effective in reducing serum calcium levels. |
| Formaldehyde sodium sulfoxylate | 5% in lavage solution (preferably combined with 5% sodium bicarbonate) | Mercury salts | Dimercaprol therapy should follow gastric lavage. |
| Sodium thiosulfate | Orally: 2 to 3 gm, or IM: 10 or 25% solution; repeat in 3 to 4 hr. | Iodine<br>Cyanide | |
| Starch | 80 gm/1000 ml water | Iodine | |

*Not approved by the FDA for IV use in children.
From Jay M. Arena, *Emergency Medicine,* April 1976. Courtesy of publisher.

TABLE 22
BROAD-SPECTRUM AND HOUSEHOLD ANTIDOTES

| *Antidote* | *Dose* | *Use* | *Reactions (to antidote) and Comments* |
|---|---|---|---|
| Charcoal, activated | 1 to 2 tbs. to glass of water or a mixture of soupy consistency | Effective for virtually all poisons (see pages 34-35), organic and inorganic compounds of large and small molecules | Broad spectrum of activity; no reaction except staining |
| Castor oil | | As a solvent (and cathartic) for *concretions* in the stomach | |
| Household antidotes | | | |
| Milk<br>Raw eggs<br>Flour | | Arsenic; mercury and other heavy metals | These are useful and readily available antidotes that can be used in an emergency; all have demulcent properties. |
| Starches | | Iodine | Same as above |
| Methylene blue | Intravenously; 1% solution given slowly (2 mg/kg) and repeat in 1 hr. if necessary orally: 3 to 5 mg/kg (action much slower) | Methemoglobinemia produced by acetanilid, aniline derivatives, chlorates, dinitrophenol, nitrites, pyridium, and more than 100 other chemicals and drugs | Perivenous infiltration can produce severe necrosis; hypertension, sweating, chest pain, confusion, nausea and vomiting, dizziness, cyanosis; hemolysis in small infants. |
| Mineral oil | | Solvent, demulcent | |
| Tannic acid | 4% in lavage solution; never use in greater concentrations | Precipitates alkaloids, certain glucosides, and many metals | Hepatotoxic; tannates formed should not be allowed to remain in the stomach; because of its hepatotoxicity, should be used cautiously and in no greater than 4% solution |
| Universal antidote (activated charcoal alone preferable) | Two parts pulverized charcoal (burnt toast);<br>One part of magnesium oxide (milk of magnesia);<br>One part tannic acid (strong tea solution) | | Overrated and ineffective; may actually be harmful in that it may give false sense of security to those who use it; mentioned here only to negate its popularity in lay journals and books |

TABLE 23
EFFECTS OF WATER AND CERTAIN SOLUTES

| | *Too Little* | *Too Much* |
|---|---|---|
| Water | Hemoconcentration<br>Thirst<br>Oliguria<br>Fever<br>Circulatory failure | Hemodilution<br>Polyuria<br>Intracranial hypertension<br>Headache<br>Weakness<br>Muscle twitchings<br>Convulsions<br>Coma<br>Death |
| Sodium | Extracellular fluid volume decreased<br>Loss of tissue elasticity<br>Microcardia<br>Hypotension<br>Circulatory failure | Extracellular fluid volume increased<br>Edema formation<br>Tendency to potassium deficiency |
| Potassium | Apathy<br>Lethargy<br>Muscle weakness<br>Electrocardiographic changes<br>Ileus or diarrhea<br>Hypopotassemia<br>Metabolic alkalosis | Hyperpotassemia<br>Electrocardiographic changes<br>Muscle weakness<br>Cardiac arrest |
| Phosphorus | Hypophosphatemia | Hyperphosphatemia<br>Hypocalcemia<br>Tetany<br>Death |
| Carbohydrate | Ketosis<br>Protoplasmic catabolism<br>Tendency to greater water and electrolyte losses | Hyperglycemia<br>Glycosuria<br>Hepatic failure<br>Death |

TABLE 24
ROUGH GUIDE TO MAINTAINING BODY WATER NEEDS
AND CORRECTING FLUID DEFICITS

| *Objective* | *Volume per sq m of body surface needed to be supplied in 24-hour period* | | |
|---|---|---|---|
| | *Normal Needs (per sq m of body surface area)* | *Moderate deficit in "average man"** | *Severe deficit in "average man"** |
| Maintenance | 1,500 ml | 2,800 ml | 2,800 ml |
| To correct moderate deficit | 900 ml | 1,600 ml | — |
| To correct severe deficit | 1,800 ml | — | 3,200 ml |
| To replace continuing losses‡ | — | X ml‡ | X ml‡ |
| Total needed, first 24 hours | | 4,400 ml + X ml | 6,000 ml + X ml |

*"Average Man" assumed to be 5′10″ tall, to weigh 155 lb. (70 kg) and to have a surface area of 1.85 $m^2$.
‡"X" equals volume lost/24 hours by *abnormal routes,* e.g., through drainage tubes, fistulas, vomiting, etc. A simple alternate and fairly accurate formula is as follows: ml of maintenance water/kg/24 hours = 100 minus (3 × age in years).

TABLE 25
ELECTROLYTE CONCENTRATIONS OF SEVERAL COMMONLY USED PARENTERAL FLUIDS

| *Solution* | *gm/liter* | *mEq/liter cations* | *mEq/liter anions* |
|---|---|---|---|
| Isotonic saline (0.9% NaCl) | 9.0 | 154 Na | 154 Cl |
| Hypotonic saline (0.45% NaCl) | 4.5 | 77 Na | 77 Cl |
| Hypertonic saline (5.0% NaCl) | 50.0 | 850 Na | 850 Cl |
| Ringer's Injection | 8.6 NaCl | 147 Na | |
| | 0.3 KCl | 4 K | 157 Cl |
| | 0.33 $CaCl_2$ | 6 Ca | |
| Sodium Lactate Injection (one-sixth molar solution) | 18.66 Na Lact | 166 Na | 166 lactate |
| Sodium bicarbonate (1.5%) | 15.0 $NaHCO_3$ | 178 Na | 178 bicarbonate |
| Lactated Ringer's Injection | 6.0 NaCl | 130 Na | 111 Cl |
| | 0.3 KCl | 4 K | 27 lactate |
| | 0.2 $CaCl_2$ | 4 Ca | |
| | 3.1 Na Lact | | |
| Potassium chloride (0.5%) | 5.0 | 67 K | 67 Cl |

power may be caused by vomiting and diarrhea; (2) increase in acid with reduction of pH by the metabolism of a poison to an acid intermediate, e.g. methanol to formic acid, retention of carbonic acid during respiratory depression and retention of metabolic acids during anuria from renal damage.

The prompt administration of polyionic solutions containing glucose often prevents the development of severe acidosis that may occur in the course of poisoning with salicylates, methyl alcohol, phenol, formalin, polymeric phosphates, etc. If severe metabolic acidosis is present, alkali therapy is indicated either as M/6 sodium lactate or 3.75% sodium bicarbonate given intravenously. The carbon dioxide of the blood can be used as an estimate of the amount of alkali which should be administered, but only enough should be given to raise the $CO_2$ content to approximately 30 vol% or 15 mEq/liter. The amounts of bicarbonate or lactate necessary to raise the carbon dioxide content of the blood are as follows:

| | *1 Vol%* | *1 mEq/liter* |
|---|---|---|
| M/6 sodium lactate | 1.8 ml/kg | 4.2 ml/kg |
| Sodium bicarbonate | 0.026 gm/kg | 0.058 gm/kg |

Tromethamine (tris-hydroxymethyl aminomethane) is a strongly alkaline organic buffer which displays distinctive properties in the treatment of acidosis. It is often superior to sodium bicarbonate for correcting metabolic acidosis. Since tromethamine (Tris) is free of sodium, it can be used in acidotic patients whose underlying disease contraindicates sodium administration. Furthermore, Tris is capable of neutralizing carbonic acid and is recommended for lowering carbon dioxide tension ($pCO_2$) in respiratory acidosis.

## The Milliequivalent

A milliequivalent is a unit of measure of the comparative weight of different compounds, elements, or groups of ions which possess the same chemical value.

$$1 \text{ mEq} = \frac{\text{atomic weight in milligrams}}{\text{valence}}$$

Values given in mg% (mg/100 ml) can be converted to mEq/liter by the following formula.

$$\text{mEq/liter} = \frac{\text{mg/100 ml} \times \text{valence}}{\text{atomic weight}}$$

TABLE 26
FACTORS FOR CONVERTING BLOOD CHEMISTRY VALUES TO MILLIEQUIVALENTS PER LITER

| | Divide by | or | Multiply by |
|---|---|---|---|
| Calcium, mg % | 2 | | 0.5 |
| Chlorides, mg % | | | |
| (from Cl) | 3.5 | | 0.286 |
| (from NaCl) | 5.8 | | 0.172 |
| Bicarbonate $HCO_3$ | | | |
| ($CO_2$, vols. %) | 2.24 | | 0.446 |
| Magnesium, mg % | 1.2 | | 0.833 |
| Phosphorus, mg % | 1.7 | | 0.58 |
| Potassium, mg % | 3.9 | | 0.257 |
| Protein, gm/100 ml | | | 2.43 |
| Sodium, mg % | 2.3 | | 0.435 |
| Sulfur, mg % | 1.6 | | 0.625 |

## ARTIFICIAL RESPIRATION

Should respiration fail, the therapeutic measure is artificial respiration, to be administered by a team or a respirator until the patient either breathes spontaneously or dies. Oxygen without carbon dioxide should be used. Drugs which stimulate the respiratory center may be indicated; however, they are relatively ineffective. Intubation, with removal of secretions to insure an adequate airway, and parenteral antibiotic therapy as prophylaxis against infection are also of considerable importance.

Because they are always available, manual methods of artificial respiration are generally employed first in an emergency. The back-pressure arm-lift Holger-Nielsen method of artificial respiration has replaced most former methods other than the mouth-to-mouth procedure. This technique differs from the prone pressure method (Schafer) in that it is a two-phase operation which actively forces air into the lungs as well as expels it. The prone pressure method forces air out but depends on the elastic recoil of the chest and internal organs to bring air into the lungs. This difference is very important in cases of deep asphyxia such as might be caused by nerve gas.

### Standard Techniques

The correct positions are for the victim to be placed face down, prone position, with elbows bent and with one hand upon the other. The cheek is placed on the hand with the face turned slightly to one side. The operator kneels on one knee (or both if more comfortable) at the head of the victim, facing him. He then places his hands on the victim's back so that the thumbs just touch and the heels of his hands are just below a line running between the armpits.

The operator then rocks forward slowly, keeping the elbows straight, until the arms are approximately vertical, exerting steady pressure upon the chest to force air out of the lungs.

The operator then rocks backward, slowly sliding his hands to the victim's arms just above the elbows, to pull air into the lungs.

Continuing to rock backward, he raises the arms until resistance and tension are felt at the victim's shoulders. Then he drops the arms and thus completes a full cycle. The cycles are repeated twelve times per minute, The expansion and compression phases being of equal length, and the release periods of minimum duration.

Evidence indicates that in the presence of resistance to pulmonary ventilation, the ancient technique of mouth-to-mouth insufflation is even more effective than the back-pressure arm-lift method. The following procedures should prove adequate.

Place victim on his back, begin rescue breathing (mouth-to-mouth). If first effort fails, sweep your fingers through his mouth to clear obstructions.

Lift the neck to tilt head as far back as possible. Hold this position. If head slumps forward, air passages will be blocked.

Take a deep breath. Open your mouth wide; seal your lips on victim's cheeks around nose. Breathe into either nose or mouth—if mouth, pinch nostrils to prevent air leakage. For child, cover both nose and mouth tightly with your mouth. Take shallow breaths for an infant. If excess air causes his abdomen to bulge, press out gently. Breathe until victim's chest rises.

Remove mouth, listen for expiration. If none, check for foreign bodies. Turn victim on side, slap his back to dislodge material in throat. Repeat breathing at least ten times per minute for adults, twenty times per minute for children.

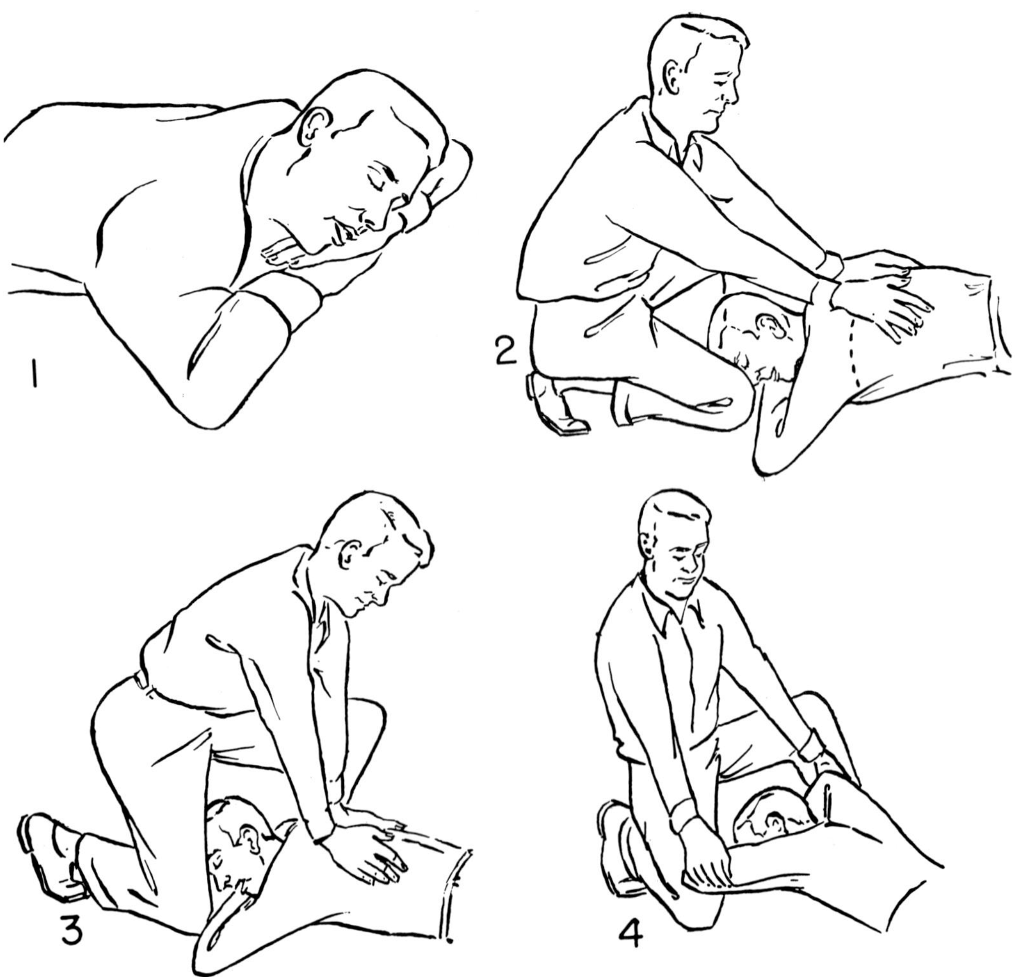


Figure 5.

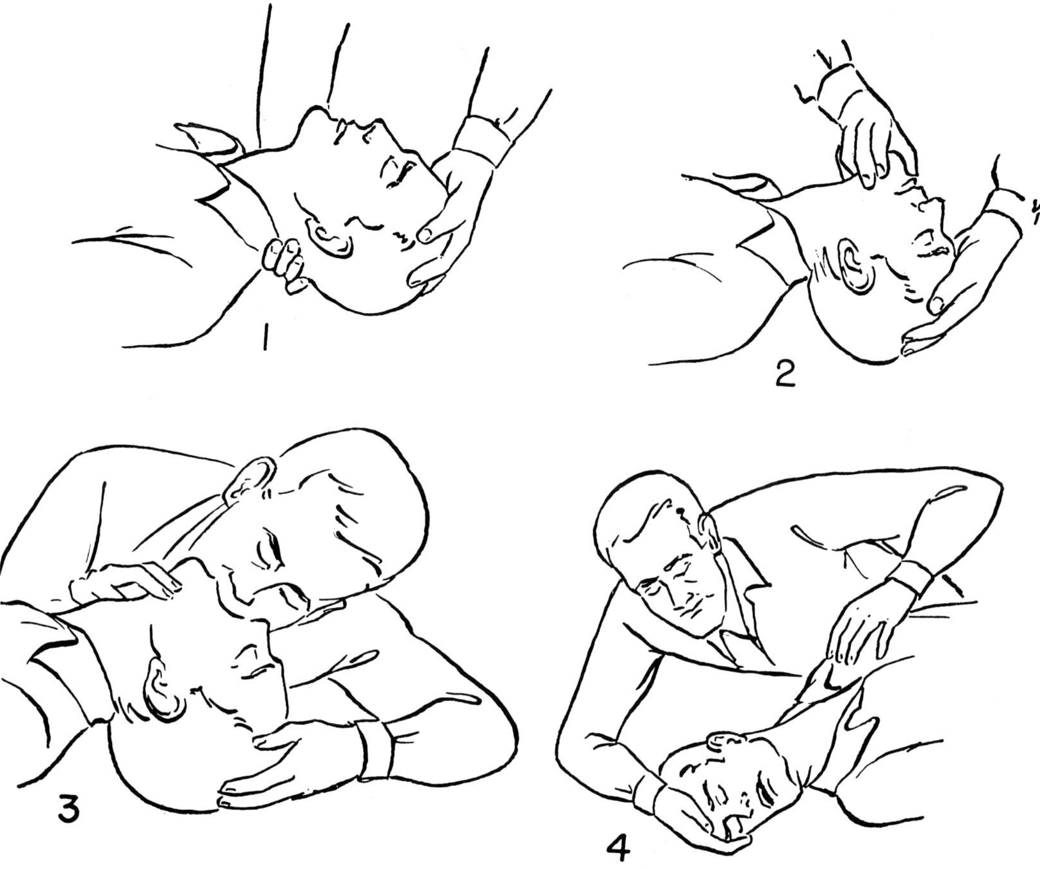


Figure 6.

## CARDIAC THERAPY

In acute poisonings, rapid failure of the heart may result because of direct myocardial damage. Cardiac standstill or ventricular fibrillation can also occur. Various arrhythmias may result from vagal overactivity, asphyxia or direct poisoning of the heart muscle. If the heart is inhibited through vagal stimulation, small doses such as 0.3 mg (1/200 gr) of atropine or scopolamine are indicated. Asphyxia should be prevented by the establishment and maintenance of an adequate respiratory exchange and an adequate circulation.

### Closed-Chest Cardiac Massage

When the circulation ceases in man because the heart is in cardiac arrest and the breathing stops, oxygenated blood is no longer supplied to the tissues. Two things are necessary: the ventilation of the lungs and the pumping of oxygenated blood to the body. The lungs may be supplied with oxygen by mouth-to-mouth insufflation, or by intubation or mask and the use of oxygen or air. Closed-chest cardiac massage circulates the oxygenated blood and maintains the patient alive.

TABLE 27
MYOCARDIOPATHY

| *Hypersensitivity Reactions* | *Chemical Compounds* |
|---|---|
| Serum Sickness | *Amanita phalloides* |
| Antivenin (all types) | Arsenic trioxide |
| Antitoxin (tetanus, botulism, etc.) | Barium |
| | Benzol |
| Drug Reactions/Overdosage | Cadmium oxide |
| | Carbon monoxide |
| Aconite | Carbon tetrachloride |
| Amphetamine | Chloroform |
| Arsphenamine | Ethanol |
| Bismuth | Favism |
| Digitalis | Fluoroacetate |
| Emetine | Halogenated hydrocarbons |
| Ephedrine | Methanol |
| Epinephrine | Nicotine |
| Ipecac | Nitroglycerine |
| Nitrites | Oxalates |
| Penicillin | Phosphorus |
| Phenylbutazone | Red Squill |
| Potassium salts* | Thallium |
| Quinidine | |
| Quinine | |
| Salicylates | |
| Sulfonamides | |
| Veratrum | |

*Morton Lite® salt substitute contains 90 per cent potassium chloride. The inadvertent use or ingestion of large amounts can produce severe hyperkalemia.

The patient in cardiac arrest should be placed in a supine position, preferably on a firm support such as the floor, a table or a bed board, and given a sharp blow to the precordium; this alone may restore cardiac activity. If it does not, provide a patent airway by inserting a tube or extending the neck and pulling the jaw up, as in mouth-to-mouth insufflation. Kneel beside the patient and place your hands on the center of his chest. To find the exact spot: locate the xiphoid and place the heel of the lower hand, with the other hand on top of it, on the sternum just above the xiphoid. Now press vertically downward, using the weight of your body, to push the sternum in for a distance of one inch to one and one-half inches. This action compresses the heart between the sternum and the vertebral column and forces the blood out of the heart and into the lungs and the systemic circulation. Now release the pressure, lifting your hands slightly. This allows the patient's chest to expand fully and the ventricles to refill. Repeat the cycle about sixty to eighty times per minute.

If you are the only person present, rapidly ventilate the patient's lungs by giving the patient three or four deep breaths, mouth-to-mouth. Then start massage and, after about a minute or a minute and a half, stop the massage and fill his lungs again with fresh air. If there is someone else present, have him ventilate the lungs simultaneously. There is no need to synchronize the two lifesaving procedures. When cardiac standstill is present, the rhythm may return spontaneously. If it does not, epinephrine (5 to 10 ml of 1:10,000 dilution) should be injected into the ventricular cavity during continued external compression. If this fails, calcium gluconate (5 to 10 ml of 10% solution) should be injected with resumption of external compression. When ventricular fibrillation is responsible for circulatory arrest, electrical defibrillation usually is necessary. Successful resuscitation becomes less likely as acidosis increases. Sodium bicar-

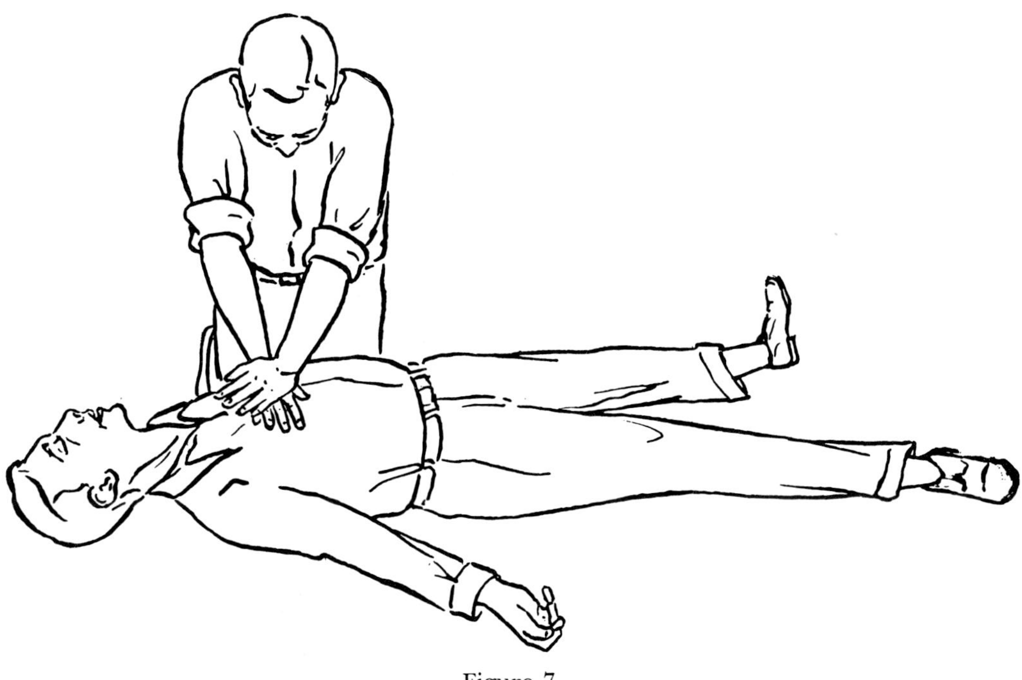

Figure 7.

bonate (44 mEq) must be given intravenously every few minutes as long as resuscitative efforts continue. *After successful resuscitation, one always should be prepared for additional episodes of circulatory arrest.*

Chronic complete heart block, unassociated with symptoms, requires no immediate treatment. Overt syncope, a brief period of asystole or ventricular fibrillation recorded electrocardiographically and congestive heart failure are the cardinal indications for treatment.

The transfer of closed-chest cardiac massage to man has been made with unusual facility due to the more favorable thoracic anatomy. The human mediastinum is fixed. The heart, particularly in the case of standstill or ventricular fibrillation, dilates and almost entirely fills the space between the sternum and thoracic spine; unless enlarged below the diaphragm, the liver escapes compression during this maneuver. The chest of the unconscious adult is remarkably flexible. Applying rhythmic, intermittent, strong vertical pressure centrally on the lower third of the sternum has resulted in maintenance of sufficient circulation to keep the brain alive in a human being whose heart remained in asystole for two hours before it resumed forcible contraction. Not only has it been possible to reestablish automatic cardiac activity from asystole, but also to provide adequate circulation in the presence of ventricular fibrillation until external defibrillation could be accomplished.

## BLOOD TRANSFUSIONS (EXCHANGE TRANSFUSIONS AND PLASMAPHERESIS)

Blood transfusion is particularly efficacious where the toxic products of the poison tend to remain in the circulating bloodstream in contrast to becoming fixed or being deposited in the viscera, bones or other tissues—in particular, the various types of drugs causing methemoglobinemia; e.g. the aniline dyes and their derivatives, such as acetanilid and phenacetin, nitrites, nitrates, bromates, chlorates, sulfanilamide, Pyridium® (phenazopyridine), nitrobenzene and related nitro compounds. The object is to supply normal hemoglobin capable of transporting oxygen. In more severe instances, exchange or exsanguination transfusions may be lifesaving, if facilities and blood are available. This procedure offers certain advantages over other methods such as hemodialysis in that it is familiar to most physicians, requires little specialized equipment and does not necessitate exceptional experience as does the safe use of hemodialysis. It has the obvious limitations that, in other than very small children, it is technically difficult and presents the hazard of blood transfusion reaction, since it may be necessary to use blood from several sources.

There are many cases of poisonings or intoxications (particularly drugs) in which plasma exchange (plasmapheresis) is useful as a therapeutic measure. The procedure rapidly removes the lethal amounts of toxins from the circulation and is particularly useful where the toxic material is nondialyzable, when dialysis facilities are not available and when time is a critical factor.

## EXTRACORPOREAL DIALYZER (ARTIFICIAL KIDNEY)

The artificial kidney in the treatment of acute drug intoxication is being used with increasing frequency and effectiveness. There is no question that some barbiturates, salicylates, bromides and many other therapeutic agents which can be toxic when ingested in large amounts may be effectively removed by dialysis. As in the evaluation of the artificial kidney for the treatment of acute renal failure, one must consider carefully whether or not conservative measures alone might be adequate. In the present state of our knowledge, we cannot always relate blood levels of these substances to the clinical status. In the patient seen forty-eight hours after the ingestion of barbiturates, who is comatose but has normal renal function and adequate ventilation and appears to be progressing satisfactorily, it is doubtful that removal of barbiturate from the blood at that point contributes enough to make the procedure worthwhile. On the other hand, the patient seen within hours after taking the drug, who has a very high blood level of barbiturate and impaired renal function, respiration and blood pressure, may profit from the removal of the toxic substance by dialysis. Between these two extremes, each case must be decided on its own merits. Recently hemodialysis has been used effectively in the treatment of acute alcohol crisis.

Contraindications, of one degree or another, to the use of the artificial kidney are (1) inexperience of the operator and inadequate knowledge of the problem to which the apparatus is to be applied; (2) bleeding, particularly bleeding from the gastrointestinal tract, since heparinization is necessary to prevent coagulation of blood in the extracorporeal circulation (it is, however, possible by "regional heparinization" to heparinize blood entering the machine, neutralizing it with protamine sulfate as it returns to the patient's venous circulation—in this way the hazards of bleeding may be minimized); and (3) destruction of platelets and white cells by the cellophane membrane during the course of hemodialysis. This is seldom of clinical significance in the individual with a normal white cell and platelet count. However, it must be considered before undertaking dialysis in patients with any disturbances in these parameters.

Hemodialysis is four to six times more effective than peritoneal dialysis and may be essential in the treatment of the more life-threatening disorders. Fortunately, blood dialysis technique is undergoing many favor-

TABLE 28
KNOWN DIALYZABLE POISONS*

Barbiturates
- Barbital
- Phenobarbital
- Amobarbital
- Pentobarbital
- Butabarbital
- Secobarbital
- Cyclobarbital

Glutethimide

Depressants, Sedatives and Tranquilizers
- Diphenylhydantoin
- Primidone
- Meprobamate
- Ethchlorvynol
- Ethinamate
- Methypyrlon
- Diphenhydramine
- Methaqualone
- Heroin
- Gallamine triethiodide†
- Paraldehyde
- Chloral hydrate
- Chlordiazepoxide

Antidepressants
- Amphetamine
- Methamphetamine
- Tricyclic secondary amines
- Tricyclic tertiary amines
- Monoamine oxidase inhibitors
- Tranylcypromine
- Pargyline
- Phenelzine
- Isocarboxazid

Alcohols
- Ethanol
- Methanol
- Isopropanol
- Ethylene glycol

Analgesics
- Acetylsalicyclic acid
- Methylsalicylate
- Acetophenetidin
- Dextropropoxyphene
- Paracetamol

Antibiotics
- Streptomycin
- Kanamycin
- Neomycin
- Vancomycin
- Penicillin
- Ampicillin
- Sulfonamides
- Cephalin
- Cephaloridine
- Chloramphenicol
- Tetracycline
- Nitrofurantoin
- Polymyxin
- Isoniazid (INH)
- Cycloserine
- Quinine
- Bacitracin

Metals
- Arsenic
- Copper
- Calcium
- Iron
- Lead
- Lithium
- Magnesium
- Mercury
- Potassium
- Sodium
- Strontium
- Zinc

Halides
- Bromide
- Chloride
- Iodide
- Fluoride

Endogenous Toxins
- Ammonia
- Uric acid
- Tritium
- Bilirubin
- Lactic acid
- Schizophrenia
- Myasthenia gravis
- Porphyria
- Cystine
- Endotoxin
- Hyperosmolar state
- Water intoxication
- Uremic toxin(s)

Miscellaneous Substances
- Thiocyanate
- Aniline
- Sodium chlorate
- Potassium chlorate
- Eucalyptus oil
- Boric acid
- Potassium dichromate
- Chromic acid
- Digoxin
- Sodium citrate
- Dinitro-ortho-cresol
- *Amanita Phalloides*
- Carbon tetrachloride
- Ergotamine
- Cyclophosphamide
- 5-Fluorouracil
- Methotrexate
- Camphor
- Trichloroethylene
- Carbon monoxide
- Chlorpropamide
- Mannitol
- Salt (sodium chloride)

* This list is complete at press time. Undoubtedly many more compounds will be found to be dialyzable as time passes and interest in this procedure increases. Agents that are highly bound to plasma protein (and hence, poorly dialyzable, at least theoretically) may actually be removed in significant quantities because of a rapid equilibrium between the bound and unbound drug fractions. It is possible, therefore, that many compounds not listed as dialyzable may very well be removed by dialysis. *Peritoneal dialysis, by rewarming the "core," has produced recovery from profound hypothermia.* The annual volume of Transactions of the American Society for Artificial Internal Organs is the best source for complete data on dialyzable chemicals and drugs.

†Excreted unchanged by the kidneys and should not be used in patients with renal damage.

able changes. Since the introduction of the short-tube clinical blood dialyzer, transfusions have not been needed. Blood heparinization can now be confined to the external pathway. Equipment is less elaborate and expensive. As a matter of fact, all of it can be carried to any room in the hospital in containers no larger than a medium-size suitcase. Treatment fluid is mixed in small, easily handled flasks at the bedside, using tap water and common available, chemicals. These advanced features should make this important and often lifesaving procedure available and operable in every hospital regardless of size for an ever-increasing number of serious diseases, poisonings, severe hypothermia and clinical emergencies. This procedure has also been used successfully in pregnancy without undue effects on the mother and fetus.

While most physicians have used the conventional membrane type of artificial kidney to clear the blood of poisons, a few have tried a simpler and more readily available approach—filtering the blood through activated charcoal immersed in normal saline. The charcoal filter adsorbs drugs and can also remove some substances that do not dialyze across membranes, either because they are strongly bound to plasma proteins or because their molecules are too large. A currently developed resin-column hemoperfusion system has been demonstrated to be technically simpler, consistently more effective and clinically superior to standard hemodialysis for acute drug intoxication (exceptionally high clearance rates have been obtained for barbiturates, glutethimide, ethchlorvynol and methaqualone). The column contains 650 gm of pyrogen-free Amberlite XAD-2 resin, which is uncharged and has a cross-linked, polystyrene macoreticular structure with particular surface attraction for high-molecular-weight, lipid-soluble molecules (Rosenbaum *et al.: New Engl J Med, 284*:874-877, 1971).

Recently it has been demonstrated that hemoperfusion using charcoal coated with an acrylic hydrogel obtained much higher drug clearances than the usual treatment methods of dialysis. Coating the charcoal with a hydrogel overcomes most of the problems previously encountered with charcoal embolism: marked thrombocytopenia, leukopenia, fibrinogen loss and pyrexia.

Complications reported in children from hemodialysis follow.

1. The disequilibrium syndrome (headache, increasing lethargy or confusion, twitching, cyanotic attacks and convulsions) which may appear during dialysis and persist during the first postdialysis day. The syndrome is considered the result of delayed clearance of urea from the cerebrospinal fluid and brain as compared with the extracellular fluid, thus creating an osmotic gradient which leads to net influx of water into the cerebral tissues with resultant cerebral edema and raised intracranial pressure (*see* Aluminum Hydroxide, page 350, as the cause for dialysis encephalopathy).
2. The urea rebound phenomenon in which there is a sharp increment in plasma urea concentration during the immediate postdialysis period.
3. Cardiac arrest. This occurrence is often difficult to attribute to the dialysis procedure itself since the depressant action on the myocardium may very well have been produced by the drug or chemical involved. However, the possibility of cardiac arrhythmias secondary to digitalis intoxication in digitalized children (with their small body size) undergoing hemodialysis must be considered because of the disproportionate removal of potassium in relation to digitalis.
4. Weight loss which reflects fluid loss and blood volume changes. Maintenance of body fluid and blood volume by methods available is necessary and critical.

## LIPID DIALYSIS

Lipid dialysis is a new technique in the treatment of poisonings by glutethimide, pentobarbital, secobarbital, phenothiazines, camphor and other lipid-soluble substances that cannot be effectively removed by hemodialysis employing an aqueous dialysate. Lipid dialysis is similar to aqueous hemodialysis, except that oil is circulated on the dialysate side of the membrane. An inexpensive and readily available, effective, safe, nontoxic and nonpyrogenic dialysate is soybean oil, U.S.P. The oil does not cross the cellophane membrane and absorbs large quantities of lipid-soluble substances.

A Klung or Kiil membrane can be easily used for lipid dialysis with only a few modifications. Two gallons of soybean oil can absorb a large quantity of the drug and compounds, and only a slow flow of the oil past the membrane is necessary for complete removal of lipid-soluble substances in each circulation of the blood through the membrane. Glutethimide is highly soluble in alcohols and lipids, but it is very poorly soluble in water.

A factor in intoxication with lipid-soluble drugs is storage of the drug in the fat tissues of the body. These drugs are rapidly deposited into lipid tissue and then gradually leak back into the bloodstream as the drug is removed. This phenomenon can produce a prolonged elevated blood level and coma even after removal of a considerable amount of the drug from the bloodstream.

## PERITONEAL DIALYSIS

Peritoneal dialysis is much more efficient than the natural kidney for ridding the body of overdoses of barbiturates and other drugs. In infants and children too small to permit adequate hemodialysis, peritoneal dialysis is the method of choice since the increased ratio of the peritoneal surface to body mass results in significantly increased efficiency. Major indications besides poisoning are acute renal failure, intractable edema, hepatic coma, hypercalcemia and chronic uremia. Contraindications are infections of the peritoneal cavity and recent or extensive abdominal surgery.

A small laporatomy incision in the right section of the mesogastric region is made and a catheter inserted with its distal tip extending about 3 cm into the peritoneal cavity. This is used as an inflow tract. A slightly larger incision is made in the left hypogastrium and two catheters, each with several openings near the tip, are inserted. The tip of one catheter is advanced to about 3 cm beyond the tip of the other. This is to enable later movement of the catheters against each other to free any fibrin or clots from occluding the openings and thus obstructing the outflow. The irrigation fluid suggested for use is as follows.

| | |
|---|---|
| Ringer's solution | 1000ml |
| Dextrose | 10 gm |
| Streptomycin | 0.5 to 1.0 gm |
| Penicillin | 10,000 units |
| Sodium citrate | (3.8%) 50 ml |

The composition of this fluid, however, should be adjusted to the individual biochemical disturbance of the patient. Tham and albumin (Albumisol®) should be added to the dialysis solution in the treatment of phenobarbital (and other drugs) intoxication. Tham, by keeping the solution alkaline, permits greater solubility, hence greater excretion of the drug, while albumin enhances excretion of phenobarbital and salicylates.

A flow of about 1 liter/hr. is recommended for adults and a proportionately slower flow should be used for children. Frequent checks of the outflow catheters are required to make sure that the lumens are not obstructed. Some physicians, on the other hand, use intermittent filling and emptying of the peritoneum by separate indwelling intake and outflow catheters.

Several laboratories have developed special electrolyte solutions and disposable apparatus which can be used with safety and simplicity and bring artificial dialysis within the reach of every physician. The solutions, known as peridial, inpersol and dianeal are available for patients with and without edema. The equipment consists of three specially designed pieces of rubber tubing. Now peritoneal dialysis can be carried out with a minimum of personnel, using a trocar and disposable equipment. It can be done at the bedside and may be started immediately when the patient enters the hospital. Available also is an automatic peritoneal dialysis system (Drake-Willock Dialysate Delivery System, Portland, Oregon) which is effective for acute as well as chronic conditions requiring dialysis.

Peritoneal dialysis involves the hazards of introducing synthetic fluids into the peritoneal cavity with the possibility of infection, adhesions, and if improperly done, even bowel perforations. Therefore, like any other treatment procedure, the risks of undertaking it must be balanced against the risks of omitting it and the expected benefits from its use.

Peritoneal dialysis in children is the only practical procedure currently available by which dialysis of an anuric infant can be accomplished. Extracorporeal hemodialysis relieves severe oliguria and removes many toxic agents from the blood but cannot be performed safely except by highly trained groups of physicians. The average capacity of the coil used for small children is about 400 ml of blood, but major fluctuations in capacity occur. If the child's blood volume is less than 1000 ml, the magnitude of potential alterations in blood volume due to change in capacity of the coil makes hemodialysis hazardous because either hypervolemia or hypovolemia may suddenly occur. Therefore, use of the extracorporeal method of hemodialysis for infants less than one year old is currently not advised.

Because of the inert semipermeable nature of the living peritoneal membrane, both the volume and electrolyte composition of extracellular fluid can be altered by the repeated instillation, equilibration and removal of solutions from the peritoneal cavity. The solutions employed have a composition similar to potassium-free extracellular fluid. Dextrose, 1.5%, is added to increase the osmolality above that found in the serum of uremic patients. The fluid has a tonicity of 360 to 380 milliosmols (mOs)/liter. Since such a solution may cause gradual dehydration, intravenous fluid therapy is usually necessary. The weight of the patient must be carefully monitored. If overhydration is to be avoided, 0.5 to 1 per cent of total body weight should be lost daily. If overhydration exists, the dialysis fluid should be made hypertonic by addition of glucose to a concentration of 4% to 7%, 550 to 660 mOs/liter, so that extracellular fluids migrate into the peritoneal cavity and are removed. Perfusing fluids must be sterile and nonirritating to the peritoneal membrane to reduce hyperemia and exudation.

An effective nonirritating peritoneal cannula with a deep helical groove punctuated at the base by many small holes is also now commercially available. The ridges surrounding the perforations prevent plugging by the omentum and thus facilitate drainage. Difficulty in placing the cannula in the peritoneal cavity because of the length and size necessitates insertion by surgical means. A small incision in the lower left quadrant permits the abdominal muscles to be spread and the peritoneum exposed and incised. With the index finger inserted along the descending colon, the cannula is guided along the colon's lateral edge and up the left paravertebral gutter. The peritoneum is then closed snugly

TABLE 29
COMPOSITION OF DIALYSIS FLUIDS

| | *Normal Serum* | *Standard Dialysis Solutions* | | *Albumisol* |
|---|---|---|---|---|
| | | *Without K* | *With K* | |
| Sodium (mEq/liter) | 140 | 140 | 140 | 142 |
| Potassium (mEq/liter) | 5 | 0 | 4.0 | 0 |
| Calcium (mEq/liter) | 5 | 3.5 | 3.5 | 0.6 |
| Magnesium (mEq/liter) | 2 | 1.5 | 1.5 | 0 |
| Glucose (%) | 0.1 | 1.5 | 1.5 | 0 |
| Albumin (%) | 5 | 0 | 0 | 5 |
| Osmolality (mOs/liter) | 280 | 372 | 380 | 280 |

about the tube, and the wound is closed in layers.

The perfusing fluid enters the abdominal cavity by gravity over fifteen to twenty minutes and remains for eighty minutes with the tube clamped. The bottle which contained the fluid is set on the floor and the cannula unclamped. Drainage and gentle siphonage empty the peritoneal cavity in about twenty minutes. The procedure is repeated every two hours, and inflow and outflow are recorded. Net water exchange is determined by weighing the patient. From 75 to 100 ml of dialyzing fluid per 100 calories expended or 1200 ml/sq. m of surface area may be introduced into the peritoneal cavity at each cycle without significant discomfort. This is equivalent to 75 to 100 ml/kg in the infant and 2000 ml in the adult.

Acute peritonitis absolutely prohibits peritoneal dialysis. Recent abdominal surgery and extensive abdominal adhesions deter but do not preclude dialysis. Reasons for institution of peritoneal dialysis in infants and small children in addition to that of poisoning are acute renal failure, acute glomerular nephritis and severe metabolic acidosis. The technic may also be used for correcting idiopathic hypercalcemia and hypernatremia as well as any type of refractory edema uncontrolled by the usual means of therapy.

Dialysis complications reported include convulsions, encephalopathies, psychotic states and transient peripheral neuropathies.

## SHOCK THERAPY

Shock, which occurs frequently in various types of poisoning, may be the result of many factors: (1) the direct vasodepressor effect of the poison or its metabolites; (2) as a nonspecific effect of metabolic disturbance or tissue hypoxia; (3) the trauma and tissue destruction associated with caustic and corrosive intoxication; and (4) the pooling and extravasation of blood and fluids into the intestinal tract as seen in arsenic, fluoride and phosphorus poisoning. Therefore, in the therapy of shock following poisoning, careful consideration is required of all the underlying factors as well as the administration of vasopressor agents and the replacement of fluids. Each type of poison is treated with whatever specific antidotes and other specific measures are available or warranted. Vasomotor stimulants should be used for vasomotor collapse only and not to support a failing circulation when blood transfusions or fluids are needed to replace diminished blood volume. Levophed (microcirculatory evidence from clinical and experimental work shows that far better results can be obtained in shock if this vasopressor is given after administration of the vasodilator, phenoxybenzamine HCl [Dibenzyline®]) is the vasopressor of choice when shock is severe and due to vasodilatation. A less severe degree of shock responds to the intramuscular use of phenylephrine (Neo-Synephrine®) 0.1 mg/kg of body weight. The free alcohol preparation of hydrocortisone (50 mg/ml of Cortef® acetate) should be used in the treatment of cardiovascular collapse which is refractory to the usual methods of therapy. It can be given in a dose of 2 to 4 mg/kg of body weight and should be diluted in no less than 250 ml of 5% glucose or physiologic saline solution. Approximately the same amounts of the succinate or phosphate esters of hydrocortisone can be administered rapidly intravenously in smaller volumes of fluid.

Early and massive doses of corticoids (25 to 50 mg/kg/day), when given as part of a total antishock regimen, may increase survival rates. The amounts that provide approximately the same anti-inflammatory effects obtained with 25 mg of cortisone or 20 mg of hydrocortisone are prednisone 5 mg; prednisolone 4 mg; methylprednisolone 4 mg; triamcinolone 4 mg; dexamethasone 0.75 mg; and betamethasone 0.6 mg. For intravenous method, use 100 mg hydrocortisone sodium succinate or 20 mg methylprednisolone sodium succinate per square meter as a slow push every six to twelve hours or placed in the IV fluids.

## DISSEMINATED INTRAVASCULAR COAGULATION (DIC)

According to clinical observations and experimental studies, disseminated intravascular coagulation (DIC) may be caused by the following.

1. Release of platelet factor 3 from thrombocytes.
2. Release of substances inducing coagulation from certain organs (lung, uterus, prostate).
3. Hemolysis, where "Erythrozytin," a lipoprotein similar to platelet factor 3, is released.
4. Blockage of the reticuloendothelial system that provides the inactivation of inductors of the coagulation and of activated coagulation products.
5. Shock conditions with disturbance of the microcirculation leading to sludge phenomenon, local hypoxia and acidosis, resulting in release of coagulation inductors.

In many cases of DIC, it is not possible to find a unique cause, and a multifactorial pathogenesis has to be postulated. In addition to the classical DIC associated with septic shock, isolated reports of this complication in exogenous intoxications have appeared in the literature, particularly after inorganic and organic acid, corrosive sublimate, dichloroethane and other poisonings. The bite of the *Loxosceles reclusa,* the brown recluse spider, has produced DIC. Other insect bites of any severity probably are capable of initiating this phenomenon.

The *therapy* of DIC consists of continuous infusions of heparin. In the case of abnormal function of kidneys, lungs or circulation, because of intravascular coagulation, *fibrinolytic therapy* should be initiated to prevent irreversible organ damage. Heparin probably should be immediately administered in all those intoxications which often lead to DIC even in the absence of decreases in thrombocytes or plasma factors, since intravascular coagulation is a severe complication which essentially contributes to a lethal outcome of exogenous intoxication.

## CRANIAL HYPERTENSION

Increased intracranial pressure can be produced by many exogenous chemicals, drugs and intoxications (lead, alcohol, arsenic, etc.), and it is, unfortunately, often an unrecognized manifestation, the treatment of which might be vital in the overall prognosis of the patient. Disturbances in the state of consciousness and the vital signs are often ascribed to a direct action of the poison instead of an increase in intracranial pressure.

Cranial decompression is best accomplished in these instances by the intravenous administration of an osmotically active solute that penetrates the brain more slowly than water can migrate out of it. Hypertonic solutions, sucrose, dextrose, albumin and sodium chloride have been used as dehydrating agents in the past. However, mannitol and urea are superior to these solutions and are now the compounds of choice in the treatment of increased intracranial pressure associated with poisoning. It has been demonstrated that each of these hypertonic solutions is able to reduce the cerebrospinal fluid pressure by more than 50 per cent within one to two hours.

Urea is usually given intravenously in a dose of 0.5 to 1.5 gm/kg of body weight. For details and methods of administration, *see* discussion of its use in Lead Encephalitis, page 265. Mannitol (a hexahydric alcohol which is filtered at the glomerulus) is preferred by some clinicians because urea solutions are unstable and cannot be sterilized by heat and without added sugar, as urea is hemolytic. Another apparent advantage of mannitol is its exclusively extracellular distribution in contrast to urea, which penetrates all cells including those of the brain. Tissue necrosis and venous thrombosis may follow areas of urea extravasation. Mannitol is used intravenously as a 20% solution in water in a recommended dose of 1.0 to 3.0 gm/kg. If necessary, mannitol or urea can be repeated several times during the course of treatment, but if they fail to control the intracranial pressure other measures should be tried (hypothermia, hyperventilation, craniectomy, etc.).

Adrenal corticosteroids are known to be effective in preventing or reversing cerebral edema. This effect, unfortunately, is often delayed for several hours, but once established it can be maintained with relative safety. A combined use of hypertonic solutions and steroids to produce early and continuous action would appear to be a logical method of initiating treatment, omitting the steroids once the early desired effects have been obtained.

## TREATMENT OF CONVULSIONS

(*See* Table 30)

Convulsions occur in the acute or terminal phase of poisoning from many chemical compounds and drugs. This ominous symptom, although frightening, does not necessarily indicate a serious outcome. Convulsions may be due primarily to the specific excitatory effect of the chemical compound such as strychnine, DDT and other chlorinated hydrocarbons, organic phosphate insecticides, etc., or they may occur secondary to nonspecific effects such as hypocalcemia, hypoglycemia, hypoxia, cerebral edema, water intoxication and metabolic disturbances.

The emergency aspect of the situation with the outside pressures is often responsible for the overtreatment of convulsions which in the long run may be more harmful than the convulsions *per se.* A calm and cautious attitude with the discerning use of anticonvulsant drugs along with the necessary supportive therapy can be far more effective than hurried, heroic measures which often are unnecessary and sometimes harmful. The drug of choice for chemically induced convulsions is a barbiturate with rapid onset and short duration of action. If intravenous therapy is indicated, the sodium salts of thiopental (Pentothal®), amobarbital (Amytal®) or pentobarbital (Nembutal®) are preferable to sodium phenobarbital because its delayed action may be responsible for overdosage. However, in the prevention of further convulsions, phenobarbital is the drug of choice because of its selective anticonvulsant properties. The intramuscular administration of a barbiturate is safer and should be used in preference to the intravenous route whenever possible.

Paraldehyde is often useful and a good therapeutic adjunct and has the added advantage in that it can be administered rectally. Intravenous or intramuscular Valium® is often the most effective drug of all. If convulsions do not respond to the above measures and are protracted, the induction of anesthesia with open drop ether may be necessary, preferably by an experienced anesthetist if at all possible. In severe cases it may be necessary to administer a skeletal muscle relaxant to prevent death from fatigue and respiratory depression.

## COMA

In the patient who is comatose, whether from poisoning or whatever the etiology, the management begins with a systematic plan of attack. A rapid, thorough physical examination to recognize anoxia, shock, recent trauma, hemorrhage and intoxication is important, since it would serve no purpose if the patient died while an exhaustive and scholarly inquiry was made.

In the course of examination, all possible

TABLE 30
TREATMENT OF CONVULSIONS

| *Drug* | *Method of Administration and Dosage* | *Advantages* | *Disadvantages* |
|---|---|---|---|
| Ether | Open drop. | Dosage easily determined. Good minute-to-minute control. No sterile precautions. | Difficult to give in presence of convulsions. Requires constant supervision by physician. |
| Thiopental sodium (Pentothal® sodium) | Give 2.5% sterile solution IV until convulsions are controlled. Maximum dose: 0.5 ml/kg. | Good minute-to-minute control. Can be given easily during convulsion. | Doses larger than recommended may cause persistent respiratory depression. Requires sterile equipment and administration. |
| Pentobarbital sodium (Nembutal® sodium) | Give 5 mg/kg gastric tube, rectally, or IV as sterile 2.5% solution at a rate not to exceed 1 ml/min until convulsions are controlled. | Good control of initial dose. | No control of effects after drug has been given. Requires sterile precautions. May produce severe respiratory depression. |
| Phenobarbital sodium | Give 1–2 mg/kg IM or gastric tube and repeat as necessary at a 30-minute interval up to a maximum of 5 mg/kg. | Effect lasts 12 to 24 hours. | Causes severe persistent respiratory depression in overdoses. |
| Succinylcholine chloride | Give 10 to 50 mg IV slowly and give artificial respiration during period of apnea. Repeat as necessary. | Will control convulsions of any type. Effect lasts only 1 to 5 minutes. Circulation not ordinarily affected. | Artificial respiration must be maintained during use. No antidote is available. Apnea may persist for several hours in some cases. |
| Trimethadione (Tridione®) | Give 1 gm IV slowly. Maximum dose: 5 gm. | Little depression of respiration. | Not effective in all types of convulsions. |
| Tribromoethanol (Avertin®) | Only by rectal instillation. 50–60 mg/kg causes drowsiness, amnesia. 70–80 mg/kg produces light unconsciousness and analgesia. | Ease of administration and pleasant induction without mental distress and respiratory irritation. | A nonvolatile anesthetic given by a route which prevents adequate control once it is administered. Contraindicated when renal or hepatic injury exists. |
| Amobarbital sodium (Amytal®) | Give 2% sterile solution. Dose range 0.4–0.8 gm. | Immediate action and lasts 3–6 hours. | Inhibits the cardiac action of the vagus. May produce severe respiratory depression. |
| Diphenylhydantoin sodium (Dilantin®) | Give slowly IV, 150–250 mg from steri-vial and repeat in 30 minutes with 100–150 mg if necessary. | Lack of marked hypnotic and narcotic activity. | Solution is highly alkaline and perivenous infiltration may cause sloughing. Not always effective and other anticonvulsants frequently must be used. Cardiac arrest has been reported following IV therapy. |
| Paraldehyde | Give 5 to 15 ml gastric tube, rectally, or IM. | Little depression of respiration. Effects last 12 hours. | Harmful in presence of hepatic disease. Old and loosely stoppered solutions can break down to acetic acid and produce serious intoxication. |
| Diazepam (Valium®) | Give 2–5 mg undiluted IV or IM. Repeat in 2 hours if necessary. | Good muscle relaxant for skeletal muscle spasm. | Hypotension. Respiratory depression or muscular weakness may occur if used with barbiturates. |

information should be obtained from anyone who can offer any. Most frequently in adults, the cause is alcoholic or other intoxication, trauma, a cerebrovascular accident or epilepsy. Diabetic acidosis, meningitis, heart failure and hemorrhage may also be responsible.

In infants and children, drug or chemical poisoning may be at fault.

The following report on the use of Ritalin® is interesting and merits further trial. Methylphenidate (Ritalin), a piperidine derivative, nullified or counteracted comatose effects of many drugs, including barbiturates, and terminated coma due to brain lesions, trauma and metabolic and other chemical disorders. The compound, usually given intravenously, restored consciousness in many instances within minutes. No significant undesirable effects were seen either in small or large doses; relapse was less likely in large doses, but consciousness could be restored after relapse with another injection.

Early cessation of coma by methylphenidate permitted complete neurological examination with cooperation from the patient. An accelerated return to consciousness also enabled patients to swallow saliva, liquids and medication, decreasing the danger of aspiration pneumonia and often obviating the use of urinary catheters and tracheostomies. Stuporous and noncomatose patients could be awakened several times a day for meals by intramuscular methylphenidate.

Drug coma caused by suicide attempt was treated in 332 patients by methylphenidate; none died and methylphenidate probably saved the lives of other comatose patients. The largest amount given was 5280 mg in eight hours and fifteen minutes. Depending upon the grade of coma, amounts varied from 30 to 200 mg. In the higher grades, dosage was repeated every twenty minutes until consciousness was restored (Col. Robert J. Hoagland, M.C.: Pharmacologic treatment of coma of diverse origin. *Am J Med Sci, 249*:623-635, 1965).

Table 31 provides clinical clues for the differential diagnosis of some of the more common types of coma and indicates the immediate treatment.

## RESPIRATORY INSUFFICIENCY

In the deeply narcotized patient, failure to establish and maintain an adequate airway often negates all other therapy. Pharyngeal and bronchial secretions should be removed with suctioning. Placing the patient in the prone position and extending the neck while pulling the mandible forward prevents the tongue from falling back into the pharynx and causing obstruction. Oropharyngeal airway and occasionally an intratracheal intubation may be necessary, but these should be removed as soon as the patient responds. If laryngospasm or laryngeal edema occurs and conservative measures fail, or if the threat of obstruction is expected to persist for more than two or three days, a tracheotomy should be done.

Prophylactic use of antibiotics and frequent postural changes are important in the prevention of hypostatic pneumonia in those with prolonged coma. Artificial respiration as well as oxygen therapy is necessary when respiratory movements lag and become inadequate. Oxygen should be administered also under any circumstances of tissue hypoxia, such as shock, whenever severe central respiratory depression occurs, in the presence of methemoglobinemia and in the cyanosis from many specific poisons. Oxygen also has a direct action in the disassociation of carboxyhemoglobin in carbon monoxide intoxication. In poisonings associated with severe central respiratory depression, oxygen therapy should be accompanied by artificial respiration to lower the blood $CO_2$ level and allow reestablishment of normal regulation of respiration.

Pulmonary edema is often the direct result of the inhalation of irritants or may follow the increased bronchial secretions caused by

TABLE 31
COMA

| | *Clinical Findings* | *Probable Etiology* | *Therapeutic Considerations* |
|---|---|---|---|
| *Coma without specific neurologic signs or meningeal irritation* | Alcohol odor to breath; hypothermia; hypotension; flushed skin; delirium; tachycardia. | Alcoholic intoxication | Supportive measures; airway; oxygen; parenteral fluids; glucose and insulin; vitamins; analeptics; prophylactic antibiotics. |
| | Slow, shallow respiration; hypothermia; hypotension; abnormal reflexes; cyanosis (occasionally). | Barbiturate intoxication | Maintain airway; oxygen as indicated; maintain fluid and electrolyte balance; prophylactic antibiotics; if severe, hemodialysis may be lifesaving. |
| | Hypotension; miosis; slow respiration; bradycardia. | Opiate poisoning | Maintain airway and fluid and electrolyte balance; naloxone hydrochloride is a specific antidote. |
| | Cherry-red skin; rapid respiration; hypotension. | Carbon monoxide poisoning | Oxygen; maintain airway; prophylactic antibiotics; general supportive measures. |
| | Dehydration; fruity odor to breath; "air hunger"; soft eyeballs; weak, rapid pulse. | Diabetic acidosis | Insulin; restoration of fluid and electrolyte balance with glucose, saline, lactate, potassium. Differentiation from insulin overdosage with hypoglycemic shock is essential. |
| | Uremic odor to breath; vascular retinopathy; history of renal disease; brownish-yellow skin; hypertension; vascular retinopathy. | Kidney failure with uremia | Rule out bilateral ureteral obstruction; careful restoration of fluid and electrolyte balance; small transfusions of sedimented red cells; calcium gluconate; prophylactic antibiotics; in acute, reversible renal failure, hemodialysis may be lifesaving. |
| | Cholemic breath; jaundice; spider angiomas; ascites; "flapping tremor"; hepatomegaly. | Hepatic decompensation | Treatment is supportive and includes glucose infusions; multivitamins; whole blood as needed; antibiotics, adrenal steroids and monosodium glutamate are also used. |
| | Cold, clammy skin; weak, rapid pulse; hypotension. | Hemorrhage | Blood replacement; plasma expanders (natural or synthetic). |
| *Coma with meningeal irritation* | Stiff neck; Kernig and Brudzinski signs; fever. | Meningitis | Specific antibiotic therapy for organism involved; general supportive measures. |
| | Stertorous breathing; stiff neck; Kernig and Brudzinski signs; hypertension; bloody spinal fluid. | Subarachnoid hemorrhage | Surgical treatment; general supportive measures. |
| *Coma with localizing neurologic signs* | History of trauma; headache; lethargy; unequal pupils. | Subdural hemorrhage | General supportive measures; surgery (if indicated); antibiotics. |
| | History of trauma; skull fracture; loss of consciousness; lucid interval followed by coma. | Epidural hemorrhage | Supportive measures; surgery. |
| | Stertorous breathing; hypertension; evidence of arteriosclerosis. | Cerebral thrombosis or hemorrhage | Supportive measures and meticulous nursing care. |

TABLE 32
CONDITIONS CAUSING COMA

A. Intracranial lesions
  1. Vascular: thrombosis, subarachnoid hemorrhage, intracerebral hemorrhage, subdural hemorrhage, epidural hematoma, embolus, venous thrombosis
  2. Cerebral contusion, concussion, laceration from trauma
  3. Tumor: primary or metastatic
  4. Infection: meningitis, encephalitis, brain abscess
  5. Encephalopathy from systemic disease (hypertension, eclampsia)
  6. Fat emboli
  7. Postictal state of epilepsy
  8. Postoperative brain edema

B. Infections
  1. Septicemia
  2. Systemic infections; cholera, malaria, pancreatitis

C. Cardiac
  1. Arrhythmias—heart block, Stokes-Adams attacks
  2. Myocardial infarction
  3. Cardiac tamponade

D. Respiratory
  1. Blocked airway
  2. Pulmonary embolus
  3. Infection
  4. $CO_2$ narcosis in severe emphysema

E. Endocrine
  1. Myxedema coma
  2. Addisonian crisis
  3. Diabetic coma
  4. Hypoglycemic coma
  5. Hyperglycemic nonketotic coma

F. Renal failure—uremia

G. Hepatic coma and acute fatty metamorphosis of liver in pregnancy

H. Syncope
  1. Vasovagal
  2. Carotid sinus irritability
  3. Cough syncope

I. Drug or toxic ingestion: barbiturates, tranquilizers, antidepressives, carbon monoxide inhalation, and many others

J. Hyperthermia or hypothermia

K. Electric shock

L. Hypersensitivity reaction—anaphylaxis

M. Shock from any cause: infection, intra-abdominal catastrophic hemorrhage

N. Pregnancy, uterine or tubal rupture, acute fatty metamorphosis of liver, toxemia

O. Hysteria and psychosis

P. Poisoning, accidental and deliberate

parasympathetic stimulants or cholinesterase inhibitors (organic phosphate compounds). In addition to the usual methods of therapy such as postural drainage, digitalization, aminophylline, etc., oxygen can be bubbled through a 20% solution of ethyl alcohol by adequate intermittent positive pressure. Evidence shows that oxygen saturated with ethyl alcohol vapor helps to collapse the foam in the bronchi and alveoli and permits better oxygen exchange.

## TOXIC HEPATITIS (DRUG-INDUCED AND CHEMICAL)*

Drug-induced hepatitis more frequently damages the liver by inducing hypersensitivity reactions and less often by acting as protoplasmic poisons. Drug-induced hepatitis differs from toxic hepatitis in that very few persons who take the drug are susceptible to hepatic damage, whereas in toxic hepatitis, all who take it are similarly affected. Other differences between drug-induced hepatitis and toxic hepatitis are (1) there is no correlation between its occurrence or severity with the amount of drug consumed; (2) there

*Material used here with permission from Coletta, D.F. and Spiegel, P.D.: Toxic and drug-induced hepatitis. *Med Sci*, December, 1966.

is no definite latent period between taking it and the occurrence of lesions; (3) the histologic pattern varies; and (4) systemic symptoms of fever, arthralgia, eosinophilia, etc. usually accompany drug-induced hepatitis.

The changes in the liver may be those of hepatocellular damage, cholestasis or both. The hepatocellular damage may be due to a hepatotoxic effect or to sensitization by the drug. Methyltestosterone and other derivatives of testosterone produce hepatic injury in man but fail to do so in experimental animals. They do, however, disturb hepatic function when given in large doses, but fail to evoke the hypersensitivity seen in other forms of drug-induced hepatitis. The fact that drug-induced hepatitis fails to produce similar lesions in animals creates problems in drug research and clinical trials. Some drugs produce characteristic liver damage in all persons given sufficiently large doses. Chloroform is an example of such a drug. Chloroform, however, is a hepatotoxin, not a sensitizing drug. There is much speculation about whether drug-induced hepatitis is the result of acquired hypersensitivity. Many drugs require conjugation with protein before they become antigenic. It is interesting to speculate whether hepatic drug reactions occur owing to conjugation in the liver and resulting hepatic sensitization.

Iproniazid produces lesions indistinguishable from those of viral hepatitis. Chloroform, on the other hand, produces a very characteristic zonal hepatic necrosis. Sulfonamides produce hepatocellular necrosis but in scattered foci with an intense inflammatory reaction in the portal areas. Phenylcinchoninic acid produces lesions similar to viral hepatitis; these occasionally involve a large area of liver parenchyma, producing massive liver necrosis. Most patients with extensive damage die. However, if healing occurs, postnecrotic cirrhosis often develops.

Some drugs produce a cholestatic lesion without hepatocellular damage. These lesions usually cause bile stasis, which is especially marked in the pericentral bile canaliculi; it is often accompanied by infiltration of the portal spaces with lymphocytes and polymorphonuclear and eosinophilic leukocytes. When these features are present without hepatocellular damage, the term "drug-induced cholestatic hepatitis" is used. However, in most cases, there is evidence of both cholestatic and hepatocellular hepatitis. Recovery is usually prompt and complete; however, some patients develop a slowly progressive periportal fibrosis which results in biliary cirrhosis. Chlorpromazine and substituted derivatives of testosterone produce a cholestatic hepatitis, but the latter drug causes no significant hepatocellular damage or inflammatory reaction. Often the onset of drug-induced hepatitis is manifested by signs of systemic hypersensitivity which are followed in a few days by jaundice and a tender liver. Sometimes liver damage occurs without jaundice. This is evidenced by BSP retention, elevated serum alkaline phosphatase, and if there is associated acute hepatocellular damage, a rise in the serum transaminase. In the hepatocellular type of drug-induced hepatitis, the laboratory findings are similar to those seen in acute viral hepatitis, i.e. bilirubinuria, hyperbilirubinemia, slight albuminuria, BSP retention and increased activity of serum enzymes. The thymol turbidity and cephalin flocculation determinations are usually elevated but may remain normal. A helpful differential diagnostic test is the high level of serum alkaline phosphatase commonly seen in drug-induced hepatitis. In cholestatic hepatitis, the laboratory findings are similar to those of extrahepatic biliary obstruction. There is an increase in serum conjugated bilirubin and bile in the urine; marked rises in serum alkaline phosphatase activity and cholesterol concentrations occur. If the laboratory studies early in the disease reveal increased serum transaminase activity before the above features, cholestatic hepatitis is likely. In addition, early eosinophilia and/or a marked increase in serum cholesterol level and in serum alkaline phosphatase activity favor the diagnosis of cholestatic hepatitis rather than of extrahepatic biliary obstructions. Some of the commonly used drugs shown to be hepatotoxins are carbutamide, 6-mercaptopurine, phenacemide, DDT, chloramphenicol, chlorambucil, diphenylhydantoin, aminosalicylic acid, PAS, tetracycline and urethane. Drugs that cause essentially an intrahepatic cholestasis are chlorpromazine, mepazine, prochlorperazine, trifluoperazine, chlordiazepoxide, chlorpropamide, Diuril®, Nostyn®, promazine, sulfonamides and erythromycin.

Many chemical substances produce toxic hepatitis regularly and the damage is often related to the dose. Acetaminophen hepatotoxicity, for example, occurs only with massive overdosage or when large amounts are taken for suicidal intent. The lesions produced are less variable than with drug-induced hepatitis and there is usually no evidence of systemic hypersensitivity reaction. Chloroform, carbon tetrachloride and phosphorus are only a few of this group. They are protoplasmic poisons that probably interfere with enzyme systems. They may impede blood flow and cause ischemic necrosis. The vascular impediment may be due to the swelling of hepatic cells or to vasoconstriction. These substances also may disturb lipid metabolism in both intrahepatic and extrahepatic fat depots. The nutritional state of the liver, preexisting liver disease and alcoholism modify the effect of the hepatotoxins. Carbon tetrachloride alters the permeability of the mitochondria, causing the loss of cellular DNA. Phosphorus has a similar effect. The cytoplasmic reticulum may be altered also. Some investigators have shown that blocking sympathetic stimuli prevents the ischemic hepatic necrosis and mitochondrial change that follow carbon tetrachloride poisoning. In addition to the zonal ischemic change produced by these toxic agents, a fatty alteration occurs and is often a striking feature. This change may be due to fatty acids driven in from the depots during sympathetic stimulation or it may be due to decreased fatty acid oxidation in the liver caused by a decrease in DPN. As stated earlier, nutritional factors play an important role in the resistance or susceptibility of the liver to hepatotoxic agents. For example, a high-fat diet enhances toxicity, whereas carbohydrate appears to protect the liver against the agents. Choline, methionine, cystine and tocopherol are substances believed to be involved in the mechanism of hepatotoxins. The exact mechanism by which these modify the action of hepatotoxins is not known, nor is it established how much protective action these substances have.

The lesions produced by hepatotoxic agents in general reveal a zonal pattern of degeneration, extensive necrosis or total necrosis with little inflammatory reaction. Fatty alteration is often a prominent feature. The zonal pattern in the carbon tetrachloride and chloroform poisoning is centrilobular, whereas in phosphorus intoxication a peripheral zonal pattern is found. In some cases, as with naphthalene poisoning, there is a diffuse massive necrosis. In many cases, the liver can be exposed to a low dose of toxin and heal without much scarring. However, repeated exposures may result in extensive irregular fibrosis. The liver function studies vary depending on the acuteness and extent of the hepatocellular damage. The results of studies are similar to those in acute viral hepatitis. The serum transaminase activity is useful in detecting acute hepatocellular damage when exposure to hepatotoxins is known or suspected. There are many other but less common causes of toxic hepatitis in which diagnostic studies assume a less significant role.

Massive doses of iron salts frequently cause a centrilobular necrosis. The primary toxic effect is on the gastrointestinal tract, resulting in severe diarrhea, gastrointestinal hemorrhage and shock. The hepatic damage may result from shock rather than from the direct toxic effect of the iron salts. Chronic iron intake is probably toxic to the liver (hemochromatosis). The effect of ethyl alcohol is still controversial. In animal experimentation, it has been shown that alcohol ingestion raises the choline requirement, increases fatty acid synthesis and mobilizes fat from the fat depots. This metabolic derangement probably potentiates the development of nutritional cirrhosis. In humans, it plays a role in the pathogenesis of Laennec's cirrhosis. Acute alcoholic poisoning, especially with strong alcoholic beverages, may result in sudden death due to brain damage rather than to hepatic toxicity. A variety of hepatic lesions has been observed in individuals with extensive burns. Experimental studies in dogs with extensive burns showed marked congestion and atrophy of hepatic parenchyma. It was noted that if tannic acid was applied to the burned area, a central hepatic necrosis ensued. A subsequent study revealed that similar changes occurred when tannic acid was injected subcutaneously in normal animals. These latter studies certainly tend to implicate tannic acid as a hepatotoxic agent, and several fatalities in humans have been reported from the use of tannic acid in barium enema mixtures. Sometimes the hepatic damage is severe, resulting in a midzonal necrosis with large eosinophilic, cytoplasmic bodies in hepatic cells, similar to that which occurs in yellow fever. It is important in extensive burn injuries not to ignore hepatic complications, since a knowledge of liver function may help in managing these patients. Moderate elevations of SGOT and SGPT levels are not uncommon. Minor elevations in thymol turbidity and cephalin flocculation studies occur in the first few days following extensive burns. The hepatic damage as associated with tannic acid application in burns is similar to those with infection secondary to extensive burns. However, little is known about the morphologic variations associated with secondary infection.

The morphologic changes in the liver secondary to radiation are not well known. However, in a few cases studied following intensive radiation, there was a marked necrosis of the bile duct epithelium, while the parenchymal cells were spared. In animals, much more is known. There is apparently considerable vascular damage manifested by edema, hyperemia and leukocytic infiltration. There is extensive necrosis of hepatic cells, with only moderate degenerative changes in the biliary epithelium. There is no explanation why these latter changes differ from those in man. It has been suggested that histamine-like substances may be released following radiation and may be the agents responsible for the necrosis. This idea was put forth because of the changes occurring following histamine injections in animals. It is interesting to note that in humans exposed to excessive atomic radiation and surviving less than six weeks, the principal findings were central congestion with atrophy of the hepatic cords and edema of the central veins. In those who survived longer, the liver showed marked fatty alteration. It is of practical interest to note that some radioactive therapeutic and diagnostic materials may injure the liver. Radioactive colloidal gold and thorium dioxide (Thorotrast®) were commonly used as therapeutic and diagnostic agents. Colloidal gold produces a midzonal necrosis in rats with considerable architectural distortion and bizarre giant cells with no fibrosis. There have been no reports of these changes occurring in man. Thorium dioxide, on the other hand, is generally believed to be hepatotoxic and carcinogenic in man. Thorium dioxide used for hepatosplenography was given in large doses. It has been estimated that about 25 per cent of the patients developed hepatic fibrosis. This dose in animals produces a focal necrosis with fibrosis. Tumors have been produced in animals with thorium dioxide, which apparently does not leave the body but remains in the phagocytic system, particularly in the Kupffer's and reticular cells of the spleen. The resulting fibrosis is due probably to the radioactivity of these phagocytic cells.

Unusual hepatic lesions are occasionally associated with pregnancy; the most frequent are those seen with toxemia and viral hepatitis. An often fatal and rapidly developing hepatic lesion may occur during the eighth or ninth month of pregnancy. This lesion has been termed "obstetric yellow atrophy," "acute fatty metamorphosis of the liver," "acute yellow atrophy," etc. Drugs or exogenous chemical factors have not been implicated.

TABLE 33
DRUG-INDUCED HEPATOTOXICITY

| | *Drug* | *Type of Reaction** | *Comments* |
|---|---|---|---|
| Anesthetic agents | Ethrane® (enflurane) | U | Hepatocellular damage reported |
| | Fluothane® (halothane) | T | Occurs in 1 in 10,000 to 1 in 20,000 patients; increased risk with multiple exposures |
| | Penthrane® (methoxyflurane) | T | Similar to halothane hepatitis reaction |
| Anti-inflammatory and antigout agents | Benemid® (probenecid) | S | Rare occurrence |
| | Butazolidin®, Azolid® (phenylbutazone) | S | Associated with repeated or long-term therapy |
| | Indocin® (indomethacin) | S | Rare occurrence of toxic hepatitis |
| | Tandearil®, Oxalid® (oxyphenbutazone) | S | Similar to phenylbutazone hepatotoxicity |
| | Zyloprim® (allopurinol) | S | May be precipitated or exacerbated by poor renal function |
| Anti-infective agents | Aminosalicylic acid (PAS) | S | Occurs in 0.5 to 3% of patients |
| | Amphotericin B | U | Acute hepatic failure with jaundice and hepatocellular dysfunction reported |
| | Atabrine® (quinacrine) | U | Rare occurrence of hepatitis |
| | Avlosulfon® (dapsone) | U | May be similar to sulfonamide reaction |
| | Cephalosporins | S | Jaundice reported with cephalexin, may occur in association with acute cephalosporin allergy |
| | Chloromycetin® (chloramphenicol) | T | Rare complication of bone marrow depression |
| | Flagyl® (metronidazole) | T, S | Jaundice and liver dysfunction reported and amebic liver abscess following metronidazole treatment of amebic colitis |
| | Griseofulvin | U | Rare occurrence |
| | Ilosone® (erythromycin estolate) | T, S | No other forms of erythromycin implicated |
| | Isoniazid (INH) | T, S | Rare occurrence, hepatitis with necrosis |
| | Macrodantin®, Furadantin®, etc (nitrofurantoin) | S, T | Obstructive jaundice has been reported |
| | Mintezol® (thiabendazole) | U | Liver function values commonly elevated; rare hepatonecrosis |

TABLE 33—*Continued*
DRUG-INDUCED HEPATOTOXICITY

| | *Drug* | *Type of Reaction* | *Comments* |
|---|---|---|---|
| Anti-infective agents | Penicillins | S | Rare; associated with acute allergic reaction; reported with penicillin G, ampicillin, oxacillin, carbenicillin |
| | Pyrazinamide (PZA) | T | Dose related; occurs in 5 to 10% of patients |
| | Rifadin®, Rimactane® (rifampin) | U | Occurs primarily when used with INH |
| | Sulfonamides | U | Occurs in 0.5% of patients receiving sulfanilamide; lower incidence with newer sulfonamides |
| | Tao® (troleandomycin) | T, S | Toxicity usually precludes use of drug |
| | Tetracyclines | U | Reported with several tetracyclines; rare reversible toxicity with oral drug; fatty infiltration with IV drug; dose-related fatalities have occurred |
| Anticonvulsant agents | Dilantin® (phenytoin, diphenylhydantoin) | S | Rare occurrence; deaths have resulted |
| | Phenobarbital | U | Rare occurrence |
| | Tegretol® (carbamazepine) | U | Rare occurrence |
| | Tridione® (trimethadione) | U | Rare occurrence of hepatitis |
| Antineoplastic agents and immunosuppressants | L-asparaginase | U | Fatty infiltration |
| | Chlorambucil (Leukeran®) | T,S | Jaundice and allergic hepatitis reported |
| | Imuran® (azathioprine) | T | May be due to reduced resistance to hepatitis virus |
| | Methotrexate | T | Dose related and reversible |
| | Mithracin® (mithramycin) | U | Elevated liver function values reported |
| | Purinethol® (mercaptopurine, 6-MP) | T | Occurs primarily with doses greater than 2.5 mg/kg/day |
| Endocrine agents | Androgens C-17-alpha-alkyl substituted steroids | T | Cholestatic jaundice reported; not seen with other testosterone derivatives |
| | Corticosteroids | U | Fatty infiltration reported; rare occurrence |
| | Estrogens | U | Hepatic porphyrias reported |
| | Oral contraceptives | U | Liver dysfunction and jaundice reported; occasional hepatocellular necrosis has occurred |
| | Propylthiouracil (PTU) | S | Rare occurrence of cholestatic hepatitis or hepatocellular jaundice |

TABLE 33—*Continued*
DRUG-INDUCED HEPATOTOXICITY

| | *Drug* | *Type of Reaction* | *Comment* |
|---|---|---|---|
| Endocrine agents | Tapazole® (methimazole) | S | Similar to PTU hepatotoxicity |
| | Sulfonylurea antidiabetic agents | U | Jaundice and cholestasis reported |
| Psychotherapeutic agents | Benzodiazepines | U | Rare occurrence of jaundice and hepatic dysfunction |
| | Monoamine oxidase inhibitor antidepressants | U | Occasional hepatitis; may range from mild to fatal |
| | Phenothiazines | S | Cholestatic jaundice reported with 2 to 3% of patients taking high-dose chlorpromazine; other phenothiazines also implicated |
| | Tricyclic antidepressants | S | Uncommon; transient jaundice; one fatality reported |
| Miscellaneous agents | Acetaminophen | T | Fatal hepatic necrosis in massive overdose |
| | Aldomet® (methyldopa) | S | Jaundice and hepatocellular damage reported |
| | Antabuse® (disulfiram) | S | Rare occurrence of acute hepatitis |
| | Aspirin | S | Associated with acute aspirin allergy |
| | Darvon®, Dolene® (propoxyphene) | S | Rare occurrence of jaundice |
| | Desferal® (deferoxamine) | T | Prolonged use may cause parenchymal damage |
| | Diamox® (acetazolamide) | U | Cholestasis with fatty infiltration reported |
| | Edecrin® (ethacrynic acid) | U | Jaundice and focal necrosis reported |
| | Hedulin®, Danilone® (phenindione) | S | Hepatocellular damage and cholestasis reported with hypersensitivity reaction |
| | Papaverine | S | Reversible toxicity; jaundice not reported |
| | Pronestyl® (procainamide) | S | One report of hepatocellular necrosis |
| | Quinidine | S | Rare occurrence of cholestasis and hepatocellular damage |
| *Key: | Tannic acid | T | Rare reports of hepatic necrosis with topical use |
| S = probably sensitization reaction, T = probably direct toxic reaction, and U = unknown mechanism. | Tham® (tromethamine) | T | Hemorrhagic necrosis reported in newborns |

From Arthur G. Lipman, reprinted from *Modern Medicine* © 1976 by Harcourt Brace Jovanovich.

TABLE 34
NEPHROTOXIC CHEMICAL COMPOUNDS

| *Metals* | *Organic Solvents* | *Glycols* |
|---|---|---|
| Mercury (organic and inorganic) | Carbon tetrachloride | Ethylene glycol |
| Bismuth | Tetrachloroethylene | Ethylene glycol dinitrite |
| Cadmium | Methanol | Ethylene dichloride |
| Lead | Cellosolve | Diethylene glycol |
| Arsine and arsenic | Miscellaneous solvents | *Diagnostic Agents* |
| Uranium | *Osmotic Agents* | Contrast agents in high concentration (pyelography and aortography); particularly vulnerable are dehydrated infants, and those with cardiac, hepatic, or renal disease. |
| Gold | Sucrose | Bunamiodyl |
| Iron | Mannitol | |
| Silver | *Physical Agents* | |
| Antimony | Radiation | |
| Copper | Heat stroke | |
| Thallium | Electroshock | |
| Beryllium | | |
| *Insecticides* | | *Miscellaneous Chemicals* |
| Chlorinated hydrocarbons | | Carbon monoxide |
| Biphenyl | | Snake venom |
| | | Ether |
| | | Poisoned mushrooms |
| *Abnormal Concentration of Physiologic Substances* | | Spider venom |
| | | Bee venom |
| Hypercalcemia (calcium) | | Creosol |
| Hyperuricemia (uric acid) | | Sodium perchlorate |
| Hypokalemia (potassium) | | Hemolysins |
| etc. | | Nephroallergens |
| | | Aniline and other methemoglobins |

## RENAL FAILURE

Oliguria and anuria may occur in the course of poisoning with a variety of compounds including carbon tetrachloride, mercury and other heavy metals, arsenicals, phosphorus, bromates and hemolytic agents such as naphthalene, benzene, etc. These substances either produce focal degenerative lesions in the tubule cells or block the tubules with hemoglobin or crystalline precipitates. In most instances renal failure is reversible, and if cellular damage has not been extensive and if the patient is able to survive the acute phase, renal function can return to normal within two weeks. Therefore, the aim of therapy is to prolong the patient's life until function returns.

## ANTIBIOTICS AND GENERAL THERAPEUTIC AGENTS

Penicillin, streptomycin, chlortetracycline, oxytetracycline and more recent antibiotics are often of considerable value in such inflammatory conditions as pneumonitis, mediastinitis, peritonitis, etc. that often follow the ingestion of certain toxic substances such as petroleum distillates, turpentine, cedar oil, lye, acids and other corrosives.

The selection of a specific antibiotic should be determined on an individual basis depending on the severity and nature of the inflammatory condition and the age of the patient. Some physicians advise giving these antibiotics even prior to the onset of signs and symptoms of infection when one is certain that substantial amounts of the particularly dangerous substances have been swallowed or aspirated in the hope of forestalling infection. Others feel that skilled and discriminating use of antibiotics excludes their "prophylactic" use except in already infected individuals, if aspiration occurs or if an indwelling catheter is necessary.

*Demulcents*

1. Olive oil 200 ml (6⅔ oz.)
2. White of egg 60 to 100 ml (2 to 3 oz.)
3. Any vegetable oil 200 ml (6⅔ oz.)
4. Milk
5. Starch water
6. Liquid petrolatum (mineral oil)
7. Butter

*To Neutralize Acids*

1. Magnesia magma (milk of magnesia) 100 to 300 ml (3 to 10 oz.)
2. Sodium bicarbonate (dilute solution)
3. Calcium hydroxide solution (limewater) 200 ml (6⅔ oz.)
4. Aluminum hydroxide gel 60 ml (2 oz.)
5. Precipitated calcium carbonate (chalk) 100 gm (3⅓ oz.)
6. Wall plaster crushed in water
7. Soap solution

*To Neutralize Alkalis*

1. Vinegar (dilute acetic acid) 100 to 200 ml (3 to 6⅔ oz.), preferably diluted with four parts of water.
2. Lemon juice 100 to 200 ml (3 to 6⅔ oz.)
3. Orange juice 100 to 300 ml (3 to 10 oz.)
4. Dilute (0.5%) hydrochloric acid 100 to 200 ml (3 to 6⅔ oz.)
5. Strong acidic antidotes are contraindicated because of the release of heat. Actually, milk, water or tea may be better than the use of any concentrated acidic substance.

*Emetics* *(Also see pages 42-45)*

1. Apomorphine hydrochloride. Adults, 6 mg (1/10 gr); children, reduce dose in proportion to age; infants, 0.03 mg/lb. Inject SC or IM.
2. Ipecac powder, 4 gm (1 tsp.); or syrup, 15 ml (½ oz.) in water. The fluidextract of ipecacuanha, which has been removed from the pharmacopeia, differs considerably from the syrup and is fourteen times more potent. They both contain the alkaloids of emetine, cephaëline and psychotrine, among others. The toxic action of emetine is well known, and severe stenosing esophagitis and several deaths have been reported from the misuse of the fluidextract. In any case, this extract, if still available, should never replace the syrup for emetic purposes.
3. Copper and zinc sulfate (not recommended).

*Sedatives*

1. Phenobarbital (PO) 0.03 to 0.1 gm (½ to 1½ gr).
2. Phenobarbital (IM) 100 to 200 mg for adults, and 1.5 to 3 mg/lb. body weight for children.
3. Sodium amytal (PO) 0.2 gm (3 gr).
4. Sodium amytal (IV) 300 to 600 mg for adults, and 1.5 to 3 mg/lb. body weight for children.
5. Pentobarbital sodium 30, 50 and 100 mg capsules; 30, 60, 120 and 200 mg suppositories. 50 mg/ml ampules. Dose same as for phenobarbital.
6. Barbital sodium 0.3 to 0.6 gm (5 to 10 gr) orally or subcutaneously.
7. Chloral hydrate 0.5 to 1 gm (7½ to 15 gr) orally.
8. Sodium bromide 0.3 to 1 gm (5 to 15 gr) orally.
9. Paraldehyde oral or rectal 0.1 ml/lb. body weight for children and 5 to 30 ml total for adults.

## TOXICOLOGY (SELECTION OF SPECIMENS IN POISONING CASES)

Of all violent deaths, those produced by poison are the most difficult to discover, to prove scientifically and to adjudicate. The cause of death in poisoning or suspected poisoning requires the cooperative efforts of the attending physician, the pathologist and the toxicologist. In many cases of death caused by a toxic agent, the determination of the causative agent is made more difficult because of a lack of complete information or because insufficient and improper samples are submitted for chemical and pathological examination.

When poisoning is suspected, a complete case history should be made available, when possible, since such information frequently can identify specific poisonous substances. In acute poisonings, the attending physician should save all gastric lavage washings and vomitus for analysis. If the patient is hospitalized, admission blood samples, twenty-four-hour urine samples and fecal excretions should likewise be preserved for chemical testing.

The pathologist participating in the investigation of a known or alleged poisoning fatality has a multifaceted responsibility. He must search for and recognize anatomic changes produced by the toxic substance, while recalling that many poisons produce no organic injury even when they are present in lethal concentration.

When death occurs the autopsy should be complete. Too many believe that an examination of the gastrointestinal tract alone is sufficient to prove poisoning. This is wrong, since the autopsy often is the only means of disclosing poison. The portion of the poison remaining in the stomach may not have affected the individual and therefore would not have been responsible for the death. Only poison which has been absorbed can be considered as being responsible for the fatality. Often in chronic poisonings, as well as in some acute cases, no indication may be found in the gastrointestinal tract. The gastrointestinal contents are valuable for chemical analysis chiefly in acute poisonings, for in such cases, a large percentage of the poison may remain unabsorbed and would be easier to detect and identify because of its high concentration in the stomach contents. However, even in some acute cases, the unabsorbed portion of the poison may be lost by vomiting and none found in the stomach contents.

Poisons may be inhaled or injected and thus may not be found in the gastrointestinal tract. It is also possible for a poisonous agent to be introduced into the stomach after death in an effort to make a homicide appear to be a suicide. In such cases, the poison would be found in the stomach contents but obviously would not have had any effect in causing the death of the individual. In all cases of poisoning, proof of absorption of the poison either by chemical identification in the organs or by evidence of pathological changes associated with the toxic substance must be obtained.

### Isolation and Separation Techniques for Identification of Poisons

1. Acetone extraction of organic substances
2. Separation of alkaloids from tissue
   a. Cation-exchange columns
   b. Acetonitrile extraction
3. Two-stage extraction
   a. Acid spot extraction—paper chromatography
   b. Protein-free filtrates—high-temperature chromatography
4. Gas chromatography

The analytical problems that confront the toxicologist in the identification of poisons are, first, that the quantity of sample is usually limited; second, the presence or absence of a large number of chemical compounds must be determined; and finally, these chemical agents are often in very low concentrations when present. With the present techniques, much time with costly equipment is often required for the analysis of even a limited number of chemical substances, which often must be selective, based on the judgment and experience of the individual toxicologist. Valuable applications of gas and paper chromatography have been found which are becoming an important tool of diagnosis because of their speed and versatility in detecting and evaluating a vast array of compounds. Of the newer techniques, gas chromatography in particular has the potential of analyzing rapidly a wide variety of chemical agents including gases, liquids and solids in complex mixtures and in extremely low concentrations. Moreover, the technique and operation of this equipment are relatively simple and inexpensive. In practice, the compound to be chromatographed is extracted with an organic solvent from blood or urine;* the solvent is then evaporated to a small volume to concentrate the material. An initial extraction of the blood or urine in the usual physiological pH range of 7.0 to 8.0 is sufficient to isolate many of the compounds of toxicological interest. Even such drugs as morphine, which tend to be quickly conjugated in the body, can be analyzed, provided an acid hydrolysis is used prior to extraction whenever a conjugated substance is suspected. A decided advantage of gas chromatography, aside from its simplicity, speed and specificity, lies in its ability to separate and detect drug metabolites simultaneously with the parent compound when they occur in the same specimen and can be extracted together. Heretofore, most procedures did not distinguish between unchanged drug and inactive metabolites. Consequently, the correlation between drug level and severity of symptoms or intoxication has not always been consistent.

*A method for detection in urine of narcotic drugs, quinine, barbiturates, amphetamines and some tranquilizers appears to be applicable to a wide range of diagnostic problems and epidemiological studies. The drugs are first absorbed on ion-exchange paper and then eluted with a series of buffer-solvent systems. An aliquot of the solvent phase is concentrated and chromatographed. A series of detection sprays have been developed to provide both sensitive detection and confirmation of positive results.

## "General Unknown" Toxicologic Tests

### *Gases*

The general pathologic picture is that of anoxia. Circumstances of death and condition of the body are important. Carbon monoxide produces typical cherry-red carboxyhemoglobin coloring of the skin. Hydrogen sulfide can be detected readily by the odor emanating from the lungs and the sulfhemoglobin present. The blood and viscera may have a greenish discoloration. In death from natural gas, only anoxia is found, but circumstances of death are frequently conclusive.

### *Metals*

In general, the heavy metals produce microscopic changes in the kidney. Most frequently encountered are bichloride of mercury and arsenic trioxide. Spectrographic identification of metals is conclusive and requires only one gram of tissue.

### *Inorganic Nonmetals*

All have a corrosive action, with principal effects seen in the stomach. This group is divided into acids (sulfuric acid), bases (ammonia and washing soda), oxidants (chlorates, potassium permanganate) and reducers (sulfites).

### *Volatiles*

In general, there are no suggestive pathologic changes. Distilled with steam, volatiles are readily identified. Action of this group of poisons varies widely. For instance, ethyl and methyl alcohol and chloral hydrate act as central nervous system depressants and produce death from anoxia. Cyanide is a respiratory enzyme poison; death occurs as a result of cardiac standstill, and the blood at autopsy is liquid. Cyanmethemoglobin has been held responsible for the bright red ecchymotic spots. Chloroform produces liver damage; so does carbon tetrachloride, which also causes lower nephron nephrosis with renal shutdown.

### *Solvents*

A few of the common solvents, such as ethanol and acetone, are water-soluble and readily identifiable in urine and in blood. Other solvents, such as trichloroethylene and benzene, have metabolites which can be detected in urine. However, many organic solvents are relatively water-insoluble. If they are present in the urine or blood, they occur in trace amounts beneath the sensitivity of detection of most conventional laboratory methods. Since no swift or universal method for the identification of unknown solvents in urine or blood has been devised, analysis of either can be very time-consuming and, therefore, unsatisfactory for most diagnostic problems.

The diagnosis of solvent poisoning or exposure can now be rapidly established by breath analysis. The analytical methods employed specifically identify the solvent and are sufficiently sensitive to permit detection hours to weeks after exposure, depending upon the amount of solvent absorbed, its rate of metabolism and its rate of excretion. Serial breath analyses after a solvent exposure allow the construction of an excretion curve which can then be compared to the excretion curves of humans previously exposed to known amounts of a given solvent. In this manner, the total body burden or total amount absorbed may be estimated. Based upon the identity of the toxic agent and the amount present within the body, a reasonable prognosis can be advanced and appropriate therapy begun. The breath samples are collected in Saran™ gas bags or glass pipettes and analyzed directly for their solvent content in a long-path-length gas cell of an infrared spectrometer or in a vapor phase chromatograph.

### *Nonvolatile Organics (including barbiturates and alkaloids)*

In the course of isolation and purification from tissue, unknown nonvolatile organic substances appear from one of five groups which are distinguished by the acidity or basicity of the organic structure. The unknown is run through a series of different reactions, each becoming more and more specific, thus eliminating "possibles" while indicating a particular type of chemical structure. Tests are started with nonspecific, sensitive reactions; then sensitive specific tests are used, the ultraviolet and infrared absorption properties are classified and finally the physical properties of the derivatives of the unknown are determined. These tests may be defined as probation, exclusion, indication, designation, differentiation and confirmation reactions.

## Toxicologic Analysis

The following listing may be used in selecting materials for toxicological examinations.

1. Brain (at least one-half) to be used for analysis for alcohol, chloroform, ether and other volatile substances; alkaloids, barbituric acid derivatives, etc.
2. Liver (at least one-half) to be used for analysis for metals (especially arsenic), barbituric acid derivatives, alkaloids, fluorides, etc.
3. Kidneys (at least one) to be used for analysis for metals.
4. Blood (at least 1 oz.) to be used for analysis for gases such as carbon monoxide. The container should be filled completely and tightly sealed. Blood may also be used for the detection and estimation of barbiturates, as well as for drowning tests. In the latter cases, separate samples should be obtained from the left and right heart chambers and placed in properly labeled dry containers. The blood should be collected with dry pipettes or syringes.

TABLE 35
INFRARED ANALYSIS OF GASES AND VAPORS IN EXPIRED AIR

| *Compound* | *Vapor Phase Chromatographic Sensitivity* (ppm)* | *Infrared Sensitivity† (ppm)* | *Infrared Analytical Wavelength (μ)* |
|---|---|---|---|
| Acetone‡ | 0.1 | 5 | 8.20 |
| Acrylonitrile | 3.0 | 5 | 10.49 |
| Amyl acetate‡ | 2.0 | 1 | 8.05 |
| Benzene‡ | 0.1 | 20 | 9.62 |
| Bromobenzene | 2.0 | 10 | 9.30 |
| Tertiary-butyl alcohol | 0.1 | 5 | 10.88 |
| Carbon dioxide‡ | 100 | 5 | 4.27 |
| Carbon monoxide‡ | 5 | 20 | 4.58 |
| Carbon tetrachloride‡ | 0.001 | 0.5 | 12.60 |
| Chloroform‡ | 0.01 | 1 | 12.95 |
| Chloropicrin | 0.5 | 2 | 11.50 |
| Cyclohexane | 0.1 | 40 | 11.60 |
| Dichlorodifluoromethane‡ (Freon-12) | 0.5 | 1 | 10.85 |
| Dioxane | 0.1 | 2 | 8.80 |
| Ethyl alcohol‡ | 0.1 | 5 | 9.37 |
| Ethyl ether‡ | 0.1 | 5 | 8.75 |
| Ethylene oxide | 0.1 | 5 | 11.48 |
| Trichloromonofluoromethane‡ (Freon-11) | 0.010 | 1 | 11.82 |
| Gasoline | 5.0 μg/liter | 5§ | 3.40 |
| Methyl alcohol‡ | 0.2 | 5 | 9.45 |
| Methyl bromide | 6 | 50 | 3.36 |
| Methyl chloride‡ | 0.2 | 30 | 3.35 |
| Methyl chloroform‡ | 0.01 | 2 | 9.20 |
| Methylene chloride‡ | 0.1 | 2 | 13.10 |
| Nitrous oxide‡ | | 25 | 7.68 |
| Perchloroethylene‡ | 0.01 | 2 | 10.92 |
| Phosgene | | 1 | 11.68 |
| Sulfur dioxide | | 15 | 8.55 |
| Toluene | 0.3 | 5 | 13.75 |
| Trichloroethylene‡ | 0.01 | 2 | 11.78 |
| Turpentine | 0.4 | 10§ | 3.40 |
| Vinyl chloride‡ | 0.1 | 10 | 10.63 |
| Vinylidene chloride‡ | 0.1 | 5 | 12.60 |
| *o*-xylene | 0.1 | 10 | 13.51 |
| *m*-xylene | 0.1 | 10 | 13.02 |
| *p*-xylene | 0.1 | 10 | 12.58 |

*Sensitivities listed are the minimum amounts detectable under current operating conditions in the laboratory. These are practical limits of detection and can be improved when necessary.

†Sensitivity is defined as the minimum concentration of the compound which will give an absorbence of at least 0.01 in a 10-meter path-length cell. Five to ten times this amount must usually be present to obtain a positive identification of the compound.

‡Materials marked have been detected in postexposure expired air.

§Aliphatic hydrocarbons can be detected at 3.40 μ but cannot usually be identified specifically at low concentrations.

From Stewart, R.D., *et al:* Diagnosis of solvent poisoning. *JAMA, 193:* 1097-1100, Sept. 1965.

5. Body fat should be preserved in suspected cases of poisoning by DDT and the newer insecticides.
6. Bone, hair and nails should be preserved for analysis in cases of chronic lead, mercury and arsenic poisoning.

7. The lungs should be preserved for analysis to determine whether the poison may have been inhaled.
8. Urine is used for analysis for barbituric acid derivatives, metals, fluorides, etc.
9. The stomach and its contents should be obtained in all cases resulting in death within a short period after the onset of symptoms. However, in order to prove absorption of the poison, at least one organ other than the stomach must be submitted for analysis. The only exception to this is in cases of death caused by mineral acids or by alkalis, because in such cases the stomach and intestinal contents are the only suitable material for analysis.

The autopsy should be performed before the body is embalmed whenever this is possible. The embalming process interferes with the detection of cyanides, alkaloids and other poisons. If the body has been embalmed prior to autopsy, a sample of the embalming fluid used should be submitted for control purposes.

The utmost care must be used in handling the organs removed from the body. They must not be placed upon any but clean surfaces or in scrupulously clean containers in order to avoid contamination.

The total weight of each of the organs removed for analysis should be recorded, and those portions of the organs to be examined should then be placed in clean glass containers provided with glass covers. If possible, metal and metal-covered containers should be avoided because of the possibility of contamination of the sample by foreign metals. Metal covers with waxed cardboard liners may be used on glass jars. It is also possible to use plastic containers or porcelain-enameled containers, if there are no breaks in the enamel. Whatever the container used, it should be sealed by means of labels or gummed tape placed over the lid and fastened to the container itself. The name or initials of the pathologist should be written on the seal at a point where it would normally be broken when the container is opened. In this way one can insure against possible tampering with the sample from the time of its collection until it is examined in the laboratory. A label or tag with the identifying data, such as the name of the deceased, date of death, date of autopsy, etc., should then be attached to the container.

If possible, a separate container should be used for each organ. However, if this is not practical, one container may be used for all the samples with the exception of the gastrointestinal contents, blood and urine. Each of these latter samples must be kept separate from all the others.

No chemical preservatives should be added since they may interfere with subsequent analytical procedures. "Dry ice" may be used for refrigeration, although it is suggested that glass containers not be placed in direct contact with such a refrigerant in order to avoid breakage due to the sudden temperature change. The samples should be submitted for analysis as quickly as possible, and a written record should be kept of the identity of the person acting as messenger. Legal proceedings require the establishment of the "chain of custody" of evidence. Therefore receipts should be obtained whenever the custody of a sample passes from one person to another.

It has been estimated that over 20 per cent of all deaths in the United States require a thorough and complete examination. To meet this challenge, the coroner should possess the three A's. He should be astute, affable and available. In addition, if at all rational or feasible, the coroner should be a physician with a high index of curiosity and some formal training in pathology. If the medical, ethical and legal needs of our society are to be properly served, this type of medical examiner, respected in his community for his specialized knowledge and integrity and adequately compensated, is worth striving for.

## TOXICOLOGICAL SCREENING TESTS*

Most of these tests may be performed on urine, plasma or gastric contents. They usually depend on the formation of a color by interaction of the toxic agent with the reagent. Therefore to reduce ambiguity it is wise always to bracket the unknown sample with, on one side, a specimen known to contain the toxic agent and, on the other side, a specimen of urine, plasma or gastric content known to be free of such agents. In many cases, the toxic plasma concentration may be too low to provide positive spot tests. Only clear fluid should be taken for the test. Centrifuging may help to separate solid material.

### *Microdiffusion*

The sample is placed in the middle (sample) ring of a Conway dish. The trapping reagent is placed in the center well. A releasing agent is added to the middle ring in such a way that it does not initially contact the sample. Water is placed in the outer (sealing) ring. The circular cover is set into the sealing ring and twisted to provide an air-tight seal. The sealed dish is gently tilted and rotated to mix the sample with the releasing agent. Volatile agents diffuse into the sealed air space and react with the trapping reagent for identification.

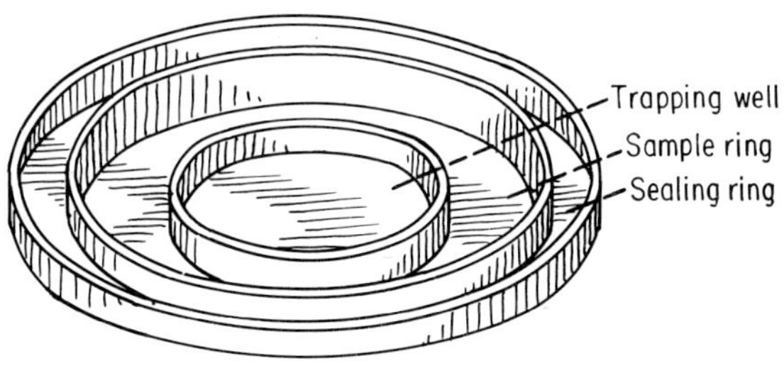


Figure 8. Conway dish for routine toxicology screening tests.

A. Test for ethyl, methyl, and isopropyl alcohol
 Trapping well: 1 ml 0.5% potassium dichromate in sulfuric acid.
 Sample well: 1 ml sample, 1 ml saturated potassium carbonate solution. Wait one hour. Green or blue color is positive.
 Since this test does not distinguish methyl and isopropyl from ethyl alcohol, further tests are necessary.

B. Tests for methyl and isopropyl alcohol
 To 5 ml of sample, add 10 ml 30% trichloracetic acid, shake and filter. Transfer 5 ml of the filtrate to a test tube and add 5% potassium permanganate solution, 1 drop at a time, until a pink color persists. Add 1 drop of 10% phosphoric acid. Allow to react for 5 minutes. Add enough solid sodium bisulfite to remove the color of the excess permanganate.
 1. Methanol test
 To 4 ml of the above solution add a little solid chromatropic acid (dihydroxynaphthalenedisulfonic acid) on the tip of a spatula. Mix. Add 3 ml concentrated sulfuric acid. Purple color is positive. This color may take 30 minutes to develop. Gentle heat (60°C water bath) hastens color development.
 2. Isopropanol test
 To the 1 ml remaining from B, add 1 drop of saturated sodium hydroxide solution followed by 1 drop of salicylaldehyde, either undiluted or in 95% ethanol. Orange color is positive. This color may take 30 minutes to develop. Gentle heat (60°C water bath) hastens color development.

C. Test for carbon monoxide
 Trapping well: 0.1% palladium chloride in dilute hydrochloric acid.
 Sample ring: 1 ml whole blood (or blood cells), 1 ml 5% silver nitrate. Wait 2 hours. Black particles or film indicate positive result.

D. Separation of diffusible anions
 This procedure is useful for separating borate, bromide, cyanide and fluoride for subsequent spot testing.

*Reproduced with the permission of Jane H. Speaker, Ph.D., Chief Toxicologist, Office of the Medical Examiner, Philadelphia, Pennsylvania.

Trapping well: 0.5N sodium hydroxide.
Sample ring: 1 ml sample, 1 ml 80% sulfuric acid, 1 ml methanol.
Keep at 100°C for two hours.
Use residue in trapping well for spot tests. Water, 1 ml, may be added to trapping well to facilitate removal of residue.

*Spot Tests*

Use white porcelain spot plates. Use three wells for each test: blank, unknown and standard.

A. Acetaminophen
 Add 1 drop of blank, sample and standard.
 Add 1 drop of concentrated hydrochloric acid.
 Keep plate at 100°C for 5 minutes.
 Add 1 drop of saturated sodium hydroxide.
 Add 1 drop of 1% o-cresol.
 Heat plate again for 1 to 5 minutes.
 Blue color is positive.

B. Borate
 Add 3 drops of blank, sample and standard.
 Add 1 drop 10% hydrochloric acid.
 Add 1 drop turmeric reagent (saturated solution of turmeric in ethyl alcohol).
 Keep spot plate at 100°C.
 Red-brown precipitate is positive.
 Add 2 drops of concentrated ammonium hydroxide.
 Blue-green solution results if borate is present.

C. Bromide
 Add 3 drops of blank, sample and standard.
 Add 3 drops glacial acetic acid.
 Add 3 drops 30% hydrogen peroxide.
 Add 1 drop 0.2% fluorescein.
 Keep spot plate at 100°C.
 Rose color is positive.

D. Cyanide
 Add 1 drop of blank, sample and standard.
 Add 1 drop of 0.5N sodium hydroxide.
 Add 5 drops of cyanide reagent (0.15% *p*-nitrobenzaldehyde and 0.17% O-dinitrobenzene in ethylene glycol monomethylether).
 Blue color (Prussian blue) is positive. (Another rapid test can be done in any laboratory. A few crystals of ferrous sulfate are added to 5 to 10 ml of gastric aspirate, then 4 to 5 drops of 20% NaOH are added to precipitate the iron. The solution is boiled, cooled, and slightly acidified with 8 to 10 drops of 10% HC1. If cyanide is present, a greenish-blue color or precipitate appears and intensifies on standing.)

E. Ethchlorvynol
 Add 1 drop of blank, sample and standard.
 Add 1 drop of concentrated sulfuric acid.
 Add 1 drop of 5% diphenylamine in chloroform.
 Red color is positive.

F. Fluoride
 Add 3 drops of blank, sample and standard.
 Add 1 drop phenolphthalein indicator
 Add 0.1 M acetic acid 1 drop at a time until pink color disappears.
 Add 5 drops fresh 2% Amadac F reagent (Burdick and Jackson Laboratories, Muskegon, Michigan).
 Blue color of positive must be distinguished from blue color of blank. Be sure to run a control.

G. Imipramine, Desipramine
 Add 3 drops of blank, sample and standard.
 Add 3 drops of imipramine reagent (equal volumes of 0.2% potassium dichromate, 20% perchloric acid [explosive hazard], 30% sulfuric acid and 35% nitric acid).
 A green or blue color is positive.

H. Iron
 Add 3 drops of blank, sample and standard.
 Add 2 drops of 2N hydrochloric acid.

Add 1 drop of 1% potassium ferrocyanide.
Blue color is positive.

I. Paraquat
Add 3 drops of blank, sample and standard.
Add some sodium dithionite crystals from the tip of a spatula.
Blue or green color is positive.

J. Parathion metabolite
Add 3 drops of blank, sample and standard.
Add 3 drops of saturated sodium hydroxide.
Yellow color is positive.

K. Phenothiazines
Add 1 drop of blank, sample and standard.
Add 1 drop of FPN reagent (5 ml 5% ferric chloride plus 45 ml 20% perchloric acid [explosive hazard] plus 50 ml 35% nitric acid).
Pink purple or blue color is positive.

L. Salicylate
Add 3 drops of blank, sample and standard.
Add 1 drop of salicylate reagent (5% ferric chloride in 1N hydrochloric acid.)
Purple or black color is positive.
Thiocyanate produces orange color.

M. Sulfanilimide antibacterials
Apply 1 drop of urine to newsprint or other paper containing wood fibers.
Add 1 drop of concentrated hydrochloric acid.
Yellow to orange color is positive.

N. Thiocyanate *See* Salicylates.

*Screening Test for Antimony, Arsenic, Bismuth and Mercury*

To 20 ml of urine in an acid-rinsed Erlenmeyer flask, add 5 ml of concentrated hydrochloric acid and an acid-washed square of copper about 5 mm on a side. Hold at 90° to 100°C for one hour. Remove copper square, rinse and inspect it.

Dark bluish sheen indicates antimony.
Dull black deposit indicates arsenic.
Shiny black deposit indicates bismuth.
Silvery deposit indicates mercury.

*Screening Test for Halongenated Hydrocarbons*

To 5 ml of sample, add 2 ml of potassium hydroxide solution and 4 ml of pyridine. Mix well. Heat at 80°C for 10 minutes. Red color in pyridine layer is positive.

The Production Identification Section of *Physicians' Desk Reference* may not always be helpful in identifying drugs, especially if they come from the street or the patient's gastrointestinal tract.

The tests above are simple, inexpensive screening tests for drug class identification that can be done rapidly in a clinic or office laboratory. The tests are not specific beyond class, and definitive biologic samples from the patient must be taken to provide final qualitative and quantitative data as to the drugs involved. Some cellar-lab and other street drugs may not react with these simple tests.*

---

*Bibliography.

Clarke, E.G.C.: *Isolation and Identification of Drugs.* London, The Pharmaceutical Press, 1969.
Curry, A.S.: *Poison Detection in Human Organs.* Springfield, Thomas, 1976.
Decker, W.J. and Treutin, J.J.: *Clin Toxicol, 4*:89-97, 1971.
Kaye, S.: *Handbook of Emergency Toxicology.* Springfield, Thomas, 1970.
Kaye, S.: *Pediatr Clin North Am, 17*:515-524, 1970.
Stewart, C.P. and Stolman, A.: *Toxicology Mechanisms and Analytical Methods.* New York, Acad Pr, 1960.
Sunshine, I.: *Methodology for Analytical Toxicology.* Cleveland, CRC Pr, 1969.

## LETHAL DOSES

Athough definitive lethal doses as reported in the literature are variable, they are, for the most part, reasonably close. The knowledge obtained from case histories and animal

TABLE 36
SCREENING TESTS FOR GENERAL DRUG CATEGORY

*Amphetamines*
Mandelin's is most specific.
Fröhde's and Marquis' also give a reaction.

*Barbiturates*
Zwikker's is most specific but less sensitive than Dille-Koppanyi's.

*Ergotamine Alkaloids*
*p*-Dimethylaminobenzaldehyde paper spot is specific for LSD and many other indole-ring compounds and may also turn up positive in patients taking Cafergot or similar drugs for migraine headache.

*Opium Alkaloids*
Marquis' is most general.
Fröhde's is a good confirming test.
Cobalt-thiocyanate is specific for cocaine, meperidine and methadone.

*Cobalt-Thiocyanate Test*
Reagent
Mix equal parts of 4% cobalt acetate in water and 4% potassium thiocyanate in water just before use.
Procedure
Add 3 to 5 drops of reagent to sample.
Reactions
Cocaine, methadone, meperidine and procaine immediately turn sky blue.
Chlorpromazine and promazine immediately turn green.

*Dille-Koppanyi's Test*
Reagents
0.1 gm of cobalt acetate in 100 ml of methanol plus 0.2 ml of acetic acid; 5 ml of *n*-butylamine in 95 ml of chloroform.
Procedure
Add 2 ml of the cobalt acetate reagent to sample in a test tube and mix, then add 1 ml of the *n*-butylamine reagent and mix.
Reaction
Barbiturates turn purple or red-violet.

*p-Dimethylaminobenzaldehyde Paper Spot Test*
Reagents
Whatman No. 1 chromatography paper dipped in a 10% solution of *p*-dimethylaminobenzaldehyde in ethyl alcohol and air-dried; 10% ferric chloride in water; absolute methyl alcohol; 50% sulfuric acid.
Procedure
Place sample on test paper and add 1 drop of ferric chloride, then enough methyl alcohol to wet the test paper. Add sulfuric acid drop by drop. If effervescence occurs, continue adding drops until it ceases, and then add 2 more drops, to a maximum of 10. The less methanol and sulfuric acid used, the more sensitive the test.
Reactions
Ergotamine alkaloids turn pink, purple or blue in the solution or on the paper within five minutes.
1 $\mu$g of LSD gives the same reaction within one minute.

*Fröhde's Test*
Reagent
0.5 gm of molybdic acid in 100 ml of concentrated sulfuric acid. The mixture should be colorless.
Procedure
Add 3 to 5 drops to sample.
Reactions
Amphetamines turn green, which changes rapidly to yellow.
Opium is stable blue, green or blue-green.

*Mandelin's Test*
Reagent
1 gm of ammonium vanadate in 100 ml of concentrated sulfuric acid.
Procedure
Dissolve a small amount of the suspect drug in 1 ml of water, then add 2 ml of reagent.
Reaction
Amphetamine and methamphetamine turns green or bluish-green.

TABLE 36—*Continued*
SCREENING TESTS FOR GENERAL DRUG CATEGORY

*Marquis' Test*
Reagent
Just before use, mix well 8 to 10 drops of 10% formaldehyde and 10 ml of concentrated sulfuric acid.
Procedure
Add 3 to 5 drops to sample.
Reactions
Acetylsalicylic acid turns raspberry red.
Amphetamines turn red-orange, which immediately darkens to brown.
Meperidine slowly turns yellow, which changes to light green, and then darkens.
Mephentermine is a stable red-orange.
Methapyrilene is red-violet.
Opium immediately turns purple.

*Zwikker's Test*
Reagents
0.5% copper sulfate in water; 5% pyridine in chloroform.
*Procedure*
Add 0.5 ml of each reagent to sample in a test tube, shake and allow layers to separate.
Reactions
Barbiturate turns purple in the bottom layer.
Thiobarbiturate turns green in the bottom layer.
Adding a drop of acetic acid should destroy or markedly reduce the intensity of color if the sample is a barbiturate.

experimentation (though animals do not always demonstrate the same reactions as humans do to the same toxic agents) is basically responsible for the general information now at hand. In spite of all the variables, there are available some fairly reliable data on the approximate minimum lethal dose (MLD) (150-pound man) for most of the common acute poisons listed in Table 38 and Table 131. The lethal dose fatal to 100 per cent or 50 per cent of animals is expressed as $LD_{100}$ or $LD_{50}$.

## POISONS AND MENTAL FUNCTION (PSYCHOSIS-HALLUCINOGENS)

Most literature on poisoning emphasizes gastrointestinal, hepatic, blood, renal and cutaneous changes, but it is important to remember that the central nervous system may also be affected. Changes in this system range from seizures (strychnine poisoning) to coma (primary as in barbiturate intoxication, or secondary as in uremia caused by heavy metal poisoning), hypoxia caused by methemoglobinemia or severe hemolytic anemia, or shock caused by a variety of severe intoxications. These changes are all readily recognized and usually correctly interpreted. On the other hand, changes in mental function in the form of emotional disorders or even psychotic behavior may also be caused by certain intoxications; these changes may be insidious or so prominent that they overshadow those in other organs, and errors in diagnosis may thereby occur. There are many compounds that cause symptoms of this type, and there is nothing to indicate that they all act via the same mechanism.

One such class of chemicals affects acetylcholine. The action of acetylcholine may be inhibited by atropine, scopolamine, stramonium (deliberate self-intoxication with Asthmador,* an old-fashioned asthma remedy containing 50.4 per cent stramonium and 4.5 per cent belladonna preparation ingested for its hallucinogenic effects) and some related synthetic drugs that are used in the treatment of Parkinson's disease. Substances which increase the amount of acetylcholine in the

*Asthmador has recently been discontinued as an over-the-counter asthma remedy in the United States.

TABLE 37

POISONOUS SUBSTANCES FOUND IN THE HOUSEHOLD*

A Glance at the Following Table Will Show What Poison the Product Probably Contains

*Polishes and Waxes for Furniture and Floors*

| *Petroleum Distillates* | | *Other Toxic Substances* | |
|---|---|---|---|
| Kerosene | Naphtha, high boiling | Antimony chloride | Isopropyl and butyl alcohols |
| Mineral seal oil | Spindle oil | Caustic alkali | Nitrobenzene |
| Mineral spirits | Summer black oil | Cellosolve | Oxalic acid |
| | | | Turpentine |

*Paint Solvents and Related Products*

| *Paint Brush Cleaners* | | *Removers of Paint, Wax,* | |
|---|---|---|---|
| *and Preservatives* | | *Lacquers, Grease Spots* | Caustic alkalis |
| Acetone | Sodium chromate | Amyl acetate | Ethyl acetate |
| Caustic alkalis | Toluol | Alcohols-amyl, butyl, ethyl | Ethylene dichloride |
| Cresols and higher phenols | Turpentine | Amylene dichloride | Kerosene |
| Dipentene | *Paints, Putty, Varnishes* | Benzene | Methyl alcohol |
| Methanol | Arsenic, Lead, Chromium, | Butyl acetate | Methylene chloride |
| Naphthalene | Iron, Titanium, Zinc | Carbon tetrachloride | Toluene |

*Cleaning, Polishing, and Bleaching Agents*

| *Dry Cleaning Fluids* | *Detergents for Dishware,* | *Metal Cleaners and Polishers* | |
|---|---|---|---|
| Acetone | *Glassware, Laundry* | *Strong Acids and Alkalis* | *Others* |
| Amyl acetate | *Strong Alkaline Solutions* | Ammonia water, caustic soda | Alkyl aryl sulfonate |
| Benzene | Sodium hydroxide | Hydrochloric acid, dilute | Oxalic acid |
| Carbon tetrachloride | Sodium metasilicate | Phosphoric acid, dilute | Potassium chlorate |
| Ethylene dichloride | Sodium perborate | Soda ash | Potassium cyanide |
| Kerosene | Sodium phosphate glass | Sulfamic acid | Thiourea |
| Methyl alcohol | Tetrasodium phosphate | Sulfuric acid, dilute | *Porcelain* |
| Naphtha, heavy petroleum | *Others* | *Stove* | Ammonium hydroxide |
| Petroleum distillates | Ethylene glycol | Naphtha | Pine oil |
| Stoddard solvent | Sodium hypochlorite | Alkalis | |
| Toluene | | | |
| Trichloroethylene | | | |

*Cosmetic Preparations* (See Sanitizing Agents Table)

| *Skin Tonics and Lotions* | *Permanent Wave Solutions* | *Hair Dyes, Tints, Colorings* | Beta-naphthol |
|---|---|---|---|
| Aluminum salts | Sodium carbonate | Ammonium nitrate; hydroxide | Cantharidin |
| Camphor or menthol | Sodium sulfite | Metallic dyes (lead or bismuth) | Glacial acetic acid |
| Methylated spirits | Thioglycolate salts | Para-phenylenediamine | Kerosene deodorized |
| Zinc phenosulfonate | *Neutralizers* | Pyrogallol | *Depilatories* |
| Zinc sulfate | Acetic acid | Sodium hypochlorite solution | Calcium thioglycollate |
| *Sun Tan Lotions* | Potassium bromate | *Shampoos* | Soluble sulfides |
| Acetone | Sodium hexametaphosphate | Denatured alcohol | Organic solvents |
| Denatured alcohol | Sodium perborate | Sodium hexametaphosphate | |
| Methyl salicylate | *Lacquers* | | *Nail Preparations* |
| Para-aminobenzoic acid esters | Denatured alcohol | | Alcohols-ethyl, isopropyl |
| *Sun-Tan Preparations* | Shellac resin | | n-butyl |

Alcohol
Sodium, methyl, ethyl-p-aminobenzoate
Titanium dioxide
Iron oxide pigment
*Hair Preparations*
*Brilliantines*
Industrial methylated spirit (contains wood naphtha)
Kerosene deodorized
*Lacquers, Plasticizers, Resins*
Dibutyl phthalate
Nitrocellulose
Sulfonamide resins
*Eyebrow pencil*
Lampblack
Petrolatum, Paraffin
*Liquid Make-up*
Triethanolamine
Titanium dioxide
Propylene glycol
Stearic or oleic acid
Color pigments

*Hair sprays*
Synthetic resins
Natural resins
Macromolecules
(potential for producing thesaurosis)
*Deodorants*
Aluminum salts
Titanium dioxide
Oxyquinoline sulfate
Zirconium salt
*Freckle Removers*
Bichloride of mercury
Bismuth
Ammoniated mercury
*Eye shadow*
Oxide pigments
Beeswax, petrolatum
Cetyl alcohol
*Perfumes*
Alcohol (up to 50%)
Essential oils
Floral odor

*Eye Cream*
Lecithin
Cholesterin
Beeswax
*Mascara*
*Cake*
Lampblack
Diethylene glycol stearate
Sulfonated castor oil
*Cream*
Triethanolamine
Lampblack
Petrolatum
Stearic acid
*Hair Lotions*
Pilocarpine
Salicylic acid
Tertiary butyl; isopropyl; ethyl alcohol

Denatured ethyl alcohol
Industrial methylated spirit
Isopropyl alcohol

Esters
Ketones
*Cuticle Removers*
Dilute caustic alkalis
*Skin Food, Cream, Masks*
Hormones
Mercury
Salicylic acid
Purified silicons
Kaolin
Zinc stearate oxide
*Lipsticks*
*Liquid*
Petroleum ether
Alcohol
Rosin
Shellac
Rhodamine B
Safranin
*Tube*
Beeswax
Tetrahydrofurfuryl acetate
Cocoa butter
Eosin dyes

*Other Types of Household Products and Chemicals*

*Antifreeze, Carburetor Cleaners*
Chlorinated benzene
Alcohols-denatured, isopropyl, methyl
Ethylene glycol
*Deodorizing Tablets*
Formaldehyde
*Anti-Rust Products*
Ammonium sulfide
Hydrofluoric acid
*Brake Fluids*
Glycols
Alcohols
Castor oil
Naphtha
Oxalic acid
*Leather Preservatives, Polishes and Dyes*
Benzene
Carnauba wax
Methanol

*Spray*
Isopropyl alcohol
Triethylene glycol
Propylene glycol
Freon propellent
*Wick*
Formaldehyde
Deodorant oils
*Shoe Cleaners and Polishes*
Aniline
Nitrobenzene

Shellac
Titanium Dioxide
Turpentine
*Jewelry and Watch Cleaners and Cements*
Ammonia
Isopropyl alcohol

*Ink, Ball-Point Pens*
Glycols (propylene, diethylene)
Dyes
*Stamping Inks*
Propylene glycol
Glycerine
Phenol
Dye
*Laundry Ink*
Aniline
*Laundry Indelible Ink*
Nigrosine dyes
Naphthas
Xylene

*Ink Eradicators*
Sodium hypochlorite
Sodium chloride
*Fire-Extinguishing Fluids*
Carbon tetrachloride
Methyl bromide
Sodium carbonate

*Plastic Menders, Glues*
Cellulose acetate
Ethylene dichloride
Formaldehyde
Nitrocellulose
*Wax Crayons*
Para red
*Spray De-Icer*
Ethylene glycol
n-propanol, $CO_2$ as propellent

*Christmas Tree Bubbling Lights*
Methylene chloride
*Cleaning Equipment*
Carbon tetrachloride
Stoddard solvent
Sodium hydroxide
Ammonia

TABLE 37—*Continued*
POISONOUS SUBSTANCES FOUND IN THE HOUSEHOLD

**Neatsfoot oil**
Talloil
Triethanolamine
*Scratch Remover*
Petroleum spirits
*Plastic*
Paraformaldehyde
*Insect Repellents*
Dimethyl phthalate
Indalone
Ethyl hexanediol
*Deodorizers*
*Cleanser Type*
Pine oil
Soap
*Refrigerator*
Charcoal, activated
*Toilet Bowl (Blocks)*
Para dichlorobenzene
Naphthalene

Nitrocellulose in ketone
Petroleum solvent
*Fire-Starting Tablets*
Methenamine
*Bluing*
*Laundry*
Borax
Trisodium phosphate
Prussian blue
*Gun*
Mercuric chloride
Potassium chlorate
*Inks*
Iron gallate
Phenol
Silver nitrate
Soda ash
Dye
*Vegetable Dye*
Rhodamine B (can cause red or pink urine after ingestion)

*Typewriter Cleaner*
Cellosolve, Methanol
*Rug Adhesives*
Latex
Sulfur
Synthetic rubber
Zinc oxide

*Drain Cleaner*
Sodium hydroxide
Sodium acid sulfate
Trichloroethane
*Bleaches*
Sodium hypochlorite
Oxalic acid
*Rug Cleaner*
Trichloroethylene
*Wallpaper Cleaner*
Kerosene
Petroleum hydrocarbons

*Thermometer Fluids*
*Clinical*—about 0.1 ml mercury
*Indoor and Outdoor*—Triethyl phosphate)
Toluene ) less than 1 ml
Xylene )
Alcohol )
*Cooking*—Methyl benzoate
Maximum) Registering— Beechwood creosote
Minimum) Registering— Ethyl alcohol
*Arctic Cooking*—Pentane
Methyl benzoate

*Formulations of household products are frequently and unexpectedly changed. Consult labels for definitive chemical ingredients. Agents with potential toxic chemicals are clearly labeled (*see* Uniform Hazardous Substance Act).

TABLE 38
LETHAL DOSES*

| *Poison* | *MLD (approximately)* | *Poison* | *MLD (approximately)* |
|---|---|---|---|
| Acetanilid | 4 gm | Chloroform | 25 ml |
| Acetic Acid | 20 ml | Cinchophen | 5 gm |
| Acetone | 100 ml | Cocaine | 0.5 gm (PO) |
| Acetylsalicylic Acid | 20 gm | Codeine | 0.8 gm |
| (Salicylates) | | Colchicine | 30 mg |
| Aconitine | 10 mg | Copper Sulfate | 15 gm |
| Alkalis | 5 gm | Curare | 50 mg |
| Amidopyrine | 15 gm | Cyanide, Hydrogen | 0.1 gm |
| Ammonia | 10 ml | Cyanide, Potassium | 0.2 gm |
| Amphetamine | 0.15 gm | Cyanide, Sodium | 0.15 gm |
| Amylene Hydrate | 30 ml | DDT§ | 15 gm |
| (Tertiary Amyl Alcohol) | | Demerol (Meperidine) | 1 gm |
| Aniline | 10 gm | Digitalis | 2 gm |
| Antihistamines | 0.1-0.5 gm | Digitoxin | 3 mg |
| Antimony | 1 gm | Dilantin | 2 gm |
| Antipyrine | 5 gm | Dinitro-Ortho-Cresol | 2 gm |
| Alphanaphthylthiourea | | Dinitrophenol | 1-3 gm |
| (ANTU) | 40 gm | Doriden (Glutethimide) | 10 gm |
| Arsenic (Trioxide) | 0.2 gm | Emetine | 0.2 gm |
| Aspidium | 20 ml | Ephedrine | 0.6 gm |
| Atropine | 0.1 gm | Epinephrine | 50 mg (SC) |
| Barbiturates | 1-6 gm (depends upon | Ergot | 1 gm |
| | derivative potency) | Ether | 25 ml (PO) |
| Barium (Soluble Salts) | 1 gm | | 100 ppm (MAC) |
| Benadryl | 0.5 gm | Ethyl Alcohol (Pure) | 300-400 ml |
| Benzene | 15 ml | Whiskey = | 40-50% alcohol |
| Benzene Hexachloride | 15 gm | Wines = | 10-20% alcohol |
| Benzine | 100 ml | Beers = | 2-6% alcohol |
| Beryllium | 0.1 gm/cu m | Ethylene Glycol | 100 ml |
| Bismuth | 15 gm | Ferrous Sulfate | 30 gm |
| Boric Acid | 10 gm | Fluoroacetate Sodium | 50 mg |
| Cadmium | 1 gm | Fluorides | 4 gm |
| Camphor | 2 gm | Food Poisoning (Botulism) | Estimated toxin 0.001 |
| Cantharidin | 30 mg | | mg |
| Carbon Disulfide | 10 ml | Formaldehyde (Formalin) | 30 ml |
| Carbon Monoxide | 40% carboxyhemo- | Hydrochloric Acid | 5 ml |
| | globin saturation | Hypochlorite | 50-75 ml |
| Carbon Tetrachloride | 4 ml | Iodides | 50 gm |
| Chloral Hydrate | 7 gm | Iodine | 2 gm |
| Chlorates | 5 gm | Ipecac (Fluidextract) | 60 ml |
| Chlordane | 8 gm | Isopropyl Alcohol | 240 ml |
| Chlorine | 500 ppm (MAC) | Kerosene | 100 ml |
| | | Lead, Soluble Salts | 10 gm |
| Lead, Tetraethyl | 0.1 gm | Phosphorus | 0.3 gm |
| Meprobamate | 30 gm | Physostigmine | 60 mg |
| Mercuric Chloride† | 0.5 gm | Picrotoxin | 0.1 gm |
| Methyl Alcohol | 75 ml | Pilocarpin | 0.13 gm |
| | 200 ppm (MAC) | Plasmochin | 0.5 gm |
| Methyl Salicylate | 30 ml | Procaine | 10 gm (PO) |
| Metrazol | 10 gm (PO) | Pyrethrins | 70 gm |
| | 2 gm (IV) | Pyribenzamine | 1 gm |
| Morphine | 0.25 gm | Quaternary Ammonium | |
| Moth Balls | | Compounds (Concentrate) | 15 ml |
| Paradichlorobenzene | 15 gm | Quinine | 20 gm |
| Naphthalene | 5 gm | Rotenone | 20-30 gm |
| Camphor | 2 gm | Santonin | 1 gm |
| Muscarine | 50 mg | Silver Nitrate | 2 gm |
| Nicotine | 60 mg | Solanine | 0.2 gm |
| Nitrates | 8 gm | Strychnine | 75 mg |
| Nitric Acid | 5 ml | Sulfide, Hydrogen | 200 ppm (MAC) |
| Nitrites | 5 gm | Sulfuric Acid | 5 ml |

TABLE 38—*Continued*
LETHAL DOSES

| *Poison* | *MLD (approximately)* | *Poison* | *MLD (approximately)* |
|---|---|---|---|
| Nitrobenzene | 2 ml | Sulfonal | 10 gm |
| Oxalates | 5 gm | Thallium | 0.3 gm |
| Paraldehyde | 100 ml | Thiocyanate | 15 gm |
| Parathion‡ | 0.1 gm | Thiourea | 10 gm |
| Permanganate | 5 gm | Toxaphene | 3 gm |
| Phenacetin | 5 gm | Tridione | 6 gm |
| Phenols | 10 ml | Turpentine | 30 ml |
| Phosphoric Acid | 8 ml | Zinc Sulfate | 15 gm |

**Also see* Table 131.
†*See* Table 52 for lethal doses of other inorganic insecticides.
‡*See* Table 49 for lethal doses of other organic phosphate insecticides.
§*See* Table 47 for lethal doses of other chlorinated hydrocarbon insecticides.

body by inhibiting or destroying cholinesterase and cause similar mental changes are physostigmine, diisopropyl fluorophosphate and some weed killers. It appears that either an excess or a deficiency of acetylcholine in the brain may cause psychiatric symptoms. The mechanism of the psychosis produced by drugs that affect acetylcholine is not known; however, acetylcholine is probably involved in the transmission of almost all nerve impulses in the central nervous system and, therefore, interference with its action might be expected to cause symptoms.

Chronic heavy metal poisoning may also mimic endogenous psychiatric disorders. The Mad-Hatter syndrome seen in chronic mercury poisoning in felt makers is the most common example. Workers develop tremors, anxiety and paranoid behavior and may also experience hallucinations.

The unsaturated indoles also cause depersonalization and disordered thinking and sometimes hallucinations. The thought disorder caused by these drugs includes a feeling of having received some great revelation or achieved some profound insight ranging from the banal to the ludicrous. One of these indoles, lysergic acid diethylamide (LSD), has received much notice as a means of producing psychoses experimentally. It is also important because it occurs in ergot, the fungus that grows on rye. Carelessly made rye flour may cause epidemics of psychosis among those who eat the bread made from it. The Heavenly Blue and Pearly Gates morning-glory seeds *(Rivea corymbosa)* and the ololiuqui seed *(Ipomoea tricolor),* a species from Mexico and Central America, contain amides of lysergic acid and have also been recently implicated. It is estimated, however, that between two hundred and five hundred seeds would need be ingested to produce a hallucination. Bufotenine and its phosphate ester, psilocybin, are also unsaturated indoles; they occur in *Amanita* mushrooms as well as in other natural products and are used by primitive peoples (and hippies) in connection with their superstitious observances. Mexico's Mazatecas Indians have for centuries known of the hallucinogenic properties of the mushroom *Psilocybe mexicana* and still ingest the plant ritually. Still another compound is harmine, which is interesting because it is related to yohimbine, a drug that produces erotic delusions and hallucinations and was the refuge of aging Don Juans in the Victorian era. Adrenolutin also causes mental changes; it is formed by the oxidation of epinephrine. Spoiled epinephrine contains it, and when sprayed into the airways in large amounts, it may produce psychosis. The fragmentary evidence currently available indicates that these indolic substances act by disrupting carbohydrate metabolism in the Krebs cycle.

Many nonindolic hallucinogenic vegetable products are also known. One of them, mescaline, may actually be converted into an indole in the body. A plant extract (and also a synthetic) mescaline comes from the peyotl cactus *(Lophophora williamsii),* which grows in

Mexico and the southwestern United States. Peyote, or the synonymous peyote button, is a thin, dried slice of the cactus. The crude cactus contains more than ten alkaloids, among which are harmine, bufotenine, lophophorine and mescaline. Peyote eating is a sacramental feature in the half-Christian, half-pagan rites of the Native American Church, which claims two hundred thousand adherents among Indians of seventeen western states. Yage, a potent brew used for centuries by Central American witch doctors, has been recently found to have more hallucinogenic effects than mescaline. Another nonindolic hallucinogen is marihuana, a common form of which is hashish. The sociologic and psychiatric problems associated with its use are well known.

LSD is by far the most powerful of the hallucinogenic drugs, having a potency approximately ten times that of psilocybin and one hundred times that of mescaline. Psychiatrists, in general, do not feel that these drugs are addictive, but they do fear the psychotic reactions and acting-out behaviors they produce and deplore their misuse. The recent observation of reappearance of LSD symptoms a month to over a year after the original use, without reingestion, is a particularly alarming phenomenon. DMT (dimethyltryptamine), a potent hallucinogen similar in effect to LSD, should not be used as a substitute for this preparation.

Dimethyltryptamine is found in the seed of *Piptadenia peregrina* and the leaves of *Pristonia amazonica.* It is perhaps possible to obtain an active form of this substance by aqueous extraction or preparing a "tea." However, it is relatively easily prepared synthetically.

The pharmacological properties of DMT, as well as those of a closely related compound, diethyltryptamine, are virtually identical with LSD. The same type of hallucinations, distortions of consciousness and bizarre behavior result from the administration of both substances. DMT differs in two important respects. The onset of a DMT psychosis is somewhat more rapid than that experienced with LSD, and the duration is somewhat shorter. In addition, DMT is not effective unless injected either intravenously or intramuscularly. This latter quality would tend to make it less attractive than LSD to casual users, but its ready availability and the relatively low cost probably would rapidly overcome that drawback among those who desire the hallucinogenic experience. There is no doubt that DMT has the same potential for psychic damage as that possessed by LSD. In fact, the pharmacological action is probably similar.

DOM or STP, a drug claimed to be an hallucinogen and reportedly in wide use in hippie circles, is a substance chemically identified as methyl dimethoxy methyl phenylethylamine (related to mescaline and amphetamine). This substance was found in tablets alleged to be STP and obtained in different parts of the country. MDA (methylenedioxyamphetamine), structurally resembling mescaline and DOM or STP, can produce serious adverse effects, although once it was thought to be a relatively "safe" hallucinogen.

Four major types of acute symptoms have been seen. These include, in decreasing frequency, hallucinations (both auditory and visual), anxiety to the point of panic, severe depression with suicidal thoughts or attempts and confusion. These symptoms may occur in patients who have taken the drug once or sixty times. They occur in persons who have taken LSD only, as well as in persons who are chronic multiple drug abusers.

A review* of the scientific literature shows 21 different reports detailing 225 patients with adverse reactions to LSD. Complications included 142 prolonged psychotic reactions, 63 nonpsychotic reactions, 11 spontaneous recurrences of LSD experiences, 28 actual or possible suicide attempts, 11 successful suicides, 4 attempted and 1 successful homicide, and 6 cases of convulsions which may have been toxic reactions.

---

*Smart, R. G. and Bateman, K.: Unfavorable reactions to LSD: A review and analysis of the available case reports. *Can Med Assoc 97*:1214-1221, 1967. (Alcoholism and Drug Addiction Research Foundation, Toronto, Ontario.)

LSD users appear to be mainly young male college students or former students, some of whom have had previous psychotic or neurotic personality problems. Unfavorable reactions occur most frequently in persons taking the drug in unprotected settings, but reactions such as suicide attempts and homicidal tendencies have occurred when the user is under supervision. Spontaneous recurrences and psychopathic reactions appear almost exclusively in very heavy users, but many of the other reactions appear after a single relatively moderate dose.

Usual responses to LSD include bizarre visual experiences such as heightening of brightness and color perception, distortions in the perception of real objects and visual delusions or hallucinations. The emotional effects are often shifting and may involve apprehension, panic, elation or depression. Prolonged psychotic episodes or at least profoundly disturbing states, often requiring treatment with tranquilizers or long-term hospitalization, have been reported. The most typical symptoms seem to be paranoid delusions, schizophrenic-like hallucinations and overwhelming fear. Prolonged psychosis is more likely in patients with previous psychiatric diagnoses but also can occur in patients without previous personality difficulties.

Pharmacological studies show that LSD is rapidly absorbed and that most of the drug is rapidly destroyed. However, some patients suffer spontaneous recurrences of parts of the LSD experience as long as one year after taking the drug. The reaction, more prevalent in persons who have taken several doses of the drug, apparently indicates that LSD or some of its effects may persist or build up sufficiently over repeated administrations to cause a recurring experience. The incidence of damage to human chromosomes *in vitro* and *in vivo* has been an ominous, but equivocal, discovery.

Panic reactions are the most frequent nonpsychotic adverse reactions to LSD. Common features are dissociation, terror, confusion and fear of going insane or not being able to return to normal.

The inexperienced user is most susceptible to the simple anxiety type of panic reaction. More serious is the toxic psychosis in which a major break with reality takes place. The user may have a frightening illusion of bodily distortion, he may try to flee or he may become paranoid and suspicious of other people. Prolonged psychotic reactions may look like endogenous schizophrenic reactions and occur most often in individuals with preexisting psychological problems.

A recently developed radioimmunoassay test for LSD is highly specific and can detect as little as 0.1 picomole of the drug in the blood or urine up to 24 hours after ingestion.

*Treatment* of the simple anxiety type of panic reaction should be nonpunitive and aimed at providing supportive care. Using the "talk down" method, the therapist reassures the patient that his distortions will end and tries to direct his attention away from the environment or the mental aberrations that have precipitated panic. Chlorpromazine (Thorazine®) is the most effective (though not the most consistent) antagonist to LSD effects. Recently diazepam (Valium) has been used for "illusionogenic" drug crises with good results.

Suicide attempts are an important complication of LSD administration. The suicide rate among persons who take the drug in unprotected surroundings is unknown, but the rate for those under supervision is low.

No deaths have been reported in man from an overdose of LSD, and it is not known whether there is an accumulation of toxic effects after a long series of doses. The acute lethal dose for man is probably many times the usual therapeutic or psychedelic dose of 100 to 300 μg, but as little as 30 μg can elicit severe toxic reactions. LSD has been known, however, to produce convulsions. This reaction is rare.

No cases of pharmacological addiction to LSD have been reported, and cases of psychological dependence have been extremely rare. Although it is suggested that LSD may encourage users to try more seriously addictive drugs, there is no evidence to date of multihabituation in LSD users.

Use or abuse of amphetamines can cause tension and anxiety progressing to depressive and paranoid psychotic symptoms. Implicated compounds include appetite-suppressing amphetamines, volatile vasoconstrictor forms and ephedrine-like agents used in treating allergies.

Physiological action on the brain is inhibition of synaptic transmission. Alertness and wakefulness result. Amphetamines produce blanching of mucous membranes, with mild peripheral effects and vasoconstriction. Muscle tone and contractility are enhanced, and fatigue is reduced. Brain stem activity and visual and auditory acuity increase, and amino oxidase is inactivated. A mild analgesic effect occurs. Blood pressure increases slightly, an effect significantly heightened by concurrent administration of atropine. Amphetamines increase blood sugar, which may account in part for appetite suppression. Neither kidney function nor endocrine secretion is altered. In addition to symptoms arising from effects on the brain, toxicity may be manifested by headache, anginal pain and cardiac arrhythmia.

Incidence of use is high in restless, tense, agitated, occasionally disorganized patients. Condition of those eventually consulting a psychiatrist may be well advanced with insomnia, anorexia, weight loss and suicide attempts. Many have symptoms similar to agitated depression of the involutional period, flight of ideas, confusion, depersonalization or hallucinations or delusions.

Phencyclidine (Sernylan®, PCP), tested in man and discarded as an anesthetic agent (ketamine is a derivative of PCP) because of its hallucinogenic properties, is being used as an anesthetic in veterinary medicine and has produced serious toxic effects in its misuse by humans. This hallucinogenic drug also known as "angel dust," "peace pills" or "elephant tranquilizer" has produced severe psychoses that are often indistinguishable from florid schizophrenic episodes. Differentiation can usually be made by the lack of a prodrome in the history and a high incidence of violent, aggressive or threatening behavior.

The diagnosis of PCP ingestion should be strongly suspected when a patient is seen with rapid onset of signs and symptoms, including drowsiness or coma, nystagmus, mild blood pressure elevation, increased deep tendon reflexes, ataxia and anxiety with marked agitation. Respiratory depression and psychiatric morbidity appear to be the most significant sequelae to phencyclidine poisoning. Rational supportive care based on a knowledge of the pharmacology of phencyclidine serves as the basis for treatment. Although these patients do not react as quickly to phenothiazines as do schizophrenics, the drugs have been used successfully. Severe and prolonged hypotension has been reported. Diazepam for convulsions and diazoxide for hypertension have been used effectively. When blood levels of PCP are observed or expected to be toxic, there are various ways of affecting the drug's distribution and excretion by taking advantage of the fact that PCP (a base) will ionize and be trapped in an acid medium. Acidification both increases urinary excretion of the drug and shifts it from the cells to the extracellular fluid.

The following procedures* should be carried out with frequent monitoring of acid-base status and serum osmolality:

1. Perform gastric lavage if patient is seen within six hours after ingestion.
2. Instill sodium sulfate, 0.3 gm/kg by nasogastric tube to promote fecal excretion.
3. Wait half an hour to permit passage of the cathartic, then begin continuous gastric suctioning and add appropriate isotonic polyionic solution to IV fluids in volume equal to suctioned material. (If oral route is used for acidification, clamp suction tube for one hour after each installation).
4. Acidify to bring blood pH intermittently to 7.2, urine to less than 5. Administer: ammonium chloride, 2.75 mEq/kg every six hours by nasogastric tube and/or

*Courtesy Alan K. Done M.D. and Regine Aronow M.D.

IV as 1 or 2% solution in saline and ascorbic acid, 2 gm every six hours in IV fluids or
cranberry juice and 1 or 2 gm of ascorbic acid orally four times a day, which may acidify urine rapidly enough if symptoms are mild in low dose toxicity.
5. Administer furosemide (Lasix) 20 to 40 mg IM or IV when urine pH falls below 5.
6. Administer IV fluids in severe cases to enhance excretion.
7. Skip steps 4, 5, and 6 consider hemodialysis or hemoperfusion in presence of renal insufficiency.

Chronic effects of PCP produce impairment of mental function (organic brain dysfunction) and behavioral deviancy (behavioral toxicity). Use haloperidol as the choice antipsychotic drug.

TABLE 39
SOURCE & COMPARATIVE STRENGTHS OF LSD AND OTHER HALLUCINOGENS (APPROXIMATE)

| | |
|---|---|
| Marihuana (leaves and tops of *Cannabis sativa,* swallowed) | 30,000 mg |
| Peyote buttons (*Lophophora williamsii*) | 30,000 mg |
| Nutmeg (*Myristica fragrans*) | 20,000 mg |
| Hashish (resin of *Cannabis sativa*) | 4,000 mg |
| Mescaline (3,4,5-trimethoxyphenylethylamine) | 400 mg |
| Psilocybin (4-phosphoryltryptamine) | 12 mg |
| MDA, DOM or STP (2,5-dimethoxy-4-methyl-phenylethylamine, methylenedioxyamphetamine) | 5 mg |
| LSD (d-lysergic acid diethylamide tartrate) | 0.1 mg |

## TOXIC EPISODES IN THE FETUS AND INFANT (MATERNAL MEDICATION AND DRUG DANGERS)

Since the placenta is known to be an ineffective barrier between the maternal and fetal circulations, any drug dangerous to the infant may be considered potentially dangerous to the fetus when given to the mother. However, many drugs toxic to infants may not reach dangerous fetal levels when administered to the mother. In general, drugs associated with jaundice should be avoided in the pregnant woman at parturition, as well as in the neonatal infant. Also, physicians should be aware of possible idiosyncrasy to certain drugs and be prepared to diagnose and treat such complications when necessary.

Circumstantial evidence is overwhelming that the nonbarbiturate sleep-inducing drug, thalidomide, has produced severe malformations of the extremities (phocomelia—"seal extremities") in numerous newborns in Germany and Western Europe. Sixteen infants are suspected of having been deformed through distribution by United States firms. The only medications known definitely to be teratogenic in the human are thalidomide, folic acid antagonists and masculinizing steroids (primarily aminopterin). Other antimetabolites are suspected but not proven to be teratogenic in human beings. Cortisone and its analogues, suspect in cleft palate, should be avoided, if possible, during the first trimester of pregnancy.

Other drugs associated with increased risk to the fetus and neonate include thiouracil, its derivatives and iodine, which can be thyrotoxic; naphthalene, methyl mercury (in food), anticonvulsants, sulfonylurea hypoglycemics, trace metals (?), synthetic vitamin K and other drugs which may cause hemolysis and associated jaundice and hyperbilirubinemia, hence increased risk of kernicterus; some substances which are metabolized by the liver (chloramphenicol) and drugs associated with hepatic toxicity (chlortetracycline, phenothiazines, anticonvulsants); sulfonamides and other drugs which cause bilirubin-albumin dissociation; agents which cause neonatal respiratory depression (morphine and derivatives); those which may produce hemorrhagic phenomena (phenothiazine derivatives, tripelennamine, barbiturates, reserpine); and certain antibiotics which may be nephrotoxic or ototoxic. Infants born to mothers who are receiving propranolol are at risk of postnatal bradycardia and hypoglycemia. Recently, reports have linked vaginal adenocarcinoma in young girls to diethylstilbestrol therapy in their mothers during pregnancy. The latest evidence not only indicates a causal relationship between cigarette smoking during pregnancy and low infant birth weight, but also points to a strong probable causal association between smoking and a higher rate of fetal and infant mortality. The eating of blighted potatoes by pregnant women, with resulting neural tube defects (NTD) in the fetus, has received much publicity of late. There is no basis for this, however. The neural tube closes during the nineteenth to the twenty-eighth day of gestation, and if there is any possibility of such an occurrence, the blighted potatoes would have to be eaten during the first month of pregnancy.

TO A HUSBAND

Before you 'pregnate her get right on the ball—
Imperfect potater makes monsters et al.—
Then show her the data how risks are not small.

To save regrets later in babes' hospital,
Advise and berate her first month, with the call:
Potater first-rater or no spud at all!

—James H. Renwick

The *Fetal Alcohol Syndrome* is only a recently recognized phenomenon. In a *New England Medical Journal* report of 633 pregnant women, 17 per cent of the heavy drinkers' children had serious birth defects as compared to 3 per cent of the babies of nondrinkers. Alcohol crosses the placenta and goes directly into the fetus. Excessive inbibing of alcohol by pregnant women has produced a variety of documented (*JAMA, 235*:1458-60, 1976) features in 41 children (*see,* Alcohol, page 210).

Toxicity of other drugs may not be recognized as yet. Although no ill effects in the fetus have been observed to date from the use of any antibiotics during pregnancy, the newer antibiotics should be used cautiously in the treatment of the pregnant woman at term. Drugs not yet standardized for use in newborns should be avoided.

The most important factor in the production of fetal malformation depends on the vulnerability of the particular structure affected (eye, heart, etc.) and the actual teratogenic agent employed. In the fetus exposed to thalidomide, it is the limb buds that are susceptible, and their period of maximum vulnerability is between the eighteenth and twenty-eighth day of gestation. There is a critical time during gestation for each organ to be affected by teratogenic agents, which coincides with greatest mitotic activity in that organ.

The concentration of a drug in the fetus is important. A large single dose taken by the mother may not be so damaging as smaller doses taken before or in early pregnancy. Indeed, the danger may not be so much from teratogenic drugs taken occasionally during pregnancy, but from the habitual taking of drugs by women of the childbearing age who may subsequently become pregnant. The woman is not sure whether she is pregnant until a month or more after actual conception, during which time the fetus is exposed to the action of the drug at a time when it is particularly susceptible.

The state of the mother, particularly her age, parity and nutrition, is important. It is possible that a dose of a teratogenic drug affecting the fetus of a malnourished woman would have no effect on the fetus of a well-nourished woman. All teratogenic agents, whether drugs, viruses or physical agents such as irradiation, have one property in common: They produce minimal disturbance in the mother.

Recently it has been demonstrated that phenobarbital can totally disrupt the normal timetable of ovulation in animals when given during the first part of the menstrual cycle. This resulted in the delayed eruption of the ovum, producing and "overripe" egg and a staggering incidence of chromosomal and congenital abnormalities in the offspring.

It is relevant to consider whether assays of

TABLE 40
PSYCHOTIC STATES ASSOCIATED WITH MISUSE OR ABUSE OF ORDINARILY

| *Compound* | | *Physical Signs* | *Level of Consciousness* | *Formal Psychiatric Aspects* |
|---|---|---|---|---|
| CNS stimulants: amphetamines, methamphetamine, mephentermine (Wyamine®), phenmetrazine (Preludin®). | | Emaciation and poor hygiene common but not universal; needle marks present in IV users; tremor noted at times. In phenmetrazine intoxication, dilated pupils with impaired light reflex and cerebellar signs noted in some cases. | No clouding of sensorium **unless other drugs (especially barbiturates and alcohol) are taken concomitantly.** Disorientation noted at times with phenmetrazine intoxication. | Amphetamine psychosis usually presents as acute paranoid psychosis in setting of clear consciousness. Auditory and visual hallucinations often present. Most patients show distractibility, flight of ideas, pressured speech, hyperalert sensitivity to environmental cues. |
| Anticholinergics: trihexyphenidyl (Artane®), belladonna, atropine. | | Widely dilated, unreactive pupils; hot dry skin; mild tachycardia; dryness of the mouth; hyperreflexia at times. | Confusion, temporal disorientation, incontinence in some cases. | Pathologic excitement, wakefulness, restlessness, pressure of speech, emotional lability, suspiciousness, fear, distortion of time sense, delusions, auditory and visual hallucinations into which the patient has no insight. |
| Barbiturates, nonbarbiturate sedatives, and minor tranquilizers: pentobarbital, secobarbital, sodium amobarbital, glutethimide, meprobamate, chlordiazepoxide, etc. | *(Intoxication)* | No specific or diagnostic signs. Ataxia, nystagmus, dysarthria, and impaired coordination are characteristic. | Depressed; orientation and concentration impaired. | Acute brain syndrome. |
| | *(Withdrawal)* | Tremulousness; **seizures and hyperthermia in severe cases.** | Clouded sensorium, impaired concentration, and disorientation. | Acute brain syndrome—often with agitation and visual or auditory hallucinations. |
| Bromides. | | Drowsiness, coma, weakness, aches and pains, dysarthria, ataxia, rash (in 25 to 30%), cyanosis (with analgesic compounds containing acetanilid), changing neurologic signs, including **focal hyperreflexia and hyporeflexia;** dehydration. | Usually depressed, with impairment of concentration and orientation. Less frequently, there is no clouding of sensorium. | **May mimic alcoholic hallucinosis, delirium, or (especially in the young) florid paranoid schizophrenia.** |
| Cough Syrups. | | No specific signs. | Variously affected. Usually somewhat depressed, at times markedly so, with confusion, disorientation, impaired concentration. | Perceptual distortions occur, as with the hallucinogens, but there is apparently a higher incidence of primary visual hallucinations, as opposed to illusory distortions. Fea- |

USEFUL DRUGS AND OTHER SUBSTANCES: DIFFERENTIATION AND TREATMENT

| *General Description* | *Course* | *Treatment* | *Laboratory Diagnosis* |
|---|---|---|---|
| Amphetamine abuse most common among young bohemians, women trying to lose weight, truck drivers, and night workers. Wyamine or Dristan inhalers are often used by prisoners. **Amphetamine abusers develop massive tolerance; doses between 200 and 1,000 mg/day are the rule.** | Patients characteristically enter a period of lassitude, sleepiness, and depression after discontinuation of the drug, but there is no true withdrawal syndrome. Clearing usually occurs within 5 to 50 days, but in schizophrenics acutely psychotic from amphetamines it may take much longer. | Psychiatric hospitalization is usually required. Visitors should be watched carefully to keep the patient from obtaining drugs. Acidification of the urine with ammonium chloride will hasten excretion. **Depression is common during clearing phase, and there is risk of suicide.** | Amphetamine in the urine may be determined by Connell's modification of methyl orange method, by paper chromatography, or by gas chromatography. |
| Agitation, confusion, hallucination, and paranoid delusions with physical signs as noted. **These patients may give a history of LSD ingestion, since anticholinergic compounds are sometimes sold as LSD.** | Clears within 2 or 3 days. | Withdrawal of drug. Sedation if required. | Paper chromatography. |
| Overdose characteristically presents picture of a straightforward sedation and depressed level of consciousness but may also present picture of intense aggressive behavior in which patient appears acutely and intensely inebriated. | Clearing rate depends on dose taken (usually within 24 to 48 hrs.). The constellation of inebriation and aggressive behavior clears after a night's sleep. | For overdose: supportive care guided by usual medical principles or, depending on severity, hemodialysis. For inebriation syndrome: hospitalization, psychiatric observation, restraint if needed, nonbarbiturate sedation if required. | Paper chromatography (urine). |
| **Syndrome resembling DT's may go on with unpredictable rapidity to seizures and death. Withdrawal should be suspected as an etiology, especially in the young, and in absence of alcoholism history.** Nurses and physicians are especially suspect. | Course depends totally on adequacy of treatment. | Prompt replacement with same preparation originally taken, in doses adequate to control symptoms (up to 1.5 gm/day of short-acting barbiturates). **Gradual reduction, by 10% daily of dose taken.** For acute emergencies, IV sodium amobarbital may be required. | None. |
| In simple intoxication the patient appears dull, sluggish, forgetful, and may be tremulous, uncoordinated, and have sluggish pupils. Patients may have auditory hallucinations in a setting of clear consciousness, be delirious, or become grossly paranoid. | Clearing occurs in four to 40 days. Some symptoms usually persist for over two weeks. **During this time, marked fluctuation in status, independent of serum bromide level, is the rule.** | Hydration and replacement of bromide with chloride: oral sodium chloride (up to 4 gm/4 hrs.), supplemented by saline (up to 4,000 ml/day); or ammonium chloride in doses up to 8 gm/day. **Addition of Mercuhydrin® (2 ml IM every 2 to 3 days) speeds excretion of the bromide ion.** | Serum bromides usually over 150 mg%. Bromide ion is detectable in urine. |
| Abusers generally take one to two bottles to obtain the desired effect. | Pharmacologic action appears to vary, lasting 6 to 18 hrs. Little is known of prolonged adverse effects. | **Observation for respiratory depression should be instituted if the patient is somnolent.** | Paper chromatography. |

TABLE 40—*Continued*

| *Compound* | *Physical Signs* | *Level of Consciousness* | *Formal Psychiatric Aspects* |
|---|---|---|---|
| | | Some patients anecdotally report feelings of CNS stimulation, but these may be idiosyncratic. | tures of organic mental syndrome may be prominent. |
| Halogenated hydrocarbons: glue, gasoline, cleaning fluids. | Tinnitus, **epileptiform seizures,** diplopia. | Somewhat depressed, but intensity of depression may vary. Paradoxical hyperactivity is frequent. | *Glue:* Lightheadedness, feelings like alcoholic intoxication, frightening visual hallucinations in about 50%. *Gasoline:* Transitory visual hallucinations, feelings of lightness, distortion of shapes, colors, space. *Cleaning fluids:* Dreamlike reverie and vivid imagery with eyes closed. |
| | | PSYCHOTIC STATES ASSOCIATED WITH THE USE OF HALLUCINOGENS, | |
| Hallucinogens **(chemical):** lysergic acid diethylamide (LSD), mescaline, psilocybin, dimethyltryptamine (DMT), diethyltryptamine (DET). | **Prominent pupillary dilation,** mild tachycardia. It has been anecdotally reported that LSD stimulates uterine contraction late in pregnancy. Chromosome breaks have been reported in human leukocytes cultured with LSD 25. | **Usually hyperalert, especially to environmental and interpersonal cues, but patients may show preoccupation with perceptual distortions.** | **Patients may show any psychiatric symptomatology, typically colored by the LSD experience; also preponderance of visual phenomena, depersonalization, and body image distortions.** Also present are changes in mood (euphoric, transcendental, or fearful), flight of ideas, distractibility, difficulty in grasping meaning of complex sentences with, at times, incoherence. |
| Hallucinogens **(natural):** peyote, morning glory seeds. | Same as with chemical hallucinogens. Nausea and vomiting may occur early in the experience. | Patient may appear somewhat unresponsive because of general discomfort from GI side effects; also, with morning glory seeds, some of the active constituents have a sedating effect. | Same as with chemical hallucinogens. Morning glory seeds sometimes produce a tendency to withdrawn behavior. |
| Datura suaveolens ("angel's trumpet"), Datura stramonium | *See* pages 544-545. | | |
| Marihuana or hashish (called "pot," "hash," "grass," "tea," etc). | **Dilation of pupils, though less intense than that seen with hallucinogens.** Increased hunger often occurs. | Both stimulation and sedation are reported. **Usually, stimulation occurs initially, mild sedation supervenes.** | Perceptual distortions (color or design), body image disturbances, depersonalization, distortion of time sense, and change in thought processes similar to those seen with hallucinogens occur, but are generally of |

| *General Description* | *Course* | *Treatment* | *Laboratory Diagnosis* |
|---|---|---|---|
| Glue intoxication is usually seen in preadolescent age groups. | The course is one of transient intoxication. However, medical sequelae are a possibility. | **Liver and kidney function should be evaluated to rule out damage. Blood should be monitored to rule out the possibility of aplastic anemia.** | None. |

MARIHUANA, AND SIMILAR AGENTS: DIFFERENTIATION AND TREATMENT*

| *General Description* | *Course* | *Treatment* | *Laboratory Diagnosis* |
|---|---|---|---|
| Acute paranoid states; acute confusional states; panic; fear of permanent change. **Homicidal or suicidal actions have occurred.** | Rapid recovery, usually within three days. | Requires only hospitalization, a supportive environment, sympathetic nursing, reassurance that symptoms result from drug ingestion. | Gas chromatography is required to identify chemical hallucinogens. |
| **Spontaneous return of perceptual distortions or feeling of depersonalization without further drug ingestion.** | May occur with intensity and frequency varying between the inconsequential and the severely incapacitating **for up to one year.** | Recurrent LSD reactions are minimally affected by phenothiazines. | |
| Chronic anxiety syndrome; psychotic states. | **Chronic anxiety syndrome may last many months after last LSD ingestion.** | Chronic anxiety is minimally responsive to phenothiazines. Psychoses respond to therapy similarly to non-drug-related psychoses. **LSD *antagonists:* Chlorpromazine in individualized doses, or sodium succinate (6 to 10 gm, IV over 10 min) can overcome a first LSD experience for several hours. Also Valium, and nicotinic acid (200 mg, IV).** | |
| Behavioral and psychiatric effects are the same as with chemical hallucinogens. Adverse reactions probably follow the same pattern, but this has not been definitively proved. | The same as with chemical hallucinogens. | The same as with chemical hallucinogens. | None at present. |
| Effects are more intense when the stronger, resinous preparations (hashish) are used; these can last over five hours when drug is eaten. Adverse reactions seem to occur less frequently than with hallucino- | Acute paranoid or depersonalization states usually clear as pharmacologic action abates. Chronic psychoses are not often seen. IV use can | Acute reactions should probably be treated in much the same way as acute reactions to hallucinogens. | Gas chromatography. |

TABLE 40—*Continued*

| *Compound* | *Physical signs* | *Level of Consciousness* | *Formal Psychiatric Aspects* |
|---|---|---|---|
| | | | lesser intensity. **Paranoid ideation is frequent.** |
| Nutmeg and mace. | Dry mouth, severe thirst, headache, tachycardia, flushing, constriction of pupils, hypothermia, abdominal pain, nausea, agitation. **Death has been known to occur in children.** | Generally depressed, with dizziness and marked impairment of concentration. **This may go on to full-blown delirium, with agitation, disorientation, and incoherence.** | Psychiatric effects are stated to be similar to those of marihuana. Delirious states and florid paranoid reactions have been noted. |
| Dried banana peel | Headache; GI symptoms of nausea, vomiting; abdominal pains and diarrhea are occasionally reported. | No sedation. | Mild alteration in intensity of color perception; altered time and tactile senses are reported, but almost universally described as mild or even barely perceptible. **Suggestion may play a great role.** |
| Cocaine (called "snow" or, when combined with heroin, "speedball"). | Pupillary dilation. Hyperthermia may be present. | Stimulation, with excitement and euphoria. | **Characteristically presents as a paranoid psychosis in a setting of clear consciousness (similar to amphetamine psychosis).** Paranoid ideation is prominent, and auditory and visual hallucinations often occur. **Tactile hallucinations (e.g., formication) are characteristic.** |

teratogenic influences can be made by easy methods. The recent literature is replete with after-the-fact reports of congenital abnormalities in infants whose mothers had taken one or another drug during pregnancy. Such reports supply numerators without denominators in that they do not record the number of cases in which use of that particular drug did not produce malformations; neither do they take into account the natural incidence of abnormalities (2% of all births). Nor do animal experiments, as yet, provide an easier approach to the problem. Attempts at comparing acute toxicity in newborn versus adult animals have often given equivocal results and many discrepancies. If a large-scale long-range all-out effort by physicians was made to keep *total* records of medications taken by pregnant women, including drugs sold "over the counter," and these complete tabulations were made retrievable, the desired information on the teratogenic effects of various drugs might soon be acquired with a considerable degree of certainty. A recent survey has shown that the average gravida uses six prescribed and four over-the-counter drugs.

The doublet "Don't make mirth of the afterbirth" is outdated, since the placental "barrier" is mythical. Every drug given to the mother by any route can be expected to be found in the fetus as soon as placentation is established. However, "placental panic" need not replace "placental pride," for in about 92 per cent of all pregnancies that terminate in a viable baby, the placenta has performed admirably. The final proof of whether a drug is likely to be teratogenic in man must be sought in man.

| *General Description* | *Course* | *Treatment* | *Laboratory Diagnosis* |
|---|---|---|---|
| gens. **Acute paranoid reactions and depersonalization states are most often seen.** | produce serious toxic effects. | | |
| The equivalent of two grated nutmegs is usually taken, but doses as large as three ounces have been reported. **Three or four hours often pass before the onset of symptoms. Often, only physical effects are experienced;** may be taken by prisoners denied access to other drugs. | Signs of intoxication usually remit within 24 to 48 hrs., **but feelings of detachment and unreality have persisted for as long as 60 hrs.** | Supportive medical care, if physical signs predominate. If psychiatric manifestations are the presenting complaint, hospitalization. Restraint if needed. **Supportive environment and, if required, nonspecific sedation for the first 72 hrs.** | None. |
| Usually a mild euphoria or feelings of tranquilization. | Intoxication usually lasts less than two hours. | None usually required. Psychotic reactions may be treated as *de novo* psychosis. Panic in response to perceptual alterations should probably be treated with simple reassurance as to their transitory nature. | None at present. |
| Patients may show symptoms of amphetamine abuse, since cocaine is costly and amphetamine is often substituted by cocaine users. | Rapid clearing of pharmacologic effects. Psychotic episodes may persist for longer periods. | Withholding of the drug; hospitalization if indicated by overall psychiatric status. | Some cocaine may be excreted unchanged in the urine. Paper chromatography. |

## ENVIRONMENTAL FETAL AND INFANT POLLUTANTS

Environmental pollutants affecting the fetus are manifold and complex, and assorted heavy metals are probably the leading and most serious pollutants. Trace metals may enter and be stored in the human body by several mechanisms. Accumulation may result from inborn metabolic errors of various transport systems. A classic example is Wilson's disease (progressive hepato-lenticular degeneration) in which copper accumulates in the liver and brain.

A second route of accumulation may be impaired excretion because of a concomitant disease such as renal failure, or because of developmental immaturity. This route is important with the fetus due to the varying rates in maturation of detoxifying and excretory systems, as well as the extent of environmental exposure.

The third route of accumulation is through ingestion or absorption of large amounts from contaminated food and water.

Known sources of mercury contamination of our environment are discharges of chlor-alkali plants, mercury catalysts in industry, fungicides used in the pulp and paper industry and in seed treatments and residues from the burning of fossil fuels. Other miscellaneous sources include medical and scientific wastes, naturally occurring geologic formations, and the processing of raw materials containing mercury. Marine paint may also add mercury to water. Agreement is general that alkylated mercury compounds are significantly more toxic than non-alkylated mercury compounds. Toxicologically and environmentally, the most important alkylated compound is methyl mercury.

Once inorganic mercury is released into the environment, methylation can occur in the

TABLE 41
MEDICATION AND THERAPY WHICH MAY AFFECT THE FETUS AND NEWBORN

| *Maternal and Newborn Medication* | *Fetal or Neonatal Effect* |
|---|---|
| Oral progestogens<br>Androgens<br>Estrogens | Masculinization and advanced bone age |
| Cortisone acetate (Cortogen® Acetate, Cortone® Acetate) | Anomalies: cleft palate (?) |
| Potassium iodide<br>Propylthiouracil<br>Methimazole (Tapazole®) | Goiter and mental retardation |
| Iophenoxic acid (Teridax®) | Elevation of PBI |
| Sodium aminopterin<br>Methotrexate® (Aminopterin) | Multiple anomalies and abortion |
| Alcohol (excessive) | Teratogenic<br>Low birth weight<br>Fetal alcohol syndrome |
| Radioactive drugs; radiation | Teratogenic<br>Carcinogenic<br>Thyroid function |
| Chlorambucil (Leukeran®) | |
| Bishydroxycoumarin (Dicumarol®)<br>Ethyl biscoumacetate (Tromexan®) Ethyl Acetate)<br>Sodium warfarin (Coumadin® Sodium, Panwarfin®, Prothromadin® | Fetal death; hemorrhage |
| Salicylates (large amounts) | Neonatal bleeding |
| Streptomycin* | Possible eighth nerve deafness |
| Sulfonamides (all types) | Kernicterus |
| Chloramphenicol (Chloromycetin®) | "Grey" syndrome; death |
| Sodium novobiocin (Albamycin® Sodium, Cathomycin® Sodium) | Hyperbilirubinemia |
| Erythromycin (Ilosone®) | Liver damage (?) |
| Nitrofurantoin (Furadantin®) | Hemolysis |
| Tetracyclines | Inhibition of bone growth<br>Discoloration and hypoplasia of teeth |
| Vitamin K analogues (in excess) | Hyperbilirubinemia |
| Ammonium chloride | Acidosis |
| Intravenous fluids (in excess) | Electrolyte abnormalities |
| Reserpine (Rauloydin®, Raurine®, Rau-Sed®, Reserpoid®, Sandril®, Serfin®, Serpasil®, Serpate®, Vio-Serpine®) | Stuffy nose; respiratory obstruction<br>Prolonged administration to patients with Huntington's chorea damages the reticular formation of the medulla oblongata |
| Hexamethonium bromide (Bistrium® Bromide) | Neonatal ileus |
| Heroin and morphine | Neonatal death |
| Phenobarbital (in excess) | Neonatal bleeding; death |
| Smoking | Birth of small babies |
| Sulphonylurea derivatives (Oral hypoglycemic agents) | Anomalies (?) |
| Phenformin hydrochloride (DBI) | Lactic acidosis (?) |
| Phenothiazines | Respiratory depression; hyperbilirubinemia (?)<br>Extrapyramidal disturbances |
| Meprobamate (Equanil®, Wyseals, Meprospan®, Meprotabs®, Miltown®) | Retarded development (?) |
| Chloroquine phosphate (Aralen® Phosphate) | Retinal damage or death (?)<br>Thrombocytopenia |
| Mepivacaine (Carbocaine®) | Neonatal asphyxia and convulsions from faulty maternal caudal anesthesia |
| Quinine | Amelia: multiple organ defects |
| Thalidomide | Phocomelia; death, hearing loss |
| Vaccination, smallpox | Fetal vaccinia |
| Vaccination, influenza | Increased anti-A and B titers in mothers |
| Antihistamines | Anomalies (?); infertility (?) |
| Thiazide diuretics | Thrombocytopenia |

TABLE 41—*Continued*

| *Maternal and Newborn Medication* | *Fetal or Neonatal Effect* |
|---|---|
| Oxygen (prematures only) | Retrolental fibroplasia |
| Digitalis (overdosage) | Myocardial toxicity |
| Breast milk | Hyperbilirubinemia (pregnanediol-steroid inhibitor of hepatic glucuronyl transferase) |
| Methyl mercury (food) | Teratogenic effects; fetal death |

*Other antibiotics that are ototoxic.

sediment of waterways through bacterial action. Methyl mercury then becomes available to the food chain, reaching humans via edible fish. Wild and domestic animals fed contaminated grains are another source of mercury contamination.

Since methyl mercury has a long retention in the human body, propensity for central nervous system damage, and known toxic effect on developing tissue, mercury poses a particular hazard for the fetus. Methyl mercury crosses the placenta easily, and may attain a 30 per cent higher concentration in fetal erythrocytes than in maternal ones.

A relationship between shellfish mercury contamination in Minamata Bay, Japan, and a cerebral palsy-like illness now seems well established. Six per cent of children born in the villages near Minamata Bay over the five-year period ending in 1959 were afflicted with mild to moderate spasticity, chorea, ataxia, coarse tremors, seizures, severe intellectual deficiencies in various combinations. Two autopsied patients showed depletion of cerebellar granular cells and damage to the cerebral cortex of a nonspecific nature, similar to the lesions seen in the adult form of fatal Minamata disease. Dying infants had high levels of mercury in their brains, livers, and kidneys approximating the levels found in adults dying of mercury poisoning. Living children who were studied had an abnormally high content of mercury in their hair (range 15 to 412 μg/gm). The dietary shellfish were believed contaminated by the effluent of a plastics plant.

Mercury can be excreted into breast milk and this can be a source of this metal for the suckling infant, especially when the mother has had long exposure to high environmental levels of mercury. Hence an acquired as well as a congenital pathogenesis may be invoked for "fetal" Minamata disease.

Further implication of methyl mercury's role as harmful to the fetal central nervous system comes from the report of an incidence of mercury poisoning during pregnancy in New Mexico. The mother's toxicity occurred from the ingestion of contaminated pork. This meat came from pigs which had been fed seed grain previously treated with a methyl mercury fungicide. The resultant fullterm boy had severe tremors which persisted for several days. His urinary mercury level during the first day of life was 2.7 parts per million (ppm). This is 100 times more than the level for normal adult urine. At six weeks of age, the infant was hypertonic and irritable, though mercury could no longer be detected in his urine. At eight months of age, he began to have myoclonic seizures, and was now hypotonic, irritable, grossly retarded and probably cortically blind. This baby had never been breast fed, providing more support that this case was actually intrauterine mercury poisoning. The mother was asymptomatic despite having elevated mercury levels during her third trimester. Ingestion of the contaminated pork was thought to have occurred between the third and sixth months of gestation.

Lead, while apparently less toxic for the fetus than mercury, may have greater implications for future generations since lead is more ubiquitous and the effects of environmentally encountered concentrations may be more subtle. For over 100 years it has been know that women employed in occupations which have heavy exposures to lead may give birth to stunted and neurologically abnormal

TABLE 42
CATEGORICAL EFFECTS OF MATERNAL DRUGS ON THE FETUS AND NEWBORN

| *Teratogens* | *Fetal Death* | *Adaption, Extra-Uterine Life* | *Withdrawal* | *Metabolic* | *Hematological* |
|---|---|---|---|---|---|
| Alcohol* | Chloral hydrate* | Anesthetic agents | Alcohol* | Alcohol (IV and oral) | Alcohol |
| Anticonvulsants | Chlorpropamide | Barbiturates | Amphetamines | Chlorpropamide | Barbiturates |
| Cancer chemotherapeutics | Dicumarol | Bromide | Anticonvulsants | Corticosteroids | Dicumarol |
| Corticosteroid | Ergot | Cholinesterase inhibitor | Barbiturates | Diuretics | Dilantin |
| Estrogens | Lead | Curare | Drugs of abuse | Hypotonic IV fluids | Diuretic |
| Hallucinogenic agents | Mercury | Diazepam | Glutethimide | Oxytocin | Hemorrhage, anemia platelet dysfunction |
| Lead | Salicylates* | Hexamethonium | Propoxyphene | Electrolyte imbalance | Hykinone |
| Mercury | | Lithium | Psychotropics | Hypoglycemia | Local anesthetic agents† |
| Ovulatory agents | THYROID | Magnesium sulfate | | Insulin | Oxytocin |
| Progestens | Iodine | Narcotics | | Tolbutamide | Promethazine |
| Psychotropics | Radioactive drugs | Oxytocin (diuretic IV fluids) | | | Quinine |
| Quinine | Radiopaque dye | Paraldehyde | | | Salicylates |
| Radiation | Thioureas | Phenothiazine | | | Sulfa drugs |
| Radioisotopes | | Pyridoxine | | | Sulfonamides |
| Tetracyclines | | Reserpine | | | Thioureas |
| Thalidomide | | Salicylates* | | | |

| *Carcinogens* | *Birth Weight* | *Seizures* | *Growth and Development* | *Mentality* | *Sexual Development* |
|---|---|---|---|---|---|
| Cancer chemotherapeutics | Alcohol* | Local anesthetic agents | Alcohol* | Alcohol* | Cancer chemotherapeutics |
| Hormones | Cigarette smoking | Magnesium sulfate | Anticonvulsants | Carbon monoxide | |
| Radiation | Corticosteroids | Oxytocin (diuretics IV fluids) | Drugs of abuse | Mercury | |
| Radioactive drugs | Drugs of abuse | Pyridoxine | | Radiation | |
| | Ovulatory agents | | | Radioisotopes | |
| | | | | Thioureas | |

* = Excessive dosages or amounts
† = Methemoglobinemia

infants. They also have had a higher stillbirth and miscarriage rate. The normal dietary intake of lead is 0.2-0.4 mg. Water is not significantly contaminated but lead pollutants in air from the burning of lead alkyl additives (anti-knock ingredients) in automotive fuels are a serious problem. In 1968, more than 500 million pounds of lead were introduced in the atmosphere from this source, and the lead concentration in the atmosphere of some urban areas is rising by five per cent per year (inhaled lead has a tenfold more toxic potential than ingested lead). Infants and growing children living in old, rundown housing, where layer after layer of lead paint has been applied for years, are particularly prone to lead poisoning from pica, and from contaminated food and water. An average-sized peeling of old paint may contain 100 mg or more of lead. In addition, minority children most likely living in such areas are often victims (approximately 15% in healthy American black males and only 1% in whites) of Glucose-6-Phosphate Dehydrogenase deficiency (G-6-PD), and, unfortunately, it has been documented that they have an increase of blood lead levels of 12% when intimately exposed.

Our environment is thoroughly contaminated with lead. It may be present in drinking water, milk, canned fruit juice, vegetation growing beside roads, toothpaste, air particulates, dirt, pencils, cigarette ash, newsprint (particularly tinted pages or sections), putty and numerous other materials in everyday use. The cumulative effect of these lead sources may be biologically significant.

Significant amounts of lead in bulk, pasteurized, homogenized milk and in canned milk products have been found. Breast milk, on the other hand, contains little or no detectable lead. Very high lead levels also occur in canned fruit juices and beverages. There is strong evidence that the containers are the major lead source, although some degree of contamination likely occurs in processing procedures (multiple steps) as well.

At contaminated levels, milk products and other foodstuffs can make a very large contribution to the child's daily lead intake. Moreover, ingestion of lead from foodstuffs rather than from paint raises some disturbing questions which so far have not been adequately answered.

1. How much exposure to lead is safe for young children? Whereas leaded paint is primarily ingested by children aged 15 to 36 months, processed milk products are fed to newborn infants, and fruit juices are fed to children aged 3 months and more. Since brain growth is most rapid during the first year of life, early absorption of lead may be particularly damaging to the central nervous system. Until this question is fully investigated, we will not have reliable information on a reasonable daily permissible intake.
2. What are the typical daily lead intakes from all sources for young children in various environments? How much is accumulated? What are the effects of, say, a moderate lead intake from foodstuffs for two years followed by ingestion of "normally safe" amounts of leaded paint?
3. How efficiently is lead in foodstuffs absorbed in the gastrointestinal system? Does calcium have a "protective" effect, in which case lead in milk may not be as toxic as lead in nondairy foods? Would iron fortified diets also have "protective" effects, as suggested by studies in weanling rats?
4. How rapidly is lead in foodstuffs absorbed, excreted and stored? Lead in foodstuffs is probably released rapidly into the bloodstream and with rapid storage this would result in transient elevated blood levels shortly after ingestion. If so, these children are much less likely to be detected than children who continuously ingest leaded paint and so have increased storage of lead in bone and relatively constant elevated blood levels.

Within the past 25 years the use of cadmium in industry has been increasing. High contents of cadmium have been reported in shellfish, seafoods, roasted peanuts and filter cigarette smoke. Of considerable interest is the finding of extremely high percentages of cadmium in some commercial phosphate fertilizers, and high levels of cadmium in plants grown after using these fertilizers. Furthermore, the cadmium content of green plants is inversely related to the distance between plants and heavily travelled highways, implying that automobile traffic may be another source of cadmium pollution.

As recently as 1969, it was believed that cadmium was absent from the fullterm human fetus. Current fetal tissue measurements using more precise techniques prove that cadmium can cross the placenta and is retained in the human fetus, reaching levels of 50 μg/kg BW or more. The concentration is maximal in the liver. Human breast milk also contains cadmium, but to a minimal degree. Animal studies have shown cadmium to be selectively retained within mammary tissues and thus prevented from incorporation in milk; this mechanism may help to protect the suckling newborn. Cadmium produces teratogenic effects in the hamster (facial, cleft and forelimb anomalies).

Animal experimentation suggests that cadmium may compete with zinc in some organs and in some enzyme systems. If this is true for humans, then a plethora of effects might be expected from cadmium in fetal tissues since zinc is one of nature's most common cofactors in biologic enzyme systems. Of pertinence in this regard is the report of environmental water pollution with both cadmium, lead and zinc in Japan. The resulting disease ("itai-itai" or ouch-ouch disease) is characterized by severe osteomalacia and renal tubular defects, occurring mostly in post menopausal women. The staples of the local diet, rice and soybean, were shown to have an average concentration of cadmium zinc, and lead, approximately twice as great as the same foods in areas where this disease is not endemic. It is theoretically possible that a high concentration of zinc could prevent many of cadmium's inhibitory effects on zinc-dependent enzyme systems. The role of the high lead concentrations in this situation is unclear.

Titanium is the third most common element to be found in the earth's crust. Biologically, titanium would be expected to be a strong reducing agent because of its tendency to lose electrons. Some algae are able to concentrate titanium up to 10,000 times, thereby having the potential to introduce large quantities of this metal into the food chain. Although titanium is generally believed nontoxic, all of the acute toxicity studies have dealt only with water insoluble titanium salts. It has been documented that half of studied fetuses and newborns have some demonstrable titanium in their tissues, confirming transplacental transport of titanium.

Nickel, widely used in industry, is found in highest concentrations in wood and steel products. It attains extremely high concentrations in cigarette smoke. In the newborn, nickel is found in highest concentrations in the lung and gastrointestinal tract. Throughout life, lung concentrations increase while gastrointestinal levels remain constant. This suggests that airborne sources of nickel are the main source of human contamination, perhaps due to smoking. Nickel is regarded as having very little toxicity. No fetal effects are known to occur.

Tin, like nickel, is widespread due to its use in industry. There are sizable amounts of tin in the air of many North American cities, less so in suburban air. Tin has never been found in the fetus or newborn, raising the question whether tin crosses the human placenta.

Vanadium, another ubiquitous metal, is concentrated in many lipids of plant and animal origin. It has been found in only one infant less than six weeks old, and never in any studied fetus. A toxic effect for vanadium on the fetus would not be predicted.

Niobium (formerly Columbium), present in soil, seawater, plants and animals, has no current wide use in industry. It has never been found in the human fetus or newborn. It has, however, been found in rat breast milk and newborn rat tissues after large amounts were fed to the mother, proving experimentally that transplacental transport is possible when maternal exposure is great.

Large amounts of arsenic are measurable in the air or water of many large American cities. Arsenic exists in two valence states. The pentavalent form is nontoxic, whereas the trivalent form is extremely dangerous. There is no reliable way currently to determine the valence state in which arsenic is present in a given sample. Since trivalent arsenic is a potent inhibitor of thiol containing enzymes, such as ketoneoxides and succinic, malic and lactic dehydrogenases, the expected effects of fetal toxicity from trivalent arsenic would be stillbirth or abortion. Obviously the pentavalent form must be the one most prevalent in the environment, but the ratio is not known.

Numerous other, but not well documented, environmental causes of fetal morbidity and birth defects are being discussed by the news media more often than in the medical literature. Some of these are:

1. The well-known herbicide, 2,4,5-Trichlorophenoxyacetic acid; (2,4,5-T) is teratogenic and fetocidal in two strains of mice and one strain of rats.
2. Nitrilotriacetic acid (NTA), as an alternative to phosphate compounds in detergents, increases the toxicity of mercury and cadmium in water, contributing to an increase in fetal abnormalities and death in mice and rats.
3. Food additives of all kinds including cyclamates, saccharin, nitrites, monosodium glutamate (MSG), food colorings (coal-tar dyes), have all been implicated in producing toxic effects in fetal animals or being carcinogenic.
4. Polychlorinated biphenyls (PCB) have wide industrial uses (electric wires, motors, plasticizers, etc.) because of their high dielectric constant and their thermal and chemical stabilities. PCB contamination is found to be almost universal, including human milk, human adipose tissue, and brain and liver of small children. Little is known about the toxic effects of PCB in humans, but an endemic poisoning ("yusho") by rice oil contaminated with PCB has been reported in Japan.
5. Birth defects linked to intensity of airport noise.
6. The recent discovery of heavily contaminated water sources with asbestos (Lake Superior) is of much public concern. It is a well-known carcinogen, and mesothelioma of the pleura and peritoneum has been linked to asbestos. The drinking of contaminated asbestos water over a period of many years raises the question of its chronic effect on the gastrointestinal tract. The fact, however, that no dust deposition of coal miners or hard-rock miners have been recorded in the GI tract or mesenteric nodes suggests that in man transmigration of ingested asbestos particles through the intestinal mucosa is not likely.
7. The average pregnant smoker has nearly twice the risk of giving birth to a low birth weight infant than does the nonsmoker. There is also a strong probable causal association between cigarette smoking and higher fetal and infant mortality.
8. There is sufficient data to establish that maternal alcoholism can cause serious aberrant fetal development. The prognosis for babies born to chronically alcoholic women is so bleak that a Seattle investigator says early termination of such pregnancies should receive serious consideration (*see* Fetal Alcohol Syndrome).

## DRUGS AND CHEMICALS IN BREAST MILK

Unbelievable as it may seem, available information derived from clinical and laboratory research about the excretion of chemicals and drugs in breast milk is scanty. There seem to be several factors responsible for this: It is almost impossible to carry out experimental observations on nursing mothers; the studies on animals are complicated; and there is great difficulty in extrapolating the data from animal to human studies. Because of the steady flow of new drugs from pharmaceutical laboratories and the ever-increasing variety of chemicals to which one is exposed—such as DDT, smoking, oral contraceptives and the like—the physician must be better informed about the available facts and become aware of new clinical discoveries and research on the risks to nursing infants from maternal medication and chemical exposure.

Fortunately, not all drugs are able to pass into the mother's milk in significant amounts. Some do, and in proportions that can jolt the baby. How much reaching the baby depends upon a number of factors. Despite the well-known fact that all products ingested by the mother are excreted in the milk in some form, general knowledge concerning excretion of drugs and chemicals in milk is quite limited. The excretion of some chemicals into the breast milk may be considerable, whereas with others only minute amounts may be found. The passage of a drug across the membrane between plasma and milk is influenced by its $pK_a$ or degree of ionization, its solubility in fats and water and the poorly understood transport mechanism. Ionized forms pass only slowly into these secretions. The concentration of acidic compounds in milk is lower than that in plasma. Nonelectrolytes, such as ethanol, urea and antipyrine, readily enter milk and reach the same concentration as in plasma independently of the pH of the milk.

One of the most searching projects about drugs and breast milk was reported from Copenhagen by F. Rasmussen in 1966. He studied the passage of drugs from blood plasma to milk in goats and cows while almost constant plasma levels were maintained by continuous intravenous infusion. Each of the drugs tested—sulfonamides, antibiotics, barbiturates, antipyrine, ethanol and urea—exhibited a constant ratio between the concentration in ultrafiltrate of milk and ultrafiltrate of blood plasma. This ratio was found to be independent of both the plasma level and the volume of milk produced during the experimental period. Therefore, the passage can be considered to have taken place by diffusion. The ratio can be changed, however, by altering the pH of the milk. The ratio of partially ionized drugs of an acidic nature is always equal to or below 1 at the normal pH of the milk (6.5 to 6.8); the ratio rises towards 1 when the pH of milk is changed towards the pH of the blood plasma (7.4). For alkaline drugs, the ratio is 1 or above, and reduced towards 1 at rising pH of the milk. At the difference of pH which exists between blood plasma and milk, this unequal distribution of weak electrolytes may be due to differences in the degree of ionization in plasma and milk respectively. Rasmussen concluded that the transfer of drugs from plasma to milk takes place by diffusion of the un-ionized, non-protein-bound fraction. The diffusion of drugs of a weak electrolyte character across the gastric, intestinal and colonic epithelia (as well as the sweat and salivary glands) appeared similar to that taking place through the mammary gland epithelium.

Like the other biological membranes, the mammary gland epithelium should be thought of as a lipid barrier with water-filled pores which can be penetrated only by water-soluble low-molecular compounds, such as urea. The un-ionized fraction of weak electrolytes of acid character constitutes a larger proportion of total content in ultrafiltrate milk than in ultrafiltrate plasma. Thus, the total concentration of such a drug will be higher in the milk than in the plasma.

Evidence regarding the physiological and endocrine factors in the initiation and maintenance of lactation is contradictory. Species differences are varied and important. Normally, lactation begins about the time of parturition or shortly thereafter. The synchronization of the onset of lactation with parturition has been explained by assuming that estrogen or progesterone produced during pregnancy inhibits the liberation of lactogen by the pituitary. Withdrawal of these hormones after parturition, therefore, permits lactogen production and induces the

TABLE 43
DRUGS EXCRETED IN HUMAN MILK

Alcohol
Allergens
Ambenonium chloride (Mytelase)
Aminophylline (theophylline with ethylenediamine)
Amphetamines
  Amphetamine sulfate (Benzedrine and numerous other trade names) and other salts of amphetamine
Dextroamphetamine sulfate
  (Dexedrine and numerous other trade names) and other salts of *d*-amphetamine
Analgesics (non-narcotic)
  Acetaminophen (Amdil, Anelix, Apamide, Elixodyne, Febrolin, Fendon, Lestemp, Lyteca syrup, Metalid, Nacetyl, Nebs, Tempra, Tylenol)
  Aspirin
  Dextropropoxyphene hydrochloride (Darvon)
  Phenacetin
  Sodium salicylate
Analgesics (narcotic)
  Mefenamic (Ponstel)
  Methadone hydrochloride (Adanon, Althose syrup, Dolophine)
  Morphine (trace)
  Heroin
Anesthetics
  Chloroform
  Cyclopropane
  Ether
Antibiotics and chemotherapeutics
  Chloramphenicol (Chloromycetin)
  Cycloserine (Seromycin)
  Erythromycin
  Flagyl
  Furadantin
  Isoniazid (more than twenty trade names)
  Mandelic acid
  Neomycin sulfate (Mycifradin, Neobiotic)
  Nitrofurantoins
  Novobiocin (Albamycin, Cathomycin)
  Para-aminosalicylic acid and salts (numerous trade names)
  Penicillin
    G
    Benzyl
  Rifampin
  Streptomycin
  Sulfonamides (breast concentration may exceed maternal plasma level; this represents a small oral dose for infant)
    sulfamethoxazole (Gantanol)
    sulfadimethoxine (Madribon)
  Tetracyclines
Antihistaminics (most pass into milk)
  Brompheniramine (Dimetane)
  Diphenhydramine hydrochloride (Benadryl)
  Methdilazine (Tacaryl)
Atropine
Barbiturates
  Amobarbital (Amytal)
  Methohexital (Brevital)
  Phenobarbital (Luminal)
  Secobarbital (Seconal)
  Thiopental (Pentothal)
Bishydroxycoumarin (Dicoumarin, Dicourmarol, Dicumarol, Melitoxin)
Bromides
Caffeine
Cortisone
Cyclophosphamide (Cytoxan)
DDT (Chlorophenothane)
Diphenylhydantoin (Dilantin)
Ephedrine and pseudoephedrine
Ergot
Estrogens
Ethyl biscoumacetate (Tromexan)
Heptachlor
Hexachlorobenzene
Imipramine hydrochloride (Tofranil)
Iodides including $^{131}$I
Iopanoic acid (Telepaque)
Isoniazid
Kepone
Laxatives and cathartics
  Aloin
  Calomel (mild mercurous chloride)
  Cascara
  Danthron (Dionone, Dorbane, Istizin)
  Rhubarb (said either not to pass or, conversely, to purge infant)
Levopropoxyphene (Novrad)
Mandelic acid
Mephenoxalone (Trepidone)
Methimazole (Tapazole)
Methocarbamol (Robaxin)
Metals, salts, minerals
  Arsenic
  Calcium
  Chloride
  Copper
  Iodides
  Lead
  Magnesium
  Mercurous chloride (see calomel)
  Mercury
  Phosphate
  Potassium
  Polychlorinated biphenyl (PCB)
  Sodium
  Sulfur
Nicotine
Papaverine
Phenylbutazone (Butazolidin)
Phenytoin (Diphenylhydantoin, Dilantin)
Propylthiouracil
Pseudoephedrine (Sudafed)
Pyrimethamine (Daraprim)
Quinidine
Quinine
Reserpine (many trade names and preparations)
Salicylates
Scopolamine (Hyoscine)
Sedatives
  Barbiturates

TABLE 43—*Continued*
DRUGS EXCRETED IN HUMAN MILK

| | |
|---|---|
| Bromides | Phenaglycodol (Ultran) |
| Chloral hydrate | Reserpine (many trade names) |
| Ethinamate (Valmid) | Trifluoperazine (Stelazine) |
| Sodium chloride | Diazepam (Valium) |
| Thiazides (insignificant amount) | Vitamins |
| Thiouracil | A, $B_1$, $B_{12}$, C, D, E, K |
| Thyroid | Folic acid |
| Tolbutamide | Niacin |
| Tranquilizers | Pantothenic acid |
| Chlorpromazine (Thorazine) | Riboflavin |
| Hydroxyzine (Atarax, Vistaril) | Thiamine |

Synonyms and combinations may be found in Wilson, Charles O. and Jones, Tony E., Eds, *American Drug Index* (Lippincott Co., 1967). Concentrations may be found in Knowles, J.A., "Excretion of Drugs In Milk—A Review," *Journal of Pediatrics, 66*:1068, 1965.

TABLE 44
ANTIMICROBIALS IN BREAST MILK
(MILK-PLASMA RATIO)

| *Antimicrobials* | *Milk-Plasma Ratio* | *Comments* |
|---|---|---|
| Aminosalicylic acid (PAS) | Data not available | Not detectable in milk |
| Ampicillin | Data not available | Maternal use may cause diarrhea and candidiasis in nursing infants; antigenic reaction possible |
| Cephalosporins | 0 | Not detectable in milk |
| Chloromycetin® (chloramphenicol) | 0.05-0.5 | About half is excreted in milk as inactive metabolite; no antibacterial activity at levels found in milk |
| Erythromycin | | |
| Oral | 0.02-0.5 | Trace amounts in breast milk |
| Intravenous | 4-6 | Intravenous form provides 10 times higher levels in milk than oral forms |
| Flagyl® (metronidazole) | 1.0 | Milk levels similar to serum levels, but no significant effects on infant reported |
| Geopen®, Pyopen® (carbenicillin) | Data not available | Milk levels too low for antibiosis; antigenic reaction possible |
| Isoniazid (INH) | 1.0 | Milk levels similar to serum levels, but no adverse effects reported |
| Kantrex® (kanamycin) | Data not available | Possibility of infant ototoxicity suggested |
| Lincocin® (lincomycin) | Data not available | Milk levels insignificant |
| Macrodantin® Furadantin® (nitrofurantoin) | 2.0 | Conflicting reports; drug is excreted in milk but has not been reported as harmful to infants |
| NegGram® (nalidixic acid) | Data not available | Levels usually insignificant; one report of hemolytic anemia in an infant with normal enzyme systems but a uremic mother |

TABLE 44—*Continued*
ANTIMICROBIALS IN BREAST MILK
(MILK-PLASMA RATIO)

| *Antimicrobials* | *Milk-plasma ratio* | *Comments* |
|---|---|---|
| Penicillin | 0.02-0.2 | Milk levels too low for antibiosis but may induce an antigenic response in a susceptible infant |
| Prostaphlin® Bactocill® (oxacillin) | 0 | Not detectable in breast milk |
| Quinine | Data not available | Milk levels insignificant |
| Streptomycin | Data not available | Maternal doses up to 1 gm per day produce no risk of infant ototoxicity; maternal renal impairment may increase milk levels up to 25 times, however, producing infant ototoxicity |
| Sulfonamides | 0.8-0.97 | Neonatal hyperbilirubinemia theoretically possible; hemolytic anemia reported in a G-6PD-deficient infant |
| Symmetrel® (amantadine) | Data not available | May produce sufficient milk levels to cause infant vomiting, skin rash, and urinary retention |
| Tetracyclines | 0.25-1.5 | No adverse effects reported; tooth staining theoretically possible |

From Arthur G. Lipman, reprinted from *Modern Medicine* © 1977 by Harcourt Brace Jovanovich.

onset of lactation. Clinically, for reasons which are not clear, estrogen may either inhibit or stimulate lactation. Estrogen does not prevent the action of lactogen when these hormones are given together, a finding indicating that the steroid hormone acts upon the pituitary and not upon the mammary glands directly. Monkeys given estrogen for long periods begin to lactate. Similarly, young virgin goats or heifers subjected to prolonged treatment with the synthetic estrogen substitute, stilbestrol, begin to lactate, and may produce large quantities of milk. Estrogen increases the lactogen content of the pituitary glands of nonparous or male rats. This action is prevented by simultaneous administration of progesterone. In cows, the volume of milk produced is increased by 30 per cent (with a corresponding increase of solids) by giving thyroxin or thyroglobulin. During lactation the amount of thyrotrophic hormone produced is increased. Lactation may occur in thyroidectomized animals, but the amount of milk is substantially reduced.

Under normal conditions, the amount of milk produced depends to a large extent on sucking, which apparently causes a reflex increase in the secretion of prolactin, and upon the frequent removal of accumulated milk from the gland, which in turn is dependent on the liberation of oxytocin. Lactogen has been used clinically in attempts to increase the milk yield in nursing women, but the results have not been convincing. Probably, deficiencies in milk production are usually caused by factors other than inadequate lactogen.

Little attention has been directed toward drug excretion in the colostrum. During the colostral phase, the mammary gland is thought to be more permeable to a number of solutes. This is borne out by the observations that zinc and iron are present in colostrum at concentrations above those in normal milk.

The composition of milk is determined by the mammary gland acting on its own. There is apparently little or no method of control from outside. Providing there is enough of it, the food of the mother can, in general, be varied to some extent without affecting the composition or volume of milk she produces. However, some deficiencies may be reflected in the milk, for example, deficiencies of the fat-soluble vitamins.

Since some of the fat in milk is derived directly from blood fat, the types of fatty acid one finds in the milk may reflect those in the mother's diet. To this extent, the latter can also affect the milk fat. Thus, abnormal iodized fats may appear in milk.

If the diet is deficient in quantity, the volume of milk is reduced, of course, but it remains equally balanced, for the underfed mother draws on the resources of her own tissues. The importance of this safety phenomenon is exemplified by what happens if the mother is not getting enough calcium. Physiologically, her system places a demand on the body's storehouse of the mineral, the bones. The organic matrix breaks down; the bones become "bendy" and, if the mother's reduced calcium intake lasts long enough, she may become permanently deformed.

One must remember that most, if not all, drugs ingested by a nursing mother are excreted in her milk, but usually in insignificant amounts. Occasionally, however, these drugs can be dangerous to the nursing infant. As examples, methemoglobin was found in a newborn infant whose mother was treated with phenobarbitone (phenobarbital) and phenytoin (diphenylhydantoin, Dilantin®) for epilepsy. This baby did well on donor's breast milk. But when put on his own mother's milk again, while she was still taking Dilantin, he became drowsy and developed a grayish-blue discoloration. However, breast milk and colostrum in another report of epileptic pregnant women on diphenylhydantoin were tested and found to contain lower concentrations than in maternal plasma, and an increase in the maternal plasma did not raise the amount of diphenylhydantoin in breast milk. There were no discernible effects produced in the nursing infants. In 1956, a number of breast-fed infants died in southeast Turkey when their mothers were poisoned by eating seed wheat treated with hexachlorobenzene, a fungistatic agent. Investigation of the Turkish incident revealed a porphyrobilinogen in the urine of affected persons. It is assumed that hexachlorobenzene, or one of its metabolites, was excreted in the mother's milk and poisoned the infants.

Since antibiotics are perhaps the most widely used group of drugs in human and veterinary medicine today, they present a particular problem. Antibiotics found in milk are more of an animal than a human problem, since the marketing of milk containing penicillin is prohibited by federal regulation; but because of the treatment with penicillin of mastitis and other infections in cows, residue of this antibiotic in milk occasionally reaches the consumer. In humans, following the intramuscular injection of 100,000 units of penicillin to nursing mothers, concentrations of penicillin in their milk of 0.015 to 0.06 unit/ml (equivalent to serum levels of 0.5 to 2.0 units/ml) have been observed. Concentrations of streptomycin in milk of puerperal women are insignificant following intramuscular injection, but they may persist for some time.

Levels of novobiocin ranging from 0.36 to 0.54 mg% have been observed in breast milk six to thirty hours after an initial oral dose of 500 mg followed by 250 mg every six hours. Corresponding blood levels ranged from 1.2 to 5.2 mg% in the mother, determined two hours after administration of the drug.

The administration of 1.0 gm of oxacillin (Prostaphlin®) orally to nursing mothers did not result in a measurable amount of the drug in their breast milk within three and three-quarters hours after ingestion. Five mothers given 500 mg of tetracycline hydrochloride orally four times daily for three days, following premature rupture of their membranes, exhibited serum values of from 0.9 to 3.2 μg/ml. Values in their milk ranged from 20 to 90 per cent of serum values with an average of 70 per cent. Levels in the infants' serum were less than 0.07 μg/ml, which is insufficient to treat an infection.

The concentration of chloramphenicol in breast milk is approximately 50 per cent of that in the serum. Blood levels of 26 to 49 μg/ml and milk levels of 16 to 25 μg/ml have been found in women treated for scrub typhus in Malaya.

TABLE 45
ADVERSE REACTIONS AND ANTIBIOTIC DOSAGE IN THE PREMATURE AND NEWBORN INFANT

| *Drug* | *Daily Dosage per kg of Body Weight* | *Route of Administration* | *Hours Between Doses* | *Caution* |
|---|---|---|---|---|
| Bacitracin | 1,000 units | Intramuscular | 12 | Nephrotoxic; store at 4° C, discard in one day |
| Chloramphenicol | 25 mg | Intramuscular, oral | 12 | Determine blood level |
| Colistins | | | | |
| Colistin sulfate | 5 mg | Oral | 6 | Nephrotoxic |
| Sodium colistimethate | 1.5 mg or less | Intramuscular | 8-12 | Nephrotoxic |
| Erythromycins | | | | |
| Erythromycin estolate | 25-40 mg | Oral | 6 | |
| Erythromycin ethylsuccinate | 25-40 mg | Oral | 6 | |
| | 10 mg | Intramuscular | 12 | |
| Kanamycin sulfate | 15 mg | Intramuscular | 12 | Ototoxic, nephrotoxic |
| Neomycin sulfate | 50 mg | Oral | 6 | Absorption may occur |
| Novobiocin | 20-25 mg | Oral | 8-12 | Inhibitor of bilirubin conjugation |
| Penicillins | | | | |
| Potassium penicillin G | 20,000 units | Intramuscular, Intravenous | 12 | Long-acting preparations contraindicated |
| Phenoxymethyl penicillin | 90,000 units | Oral | 8 | |
| Polymyxin B sulfate | 1.5 mg or less | Intramuscular | 8-12 | Nephrotoxic |
| Streptomycin sulfate | 10-20 mg | Intramuscular | 12 | Not longer than ten days |
| Tetracyclines | | | | |
| Chlortetracycline, | 15 mg | Intramuscular, Intravenous | 12 | Growth arrest, staining of teeth, enamel hypoplasia |
| Demethylchlortetracycline, Oxytetracycline, Rolitetracycline, Tetracycline, Tetracycline phosphate complex | 100 mg | Oral | 6 | |

Among other antibacterial agents, sulfanilamide and sulfapyridine in doses of 2 and 3 gm/day produced milk levels of 3 to 13 mg/100 ml. The levels in milk are approximately equal to those in the maternal serum. When 3 gm of nonabsorbable sulfathiazole was administered to one group, the milk contained only 0.5 mg%.

Isoniazid appears in breast milk in approximately the same concentrations as it does in the maternal serum. A linear relationship exists between the dose of INH administered and the milk-serum concentrations. Rifampin, a recently developed drug used in the treatment of tuberculosis, diffuses readily in breast milk.

As much as 27 per cent of a 10 to 30 mc tracer dose of radioactive iodine administered to a lactating woman may cross the plasma-milk barrier. The major portion appears in milk within the first twenty-four hours with smaller traces persisting for several days. This is enough to produce a significant suppressive effect on the infant's developing thyroid gland; therefore breast feeding should be discontinued for a week. Thiouracil given to a lactating woman appears in her milk in a higher concentration than in her blood or urine and could possibly produce goiter in the nursing infant.

If techniques using technetium 99 are required in nursing mothers, a breast pump should be used for at least three days after administration of the isotope. Studies in a twenty-four-year-old nursing mother undergoing a brain scan showed that a significant amount of radioactive isotope remained in the breast milk for at least twenty-four hours after administration, and small amounts were detectable after forty-six hours. By the third day, no radioactivity was detected in the milk.

Atropine is contraindicated for nursing mothers because it decreases milk production and may cause intoxication of the infant. However, only minute amounts of atropine (less than 0.1 mg/100 ml) have been detected in milk when therapeutic doses of 600 mg were taken *orally* by lactating women.

Diazepam (Valium) and its active metabolite, desmethyldiazepam, passes from mother's blood into breast milk. Since neonates metabolize diazepam more slowly than adults, continued medication of a lactating mother could lead to accumulation of the drug in the infant. Theoretically, this accumulation could reach toxic levels.

Nine breast-feeding mothers were given diazepam after delivery because of persistent hypertension. Appreciable amounts of active substances were detected in one infant ten days after the mother received a single dose during labor. Three mild cases of jaundice were the only adverse clinical effects observed (Cole and Hailey: *Arch Dis Child, 50*:741, 1975). Bromides, anthraquinones (cascara, senna, aloe, danthron Dorbane®), metronidazole (Flagyl®) and ergot ingested by the mother are secreted in her milk and may give rise to symptoms in the infant when doses larger than average or usual, are prescribed or taken. Compounds that are detoxified by the same mechanism that conjugates free bilirubin would be particularly hazardous for the icteric nursing infant.

On the other hand, only small amounts, too little to be of clinical significance, of morphine, codeine, glutethimide, scopolamine, phenolphthalein, sulfonamides, antibiotics, nitrofurantoin, tolbutamide (Orinase®), mandelic acid, iodides, quinine, salicylates and many psychotherapeutic drugs are found in milk. Hence, these drugs are ordinarily not contraindicated for the nursing mother, except when they are prescribed in unusually large dosage, as might be the case of the nursing mother with rheumatoid arthritis who takes very large doses of salicylates each day. Caffeine may pass into milk, but it does not seem to affect the baby; about 1 per cent of that ingested is found in the infant. There is little risk of digoxin getting into breast milk (less than a therapeutic dose) when the nursing mother is on the drug.

It is well documented that reserpine in the parturient mother causes severe and sometimes serious nasal stuffiness and blockage in her newborn. If the mother continues to take this drug, it could very possibly produce the same symptoms in the nursing infant.

Breast-feeding alone cannot provide the optimal amount of flouride for prevention of dental caries. It has been demonstrated that lactating women who were drinking water containing 0.55 ppm of fluoride have a level of only a little above 0.1 ppm in their breast milk.

In regard to alcohol, moderate amounts (say, one or two cocktails a day) are not harmful to the nursing mother or infant. A woman who drinks too much would probably not desire to nurse. In some cases, the emotional security and gratification she derives from drink could outweigh the disadvantages.* Barbiturates in usual doses excreted in breast milk have never been found to affect the nursing infant.

Cigarette smoking raises a question for the lactating mother deserving of special attention. Smoking may reduce the volume of milk excreted, and that is a problem in itself. Lactating women who smoke from ten to twenty cigarettes a day pass along from 0.4 to 0.5 mg of nicotine in each liter of milk. Applying Clark's rule, this is the equivalent of 6 to 7.5 mg of nicotine in the adult. While this is but one-tenth the lethal dose, 4 mg taken orally have been known to produce alarming symptoms in adults. This is, of course, less than the heavy-smoker mother passes on to her infant. It has been found recently that all other factors being comparable, women who smoke excessively have smaller babies than nonsmokers.

The most active component of marihuana (tetrahydrocannabinol) is fat-soluble, and it is likely to appear in breast milk. However, the long-range effects on the infant of this toxin have not as yet been documented but the potential for ill effects exists.

Oral contraceptives pose a special problem of their own for the nursing mother. Little is known about the excretion of hormones in milk. The excretion in milk of ingested thyroid drugs has not been well documented. Studies on lactating rats given cortisone revealed a significant retardation of growth and development in litters suckled by rats receiving 20 mg of cortisone per day, but valid human data are lacking. It is reasonable to expect that the continued use of hormone combinations such as the oral contraceptives would have unbalancing effects on the developing endocrine system of a suckling baby.

From a practical standpoint, oral contraceptives, that is, progestin-estrogen combinations of drugs, might inhibit lactation. However, the exact effect of such a regimen on lactation depends on how early the drug is given during the puerperium and how large the dose is. Diminished lactation is most apt to result when oral contraceptive therapy is started early in the postpartum period. The possibility of diminished lactation is reduced when oral contraceptive preparations containing smaller doses of progestogen are used later. Data concerning the effects of the sequential oral contraceptives on lactation are lacking. Since the control of lactation involves prolactin (luteotrophic hormone), any agent that suppresses gonadotropins may be considered to have a potential for inhibiting lactation. The entire endocrine system is such a delicately balanced, interdependent galaxy of metabolic phenomena that it is not reasonable to expect that the infant could withstand without harm the daily jolt of estrogen and progesterone in his diet. Gynecomastia has been reported in one nursing male infant whose mother was taking norethynodrel with mestranol. The long-range effects of oral contraceptives on a nursing infant could be considerable.

The nursing mother, like everyone else, is exposed to environmental toxicants. The facts that DDT is present in all human milk and that breast milk contains more DDT than does cow's milk have been recognized for years. However, there has been no increase in these values, even though many studies show considerable variations in their reports. A review of the literature reveals that since DDT was first reported in human milk in 1950 at a mean concentration of 0.13 ppm, it apparent-

---

*A reversible pseudo-Cushing syndrome in infants through excessive alcohol drinking by their lactating mothers has been reported. The normal rhythm of ACTH secretion is deranged, but whether this effect is primarily on the hypothalamus or pituitary is not clear.

ly has been declining. In 1960 through 1961, a study showed a level of 0.08 ppm; in 1968, the level was 0.03 to 0.04 ppm. A similar apparent decline in the level of DDT in cow's milk has been noted over the years.

The medical importance of DDT in human milk depends entirely on the amount received by babies. Whether human or cow's milk contains more is irrelevant. Any calculation should be made in terms of DDT, because DDE and other related derivatives present in milk are very much less toxic. An infant consumes about 0.6 liter of milk per day. Taking this value and a DDT concentration of 0.08 ppm, a daily intake of 0.048 mg for the average infant may be calculated. If this is divided by 3.36 kg (the average weight of babies at birth), one obtains a value of 0.014 mg/kg/day rather than the oft-quoted value of 0.02 mg/kg/day. As the infant grows, the intake on a per-kilogram basis probably decreases slightly. Therefore, the average daily intake of breast-fed infants in this country is little, if any, greater than the permissible rate set by the World Health Organization and the Food and Agriculture Organization after years of study.

The general conclusion can be made that nearly all compounds ingested by the lactating mother are excreted in her milk to some degree in some form, though in most instances in such small amounts as to be barely detectable and insignificantly hazardous. However, the following drugs should be avoided while breast-feeding: any drug or chemical in excessive amounts, diuretics (insignificant amount for chlorothiazide), atropine, reserpine, steroids, radioactive preparations, hallucinogens, anticoagulants, bromides, antithyroid drugs, anthraquinones, dihydrotachysterol, antimetabolites and perhaps oral contraceptives. Breast-feeding should be contraindicated in mothers with illnesses which require large doses of any drug and also in those using a new and unusual drug. These limitations, however, should in no way discourage the majority of mothers requiring medication who want to breast-feed. When the possibility of potential harm for the nursing infant exists, the offending drug can usually be discontinued, or the chemical removed from the mother's immediate environment.

## Drug Bilirubin-Albumin Binding*

The clinical risk of free bilirubin from any drug is dependent on the drug concentration itself, whether it is totally or partially competitive for binding, the *in vivo* bilirubin albumin ratio, the simultaneous existence of other local conditions, i.e. acidosis and hypothermia, and the presence or absence of other competitive anions.

For the physician administering drugs to newborn infants, the temptation to try a new agent with a slightly different structure (common among antibiotics) should be avoided unless its precise status with respect to bilirubin-albumin is known. A structural relationship is not a guarantee of similar bindings characteristics, *viz.,* salicylate dis-

*Data from Stern, L.: Drug interactions—part II: Drugs, the newborn infant, and the binding of bilirubin to albumin, *Pediatrics, 49*:6, 916-18; and Chan, G.: *The Binding of Bilirubin to Albumin* (Thesis).

TABLE 46
DRUGS CAPABLE OF IN VITRO DISPLACEMENT OF BILIRUBIN FROM ALBUMIN IN THE NEWBORN

Caffeine Sodium Benzoate
Sodium Salicylate
Diazepam (Valium)
Tolbutamide (Orinase)
Sulfisoxazole (Gantrisin®)

Furosemide (Lasix)
Sodium Oxacillin (Prostaphlin)
Hydrocortisone
Gentamycin (Geramycin)
Digoxin
Sodium Meralluride (Mercuhydrin)
Sulfadiazine

(Generic and trade names are listed in order of quantitative displacement exhibited; concentrations of drugs used were those of *in vivo* levels resulting from manufacturers' recommended dosages.)

* Injectable preparation only.

places; salicylamide does not. Similarly, oxacillin displaces, but methicillin and penicillin G do not. Any drug used in the newborn must have, in addition to its other metabolic and pharmacokinetic data, some form of study to determine its capacity to displace bilirubin from albumin.

Drugs may reach the newborn not only directly, but also via breast milk of a nursing mother, as well as via cord blood if administered just prior to or during labor e.g. psychotropic, sedative and tranquilizing agents. At present, neither the Food and Drug Administration nor its Canadian counterpart, the Food and Drug Directorate, requires information on albumin-bilirubin displacement from the manufacturer for licensing a drug. The information is not difficult to obtain and should be made mandatory for every drug that could be used in the neonatal period.

## Summary

In the preceding pages, a number of modalities of treatment and general considerations of poisoning have been outlined. However, when confronted with a poisoned victim, it is imperative that one must *treat the patient—not the poison.* As noted in other sections of this book, the truly useful and effective antidotes for poisons can be counted on the fingers of the hands. Even the use of some of these are equivocal, and certainly there is no serious urgency in using antidotes before the patient is stabilized with symptomatic and supportive treatment. Therefore, in concluding this first section on poisoning, it is axiomatic to emphasize to first *treat the patient—not the poison.*

## Chapter 2

# INSECTICIDES

In the past two decades a whole new group of agricultural chemicals has been introduced to control crop-destroying insects, diseases and weeds. As a result, the yields of food crops per acre have reached new high levels. The general acceptance of the use of these chemicals in agriculture and in the home and the recognition of their usefulness and even necessity have perhaps been responsible for frequent neglect of their toxicity to man and domestic animals. To aid in prevention of poisoning by these agents, federal and state legislation has been enacted. The Federal Insecticide, Fungicide and Rodenticide Act of 1947 requires the registration and proper labeling of every new pesticide agent before it is shipped in interstate commerce. The Miller Pesticide Amendment to the Federal Food, Drug and Cosmetic Act provides for the establishment of tolerance levels, i.e. the maximum quantities which can be present on raw agricultural products. Most states have legislation concerning pesticides, generally requiring the licensing of each substance before it can be sold. State laws usually follow the same pattern as federal laws to avoid conflict with respect to labeling. Unfortunately the requirements differ greatly in various states, and uniformity in state laws is badly needed.

The National Agricultural Association has established a network of more than forty trained decontamination teams located in all parts of the United States. The network is prepared to provide the necessary advice and assistance whenever *Class B poison pesticide chemicals* are involved in transportation or warehouse accidents. A Class B poison pesticide is identified by the skull-and-crossbones poison symbol on the label. The network can be contacted on one emergency telephone number, 800-424-9300. Contact this network only when poison pesticides are involved.

Chemically the important insecticides can be divided into four major groups: synthetic organic, inorganic, biological and botanic.

A. Synthetic organic insecticides
   1. Chlorobenzene derivatives
      a. DDT* Dichlorodiphenyltrichloroethane
      b. TDE Tetrachlorodiphenylethane
      c. DFDT Difluorodiphenyltrichloroethane
      d. Dimite dichlorodiphenylethanol
      e. DMC Dichlorodiphenyl methyl carbinol
      f. Methoxychlor
      g. Neotrane
      h. Ovotran
      i. Dilan
   2. Indane derivatives
      a. Chlordane
      b. Heptachlor
      c. Aldrin
      d. Dieldrin
      e. Endrin
      f. Diendrin
      g. Kepone (Chlordecone)
   3. Benzene hexachloride (Lindane)
   4. Chlorinated camphene (Toxaphene)
   5. Phosphate esters
      a. Chlorothion

---

*Final federal notices of cancellation were issued for the remaining uses of DDT, except for public health and quarantine purposes and three major agricultural uses, on June 14, 1972. The ban became effective January 1, 1973.

b. Diazinon
c. DFP Diisopropylfluorophosphate
d. EPN
e. Leptophos
f. Malathion
g. Metacide
h. OMPA Octamethylpyrophosphoramide
i. Para-oxon
j. Parathion
k. Potosan
l. Systox
m. TEPP Tetraethylpyrophosphate
n. Thio-TEPP

6. Carbamates

B. Inorganic chemical-type insecticides
1. Arsenic compounds
2. Fluorides
3. Thallium
4. Selenium
5. Metaldehyde
6. Mercury
7. Phosphorus
8. Sodium borate
9. Hydrocyanic acid (Cyanide)
10. Antimony

C. Insecticides from botanical sources
1. Nicotine
2. Pyrethrin
3. Ryania
4. Rotenone
5. Sabadilla

D. Biological pesticides

## SYNTHETIC ORGANIC INSECTICIDES

*Chlorobenzene Derivatives*

These chemicals are soluble in fat but not in water and are soluble weeks to months after application. DDT and its metabolites accumulate and persist in body fat for long periods of time. The amounts of these substances present in the body fat of United States residents are higher than those found in Canada, Europe, England, France and West Germany, but about the same as for Hungary. However, they evidently are not accumulating beyond tolerable levels in fat tissue of the general population. Analysis of fat samples obtained from autopsies shows that only lindane, dieldrin and DDT are regularly recognizable. Accumulation of lindane and dieldrin is insignificant, ranging between 0.1 and 1 ppm. Mean accumulation of DDT is 2.9 ppm. Low chronic intakes of DDT from sprayed foods soon reach an equilibrium in which excretion is equal to intake. The absorbed pesticide is partitioned between adipose tissue and blood, where it is partly converted to a much less toxic dehydrochloride, DDE. Mean DDE accumulation in fat tissue is 7.4 ppm. During chronic intake, DDT conversion into DDE exceeds DDT intake so that the DDE percentage slowly and continuously rises. Some DDT is converted directly to an acetic derivation DDA, conjugated in the liver and excreted in bile and urine. A large portion of ingested DDT is never absorbed and is excreted in the feces. Pesticides have been found in seals and penguins in Antarctica and in animals in the Far North, but scientists still do not know how the pesticide traces were carried to these regions.

Commercial preparations consist of these insecticides in technically pure form, in dry mixtures of several types or in solutions of one or more inorganic solvents such as kerosene, benzene or other petroleum derivatives. The solvents are themselves toxic and can further increase the involvement of the central nervous system, causing stimulation with symptoms of restlessness, hyperirritability, incoordination, muscle spasms, tremors and clonic and tonic convulsions, followed by depression, collapse, cyanosis, labored respiration and death due to respiratory failure.

Following ingestion of toxic doses, salivation, nausea, vomiting and abdominal pain may occur. After absorption through the skin or by inhalation, symptoms may include irritation of the eyes, nose, and throat, blurring of vision, cough, pulmonary edema and dermatitis.

In chronic poisoning the symptoms are anorexia, loss of weight, liver and kidney damage and emaciation, in addition to disturbances of the central nervous system and skin irritation.

Cerebral dysfunction (fatigue, dullness, blurred vision, headache, ataxia) from small amounts of DDT in highly sensitive individuals has been documented and may occur more frequently than previously recognized. When the diagnosis is in doubt, the urine can be examined for the presence of DDA (bis [*p*-chlorophenyl] acetic acid).

*Treatment.* If ingested, the material must be removed from the gastrointestinal tract by gastric lavage followed by saline cathartics. Fats and oils, such as oil purgatives, demulcents and evacuants, as well as milk, should be avoided because they increase the rate of absorption of chlorinated hydrocarbons. Epinephrine and related compounds should also be avoided, as they may induce ventricular fibrillation by sensitizing the myocardium. In case of skin contamination, prompt washing with soap and water is required to prevent skin irritation and reduce systemic absorption. Contaminated clothing should always be removed immediately and the patient showered, with particular attention being given to the hair and fingernails.

If muscular twitching or tremors develop, phenobarbital sodium should be administered. For treatment of convulsive states, the more rapid, shorter-acting barbiturates, such as pentobarbital sodium, are indicated. Maintaining clear air passages and the use of oxygen therapy are important therapeutic measures.

In the event of suspected liver or kidney damage, a low-fat, high-carbohydrate and high-protein diet should be given together with other appropriate measures.

### *Indane Derivatives*

These derivatives are synthetic fat-soluble, but water-insoluble, chemicals which either singly or in mixtures in the form of dusts, wettable powders or solutions are used as insecticides for the control of flies, mosquitoes and field insects. Aldrin is the most toxic of these, being two to four times as toxic in animals as chlordane. The other derivatives have intermediate toxicity. Symptoms in man can occur after ingestion of or skin contamination with 15 to 50 mg/kg of body weight of these preparations. Acute poisoning from the ingestion, inhalation or skin contamination is characterized by hyperexcitability, tremors, restlessness, ataxia and tonic and clonic convulsions. Since liver function in animals is impaired well below lethal levels, the toxicity of these derivatives is enhanced in humans with previous liver damage.

Recent studies by the National Cancer Institute add to already substantial evidence that heptachlor causes malignant tumors in mice and rats and therefore poses a cancer hazard to man (Chlordane contains about 10% heptachlor). Studies by the Food and Drug Administration indicate that more than 70 per cent of all meat, fish, poultry and dairy products in the United States contains residues of these pesticides. Heptachlor and chlordane were also present in the fatty tissues of more than 97 per cent of the people tested by the EPA in 1973. Heptachlor occurs in mothers' milk and can be transmitted to the human fetus. Because these chemicals are so widespread, the major sources of human exposure are largely unavoidable by individual action. The Environmental Protection Agency has announced its intention of suspending the production of heptachlor and chlordane, both of which have been incriminated in producing blood dyscrasias in humans.

Kepone, an ant and roach pesticide, has produced brain and liver damage in workers exposed to high levels, and it has been found in breast milk of mothers in Georgia, Alabama and North Carolina. The complex neurological disorder was characterized by insidious onset of tremors, chest pain, weight loss, mental changes, arthralgia, skin rash, opsoclonus, muscle weakness, gait ataxia, incoordination and slurred speech.

*Treatment* (*see* Chlorobenzene).

### *Benzene Hexachloride (Lindane)**

This chemical is widely used in the control of cotton insects as well as DDT-resistant insects and in thermal insecticide vaporizers. The signs of acute poisoning are vomiting and diarrhea, excitability, loss of equilibrium and convulsions. Recovery is likely unless the material involved contains an organic solvent, in which case dyspnea, cyanosis and circulatory failure may follow rapidly. Exposure to smaller amounts by skin contamination leads to nausea, dizziness, headaches, tremors and muscular weakness. Contact with the vaporized fumes can produce, in addition to the above symptoms irritation of the eyes, nose and throat. Such symptoms clear up promptly upon removal from further exposure. Aplastic anemia, an ominous effect, has been documented. In experimental animals, liver necrosis is the most significant pathological finding, and although chronic poisoning has not been reported in man, the possibility of liver damage in the constantly exposed should be kept in mind. Kwell® and Gamene® are specific agents containing gamma benzene hexachloride approved by the FDA for marketing for the eradication of scabies and head lice. Now, there are reports of convulsions and coma occurring in small children with extensive use of these preparations, which probably should be washed off soon after application, rather than left on for the entire day.

*Treatment* (*see* Chlorobenzene).

*Lindane is the accepted common name for essentially pure gamma isomer of benzene hexachloride, however, there are other isomers and therefore the two are not necessarily synonymous compounds.

### *Chlorinated Camphene (Toxaphene)*

This is a relatively slow acting residual fat-soluble but not water-soluble insecticide, which is formulated for use as a dust, emulsion spray or wettable powder. It can be used against many insects, ticks and mites.

Toxaphene has a faint, pleasant terpene odor; it is tasteless and does not have an appreciable irritating effect on mucous membranes. Poisoning by this insecticide has been mainly by accidental ingestion where the toxaphene has been left in unlabeled containers. Other potential exposures are by inhalation or absorption through the skin.

Symptoms of acute intoxication are the result of diffuse stimulation of the cerebrospinal axis with generalized convulsions. With a lethal dose, there may be a series of severe convulsions, and death results from anoxia and respiratory failure.

When toxaphene has been ingested, the stomach should be lavaged and this is followed by a saline cathartic. There is a definite contraindication to the use of oily cathartics and fatty substances as they facilitate and increase the absorption of the toxaphene. Barbiturates, such as phenobarbital sodium, should be given parenterally early in an attempt to prevent convulsions. After the onset of generalized convulsions, the fast-acting pentobarbital sodium should be given intravenously even to the extent of giving a full anesthetic dose. Sedation should be continued for several hours. Other than a period of weakness and lassitude, there have been no residual manifestations after recovery nor have there been any reported effects from exposure to small amounts over a long period of time.

### *Phosphate Esters*

These highly toxic compounds, discovered by the Germans during World War II in their search for lethal gases, have come into widespread use throughout the world for eradication of distinctive insects, particularly

TABLE 47
ESTIMATED LETHAL DOSES OF CHLORINATED HYDROCARBON INSECTICIDES

| *Common Name* | *Chemical Name* | *Estimated Fatal Oral Dose (gm/70 kg)* | *Treatment* |
|---|---|---|---|
| Chlorophenothane; DDT | Trichloro-bis- (p-chlorophenyl) ethane | 30 | Phenobarbital or Pentobarbital |
| Toxaphene | Chlorinated camphene | 5 | Phenobarbital or Pentobarbital |
| Benzene hexachloride (BHC) | Hexachlorocyclohexane | 28 | Phenobarbital or Pentobarbital |
| Lindane | Gamma isomer of benzene hexachloride | 15 | Phenobarbital or Pentobarbital |
| Chlordane | Octachloro-hexahydro-methanoindene | 6–60 | Phenobarbital or Pentobarbital |
| Aldrin | Hexachloro-hexahydro-dimethanonaphthalene | 5 | Phenobarbital or Pentobarbital |
| Dieldrin | Hexachloro-epoxy-octahydro-dimethanonaphthalene | 5 | Phenobarbital or Pentobarbital |
| Methoxychlor | Trichloro-bis (p-methoxyphenyl) ethane | 350 | ———— |

the soft-bodied ones. These insecticides have high mammalian toxicity, except malathion and chlorthion, and are readily absorbed from the skin, lungs and gastrointestinal tract, thus increasing the possibility of acute poisoning during their application and use. Investigators have demonstrated that the hazard from respiratory exposures may be three times as great as that from oral exposure and ten or more times greater than from dermal absorption. Contaminated clothing, nevertheless, can produce symptoms as an unsuspected source. Six children were made ill from wearing newly acquired jeans that had been contaminated on a transport truck eight months previously.

All of the organic phosphate group of insecticides have essentially the same mechanism of action. These products are also known to break down into toxic components and accumulations, probably as a result of aging, weathering, plant alteration or other degradation. The most likely suspect is the oxygen analog of parathion, para-oxon, a cholinesterase-inhibiting compound with cutaneous toxicity ten times that of parathion. S-phenyl and S-ethyl isomers are also implicated. Parathion, generally considered to decompose rapidly after application, can persist to become a water contaminant (wells) under certain circumstances. It owes its toxicity to an ability to inhibit cholinesterase, the enzyme that normally detoxifies acetylcholine. Some organic phosphates undergo metabolic conversion to yield cholinergic metabolites. Thus the insecticidal thiophosphates undergo metabolic change in the liver, which consists of replacement of sulfur by oxygen. The resulting oxygen analog is the inhibitor of cholinesterase. The end result of the inhibition of cholinesterase activity is accumulation of unhydrolyzed acetylcholine. The resulting symptoms resemble those that would expectedly be found from excessive and continued stimulation of the central nervous system and structures innervated by the parasympathetic and somatic motor nerves. The clinical manifestations of poisoning consist of weakness, unsteadiness, blurred vision and a sense of constriction of the chest. These symptoms are followed by vomiting, abdominal cramps, diarrhea, salivation, lacrimation, profuse sweating, tremors of the extremities and difficulty in breathing. A disagreeable garlicky odor is often associated with malathion intoxication. Pinpoint and nonreactive pupils are observed, and secretions accumulate in the respiratory passages. Cyanosis may occur as well as severe muscular fibrillations, coma and convulsions. Severe hypoglycemia has been reported in a child of eight months who died, and it has also been produced experimentally in animals. Death is associated with respiratory failure. After lethal doses, the onset of symptoms usually is extremely rapid and death generally occurs within twenty-four hours. After sublethal doses, reversal of the inhibition of cholinesterase and disappearance of the symptoms follow, but the rate varies from a few hours to several days with different compounds.

The medical aspects of poisoning by insecticidal organic phosphates consist of prevention, detection and treatment. Prevention can be accomplished by education of persons (farmers and florists) occupationally exposed to the compounds concerning the dangers of skin contamination, inhalation and ingestion. Protective clothing should be worn, and contaminated skin should be washed immediately.

Detection of poisoning by organic phosphates depends on recognition of the characteristic symptoms of acetylcholine poisoning. Exposure to amounts of organic phosphates too low to produce symptoms can be detected by periodic measurement of blood cholinesterase.

A more valid guide for those who are frequently or continually exposed to the organic phosphates is the use of preexposure value of cholinesterase activity, if available, and if not, the use of a chart of mean value, to determine the degree of inhibition of cholinesterase and intoxication present. A depressed cholinesterase level is not, by definition, an illness. The cholinesterase is used as an indicator of exposure with absorption of the inhibitor and as such is a very valuable measurement. Marked depression of the cholinesterase activity of the blood occurs first, before symptoms appear.

In cases of illness where organic phosphate intoxication is suspected, plasma and red cell cholinesterase determinations should be made. The cholinesterase found in erythrocytes is a truer reflection of the cholinesterase content of the central nervous system and is, therefore, more important in evaluating the significance of the exposure to a cholinesterase inhibitor.

As a general rule, for persons working on

TABLE 48
ORGANIC PHOSPHATE ESTER POISONING SYMPTOMS

| *Muscarine Effects* | *Nicotinic Effects* | *Central Nervous System* |
|---|---|---|
| (Autonomic nervous system) | (Striated muscles) | |
| **G-I tract** | Incoordination | Giddiness, anxiety, apathy and confusion |
| Vomiting | Muscle twitchings, tremors and weakness | Convulsions |
| Diarrhea | Paralysis | Ataxia |
| Abdominal pain (tenesmus) | Pallor and occasionally hypertension | Coma |
| Fecal incontinence | | Depression of respiratory and circulatory centers |
| **Respiratory tract** | | Death may follow interference with respiration through any combination of the following four mechanisms: |
| Tightness in chest | | 1. bronchial constriction |
| Increased bronchial secretions | | 2. excessive respiratory tract secretions |
| Cough, dyspnea, cyanosis | | 3. paralysis of the muscles of respiration |
| Pulmonary edema | | 4. failure of the respiratory center |
| *Other cholinergic symptoms* | | |
| Increased sweating, salivation and tearing | | |
| Pinpoint pupils (miosis) | | |
| Bradycardia and hypertension | | |
| Urinary frequency and incontinence | | |

the ground (as opposed to pilots), a decrease of 40 per cent in red cell cholinesterase is a danger signal and a decrease of 60 per cent from the preexposure concentration is an indication for removal from work. If pre-exposure values are not available, the mean value as obtained from a prepared chart should be used until the individual's own normal value can be determined. The normal range of red blood cell cholinesterase activity ($\Delta$pH/hr) is 0.39 to 1.02 for men and 0.34 to 1.10 for women. The normal range of the enzyme activity ($\Delta$pH/hr) of plasma is 0.44 to 1.63 for men and 0.24 to 1.54 for women. The asymptomatic person removed from work may continue working if unexposed to cholinesterase inhibitors. He may return to a job with possible exposure only when his red cell cholinesterase reaches 50 per cent of his normal or of the normal mean value (by chart), if his normal is unknown.

Unopette® #5820 is a unit for testing for organic phosphate poisoning (cholinesterase). It consists of two reservoirs with premeasured amounts of bromthymol blue and saline, a pipette for collecting blood, a prefilled pipette with a stabilized volume of acetylcholine chloride substrate and a color comparison chart (Becton, Dickinson and Company, Rutherford, New Jersey 07070). Analyzing urinary metabolite levels, para-nitrophenol (PNP) and correlating increased levels, is a good index of varying degrees of exposure and potential toxicity to parathion. Although the excretion of para-nitrophenol may be detected at levels of absorption too low to produce a detectable level on blood cholinesterase, there is a good similarity between the two parameters. The occurrence of aminoaciduria in 55 per cent and glycosuria in 30 per cent of one series has been reported.

The present method of *treatment* of acute

TABLE 49
ACUTE TOXICITY OF ORGANIC PHOSPHORUS-CONTAINING INSECTICIDES

| *Common Name* | *Chemical Name* | *Comparative Toxicity* | *Estimated Fatal Oral Dose (gm/70 kg)* |
|---|---|---|---|
| TEPP | Tetraethylpyrophosphate | Highly toxic | 0.05 |
| OMPA | Octamethyl pyrophosphoramide | Highly toxic | 0.2 |
| Dipterex | Dimethyl-1-hydroxy-2,2,2-trichloroethylphosphonate | Moderately toxic | 25.0 |
| Chlorthion | p-Nitro-m-chlorophenyl dimethylthiophosphate | Slightly toxic | 60.0 |
| Di-syston* (Disolfton) | Diethyl-S-2-ethyl-2-mercaptoethyl phosphorodithioate | Highly toxic | 0.2 |
| Co-Ral | Diethyl-O-(3-chloro-4-methyl-7-coumarinyl) phosphorothioate | Moderately toxic | 10.0 |
| Phosdrin | Dimethyl-O-(1-methyl-2-carbomethoxyvinyl) phosphate | Highly toxic | 0.15 |
| Parathion | Diethyl-p-nitrophenyl monothiophosphate | Highly toxic | 0.1 |
| Methyl parathion | Dimethyl-p-nitrophenyl thiophosphate | Highly toxic | 0.15 |
| Malathion** | Dimethyl-S-(1,2-bis-carboethoxy) ethyl phosphorodithioate | Slightly toxic | 60.0 |
| Systox | Diethyl-O-ethylmercapto-ethyl phosphorothioate | Highly toxic | 0.1 |
| EPN | Ethyl-p-nitrophenyl thionobenzenephosphonate | Highly toxic | 0.3 |
| Diazinon | Diethyl-O-(2-isopropyl-6-methyl-4-pyrimidyl) phosphorothioate | Moderately toxic | 25.0 |
| Guthion | Dimethyl S-(4-oxo-1,2,3-benzotriazinyl-3-methyl) phosphorodithioate | Highly toxic | 0.2 |
| Trithion | S-(p-chlorophenylthio)-methyl-O,O-diethyl phosphorodithioate | Highly toxic | 0.6 |

*Trade name Scope® is also used for a popular mouthwash. This should be kept in mind when inquiries are made on Scope.

**The only organic phosphate insecticide approved for household use.

poisoning by organic phosphates consists of supporting respiration and administering atropine. Metaraminol (Aramine®) bitartrate enhances the antagonistic action of atropine against acetylcholine, lessens its side-effects and should also be used in doses about twice that of atropine. Artificial respiration or the administration of oxygen, when possible, should be maintained as long as signs of respiratory embarrassment persist, and the respiratory tract should be kept clear of secretions. Atropine is the specific antidote for organic phosphate poisoning but should not be used until *cyanosis* has been overcome since atropine produces ventricular fibrillations in the presence of hypoxia. The initial dose usually is 2 mg, but in severe cases 4 or 6 mg can be given intramuscularly or intravenously. This dose is over ten times the amount which is administered for other conditions in which atropine is considered for therapy. Initially the interval between doses is fifteen to thirty minutes; repeated doses are given less frequently. A total dosage of 20 to 30 mg may be required during the first twenty-four hours, and much larger doses are sometimes necessary. A total of over 300 mg (600 mg in one instance) of atropine has been administered in several documented cases. Although specific against the parasympathetic effects of the poison, this does not help the muscular weakness and other nicotine actions. Therefore, artificial respiration for many hours may be necessary. Suction to clear the airway and positive-pressure oxygen should be given if pulmonary edema occurs. The use of a respirator may prove lifesaving. Respiratory depression contraindicates the use of morphine. Pronounced changes in electrolytes and serum pH may require adequate amounts of electrolytes and sodium bicarbonate intravenously.

Parenteral diphenhydramine (Benadryl®) has been used as an anticholinergic agent instead of atropine in Colombia, South America for organic phosphate poisoning with good results (Valencia, C. et al.: *Antioquia Médica, 20, 5*:249-56, 1970).

The availability now of the previously investigational oximes in the treatment of organic phosphate ester poisoning provides specific antidotes that only supplement atropine therapy but should never supplant it. These compounds function by regenerating active cholinesterase from the inhibited enzyme complex and are called cholinesterase reactivators. The oximes are capable of breaking this phosphate binding because of the presence of complementary active sites on the molecules of inhibited cholinesterase and the oxime. It has been demonstrated that reactivation of acetylcholinesterase occurs rapidly within ten to fifteen minutes; cholinesterase in plasma, on the other hand, requires twelve to fifteen days to return to normal levels.

Pralidoxime iodide (2-PAM iodide or 2-pyridine aldoxime methyliodide) can be given for moderate to severe intoxication in doses of 1 to 2 gm IV (also IM and SC) slowly as a 5% solution in isotonic saline. For children, 25 to 50 mg/kg should be adequate. These doses can be repeated at ten- to twelve-hour intervals as necessary for those whose symptoms persist or recur. More recently, DAM (diacetyl monoxime) and Protopam® (pralidoxime chloride—2-PAM chloride) and 2-pyridine aldoxime methylchloride have been found to be effective cholinesterase reactivators. The dosage used for Protopam is identical to that of the iodide compound. The use of these drugs does not preclude the use of atropine, as they have no direct immediate effect on the excess acetylcholine. They do, however, seem to reduce tolerance to the atropine, and smaller, more conventional amounts of atropine may be given. No serious side-effects or toxicity have been reported thus far, although brief episodes of dizziness, blurred vision, diplopia, headache, nausea and tachycardia are occasional complaints in conscious patients. Rapid administration has produced serious laryngeal and glottic edema. Pralidoxime iodide can be obtained from the Borden Company, 5000 Langdon Street, Philadelphia, Pennsylvania, and pralidoxime chloride from Ayerst Laboratories, 685 Third Avenue, New York, New York, 10017.

The following outline of comprehensive procedures should be of considerable aid in the *treatment* of the various degrees of this type of poisoning.

VERY SEVERE CASE (coma, cyanosis, respiratory embarrassment). Throughout procedures 1 to 5, the operator should take precautions against his own exposure to the toxic agent, such as wearing rubber gloves if extensive skin contact is involved.

1. *Removal of secretions and maintenance of a patent airway.* Place the patient in a prone position with head down and to one side, mandible elevated and tongue pulled forward; clear the mouth and pharynx with finger or suction. Use an oropharyngeal or nasopharyngeal airway or endotracheal intubation if airway obstruction persists.
2. *Artificial respiration.* Use a positive-pressure method because of restricted airway. Once spontaneous respiration has been restored, 50% oxygen inhalation may be beneficial.
3. *Atropine administration.* As soon as cyanosis has been overcome, give 2 to 4 mg of atropine intravenously. Repeat this dose at five- to ten-minute intervals until signs of atropinization appear (Dry, flushed skin and tachycardia as high as 140 beats per minute. Cessation of oral and tracheal secretions may be a better criteria). A mild degree of atropinization should be maintained for at least forty-eight hours. The interdiction of atropine in a cyanotic patient is because of the possibility of inducing ventricular fibrillation. Parenteral administration of metaraminol (Aramine) at a dose of 2 to 4 mg to children and 10 mg to adults may be combined with atropine since the side-effects of the latter drug are reduced or obviated by administering it with the long-acting sympathomimetic pressor drug.
4. *Protopam (pralidoxime chloride) administration.* Inject an initial dose (adults) of 1000 mg *slowly,* intravenously at a rate not in excess of 500 mg/min. It may be given, if preferred, as an infusion in 250 ml of saline over a thirty-minute period. After about an hour, a second dose of 1000 mg is indicated if muscle weakness has not been relieved. After an overwhelming exposure to, or ingestion of, the toxic agent, these doses may be doubled. For children, the dose may be 25 to 50 mg/kg (melphalan alidoxime can be used in the same dosage). If intravenous administration is not feasible, intramuscular or subcutaneous injection should be used. Additional doses may be given cautiously if muscular weakness persists, but Protopam is itself a weak anticholinesterase and facilities for artificial respiration should be maintained in readiness. Treatment is most effective if given within a few hours after poisoning by an anticholinesterase. At least in the case of parathion, little is accomplished if the drug is administered more than thirty-six hours after exposure has occurred. Presumably a similar time relationship holds for other anticholinesterases. In severe cases, it may be desirable to monitor the effect of therapy electrocardiographically because of the likelihood of heart block due to the anticholinesterase.
5. *Termination of exposure.* Remove clothing and wash contaminated skin thoroughly with a generous amount of soap or detergent and water, but avoid skin abrasion. If available, washing soda or baking soda may be added to the wash water to accelerate the hydrolysis of the phosphate ester. Then wash with alcohol, since many of the poisons in question are more soluble in alcohol than in water. Wash eyes repeatedly with physiologic saline, if available, or tap water. Use gastric lavage if ingestion or inhalation (which may lead to ingestion) has occurred. If the stomach is distended, empty it with a Levine tube. Since PAM reduces peristalsis so that the intestines are not cleared at the normal rate, a saline cathartic should be left in the stomach.
6. *Alleviation of convulsions, if these interfere with respiration.* Give sodium thiopental (2.5% solution) intravenously with more than the usual care; poisoning by anticholines-

terases sensitizes the medullary centers to depression by barbiturates.

7. *Contraindicated drugs.* As noted above, atropine should not be used until cyanosis has been corrected. Morphine, theophylline, aminophylline and succinylcholine are contraindicated. Tranquilizers of the reserpine or phenothiazine type are to be avoided.
8. *Continued observation.* Watch the patient continuously for not less than twenty-four hours since serious and sometimes fatal relapse can occur due to the continuing absorption of the poison or to dissipation of the effect of the antidotes. After severe poisoning, reasonably close observation is indicated for an additional forty-eight to seventy-two hours. Close medical supervision should be continued for at least twenty-four hours after the patient appears to be out of danger. After discharge, the patient must avoid exposure to phosphate ester insecticides for several weeks because of increased sensitivity.
9. All equipment used for application or handling should be thoroughly decontaminated.

Moderately Severe Case (excessive sweating, lacrimation, salivation, diarrhea, tightness of chest). The procedures described in paragraphs 1 and 2 are not required, but equipment for artificial respiration should be at hand in case the severity of symptoms increases. Probably only one dose of Protopam (pralidoxime chloride) is necessary. Otherwise, the procedures given above apply.

Mild Case (headache, blurred vision, mild muscarinic signs). Termination of exposure is essential since a mild case may become severe due to absorption of poison from unsuspected areas of contamination. A single oral dose of 1000 to 2000 mg (2 to 4 tablets) of Protopam usually gives full remission of symptoms within an hour or less. This dose may be repeated after three hours if necessary. The patient must be kept under medical supervision for at least twenty-four hours.

Prophylactic Use. Prophylactic use of Protopam in connection with exposure to phosphate ester insecticides and chemicals may be attempted by experienced physicians if all of the following conditions are met: (1) The contemplated exposures are discrete periods of not longer than a working day and are not repeated within less than a week. (2) No relaxation of proper safety precautions, such as respirator, protective clothing, decontamination, etc., is tolerated. (3) All subjects remain for forty-eight hours after exposure within reach of the prescribing physician or of another physician who is experienced in the treatment of intoxication due to phosphate ester anticholinesterases. This is because the onset of action of many of these poisons is slow and continuing absorption may occur after the exposure period is passed. Under these circumstances, Protopam may be prescribed in doses of 3000 mg (6 tablets) for not more than four to five doses. The first dose may be taken just before exposure, the second just after the conclusion of exposure or five hours after the first dose, whichever comes first. Further doses would be indicated only if signs or symptoms should appear. The prophylactic use of Protopam is a safer procedure than such use of atropine since it is less likely to suppress premonitory symptoms and signs of severe poisoning. Continued prophylactic use of Protopam, however, should not be attempted at present because of the lack of information on the toxicity of the drug when given over a prolonged period.

Devices for personal protection during exposure to the toxic organophosphate compounds are of limited value. These materials are usually applied in hot summer weather when it would be impractical to recommend the use of impervious clothing. Rubber gloves are frequently contaminated inside and may themselves serve as a focus of absorption. Respirators are typically ill-fitting and thus inefficient. In some cases, use of proper gloves, boots, aprons and possibly even respirators may be indicated, but these should not be depended on nor used without a clear understanding of their shortcomings.

Common errors of treatment are failure to decontaminate the patient, failure to obtain and maintain an open airway, inadequate artificial respiration, insufficient atropine, failure to use the specific oximes and failure to provide for fluid and electrolyte losses.

A study of sequelae (*J Occup Med, 8*:5-20, 1966) on 114 individuals known poisoned with organic phosphate insecticides revealed that 43 had complaints which persisted more than six months after poisoning and that 33 had persistent complaints. Eight individuals complained of continued disturbed vision; 6 attributed it to the acute episode. In 4 the difficulty involved only near vision and was diagnosed as presbyopia. Seven individuals had symptoms of peptic ulcer at some time subsequent to poisoning, but the time relationships and the existence of a variety of family and job stresses made it improbable that the pesticide poisoning played a major role. Headaches in 7 individuals had no consistent pattern. Two coronary occlusions had occurred, but no causal relationship was apparent. Ten individuals had persistent symptoms that seemed primarily referable to the central nervous system; none felt that this problem was a result of acute poisoning. Intolerance of the odor of pesticide preparations was mentioned by 20 subjects. Cholinesterase activity in the red blood cells and plasma was determined for 110 of the group. The major finding of interest was the distribution of pseudocholinesterase levels, which showed more than the expected proportion of higher levels of activity. A study of this type would have detected serious sequelae of high incidence, but would not reveal minor aftereffects of those of low incidence.

EPN and leptophos are particularly neurotoxic compounds by causing degenerative changes in the myelin sheaths of nerves, producing partial paralysis, incoordination and ataxia. These symptoms usually develop one to two weeks after heavy exposure, but they may not show up for months, and multiple sclerosis or encephalitis is often misdiagnosed.

Antiflea dog and cat collars have become popular agents in the United States. Many contain dichlorvos-DDVP, 2,2-dichlorovinyl dimethyl phosphate (Vapona®) and related compounds. These collars have merit in that they are usually effective. However, they have been reported to cause skin irritation to the animal, his owner or both. The use of organophosphates either orally or topically, or the administration of anesthetics to animals wearing or having recently worn these collars, may result in intoxication. These collars should be worn loosely about the neck and they should be removed while bathing the animal, since the compound is water-soluble and can be spread. This insecticide is also widely used now in a hang-up fly repellent and killer strip. There is substantial evidence to prove the safety of these strips with the recommended use rate of one strip/1000 cu. ft. of house space.

### *Carbamates (Carbaryl, Sevin®)*

Carbamates are used as a wide-spectrum insecticide, miticide and aphicide against insect pests of fruits, nuts, vegetables, forage crops, cotton and forest and range lands. They are manufactured as flowable formulations, dusts and wettable powders and are absorbed by all portals including the skin. Concentrates may produce skin irritation as well as systemic poisoning. These compounds should not be confused with the fungicide dithiocarbamates, which are regarded as rather innocuous agents.

The carbamates are reversible inhibitors of cholinesterase. This reversal is often so rapid that measurements of blood cholinesterase of exposed animals or humans are likely to be inaccurate and always in the direction of appearing to be normal. A technique that minimizes reactivation should be used for diagnosis. The compound is promptly metabolized and the naphthalene half is excreted in the urine as β-naphthol, largely in a conjugated form. The presence of an unusual concentration β-naphthol in the urine, which is present normally only in traces, should make one suspicious of carbamate intoxication.

Since these insecticides are cholinesterase inhibitors, the symptoms are not unlike those that occur with the phosphate esters as discussed above or with other cholinesterase-inhibiting agents that are capable of producing effects from acetylcholine "excess." Depending, of course, on the exposure and concentration, the symptoms are not as severe as in those seen with organic phosphate poisoning. Carbamates do not effectively

TABLE 50
INSECTICIDES

| *Trade Name* | *Common Name* |
|---|---|
| Aldrin | aldrin |
| Baytex (Entex) | fenethion |
| Chlorobenzilate | chlorobenzilate |
| Co-Ral | coumaphos |
| Chlordane | chlordane |
| Cygon | dimethoate |
| DDD | TDE |
| DDT | DDT |
| DDVP | dichlorvos |
| Delnav | dioxathion |
| Diazinon | diazinon |
| Dibrom | naled |
| Dieldrin | dieldrin |
| Dipterex | trichlorfon |
| Di-Syston | disolfoton |
| Dylox | trichlorfon |
| EPN or EPN 300 | EPN |
| Entex (Baytex) | fenethion |
| Ethion | ethion |
| Ethyl Guthion | azinphosethyl |
| gamma BHC | lindane |
| Guthion (methyl) | azinphosmethyl |
| Heptachlor | heptachlor |
| Kelthane | dicofol |
| Korlan | ronnel |
| Lannate | methomyl |
| Lindane | lindane |
| Malathion | malathion |
| Marlate | methoxychlor |
| Methoxychlor (Methoxy DDT) | methoxychlor |
| Methyl parathion | methyl parathion |
| Mirex | mirex |
| Morocide | binapacryl |
| Neguvon | trichlorfon |
| Ovatran | ovex |
| Parathion (Niran, Thiophos) | parathion |
| Phosdrin | mevinphos |
| Phosphamidon | phosphamidon |
| Rhothane | TDE |
| Rogor | dimethoate |
| Ronnel | ronnel |
| Sevin | carbaryl |
| Systox | demeton |
| TDE | TDE |
| Tedion | tetradifon |
| TEPP | tepp |
| Thimet | phorate |
| Vapona | dimethyl phosphate |

penetrate the CNS as do the organophosphates; therefore they produce limited CNS toxicity.

*Treatment* is identical to that as outlined for phosphate esters with the exception of the use of the so-called cholinesterase reactivators (pralidoxime iodide or chloride), which are contraindicated because of the rapid reversible inhibition of cholinesterase that occurs. Animal studies have also demonstrated their harmful effects, especially with carbaryl (less so with other carbamates), and until further evidence to the contrary is forthcoming, these oximes should not be used. CNS depressants such as reserpine, chlordiazepoxide, phenobarbital, etc. potentiate carbaryl poisoning and should be avoided. *Lannate* (methomyl thioacetimidate), a cholinesterase inhibitor, is used especially for insect control on cabbage, broccoli, cauliflower and chrysanthemums. The *treatment* is identical to that above, again omitting the use of the pralidoximes.

## INORGANIC CHEMICAL-TYPE INSECTICIDES

### *Arsenic Poisoning*

Arsenic is used in insecticides, ant poisons, weed killers, wallpaper, paint, ceramics and glass. The inorganic arsenicals such as arsenic trioxide or one of its salts are more toxic than the organic compounds (used in protozoal infections and formerly in syphilis), which rarely produce chronic poisoning but are capable of doing so. The action of acids on metals in the presence of arsenic forms arsine gas, the arsenical analogue of ammonia, a fantastically toxic gas: 30 ppm by inhalation can give rise to symptoms. Arsenic presumably causes toxicity by combining with sulfhydryl (-SH) enzymes and interfering with cellular oxidative processes. In this respect, arsenic behaves rather like a heavy metal, although chemically it is more ambiguous, lying somewhere between phosphorus and antimony and in most respects is not metallic at all. When ingested, arsenic trioxide appears as a barium-like radiopaque material on roentgenograms of the abdomen. This can lead to an early diagnosis and much valuable time saved in instituting early treatment even before chemical confirmation. Its soluble compounds are readily absorbed via skin and mucous membranes and only slowly eliminated so that repeated doses are cumulative. The fatal dose of arsenic trioxide is 120 mg (2 gr). The allowable food residue is limited by federal law to 0.65 mg (1/100 gr)/lb. Because of the widespread use of health food preparations (kelp tablets), attention is drawn to this possible unsuspected source of arsenic.

The reported upper limits of arsenic content (as $As_2O_3$/100 gm of tissue) in adult autopsy material are as follows.

| | |
|---|---|
| 0.0050 mg | liver |
| 0.0048 mg | kidney |
| 0.01 mg | hair |
| 0.0048 mg | brain |

Symptomatology is entirely dependent on the amount ingested or inhaled. When massive amounts of arsenic are ingested, initial symptoms are violent gastroenteritis with vomiting and copious watery or bloody diarrhea and burning esophageal pain. There is a sweetish metallic taste in the mouth with garlicky odor of breath and stools. Later the skin becomes cold and clammy. There is generalized weakness and the blood pressure falls. Ventricular fibrillation has been documented. Convulsions and coma are the terminal signs and death is from circulatory failure. If death is not immediate, jaundice, oliguria or anuria appears after one to three days. Inhalation of arsenic dusts may cause lassitude, dyspnea, cyanosis, cough with foamy sputum and pulmonary edema.

Skin involvement may be varied and complicated with erythema, eczema, pigmentation (melanosis), scaling and desquamation and keratosis (palms and soles). Other manifestations are brittle and deformed nails, with transverse ridges (Aldrich-Mees' lines), loss of hair and nails and localized subcutaneous edema, especially of the eyelids. Encephalopathies occur but peripheral neuritis is more common. Sensation is involved first, but eventually paralysis and muscular atrophy appear, usually in the legs. Protein-losing enteropathy has been reported. Pancytopenia is a prominent feature, characterized by an absolute neutropenia and a white cell count of less than 1000. The number of lymphocytes is also decreased, but less strikingly. Patients have relative eosinophilia. Normoblasts are seen more frequently than myeloid immaturity. Thrombopenia occurs in one-half of the patients, but no significant bleeding results.

Peripheral blood smears show varying degrees of anisopoikilocytosis. Erythrocytes are basically normocytic and normochromic but sometimes show a mild degree of hypochromasia. Regenerative macrocytes may be demonstrated. Degree of polychromasia corresponds with level of reticulocytosis. Basophilic stippling is a prominent feature and is seen in most cases.

Bone marrow examination may reveal partial maturation, arrest of myelopoietic elements at the myelocyte level or a decrease in myelocytes, metamyelocytes and neutrophils without a corresponding increase in the number of stem cells or progranulocytes. The most striking feature is an increase in erythropoiesis, which is predominantly normoblastic but may include a few megaloblastoid forms. Occasionally, binucleated red cell precursors are present, and the number of mitotic figures may be increased. Karyorrhexis, producing an irregular pyknotic nucleus, may be prominent in polychromic or orthochromic normoblasts. Megaloblastic anemia and folic acid deficiency have also been reported in chronic arsenic poisoning.

An analysis of the patient's urine should be performed if the substance is not demonstrable in the gastric contents, especially if there is a history of vomiting. Gutzeit's qualitative procedure for arsenic is simple and rapid and gives a positive color reaction with as little as 5 to 10 μg of arsenic. This test can be done by placing 5 ml of urine in a test tube and adding a few drops of sulfuric acid and a few granules of zinc. Cover the top of the tube with filter paper containing a drop or two of silver nitrate solution. Browning or blackening of the silver nitrate occurs if arsine is being liberated. The general measures to adopt for arsenic poisoning are to keep the patient recumbent and warm and to hospitalize him as soon a possible. Every effort should be made to remove arsenic from the stomach by thorough lavage, using warm water and milk (as a demulcent) followed by a saline cathartic. If the patient is seen immediately after ingesting arsenic, the oral administration of a mixture of 30 ml of tincture of ferric chloride and 30 gm of sodium carbonate in 120 ml of water is an effective antidotal solution. However, care should be taken to remove the resulting precipitate as completely as possible by gastric lavage. Intensive hydration should be instituted in order to maintain fluid balance and to prevent shock.

The specific *treatment* is dimercaprol (BAL) utilized as a general antidote to sulfhydryl injury by arsenic and heavy metals. The dosage is 2.5 to 5.0 mg/kg of body weight by intramuscular injection every four to six hours for two days, and then twice daily for the next ten days or until recovery is complete. Children can be treated in the same fashion for they tolerate BAL as well as do adults.

D-penicillamine should be considered as adjunct therapy to BAL if results are unsatisfactory. One hundred mg/kg/day orally in four divided doses preceding meals to a maximum dose of 1 gm/day for five days can be given. Three to five days of observation should follow with reinstitution of therapy if symptoms recur. When the 24-hour urinary arsenic excretion has fallen below 50 μg/24 hours, further chelation therapy would not be necessary. At intervals it is well to test the urine, stools and blood to gauge how rapidly arsenic is being eliminated and how effective is the course of treatment. Antiarrhythmic drugs should be used when indicated. In concomitant renal failure, hemodialysis can produce dramatically good results.

### *Arsine*

Arsine ($AsH_3$) is an extremely poisonous colorless inflammable gas. It can be evolved whenever ores contaminated with arsenic come in contact either with hydrogen ions from the action of acid on metal or with aluminum used as a finely divided wetted dross (which probably evolves hydrogen by electrolysis or hydrolysis). Most cases of arsine poisoning are found in the metallurgic industries. Ships carrying ferrosilicon, which is used in the iron industry, should follow established safety regulations. When this product is exposed to extreme dampness, toxic amounts of arsine gas as well as phosphine are emitted.

Symptoms include nausea, vomiting and abdominal cramps; hemolysis, hemoglobinuria and jaundice; and oliguria, anuria and uremia due to blocking of renal tubules by products of hemoglobin breakdown.

Toxic effects can generally be explained by the RBC destruction, but the damaging effect on liver, spleen, kidneys, lungs, etc. is also direct and severe. EKG changes are felt to be of importance in diagnosis of even minimal exposure cases. Immediate measures are required if the hemolytic and toxic effects of arsine gas are to be overcome. Patients receiving sublethal amounts of the arsine recover without apparent sequelae. Those receiving a lethal dose are doomed in spite of therapy. Early exchange transfusion has been advocated. Dimercaprol, although usually ineffective, should be used.

The true solution to this problem lies in prevention: adequate ventilation, education and efficient warning devices—these are essential in any industry where arsine gas is a possibility. The odor cannot always be relied upon for detection of the gas even though it often has an offensive smell resembling that of onions or carbide, which should arouse suspicion.

### *Fluoride*

Fluoride salts and compounds are rapidly absorbed and slowly excreted. Intoxication is most frequently due to accidental ingestion of an insecticide such as "roach powder," generally kept in the kitchen and containing 30 to 90 per cent of sodium fluoride. Roach powder has been substituted for baking powder in a pancake batter, and once in an institutional kitchen, it was mistaken for powdered milk and mixed—17 pounds of it—with 10 gallons of scrambled eggs. This resulted in 47 fatalities in a group of 263 persons who did not mind the salty or soapy taste of the eggs. It is unlikely that the ingestion of large numbers of vitamin-fluoride tablets would produce any serious toxicity (*see* Vitamins).

The initial symptoms following ingestion are intense epigastric pain, dysphagia, salivation, nausea, hematemesis, hematuria and diarrhea. It is possible that corrosive hydrogen fluoride is formed in the acid medium of the stomach; in fact, such gastric contents have been known to etch glass and produce superficial and deep ulcerations of the esophagus, mucous membranes and skin. Vomiting and diarrhea, fortunately, often eliminate much of the poison, but there is ready absorption of the soluble fluoride salts from the gastrointestinal tract.

Fluoride is a general protoplasmic poison, probably because of its capacity to inactivate several proteolytic and glycolytic enzymes, and death has occurred within a few minutes after ingestion. Fluoride ion also binds blood calcium as calcium fluoride, which is an insoluble compound. As ionized blood calcium falls, the patient shows signs of increasing excitability of skeletal muscles, a positive Chvostek sign, hyperactive reflexes, painful spasms (especially of the extremities), weakness and then full-blown tetanic contractures alternating at times with paresis. The onset of tetany is usually delayed three to five hours. The clinical picture, in part, appears to be due to these consequences of hypocalcemia. Chemical binding with potassium and magnesium followed by relocation to intracellular and intraosseous sites can produce hypokalemia and hypomagnesemia, which if severe enough, could produce myocardial irritability and ventricular fibrillation.

The respiratory center is at first stimulated, but eventually becomes depressed, and death may result from respiratory paralysis. Death may also be due to shock because of the combined effects of excessive fluid loss as a result of violent emesis, profuse salivation and perspiration and the toxic effect of the fluoride ion on heart muscle, causing cardiac arrhythmias and myocardial failure. If death occurs, the pathologic findings include congestion and hemorrhagic infiltration of all the organs and hydropic degeneration of the kidneys and liver.

The lethal dose of sodium fluoride* is surprisingly large, about 5 gm, but a dose as low as 2 gm has been recorded as fatal. The estimated fatal dose for an adult is 50 to 225 mg/kg. Chronic intake of more than 6 mg/day of fluoride (13.2 mg NaF) produces fluorosis (severe mottling of the enamel of teeth). Doses in the range of 25 to 50 mg may cause acute gastroenteritis. Bone is an accumulator of excess fluoride when ingestion exceeds 5 mg daily. Skeletal fluorosis has been reported with ingestions of 10 to 15 mg daily, particularly under conditions of high industrial fluoride contamination.

Nutritional surveys continue to show dental caries as the foremost nutritional disease for all age groups beyond infancy. The administration of fluoride is an effective means of reducing the incidence of dental caries. Physicians caring for infants and children in regions of the country where commercial waters are not fluoridated and the natural water contains a low level of fluoride (0.5 ppm) should see that sufficient fluoride is prescribed to provide an intake of 0.5 mg/day for children up to three years of age and 1.0 mg/day after age three years. Tea, which is naturally high in fluoride, has approximately 0.5 mg/prepared cup.

*Treatment* consists essentially of making use of the characteristic insolubility of calcium fluoride by binding as much fluoride ion as possible with calcium, per os or intravenously. The patient should be made to drink limewater (0.15% calcium hydroxide), calcium chloride solution (1 tsp./qt. of water) or milk. Milk acts both as a demulcent and as a fluoride "binder." This should be followed by gentle gastric lavage with any of the same fluids. Even in the absence of signs of muscular hyperirritability, the victim should receive a slow intravenous injection of 10 ml (5 ml for children) of either 10% calcium gluconate or calcium chloride, and more should be available in a syringe for use at the first signs of muscular spasm. (The injection of calcium chloride should be particularly slow.) Calcium solution should also be used to wash away corrosive vomitus and excreta from the skin. For hydrofluoric acid burn of the skin, wash thoroughly with cold water and apply magnesium oxide paste. Parenteral potassium and magnesium should be administered according to serum measurements or to the electrocardiographic signs of hypokalemia or hypomagnesemia. If severe cardiac irritability and arrhythmias develop, intracardiac pacemaking should be considered as well as pharmacologic agents (lidocaine, etc.) to reduce myocardial irritability. In case of shock parenteral fluids should be given as necessary. In the presence of normal renal function, maintenance of an adequate urine output is the most effective way to assure removal of fluoride from the body. Hemodialysis may be useful in a patient with compromised renal function but is not indicated in the presence of a normal renal function and urine output.

### *Thallium*

Poisoning from thallium is still encountered in the United States, even though since 1960 the content of thallium in pesticides for household use has been limited by the

*2.2 mg sodium fluoride contains 1 mg fluoride.

Department of Agriculture to 1 per cent and finally removed from the market altogether in 1965. The known thallium trade-named products once sold for use against roaches, water bugs, moles, ants, silverfish, mice, rats and other pests numbered at least forty-four, and probably more were available as noninterstate agents. Unfortunately, products containing thallium can still be found on home and store shelves and its use in industry is increasing. Because of its high refractive index, it is incorporated into the manufacturing of optical lens and in imitation precious jewelry. It is used in alloys along with silver as a catalyst in a number of organic reactions and has also been included in fireworks.

Of seventy-two confirmed cases of thallium poisoning in southern Texas, nine children died and twenty-six (50%) had permanent central nervous system sequelae consisting of abnormal reflexes, ataxia, tremors, psychosis and mental retardation. The use of this toxic compound as a pesticide should remain replaced by other substances which are effective yet safer for children. Thallium salts were used widely as rodenticides, insecticides (ants) and depilatories. Poisoning most often resulted from the accidental ingestion of rodent or ant bait which consisted of thallium sulfate or acetate mixed with grain, bread crumbs, honey or syrup. Thallium, unfortunately, is tasteless and odorless, so that its presence was entirely masked in the sugary products and pastes in which it was often concealed to kill pests. Chronic poisoning can come from skin absorption as well as ingestion.

Thallium compounds induce degenerative changes in all cells. The cells most susceptible are those of the hair follicles, followed by those of the central nervous system. The fatal dose is approximately 1 gm of absorbed thallium. The minimum lethal dose is 12 mg/kg of body weight. A dose of 1 oz. (30 gm) of a 1% preparation can be lethal for a 25 kg (55 lb.) child.

Neurologic and gastrointestinal symptoms may dominate the clinical picture, but the pathognomonic sign is *alopecia,* which may begin as early as seven days after exposure but usually not until the second or third week or later. The evidences of poisoning appear in one to fourteen days; these include pain and paresthesia in the extremities, ptosis, fever, conjunctivitis, abdominal pain, nausea, hematemesis, bloody diarrhea and loss of hair. Progression of poisoning is indicated by the appearance of lethargy, tremors, choreiform movements, ataxia, convulsions and cyanosis. Signs of pulmonary edema and pneumonia may precede death from respiratory failure.

Alopecia is invariably present in chronic poisoning and occasionally seen with other chemicals and drugs (*see* Table 51). Atrophic changes in the skin and nails, salivation, pigmentation of the gums and renal damage may occur along with the acute symptoms mentioned above.

Psychotic symptoms may lead one to miss the diagnosis. The patient may be nervous, anxious or depressed. Impaired memory, sloppiness and gradually deteriorating work performance indicate organic brain damage.

Laboratory Tests. The best means of confirming the diagnosis of thallotoxicosis is to demonstrate the presence of thallium in the urine.* Even traces of thallium in the urine should be considered abnormal and may still be detectable many weeks after ingestion.

Thallium salts are radiopaque and sometimes lead to opacities in the liver in abdominal roentgenograms. This finding may clarify a difficult differential diagnosis.

*Treatment.* The ingested poison should be removed immediately by thorough gastric lavage. If this procedure cannot be done readily, then vomiting should be induced by an emetic or by pharyngeal stimulation. Any thallium-containing material which may remain on the skin should be washed off completely with soap and water. Activated

*Combine a few drops of urine with 3 drops of saturated bromine water, 3 drops of sulfosalicylic acid, 1 drop of reagent grade hydrochloric acid, 2 drops of a solution of 0.05 gm of rhodamine B in 100 ml of concentrated hydrochloric acid; mix; add 1 ml of reagent grade benzene, then shake, centrifuge, and examine the benzene layer. A bright yellow or fluorescent red color is a positive test.

TABLE 51
CHEMICALS AND DRUGS PRODUCING ALOPECIA

| | |
|---|---|
| Allopurinol | Methimazole |
| α-methyl dopa | Methotrexate |
| Anticoagulants | Norethindrone acetate |
| Arsenic | Oral contraceptives |
| Aspirin | Propylthiouracil* |
| Amphetamines | Quinacrine |
| Clofibrate | Selenium sulfide |
| Cyclophosphamide | Sodium warfarin |
| Diphenylhydantoin | Thallium |
| 5-Fluorouracil | Trimethadione |
| Gentamicin | Triparanol |
| Gold salts | Uracil mustard |
| Heparin | Vinblastine |
| Iodine* | Vincristine |
| Levodopa | Vitamin A |
| Mepesulfate | |
| Mephenytoin | |

*Alopecia can occur in spontaneous hypothyroidism.
Reprinted by permission of The Medical Letter, Inc., 56 Harrison Street, New Rochelle, New York, 10801.

charcoal by mouth in dosage of 0.5 gm/kg twice a day for at least five days, along with potassium chloride 3 to 5 gm daily orally for five to ten days, have been found effective adjuncts to therapy.

BAL may be employed as a detoxification agent, but the reports of its value are equivocal. In maximal dosages, however, the results have been encouraging and further trial is needed.

Prussian blue (ferric ferrocyanide) has been reported to be effective in animals and humans by markedly increasing the excretion of thallium from the intestinal tract. Soluble ferric ferrocyanide 125 mg/kg twice a day with 50 ml of 15% mannitol is given by duodenal tube. This therapy should be continued until urinary excretion of thallium is 0.5 mg or lower/day.

Dithizon (diphenylthio-carbazone), a chelating agent, 10 mg/kg orally dissolved in 100 ml of 10% glucose solution twice daily for five days, has been tried with equivocal results. As yet, however, no preparation of dithizon is marketed for therapeutic use. Chemical supply houses include in their catalogs explanatory statements indicating that they are uncertain of the purity of this agent and that it is sold for chemical and investigational purposes only. Because of its diabetogenic effect on animals, dithizon, if tried, should be used with caution.

Trihexyphenidyl (Artane®) may be useful in controlling the distressing tremors and severe ataxia that accompany thallium intoxication.

For chronic poisoning, it is imperative to eliminate further exposure in addition to the above therapy.

Other forms of treatment which have been proposed are now largely discarded. Pilocarpine has been used in an attempt to promote sweat gland excretion of thallium, but there is no experimental or clinical evidence of its efficacy. Sodium iodide parenterally has been suggested in the hope of converting a toxic soluble thallium to a nonsoluble state. While theoretically feasible, the clinical use of such therapy has been unsuccessful except as a lavage soon after ingestion. Cystine increases the renal excretion of thallium in laboratory animals and tends to protect them from chronic intoxication. Yet with animals acutely poisoned, neither cystine nor methionine have been found effective and there is no well-documented evidence to support the clinical use of these agents. Various resins and diuretics which have been tried so far have not produced any increase in thallium excretion nor protected experimental animals. Oral potassium chloride effectively releases tissue thallium but aggravates symptoms by increasing plasma thallium content.

## *Selenium*

Selenium poisoning is not common in humans. The presence of this nonmetallic element of the sulfur group in the soil, however, may give rise to accumulation in plants and these in turn may cause symptoms and even death in grazing animals (loco disease). Such extremes in the selenium intake of animals are due to the fact that the plants consumed by the animals are often of local origin and there are great geographical variations in the amount of selenium in the soil that is available for uptake by the plants.

In contrast to animals, the human population generally draws its foods from several different regions of the country. There is no evidence at this time to suggest that the food supply in the United States contains either too little or too much selenium. There is reason, however, to suspect that indiscriminate selenium supplementation of the diet is potentially hazardous. A well-balanced diet is the best way to obtain not only selenium but all of the other nutritionally essential trace elements as well. The 150 μg/day of selenium furnished by the average American diet is sufficient. The best sources of the element are organ and muscle meats and seafoods. Most fruits and vegetables, except for garlic, mushrooms and asparagus, are generally poor sources of selenium. The effect of low levels of selenium in the soil of some areas is canceled by interregional food shipments and the addition of selenium to swine and poultry feed.

Since selenium is used in the manufacture of photoelectric cells, glass and other products, constant exposure may lead to chronic poisoning. This is characterized by pallor, garlicky odor to the breath, metallic taste, gastrointestinal disturbances, irritation of the nose and throat, conjunctivitis, lacrimation, dermatitis, drowsiness and constriction of the chest. The urine may contain albumin, urobilinogen, urobilin and porphyrin, and there may be a profound anemia with leukocytosis.

*Treatment* consists of removal from the occupational environment, a selenium-free diet and bromobenzene (*see* page 33).

## *Metaldehyde*

Metaldehyde is a tasteless water-insoluble solid that is a polymerization product of acetaldehyde. It is often combined with calcium arsenate and used for slug and snail bait. Metaldehyde is also marketed in the form of tablets as fuel for small heaters; emitted vapors are also a source of poisoning in situations where poor ventilation exists. Children have been poisoned by eating this bait and the fuel tablets, which they mistake for candy. Ingestion causes salivation, nausea, abdominal pain, severe vomiting, numbness in the legs and ataxia. The face becomes flushed, the temperature elevated, and muscular rigidity, twitching and choreiform movements may occur. In fatal cases there are convulsions, coma and death from respiratory failure. The *treatment* consists of immediate gastric lavage and supportive therapy. Analeptics or sedatives should be used if indicated by the condition of the patient. Parenteral chlorpromazine (Thorazine) and calcium gluconate may also be effective therapy.

## *Mercury*

Mercury is a highly toxic, silver-white, liquid metal which is slightly volatile at ordinary temperature, being readily absorbed by the inhalation of its fumes. Mercury salts are widely used in medicine as cathartics, antiseptics and diuretics, in cosmetics as a skin and hair bleach and preservative, and in agriculture and industry in the form of dusting or wettable powder and fumigants. Since every known form of mercury compound is potentially dangerous (organic mercurials, because they are poorly absorbed, are often less toxic than the inorganic), the opportunity for accidental intoxication is widespread.

The chemical form of mercury is an important determinant of toxicity. Three basic forms are encountered.

1. Free metal; found in barometers, thermometers and medical instruments.
2. Inorganic salts; antiseptics, obsolete cathartics (calomel) and pigments.
3. Organic salts; diuretics, antiseptics and fungicides.

Ingestion of the *free metal* from broken thermometers or instruments constitutes *little* threat to health since it is not absorbed from the GI tract. Mercury vapor, however, is a hazard. Chronic exposure may occur in laboratories where spilled metal is not cleaned up. After mercury vapor is inhaled, mercury appears in the blood partly unchanged and partially oxidized. Elemental mercury is therefore in position to diffuse into the tissues by crossing cell membranes. This movement is enhanced by the lack of charge of the elemental mercury and by its liquid solubility. It is likely that this phenomenon accounts for the fact that the brain retains ten times more mercury after exposure to mercury vapor than when an equal amount of mercuric salt is administered. In animal experiments, mercury concentrates in the cerebellum, hypothalamus, areas adjacent to the lateral ventricles and the area postrema. Mercuric chloride (an antiseptic) is extremely toxic if ingested, but less soluble antiseptics like mercurochrome and thiomerosol are relatively safe. Organic mercurials, especially the alkyl derivatives used to treat seeds and created by environmental pollution, are lipid-soluble and readily cross biologic membranes including the placenta and are highly toxic. Acute poisoning, however, occurs most frequently on the farm or in the home from food (fish) contamination or water pollution, while the subacute and chronic forms are more common in industry and medicine.

The mercuric ion has a specific affinity for the sulfhydryl groups of intracellular proteins and, in addition, very effectively precipitates protein substances. Solutions of mercuric salts are also markedly corrosive. The most dangerous of these when swallowed is mercuric chloride. Acute poisoning, accidental or willful, is frequently caused by the ingestion of this compound, even though it is manufactured as a deep blue coffin-shaped tablet labeled "poison."

Acute mercury vapor poisoning from a freshly painted gas heater has been responsible for the death of three children. Mercury fume hazards have also been reported from scraping marine antifouling paint from boats, the operation of an electric display sign and in workers manufacturing costume jewelry.

Metallic mercury, since it is not absorbed, is nontoxic. Rhazes (A.D. 865 to 923) clearly established the innocuous nature of this heavy metal in an experimental study of the gastrointestinal tract of a monkey. The occasional ingestion, then, of this compound by children from broken or cracked thermometers should give no great concern. Mercury droplets can be picked up by a piece of clean copper.

Embolization has been reported now that metallic mercury is being used instead of mineral oil as the anaerobic seal and mixing agent in syringes used for blood gas analyses. This hazard of parenteral absorption during blood sampling should be kept in mind. The willful or accidental subcutaneous injection of mercury, contrary to previous beliefs of being nontoxic, can produce serious symptoms and death.

Phenyl mercuric propionate to prevent mold growth is used as an antimildew additive and incorporated in many of the water base paints that are prepared for outdoor use today. It is a source of potential danger of mercury intoxication either from ingestion or inhalation of its toxic vapors.

Warkany, Hubbard, and others have assembled convincing data that most, if not all, instances of acrodynia are the result of an unusual sensitivity or idiosyncrasy to mercury (calomel, mercurous chloride in teething powders or lotions, mercurial ointments, vaporization of mercury in paint used in a poorly ventilated room, etc.). Copper intoxication can also produce acrodynia.

Within a few minutes to half an hour following ingestion, the patient develops symptoms of an acute gastrointestinal inflammation. He complains of a metallic taste, thirst, nausea, retching and pain in the pharynx and abdomen, followed by vomiting of blood-stained material. Later, with tenesmus and bloody diarrhea, the clinical picture is that of hemorrhagic gastritis and colitis, with continuous or intermittent suppression of urine, uremia and circulatory collapse. The corrosive preparations of mercury cause immediate necrosis of the buccal, pharyngeal and gastrointestinal mucosa. The patient may die within hours if vomiting is severe enough to produce electrolyte losses leading to peripheral vascular collapse.

The second phase of poisoning, which develops in a patient surviving one to three days, is characterized by stomatitis, gastritis, colitis and severe renal tubular degeneration. It is seen even with noncorrosive (mercurous or monovalent) preparations of mercury, regardless of the portal of entry. Death at this time is usually the result of irreversible renal failure.

Chronic intoxication with inorganic mercurials results in salivation, loosening of the teeth, fetor oris, gingivitis and ulceration of the mouth. The characteristic neurologic symptoms are (1) erethism (a mental state of fatigability), easy embarrassment, irritability, apprehension and withdrawal; and (2) tremors of the hands, feet, tongue and lip, staggering and slurred speech. Such an intoxication can occur from industrial exposure to metallic mercury or its vapors, fingerprint photography, gilding, and formerly from the carrotting process in making felt for hats—the "mad hatters."

Chronic exposure to organic mercurials, in contrast, has a predilection to affect the central nervous system. Lesions of the spinal cord producing a clinical and pathologic resemblance to amyotrophic lateral sclerosis have been reported.

Organic compounds have low dissociation constants and are excreted by the kidney. An effective concentration of mercurial ions is only obtained in the kidney where sulfhydryl enzymes essential in the tubular reabsorption process are inhibited. This mechanism may partially account for the clinical differences between chronic exposure to inorganic and to organic mercurials; perhaps the blood-brain barrier is more permeable to the latter. It does not, however, satisfactorily explain why some patients, following prolonged exposure, have no symptoms of mercurialism, others react quickly to relatively slight exposure but have a short benign course and still others have a protracted siege of systemic and neurologic disability.

Death has resulted from as little as 0.5 gm of mercury, although the lethal dose for adults is between 1 and 4 gm. Absorption through the gastrointestinal tract is so quick and complete that the outcome depends greatly upon what happens during the first fifteen minutes or so, particularly in respect to vomiting or the possibility of rapid gastric lavage.

A technique for the quantitative determination of the mercury content of urine has been worked out using x-ray spectrochemical analysis. The time required to complete the analysis is only a fraction of the time required by classic procedures. Measurements have been made on concentrations as low as 3 mg of mercury in 100 ml of urine (one-tenth the clinically maximum allowable concentration). The technique involves destruction of the organic matter with potassium permanganate in a sulfuric acid solution of the sample. The mercury is precipitated as the sulfide with thioacetamide in the presence of copper as a collector. The precipitate is then collected on a millipore filter and directly analyzed in the x-ray spectrometer. This rapid method can be extremely helpful in making a correct early diagnosis of mercury poisoning when doubt exists. The amount of mercury excreted in the urine, (abnormal value greater than 10 mg/24 hr.), however, seemingly bears no direct relationship to the severity of symptoms. One must conclude that the response to mercurial exposure is to a great extent based, as it is with drugs in general, on individual sensitivity. The mercury level in the blood is a less reliable indicator of degree of exposure than the mercury level of the urine. There is a rapid loss of mercury from the bloodstream after absorption and the variation of mercury level in the blood in different individuals is greater than the variation in mercury levels of the urine. In individual cases, correlation between mercury levels in the urine or blood and symptoms of poisoning is poor. Some with signs of poisoning may have lower mercury levels in the urine or blood than those without signs of poisoning. The diagnosis of mercury poisoning must be based on the history of exposure and physical examination, with secondary reliance on mercury level in the urine or blood or both. Salivary (parotid) excretion of mercury has been found to be two-fifths and one-tenth of the blood and urinary mercury concentrations respectively, and this could be used as another simple and useful parameter of exposure and excretion.

The *treatment* of mercury poisoning aims at the precipitation and removal of mercury from the gastrointestinal tract, the inactivation of absorbed mercuric ions and general supportive measures to maintain electrolyte and fluid balance. To be successful, treatment must be prompt and intensive. The administration of egg white or milk may be helpful by precipitating mercury and thus delaying its absorption. Better results are produced by immediate gastric lavage with egg white solution (two egg whites mixed with glass of milk [preferable] or water) or with 5% sodium formaldehyde sulfoxylate (which reduces mercuric chloride to metallic mercury). The sodium formaldehyde sulfoxylate can also be mixed with a 3% solution of sodium bicarbonate. About 200 ml of the solution should be left in the stomach. In the absence of this compound, a 2% to 5% solution of sodium bicarbonate can be used. Also recommended is 15 to 30 gm of sodium or magnesium sulfate in 6 to 8 oz. of water, unless there is diarrhea.

To inactivate the mercury already absorbed, therapy with BAL, which has a greater affinity for the mercuric ion than do the sulfhydryl groups, is instituted as promptly as possible. There is some difference of opinion as to the dosage to be administered. Gleason and associates recommended giving 3.0 mg of BAL per kilogram of body weight every four hours for six injections on the first two days, the same dose every six hours on the third day, then 3.0 mg/kg every twelve hours until recovery occurs. If intoxication is mild, 2.5 mg/kg is recommended. Other clinicians use as much as 5.0 mg/kg initially, followed by 2.5 mg/kg every three hours for the first twenty-four hours in cases of severe poisoning (*see* BAL, p. 32).

Shock due to peripheral vascular collapse is treated by whole blood or plasma and infusions of dextrose and saline solution.

Renal insufficiency is managed by the usual therapy for acute renal failure. Spironolactone (Aldactone®) in experimental animals (rats) has prevented renal tubular necrosis by mercuric chloride when well-tolerated amounts of the drugs were given beforehand.

It has been shown in experiments that D-penicillamine is effective in protecting the rat from lethal effects of mercuric chloride. Interest in the sulfhydryl amino acid penicillamine (beta, beta-dimethylcysteine) and its derivatives has led to work suggesting that these new agents may be of value in the treatment of heavy metal intoxication. It has been demonstrated that penicillamine (0.6 to 1.0 gm daily) increases the urinary excretion of copper in people with an accumulation of excess copper in the tissues (Wilson's disease). D-penicillamine reduces the excretion of cystine in the urine of patients with cystinuria and cystine calculi. This action appears to be the result of the formation of a mixed penicillamine-cysteine disulfide which is more soluble than cystine. Its value in cystinosis has not been fully established. Its use, however, has great possibilities and should be encouraged. The drug is reported to cause the dissociation of some macroglobulins such as those present in rheumatoid arthritis and also to reduce the viscosity of the plasma in macroglobulinemia, diminishing the load on the heart and improving the peripheral circulation. IgA deficiency induced by D-penicillamine (and phenytoin) has been recently reported. The compound has also been shown to increase lead and iron excretion in humans with lead intoxication and hemosiderosis.

A protective action in rats against the lethal effects of mercuric chloride has also been demonstrated for DL-penicillamine and more recently, for N-acetyl-DL-penicillamine. Of the three compounds, the last, N-acetyl-DL-penicillamine, appears to be the most effective since this compound is more active and less toxic in protecting rats from the lethal effects of mercuric chloride.

The greater protective action of N-acetyl-DL-penicillamine may be due to greater stability of the N-acetyl-DL-penicillamine-mercury complex (the presence of the acetyl radical protects the amino group from metabolic reaction or degradation) or to the fact that the N-acetyl compound penetrates cells to a greater extent than does penicillamine.

The greater toxicity of DL-penicillamine over D-penicillamine or N-acetyl-DL-penicillamine seems to be associated with the L-penicillamine isomer. Growth in rats and in some microorganisms has been inhibited by the L isomer; this may possibly be related to the anti-vitamin-$B_6$ activity of L-penicillamine.

The mechanism underlying the protective action of the penicillamine derivatives is as yet unknown. The exact structure of the resulting metal-penicillamine derivative compounds has not yet been determined. It is interesting that BAL (2,3-dimercaptopropanol) is a dithiol, while penicillamine and its derivatives are monothiols. BAL is an effective antidote in heavy metal intoxication because its two sulfhydryl groups successfully compete with tissue enzyme sulfhydryl groups for the offending metal to form a more stable ring with the metal. No doubt the sulfhydryl grouping of the penicillamine derivatives plays an important role in protection against heavy metals. However, the exact mechanism is probably more complex than direct reaction between sulfhydryl and metal, for other monothiols such as cysteine and glutathione are not as protective as the penicillamine derivatives.

BAL is somewhat more effective than D-penicillamine and DL-penicillamine in protecting rats against the lethal effects of mercuric chloride. The oral effectiveness of the penicillamine derivatives is given as an advantage of these compounds over BAL. However, since severe vomiting is an almost constant early manifestation of heavy metal intoxication, an oral antidote might not be too advantageous. Nevertheless, these investigations of the penicillamine derivatives are a valuable contribution to basic knowledge about poisoning. Further clinical evaluation may permit the addition of these compounds to the too small list of already existing antidotes. D-penicillamine (Cuprimine®) is the only preparation available at present. The dose for older children and adults is 250 mg four times daily. For infants six months of age and young children, the daily dose of 250 mg should be dissolved in fruit juices.

The numerous side-effects in humans attributed to penicillamine therapy, which include fever, drowsiness, stupor, headache, anorexia, nausea, vomiting, myalgia, conjunctivitis, skin eruptions, nephropathy (nephrosis) on the basis of allergic glomerulitis, neutrophilic agranulocytosis (cytotoxic effect), leukopenia and thrombocytopenia, generally have been considered to be insufficiently severe to warrant more than temporary interruption of therapy. The report of reversible optic axial neuritis, probably due to metabolic antagonism between penicillamine and pyridoxine, would appear to justify therapeutic pyridoxine supplementation as a preventive measure. Taste dysfunction (hypergeusia) rarely occurs and is reported to respond best to oral copper salts. Patients who are sensitive to penicillin may have a similar reaction to penicillamine.

### *Methyl Mercury (in fish and humans)*

Physicians have long been accustomed to using inorganic mercury (Hg) compounds for a variety of medicinal reasons. Many were therefore not particularly impressed by the sudden revelation that fish in lakes and streams throughout the country contained an abnormally high percentage of mercury. In most instances, the source of contamination appeared to be the agricultural fungicides and the metallic Hg discharged into the water by such industries as those producing chlorine and alkali. For every ton of chlorine produced, nearly half a pound of mercury escapes into the environment. Based on projected chlorine tonnage, this adds up to 3300 lb./day, or 1.2 million lb./year. Mercury also enters the ocean from volcanoes. At present, about 10,000 tons of mercury flow into the sea each year; about one half of this is of natural origin and the other half is from industrial sources. In agriculture, we use an additional million lb./year as fungicides protecting our seed grain and as pesticides sprayed on plants.

It was not generally known that the relatively inoffensive metal is converted, before entering the algae-fish-human food chain, into one of the most potent and insidious poisons in existence, namely organic methyl mercury. This biological methylation is accomplished by bacteria called *Methanobacterium omelanskii* living in the bottom mud. These bacteria are then eaten by plankton, which in turn are eaten by fish. Contaminated species include pike, pickerel, perch, walleye, muskie and white bass. Methylation is carried out under mostly anaerobic conditions and is facilitated by the presence of raw sewage discharged into the water by industrial and municipal sources. Eating contaminated meat (from the inadvertent feeding to hogs of grain treated with alkyl mercury) has produced serious human mercury poisoning in this country.

Methyl mercury, unlike inorganic Hg compounds, is an extremely subtle, difficult-to-detect and long-lasting poison. It is bound by hemoglobin in the red blood cells and circulates in this form for months. When it reaches the intestinal tract, most of it is readsorbed into blood and excreted at the rate of only 1 per cent per day, mostly in the feces; the estimated half-life in man is seventy days and in fish two hundred days. It passes easily into the central nervous system, where it selectively and irreversibly damages the cells of the granular layer in the cerebellum, the cerebral cortex and the calcarine cortex. It swiftly passes the placental barrier and accumulates in the fetal brain and blood, building up to 30 per cent higher red blood cell levels than in the mother. It appears, further, to be more cumulative in female than in male blood and to be especially injurious to the central nervous system of infants and children.

The manifestations of methyl mercury poisoning typically appear several weeks or months, perhaps years, after ingestion or absorption of a toxic dose. Stemming chiefly from CNS involvement, they include any or all of the following.

1. Paresthesia of the mouth, lips, tongue, hands, feet, fingers and toes.
2. Constriction of visual fields, with abnormal "blind spots" ("tunnel vision").
3. Hearing difficulty, especially in picking out one voice from a group.
4. Speech disorders, such as loud, explosive sounds, difficulty in articulating words and swallowing.
5. Neurasthenia, including weakness, fatigue and inability to concentrate.
6. Inability to write, read or recall basic things such as the alphabet, familiar addresses, numbers, etc.
7. Emotional instability, fits of anger, depression and agitation.
8. Ataxia, including dysdiadochocinesia; stumbling gait; clumsiness in handling familiar objects such as forks, buttons and shoelaces; grotesque, wholly uncoordinated movements; spasticity; rigidity; and paralysis.
9. Stupor, coma and death in extreme cases.

The first known cases of human poisoning from fish contaminated with methyl mercury were reported in Japan, on the island of Kyushu, around Minamata Bay. Between 1953 and 1970, more than 121 poisonings were reported in this area, with 46 deaths recorded. The victims had eaten large quantities of fish and shellfish containing an estimated 10 to 20 parts per million (ppm) of methyl mercury chloride. This chemical had been discharged directly into the bay and the river feeding it by a plant manufacturing plastics from vinyl chloride and acetaldehyde.

In 1964, a similar outbreak of poisonings occurred at Niigata, Japan, along the lower Agano River. At this site, 43 cases, including 6 deaths, were officially documented; however, 120 persons were affected, showing one or more symptoms together with an abnormal methyl mercury blood level. Many of these persons died later of secondary illnesses, such as pneumonia and inanition.

Much work has been done in Sweden on the medical aspects of methyl mercury contamination of fish. A number of lakes have been found to contain fish with 0.5 to 1 ppm or more of Hg, including Sweden's largest, Lake Väner, 5585 square kilometers, about 200 miles west of Stockholm. Such fish have also been found in the coastal waters in the Baltic

Sea for several hundred miles north and south of Stockholm and in parts of the Kattegat Strait between Sweden and Denmark. Wild fowl are also seriously contaminated.

Intensive investigations of Hg levels in wild fowl, fish and human beings also have been carried out in Canada. In 1970, the Canadian government informed United States authorities that fish caught in the Great Lakes and adjacent waters had Hg (virtually 100% methyl mercury) levels up to 2.8 ppm. More recently, levels up to 9 ppm have been found in a few specimens. A chemical plant in Sarnia, Ontario, was estimated to be discharging up to 200 lb. of "waste" metallic Hg daily into the St. Clair River, which flows between Lake Huron and Lake Erie.

Studies done in Sweden, Finland, Japan, Canada and the United States of people who eat little or no fish, contaminated or uncontaminated, are in close agreement in setting "normal" human blood levels of Hg. These are approximately 5 parts per billion (ppb) in whole blood and approximately 10 ppb in red blood cells. "Normal" levels of Hg in human hair are not as well established, but probably range up to about 10 ppm.

Values much higher than any of these, however, have been found in many persons with no detectable symptoms of poisoning, although they have regularly eaten contaminated fish in fairly large quantities.

The average tuna must contain less than 0.5 mg/kg by FDA regulation. Tuna with a higher level is discarded by the canning industry. Since the $LD_{50}$ of mercury for humans is approximately 500 mg, it would be necessary to consume about 2200 lb. of tuna to be poisoned. Many scientists recommend, for safety, that a whole blood level of approximately 100 ppb should not be exceeded. This would correspond to a daily intake of 0.1 mg of Hg, or about 100 gm of fish containing 1 ppb (mg/kg) of Hg. The "safe" weekly limit would thus be, assuming the same fish content of 1 ppb, about 700 gm (1½ lb.), or three goodly portions of fish a week. For fish containing 2 ppb, the weekly limit would be ¾ lb. At 3 ppb, the limit would be ½ lb., or one meal per week. This assumes that all of the fish flesh contains the same amount of Hg and that human intestinal absorption is complete.

The above assumptions are theoretical, since no cases of human poisoning have been reported except those in Japan, which, unfortunately, were incompletely studied. Moreover, we have dealt so far only with the question of clinically detectable symptoms in adults. There remain more insidious questions about which we know very little.

In Sweden, it has been demonstrated in five instances that fetal red blood cells at birth had an average concentration of Hg 28 per cent higher than that of the mother. Moreover, the higher the maternal red blood cell level, the faster the rate of increase in fetal red blood cell Hg levels; in other words, the rise in fetal red blood cell levels is disproportionately rapid at higher maternal levels. The accentuated effects of methyl mercury on the fetus are attested by the fact that in nineteen Minamata cases of infantile cerebral paresis, the mothers showed no typical clinical symptoms of poisoning except for some complaints of numbness during pregnancy, although they were all heavy fish eaters. On the basis of these facts, it must be recommended, pending further studies, that pregnant women abstain from eating fish contaminated with methyl mercury.

The second question, about which we know even less, is that of the effects of methyl mercury on genetics. It has been shown that methyl mercury is 1000 times more potent in causing genetic damage than the next most powerful agent known, colchicine. In experiments on fruit flies (Drosophila) and onion root cells (Allium cepa), methyl mercury was found to inhibit mitosis and chromosome breakage in extremely low doses of 0.1 ppm or less. Injected intraperitoneally into mice in sublethal doses, it caused a decreased fertility rate; in pregnant female mice there was a higher rate of litter resorption and an increased percentage of fetuses born dead. Potential teratogenetic effects were also observed which appear to be corroborated by data from Minamata. Finally, a preliminary report indicates a significantly higher frequency of lymphocyte chromosome breakage among Swedes eating fish three times a week than among control subjects. A complete clarification of these findings may not appear until after several generations have passed.

It has been estimated that even after mercury contamination has ceased, a body of water may remain polluted for ten to one hundred years. No satisfactory method of reducing the pollution has yet been found. The proposed "solution" of dredging appears to be ineffective; no decrease in Hg levels of either shellfish or bottom mud was noted in Minamata Bay after dredging. Another method, dumping of sludge from ore concentration plants into streams and lakes in order to chemically inactivate both metallic Hg and methyl mercury, has shown promise after a small-scale trial in Sweden. It is unlikely that larger bodies of water, especially swiftly flowing rivers, can benefit from this treatment. A polystyrene resin containing sulfur has been found to greatly accelerate the time it takes for mice to excrete methyl mercury, and experiments are now being made with resin in stopping the passage of mercury in the food chains. It has been found that selenium counteracts the toxic effects of methyl mercury, but the amount of selenium available in sea water is insufficient to cope with gross contamination such as occurred in Minamata Bay.

### *Phosphorus*

Phosphorus exists in two forms: a red, granular, insoluble, nonabsorbed form which is nontoxic, and a yellow or white waxy form which is highly poisonous and burns on contact with water or even moist air, leaving a garlic-like odor.

This chemical is used in insect and rodent poisons, fireworks and fertilizer manufacture. Matches on the United States market now contain phosphorus trisulfide, which is very unreactive chemically, thus eliminating the danger of poisoning that existed in the past when yellow phosphorus was used in the heads of matches.

After ingestion, phosphorus exerts a toxic action locally in the digestive tract and is then absorbed with later injury to liver and muscle; the heart, kidney and nervous system are also damaged. Gastric symptoms may be immediate or delayed for some hours, but then abdominal pain, nausea, vomiting and diarrhea ensue. The vomitus has an odor of garlic and is luminescent. A symptom-free period of one to three days may then follow, marked by minor complaints such as eructation, nausea and thirst, before intensified symptoms reappear as a result of widespread organic and systemic effects. Death may also occur from vascular collapse or from acute damage to the myocardium owing to a direct toxic action within twelve hours.

Nausea, protracted vomiting (with streaking of blood), bloody diarrhea, jaundice, pruritis and abdominal tenderness in the region of an enlarged liver indicate hepatic degeneration. Delirium, convulsions, coma and sudden collapse suggest acute yellow atrophy. Hepatic insufficiency is further evidenced by a decrease in blood sugar (failure of glycogenolysis), hypoprothrombinemia and increased coagulation time. These abnormalities and direct damage to the walls of blood vessels are responsible for ecchymoses and petechiae of the skin, mucous membranes and viscera. The hepatic insult is reflected by a lessened urea content and the presence of amino acids in the urine, especially leucine and tyrosine. An early hyperglobulinemia, attributed to hepatic change and dehydration from continued vomiting or diarrhea, may persist even after efficient hydration.

The kidney is injured; the urine is scanty, phosphorescent and bloody and contains droplets of free fat and albumin. Death may follow in one or two days with acute renal shutdown and peripheral vascular collapse.

There are individual peculiarities in the toxic response. In a healthy adult, 50 to 60 mg may produce decidedly dangerous or fatal symptoms. Yet recovery has been reported after doses up to 400 mg. High mortality is expected if the poison is in a liquid vehicle (especially alcohol).

The oral ingestion of phosphorus presents an emergency which demands early diagnosis and immediate *treatment.* A history of ingestion of a phosphorus-containing substance, the garlic odor in vomitus or feces, the recovery or demonstration of phosphorus in them and the presence of the characteristic toxic symptoms serve as diagnostic criteria.

Gastric lavage should invariably be done if the patient is seen within the first five hours. If shock is imminent, gastric lavage may intensify circulatory failure and should therefore be used with caution. Copper sulfate (0.25 to 0.3 gm in a glass of water) forms an insoluble coating of copper phosphide. Potassium permanganate (1:5000 solution) or 2% hydrogen peroxide are effective as oxidizing agents and as aids in mechanical removal. At least 4 liters are recommended to remove the element thoroughly from the stomach, followed by activated charcoal, which should be instilled before the lavage tube is removed. Mineral oil or petrolatum has been given by mouth (or stomach tube) as a solvent to prevent absorption of phosphorus and to hasten its elimination; a dose of 200 to 250 ml is given at first and then doses of 30 to 40 ml every three hours for the first forty-eight hours. However, absorption can be increased by other fats and oils. A cathartic of magnésium sulfate after gastric lavage helps to cleanse the bowel of phosphorus, but purgation, by its dehydrating and diarrheal effects, may place an extra load on the circulatory system and should be avoided.

The supportive measures are directed at the prevention or treatment of acidosis, dehydration, shock and relief of pain. Fluid and electrolytes are given to maintain balance. For protection of the liver, large quantities of glucose by mouth (if possible) and vein are helpful. Vitamin K is indicated if the blood prothrombin level is low. Vitamin B complex, thiamine and ascorbic acid are regarded as useful supplements. The indications for blood transfusion must be carefully evaluated, for the main defect is poor venous return. Cutaneous burns should be washed with copious amounts of water or with a 1% solution of cupric sulfate, which forms a coat of black cupric phosphide.

Even with energetic treatment the mortality is near 50 per cent.

### *Phosphine*

The action of water or acids on phosphides or metals liberates phosphine ($PH_3$) if phosphorus is present as a contaminant. The prolonged inhalation of this gas can cause vomiting, fall in blood pressure, dyspnea, pulmonary edema, circulatory collapse, convulsions and coma.

*Treatment* is symptomatic and supportive. Exposure to the gas must be terminated at once and the use of contaminated water for drinking or bathing should be forbidden. There is no known specific antidote.

### *Borate, Sodium (Borax-Boric Acid)*

Boric acid is a white crystalline powder used as an antiseptic (properties of which are insignificant; there is no evidence that the isotonicity of a saturated solution is superior to a saline solution), food preservative and as a buffering and fungistatic agent in talcum powder. There is no question that indiscriminate use of boric acid over large areas of broken skin or mucous membrane is dangerous. However, the small amount present in baby powders is safe for normal use.

A recent report reviewed 83 fatal and 89 nonfatal cases of boric acid poisoning which have been documented in the literature. That there are more, recognized and unrecognized, there can be little doubt. While boric acid is relatively safe when properly used, its presence in hospitals always poses the threat of accidental substitution. The risk, albeit slight, seems unnecessary when the value of the product is questionable at best, and safer substitutes can be found. The Subcommittee on Accidental Poisoning of the American Academy of Pediatrics recommended that hospitals exercise rigid controls over the use of boric acid and that it be eliminated from newborn nurseries and pediatric sections of all hospitals. Such steps certainly should be undertaken as a minimum. Numerous institutions have gone further and have eliminated boric acid entirely. This would certainly provide the greatest degree of safety without significantly affecting the quality of patient care. "Perhaps it is not mere rhetorical coincidence that the major source of boron compound comes from Death Valley."

Sodium borate is used as an antiseptic, cleaning agent and insecticide spray and dust. Sodium perborate is used as a mouthwash and dentifrice. The lethal dose of these agents, which are alkaline, is estimated to be between 15 to 30 gm. They are toxic to all cells, and since the highest concentrations are reached during excretion, the kidneys are more seriously damaged than other organs such as liver and brain. Intracytoplasmic inclusion bodies have been reported in the acinar cells of the pancreas.

The principal manifestations of poisoning are erythema and exfoliation of the skin ("boiled lobster" appearance), fever, vomiting, inanition, dehydration, anuria and convulsions. Preceding the above symptoms, chronic intoxication from ingestion or absorption causes alopecia, weight loss and mild diarrhea. The local use as a mouthwash of sodium perborate in high concentrations may cause chemical stomatitis of variable degrees depending on the length of its use.

The presence of these compounds can be detected by applying a drop of urine, acidified with hydrochloric acid, to turmeric paper (impregnated with dye curcumin from turmeric plant), a chemical indicator. On contact a brownish-red color is produced

In the *treatment,* if the borates have been ingested, these should be removed immediately by either gastric lavage or emesis followed by catharsis. If symptoms are due to absorption, it is imperative that the product involved be removed from the skin or mucous membranes by thorough washing and that their use be immediately discontinued. Intravenous 10% glucose in water induces diuresis and is reported to exert a "binding" effect on circulating borate ions. Convulsions are controlled by pentobarbital or inhalation anesthesia. Exchange transfusion, artificial kidney or peritoneal dialysis may be lifesaving procedures in extreme cases. For infants critically ill from boric acid poisoning, peritoneal dialysis is as effective as exchange transfusions (four hours of peritoneal dialysis removes approximately the same amount of boric acid as a single exchange transfusion), is the treatment of choice and should be considered in the treatment of poisoning caused by other water-soluble toxic substances.

### *Hydrocyanic Acid* (Also see *Cyanide*)

Hydrocyanic acid and its sodium and potassium salts are among the most potent and rapidly acting poisons known. The acid is extremely volatile, producing a deadly gas, hydrogen cyanide, with a distinctive odor of bitter almonds. Cyanides are present in rodenticides and seeds of apple, peach, plum, cherry and chokeberry. Cyanide compounds are widely used in industry in ore-extracting processes, electroplating and polishing metals, photography and the fumigation of ships and warehouses. Special ventilating devices are necessary to avoid poisoning. Acrylonitrile is employed in the synthetic production of rubber. Cyanide is also used as a fertilizer and as a source of hydrogen cyanide.

The cyanide ion produces cellular anoxia by reversibly inhibiting those oxidizing enzymes which contain ferric ($3^+$) iron, particularly cytochrome oxidase. Death then occurs from tissue asphyxia, notably of the central nervous system. Hemoglobin, the largest body store of iron, is in the ferrous ($2^+$) state and does not react with cyanide.

Cyanides are rapidly absorbed from the skin and all mucosal surfaces and are most dangerous when inhaled, because toxic amounts are absorbed with great rapidity through the bronchial mucosa and alveoli.

The lethal dose of the absolute acid is about 50 mg; that of the potassium or sodium salt, 200 to 300 mg. Breathing air containing a concentration of 0.2 to 0.3 mg/liter is almost immediately fatal, while 0.13 mg/liter (130 ppm) would be fatal after an hour.

Following the inhalation of toxic amounts, symptoms usually appear within a few seconds, whereas they take a few minutes to appear following oral ingestion or skin contamination by the salts. If large amounts have been absorbed, collapse is usually instantaneous, the patient falling unconscious, often with a loud cry and convulsions, and dying almost immediately. This is known as the "apoplectic form" of cyanide poisoning.

With smaller doses, the patient complains of weakness, giddiness, headache, nausea, vomiting and palpitations. With the rise of the cyanide level of the blood, ataxia develops and is followed by convulsions, coma, and death. Diagnosis is usually made by the history, the abrupt, catastrophic onset and the bitter almond odor to the breath.

Fortunately, the affinity of cyanide for substances containing ferric iron is reversible, and this suggested the possibility of converting hemoglobin to methemoglobin (containing ferric iron), which would then compete for the cyanide ion to form cyanmethemoglobin, sparing the more essential enzyme systems. Methemoglobin can be produced either by inhalation of amyl nitrite or injection of sodium nitrite intravenously. Furthermore, if thiosulfate is made available, the relatively nontoxic thiocyanate is formed and excreted.

To be of any value, *treatment* must be immediate. Although death may take place within minutes, it may not occur for as much as three hours even when no treatment is given; there is thus a chance to save the patient as long as clinical death has not yet occurred.

While the intravenous solutions are being prepared, amyl nitrite pearls are crushed, one at a time, enveloped by a gauze pad or handkerchief and held about one inch from the patient's nostrils for fifteen to thirty seconds per minute. Artificial respiration is begun immediately if breathing has ceased or is labored. Meanwhile, contaminated clothing is quickly removed and skin areas thoroughly washed with soap and water. If poisoning is the result of ingestion, gastric lavage becomes mandatory; a 1:5000 solution of potassium permanganate is used for this purpose.

As soon as it is prepared, 10 ml of a 3% solution of sodium nitrite is injected intravenously within two or four minutes. If sterile materials are not available, nonsterile ones should be used. This is followed immediately by the injection of 50 ml of a 25% solution of sodium thiosulfate at the same rate and through the same needle. Once the solutions are injected amyl nitrite inhalation is discontinued. Should a sharp drop in blood pressure occur (an occasional effect of nitrite administration), epinephrine or ephedrine may be administered (for dosages in children, *see* p. 36). For moderate hypotension, slow the nitrite injection and place the patient in Trendelenburg position. In Europe, dicobalt tetracemate (Kelocyanor®) is replacing the nitrite-thiosulfate regimen. Two 20 ml ampuls of 1.5% solution are injected intravenously and followed by 20 ml of 50% glucose. Cobalt forms a chelate compound and the end product is vitamin $B_{12}$. This agent is not approved for United States use.

The patient is observed for the next twenty-four to forty-eight hours, and if the signs of intoxication persist or reappear, injection of both substances should be repeated in the same manner, using only half the dosage. Some have repeated the injections after two hours as a prophylactic measure, even if the patient appeared improved.

In the past, methylene blue has been employed, although its action in the formation of methemoglobin was much slower. Oxygen is a readily available therapeutic and specific agent, and its use in cyanide poisoning should not be neglected. Experimental data show that a high oxygen tension blocks the respiratory gasp reaction to intravenous cyanide in man, partially revises elecrocardiographic anoxic changes in dogs and protects goldfish from lethal doses. Probably oxygen should be used even after administration of nitrites and thiosulfate, as the methemoglobinemia induced by this treatment reduces the ability of blood to carry oxygen to the brain. Whole blood transfusions may be necessary if the nitrite-induced methemoglobinemia becomes too severe.

Since the success of therapy for cyanide poisoning is predicated upon speed, emergency kits containing amyl nitrite pearls and ampules of the necessary doses of sodium nitrite and thiosulfate, together with a large bore gastric tube, sterile syringes and needles, gauze pads, ampule file and a tourniquet should be available for immediate use wherever there is a possibility of intoxication. A complete cyanide antidote package can be purchased from the Eli Lilly Company, stock number M76 (*see* pp. 235 through 237 for more detailed discussion of Cyanide Poisoning and therapy).

## *Antimony*

Antimony and its compounds are used in alloys, type metal, batteries, foil, ceramics, safety matches, ant paste, textiles and medicinals (tartar emetic, Fuadin®, antimony sulfide, etc.). "Butter of antimony" is antimony trichloride. Metals containing antimony, when treated with acids, release antimony hydride (stibine), a colorless gas which can cause hemolysis of the red blood cells and involvement of the central nervous system. Antimony is strongly irritating to tissues and mucous membranes. The lethal dose is between 100 and 200 mg, and deaths are mainly due to massive or overdosage of drugs and rarely occur from the industrial environment or occupations where fume and dust exposure may cause chronic poisoning. Chronic antimony poisoning is very similar to chronic arsenic poisoning, with symptoms of itchy skin, pustules, stomatitis, conjunctivitis, laryngitis, headache, anorexia, weight loss and anemia. In acute poisoning from ingestion, the symptoms are chiefly gastrointestinal such as nausea, vomiting and severe diarrhea with mucus and later with blood. Hemorrhagic nephritis and hepatitis may occur concomitantly or follow the gastrointestinal manifestations later. The inhalation of stibine can cause severe headaches, weakness, nausea, vomiting and anemia. Pertinent laboratory findings may show profound anemia with reduction of the red blood cells, and up to 25 per cent of the total white cells are eosinophils and agranulocytes. The urine may contain red blood cells and hemoglobin.

The *treatment* in ingestion poisoning should consist of immediate gastric lavage or emesis and catharsis. A 1% sodium bicarbonate solution (3 level tsp./qt. of water) is an effective lavage solution. This should be followed by demulcents. Morphine 15 mg (¼ gr) may be used to control severe pain. Administer BAL quickly and, in general, treat as for arsenic poisoning. In the chronic form of intoxication, it is imperative that further exposure be eliminated. In prevention, adequate fume and dust control is necessary to prevent the maximum allowable concentration (MAC) from being exceeded.

TABLE 52
ACUTE TOXICITY TO MAN OF SOME INORGANIC INSECTICIDES

| *Common Name* | *Chemical Name* | *Estimated Fatal Oral Dosage (gm/70 kg)* | *Antidote* |
|---|---|---|---|
| Sodium fluoride | Sodium fluoride | 1.0 | |
| Arsenic trioxide | Arsenic trioxide | 0.1 | Dimercaprol |
| Paris green | Copper acetoarsenite | 0.1 | Dimercaprol |
| Tartar emetic | Antimony potassium tartrate | 0.15 | Dimercaprol |
| Corrosive sublimate | Mercuric chloride | 0.5 | Dimercaprol |
| Borax | Sodium borate | 8.0 | |
| Sodium selenate | Sodium selenate | 0.2 | |
| Hydrogen cyanide | Cyanide | 0.3 | Sodium nitrite and Sodium thiosulfate |

## INSECTICIDES FROM BOTANICAL SOURCES

### *Nicotine*

Nicotine, the chief alkaloid of tobacco, is one of the most toxic and rapidly acting poisons. Tolerance fortunately develops with repeated administration in small doses, as with smokers and tobacco chewers. Dangerous exposure may occur during manufacture and use of nicotine-containing insecticides and when the alkaloid has been ingested in attempted suicide. Death has followed the lay use of tobacco infusions as enemas in the treatment of intestinal parasites in children.

Absorption of nicotine takes place in the alimentary and respiratory tracts as well as through the intact skin. The fatal dose varies widely: As little as 4 mg may produce marked symptoms, while one patient ingested 2 gm and survived. About 40 mg is generally fatal. Cigarette tobacco varies in its nicotine content, but regular (not low-tar) blends contain 15 to 20 mg for each cigarette. Cigars vary from 15 to 40 mg.

Nicotine is not readily absorbed in the stomach from ingested tobacco, as when children swallow cigarettes, and the initial stimulus to vomiting usually removes most of it before much harm is done by an otherwise serious dose.

The ingested alkaloid exerts a direct, rapid, caustic action causing a hot, burning sensation in the mouth, throat, esophagus and stomach; but the systemic effects after absorption are of much greater significance. Nicotine initially and transiently stimulates all sympathetic and parasympathetic ganglion cells. This is rapidly followed by a more persistent depression and paralysis. The ganglion cells are first made more sensitive to and then resistant to acetylcholine. A similar dual action is exerted on skeletal muscle (curariform effects) and on the central nervous system.

The effect of nicotine on respiration is a curare-like action paralyzing the respiratory muscles. This is reflex in origin, with a direct ganglionic blocking action providing the mechanism of respiratory arrest and death with toxic doses. The initial effect of nicotine on the cardiovascular system is a slowing of the heart rate, followed by cardiac acceleration, a rise in blood pressure and a rapid hypotension. There is evidence of increased coronary blood flow and a marked vasoconstriction of the peripheral vessels.

The effects of nicotine on the body are thus complex and unpredictable, and they vary with dosage. Symptoms following a relatively small dose are transient and consist of salivation, nausea, perhaps vomiting, diarrhea, bradycardia and dizziness. In severe acute poisoning with pure alkaloid, the patient may collapse and die within minutes from overwhelming paralysis. Where death is delayed, abdominal pain is marked, diarrhea severe and a cold sweat prominent. Mental confusion, giddiness, restlessness, muscular weakness and disturbed vision and hearing are followed by a loss of coordinating power and partial or complete unconsciousness. Blood pressure may initially be raised and respiration stimulated, but a fall in blood pressure, a rapid, irregular pulse and labored breathing follow shortly. Clonic convulsions are followed by collapse and complete muscle relaxation. Reflexes disappear; respiration becomes slow and weak, then ceases.

Green-tobacco sickness is a self-limited illness of short duration characterized by pallor, vomiting and prostration. The condition occurs principally in young men who handle uncured tobacco leaves in the field and is correlated with cropping (picking) the tobacco while it is wet; the absorption of nicotine from the tobacco leaf is the probable cause. Some of the victims likened the experience to extreme seasickness. Pesticides are not incriminated, and antihistamines with antiemetic properties (Dramamine®, meclizine) are effective agents. Cigarette smokers and older tobacco harvesters are apparently immune to this phenomenon.

*Treatment.* Since nicotine is completely eliminated in sixteen hours, the patient may survive if he can be sustained over that period. Artificial respiration and oxygen are most urgent in severe poisoning, for death usually results from respiratory failure due to paralysis of the respiratory muscles. The use of a positive-pressure resuscitator throughout the period of respiratory failure may prevent death.

Immediate steps are taken to remove the poison. If it entered through the skin, garments are removed and the skin washed copiously with water and scrubbed with soap. For ingestion of nicotine, gastric lavage with potassium permanganate solution (1:5000 to 1:10,000) helps to remove and oxidize any nicotine left in the stomach. This should be followed by the administration of activated charcoal. Convulsions should be controlled with pentobarbital or, if necessary, with ether anesthesia. Ephedrine may be helpful for the hypotension. Many of the visceral manifestations can be controlled by combinations of autonomic blocking drugs such as atropine and Dibenzyline. Caramiphen (Panparnit®) hydrochloride and diethazine (Diparcol®) are more complex compounds that have been found to be very effective in experimental nicotine poisoning. Their value in humans has not yet been documented, but they are available as oral preparations and deserve clinical trial.

### *Pyrethrins and Cinerins (Pyrethrum-Allethrin)*

Pyrethrum is one of the oldest insecticides known to man. The constituents that are active as insecticides are esters called pyrethrins and cinerins. The ground flowers of the plant are used undiluted or mixed with inert diluents or other insecticides as household and horticultural dusts. Liquid extracts employing kerosene or other organic solvents are used in preparing agricultural, livestock and household sprays. Contact with the skin may cause dermatitis in sensitive persons and in about 50 per cent of those who are sensitive to ragweed. The dermatitis is of an erythematous, vesicular, papular and anaphylactic type and may be associated with eosinophilia. In allergic individuals, asthma and rhinitis may be produced, and hypersensitivity pneumonitis has been reported. Modern, refined pyrethrins have insignificant allergenic properties and the problems of allergy have lessened.

Pyrethrin insecticides are capable of causing nausea, vomiting, gastroenteritis with diarrhea (which may respond to atropine therapy), hyperexcitability, incoordination, tremors, muscular paralysis and death due to respiratory failure. However, severe poisoning from pyrethrin insecticides is rare and is more often due to the other ingredients, such as the petroleum solvent base, which are present in these agents. Nevertheless, pyrethrins should be washed from the skin and eyes, as they can cause severe local irritation.

Allethrin is a botanical insecticide having a low order of toxicity. It has recently been demonstrated to have a high repellent potency against mosquitoes, which may make this compound a suitable insect repellent.

### *Ryania*

Ryania and its alkaloids, ryanine and ryanodine, belong to a genus of tropical American shrubs and trees of the Flacourtiaceae family and are employed in a variety of insecticide powders. The $LD_{50}$ in rats is 750 mg/kg.

Symptoms of poisoning consist of generalized weakness, deep and slow respiration, vomiting, tremors, convulsions, coma and death in severe intoxication.

*Treatment* is similar to that for rotenone and is mainly supportive and symptomatic.

### *Rotenone*

The ground roots and extracts of the roots of rotenone-bearing plants *(Derris and Lonchocarpus)* are used as insecticides. They are prepared as dusts with inert diluents or with other insecticides as washes and dips against animal ectoparasites; as agricultural, horticultural and household sprays; and as emulsions, lotions and ointments for treatment of head lice, scabies and as a palliative for chigger bites. Local effects reported after exposure to *Derris* have included conjunctivitis, dermatitis, pharyngitis and rhinitis. In the finely divided form it is irritating to the skin of experimental animals, and in the undiluted form it is irritating to the conjunctiva and produces numbness of the mucosa of the nose and throat which persists for several hours. Orally it is a gastrointestinal irritant and produces nausea and vomiting promptly after ingestion. The local effects on the intestinal tract together with a stimulant effect on the emetic center tend to force expulsion of the material before absorption occurs. It is much more toxic when it is inhaled and can cause convulsions and death due to respiratory failure. *Treatment* of rotenone poisoning is largely symptomatic and supportive and consists of removal of the material from the skin and gastrointestinal tract. Oily cathartics should not be used to aid in the removal of rotenone from the gastrointestinal tract since absorption may be increased by their use.

### *Sabadilla*

Sabadilla is a melanthaceous plant of Mexico, the source of cevadine, a violent emetocathartic. Poisoning may cause intense irritation of the gastrointestinal tract with severe vomiting and diarrhea. *Treatment* is symptomatic and includes demulcent drinks after gastric lavage and activated charcoal.

TABLE 53
TOXICITY OF INSECTICIDES OF BOTANIC ORIGIN TO MAN

| *Common Name* | *Toxic Constituents* | *Comparative Toxicity* | *Estimated Fatal Oral Dose (gm/70 kg)* |
|---|---|---|---|
| Pyrethrum | Pyrethrins and cinerins | Slightly toxic | 50 |
| Derris | Rotenone | Slightly toxic | 10 to 100 |
| Allethrin | Allyl cinerin | Slightly toxic | — |
| Tobacco | Nicotine | Highly toxic | 0.07 |

## BIOLOGICAL PESTICIDES

The biological control of insect pests and weeds has been practiced since ancient times, when the Chinese placed nests of predacious ants in their mandarin orange groves to help keep down insect pests; the ants were even provided with bridges of bamboo rods between trees. One of the most successful early biological control experiments in the United States was the introduction of the vedalia beetle into California to combat the cottony/cushion scale. The ecologic basis of regulation in the "balance of nature," mass production culture and colonization of natural enemies of pests, quarantine handling, insect pathology and the use of microorganisms to manipulate insect population and weed control is just now being unraveled. The benefits of biological control, whether natural or induced, are gaining greater recognition and support, mainly because they are safer than chemical pesticides. Pheromone is a substance secreted externally (unlike internal secretion of a hormone) that influences the behavior of other animals of the same species. These pheromones are used as a means of chemical communication that help to regulate the organism's external environment by influencing other animals.

The modern strategy of pest management calls for integrated programs that combine the judicious use of conventional chemical insecticides with various biological, biochemical or microbial agents that specifically control certain pests. Researchers have synthesized analogues of insect juvenile hormones that interfere with metamorphosis and female sex pheromones that lure males to traps or cause such confusion that they are unable to find mates. Entomogenous viruses, bacteria and parasites that only affect certain insects are being used in some experimental control programs and the sterilization of males by means of irradiation continues to be a highly effective method of reducing the population of screwworms that cause extensive morbidity and mortality in cattle and other livestock.

## Chemtrec and PSTN

Two widely known emergency services, the Chemical Transportation Emergency Center (CHEMTREC) and the Pesticide Safety Team Network (PSTN), have combined their communication links to provide a more unified system to deal with chemical-pesticide-related accidents.

The PSTN was organized in March of 1970 to provide emergency assistance in the event of a pesticide spill or accident during transportation. It is a cooperative voluntary program operated as a public service by the National Agricultural Chemical Association and fourteen member companies.

TABLE 54
INSECTICIDES

| *Trade Name** | *Harmful Ingredients* | *Treatment Reference Page Number* |
|---|---|---|
| Aceteen Stops Termites | Arsenic Trioxide | |
| Acme All Round Insect Bomb | Pyrethrins, Rotenone | |
| Acme Emo-Nik | Nicotine | |
| Acme Flybait | Malathion | |
| Aerosect Ant Preventive | Pyrethrins | |
| Aerosect Fly Spray | Pyrethrins | |
| Afcophene | Toxaphene | |
| Agicide Dog and Cat Flea Powder | Rotenone | |
| Agicide Fly Spray | Methoxychlor | |
| Agicide Houseplant Aerosol Bomb | Pyrethrins, Rotenone | |
| Agicide Maggott Killer | Aldrin | |
| Agicide Roach and Ant Powder | Lindane | |
| Agicide Rose Aerosol Bomb | Pyrethrins, Rotenone | See Index |
| Agicide Sabadust | Sabadilla, Alkaloids | |
| Agritox Agrithion Dust | Malathion | |
| Agritox Cryolite Dust | Sodium Fluoaluminate | |
| Air-Tox Household Aerosol Bomb | Pyrethrins, Rotenone | |
| Alco Fly Cake | Parathion | |
| Alkron | Parathion | |
| All-Plan | Aldrin | |
| Alltox 5 Bait | Toxaphene | |
| Ant-Foil | Sodium Fluoride | |
| Ant-Not Ant Trap | Thallium Sulfate | |
| Antrol African Violet & House Plant Bomb | Pyrethrins, Rotenone | |
| Antrol Ant Killer | Sodium Arsenite | |
| Antrol Ant Spray | Chlordane | |
| Antrol Ant Syrup | Sodium Arsenite | |
| Antrol Ant Trap | Thallium Sulfate | |

*All products listed below are registered trademarks. Since trade names and formulations are frequently and unexpectedly changed, consult labels for definitive contents. Thallium has been removed from the market, but since many of these products are perhaps still available on shelves of retail stores, they have not been deleted from this listing.

TABLE 54—*Continued*
INSECTICIDES

| *Trade Name** | *Harmful Ingredients* | *Treatment Reference Page Number* |
|---|---|---|
| Antrol Lawntrol Granules | Naphthalene | |
| Ant-Roach Killer | Chlordane | |
| Ant-X Ant Traps | Thallium | |
| Ant-X Jelly Bait | Thallium | |
| Aphamite | Parathion | |
| Aqualin Herbicide | Acrolein | |
| Arab U-Do-It Termite Control | Chlordane, Lindane | |
| Arwell Fly Spray | Pyrethrins | |
| Arwell Roach Spray | Chlordane | |
| Arwell Super Spray | Pyrethrins | |
| ASL Spray Base | Malathion | |
| Atox | Rotenone | |
| Bab-O-Ant & Roach Killer | Diazinon | |
| Bab-O-Fly and Mosquito Killer | DDT | |
| Bacikicide | Pyrethrins | |
| Banafly Bait | Diazinon | |
| Barco Animal and Dairy Spray | Petroleum Distillates | |
| Barekil | Nicotine | |
| Beacon Ant Killer | Thallium Sulfate | |
| Bee Brand Ant and Flea Killer | Rotenone | |
| Benesan | Lindane | |
| Benexane 5 | Lindane | |
| Benexane 50 | Gamma BHC | |
| Benzahex | Gamma BHC | |
| Benzex | Gamma BHC | *See Index* |
| Berlou Instant Spray Moth Proofer | Petroleum Distillates | |
| B-Hex | Gamma BHC | |
| Bidrin | Phosphate Ester | |
| Bif Ant and Roach Spray | Chlordane | |
| Bif Insecticide Powder | Chlordane | |
| Bif Stinky Control Fluid | DDT | |
| Bin-Fume | Carbon Tetrachloride | |
| Bin-Treat | Lindane | |
| Black Flag Bug Killer | Pyrethrins | |
| Black Flag Flea-Tick & Louse Powder | Pyrethrins, Rotenone | |
| Black Flag Moth Ded | Paradichlorobenzene | |
| Black Flag Special Roach Spray | Chlordane | |
| Black Leaf 11 36 Insect Killer | DDT | |
| Black Leaf | Nicotine | |
| Black Leaf CPR Insect Killer | Pyrethrins | |
| Black Leaf Mash-nic Powder | Nicotine | |
| Black Leaf Pyrenone Insect Killer | Pyrethrins | |
| Black Leaf Slug & Snail Pellets | Calcium Arsenate | |
| Bladex | TEPP | |
| Boncep | Copper Sulfate | |
| Bonide Ant Dust | Chlordane | |
| Bonkil Insecticide Powder | DDT | |
| Bonide Lintox | Lindane | |
| Bonide Outdoor and Garden Spray | Malathion | |
| Bonide Ryatox | Ryania | |
| Bontox | DDT | |
| Bontano Liquid Spray | Rotenone, Pyrethrins | |
| Bouquet-Aire Hang-Up Cakes | Paradichlorobenzene | |

TABLE 54—*Continued*
INSECTICIDES

| *Trade Name** | *Harmful Ingredients* | *Treatment Reference Page Number* |
|---|---|---|
| Brayton Dairy Farm Spray | Pyrethrins | |
| Brayton E-M Farm Insecticide | Malathion | |
| Brayton's Fly Killer | Pyrethrins | |
| Brayton's KO Fly Killer | Pyrenone Concentrate | |
| Brayton's P-B Insecticide | Pyrethrins | |
| Brayton's Residual Insecticide | DDT | |
| Breck's Ant & Earwig Spray | Chlordane | |
| Breck's Ant Spray | Pyrethrins | |
| Bridgeport Moth Bomb | Methoxychlor | |
| Bridgeport No. 137 Moth Bomb | Methoxychlor | |
| Bridgeport No. 424 Mothproofer | DDT | |
| Brulin's Insecticide Aerosol | Pyrethrins | |
| Brulin's Insect Spray | Pyrethrins | |
| Brulin's Liquid No-Tox | Pyrethrins | |
| Brulin's Moth Spray | DDT | |
| Brulin's Roach & Ant Toxicant | Malathion | |
| Brulin's 4-X Concentrate | DDT | |
| Bug-Ant Doom | Pyrethrins | |
| Bug-A-Way | Petroleum Distillates, Pyrethrins | |
| Bug Bomb | Petroleum Distillates | |
| Bug Butcher | Aldrin, Naphthalene | |
| Bug-Geta Snail Bait Meal | Calcium Arsenate | |
| Bug-Kill Pellets | Gamma BHC | |
| Carac Ant and Lawn Grub Killers | Chlordane | |
| Carac Kills All Insecticide | Malathion | *See Index* |
| Certo-Kill | DDT | |
| Chapman Roach and Pest Killer | Chlordane | |
| Check Pest Livestock Spray | Toxaphene | |
| Check Pest Outdoor Insecticide | Lindane, Chlordane | |
| Check Pest Systemic Insecticide | Octamethyl Pyrophosphoramide | |
| Chem-Chlor | Lindane, Chlordane | |
| Chem-Drin | Wettable Chlordane Powder | |
| Chem-Fog | DDT | |
| Chem-Hex | Gamma BHC | |
| Chem-Klor | Chlordane | |
| Chem-Lin | Lindane | |
| Chem-Mite | Rotenone | |
| Chemform Home Termite Concoction | DDT, Chlordane | |
| Chemform Turfacide | Dieldrin Granules | |
| Chlordust | Chlordane | |
| Chlorkil | Chlordane | |
| Chlorocide | Chlordane | |
| C-I-L Louse Powder | Rotenone | |
| Chlorgran | Chlordane | |
| College Brand Household Spray | DDT | |
| Comon Sense Cockroach Preparation | Phosphorus | |
| Common Sense Insect Spray | Pyrethrins | |
| Common Sense Insect Spray, Plain | Pyrethrins | |
| Cook's Real-Kill Mothproofer | DDT | |
| Co-Op One Shot Dust | Parathion | |
| Co-Op 70-30 Dust | Sodium Fluoaluminate | |
| Cornell Cattle Spray | Pyrethrins | |
| Cornell Residual Household Spray | DDT | |

TABLE 54—*Continued*
INSECTICIDES

| *Trade Name** | *Harmful Ingredients* | *Treatment Reference Page Number* |
|---|---|---|
| Corn King Dairyland Fly Spray | Petroleum Distillates | |
| Corn King Dead-White | Lindane | |
| Corn King De-Louser Powder | Malathion | |
| Corn King Fly Mort | Malathion | |
| Corn King Fly Spray | Petroleum Distillates | |
| Corn King Verm-O-Phen Granules | Phenothiazine | |
| Corothion | Parathion | |
| Cotton States Fly Spray & Repellent | Pyrethrins | |
| Cowley Spray | Methoxychlor | |
| CPR Liquid Base | Pyrethrins, Rotenone | |
| CPR-GP Plant Spray | Pyrethrins, Rotenone | |
| Crane's Moth-Ex Junior | Lindane, Benzene Hexachloride | |
| Cross Country Fire Ant Killer | Dieldrin | |
| Cured Flea Duster | Rotenone | |
| Dairy-Mist Fly Spray Concentrate | DDT | |
| Dampo | DDT | |
| Dawson #3 Insecticide | Malathion | |
| Dawson #4 Insecticide | DDT | |
| D & P Cinch-Tox | DDT, Chlordane | |
| D & P Slug Tox | Calcium Arsenate | |
| D & P Trispray | Nicotine | |
| Debrom | Organic Phosphate | |
| Ded-Tox Dust | DDT | |
| Dee-Dex | DDT | |
| Dee-Dex "25" | DDT | See Index |
| Delcro Shampoo for Dogs | Rotenone | |
| Denoxo | DDT | |
| Deroxide | Rotenone | |
| Destruol Antroach Dust | Chlordane | |
| D-D Soil Fumigant† | Dichloropropene-Dichloropropane Mixture | |
| Dianol Insect Killing House Spray | TDE, Chlordane | |
| Diazinon | Diethyl-Isopropyl Methyl Pyrimidyl Thiophosphate | |
| Didimac | DDT | |
| Die Fly | Dichlorovinylphosphate | |
| Dieldrec | Dieldrin | |
| Dipterex | Dimethyl Hydroxy Trichloroethyl Phosphonate | |
| Dithio | TEPP | |
| Dithiono | TEPP | |
| Dow Grain Bin Spray | DDT | |
| Dro Rose and Ornamental Plant Spray | Pyrethrins | |
| Dro Snosphra | Carbon Tetrachloride | |
| Du-Kill | Pyrethrins | |
| Duricide DDT | DDT | |
| Dustox | Rotenone | |
| Dyocide 8 | DDT | |
| Dyohex Dust | Gamma BHC | |
| Dyochlor Powder | Chlordane | |

†Is highly toxic to mammals by ingestion and inhalation and less so by dermal absorption. Its odor and intense irritation to eyes, skin, and respiratory tract, warn of danger and reduce the exposure hazard. Author knows of death of one adult from accidental ingestion.

TABLE 54—*Continued*
INSECTICIDES

| *Trade Name** | *Harmful Ingredients* | *Treatment Reference Page Number* |
|---|---|---|
| Elco-Cide | Chlordane, DDT | *See Index* |
| Elco Roach and Ant Powder | Sodium Fluoride | |
| Emo-Nik | Nicotine | |
| Emulsa Chlor | Chlordane | |
| End-O-Pest Arc Ant & Lawn Insect Dust | Chlordane | |
| End-O-Pest Arc for Ants & Lawn Insects | Chlordane | |
| End-O-Pest Evergreen & Ornamental Spray | Malathion | |
| End-O-Pest Mosquito Killer | Malathion, DDT | |
| End-O-Pest Rose Dust | DDT | |
| Engo | Chlordane | |
| ERL | Nicotine | |
| Falcon Roach Powder | Sodium Fluoride | |
| Farm & Garden Brand Aphis Dust or Spray | Lindane | |
| Farm & Garden Brand Chlordane Dust | Chlordane | |
| Fasco Bur-Gam Dust | Lindane | |
| Fasco Fly Flakes | Malathion | |
| Fasco Master Lice Powder | Sodium Fluoride | |
| Fasco Ant Poison | Sodium Arsenite | |
| Flag Cryolite Dust | Sodium Fluoaluminate | |
| Flea-Foil Flea Powder | DDT | |
| Flea-Go | Lindane | |
| Flea-Not Powder | Rotenone | |
| Flit Aerosol Fly Mosquito Killer | DDT | |
| Flit Aerosol House and Garden Insect Killer | Pyrethrins | |
| Flit Bug Killer | Chlordane | |
| Flit Bug Killer Pressurized | Lindane | |
| Flit Fly and Mosquito Killer | DDT | |
| Flit Moth Proofer | DDT | |
| Flit Roach and Ant Killer | Dieldrin | |
| Flit Roach and Ant Killer Pressurized | Dieldrin | |
| Florbait | Malathion | |
| Flower Guard | Pyrethrins | |
| Fly Dair | Pyrethrins | |
| Fly Doom Spray | Pyrethrins | |
| Fly-Dy | Pyrethrins | |
| Fly-B-Gon Insect Spray | Gamma BHC | |
| Fly Hot Foot | Malathion | |
| Fly Hot Lunch | Malathion | |
| Fly Jinx Insect Spray | Pyrethrins | |
| Foliafume | Pyrethrins, Rotenone | |
| French's Flea Powder for Dogs | Pyrethrins | |
| Fuedeth Roach Powder | Sodium Fluoride | |
| Gamtox Mosquito Cone | Gamma BHC | |
| Gator Roach Hive | Lead Arsenate | |
| Geller's Roach Fel | Chlordane | |
| Genidust D-10 Dust | DDT | |
| Geniphene | Toxaphene | |
| Genithion P-25 Dust Base | Parathion | |
| Genitol | DDT | |
| G. C. Flykiller | Dipterex | |

TABLE 54—*Continued*
INSECTICIDES

| *Trade Name** | *Harmful Ingredients* | *Treatment Reference Page Number* |
|---|---|---|
| G.L.F. Dust #8A | Parathion | |
| G.L.F Dust #10 | Parathion | |
| G.L.F. Dust #30A | Malathion | |
| G.L.F. Dust #33 | Endrin | |
| G.L.F Dust #34 | Heptachlor | |
| G.L.F. Dust #61 | Malathion | |
| Globe Flea Bomb and Deodorant | Pyrethrins, Malathion | |
| Globe Liquid Grub Killer | Naphthalene | |
| Globe Sud-N-Deth Fly Bait | Dichlorovinylphosphate | |
| Go-Nex | DDT | |
| Green Cross Slug Bait | Calcium Arsenate | |
| Green Light Fire Ant Killer | Heptachlor | |
| Green Light Fly and Mosquito Bomb | Pyrethrins | |
| Green Light Oil for Scale | Petroleum Oils | |
| Green Light Roach and Ant Killer | Malathion | |
| Gulfspray Aerosol Bomb | Pyrethrins | |
| Gulfspray Cone Aerosol Insecticide | Pyrethrins | |
| GTA Ant Base | Thallium Sulfate | |
| Gy-Phene | Toxaphene | |
| Gy-Tet | TEPP | |
| Handy Killer | Arsenic | |
| Harris Roach Tablets | 60% Boric Acid | |
| Haviland 3D Insecticide | DDT | |
| Hep Ant & Roach Killer | Malathion | |
| Hep Bug Killer | Malathion | *See Index* |
| Hep 5% Insect Killer | DDT | |
| Heptagran | Heptachlor | |
| Heptal | Heptachlor, Aldrin | |
| (Dr.) Hess Powdered Louse Killer | Rotenone | |
| Hubklor Dust | Chlordane | |
| Huntington Roach Spray | Chlordane | |
| Huntington Vaporizing Fluid | Pyrethrins | |
| Hy-Tox Fly Bait | Malathion | |
| Impregno | Pyrethrins | |
| Insecto-Fog | Malathion | |
| Isotox Dairy Spray | Lindane | |
| Isotox Garden Dust | Lindane | |
| Itso Insect Killer | Pyrethrins | |
| Jap Beetle Killer | DDT | |
| Jitter Bug Insect Repellent | Hydrogenated Rotenone | |
| Johnson's Super No-Roach Killer | Malathion | |
| Kalite | Rotenone | |
| Kayo Bug Killer | Calcium Arsenate | |
| Kellogg's Ant Paste | Arsenic | |
| Ketokil No. 2 | DDT | |
| Killer | TEPP | |
| Killer Dust D-10 | DDT | |
| Killer Dust Tox | Toxaphene | |
| Kil-Mor Roach Ant Killer | Chlordane | |
| Kill-Ogen Instant Spray | Pyrethrins, Rotenone | |

TABLE 54—*Continued*
INSECTICIDES

| *Trade Name** | *Harmful Ingredients* | *Treatment Reference Page Number* |
|---|---|---|
| Kilmite | TEPP | |
| King Special Bug Killer | Arsenic | |
| King Warble Fly Spray | Rotenone | |
| Klane | Chlordane | |
| Klenzade Fly Spray | Pyrethrins | |
| Klenzade Roach Spray Ins-40 | Pyrethrins | |
| Knoxout Farm Insecticide | Lindane | |
| Knoxout Insect Spray and Powder | DDT | |
| Kolocide | Lindane, DDT | |
| Kolorsmear Screw-Worm Remedy | Lindane | |
| Kolotex | Arsenic | |
| Korlan 12 E | Trichlorophenyl | |
| Korlan 25 W | Trichlorophenyl | |
| Korlan 24 E | Trichlorophenyl | |
| Kritter Kote | Crude Petroleum | |
| Kritter Spray | Petroleum Distillates | |
| Kryfax | Sodium Fluoaluminate | |
| Kryocide | Sodium Fluoaluminate | |
| Krytox | Sodium Fluoaluminate | |
| Lebanon Japanese Beetle Spray | DDT, Chlordane | |
| Lebanon Klor Dust | Chlordane | |
| Lestox Fly Spray | Pyrethrins | |
| Lethalaire G-57 | DDT | |
| Lexone Insecticide | Gamma BHC | |
| Lindex Dust No. 10 | Lindane | See Index |
| Lintodd No. 102 | Lindane | |
| Lintox | Lindane | |
| Little David Insect Spray | DDT | |
| Lorenz Activated Knockdown Concoction | Pyrethrins | |
| Lucide | Chlordane | |
| Mackodiel | Dieldrin | |
| Mack-O-White | Malathion | |
| Magikil Ant and Roach Duster | Thallium Sulfate | |
| Magikil Jelly Ant Bait | Thallium Sulfate | |
| Magik-Mist Insecticide | DDT, Pyrethrins | |
| Malafog | Malathion | |
| Malanox Residual Bait Spray Concentrate | Malathion | |
| Marlate | Methoxychlor | |
| Martin's Mar-Chlor | Chlordane | |
| Martin's Mar-Termino | Chlordane | |
| Martin's Stock Tox | Toxaphene | |
| Mash-Nic Powder | Nicotine | |
| Metacide | Parathion | |
| Metag Agricultural Bait | Calcium Arsenate | |
| Methanox Residual Fly Spray Concentrate | Petroleum Solvent | |
| Metho-Penn | Methoxychlor | |
| Methoxide | Methoxychlor | |
| Methoxlin Insect Spray | Methoxychlor, Lindane | |
| Midland Insecto-LOH 68 | Chlordane | |
| Midland Mill-O-Cide Formula B-9 | Pyrethrins | |
| Midland Ware-O-Cide Super Strength | Chlordane | |
| Miller's Chlorospra | Chlordane | |

TABLE 54—*Continued*
INSECTICIDES

| *Trade Name** | *Harmful Ingredients* | *Treatment Reference Page Number* |
|---|---|---|
| Miller's DDT Household Spray | DDT | |
| Miller's Fly-Ro-Cide | DDT, Chlordane | |
| Miller's Methoxo | Methoxychlor | |
| Miller's Paraspra | Parathion | |
| Miller's Pestkil | Toxaphene, Lindane | |
| Miller's Malaspra | Malathion | |
| Miller's Rotefive | Rotenone | |
| Miller's Rotefour | Rotenone | |
| Miller's Spray-O-Cide | DDT | |
| Miller's Texaspra | Toxaphene | |
| Miracle Kill Roach Death | Thallium Sulfate | |
| Mirasect | Sodium Fluoride | |
| Mission Brand Ant Powder | Lindane, DDT | |
| Mission Brand Ant Roach Killer | Potassium Cyanide | |
| Mission Brand Tix-Toc | Toxaphene, BHC | |
| Monsanto Niran | Parathion | |
| Monsanto Santobane | DDT | |
| Mop-N-Mix | Calcium Arsenate | |
| Mothene | DDT | |
| Mulch-Rite | Nicotine | |
| Multi-Tox C | Chlordane, DDT | |
| Multi-Tox L | Lindane, DDT | |
| Mysterious Roach Killer Outfit | Pyrethrum, DDT | |
| N-K Seed Protectant | Heptachlor | |
| Na-Klor Dust | Chlordane | See Index |
| Nemagon Soil Fumigant | Dichloropropane | |
| New Larvex | DDT | |
| Niagara Chlorkil Spray | Chlordane | |
| Niagara Kalophoskil 1 Dust | Parathion | |
| Niagara Phoskil Spray | Parathion | |
| Niagara Quik-Kil Poison | Calcium Arsenate | |
| Niagara Ro-Kil Spray | Rotenone | |
| Niagara Thiodan 4 Dust | Indane Derivative | |
| Niagara Thiodan Miscible | Indane Derivative | |
| Niagara Toxakil Dust | Toxaphene | |
| Nico-Dust 10 | Nicotine | |
| Nico-Fume Liquid | Nicotine | |
| Nico-Mulsion | Nicotine | |
| Nicotrol | Nicotine | |
| Nicotrox 10-X | Nicotine | |
| Niocide 10 Dust | Nicotine | |
| Nip-An-Tuck Roach Powder | Sodium Fluoride | |
| No Ro | Chlordane | |
| Nott's 3-Way Bulb Saver | Naphthalene | |
| Nott Roach Powder | Sodium Fluoride | |
| Nox-Kwik High Test Insecticide | Pyrethrins | |
| O.K. Plant Spray | Nicotine | |
| Omnicide | Pyrethrins | |
| Ompa Aerosol | Octamethyl Pyrophosphoramide | |
| Orchard Brand 400 Spray Powder | Rotenone | |
| Ortho C-40 Dust | Sodium Fluoaluminate | |
| Ortho Earwig Bait | Sodium Fluosilicate | |

TABLE 54—*Continued*
INSECTICIDES

| *Trade Name** | *Harmful Ingredients* | *Treatment Reference Page Number* |
|---|---|---|
| Ortho Fly Killer Dry Bait | Malathion | |
| Ortho Fly Killer M | Malathion | |
| Orthophos 4 Spray | Parathion | |
| Pan-thion Spray | Parathion | |
| Para-Denoxo | Parathion | |
| Paradust | Parathion | |
| Paraflow | Parathion | |
| Para-Sul | Parathion | |
| Parawet | Parathion | |
| Parson's Cal-C-Nate | Arsenic | |
| Parson's Insecticide Dust | Rotenone | |
| Parson's Kal-Zoo Ant & Roach Dust | Chlordane | |
| Parson's Tomato Dust | Methoxychlor | |
| Patco Pestkill | Dieldrin | |
| Patterson's Fly Bye | Malathion | |
| Patterson's Household Fly Spray | DDT | |
| P*Forty | Sodium Selenate | |
| Pearson's Kwik-Kill Bait | Calcium Arsenate | |
| Penco Cryocide | Sodium Fluoaluminate | |
| Penco-D-Phos | Parathion | |
| Penco-Hi-Gam | Lindane | |
| Penco Pencal | Tricalcium Arsenate | |
| Penco Super Seventy | Sodium Fluoaluminate | |
| Penick Roach Insecticide No. 2 | DDT | |
| Penn-Dane | Lindane | |
| Penphos | Parathion | *See Index* |
| Pescocide A | Sodium Arsenite | |
| Pest-B-Gon Spray | DDT | |
| Pestroy | DDT | |
| Peterman Ant Food | Sodium Fluoride | |
| Peterman Roach Food | Sodium Fluoride | |
| Peterman Roach Powder & Paste | Sodium Fluoride | |
| Petox | Pyrethrins | |
| Phoenix Brand Delnar Cotton Spray | 2, 3,-p-Dioxanedithiol-bis | |
| Phosfume | Parathion | |
| Phoskil | Parathion | |
| Phosvex | TEPP | |
| Pied Piper Chlor-O-Cide | Chlordane | |
| Pied Piper Dog Shampoo | Chlordane | |
| Pied Piper Roachicide | Sodium Fluoride | |
| Plan-A-Diel | Dieldrin | |
| Plane Dane | Chlordane | |
| Planeto | Chlordane | |
| Plan-O-Lin | Parathion | |
| Planters Save-A-Root | Parathion | |
| Planters Special Insect Spray | Rotenone | |
| Planters Special Jap Beetle Killer | Methoxychlor | |
| Planters Termitox | Chlordane | |
| Planters Truk-Dust | DDT | |
| Planthion Aerosol | Parathion | |
| Port Brand Kryolite Dust | Sodium Fluoaluminate | |
| Port Brand Tepp-Tone Emulsion | TEPP | |
| Prentox Roach Powder | Chlordane | |

TABLE 54—*Continued*
INSECTICIDES

| *Trade Name** | *Harmful Ingredients* | *Treatment Reference Page Number* |
|---|---|---|
| PSC Co-Op Slug Pellets | Calcium Arsenate | |
| PSC Co-Op Weevil Bait | Sodium Fluosilicate | |
| Pyfos | TEPP | |
| Pyro-Phos | TEPP | |
| Pyrosect | Pyrethrins | |
| | | |
| Raid Roach and Ant Killer | Dieldrin | |
| Raid Bug Killer | Pyrethrins | |
| Raid Insect Spray | Dieldrin | |
| Real-Kill Bug Killer | Dieldrin, DDVP | |
| Red Devil Dust | Sabadilla Alkaloid | |
| Repel-X-Fly Spray Concentrate | Pyrethrins | |
| Residol | DDT | |
| Rid Roach | Sodium Fluoride | |
| Ridsect Household Spray | Pyrethrins | |
| Roachkil Insect Spray | Chlordane | |
| Roach Doom | Sodium Fluoride | |
| Roach Go Insect Spray | Chlordane | |
| Roach Salt | Sodium Fluoride | |
| Rohm & Haas Mosquito Larvicide No. 30 | DDT | |
| Ro-Kil Spray | Rotenone | |
| Ro-Ko Liquid Spray | Rotenone | |
| Rotenox | Rotenone | |
| Rotocide | Rotenone | |
| Roto-Dust | Rotenone | |
| Rotrate 5 | Rotenone | *See Index* |
| Run Roach | Pyrethrins | |
| Ryanicide 100 | Ryania | |
| Ryatox | Ryania | |
| | | |
| Salp | Sodium Antimony Lactophenate | |
| (Dr.) Salsbury's Nic-Sal | Nicotine | |
| (Dr.) Salsbury's Pest Spray | Lethane | |
| (Dr.) Salsbury's Vapor-Roost | Gamma BHC | |
| Sani-Deth Multi-Purpose Spray | Petroleum Distillates | |
| Sani-Deth Will-Kill Water Bug Death | DDT | |
| Saphex Fly Spray | Pyrethrins | |
| Sapho 25% C.P.R. Insecticide Dust | Pyrethrins, Rotenone | |
| Sapho Insect Powder | Pyrethrins | |
| Security Brand New 3-Way Tobacco Dust | Parathion | |
| Security Brand Powdered Cube | Rotenone | |
| Security Poison | Tricalcium Arsenate | |
| Sel-Kaps | Sodium Selenate | |
| Sel-Tox | Sodium Selenate | |
| Skookon | Pyrethrin Concoction | |
| Slug-a-Bug | Pyrethrins | |
| Slug-a-Bug Aerosol | Pyrethrins | |
| Smo-Cloud | Methoxychlor | |
| Smo-Cloud Bug Killer | Lindane | |
| Snarol Meal | Tricalcium Arsenate | |
| Snoflake Moth Spray | Carbon Tetrachloride | |
| Sodite | Arsenic | |
| Solution 45 Insect Killer | Pyrethrins | |
| Special Outdoor Fogging | | |

TABLE 54—*Continued*
INSECTICIDES

| *Trade Name** | *Harmful Ingredients* | *Treatment Reference Page Number* |
|---|---|---|
| Concoction No. 11 | Diazinon | |
| Spray-Trol Brand MelaOTrol | Malathion | |
| Spray-Trol Brand Super Trol | Pyrethrins | |
| Sprayway Tru-Nox Insect Spray | Pyrethrins | |
| Stabchlor | Chlordane | |
| Stay-Dee Dusting Powder | DDT | |
| Steamship Vaposector | Petroleum Hydrocarbons | |
| Sterminate Aerosol | Pyrethrins | |
| Super-Five | DDT | |
| Sweeney's Ant-Go | Sodium Arsenite | |
| Swift's Gold Bear Grand Fly Spray | Malathion | |
| Swift's Gold Bear A-2-E | Heptachlor | |
| Swift's Gold Bear B-1-E | Petroleum Hydrocarbons | |
| Swift's Gold Bear D-2-E | DDT | |
| Swift's Gold Bear D-B-E | DDT | |
| Synklor | Chlordane | |
| Tabu-X-Spray | Petroleum Hydrocarbons | |
| Tat Ant Trap | Thallium Sulfate | |
| Tat-Chloro-40 | Chlordane | |
| Telodrin | Aldrin | |
| Teppcide | TEPP | |
| Terminix BTL | Chlordane | |
| Terminix OG6 Concentrate | Chlordane, Dieldrin | |
| Tetron | TEPP | |
| Tetrox | TEPP | See Index |
| Thiophos | Parathion | |
| Thiotep | TEPP | |
| Tok-Tik | Toxaphene | |
| Top | DDT | |
| Tornado Roach & Pest Killer | Chlordane | |
| Tox-Plan | Toxaphene | |
| Toxane | Toxaphene, Lindane | |
| Tox-Sol | Toxaphene | |
| Tree-Mist | DDT | |
| Tri-Excel Dust Concoction | Rotenone, Pyrethrins | |
| Tri-Ogen Rose Bomb | Pyrethrins, Rotenone | |
| Tri-Spray | Nicotine | |
| Trolene | Phosphordithioate | |
| Twenty X-N | Nicotine | |
| Twin Light Dieldrin-Thane Dust | Dieldrin | |
| Twin Light Gam Dust No. 1 | Lindane | |
| Twin Light Granular Chloro Dust | Chlordane | |
| Twin Light Malathion-Perthane Dust | Malathion | |
| Twin Light Nu Spray | DDT | |
| Twin Light Para Dust No. 1 | Parathion | |
| Twin Light Sabadust | Sabadilla Seed | |
| Vapomite 1-3 Dust | TEPP | |
| Vapona | DDVP (Phosphate Ester) | |
| Vapophos Citrus Spray | Parathion | |
| Vapophos Dust | Parathion | |
| Vapophos Liquid Spray | Parathion | |
| Vaposector | Pyrethrins | |

TABLE 54—*Continued*
INSECTICIDES

| *Trade Name** | *Harmful Ingredients* | *Treatment Reference Page Number* |
|---|---|---|
| Vapotone | TEPP | *See Index* |
| Vintox | Sodium Arsenite | |
| Volk Isotox Spray | Lindane, DDT | |
| Westicide | Malathion | |
| West Rid-All | Lindane | |
| Will-Kill Bug Killer | Chlordane | |
| Wilsonol | Nicotine | |
| Winru Pyrenone Fly Spray | Pyrethrins | |

The 24-hour toll-free answering service (800-424-9300) currently provided by CHEMTREC serves as a direct link to relay requests for assistance to one of the ten PSTN area coordinators across the country. The person requesting assistance for an appropriate pesticide problem is contacted by the PSTN coordinator in a matter of minutes with instructions for necessary actions. The coordinator also determines whether to dispatch a safety team to the scene.

Should a poison control center need assistance with a nontransportation chemical or pesticide problem, first try to get the information from a larger center or the clearinghouse. Should those sources fail, the CHEMTREC-PSTN number may be called, but in no case should the emergency number be given to the public or patient. Any help available should go through the poison control center personnel.

## Miscellaneous Insecticides (Combination Sprays and Powders)

This group of household agents contains many of the better known fly and mosquito sprays. Most of the products in the following list are special formulations having several substances, each intended to endow the product with some desirable quality.

In addition to chemicals from the classes already discussed, many of these products contain certain compounds said to synergize the effectiveness of the other insecticides. These include piperonyl cyclonene, piperonyl butoxide, sulfoxide, n-propyl isomer and n-octyl bicycloheptene dicarboximide. All of these chemicals are considered essentially nontoxic in the amounts usually present in these formulations. They may, however, enhance the pharmacologic effect of drugs and potentiate the toxicity of environmental agents.

Other substances in this class are effective both as activators for the botanical derivatives (pyrethrum and rotenone) and as insecticides with a toxic action of their own. Most prominent among these are Thanite® (isobornyl thiocyanoacetate) and the lethanes, including Lethane-384® (beta-butoxy-beta thiocyano diethyl ether).

While these aliphatic thiocyanates (rhodanates) are toxic in high concentrations, they are not likely to be dangerous in the amounts present in most of these preparations. Generally, toxicity associated wih these products is due less to the insecticidal ingredients than to the petroleum solvent base (*see* discussion of Organic Thiocyanates).

TABLE 55
MISCELLANEOUS INSECTICIDES
(COMBINATION SPRAYS AND POWDERS)

| *Trade Name** | *Harmful Ingredients* | *Treatment Reference Page Number* |
|---|---|---|
| Agicide Aerosol Bombs | DDT, Methoxychlor, Allethrin, Aromatic Oil | |
| A.M.R. Insect Killer | DDT, Allethrin, Isobornyl Thiocyanoacetate | |
| Antrol Ant Powder | Chlordane, Pyrethrins, Piperonyl Cyclonene | |
| Antrol Push Button Ant and Roach Bomb | Lindane, Pyrethrins, Piperonyl Butoxide | |
| Antrol Rush Spray Flower Bomb | Lindane, Rotenone, Rotenoids | |
| Arwell Moth & Insect Spray | DDT, Lethane, Pyrethrins | |
| Black Flag Bug Killer | G-Isomer of BHC, Pyrethrins, Petroleum Distillates | |
| Black Flag Insecticide Powder | Chlordane, Piperonyl Cyclonene, Pyrethrins | |
| Black Flag Insect Spray | DDT, Methylated Naphthalenes, Beta-Butoxy-Beta Thiocyano Diethyl Ether | |
| Black Flag Push Button Aerosol Insect Killer | DDT, Allethrin, Piperonyl Butoxide | |
| Black Flag Push Button Flower Bomb | Lindane, Rotenone, Rotenoids | |
| Black Flag Push Button Roach and Ant Killer | Lindane, Pyrethrins, Piperonyl Butoxide | |
| Black Leaf | DDT, Parathion | |
| Black Leaf Spray | Methoxychlor, Pyrethrins, Isobornyl Thiocyanoacetate | |
| Bonide Roton Fly Spray | Beta-Butoxy-Beta Thiocyano Diethyl Ether | |
| Bridgeport Aer-A-Sol Insecticide | Pyrethrins, Terpene Polychlorinates | |
| Bridgeport No. 400 Aer-A-Sol Insecticide | Pyrethrins, DDT, Beta-Butoxy-Beta Thiocyano Diethyl Ether | |
| Bridgeport No. 12 Bug Bomb | DDT, Beta-Butoxy-Beta Thiocyano Diethyl Ether, Allethrin | |
| Bright Sail Insect Killer | DDT, Allethrin, N-Octyl Bicycloheptene Dicarboximide, Petroleum Distillates | |
| Brildane | Lindane, Piperonyl Butoxide, Pyrethrins | |
| Bug Blast Aerosol | Methoxychlor, Allethrin, N-Octyl Bicycloheptene Dicarboximide, Pyrethrins | |
| Bug-Dust | Rotenone, Dusting Sulfur | |
| Chaperone Insect Killer | DDT, Pyrethrins | *See Index* |
| Chemform Fly & Mosquito Aerosol Bomb | DDT, N-Octyl Bicycloheptene Dicarboximide, Allethrin | |
| College Brand Powdered Insecticide | DDT, Pyrethrins | |
| Cook's Push Button Real-Kill Insect Bomb | Pyrethrins, Piperonyl Butoxide, Allethrin, N-Octyl Bicycloheptene Dicarboximide, Methoxychlor | |
| Cook-Kill Bug Killer | Chlordane, Pyrethrins, Piperonyl Butoxide | |
| Cornell Household Aerosol Spray Insecticide | DDT, Piperonyl Butoxide, Pyrethrins | |
| Done-Died Perfumed Moth Killer | N-Octyl Bicycloheptene Dicarboximide, Methoxychlor, Allethrin | |
| Doomsday | Pyrethrins, Allethrin, Terpene Polychlorinates | |
| D & P Bulb Saver | DDT, Sulfur, Ferbam | |
| D & P Fruit Spray | Gamma BHC, DDT, Ferbam, Sulfur | |
| Dwin Aerosol Insect Killer | Allethrin, Pyrethrins, Sulfoxide Tech. | |
| Eastern States Aerosol Insecticide | Pyrethrins, DDT, Piperonyl Butoxide, Methyl Naphthalene | |
| Fast Kill Bug Killer | Chlordane, Pyrethrins | |
| Flit | DDT, Isobornyl Thiocyanoacetate, Petroleum Distillates | |
| Flit Aerosol Insect Spray | Pyrethrins, DDT, Piperonyl Butoxide | |
| Flit Bug Killer | G-isomer of BHC, Technical Chlordane, Pyrethrins | |
| Flit with 5% DDT | DDT, Isobornyl Thiocyanoacetate, Aliphatic Thiocyanates | |
| Flit Double Action Insect Spray Aerosol | Pyrethrins, DDT, Beta-Butoxy-Beta Thiocyano Diethyl Ether | |
| Flor-A-Bomb | Pyrethrins, Isothymoxychloroethyl Ether, Methylene Chloride | |
| Fly-Ded | DDT, Allethrin | |
| Flyded Aerosol Insect Killer | DDT, Lethane, Piperonyl Butoxide, Allethrin | |
| Flyded Insect Spray | DDT, Methylated Naphthalenes, Beta-Butoxy-Beta Thiocyano Diethyl Ether | |
| Fly-Tox Aerosol Insect Bomb | Pyrethrum, DDT | |
| Fort Dodge Flea and Louse Powder | Rotenone, Isobornyl Thiocyanoacetate | |

TABLE 55—*Continued*
MISCELLANEOUS INSECTICIDES
(COMBINATION SPRAYS AND POWDERS)

| *Trade Name** | *Harmful Ingredients* | *Treatment Reference Page Number* |
|---|---|---|
| Geller's Cedarized Insecticide | Pyrethrins, Allethrin, Methoxychlor | |
| G & O Plant Spray | Pyrethrins, Nicotine Sulfate, Cresylic Acid | |
| Green Cross Residual Household Spray | Lindane, Lethane, Pyrethrins | |
| Gulf Roach & Ant Killer | Pyrethrins, Chlordane | |
| Gulfspray | Tech. Piperonyl Butoxide, Methoxychlor Distillates | |
| Gy-Zip | Methoxychlor, Piperonyl Butoxide, Pyrethrins | |
| Hep Surface Spray | Pyrethrins, Dieldrin, Tech. Piperonyl Butoxide | |
| Hess Bomb | DDT, Pyrethrins, Piperonyl Butoxide | |
| Hil Flea Powder | Rotenone, Dichlorophene, Trichlorophenol | |
| Howard Insect Aerosol Bomb | Lethane, Pyrethrins, Piperonyl Butoxide | |
| Hydromix Garden Insecticide | Malathion, Methoxychlor | |
| Hydromix Lawn and Termite Spray | Naphthalene | |
| Hy-Tox Insect Spray | Malathion, Methoxychlor | |
| Isto Insect Killer | Lindane, Pyrethrins | |
| Kan-Kil | Pyrethrins, Terpene, Polychlorinates, Tech. Piperonyl Butoxide | |
| Kilspray Aerosol Insecticide | Pyrethrins, DDT, Piperonyl Butoxide | |
| Magik-Mist Year Round Insecticide | DDT, Pyrethrins, Methoxychlor | |
| Magik Rid | Allethrin, N-Octyl Bicycloheptene Dicarboximide, Ethylene Glycol | |
| Martin's Multi Kill | DDT, Chlordane, Pyrethrins | |
| Mission Brand Pesticide Spray | Chlordane, Pyrethrins | |
| Moth-Ded Mothproofing Spray | DDT, Methylated Naphthalenes, Piperonyl Butoxide | |
| Moth-Ded Button Moth Proofer | DDT, Methoxychlor, Methylated Naphthalenes | |
| NIC Odorless Fly Killer | Allethrin, N-Octyl Bicycloheptene Dicarboximide, Methoxychlor | |
| Nip & Tuck Roach Powder | DDT, Sodium Fluoride, Pyrethrins | *See Index* |
| Omnicide "BB" | Pyrethrins, Piperonyl Butoxide, Chlordane | |
| Ortho Fly Spray | Pyrethrins, Piperonyl Butoxide, Thanite | |
| P-51 Fast Kill Insect Spray | DDT, Allethrin, N-Octyl Bicycloheptene Dicarboximide | |
| Parsons Kilane Contact and Residual Spray | Isobornyl Thiocyanoacetate, Ethylhexanediol, Chlordane | |
| Parsons Louse Dust | Naphthalene, Sulfur, Rotenone, Rotenoids | |
| Parsons Mosquito Yard Spray | Methoxychlor, Ethylhexanediol, Pyrethrins | |
| Pestene Insecticide Powder | DDT, Pyrethrins | |
| Pied Piper Household Insecticide Containing DDT | DDT, Thanite, Paradichlorobenzene | |
| Pi-Co | Naphthalene 98.5% | |
| Pratt's D-X Insect Spray | Rotenone, Rotenoids, Piperonyl Cyclonene, Pyrethrins, Pine Oil | |
| Pratt's Surfispray | DDT, Pyrethrins, Piperonyl Butoxide | |
| Quick Action Gulfspray | Pyrethrins, Piperonyl Butoxide, Methoxychlor | |
| Raid Bug Killer | Methoxychlor, Pyrethrins, Rotenone | |
| Raid Insect Spray | Pyrethrins, N-Octyl Bicycloheptene Dicarboximide | |
| Ridsect Aerosol | DDT, Piperonyl Butoxide, Lethane | |
| Roachkil Insect Spray | Chlordane, Pyrethrins | |
| Sapho Flower and Garden Aerosol | Pyrethrins, Piperonyl Cyclonene, Methoxychlor | |
| Sapho Insect Bombs | DDT, Piperonyl Butoxide, Pyrethrins | |
| Sla Cedarized Spray | Pyrethrins, Allethrin, N-Octyl Bicycloheptene Dicarboximide | |
| Sprayway Bug-Go Insect Spray | DDT, Pyrethrins, Piperonyl | |
| Sprayway Fast Kill Bug Killer | Chlordane, Piperonyl Butoxide | |
| Termitine | DDT-Cresylic Acid, Orthodichlorobenzene | |
| Tetrakote | Pyrethrins, Ethylene Tetrachloride | |
| Triclane Household Spray | DDT, Pyrethrins | |

*All products listed below are registered trademarks. Since trade names and formulations are frequently and unexpectedly changed, consult labels for definitive contents as some products may be obsolete.

*Chapter 3*

# RODENTICIDES, FUNGICIDES, HERBICIDES, FUMIGANTS AND REPELLENTS

## RODENTICIDES

The rodenticides in common use are inorganic salts and synthetic and naturally occurring organic compounds.

A. Inorganic compounds
   1. Arsenic (*see* Chap. 2)
   2. Thallium (*see* Chap. 2)
   3. Phosphorus (*see* Chap. 2)
   4. Barium carbonate
   5. Zinc phosphide
   6. Vacor (N-3 pyridylmethyl-N'-*p*-nitrophenyl urea)

B. Organic compounds
   1. Sodium fluoroacetate (1080)
   2. Alphanaphthylthiourea (ANTU)
   3. Warfarin (Pival, Valone)
   4. Red squill
   5. Strychnine sulfate
   6. Dicarboximide

### *Barium*

The chief soluble salts are chloride and nitrate; however, carbonate, sulfide hydrate and fluosilicate are soluble in sufficient degree to cause poisoning. Barium carbonate, hydroxide and chloride are used in rodenticides and pesticides. The sulfide is sometimes used in depilatories. Barium sulfate used as a radiopaque medium is insoluble and, when pure, is harmless.

The toxic action of the barium ion results in severe gastrointestinal symptoms, cardiovascular irregularities and respiratory difficulties. The chief manifestations are vomiting, diarrhea, fibrillary muscular tremors, weakness, paresis, anxiety, dyspnea, irregularity of the heart, convulsions and death from cardiac and respiratory failure. Severe hypokalemia often results and may be responsible for some of the symptoms mentioned associated with this disorder. The EKG may be helpful in showing ectopic beats or other disturbances.

*Treatment* consists of prompt gastric lavage or emesis for removal of ingested agents. A 2% to 5% solution of either magnesium sulfate (Epsom salt) or of sodium sulfate (Glauber's salt) should be given as the lavage solution to inactivate the barium by forming its insoluble and nontoxic sulfate salt, and lavage should be maintained until the return is clear.

As an antidote to precipitate the barium ion, give 10 ml of 10% sodium sulfate slowly intravenously and repeat every thirty minutes until symptoms subside, or in less severe poisoning, 30 gm (1 oz.) of sodium sulfate in 250 ml (8 oz.) of water can be given by mouth and repeated in one hour. If symptoms have appeared, this can be given by gastric tube. Artificial respiration and oxygen should be used for respiratory paralysis until the antidote is given and normal respiration has returned.

Barium sulfide, on contact with gastric acid, produces hydrogen sulfide which, like cyanide, can inhibit oxidative respiratory enzymes and cause tissue anoxia. Based on animal studies, administration of amyl nitrite by inhalation and 10 ml of a 3% solution of sodium nitrite, slowly intravenously (forms methemoglobin which in turn inactivates the sulfide as sulfmethemoglobin), may be beneficial in preventing severe anoxia. For the control of ventricular arrhythmias, procainamide hydrochloride in oral doses of 100 to 250 mg can be given to a two– or three-year-old child and 50 to 150 mg in 10% solution intramuscularly or intravenously. (Propranolol hydrochloride [Inderal®] has also been experimentally effective for this purpose.) Adult doses are two to three times as large. Intravenous administration should be made slowly to minimize the possibility of cardiac standstill. Potassium therapy is absolutely essential for the hypokalemia that occurs. Atropine subcutaneously is effective for abdominal pain, but for severe colic, morphine may be necessary. Prognosis is excellent if proper antidote and therapy are given before symptoms become severe. Survival for more than twenty-four hours has almost always been followed by recovery without sequelae.

## *Zinc Phosphide*

This compound is a crystalline, gray powder of a pungent phosphorus-like odor. It releases phosphine on contact with water, the inhalation of which can cause restlessness, tremors, fatigue and drowsiness.

Zinc phosphide is not available as a household agent, nor is it widely used as a rodenticide by pest control operators, government control officials or farmers for rodent control because of its high toxicity and strong odor. Most domestic animals do not touch baits containing this agent, but rodents seem to like the rotten fish odor and readily accept this type of bait. Inhalation of zinc phosphide dust is followed in several hours by vomiting, diarrhea, cyanosis, rapid pulse, fever, irritability and shock. The breath and black stomach contents or vomitus smell of phosphine.

The *treatment* is mainly symptomatic for poisoning from inhalation; however, if ingestion has occurred the stomach should be lavaged. Potassium permanganate 1:5000 solution should be used in the last washing to oxidize any remaining phosphide present.

## *VACOR (N-3 Pyridylmethyl-N'-p-nitrophenyl Urea)*

VACOR™ RatKiller, DLP-787 2% Bait and DLP-787 10% House Mouse Tracking Powder contain the active ingredient N-3 pyridylmethyl-N'-*p*-nitrophenyl urea, a single-dose, quick-kill rodenticide. They are used for the control of the Norway and roof rats and the house mouse.

VACOR RatKiller is sold over-the-counter in retail outlets. Both DLP-787 2% Bait and DLP-787 10% House Mouse Tracking Powder are available only to pest control operators.

| *Product* | *Physical Appearance* | *Toxicity* ($LD_{50}$) *Albino Rats* | *Albino Mice* |
|---|---|---|---|
| VACOR RatKiller (2% Active Ingredient) | Yellow; resembles corn meal | 580 mg/kg | —— |
| DLP-787 2% Bait | Yellow; resembles corn meal | 580 mg/kg | 4120 mg/kg |
| DLP-787 10% House Mouse Tracking Powder | Pale light green powder | —— | 1050 mg/kg |

All three products should be handled and treated as though they are toxic to humans. Minimum lethal dose for humans is not known. Toxicity studies on other animals using RH-787 Technical Material (100% active ingredient) indicates $LD_{50}$ for dogs is greater than 4 gm/kg and for Rhesus monkeys 2 to 4 gm/kg.

VACOR or DLP-787 *does not* have an anticoagulant effect in animals or man. Exact mechanism of action is unknown. It does interfere with nicotinamide metabolism in rats. Previously unrecognized diabetes mellitus and autonomic nervous system dysfunction have been observed in several instances in humans after ingestion of VACOR. Human exposure data is limited. The minimum lethal dose for man is not known, but the diabetogenic effect has occurred after ingestion of a single package (30 gm). If unrecognized and untreated, this condition could be fatal.

SIGNS AND SYMPTOMS. Variable, depending on dose, individual and treatment.

**Initial:** (May be delayed in onset 4 to 48 hours)

- Nausea
- Vomiting
- Abdominal pains/cramping
- Chills or chilliness
- Mental confusion

**Intermediate:**

- Anorexia
- General body aches, particularly in limbs
- Dilated pupils
- Dehydration
- Chest Pain
- Glycosuria and elevated blood glucose
- Diabetic-type keto acidosis
- Dysphagia
- Leukocytosis
- Gastrointestinal dystonia
- Urinary retention/bladder dysfunction
- Cardiovascular involvement with arrhythmias
- Postural hypotension
- Peripheral neuropathy, nonspecific
- Fine tremors of extremities
- Muscular weakness
- Elevated serum amylase and lipase
- Temporary blindness (in dogs)
- Plantar hyperesthesia

**Late:**

- Severe autonomic dysfunction
- Cardiovascular collapse
- Respiratory failure
- Coma
- Death

*Treatment.*

1. Prompt emptying of the stomach by induced emesis followed by gastric lavage is indicated for all ingestions of VACOR or DLP-787 as early as possible. This should be followed by 30 ml of mineral oil plus a cathartic. Emesis and lavage is warranted up to twelve hours postingestion.
2. Niacinamide (nicotinamide) has been demonstrated to be an effective antidote in rats if administered shortly after exposure. It is recommended as an antidote for any significant human exposures.
   a. It is recommended that 500 mg of niacinamide U.S.P. (nicotinamide) be given intramuscularly or intravenously immediately. Then give 100 to 200 mg IM or IV every four hours for up to forty-eight hours. If signs of toxicity develop (as noted above), increase frequency of injection to every two hours. Do not exceed 3 gm/day for adult. Administer one half of adult dose to small children.
   b. When patient is able to take medication by mouth, continue to give 100 mg of niacinamide PO three to five times daily for the next two weeks.
3. If patient develops signs of diabetes mellitus as a result of VACOR ingestion, indications are that it will respond to appropriate insulin therapy. Close observation for development of keto acidosis and autonomic nervous system dysfunction is warranted. The diabetes may be "brittle" and persistent.
4. Other treatment should be symptomatic and supportive.
5. In the event of *human* VACOR ingestion, notify the following.

Corporate Medical Director
Rohm and Haas Company
Independence Mall West
Philadelphia, Pennsylvania 19105

Telephone—(215) 592-2912 Business Hours
(215) 592-3000 After Hours

### *Fluoroacetate (Fluoroacetamide 1080)*

This compound is a highly toxic and a very effective rodenticide. Because of its extreme toxicity to most forms of life and the lack of specific antidotes, it is not available for household or general use. It is sold only to licensed pest control operators and others qualified by training and experience in rodent control procedures. It occurs naturally as a constituent of *Dichapetalum cymosum* (Gifblaar), a plant found in South Africa where it has caused poisoning of livestock. The synthetic sodium salt is water-soluble, and the estimated lethal dose is between 50 and 100 mg (¾ to 1½ gr). Fluoroacetate in the body forms fluorotricarboxylic acid which blocks cellular metabolism and acts predominately on the heart and the central nervous system.

Sodium fluoroacetate and some closely related compounds have a unique mode of action. The toxicity is apparently not due to its fluoride content, as the clinical toxicity and pathological findings are quite distinct from those in fluoride poisoning. The biochemical action of this material appears to come by formation of a fluorocitrate compound that inhibits the reactions of the Krebs cycle. For this reason, there is often a delay of a few hours in the onset of its action that is related to the need to metabolize the fluoroacetate.

The symptoms of poisoning in man appear primarily related to the central nervous system (CNS) and the cardiovascular system. The CNS effects are usually agitation, depressed consciousness, seizures and eventually coma. The cardiovascular effects, which often result in death, appear to take the following course: First, there is tachycardia and increase in amplitude of T waves, followed by ST elevation and irregular rhythm with premature ventricular contractions that may progress to a bigeminal pattern. Finally, in adults, there may be ventricular tachycardia and fibrillation leading to death. In children, the final stage is usually heart failure and cardiac standstill rather than ventricular fibrillation.

*Treatment* for sodium fluoroacetate poisoning is mainly symptomatic. Immediate emesis and gastric lavage followed by oral doses of magnesium sulfate are useful. Administration of certain compounds capable of supplying acetate ions has shown antidotal effects (prevention or reversal of pulsus atlernans or electric alternans on the EEG) in animals including monkeys. The choice drugs are monoacetin (glyceryl monoacetate 0.24 gm/kg) and a combination of sodium acetate and ethanol (0.12 gm/kg of each), but reports of their use in humans have rarely appeared in the literature. If parenteral administration is not feasible, a mixture of 100 ml of undiluted monoacetin in 500 ml of water can be given orally and repeated in an hour. A single dose of magnesium sulfate (800 mg/kg) given intramuscularly as a 50% solution has saved the lives of rats dosed with lethal amounts of sodium fluoroacetate. Oily cathartics and epinephrine should not be used. Complete quiet and rest are indicated. Barbiturates to the point of anesthesia have proved disappointing when used as antidotes against this poison, but of course are useful in controlling convulsions. Slow intravenous injection of procainamide is a useful measure to restore normal rhythm in ventricular fibrillation.

### *Alphanaphthylthiourea (ANTU)*

This compound was developed after it was found to be an active rodenticide while being fairly innocuous to humans. The only drawback to its use is that some species of rats are not sensitive to it, while others develop resistance rapidly.

ANTU is a stable, odorless, slightly bitter, blue-gray powder that is highly insoluble in water. ANTU is not greatly toxic to man except possibly in large amounts. The mean lethal oral dose is 4 gm/kg in monkeys. Due to the action of ANTU on pulmonary capillaries, pulmonary edema and pleural effusion have been found in experimental animals.

Symptoms, if they occur, pertain to the respiratory tract. Dyspnea, rales and cyanosis may occur if pulmonary edema or pleural effusion develops. Hypothermia may be a prominent symptom. ANTU may possess antithyroid activity in chronic sublethal exposures. The skin is generally not affected with exposure or handling. Since this chemical is practically insoluble, *treatment* consists of prompt gastric lavage with tap water or an emetic. This should be followed with a saline cathartic such as sodium sulfate, 15 to 30 gm in water. Since ANTU is readily absorbed in oil, mineral oil and fat ingestion should be avoided. Intravenous fluids should be given with caution because of the danger of precipitating pulmonary edema. If this develops, positive-pressure oxygen, postural drainage and antibiotics are necessary.

### *Warfarin (Pival, Valone)*

These related synthetic anticoagulant compounds produce a reversible and controllable hypoprothrombinemia and capillary injury. These are ideal rodenticides in that they are fairly safe as far as humans are concerned. The dangerous dose is approximately 100 mg (1½ gr) daily. This represents the ingestion of about 0.5 kg (1 lb.) of rat bait. Warfarin inhibits prothrombin synthesis, but the liver contains a sufficient reserve, and this inhibition must continue until the reserve is depleted for specific symptoms to appear. The pathogenic manifestation of poisoning by these agents is bleeding. The toxicity of a single large dose, however, is slight, and only when it is taken over a period of several days or on repeated ingestions does the bleeding tendency appear. However, percutaneous absorption from the continual handling of warfarin solutions or mixtures can produce the same effects. There may be epistaxis, massive purpura or petechiae at the knees and elbows, weakness, pallor, hematuria and rectal bleeding. The bleeding and clotting time and plasma prothrombin determinations are prolonged in serious poisoning.

*Treatment* consists of gastric lavage if more than 0.5 gm has been ingested and if no more than two or three hours have elapsed. This should be followed by sodium sulfate catharsis. If bleeding occurs or if the prothrombin time is prolonged more than twice normal, vitamin K, natural or synthetic, should be given intramuscularly or intravenously in a dose of 50 to 100 mg to an adult or 10 to 20 mg to a small child. If hemoglobin is below 60% (10 gm/100 ml blood) or if the bleeding is severe, 500 ml (1 pt.) of fresh whole blood should be given. This may be repeated if necessary or until the anemia is corrected.

### *Red Squill*

This botanic substance contains cardiac glycosides and is one of the least toxic of the rodenticides. In excessive doses it increases the irritability of the ventricular muscle, resulting first in extrasystoles, then ventricular tachycardia and eventually ventricular fibrillation. It is also an irritant and central-acting emetic. The symptoms from acute poisoning are nausea, vomiting and diarrhea, abdominal pains, scotomata, cardiac irregularities, convulsions and death from ventricular fibrillation.

In the *treatment,* delay in absorption of the ingested material can be accomplished by giving milk to drink, after which the stomach should be lavaged. Quinidine sulfate 0.2 gm orally reduces myocardial irritability. Epinephrine or other stimulants should not be given as they may induce ventricular fibrillation.

### *Strychnine*

Strychnine is a rodent bait as well as a component of various tonics and cathartic pills which are brightly colored and sugarcoated and very attractive to young children. Unfortunately these are found in some homes and are often carelessly left about where infants can get them. The lethal dose varies considerably, but deaths have been reported from as little as 5 or 10 mg, although the $LD_{50}$ in man is probably 100 to 120 mg. Strychnine differs from most alkaloids in that it is absorbed from the stomach and symptoms appear quite readily from ingestion. This potent alkaloid acts in the body primarily as a central nervous system stimulant. There is greatly increased reflex excitability in the spinal cord which results in a loss of the normal inhibition of spread of motor cell stimulation so that all muscles contract simultaneously. This leads to the characteristic strychnine convulsion. All skeletal muscles partake in it, and the stronger partners of antagonistic groups exert dominance in determining the posture assumed. Thus it is that the victim shows extensive rigidity of the trunk (opisthotonus) which may be so extreme that only the heels and the crown of the head are in contact with the ground. The forearms are usually flexed across the chest. The facial muscles also show a typical tetanic spasm which gives the risus sardonicus expression to the features. The diaphragmatic and thoracic muscles are likewise involved, and as a result, respiration ceases during the seizure. The venous congestion, blue-black cyanosis, bulging eyes, dilated pupils and facial grimace of these patients are not easily forgotten once witnessed. In addition, the person is acutely conscious throughout, and the pain is intense. There is usually experienced terrifying fright, the feeling of impending death and the sensation of being hurled through space. The convulsion lasts from one-half to two minutes and is followed by a period of relaxation. When respiration is resumed, cyanosis disappears and circulation improves. These convulsions occur at intervals of five to fifteen minutes, varying with the type and intensity of external stimuli. Profound metabolic acidosis has been documented with seizures. Death due to respiratory failure and asphyxia ensues unless these seizures are controlled before great damage is done to the vital centers of the medulla.

The symptoms, which usually appear within ten to twenty minutes after ingestion of the poison, are often preceded by restlessness, mental anxiety and twitching of the fingers, hands and face.

The two aims of *treatment* are toward the prevention of convulsions and the removal or neutralization of the poison. The patient should be in bed in a dark room, free from noise and disturbance. If much twitching and convulsions have not occurred, a chemical antidote should be administered, such as tannic acid, 1 gm or 1 tsp. in half a glass of water; tincture of iodine or compound solution of iodine, 1 or 2 ml in a glass of water; strong tea, potassium permanganate, 0.25 gm (4 gr) in a glass of water; and activated charcoal. One gm of charcoal absorbs more than 950 mg of strychnine. It is probably the best therapeutic measure available and should be used immediately, for to be effective it must be given early in the treatment. The stomach should then be emptied by lavage or emesis. Fatal convulsions may be precipitated by attempts at gastric lavage unless barbiturate sedation is instituted beforehand.

In the presence of seizures or threatened convulsions, the administration of short-acting sedatives is paramount. Intravenous and rectal instillation of one of the barbiturates is necessary to control the convulsions. Parenteral diazepam has been used successfully and may be even more effective for this purpose. Muscle relaxants, such as intravenous mephenesin, are reported to be useful adjuncts in therapy. They reduce the muscular rigidity and allow normal respiratory movements to continue. The antagonism between strychnine and mephenesin is more complete than that with the barbiturates, and in addition, mephenesin does not depress the central nervous system. Artificial respiration, oxygen and other supportive measures are mandatory in treatment. Morphine should not be used at any time in the treatment, for it further depresses an already precariously depressed respiration and acts as a spinal cord stimulant which synergizes with the stimulation from strychnine. Parenteral bicarbonate should be administered for metabolic acidosis if it occurs.

### *Dicarboximide (Raticate)®*

This compound 5-(a-hydroxy-a-2-pyridylbenzyl) -7-(a-2-pyridylbenzylidene) -5-norbornene-2,3-dicarboximide (Tavolek Laboratories, Fort Washington, Pennsylvania) is a specific toxicant only to the Norway or brown rat. It does not have a similar effect, even at extremely high doses, on mice or other species studied for toxicity, such as domestic animals, poultry, household pets and numerous wild animals, including monkeys and other primates. The substance seems to exhibit a very low toxicity to the human. It is not available for general use.

Poisoned rats exhibit restlessness, ataxia, weakness of hindquarters and labored breathing. The ears, eyes, feet and tail are strikingly blanched, and death follows, usually with mild convulsions. Death may be due to the simultaneous vasoconstrictor effects on multiple systems and organs.

TABLE 56
ESTIMATED FATAL DOSES OF RODENTICIDES TO MAN

| *Common Name* | *Chemical Name* | *Comparative Toxicity* | *Estimated Fatal Oral Dose (gm/70 kg)* | *Antidote* |
|---|---|---|---|---|
| Thallium sulfate | Thallium sulfate | Highly toxic | 1 | |
| Barium carbonate | Barium carbonate | Moderately toxic | 5 | Magnesium sulfate |
| Strychnine sulfate | Strychnine sulfate | Highly toxic | 0.1 | Barbiturates, mephenesin |
| ANTU | Alphanaphthyl-thiourea | Slightly toxic | 7 to 10 | |
| 1080 | Sodium fluoroacetate | Highly toxic | 0.15 | |
| Warfarin | Acetonylbenzyl hydroxycoumarin | Slightly toxic | 0.5 | Vitamin K |
| VACOR® | N-3 Pyridylmethyl-N-*p*-nitrophenyl urea | Moderately toxic | ? ($LD_{50}$ for dogs 4 gm/kg) | Niacinamide U.S.P. |

## FUNGICIDES

These chemicals employed to eradicate fungi and protect materials from rot and decay include a large number of inorganic and organic compounds. Some are highly toxic to humans, while others are of little danger under ordinary circumstances. Among the most commonly used substances for this purpose are the following.

1. Mercury compounds (*see* Chap. 2)
2. Copper compounds
3. Pentachlorophenol
4. Dithiocarbamates
5. Tetramethylthiuram disulfide (Thiram)
6. Hexachlorobenzene
7. Dodine

### *Copper Compounds (Copper Chloride, Oxide, Sulfate, Phosphate, Silicate, etc.)*

These salts applied locally or absorbed from the gastrointestinal tract or through the skin can cause toxic effects. Direct contact with the skin may give rise to an itching papulovesicular and eczematoid lesion, which on continued contact may result in some degree of necrosis. Copper dust or salts splashed in the eye can cause severe conjunctivitis, edema of the lids and even ulceration of the cornea. Prolonged inhalation of these compounds can produce severe congestion of the nasal mucosa with rhinitis and possible sloughing and ulceration. The ingestion of large doses causes violent vomiting. (Copper sulfate is often used as an emetic in European countries but rarely in the United States. The ordinary emetic dose is 0.25 gm as a 1% solution.) The violent vomiting usually results in removal of most of the poison. However, systemic absorption may result in blue discoloration of the gums and tongue, hemolytic anemia, hemorrhagic gastritis, colic and diarrhea with bloody stools. In more protracted cases, liver and kidney damage with severe anemia may follow. Finally the patient becomes somnolent and comatose and dies from circulatory failure.

Contaminated dialysis caused by copper that was released from copper tubing in the dialysate-making equipment has produced acute hemolysis in three reported episodes of hemodialysis. Copper cooking vessels or piping do not impart significant quantities of copper to water or food. However, foods are not usually prepared in copper vessels due to the catalytic properties of this element. Vitamin C is rapidly destroyed if foods containing this vitamin are heated in the presence of copper. Beverages prepared or stored in brass containers may become contaminated by copper ions and cause nausea and vomiting as well as other toxic manifestations.

The stains in water supply attributed to copper are more likely to be an accumulation of iron and calcium deposits. The federal government has set a maximum limit to the copper content of potable water at 0.2 mg/liter. Since the absorption of copper is limited, its toxicity to animals is low. However, significant increase of copper in the water supply can color shampooed hair green. In copper workers, green hair may develop as a result of environmental exposure. Severe hemolytic anemia may require blood transfusions.

Copper is a vital constituent of a number of enzymes, including ascorbic acid oxidase, lactase and tyrosinase, and is considered to be an essential mineral. Most diets supply 2 to 5 mg of copper/day, an amount adequate to meet all needs.

*Treatment.* Dilute solutions (1%) of potassium ferrocyanide (forms insoluble copper ferrocyanide), sodium carbonate, milk or egg white should be given quickly to precipitate the copper, and the stomach should then be cleansed by gastric lavage or emesis. Intravenous and oral calcium edathamil is a good antidote for copper poisoning and should be given after the stomach has been emptied. BAL and penicillamine are additional useful agents that can be tried. Symptomatic and supportive treatment of pain, dehydration, nephritis and coma may be necessary. Peritoneal dialysis with an albumin (Albumisol®) enriched dialysis fluid has been used effectively for renal failure.

### *Pentachlorophenol*

Pentachlorophenol is a weed killer and insecticide as well as a preservative of wood against fungi. It has been reported to have mutagenic effects, and the fatal dose for laboratory animals varies from 30 to 100 mg/kg according to the solvent, route of administration and animal species. This compound is severely irritating to the skin and respiratory and gastrointestinal mucosa. The pharmacologic action is similar to that of the dinitrophenols and consists of an increase in the metabolic rate, leading to a marked elevation of body temperature. The main action of the chemical is a rapid uncoupling of oxidation and phosphorylation cycles. Systemic poisoning, although rare, can produce convulsions and late liver or kidney damage, fever, collapse and occasionally death.

Use of pentachlorophenol (PCP) as a fungistatic agent to launder diapers and infants' bed linen caused, in nine neonates, an unusual illness characterized by fever, tachycardia, excessive sweating and dyspnea, with hepatomegaly in six and splenomegaly in two of them. The sweating was out of proportion to the fever and suggested increased metabolic rates in the sick babies. PCP was identified in serum and urine of the affected infants, two of whom died. Six, who received exchange transfusions, recovered rapidly; one recovered without tranfusion. Exchange transfusion proved to be a fortunate choice since phenols are not stored in the tissues to any great extent and blood levels correlate well with the severity of the poisoning. The experience with PCP should alert others to the possibility that this or some other water-soluble toxic chemical may cause similar outbreaks in nurseries.

*Treatment.* It is important that this substance be thoroughly removed from the skin by adequate cleansing with soap and water. The use of an emetic or gastric lavage for ingestion, if it occurs, is imperative; otherwise, the treatment is symptomatic and supportive.

### *Dithiocarbamates (Thiocarbamates)*

Dithiocarbamates (ferbam, ziram, maneb, zineb, nabam) are fungistatic agents available as sprays, dusts and wettable powders and are used mainly on fruit crops and tobacco and often on vegetables and ornamental plants. The exact dosage necessary to produce poisoning in man is not known for any of these compounds. Most applicators consider the dithiocarbamates to be essentially harmless since they have experienced no more serious symptoms than mild conjunctivitis, rhinitis, pharyngitis and bronchitis as well as an insignificant dermatitis as a result of rather heavy exposures. There is some evidence that many of the primary disturbances from formulations of these substances may be due to the vehicles used, as well as to the active ingredients. Sulfhemoglobinemia, Heinz body formation and acute hemolytic anemia have been reported following skin contact and possible ingestion of zineb in an individual with G-6-PD deficiency.

*Treatment.* If symptoms appear, the applicator should cease the method of spraying and remove himself from the environment. Alcohol greatly increases the toxicity of the thiocarbamates and therefore should be avoided. Otherwise treatment would be symptomatic.

### *Tetramethylthiuram Disulfide (Thiram)*

This compound is the methyl analogue of disulfiram (Antabuse®) and is used as an agricultural fungicide as well as insecticide and repellent against the Japanese beetle. The lethal dose has been estimated to be 0.5 gm/kg. Thiram is a moderately severe irritant of the mucous membranes and a mild irritant of intact skin. The toxicity is increased in the presence of fats, oils and fat solvents, which promote absorption.

The principal manifestations of poisoning are sensation of heat, flushing, vasodilation, nausea, vomiting, severe diarrhea, anorexia and loss of weight. In addition there may be hyperexcitability, ataxia, hypotension, hypothermia, weakness and flaccid paralysis. Contact dermatitis may be severe and incapacitating.

*Treatment* consists of immediate gastric lavage and symptomatic and supportive treatment for various gastrointestinal symptoms and neurological complications. Fats, oils and lipid solvents should be avoided and alcohol strictly prohibited for one to two weeks. Skin contacts should be thoroughly washed.

### *Hexachlorobenzene ($C_6$ $Cl_6$)*

Hexachlorobenzene was introduced as a fungicide in 1954 and is an entirely different chemical from the insecticide hexachlorocyclohexane ($C_6H_6Cl_6$) (*see* Benzene hexachloride [Lindane]). The oral lethal dose in guinea pigs is reported to be greater than 3 gm/kg. Prolonged skin contact has caused exfoliation to occur, but very little is known of its systemic effects.

Hexachlorobenzene has produced more than three thousand cases of acquired toxic porphyria cutanea tarda in the southeastern region of Turkey. (Other substances capable of producing this condition are alcohol, estrogens, sulfonmethane [Sulfonal] and chloroquine.) The outbreak was traced to the consumption of wheat as food, contrary to plan, after it had been prepared for seed planting by treating it with hexachlorobenzene for its fungicidal properties. The porphyrinogenic nature of this halogenated benzene has subsequently been demonstrated in animal experiments. This concept that some forms of porphyria cutanea tarda may be acquired rather than inherited is not new, but the report from Turkey provides the first direct evidence, implicating a specific toxin to which the afflicted patients were exposed. In spite of these observations, the various syndromes of human porphyria have been demonstrated beyond reasonable doubt to be due to a genetic transmission of a metabolic defect and the possibility of a hereditary pattern, though unlikely in such an explosive occurrence as this of a relatively rare disease, should not be entirely discounted until proven otherwise.

### *Dodine*

Dodine (n-dodecylguanide acetate) is a cationic surface-active agricultural fungicide. The most conspicuous acute toxic action of the dry material or concentrated solutions is a pronounced irritant effect on the skin and mucous membranes. Unless large amounts are ingested, systemic symptoms are unlikely to occur.

*Treatment* consists of removal from the skin, mucous membranes or eyes with large quantities of water. In case of ingestion, the stomach should be emptied by emesis or gastric lavage.

## HERBICIDES

Weed control is accomplished at present by the use of general contact weed killers and selective herbicides. The chemicals used are of two main classes: those which are toxic to all plants with which they come in contact, as well as to humans and animals; and those which are toxic only to certain types of weeds and which are not dangerous to man and animals. The contact weed killers in common use are the following.

1. Sodium chlorate
2. Dinitrophenol derivatives
3. Potassium cyanate
4. Sodium arsenite
5. Caustic acids and alkalis
6. Petroleum distillates (Diesel oil, Crude oil, etc.)
7. Trifluralin (Treflan®)
8. Diquat, Paraquat

The selective herbicides or hormone-type weed killers are plant growth regulators and as a group are relatively nontoxic. They include alphanaphthalene acetic acid, dalapon sodium (2-2 dichloropropionic acid), aminotriazole (amizol, ATA), maleic hydrazide (MH-30) and the salts of chlorinated phenoxyacetic acid (2,4-D, 2,4,5-T and MCPA).* Dioxin (tetrachlorodibenzo-*p*-dioxin) is a highly toxic impurity formed during production of 2,4,5-T and trichlorophenol. Its effects are cumulative with acne, bone marrow depression, liver disease and CNS symptoms. It is also a carcinogen in animals.

These compounds are sold as dry salts, pastes, emulsifiable concentrates, water-wettable powders and dusts varying in strength of active ingredients from 2 to 98 per cent. A wide variety of solvents have been used with these compounds and must be considered in case of poisoning.

If ingested, all of these products should be removed from the stomach, by lavage or emesis. Quinidine may be necessary if a myotonia-like state and ventricular fibrillation occur in 2,4-D, 2,4,5-T and MCPA intoxication; chronic exposure can produce aplastic anemia, which may require blood transfusions and steroid therapy. Antipyretics with alcohol sponging should be used for hyperpyrexia. Persons allergic to phenols may experience sensitivity to the phenolic agents, but otherwise they are nonirritating to the skin except in solid or concentrated form. If this be the case, the skin, eye and mucous membranes should be thoroughly washed with water.

### *Sodium Chlorate (Bromates)*

Sodium and potassium chlorates are water-soluble and act as mild oxidizing agents, and because of this action, the potassium salt was used often in the past as an ingredient in mouthwashes and gargles. The sodium salt is used for weed control and soil sterilizers. It is a

*2,4-D is Dichlorophenoxyacetic acid.
2,4,5-T is Trichlorophenoxyacetic acid.
MCPA is Methyl-4-Chlorophenoxyacetic acid.

colorless, odorless crystal with a slightly saline taste. While moderately toxic, its main danger is that of combustion. Because of its strong oxidizing properties, it starts to release oxygen when heated. Contaminated clothing and treated dry vegetation can become a fire hazard by exposure to any combustible material. Since sodium chlorate is readily soluble in water, laundering removes the danger associated with clothing. Sodium chlorate should never be mixed with or stored near organic compounds, oils, sulfur, sulfides, powdered metals, ammonium salts or phosphorus. If mixed with these compounds, it may produce ignition, an explosion or toxic gases depending on the combination of the materials. The lethal dose is about 15 gm for adults and 2 gm for children. Bromates are used as neutralizers in hair waves. The fatal dose is estimated to be 4 gm. The chlorate or bromate ions are irritating to mucous membranes in concentrated solution; after absorption they produce methemoglobinemia by virtue of their oxidizing properties. However, the salts are not reduced in the process but act as a catalyst, so that only small amounts can still produce severe methemoglobinemia.

Symptoms in acute poisoning are chiefly gastrointestinal with nausea, vomiting, abdominal pain and diarrhea. Concomitantly or later hemolysis, cyanosis, anuria, coma and convulsions may occur. Continued use of doses less than necessary to produce acute symptoms may lead to anorexia and weight loss. Deafness and renal failure have been reported with potassium bromate poisoning.

*Treatment.* Remove material from the stomach by gastric lavage with 1% sodium thiosulfate (carefully remove all of the solution) or emesis. Give milk or other demulcents to relieve gastric irritation. Force fluids to 2 to 4 liters daily if urine output is adequate; 100 to 500 ml of sodium thiosulfate can be given intravenously. In serious intoxication hemodialysis or peritoneal lavage should be used. Cyanosis and methemoglobin levels of 40% and above require oxygen and whole blood replacement transfusion. Do not use methylene blue for methemoglobinemia because this dye may enhance the toxicity of either chlorate or bromate. Dialysis should be used for any serious poisoning.

### *Dinitrophenol Derivatives*

A number of dinitrophenols, alone or as salts of aliphatic amines (triethanolamine hydroxide), are used in dormant sprays for the control of mites, aphids and other pests over the wintering stages. They are more extensively used, however, as eradicant herbicides in such locations as roadsides, rights-of-way or as selective weed killers in fields and pastures.

The principal manifestations of poisoning with the dinitro derivatives are elevation of body temperature and increased respiration, pulse and oxygen consumption due to the stimulation of metabolism of all body cells. In acute poisoning from skin contamination, ingestion or inhalation, symptoms are frequently of sudden onset up to two days after cessation of exposure and include high fever, prostration, thirst, nausea, vomiting, excessive perspiration and difficulty in breathing. Later, symptoms progress to anoxia with cyanosis and acidosis, and finally muscular tremors and coma. Chronic poisoning has not been reported following agricultural exposure. Medicinal use (now abandoned) to induce weight loss has been accompanied by the following toxic reactions: skin eruptions, peripheral neuritis, liver and kidney damage, granulocytopenia, and rarely, cataract formation. The fatal adult oral dose is 1 to 3 gm. *Treatment* consists of gastric lavage with large volumes of sodium bicarbonate solution if ingestion occurs. For skin contamination, the skin should be thoroughly washed with a weak alkaline solution. No attempt should be made to remove the deeply penetrated persistent stain from the skin or hair. Oxygen and circulatory stimulants should be administered and the temperature reduced by alcohol sponging or ice packs to the body. Atropine is definitely contraindicated and antipyretics are usually not effective. Infusion of isotonic saline to replace the fluids and electrolytes lost by sweating, as well as specific fluid therapy for acidosis, may be necessary.

### *Potassium Cyanate*

Unlike the cyanides, this compound is relatively nontoxic to man and animals. Most instances of poisoning have been associated with the therapeutic administration of potassium thiocyanate for hypertension and not from cyanate, which has an estimated lethal dose of approximately 50 gm. *Treatment* consists of emptying the stomach by gastric lavage or emesis and supportive measures, particularly for hypotension if it occurred.

### *Trifluralin (Treflan)*

Trifluralin, a herbicide, is a yellow-orange solid which is almost insoluble in water, but freely soluble in acetone, Stoddard solvent and xylene. Trifluralin is poorly absorbed after oral administration, with 78 per cent being excreted in the feces and 22 per cent in the urine, mostly within the first twenty-four hours. It has an acute oral $LD_{50}$ of 5000 mg/kg in rats; acute oral $LD_{50}$ was greater than 2000 mg/kg in the mouse, adult and weanling rat, rabbit, dog and chicken. Rats were not injured after inhaling 2.8 mg/liter/hour in air. The percutaneous $LD_{50}$ on rabbits' skin was greater than 2500 mg/kg. In chronic toxicity studies, rats fed diets containing trifluralin at levels of 2000 ppm for two years showed no pathologic changes.

Symptoms may be produced by the solvents used in formulations of this herbicide; otherwise no definitive symptoms have been noted so far.

*Treatment.* Induce emesis or perform gastric lavage. Give milk, demulcents and saline cathartic. As most formulations of this herbicide contain aromatic hydrocarbon solvents or Stoddard solvent (mineral spirits), treatment depends also upon the type and amount of solvent present in various formulations. Symptomatic and supportive therapy, in general, is all that is necessary.

### *Diquat (1,1-ethylene 2,2-dipyridylium dibromide)*

Diquat is a quaternary ammonium compound used as a herbicide, desiccant and defoliant for plants. The concentrate is corrosive and a primary skin irritant. The amount of diquat ion which would cause death in man following a single oral dose has been estimated at 6 to 12 gm. It has an acute oral $LD_{50}$ value of 30 mg/kg in cows, 190 mg/kg in rabbits and 400 to 440 mg/kg in rats. Acute (single) dermal application of 500 mg/kg produced no evident effects in rabbits. However, repeated contact may increase danger of skin absorption. Diquat may be absorbed following oral ingestion, dermal exposure or inhalation of spray mists. Over 90 per cent of an oral dose is recovered from the feces in two days, indicating minimal absorption from the gastrointestinal tract. It is water-soluble, with urinary excretion of that portion which is absorbed.

INGESTION. Concentrated solutions of diquat cause severe irritation to the mucous membranes of the mouth, pharynx, esophagus and stomach. This may be followed by ulceration and perforation. There is usually recurrent vomiting and, after large doses, restlessness and hyperexcitability. In animals, death from diquat poisoning is accompanied by thickening of the alveolar lining of the lungs and by gross abdominal distention due to retention of gas and fluid and paralytic ileus. Intraperitoneal doses of 500 mg/kg in rats produced cyanosis, convulsions and death within two hours.

INHALATION. Exposure to spray mists may cause skin irritation, nasal bleeding, irritation and inflammation of the mouth and upper respiratory tract, cough and chest pain.

SKIN. Contact with the concentrate may cause severe skin irritation and burning. Contact with dilute liquid or dust formulations of diquat may result in reversible skin irritation. Systemic toxicity, with symptoms similar to those following ingestion, may occur from skin absorption, especially with repeated contact.

EYES. Contact with dilute liquid or dust formulations may cause reversible eye irritation. More severe irritation would be expected from the concentrate. No effects were produced by application of 0.1 ml of a 10% solution to the eyes of rabbits.

*Treatment.* Dilute at once with milk, mild soap (not detergent) solution, egg whites or water. Induce emesis (unless corrosive damage evident). Perform careful gastric lavage (avoid aspiration) with milk, mild soap solution, or water; instill 1 to 2 liters of 7% suspension of bentonite, which is capable of removing cationic substances from solution by a cation-exchange mechanism. Give demulcents. Maintain respiration (oxygen [cautiously] for dyspnea or cyanosis). Maintain high fluid intake and induce osmotic diuresis to aid excretion. Keep patient quiet. Test urine for diquat especially in the twenty-four- to forty-eight-hour period following exposure. If urine (or blood) shows appreciable quantities of diquat, keep the patient at rest and under medical observation for at least two weeks. Symptomatic and supportive treatment for hyperexcitability, shock and ileus are indicated.

SKIN. Wash thoroughly with soap and water. Healing time may be somewhat delayed. If the skin exposure is massive or prolonged, animal studies have suggested that symptoms would be similar to those seen following ingestion and should be treated accordingly.

EYES. Wash with large quantities of water. Consult ophthalmologist if necessary.

### *Paraquat (1,1-dimethyl 4,4[1] bi-pyridylium chloride)*

Fortunately the herbicide, paraquat, which is produced in a 30% concentrated aqueous solution, is not found on regular garden supply shelves. Serious paraquat poisoning in human beings has occurred only following ingestion or parenteral administration. Exposure to paraquat by skin, eye or inhalation has resulted in local irritation or inflammation of varying degree, sometimes severe. The $LD_{50}$ is twice that of diquat.

In cases of paraquat ingestion, there is usually an immediate burning discomfort of the mouth and pharynx due to the severe irritating effect of the formulation. This is generally followed by repeated vomiting. If the dose was large (6 to 8 oz.) the lungs, kidneys, liver and adrenals may be severely affected initially, followed by possibly fatal pulmonary edema within twenty-four to seventy-two hours. When lesser amounts are taken, a decrease in urine volume due to acute renal failure may occur from one to six days following ingestion. Jaundice is sometimes noted. BUN and serum creatinine levels are characteristically elevated during this time. Temperature and blood pressure are usually normal. Depending upon the amount of paraquat ingested, some pulmonary edema may also be present. This initial phase is followed by a latent period sometimes lasting as long as two weeks, during which time the patient feels well and kidney function generally improves. However, pulmonary changes may occur which are clinically manifested by generalized rales and decreased pulmonary function. Diminished gas exchange in the lungs occurs, and a continual decline in the arterial oxygen partial pressure is typically seen. Lung x-rays show progressive fine granular changes.* Respiratory distress occurs, the patient becomes cyanotic and death ensues from respiratory failure. The pulmonary changes are due to a proliferative alveolitis, in which the alveolar walls become thickened and alveolar spaces congested by invading neutrophils, lymphocytes, macrophages, fibroblasts and an increased cellularity of the alveolar wall itself. In fatal cases, formation of hyaline membrane, loss of pulmonary surfactant and fibrosis have also been noted. Fatal aplastic anemia has been documented.

Dermal exposure to the concentrate may result in severe skin irritation. Dilute spray solutions may produce slight to moderate irritation if left in prolonged contact. Dermal absorption is apparently slight and no confirmed cases of systemic poisoning in man have been reported from dermal exposure to

*At present paraquat-induced lung damage for users of mexican marihuana has not been reported in humans.

either concentrate or dilute spray. Fingernails or toenails which have been exposed to the concentrate crack and shed, followed by normal regrowth. Nail contact with dilute spray solution may lead to the formation of white spots which gradually grow out.

Paraquat has an extremely low vapor pressure and thus, there is no vapor hazard. No cases of acute systemic poisoning in man have been reported as a result of inhaling paraquat spray. Agricultural spray droplets are usually too large to reach the alveoli. However, those droplets that are inhaled are deposited in the upper respiratory tract and may cause nosebleed, sorethroat, headache and coughing if exposure is excessive. These effects are due to the local irritant action of paraquat and reverse if the exposure is discontinued. A mask capable of filtering particles is effective in screening paraquat mist and should be used when exposure to spray mist can occur.

Liquid concentrate in the eyes may cause severe inflammation which develops gradually, reaching its maximum after twelve to twenty-four hours. There may be extensive stripping of superficial areas of corneal and conjunctival epithelium. Although healing may be slow, the injury is superficial and, even in severe cases, recovery is usually complete, given proper medical care. All cases of eye injury should be seen by a specialist as soon as possible.

*Treatment.* Induce vomiting with syrup of ipecac or perform gastric lavage if vomiting has not occurred. If lavage is performed, care must be taken as paraquat may be corrosive to the esophagus.

Immediately following vomiting or lavage, give approximately 200 to 500 ml of a 30% aqueous suspension of an adsorbent clay (such as Robinson's Bentonite® U.S.P. or Robinson's Fuller's Earth® U.S.P.) plus an effective dose of cathartic, e.g. magnesium sulfate, to remove paraquat from the *entire* GI tract. Repeat as often as practical (every two to four hours for several days until paraquat can no longer be detected in blood, urine or dialysate). If bentonite or fuller's earth is not immediately available, an adsorbent such as powdered activated charcoal should be used until better clays are obtained. Oxygen should be used sparingly and cautiously for dyspnea or cyanosis since it may aggravate the lung lesions. Forced diuresis should be started as soon as possible to remove paraquat from the blood. If renal function is impaired, hemodialysis or peritoneal dialysis may be of value. Use of both forced diuresis and hemodialysis together may aid in hastening the removal of paraquat. Monitor the patient's BUN and serum creatinine levels since these are early indicators of systemic poisoning and are useful to determine the patient's progress. Also, obtain daily chest x-rays, arterial oxygen partial pressure, pulmonary function studies and chest auscultation. Obtain urine, blood and dialysate samples initially and at least daily to monitor the elimination of paraquat.

For skin contamination, clothing should be removed and the skin thoroughly washed with soap and water for several minutes. If the eyes are involved, they should be irrigated immediately for ten to fifteen minutes and then seen by an ophthalmologist.

## FUMIGANTS AND REPELLENTS

1. Cyanides
2. Carbon tetrachloride
3. Naphthalene
4. Paradichlorobenzene
5. Methyl bromide, chloride, and iodide
6. Dimethylphthalate
7. Indalone
8. Diethyltoluamide

These agents include a wide variety of chemical compounds, many of which are highly toxic when ingested or inhaled. The least dangerous ones are those repellents intended for local application to the skin, including dimethylphthalate, indalone, etc. The most toxic types are the soil fumigants such as the cyanides and the halogenated

TABLE 57
RELATIVE TOXICITY OF HERBICIDES TO MAMMALS*

| *Common Name or Designation* | *Trade Name*† | *$LD_{50}$ mg/kg* | *Toxicity‡ Rating* | *Dermal Response Rating§* |
|---|---|---|---|---|
| Sodium arsenite | Atlas A, Triox | 10 | 5 | 1-2 |
| Methyl bromide | Various brands | 17 ppm (air) | 5 | 2 |
| DNBP | Sinox, Dow General | 30 | 5 | 1 |
| Endothal | Endothal, Aquathol | 35 | 5 | 3 |
| Calcium arsenate | Various brands | 35 | 5 | 4 |
| PMA | PMAS, Tat-C-Lect | 40 | 5 | 2 |
| DNBP (amine) | Premerge, Sinox PE | 40 | 5 | 1 |
| Acrolein | Aqualin | 46 | 5 | 2 |
| Kerosene | Various brands | — | 4 | — |
| KOCN | Various brands | 85 | 4 | — |
| Paraquat | Paraquat | 157 | 4 | — |
| Gasoline | Various brands | — | 4 | — |
| Aromatic solvents | Various brands | — | 4 | — |
| PCP (Na salt) | Weedbeads | 210 | 4 | 1 |
| SMDC | Vapam | 285 | 4 | 3 |
| 2, 4, 5-T | Various brands | 300 | 4 | 4 |
| Copper sulfate | Various brands | 300 | 4 | — |
| ——— | Ortho C-56 | 300 | 4 | 1-2 |
| Diallate | Avadex | 395 | 4 | — |
| Diquat | Diquat | 400 | 4 | — |
| CMA | Super-Dal-E-Rad | 440 | 4 | — |
| Silvex | Kuron, Weedone-TP | 500 | 4 | 4 |
| 2, 4-DB | Butyrac, Butoxone | 500 | 4 | — |
| 2, 4-D | Various brands | 500 | 4 | 4 |
| DMTT | Mylone | 500 | 4 | 4 |
| Petroleum solvents | Various brands | — | 4 | 1 |
| Bandane | Bandane | 540 | 3 | — |
| Swep | Swep | 552 | 3 | — |
| DSMA | Sodar, Ansar, Methar | 600 | 3 | 5 |
| MCPP | Mecoprop, Mecopex | 650 | 3 | — |
| PBA | Benzac, Zobar | 700 | 3 | — |
| CDAA | Randox | 700 | 3 | 2 |
| MCPA | Various brands | 700 | 3 | 4 |
| MSMA | Weed-E-Rad, Ansar | 700 | 3 | — |
| MAMA | Ansar, Methar | 720 | 3 | — |
| Aspirin | (For comparison) | 750 | 3 | — |
| Bensulide | Betasan, Presan | 770 | 3 | — |
| 2, 4-DEP | Falone | 850 | 4 | — |
| CDEC | Vegadex | 850 | 4 | 3 |
| Cypromid | Clobber | 900 | 4 | — |

* Laboratory animals (adult white rat usually).
†All products listed below are registered trademarks.
‡Numerical toxicity rating is based on a modification of the classification of pesticides in the Federal Insecticide, Fungicide, and Rodenticide Act and from *Clinical Toxicology of Commercial Products* by Gleason, M.N., Gosselin, R.E., and Hodge, H.D. Williams and Wilkins Co., Baltimore, Md., 1976.

| *Toxicity Rating* | *Class* | *$LD_{50}$ (mg/kg)* | *Probable Lethal Dose for 150 lb. man* |
|---|---|---|---|
| 1 | Extremely toxic | Less than 5 | A taste (less than 7 drops) |
| 2 | Very toxic | 5 to 49 | 7 drops to 1 teaspoonful |
| 3 | Moderately toxic | 50 to 499 | 1 teaspoonful to 1 ounce |
| 4 | Slightly toxic | 500 to 4999 | 1 ounce to 1 pint (1 pound) |
| 5 | Almost nontoxic | 5000 to 14,999 | 1 pint to 1 quart |
| 6 | Nontoxic | 15,000 and above | More than 1 quart |

§Numerical rating is based on the following classification:
1. Absorbed and poisonous
2. Causes burns and blisters
3. Moderately irritating
4. Mildly irritating
5. Nonirritating

TABLE 57—*Continued*
RELATIVE TOXICITY OF HERBICIDES TO MAMMALS

| *Common Name or Designation* | *Trade Name* | *$LD_{50}$ mg/kg* | *Toxicity Rating* | *Dermal Response Rating* |
|---|---|---|---|---|
| Diphenamid | Dymid, Enide | 960 | 4 | — |
| Cacodylic acid | Ansar 560, 120 | 1000 | 4 | — |
| ——————— | Patoran | 1000 | 4 | — |
| Sesone | Sesone | 1000 | 4 | — |
| Erbon | Baron, Novon | 1000 | 4 | 3 |
| DMPA | Zytron | 1000 | 4 | — |
| Dicamba | Banvel D | 1040 | 4 | — |
| Pebulate | Tillam | 1120 | 4 | — |
| HCA | HCA Weed Killer | 1290 | 4 | — |
| Barban | Carbyne | 1350 | 4 | — |
| Dichlone | Phygon | 1380 | 4 | 3 |
| Propanil | Stam F-34, Rogue | 1384 | 4 | — |
| Calcium cyanamide | Aero-Cyanamide | 1400 | 4 | — |
| Linuron | Lorox | 1500 | 4 | — |
| AMS | Ammate | 1600 | 4 | 5 |
| EPTC | Eptam | 1630 | 4 | — |
| 2, 3, 6—TBA | Tryben, Benzac | 1644 | 4 | 5 |
| NPA | Alanap (Na salt) | 1770 | 4 | — |
| Vernolate | Vernam | 1780 | 4 | — |
| Monuron—TCA | Urox | 2300 | 4 | — |
| MH (amine) | MH-30 | 2340 | 4 | — |
| Norea | Herban | 2500 | 4 | — |
| Borate | Borax, Borassu | 2500 | 4 | 4 |
| Dichlobenil | Casoron | 2710 | 4 | — |
| Prometone | Prometone | 2980 | 4 | — |
| Fenac | Fenac | 3000 | 4 | — |
| DCPA | Dacthal | 3000 | 4 | 5 |
| IPC | Propham | 3000 | 4 | — |
| Atrazine | Atrazine | 3080 | 4 | 5 |
| DCMA | Dicryl | 3160 | 4 | — |
| ISOCIL | Hyvar | 3250 | 4 | — |
| Table salt | (for comparison) | 3320 | 4 | — |
| TCA | Various brands | 3370 | 4 | 2 |
| Diuron | Karmex | 3400 | 4 | 4 |
| Amiben | Amiben, Vegiben | 3500 | 4 | — |
| Monuron | Telvar | 3500 | 4 | 4 |
| Pyrazon | Pyramin | 3600 | 4 | — |
| Trifluralin | Treflan | 3700 | 4 | — |
| Chloroxuron | Tenoran | 3700 | 4 | — |
| Prometryne | Caparol | 3750 | 4 | — |
| Fenuron—TCA | Urab | 4000 | 4 | — |
| Amitrole-T | Amitrol-T, Cytrol | 5000 | 4-5 | — |
| CIPC | Chloro-IPC | 5000 | 5 | — |
| Siduron | Tupersan | 5000 | 5 | — |
| Simazine | Simazine | 5000 | 4 | 5 |
| Propazine | Propazine | 5000 | 4 | — |
| Bromacil | Hyvar X | 5200 | 5 | — |
| Fenuron | Dybar | 6400 | 5 | 4 |
| DCU | Crag | 6680 | 5 | — |
| Picloram | Tordon | 8200 | 5 | — |
| ——————— | Cotoran | 8900 | 5 | — |
| Dalapon | Dowpon | 9300 | 4 | 4 |
| Benefin | Balan | 10,000 | 4 | — |
| Solan | Solan | 10,000 | 5 | — |
| Sodium chlorate | Atlacide | 12,000 | 5 | 4 |
| Amitrole | Amino Triazole, Weedazol | 15,000 | 6 | 4 |
| ——————— | Azak | 34,600 | 6 | — |

hydrocarbons. Naphthalene and paradichlorobenzene are important because of their wide use in the home as a moth repellent.

### *Carbon Tetrachloride*

Carbon tetrachloride is a volatile colorless fluid with an odor similar to chloroform, to which it is chemically closely related. It decomposes to phosgene on heating. It is mainly used as a nonflammable solvent and cleaner in factories, garages, household floor waxes and cleaners. Carbon tetrachloride is still an important ingredient in fire extinguisher fluids and insecticide spray, but its use as an anthelmintic has been almost universally discarded. Over half the carbon tetrachloride produced in the United States is used in the manufacture of other chemicals such as the Freon™ propellants and refrigerants.

IDENTIFICATION OF CARBON TETRACHLORIDE.

1. Odor of carbon tetrachloride on the breath or in the vomitus.
2. Positive Fehling's test for sugar in the urine.
3. Isonitrile test: Place a small amount of suspected liquid in 10 ml of distillate. Then add 1 ml of purified aniline and 2 ml of 20% sodium hydroxide and gently heat this mixture for several minutes. A positive result produces a foul (skunk) odor of phenylisonitrile. Other chlorinated hydrocarbons such as chloroform, trichloroethylene and chloral hydrate also give a positive reaction.
4. Pyridine test: To 1 ml of suspected fluid or 10 ml of distillate add 5 ml of sodium hydroxide and 5 ml of purified pyridine. Gently heat for five to ten minutes on a steam bath. A pink-red color may indicate carbon tetrachloride. Chloral hydrate, chloroform or other chlorinated hydrocarbons also give similar reactions. If distillate or solution is very dilute, first concentrate it by extraction with n-heptane and then do test on this.
5. Microdiffusion test may be employed directly on biologic specimen.
   a. Reflux two hours with sodium hydroxide and titrate for organic-bound chlorides.
   b. Beilstein test: Burns with a green flame with CuO heated on a copper wire. (All chlorinated hydrocarbons yield green flame.)
6. Quantitative analysis of blood or expired breath or both can be determined rapidly by a simple infrared method (*J Occup Med, 3:* 586 to 590, 1961; and *J Lab Clin Med. 56:* 148 to 156, 1960). When the concentration of carbon tetrachloride in the blood drops below the level of detection by infrared spectroscopy, the compound is still readily detectable in the exhaled breath several weeks after a significant exposure. Breath analyses, therefore, not only afford the physician a rapid, specific means of establishing the diagnosis, but also indicate the magnitude of the hazard.

Intoxication follows inhalation, ingestion or absorption of the substance through the skin, and as little as one teaspoonful has been known to cause death. Alcohol taken in the course of exposure, or shortly after, greatly potentiates the toxic effects, and an otherwise minimal exposure can produce severe poisoning. The presence of fat in the small intestine also seems to favor more severe intoxication. The greatest number of acute poisonings follow its use in a poorly ventilated room and are due to inhalation. The MAC in air is 25 ppm or the equivalent of 250 ml (½ pt.) evaporated in a room size 50 x 50 x 15 ft. In mild reactions, no more than intestinal cramps and diarrhea may develop some time after exposure; the pain may be severe, however, and mimic an acute abdomen. The immediate results of more severe intoxication are drowsiness and sluggishness. Nausea, vertigo, vomiting, headache and malaise accompany the drowsy state. If alcohol has been ingested at the same time or shortly after exposure, unconsciousness can quickly follow. Frank respiratory failure and ventricular arrhythmia may occur. Stimulants such as epinephrine or ephedrine therefore should not be used as they may induce ventricular fibrillation.

If a patient is seen shortly after inhaling the agent, he should be removed to fresh air and, if indicated, given artificial respiration. If the solvent was swallowed, immediate gastric lavage should be performed with tap water and magnesium sulfate given orally. Liquid with a high fat content, such as milk, is definitely contraindicated.

Renal (acute tubular necrosis) and hepatic failure are the complications to be feared. If mild, no more than oliguria lasting a few days may follow. In more severe involvement, complete anuria may set in following a few days or a week or more of oliguria with red cells and albumin present in the scanty urine. Hypertension, acidosis and terminal uremia develop if kidney function is not restored. A toxic hepatitis may exist, producing only a subclinical jaundice, or severe hepatic necrosis may result in progressive jaundice leading to hepatic coma. Edema of the brain with small confluent hemorrhages with a predilection for the pons and cerebellum has been reported.

Mortality in this condition has, in the past, reached as high as 90 per cent in severe intoxication, but there is no doubt that with early recognition and careful treatment many patients will survive, providing that hepatorenal necrosis is not so severe as to preclude recovery.

*Treatment* is primarily supportive and is directed to tiding the patient over the period of oliguria or anuria. Recent investigation has suggested that mannitol infusion, begun within twelve to twenty-four hours of the renal insult, may prevent progression of functional to organic renal failure. For an adult, 50 gm are given intravenously as a loading dose over a six-hour period. Thereafter, 25 gm should be administered every six hours for five days or until the carbon tetrachloride in the expired air is lowered to a low concentration or refractory oliguria has developed. Forcing fluids to stimulate kidney recovery is dangerous and may have been a cause of death. Since death has frequently been due to pulmonary edema or hyperkalemia, careful attention must be given to maintenance of fluid and electrolyte balance. During the period of anuria, fluids should be limited to about 800 ml/day plus the estimated loss by perspiration, diarrhea, vomitus, etc. This is best given as 10% glucose, which also serves to spare body proteins and lessen the possibility of high serum levels of potassium. Hyperkalemia can be promptly but temporarily reduced by administering intravenously hypertonic glucose with insulin, or with molar sodium lactate which is the treatment of choice; intravenous calcium gluconate alleviates the effects of elevated serum potassium. In exceptional cases artificial dialysis is necessary. Sulfhydryl compounds have been reported as being beneficial. Methionine and cysteine can be given in a dosage of 10 to 15 gm/day. Recently the experimental administration of nicotinic acid or tryptophan to animals has protected against lethal doses of carbon tetrachloride.

Profound diuresis frequently accompanies renal recovery; significant losses of sodium, potassium and chloride may occur, requiring careful replacement as indicated. Treatment of the liver damage is similar to that of acute hepatitis and is primarily supportive. A high-carbohydrate diet is beneficial.

Prophylaxis is of the utmost importance and is the only certain way to eliminate poisoning. Substitutes that are less toxic are available for all the possible uses of "carbon tet." Methyl chloroform is a solvent compound nearly as efficient as carbon tetrachloride and is considerably safer to use. MAC is 250 ppm. It is nonflammable, has a pleasant odor, is relatively noninjurious to kidney and liver and is considered only slightly toxic under normal circumstances. Perchloroethylene and trichloroethylene are other safer solvents. If the use of carbon tetrachloride is unavoidable, adequate ventilation to permit rapid removal of vapors and abstinence from alcohol are mandatory. Other halogenated hydrocarbons (allyl bromide and chloride, ethyl bromide and chloride, etc.) are treated in a similar fashion.

*Naphthalene*

Naphthalene, a constituent of coal tar, is a white scaly powder that volatilizes easily at ordinary temperature. It is used as a moth repellent in the form of mothballs, moth flakes, deodorant cakes, etc. However, it has been used in the past as an antiseptic and anthelmintic. It plays an important role in the chemical industry as a synthetic intermediate.

The toxicity of naphthalene is not generally appreciated, so it is often left around for infants and children to ingest in the belief that it is candy. The result can be a severe and rapidly progressive hemolytic anemia. The lethal dose of ingested naphthalene is approximately 2 gm. Only recently has the hazard of naphthalene poisoning from transcutaneous absorption and from inhalation of its vapors been emphasized. It is not generally known to parents and homemakers that naphthalene is not appreciably soluble in water and may remain in a garment or blanket in spite of thorough washing. The fact that the chemical is very soluble in oil makes the storing of baby clothes in naphthalene balls or crystals especially dangerous, because the baby oil commonly rubbed on the skin of infants acts as a solvent for the toxic substance which can then be adsorbed through the child's skin.

In twenty-one newborns, a rather severe form of hemolytic anemia, associated with jaundice and kernicterus and produced from the inhalation of naphthalene used in blankets and woolen clothing stored for the summer, was reported from Greece. The potential dangers to the neonate from the use of clothing stored with mothballs, particularly in the black and ethnic groups most likely to have glucose-6-phosphate dehydrogenase (G-6-PD) enzymic deficiency, should be well documented and eliminated. The toxic agent responsible for hemolysis is not naphthalene but its metabolic products α– and β-naphthol and naphthoquinone. These substances require conjugation with glucuronic acid for their excretion. It is reasonable, therefore, to assume that newborn infants, because of their limited conjugating capacity, are more susceptible to the toxic action of these compounds.

Naphthalene itself is not hemolytic, either when injected directly into the bloodstream or when added to a suspension of erythocytes. Hemolysis is due to primaquine-like sensitivity reaction, which has been shown to occur in those individuals who have a hereditary genetically induced deficiency (Mendelian recessive) of glucose-6-phosphate dehydrogenase. In addition to naphthalene, sulfonamides, acetophenetidin, synthetic water-soluble vitamin K compounds, as well as other drugs and the fava bean, produce hemolytic anemia in subjects who have this enzyme deficiency. The defect can be identified by various tests of the blood as described in the detailed discussion of G-6-PD enzymic deficiency (*see* pages 336 through 344).

Hemolysis does not occur until three to seven days after ingestion. The symptomatology is that associated with any acute and rapid destruction of red blood cells. Premonitory symptoms include fever, pallor, lethargy, abdominal pain, diarrhea, anorexia, vomiting and headache. Jaundice is absent or slight, the liver is moderately enlarged and the spleen generally is not palpable.

The urine is dark or port wine in color and, as a rule, free of red blood cells; albumin and casts are usually present. Early in the course of the illness, the urine contains an odor of moth balls and gives a positive reaction for hemoglobin.

Anemia is usually profound. An examination of the blood smear shows anisocytosis, microspherocytosis, polychromatophilia and fragmentation of erythrocytes with the appearance of irregular, jagged borders to the red cells. The hemoglobin is concentrated to one side of the red cell. Heinz bodies can be demonstrated in the red cells at an early stage. (These are minute, peripheral particles that stain with cresyl blue and are numerous just before the hemoglobin falls in hemolytic anemia due to chemical poisoning. Presumably they consist of denatured proteins and lipoproteins produced by irreversible injury of red blood cells.) Hemoglobinemia and hemoglobinuria are present in most cases, but there is no rise in methemoglobin or sulfhemoglobin. Tests for isohemagglutinins, autohemagglutinins, cold agglutinins and cold and warm hemolysins are negative. The fragility of the erythrocytes to hypotonic saline is increased.

*Treatment.* If ingested, remove immediately with gastric lavage or emesis. Follow by saline cathartic. Avoid alcohol, milk, oil or fatty meal. Force fluids to stimulate diuresis, sodium bicarbonate, 5 gm (less for children), are given orally every four hours as necessary to maintain an alkaline urine to prevent the precipitation of acid hematin crystals and subsequent blocking of the renal tubules. Give repeated small blood transfusions if indicated until hemoglobin is 60 to 80 per cent of normal. Cortisone therapy may be beneficial in reducing the hemolytic process.

In prevention, naphthalene products should be kept out of the hands and clothes (infants' diapers) of children.

### *Paradichlorobenzene (Dichlorocide)*

This common mothproofing compound is less dangerous than naphthalene. There is no definite information as to the toxic dose (ingestion of 20 gm has been tolerated by man). The para compound is a white solid, while orthodichlorobenzene is a liquid. Besides its extensive use for household moth control, it is also employed for control of termites, powerpost borers and as a toilet bowl cake deodorant. Naphthalene is usually the main ingredient in "balls" and "flakes," while paradichlorobenzene is usually the main ingredient in "crystals," "nuggets" and "cakes." However, this may not always be the case, and obviously an attempt should always be made to verify the ingredients. One way to accomplish this is to keep reference samples of each in the emergency room and compare the odor of the unknown moth repellent with these samples. Other helpful clues are surface appearance and solubility. Naphthalene products look dry and are slowly soluble in unheated ethanol. Paradichlorobenzene products look wet and oily and are rapidly soluble in unheated ethanol.

When ingested, it may cause nausea, vomiting, diarrhea, abdominal pain and liver or kidney damage. The vapors and sprays are irritating to the eyes, nose and throat, but the effects seem to quickly disappear. Methemoglobinemia may occur and allergic purpura has been reported.

*Treatment.* General measures for removing the substance from the stomach, followed by symptomatic treatment are required (*See* Naphthalene).

### *Methyl Bromide, Chloride and Iodide*

These volatile liquid compounds are all gaseous at ordinary temperatures and are used as refrigerants, in synthesis and as fumigants in disinfestation of fruits and stored grain. In addition, methyl bromide is used with carbon tetrachloride in fire extinguishers and as a total herbage destroying agent for golf and bowling greens. During the years 1957 through 1964, a total of 166 cases with 5 deaths occurred in California from occupational exposures. These compounds are depressants of the chloroform type and therefore are dangerous, not only because of the CNS depression but also because of possible myocardial involvement and liver and kidney damage. Methyl chloride does not remain inert in the body but is changed to methyl alcohol and sodium chloride. A similar change occurs with methyl bromide and iodide, except that the corresponding halogen salts are formed. The methyl alcohol is incompletely changed to formic acid, which is very toxic. Formates are invariably found in the urine. The principal manifestations in acute poisoning depend on the amount ingested or the concentration inhaled or absorbed. If the amount is large or the concentration high, nausea, vomiting, vertigo, weakness, drowsiness, hypotension, coma, convulsions and pulmonary edema may occur after a latent period of one to four hours.

After exposure to lower concentrations, symptoms are less severe and may be delayed twelve to twenty-four hours. Skin contact causes erythema and vesiculation. In chronic poisoning from constant skin absorption or from inhalation of concentrations slightly higher than the MAC, visual disturbances, muscular weakness, confusion, hallucinations, somnolence and bronchospasm are common symptoms. The MAC is 20 ppm for methyl bromide and 100 ppm for methyl chloride and iodide. Since these agents are practically odorless and tasteless, it is not apparent to the user when a toxic atmosphere is encountered. It is essential therefore that respiratory as well as dermal protection be taken at all times.

Laboratory tests are not too useful for detecting a case of sublethal systemic intoxication. The white blood cell count is usually moderately elevated, while albumin, casts and red blood cells may appear in the urine. Blood glucose, urea and bilirubin levels are unchanged, but the blood bromide level likely stays above normal for a long period of time. Traces of methyl alcohol may be evident in the blood or urine.

*Treatment.* If ingestion has occurred, the stomach should be emptied immediately by gastric lavage or emesis. Otherwise acute poisoning is treated by removal from the source of exposure, using artificial respiration and oxygen if necessary, and treating convulsions or shock if they occur. Quickly remove any contaminated clothing (methyl bromide is capable of penetrating ordinary rubber gloves) and wash skin thoroughly with water. Any severe acidosis must be treated cautiously with alkali. It is essential that the patient be kept under observation for twenty-four to forty-eight hours as symptoms may not appear initially. BAL therapy might be considered at this time since it has been found effective experimentally. Hemodialysis hastens the removal of methyl alcohol and its metabolite, formic acid, and may be indicated in serious intoxication when these syntheses occur with methyl chloride.

### *Dimethylphthalate and Indalone®*

These insect repellents are intended for application to human skin and are the least dangerous of the compounds used for this purpose. Accidental ingestion in one reported case, however, resulted in an immediate burning sensation of the lips, tongue and mouth, followed two hours later by a deep coma. The patient improved rapidly after gastric lavage and intravenous dextrose solution.

### *Diethyltoluamide (Deet)*

For skin application, the better repellents of mosquitoes are deet, chlorodiethyl benzamide, ethyl hexanediol, dimethylphthalate, dimethyl carbamate and butopyronoxyl. Butyl ethyl propanediol, ethyl hexanediol and deet are effective repellents for treatment of clothing for protection against mosquitoes.

Several isomers of deet have been used in commercial insect repellent agents. The meta-form has been found to be most useful, and the acute oral $LD_{50}$ in rats is 2.0 gm/kg. The ortho-isomer is most toxic while the para-isomer is less so. Toxic manifestations in experimental animals include loss of righting reflexes, staggering, labored respiration, central nervous system depression, convulsions and coma. Undiluted material is a moderate to severe irritant to the eye. In man, dermal application of undiluted material and 50% solutions caused no primary irritation or skin sensitivity, but in rabbits erythema and desquamation occurred.

Ingestion of this product necessitates the use of an emetic or gastric lavage. The remainder of the *treatment* should be symptomatic and supportive.

TABLE 58
RODENTICIDES, HERBICIDES, FUNGICIDES

| *Trade Name** | *Harmful Ingredients* | *Treatment Reference Page Number* |
|---|---|---|
| Acme Garden Fungicide | Captan, Karathane | |
| Acme Weed Killer | Arsenic | |
| ACP Brush Killer | 2 4 5-T - 2 4 - D Acids | |
| ACP Grass Killer | Sodium Trichloroacetate | |
| Acteen Stops Weeds | Arsenic Trioxide | |
| Aerocyanate | Potassium Cyanate | |
| Agicide Crab Grass Killer | Potassium Cyanate | |
| Agicide Rat and Mouse Bait | Warfarin | |
| Agicide Weed Wilt | 2 4-D | |
| Agicide Yellow Dot Fungicide | Zinc Ethylene Bisdithio Carbamate | |
| Agro | Phenyl Mercury Urea | |
| Allen Tomato Dust | Copper | |
| Allen Weed (Potato Vine) Killer | Sodium Arsenite | |
| A-Mean | 2 4-D Amine Salts | |
| Ammate X Herbicide | Ammonium Sulfamate | |
| Anap | N-Naphthyl Phthalmic Acid | |
| Antirot | Pentachlorophenol | |
| Antrol | Arsenic | |
| Arab Rat & Mouse Killer | Arsenic | |
| Arasan | Tetramethylthiuram Disulfide, Thiram | |
| Arwell Rat & Mouse Bait | Pival | |
| Artox | Disodium Methyl Arsenate | |
| Atlacide Weed Killer | Sodium Chlorate | |
| Atlas A | Sodium Arsenite | |
| Avon Annalos Weed Killer | Petroleum Oil | |
| Banarat Bits | Warfarin | |
| Banarat Premix | Warfarin | |
| Basicop | Copper Sulfate, Tribasic | |
| Black Flag Rat & Mouse Killer | Warfarin | |
| Black Leaf Crabgrass Killer | Potassium Cyanate | |
| Black Leaf Mousekiller Bait | Warfarin | *See Index* |
| Black Leaf Ready Mixed Bait | Warfarin | |
| Black Leaf Weedkiller (Arsenical) | Arsenic Trioxide | |
| Black Panther Rat & Mouse Killer | Warfarin | |
| Blue Death Rat Killer | Phosphorus | |
| Bontu Prep. Rat Baits | ANTU | |
| Bontu Rat Powder | ANTU | |
| Bramblicide Brushkiller | 2 4 5-T Pentyl Esters | |
| Bramble Weedicide | 2 4 5-T Pentyl Esters | |
| Brayton's Raticide Cereal Bait | Warfarin | |
| Brown Rat Poison | Naphthylthiourea | |
| Brush-Bane | 2 4 5-T - 2 4-D | |
| Brush-Kil | 2 4 5-T - 2 4-D | |
| Brushoff | 2 4 5-T - 2 4-D | |
| Bruweed | 2 4 5-T - 2 4-D | |
| Bug-A-Boo Moth Crystals | Paradichlorobenzene | |
| Bug-Getta | Arsenic | |
| Caddy | Cadmium Chloride | |
| Calgreen | Copper Arsenite, Calcium Arsenate | |
| Calo-chlor | Mercuric Chloride, Mercurous Chloride | |
| Carac Lawn Weed Killer | 2 4-D | |
| Carac Crabgrass Killer | Phenyl Mercuric Acetate | |
| Ceresan | Ethyl Mercury Phosphate | |
| Ceresan-M | Ethyl Mercury P-Toluene Sulfonanilide | |
| Chem-Sect Brand Rat Powder | Red Squill | |
| Chemrat | Pival | |
| Chem San | Sodium Arsenite | |

*All products listed below are registered trademarks. Since trade names and formulations are frequently and unexpectedly changed, consult labels for difinitive contents as some products may be obsolete.

TABLE 58—*Continued*
RODENTICIDES, HERBICIDES, FUNGICIDES

| *Trade Name** | *Harmful Ingredients* | *Treatment Reference Page Number* |
|---|---|---|
| Chem-Weed P.I. & Brush Killer | 2 4 5-T - 2 4-D | |
| Cherry Coposil Fungicide | Copper | |
| Chipman Fungicide Dust | Copper Hydroxysulfate | |
| Chipman Grain Fumigant | Ethylene Dibromide | |
| Chipman Top Killer | Arsenic | |
| Chipman Toxaphene 8L | Toxaphene | |
| Chlorax-40 | Sodium Chlorate | |
| C-L-L Brush Killer | 2 4 5-T - 2 4-D | |
| Claire Insect Repellent | Ethylhexanediol | |
| Cleartox | Pentachlorophenol | |
| Click (Para) Crystals | Paradichlorobenzene | |
| College Brand Blight Dust | Copper | |
| College Brand Rodenticide | ANTU | |
| Common Sense Rat Preparation | Phosphorus | |
| Contax Weed Killer | Dinitro Phenol Derivatives | |
| Copper Hydro-Bordo | Copper Hydroxysulfate | |
| Copper-A Dust | Copper | |
| Copper-Cure | Copper Naphthenate | |
| Coppo-Clear | Zinc Naphthenate | |
| Coppo-Regular | Copper Naphthenate | |
| Cornell Penta-Gard | Pentachlorophenol | |
| Cornell WO 5 Rodenticide | Warfarin | |
| Crab-Erad Crabtex | Disodium Methyl Arsenate | |
| Crab Fruit Fungicide | Glyoxalidine Derivative | |
| Crab-Not Powder | Potassium Cyanate | |
| Crab-Not Special | Potassium Cyanate, 2 4-D | |
| Cross Country Crabgrass Killer | Potassium Cyanate | |
| Cupro-K | Copper Oxychloride | |
| Cyano Gas A Dust | Calcium Cyanide | |
| Cymag | Sodium Cyanide | *See Index* |
| D & P Double O Crab Grass Killer | Potassium Cyanate | |
| D & P Liquid Fungicide | Potassium Thiosulfate | |
| D & P Tomato Dust | Copper, Calcium Arsenate | |
| D & P Weedkiller | Sodium Arsenite | |
| Dowfume MC-2 | Methyl Bromide | |
| Dowfume V, C, F, G, H, J, 75, 80-20 | Carbon Tetrachloride, Carbon Bisulfide, Ethylene Dichloride | |
| Dow Brush Killer | 2 4-D, 2 4 5-T Butyl Esters | |
| Dow Seed Protectant | Zinc Trichlorophenate | |
| DuPont Liquid Fungicide | Zinc Ethylene Bisdithio Carbamate | |
| DuPont Lawn Weeder | 2 4-D | |
| DuPont Liquid 241 | Phenyl Mercuric and Ethyl Mercuric Acetates | |
| Dust-A-Way Crab Grass Dust | Potassium Cyanate | |
| Eastern States Duocide Mixed Bait | Pival | |
| Easy Monday Mothproofer | DDT | |
| E-D Bee | Ethylene Dibromide | |
| Electric Paste | Phosphorus, Arsenic | |
| El Rey Mouse Bait | Strychnine | |
| End-O-Pest Crabgrass Killer | Potassium Cyanate | |
| End-O-Weed Weed Killer | 2 4-D Esters | |
| Erco Brush Kill | 2 4-D, 2 4 5-T | |
| Ercocide | Sodium Chlorate | |
| Esso Weed Killers | Petroleum Oil | |
| Estercide Weed Killers | 2 4-D, 2 4 5-T Esters | |
| Esteron Weed & Brush Killers | 2 4-D, 2 4 5-T Esters | |
| Expello Moth Baglets | Paradichlorobenzene | |
| Expello Moth Proofer & Wool Wash | Dichlorobenzyl Triphenyl Phosphonium Cl | |
| Expello Moth Vapors | Paradichlorobenzene | |
| Ex-L Pellets | Paradichlorobenzene | |

TABLE 58—*Continued*
RODENTICIDES, HERBICIDES, FUNGICIDES

| *Trade Name** | *Harmful Ingredients* | *Treatment Reference Page Number* |
|---|---|---|
| F & B Weed Killer | Sodium Arsenite | *See Index* |
| Farmrite Crab Grass Killer | Phenyl Mercury Triethanol-Ammonium Lactate | |
| Farmrite 21-10 Dust | Zineb | |
| Farmrite Tomato Blight Dust | Basic Copper Sulfate | |
| Fasco Cuminoil Emulsion | Copper, Petroleum Oil | |
| Fasco Fume | Ethylene Dibromide | |
| Fasco Peach Dust | Lead Arsenate, Sulfur | |
| Fasco Wy-Hoe | Isopropyl-N-Carbamate | |
| Fatal Prepared Rat & Mouse Bait | Warfarin | |
| Ferradow | Ferbam | |
| Field Rat Powder | Zinc Phosphide | |
| Flight Brand Melon Dust | Zineb | |
| Flit Moth Proofer | Chlorinated Terpenes | |
| Floratox Herbicide | Pentachlorophenol | |
| Floratox Weed Killer | 2 4-D Amine Salt | |
| Four X-D | 2 4-D | |
| Fulex Blue Label | Aramite | |
| Fulex Green Label | Lindane | |
| Fulex Red Label | Parathion | |
| Fumo-Gas | Ethylene Dibromide | |
| Fung Chex | Mercuric and Mercurous Chloride | |
| Fungtrogen | Copper | |
| Galltox | Phenyl Mercuric Ammonium Acetate | |
| G & O Moth Deodorant Nuggets | Paradichlorobenzene | |
| Geller's Moth Proofer | DDT, Petroleum Distillates | |
| Geigy Lo-V Brush Killer | 2 4 5-T Esters | |
| Geigy Potato Vine & Weed Killer | Sodium Arsenite | |
| Geigy Rat & Mouse Bait | Warfarin | |
| Go-Crab | Potassium Cyanate | |
| Golf Brand Weed Killer | Phenyl Mercuric Acetate | |
| Golf Crabgrass Preventer | Calcium Propyl Arsonate | |
| Gopher Death | Strychnine | |
| Gopher Go | Strychnine | |
| Grainfume | Carbon Tetrachloride, Carbon Disulfide | |
| Green Cross Basi-Cop | Basic Copper Sulfate | |
| Green Cross Brushkil 64 | 2 4 5-T, 2 4-D Esters | |
| Green Cross Couchgrass Killer | Sodium Trichloroacetate | |
| Green Cross Crabgrass Killer | Potassium Cyanate | |
| Green Cross Fruit Fungicide | Glyoxalidine Derivative | |
| Green Cross Karbam Black Fungicide | Ferbam | |
| Green Cross Potato Top Killer | Arsenic Trioxide | |
| Green Cross Rat & Mouse Bait | Pival | |
| Green Cross San Seed Disinfectant | Phenyl Mercuric Acetate | |
| Green Cross Tantoo | Dimethyl Phthalate | |
| Green Cross Tantoo Bomb | Ethylhexanediol | |
| Green Cross Weed-No-More Dust | 2 4-D | |
| G. T. A. Bait for Rats, Mice | Thallium Sulfate | |
| Gy-Cop | Basic Copper Sulfate | |
| Hammond Do-Di Lawn Weed Killer | 2 4-D | |
| Hammond Tomato Dust | Basic Copper Sulfate | |
| Hammond Weed Killer | Phenyl Mercuric Acetate | |
| Hess, (Dr.) Anturat | ANTU | |
| Hess, (Dr.) Rat & Mouse Killer | Pival | |
| Hess, (Dr.) Warfarat | Warfarin | |
| Hot Spring Buttons | Strychnine | |
| Howard Rat Kill Cone | Warfarin | |
| Howard Ready-To-Use Rat Kill | Warfarin | |
| Howard Warficide Rat Kill | Warfarin | |
| Hubbard Blight Control Dust | Copper | |
| Hydromix Crabgrass Killer | Disodium Methyl Arsenate | |

TABLE 58—*Continued*
RODENTICIDES, HERBICIDES, FUNGICIDES

| *Trade Name** | *Harmful Ingredients* | *Treatment Reference Page Number* |
|---|---|---|
| Hydromix Crabgrass & Weed Preventer | 2 4-D Salt | |
| Ideal Brand Perk | Sulfur, Copper, Zinc | |
| Infuco 80-20 Fumigant | Carbon Tetrachloride, Carbon Bisulfide | |
| J-O Paste | Phosphorus | |
| Karmex Herbicide DL | Dichlorophenyl Dimethylurea | |
| Karmex Herbicide W | Chlorophenyl Dimethylurea | |
| Kayo Killer | Copper, Calcium Arsenate | |
| Kelly's Red-Mix Rat & Mouse Killer | Warfarin | |
| Kilbrush Brush Killer (Bonide) | 2 4-D, Triethanolamide | |
| Killer Blightex | Tribasic Copper Sulfate | |
| Kilmice | Strychnine Sulfate | |
| Killer Kane Kartridges | 2 4-D | |
| Killer Katz | Warfarin | |
| Kill Wood Dust | 2 4-D Esters | |
| Kil-Mor Moth Proofer | Terpene Polychlorinates | |
| Kilz-Moths | Paradichlorobenzene | |
| Kling-Tite Dry | Alpha Naphthalene Acetic Acid | |
| Klinzmoth Flakes | Naphthalene & Paradichlorobenzene | |
| Koneprox | Copper Oxychloride | |
| Konex | Pentachlorophenol | |
| Kopper Moth Balls | Naphthalene | |
| Knoxweed Contact Weed Killer | Dinitro Butyl Phenol | |
| Krab Crabgrass Killer (Bonide) | Potassium Cyanate | |
| K-R-O Powder | Red Squill | |
| K-R-O Rat & Mouse Killer | Warfarin | |
| K-R-O Ready Mixed Bis-Kit | Red Squill | |
| Kuron | 2 4 5-T | |
| Larvatox | Zinc Fluosilicate | |
| Larvex | Sodium Aluminum Silicofluorate | *See Index* |
| Lebanon Arisod Grass & Weed Killer | Sodium Arsenite | |
| Lebanon Bait Kills Rats and Mice | Warfarin | |
| Lebanon Brush Killer | 2 4 5-T, 2 4-D | |
| Lebanon Crab Grass Killer | Potassium Cyanate | |
| Lebanon Parafume Moth Crystals | Paradichlorobenzene | |
| Lebanon Tomato Blight Dust | Basic Copper Sulfate | |
| Lignasan | Ethyl Mercury Phosphate | |
| Lovester | 2 4 5-T | |
| Lo-Voi Brush Killer | 2 4-D, 2 4 5-T | |
| Low-Dee | 2 4-D | |
| Lumber Last | Pentachlorophenol | |
| Magclor Defoliant | Magnesium Chlorate | |
| Magitrack Mouse Duster | DDT | |
| Martin's Mar-Fin Ready Bait | Warfarin | |
| Martin's Mar Penta | Pentachlorophenol | |
| Martin's Rat Stop Liquid | Thallium Sulfate | |
| Martin's Wonderiex | Phenol, Oil | |
| Melsan | Ethyl Mercury Phosphate | |
| Mema | Methoxy Ethyl Mercuric Acetate | |
| Mergamma | Phenyl Mercury Urea | |
| Mersolite-8 | Phenyl Mercuric Acetate | |
| Methate | Disodium Methyl Arsenate | |
| Methar | Disodium Methyl Arsenate | |
| Mice & Rat Doom | Warfarin | |
| Mice Doom Pellets | Strychnine | |
| M.G.K. Repellant 11 | 2-Butylene, Tetrahydrofurfural | |
| MH-30 | Maleic Hydrazide | |
| Micro-Bu Cop | Copper | |
| Micro Penta | Pentachlorophenol | |
| Miller's Bordo | Copper | |
| Miller's Microcop | Tribasic Copper Sulfate | |

TABLE 58—*Continued*
RODENTICIDES, HERBICIDES, FUNGICIDES

| *Trade Name** | *Harmful Ingredients* | *Treatment Reference Page Number* |
|---|---|---|
| Miller's Postreat | Mercury Bichloride | |
| Millfume | Carbon Tetrachloride | |
| Mission Brand Gam-O-Sam | Lindane, Mercury | |
| Mission Brand Weedkiller | Potassium Cyanate | |
| Mo-Go | Strychnine Sulfate | |
| Mole Nots | Strychnine Sulfate | |
| Mologen | Strychnine Sulfate | |
| Monsanto Santochlor | Paradichlorobenzene | |
| Moth Chaser | Naphthalene | |
| Moth-Ray | Paradichlorobenzene | |
| Moth-Tox | Paradichlorobenzene | |
| Mouse Lure | Strychnine | |
| Mouse Nots | Strychnine Sulfate | |
| Mouse Seed | Strychnine | |
| Myerkill | Warfarin | |
| Neutro Cop | Copper | |
| Niagara Brush Killer | 2 4-D, 2 4 5-T | |
| Niagara Copodust | Copper Oxychloride Sulfate | |
| Niagara Copotex | Calcium Arsenate | |
| No-Bunt | Ferbam | |
| Nodar | Paradichlorobenzene | |
| No Moth | Paradichlorobenzene | |
| Nott's Rat-TU | ANTU | |
| Nu Leaf Dust | Ferbam | |
| Omazene | Copper Dihydrazinium Sulfate | |
| Ortho Aquatic Weed Killer | Petroleum Oil | |
| Ortho Brush Killer | 2 4 5-T Esters | |
| Orthocide Garden Fungicide | Captan | |
| Ortho-Cop Fungicide | Copper | *See Index* |
| Ortho Crab Grass Killer | Phenyl Mercuric Acetate | |
| Ortho Defoliant Weed Killer | Sodium Chlorate | |
| Ortho Grass Killer | Isopropyl N-Phenyl Carbamate | |
| Panoram | Tetramethylthiuram Disulfide | |
| Paradize Moth Balls | Naphthalene | |
| Paradize Nuggets | Paradichlorobenzene | |
| Paradow | Paradichlorobenzene | |
| Paris Green | Arsenic | |
| Parson Moth Crystals | Paradichlorobenzene | |
| Parson's Rat Killer | Warfarin | |
| Parson's Weed Killer | 2 4-D Esters | |
| Parson's Wood Preservative | Pentachlorophenol | |
| Patterson's Mole & Gopher Killer | Warfarin | |
| Patterson's Rat & Mouse Killer | Pival, Warfarin | |
| Patterson's Super Brushkiller | 2 4-D, 2 4 5-T | |
| Patterson's Weed Killer | 2 4-D, 2 4 5-T | |
| Penco Penite 6X | Sodium Arsenite | |
| Penco Pentrete | Phenyl Mercuric Ammonium Acetate | |
| Penta-Core | Pentachlorophenol | |
| Penta-Five | Pentachlorophenol | |
| Penta Plus-40 | Pentachlorophenol | |
| Penta-Preservative | Pentachlorophenol | |
| Penta-Kill | Pentachlorophenol | |
| Penta Weed Killer Concentrate | Pentachlorophenol | |
| Permatox-A | Pentachlorophenol | |
| Per-Mo Mothproofing Spray | Magnesium Silicofluoride | |
| Pfeuger Shoo Fly Insect Repellent | Ethylhexanediol | |
| Phytocide | Pentachlorophenol | |
| Pied Piper for Rats & Mice | ANTU, Warfarin | |
| Pied Piper Kwik-Kill Mouse Seed | Strychnine | |
| Pied Piper Moth Crystals | Paradichlorobenzene | |

TABLE 58—*Continued*
RODENTICIDES, HERBICIDES, FUNGICIDES

| *Trade Name** | *Harmful Ingredients* | *Treatment Reference Page Number* |
|---|---|---|
| Pied Piper Rodenticide | Red Squill | |
| Pied Piper Brush Killer | 2 4-D, 2 4 5-T | |
| Pittsburgh Weed Killer | 2 4-D | |
| Pivalyn Packets | Pival | |
| Plan-O-Weed | 2 4-D | |
| Planter's Blue Mold Dust | Ferbam | |
| Planter's Rat & Mouse Bait | Warfarin | |
| Pluraturf Crabgrass Killer | Phenyl Mercuric Acetates | |
| Polar Moth Balls | Naphthalene | |
| Polar Moth Flakes | Naphthalene | |
| Polar Moth Rings | Naphthalene | |
| Port Brand Than-O-Dust | Zineb | |
| Poulins Rat Doom | Arsenic | |
| Powco Brush Killer | 2 4-D, 2 4 5-T | |
| Pratt's 622 Insect Repellent | Dimethyl Phthalate | |
| Pratt's Weed Killer | Sodium Arsenite | |
| Pratt's Tomato Dust | Copper Sulfate | |
| Premerge | Dinitrobutylphenol | |
| Pro-Tex Moth Balls | Naphthalene | |
| PSC Co-Op Cuprocide Dust | Cuprous Oxide | |
| PSC Co-Op Weed Killer | 2 4-D Esters | |
| Puraturf Crabgrass Killer | Phenyl Mercuric Triethanol | |
| Pure Para | Paradichlorobenzene | |
| Rat and Mouse Controller Paste | Thallium | |
| Rataway | Warfarin | |
| Rat-B-Gon Rat & Mice Bait | Warfarin | |
| Rat-Deth | Warfarin | |
| Rat-Kill | Warfarin | |
| Rat-Nip | Phosphorus | *See Index* |
| Rat-Nix | Warfarin | |
| Rat-Nots | Red Squill | |
| Rat-O-Cide No. 2 | Warfarin | |
| Rat-O-Cide Rat Bait | Red Squill | |
| Rat-Ola | Warfarin | |
| Ratorex | Warfarin | |
| Rat-Pak | Red Squill | |
| Rat-Seed | Strychnine | |
| Rat-Snax | Red Squill | |
| Rat-Trol Bait | Warfarin | |
| Rat's End | Red Squill | |
| Rax-Powder | Warfarin | |
| Real Kill Mothkiller | Naphthalene | |
| Red Seal Rodenticide | Arsenic | |
| Red Star Crabgrass Killer | Disodium Methyl Arsenate | |
| Reliable Moth Balls & Flakes | Naphthalene | |
| Repel-A-Mist | Ethylhexanediol | |
| Richfield Weedkiller "A" | Petroleum Hydrocarbons | |
| Rid-O-Moth Flakes & Balls | Naphthalene | |
| Rid-O-Moth Nuggets & Crystals | Paradichlorobenzene | |
| Rid-O-Weed | 2 4-D | |
| Rockland Brush Killer | 2 4-D, 2 4 5-T | |
| Rockland Weed Killer | Sodium Arsenite | |
| Rodene | Red Squill | |
| Rodent-Rid | Pival | |
| Rodent-Vev | Pival | |
| R-Deth Grain Killer | Warfarin | |
| Rodine | Red Squill | |
| Ro-Do | Warfarin | |
| Rose Rat Killer | Arsenic Trioxide | |
| Roxex | Arsenic Trioxide | |

TABLE 58—*Continued*
RODENTICIDES, HERBICIDES, FUNGICIDES

| *Trade Name** | *Harmful Ingredients* | *Treatment Reference Page Number* |
|---|---|---|
| Rough & Ready Mouse Mix | Warfarin | *See Index* |
| Rough & Ready Rat Bait | Red Squill | |
| Rough & Ready Rat Paste | Red Squill | |
| Rough on Rats | Arsenic | |
| Rot Not | Copper Naphthenate | |
| Rutgers 612 | Ethylhexanediol | |
| Safite Rodenticides | Warfarin | |
| Sage Savers | Naphthalene | |
| Sapho Crystals | Paradichlorobenzene | |
| Sapho 622 Repulseur Liquid and Cream | Dimethyl Phthalate | |
| Sanaseed Mouse Seed | Strychnine Sulfate | |
| Scutl | Phenyl Mercuric Salts of Acetic, Propionic and Naphthyl Phthalamic Acids | |
| Seal Treat Preservative | Pentachlorophenol | |
| Senco Corn Mix | Thallium Sulfate | |
| Senco Microfine Powder | Arsenic Trioxide | |
| Senco Paste | Phosphorus | |
| Senco Poison Oat Kernels | Strychnine Sulfate | |
| Setrete | Phenyl Mercuric Ammonium Complex | |
| Shaple Rat & Mouse Killer | Warfarin | |
| Shed-A-Leaf | Sodium Chlorate | |
| Shirlan | Salicylanilide | |
| Silvex | 2 4-5-T | |
| Singletary's Pest Control | Arsenic | |
| Sla-Rat Prepared | Warfarin | |
| Snow White Flakes | Paradichlorobenzene | |
| Snowflake Moth Spray | Carbon Tetrachloride | |
| Sodar | Disodium Methyl Arsenate | |
| Speckman Durotox | Pentachlorophenol | |
| Speckman Naptox | Copper Naphthenate | |
| Speckman Permite | Pentachlorophenol | |
| Speckman Deth-Bait | Warfarin | |
| Spotrete | Tetraethylthiuram Disulfide | |
| Spray-Trol Brand Para-Trol | Paradichlorobenzene | |
| Spray-Trol Brand Rodent-Trol | Warfarin | |
| Sprayway Moth Proofer | Parachloroaniline Oleate | |
| Sprayway X-M Insect Repellent | Ethylhexanediol | |
| STAC Weed Killer | Trichloroacetic Acid | |
| Sta-Klor | TCA Chlorate | |
| Stantox | 2 4-D, 2 4 5-T | |
| Stauffer's Brush Killer | 2 4-D, 2 4 5-T | |
| Stauffer's Brush Killer-Ready To Use | Warfarin | |
| Stauffer's Rodent Bait Cone | Warfarin | |
| Stauffer's Weed Killer | 2 4-D, 2 4 5-T | |
| Stop-Rat | Pentachlorophenol | |
| Superlarvex Mothproofer | Sodium Aluminum Ammonium Fluosilicates | |
| Swan Brand Dry Insecticide | Naphthalene | |
| Sweeny's Poison Wheat | Strychnine Sulfate | |
| Swift's Gold Bear Brand Brush Killer | 2 4-D, 2 4 5-T | |
| Tag Fungicide | Phenylmercuric Acetate | |
| Tat Insect Repellent | Dimethyl Phthalate | |
| Telvar Weed Killer | Dichorophenyl Dimethylurea | |
| Ten-Twenty Brush Killer | 2 4-D, 2 4 5-T Esters | |
| Terratox Weed Killer | Sodium Chlorate | |
| Terro Ant Killer | Arsenic | |
| Tetrafume Grain Fumigant | Carbon Tetrachloride | |
| Tetrakil Grain Fumigant | Carbon Tetrachloride | |
| T-H Spot Fumigant | Carbon Tetrachloride | |
| Timbertox | Pentachlorophenol | |
| Topzol Rat Baits | Red Squill | |

TABLE 58—*Continued*
RODENTICIDES, HERBICIDES, FUNGICIDES

| *Trade Name* | *Harmful Ingredients* | *Treatment Reference Page Number* |
|---|---|---|
| Topzol Rat Killing Syrup | Red Squill | |
| Tri-Cop | Copper | |
| Trikop | Copper | |
| Triox | Arsenic Trioxide | |
| Trioxone | 2 4-D, 2 4 5-T Esters | |
| Triple D-Dust 5 | DDD | |
| Triple-X Rat Poison | Red Squill | |
| Trox | Copper | |
| Tumbleweed | Sodium Chlorate | |
| Twin Light Rat-Away | Warfarin | |
| United Chemical Clorblor Weed Killer | Sodium Chlorate | |
| United Chemical Ester Weed Killer | 2 4-D Esters | |
| United Chemical Garden Unifume | Ethylene Dibromide | |
| United Chemical General Weed Killer | Dinitro-O-Secondary Butyl Phenol | |
| U.S. Sanitary Specialities Moth Flakes | Naphthalene | |
| U.S. Sulfur Fumigating Candles | Refined Sulfur | |
| University Brand Grain Fumigant | Carbon Tetrachloride | |
| Verdasan | Mercury | |
| Vintox | Sodium Arsenite | |
| Voo-Doo 42 | Warfarin | |
| Voo-Doo White Magic Mouse Killer | DDT | |
| Warficide Rat Killer | Warfarin | |
| Weed A Bomb | 2 4-D Ester | |
| Weeder 64 | 2 4-D Alkanolamine | |
| Weed-B-Gon | 2 4-D Dimethyl Amine | *See Index* |
| Weed-Bane | 2 4-D | |
| Weeded | Sodium Metarsenite | |
| Weedeth | 2 4-D Salt | |
| Weedicide | 2 4-D Salts | |
| Weed-No-More | 2 4-D Ester | |
| Weednox | Sodium Arsenite | |
| Weedane Aero-Concoction | 2 4-D Ester | |
| Weedone Sodar | Disodium Methyl Arsonate | |
| Weedster | 2 4-D Ester | |
| Wekill | 2 4 5-T Ester | |
| Wilson Elect-O-Weed | 2 4-D | |
| Wilson's Tri Rose | Copper Ammonium Complex, Nicotine | |
| Wonder Rodenticide | Warfarin | |
| WW 42 | Warfarin | |
| X-It Rat and Mouse Poison | Arsenic | |
| XXX (Triple) Alcufe Fungicide | Copper Salts | |
| XXX (Triple) DDT Spray | DDT | |
| XXX (Triple) Endrin Spray | Endrin | |
| XXX (Triple) Flowable 75 | Petroleum Oil | |
| XXX (Triple) Liquid Thrip-Tox | Sabadilla Alkaloids | |
| XXX (Triple) Tox-R | Rotenone | |
| XXX (Triple) Unicide 60 | Petroleum Oil | |
| XXX (Triple) Vigrocide | Colloidal Sulfur, Zinc Sulfide | |
| XXX (Triple) Zinc Nutraspray 20 | Zinc Salts | |
| Zelio | Thallium | |
| Zotox Crab Grass Killer | Arsenic Acid | |
| Zurd Rodenticide | Warfarin | |

*Chapter 4*

# INDUSTRIAL HAZARDS

A. Nitrogen compounds
   1. Aniline (Dimethylaniline, Nitroaniline, Toluidine, Nitrobenzenes)
   2. Trinitrotoluene (TNT)

B. Halogenated hydrocarbons
   1. Carbon tetrachloride
   2. Tetrachloroethylene
   3. Trichloroethylene
   4. Trichloromethane (Chloroform)
   5. Trichloroethane
   6. Tetrachloroethane
   7. Ethylene dichloride
   8. Ethylene chlorohydrin
   9. Chlorinated naphthalene and Biphenyl

C. Alcohols and Glycols
   1. Ethyl alcohol
   2. Methyl alcohol
   3. Glycol; Ethylene, Diethylene, Hexylene and Propylene

D. Aldehydes, Ketones, Ethers and Esters
   1. Dimethyl sulfate
   2. Tri-Ortho-Cresyl-phosphate
   3. Acetaldehyde, Paraldehyde, Metaldehyde, and Acrylaldehyde
   4. Acetone
   5. Dioxane
   6. Amyl acetate

E. Hydrocarbons
   1. Petroleum distillates (Kerosene, Gasoline, Solvent distillate, etc.)
   2. Benzene
   3. Naphthalene
   4. Turpentine

F. Corrosives
   1. Acids
      a. Miscellaneous acids and acid-like corrosives
      b. Hydrofluoric acid
      c. Oxalic acid
   2. Alkalis
      a. Chlorinated alkalis
      b. Sodium and Potassium carbonate
      c. Ammonia and Ammonium hydroxide
   3. Gases
      a. Fluorine and derivatives
      b. Cyanide, Hydrogen and derivatives
      c. Sulfides, Mercaptans and Carbon disulfide
      d. Carbon monoxide
      e. Carbon dioxide
      f. Sulfur dioxide
      g. Methyl chloride and bromide
      h. Carbon tetrachloride
      i. Formaldehyde
      j. Gasoline vapor
      k. Chlorine
      l. Oxygen
      m. Nitrogen oxides
      n. Mace
      o. Phosgene (Carbonyl chloride)

G. Metallic poisons
   1. Antimony and Stibine
   2. Arsenic and Arsine
   3. Beryllium
   4. Cadmium
   5. Chromium
   6. Lead
   7. Manganese
   8. Mercury

9. Nickel and Nickel carbonyl
10. Phosphorus, Phosphine and Phosphides
11. Zinc
12. Trace metals
13. Tin
14. Titanium tetrachloride

## NITROGEN COMPOUNDS

*Aniline and Derivatives (Dimethylaniline, Nitroaniline, Toluidine)*

Aniline is amino benzol, a colorless oily fluid with a characteristic odor. Upon exposure to air, it assumes a brownish color. This chemical is the starting point for the manufacture of many dyes and drugs. Its principal use is in printing inks, cloth marking inks, paints, paint removers and the synthesis of dyes. Industrial poisoning is usually complicated by the fact that the aniline is impure and contains other toxic substances. The derivatives are used in the synthesis of other chemicals. Aniline dye poisonings are fairly numerous in infants and children. Newborn infants have been poisoned by contact with diapers freshly stamped with material containing aniline dye and even by inhaling fumes from such diapers. Sufficient aniline dyes may be absorbed from shoe polish to cause symptoms. Toluidine blue (tolonium chloride, Blutene®) is a basic cationic dye similar in structure to azure A, methylene blue and Gentian Violet. It is used for menorrhagia; its antihemorrhagic effects are presumably due to heparin inhibition. Side-effects include nausea, vomiting, diarrhea, abdominal pain, dysuria, blue-green urine and hematuria.

Though ingestion of wax crayons by children is a relatively common occurrence, toxic effects are uncommon. This is in part due to the extreme indigestibility of the crayons, with consequent lack of absorption, and also to a factor of individual sensitivity. Dyes are not used in concentrations greater than 0.5%, and it is almost impossible to leach out these dyes from the wax.

The dyes, from the standpoint of toxicity, are those containing either para-nitroaniline or benzidine as one of the manufacturing components. Both of these compounds are known methemoglobin forming agents and may be present in orange, orange-red, yellow or violet crayons. Rare cases have been reported where children have become cyanosed after the ingestion of these particular colored crayons. Glucose-6-phosphate-dehydrogenase-deficient (G-6-PD) individuals are, however particularly susceptible to these compounds. Cyanosis is the first manifestation and can appear as early as ten minutes or as late as eight hours after ingestion. Symptoms include headache, mental confusion, nausea and vertigo. The blood may show methemoglobinemia associated with leukocytosis and the appearance of Heinz bodies.

Although recovery has followed ingestion of 30 gm, deaths have been reported from as little as 1 gm. The MAC in air of aniline and its derivatives is 5 ppm.

Symptoms are due to an intermediate oxidation product which changes hemoglobin to methemoglobin. If intense methemoglobinemia results, severe damage to the cells of the central nervous system occurs. Pathological findings include hemolysis, chocolate color of the blood, and injury to liver, spleen, kidney and bladder wall. β-Naphthylamine, a contaminant of commercial aniline, is capable of causing papilloma in the bladder wall after constant exposure. These often become malignant if not removed.

The clinical picture of poisoning is dependent on the intensity of exposure and possible sensitization. Direct contact of aniline with the skin may cause dermatitis.

Moderate exposure may cause only cyanosis of the lips, ears and cheeks without any subjective symptoms. In severe cases the cyanosis is quite marked with oppression in the chest, palpitation, headache, vertigo, chills, nausea and vomiting. Infants particularly are apathetic and dyspneic and may have convulsions and finally coma. In chronic poisoning from inhalation or skin absorption, mild cyanosis may be detected along with anorexia, weight loss, weakness, headache, vertigo, irritability, anemia and Heinz body formation in the erythrocytes. Methemoglobin production runs parallel with the oxidative degradation of hemoglobin, but Heinz body formation can occur without necessarily going through the stage of methemoglobin. N-acetyl-*p*-aminophenol (the chief metabolite of aniline) may be detected in the urine. Spectrophotometric methods for determination of methemoglobin can be used to monitor levels well below that at which cyanosis is clinically evident. The hemoglobin level is typically normal, whereas the blood oxygen-carrying capacity is measurably low. This difference is also a sensitive index of methemoglobinemia. The urine is almost always dark and often compatible with intravascular hemolysis, methemoglobinuria and renal injury.

*Treatment* should be directed against further absorption by removing the patient to fresh air. The skin, if contaminated, must be washed thoroughly with vinegar (5% acetic acid) and then soap and water. If ingestion has occurred, the stomach should be lavaged with weak acetic acid. This should be followed by liquid petrolatum, which binds the aniline, and a saline cathartic. If cyanosis is alarming, methylene blue should be given slowly, preventing perivenous infiltraton if at all possible, as a 1% solution, injected intravenously over a five-minute period in dosage of 0.2 ml/kg of body weight. This can be repeated in one hour if a concentration of methemoglobin above 40% persists. Oxygen therapy is paramount for anoxia and respiratory distress. Analeptics, artificial respiration and blood transfusions or washed red cells in saline may be necessary as adjunct therapy. In very severe or serious aniline poisoning, hemodialysis should be used and continued until significant chemical change or definite clinical improvement, including improved skin color, has occurred.

### *Nitrobenzene*

Nitrobenzene poisoning is in most respects similar to aniline intoxication. Aniline is obtained from the reduction of nitrobenzene, and the two chemicals are often used in the same industrial process. This compound is used in shoe dyes and as an artificial flavor in foods, soap and perfume because its odor is like that of oil of bitter almonds. It is a volatile yellowish fluid. The vapors are more toxic than the fluid itself. Nitrobenzene is not only a blood and cardiac intoxicant like aniline but is also a central nervous system depressant. The depression may be preceded by stimulation. Symptoms are often delayed in onset for hours if the poison is swallowed but are prompt and severe when they do appear. Symptoms from inhaling nitrobenzene occur immediately. The patient behaves as if he were inebriated. There is then noted headache, vertigo, nausea, vomiting, depressed respiration, disturbed vision, stupor, coma and death from respiratory failure. The skin is bluish gray or intensely cyanotic. The blood is chocolate-colored from methemoglobin and nitrobenzene-hemoglobin and may show evidence of an acute hemolytic crisis. The urine is dark, and both the urine and vomitus have the odor of oil of bitter almonds. Chronic poisoning is characterized by bladder distress, cyanosis, disturbed vision, peripheral neuritis, anemia and weight loss. Benign and malignant bladder tumors apparently occur as in the case of chronic aniline poisoning.

*Treatment* is similar to that for aniline poisoning.

### *Trinitrotoluene (TNT)*

Trinitrotoluene is a yellow crystalline compound used in the munitions industry as an explosive. (Dinitrophenol is a synthetic by-product from the manufacture of trinitrotoluene.) The fatal toxic dose has been estimated to be between 1 and 2 gm. The MAC in air is 1.5 mg/cu. m. The pathological manifestations are acute yellow atrophy of the liver, petechial hemorrhages, aplasia of the bone marrow and nephritis.

The principal symptom of poisoning is jaundice. There is a yellow discoloration of the skin, nails and hair. In addition, a severe irritation and erythema of the skin, often resulting in eczematoid lesions, may be present. One of the most conspicuous signs is cyanosis due to methemoglobinemia, which is first manifested in the fingertips, lips and ears. Associated with the cyanosis are headache, fatigue, lassitude and drowsiness. In severe cases there may be anuria, delirium, convulsions and coma. Among the first symptoms of incipient poisoning are the gastrointestinal disorders, i.e. nausea, vomiting, diarrhea and anorexia.

*Treatment.* Ingested trinitrotoluene should be removed immediately by emesis or gastric lavage. This should be followed by a saline purge. For skin contamination, thorough washing with soap and water is imperative (*see* Chap. 1 for treatment of methemoglobinemia). Supportive measures for possible or actual liver damage should be included.

## HALOGENATED HYDROCARBONS

### *Carbon Tetrachloride (see page 189)*

### *Tetrachloroethylene (Perchloroethylene)*

Tetrachloroethylene, a colorless, nonflammable liquid with a somewhat ethereal odor, is now used extensively in industry as a solvent and dry-cleaning agent. It is administered occasionally in humans (and animals) as an anthelmintic in therapeutic adult oral doses up to 4 ml.

It is readily absorbed through the lungs and to a much smaller degree through skin or mucous membranes or following ingestion. The threshold limit value is 100 ppm compared to 25 ppm for carbon tetrachloride. In humans, at 200 ppm, light narcosis is produced in a few minutes. The oral lethal dose in laboratory animals varies between 4 to 25 ml/kg, while the MAC is 5000 to 6000 ppm.

Tetrachloroethylene, when heated to decomposition (over 140°C), produces corrosive products such as hydrochloric acid, free chlorine and phosgene.

Symptoms consist of irritation of the eyes, skin and mucous membranes. Inhalation produces cough, pulmonary edema, salivation, perspiration, confusion, vertigo and an alcohol-like intoxication. In addition, with unusually large amounts, there may be headache, excitement, weakness, nausea, vomiting, weak pulse and stupor with anesthesia. Ingestion causes systemic manifestations similar to those of inhalation as well as severe gastrointestinal irritation with nausea, vomiting, abdominal cramps, diarrhea and bloody stools. Renal and hepatic injury occurs infrequently. Teratogenic effects and liver cancer have been recently found in laboratory studies on mice.

*Treatment* consists of terminating exposure immediately and maintaining respiration with oxygen and artificial respiration if necessary. Induce emesis or perform gastric lavage, if ingested, and follow with saline cathartic. Do not give epinephrine, fats or oils. Wash eyes and skin thoroughy with water (adding soap for skin), if indicated, and remove contaminated clothing.

Hemodialysis or peritoneal dialysis for renal failure, which is reversible, can be a lifesaving procedure.

### *Trichloroethylene*

This is a nonflammable liquid which is practically insoluble in water, but soluble with ether or chloroform. Trichloroethylene is used as an industrial solvent, household cleaner and as an inhalation anesthetic. The MAC is 200 ppm at which level the odor should be detectable. The most striking effect of trichloroethylene is the depression of the central nervous system. The heart, liver and kidneys are also affected and the presence of tetrachloroethane as a contaminant in commercial trichloroethylene increases the cellular damage. Solvents which are paramount in the use of trichloroethylene can produce more toxic effects than the chemical itself.

The symptoms of poisoning depend on the type of exposure and concentration. Exposure to trichloroethylene can be checked by determining the concentration of trichloroacetic acid in the urine. At 40 to 75 mg/liter, 50 per cent of workers show toxic effects. The principal manifestations are headache, vertigo, paresthesia and drowsiness, stupor, unconsciousness and coma. Exposure to its vapors causes irritation of the mucous membranes with resultant conjunctivitis and rhinitis. Skin contact produces severe erythema and vesiculation followed by exfoliation. Ingestion causes a burning sensation in the mouth, nausea, vomiting and abdominal pain. Ventricular arrhythmia including ventricular fibrillation is not uncommon and may be precipitated by the administration of epinephrine.

*Treatment* consists, above all, of moving the patient from the exposure to fresh air, and removing all contaminated clothing. Artificial respiration and oxygen should be used for respiratory failure. In case of ingestion, the stomach should be lavaged, followed by a saline cathartic. Epinephrine or other stimulants should not be used.

### *Trichloromethane (Chloroform, $CHCl_3$)*

The primary effect of chloroform is central nervous system depression with inebriation, anesthesia and narcosis. Although now rarely used for anesthesia, over 250 million lb. of chloroform were produced in the United States in 1973 for industrial use.

Chloroform can be absorbed through the lung, from the gastrointestinal tract, and to some extent, through the skin. The inhalation route is, of course, the primary source of chloroform absorption in man. Inhalation toxicology of $CHCl_3$ in animals has been summarized by von Oettingen (1955). Mice exposed to 8000 ppm of $CHCl_3$ died after three hours of exposure, rabbits died after a two-hour exposure to 12,500 ppm, while dogs survived much higher concentrations. Acute chloroform exposure may result in death by respiratory arrest. The primary toxic response at lower levels of exposure is hepatotoxicity leading to fatty liver and centrilobular necrosis.

Kidney damage may also occur in animals after acute poisoning, primarily in the convoluted tubules, but it may also affect the epithelium of Henle's loops. Watrous and Plaa (1972) demonstrated that chloroform as well as carbon tetrachloride partially inhibited the accumulation of *p*-aminohippuric acid in rat kidney slices, indicating an effect of these solvents on the active transport of *p*-aminohippuric acid after small doses were given to rats one day prior to sacrifice. Cohen and Hood (1969), utilizing low-temperature autoradiography, demonstrated the long-term retention of $CHCl_3$ in body fat, with an increased radioactivity occurring in liver during the postexposure period. Thin-layer chromatography also established the presence of two nonvolatile metabolites in liver.

Van Dyke and coworkers (1964) had demonstrated that after a single injection of $^{14}C$-labeled chloroform, $^{14}CO_2$ appeared in the expired air in less than one hour and was still being expired twelve hours later, with 4 to 5 per cent of the total dose being exhaled as $^{14}CO_2$, and up to 2 per cent of $^{14}C$-labeled metabolites appearing in the urine. This represents considerable metabolism of a type of compound usually thought of as biologically stable. In this same study utilizing $^{36}Cl$-labeled chloroform, measurable but variable quantities of labeled compounds appeared in the urine, largely in the inorganic form.

Dingell and Heimberg (1968) reported a 40

per cent inhibition of microsomal drug-metabolizing enzyme activity in rats fed 1.05 ml/kg of $CHCl_3$ twenty-four hours prior to sacrifice. This may be related to the degree of hepatic necrosis produced by $CHCl_3$ or to a more subtle effect on the microsomal enzyme system. That this oxidizing system is involved in the metabolism of $CHCl_3$ would be expected because of its structural relationship to $CCl_4$, where considerable evidence has been developed that implicates this enzyme system with metabolism and toxicity. In the case of $CHCl_3$, Scholler (1970) also reports that the hepatotoxicity of $CHCl_3$ in rats is markedly enhanced by pretreatment with phenobarbital, a known inducer of microsomal oxidizing system.

It is becoming more apparent that, in a number of instances, the toxic response to seemingly inert chemicals may be related to the metabolism of these compounds and the production of small quantities of unknown metabolites that can have a profound effect on important biologic processes.

The National Cancer Institute has found that chloroform causes hepatocellular carcinoma in both male and female mice and kidney tumors in rats.

Definitive signs, symptoms and treatment of poisoning are similar to those outlined for other halogenated hydrocarbons.

### *Trichloroethane (Methyl Chloroform)*

1,1,1 and 1,1,2 trichloroethane (methyl chloroform and beta-trichloroethane) are widely used commercial solvents with an estimated lethal human dose of 500 to 5000 mg/kg. These compounds are rapidly absorbed from the lungs and gastrointestinal tract. In humans, exposure to vapor concentrations near 2000 ppm for five minutes causes equilibrium disturbances and anesthetic effects (narcosis). MAC is 350 ppm. Breath analysis with gas chromatographic techniques offers specific sensitivity and can be used for rapid diagnosis and to detect the compound in the breath for days following vapor exposure.

Symptoms and signs are irritation of the eyes, mucous membranes and lungs. Inhalation or ingestion could produce central nervous system depression, headache, lassitude, incoordination, vertigo, hypotension, anesthesia and coma. Cardiac arrhythmias due to sensitized myocardium may occur. Heavy exposure can cause hepatic and renal injury. Death is usually due to respiratory arrest or peripheral vascular collapse. Lethal blood level is 10 to 100 mg%.

*Treatment.* Ingested trichloroethane should be removed immediately by emesis or gastric lavage. For inhalation, remove from exposure, administer oxygen and maintain respiration. Flush eye or skin contact thoroughly with water. Avoid alcohol and the use of epinephrine or related sympathomimetic stimulants due to the danger of inducing ventricular fibrillation.

### *Tetrachloroethane*

This is the most toxic of the chlorinated hydrocarbons. The MAC is 5 ppm. It is used as an industrial solvent and occurs as a contaminant in the halogenated hydrocarbons. Tetrachloroethane causes prolonged narcosis, nephritis and severe toxic hepatitis with acute yellow atrophy of the liver. An increase in the large mononuclear cells above 12 per cent in the differential blood smear often indicates significant exposure. Symptoms and *treatment* are similar to those for carbon tetrachloride poisoning.

### *Ethylene Dichloride*

This compound is used as a solvent in the plastic, rubber and insecticide industries and in plastic and rubber cement for household use and hobby craft. The MAC in air is 100 ppm and the ingestion of 5 ml has caused fatalities. By oral route or by inhalation, ethylene dichloride causes severe central nervous system depression. All reported deaths from ingestion have shown acute hemorrhagic gastroenteritis, hepatitis, nephritis and petechial hemorrhages in the brain. Initial symptoms are hypotension, cyanosis, vomiting, diarrhea, pulmonary edema and coma. Jaundice, oliguria and anemia may occur later in the course, if the patient survives.

*Treatment* is similar to that for carbon tetrachloride poisoning.

### *Ethylene Chlorohydrin*

This is a colorless, aromatic liquid which evaporates readily at room temperature. It is used as a solvent in the chemical and textile industries and to speed the germination of seeds and potatoes. Ethylene oxide, used as a fumigant in the food industry and for sterilizing medical equipment, is converted to ethylene chlorohydrin in the presence of moisture and chloride ions. The MAC in air is 2 ppm. Depression of the central nervous system and tissue damage of heart, lungs, liver and kidney follow prolonged exposure. Impaired DNA in living cells has been reported.

Unfortunately, ethylene chlorohydrin does not have an odor nor does it cause much irritation of the nose and throat. Symptoms arise soon after exposure and include nausea, vomiting, headache, vertigo, delirium, hypotension, slow respiration, fasciculation of muscles, cyanosis and coma. Death, when it occurs, is due to respiratory and circulatory failure.

*Treatment* is similar to that for trichloroethylene poisoning.

### *Chlorinated Naphthalene and Polychlorinated Biphenyl*

These compounds are used as high-temperature dielectrics for electric wires, motors, transformers, other electrical equipment and plasticizers. They produce skin irritation, acne, nephritis, and necrosis of the liver. The MAC for industrial exposure is 1 mg/cu. m. Symptoms occur from prolonged exposure and consist of acneiform eruption, anorexia, nausea, lethargy, jaundice, hepatomegaly and weakness progressing to comatose state.

The characteristic properties of PCB which make it desirable for industrial use are the high dielectric constant and the thermal and chemical stabilities. The stability of these compounds, on the other hand, combined with the fact that PCB is readily taken up by living organisms and accumulated at higher levels of the food web, causes problems in the environment. PCB contamination is found to be almost universal, including human milk, human adipose tissue and brain and liver of small children. Little is known about the toxic effects of PCB in humans, but rhesus monkeys given 25 ppm showed signs of PCB intoxication, including hair loss, edema of the face, skin redness and acne, and gave birth to underweight offspring even when taken off the diets. Infants exposed *in utero* to PCB had extensive stillbirths and birth defects.

In 1968, PCB leaked into rice bran oil consumed by people in Japan. As little as 500mg ingested over a fifty-day period prompted symptoms and even liver damage in some victims ("Yusho").

The clinical picture included acneiform eruption; distinctive hair follicles; pigmentation of skin, nails, conjunctiva and oral mucosa and hypersecretion from Meibomian glands. Systemic symptoms included anorexia, general fatigue, weight loss and impotence. Over 1000 persons were affected.

The present recommendation of the FDA is that food products should not contain more than 5 ppm of PCB.

The Monsanto Company, the only manufacturer of PCB in the United States, has announced that it will stop producing this compound.

The *treatment* is mainly supportive and symptomatic in the prevention of latent liver damage. It is absolutely essential that further exposure be eliminated.

# ALCOHOLS AND GLYCOLS

## *Alcohol, Ethyl (Ethanol, Grain Alcohol)*

Alcohol is a primary and continuous depressant of the central nervous system and has the same general properties of the methane series. The range between a dose which produces anesthesia and one which impairs actual functions is small. The toxic potentialities of the imbibing of alcoholic beverages in children should never be overlooked or minimized. Many have been made seriously ill, and a number of deaths have been reported from ingestion when children were unsupervised and had easy access to these products. The fatal dose is from 250 to 500 gm of alcohol (500 to 1000 ml of whiskey). Continuous alcohol sponging of a febrile infant has produced severe intoxication (hypoglycemia, coma) and even death from inhalation of alcohol vapors. In chronic poisoning there are degenerative changes in liver, kidney and brain, gastritis and eventually cirrhosis of the liver. In acute poisoning, however, there is rather severe edema of the brain and gastrointestinal tract with hyperemia.

Alcohol is readily absorbed from the stomach and intestinal tract. Approximately 90 to 98 per cent of the amount absorbed is completely oxidized while the remaining 2 to 10 per cent is eliminated primarily through the kidneys and lungs. Insignificant fractions are excreted in bile, sweat, tears, saliva, and gastric juice. In the metabolism of alcohol, oxidation to acetaldehyde occurs first. This reaction is catalyzed by alcohol dehydrogenase, a zinc-containing enzyme found primarily in the liver but also found in the kidney. Small amounts of acetaldehyde are converted to condensation products such as acetoacetic acid or beta-hydroxybutyrate, but the major pathway involves its further oxidation to the key intermediate, acetylcoenzyme A (acetyl-CoA). This compound may be further broken down to acetate; it has been shown that blood acetate levels increase appreciably after human ethanol ingestion. The acetate portion of acetyl-CoA can be oxidized completely to carbon dioxide and water or converted through the citric acid cycle to other biologically important compounds as fatty acids. When alcohol is oxidized to acetaldehyde and then to acetyl-CoA, diphosphopyridine nucleotide (DPN) acts as the cofactor and hydrogen acceptor. The hydrogen molecules are transferred from alcohol or acetaldehyde to DPN to form reduced DPN or DPNH. Oxidation beyond acetaldehyde can be blocked by disulfiram (Antabuse), butyraldoxime, cyanamide, chlorpropamide (Diabinese®) and by tolbutamide (Orinase). For other common drug interactions with ethanol, *see* Table 60, page 214.

Ethanol is the most common cause of elevated plasma osmolality, and if it is normal or only slightly elevated, coma is not likely due to alcohol. In one large series with serum osmolalities of 320 mOsm/kg (considered as a test for blood alcohol of 50 mg/100 ml), 90 per cent were positive for alcohol. Gamma glutamyl transferase (GGT), an enzyme in the liver cytoplasma and bile ducts, is raised considerably (ten to twenty times normal) in more than 80 per cent of people who drink heavily, whether alcoholics or not. Normal values are about 45 U./liter for men and 30 U./liter for women.

In children, hypoglycemia and convulsions have been frequently reported following large ingestion of alcohol. Factors responsible for this reaction are not clearly understood. There is great experimental variability in the effects of alcohol on carbohydrate metabolism. Acting as a metabolic poison, however, it is possible that alcohol could interfere with gluconeogenesis (from amino acids) or inhibit glycogenolysis. At any rate, if hypoglycemia occurs, it should be treated promptly with parenteral glucose. Glucagon does not terminate the hypoglycemia, probably because of exhaustion of hepatic glycogen.

The signs of alcoholic intoxication can be

simulated by the effects of drugs and many diseases such as diabetic coma, subdural hematoma, etc. The odor of the breath is a notoriously misleading index as to whether the suspect has taken sufficient alcohol to cause his symptoms, and indeed it is a poor guide for any intoxication at all.

With the use of ethanol in hyperalimentation regimens and for the inhibition of premature labor, there is increased opportunity for exposure of the fetus to this potentially toxic substance.

Ethanol is known to cross the placental barrier freely and is distributed throughout the water phase of the fetus. Cord blood levels are slightly below maternal levels. Alcohol dehydrogenase activity is known to be low in human fetal liver and reaches 20 per cent of adult activity at term. There is a reduced rate of ethanol clearance in premature infants compared to adults. This reduced rate is believed to represent the combination of an increased percentage of total body water and a low level of hepatic alcohol dehydrogenase activity. The *fetal alcohol syndrome* (FAS) from excessive or even modest alcohol imbibition by women, particularly during the early stages of pregnancy, can produce the following features in the fetus and newborn.

1. Prenatal growth deficiencies affecting body length more severely than weight.
2. Postnatal growth deficiency, often of such a degree that these infants were considered not to thrive.
3. Delay of both gross and fine motor development, with mental retardation of varying degrees.
4. Craniofacial anomalies, e.g. microcephaly, short palpebral fissures, microphthalmia, epicanthal folds, maxillary hypoplasia, cleft palate and micrognathia.
5. Joint anomalies, such as restriction of joint movement and an altered palmar crease pattern.
6. Cardiac anomalies, such as ventricular septal defect, or miscellaneous defects, such as capillary hemangiomas and anomalous external genitalia.

Ethanol is known to be a potent CNS and respiratory depressant with shallow respiration and general CNS depression manifested by lethargy, poor tone and abnormal reflexes. Hiccups are a prominent clinical sign and gastric irritation produces vomiting. In addition, there can be irritability, jitteriness, apnea, temperature instability and hypoglycemia as complications of acute intoxication. Clinical differentiation from sepsis can be difficult. Acute exposure to ethanol has also been shown to influence bone marrow structure in the neonate and to alter bilirubin metabolism.

Symptoms vary with the alcohol level of the blood.* At levels of 0.05% to 0.15%, there is slight muscular incoordination and visual impairment and a slowing of the reaction time. Levels of 0.15% to 0.3% show slurring of speech, definite visual impairment, muscular incoordination and sensory loss. In levels of 0.3% to 0.5%, there is marked muscular incoordination, sensory loss, blurred or double vision and approaching stupor, while at 0.5% concentration there is coma, slowed and labored respiration, decreased reflexes and sensory loss. Deaths occur in this range (Winek, C.L.: Post-mortem Synthesis and Diffusion of Ethanol. In *Toxicology Annual.* New York, Dekker, 1975.). The generally accepted average rate of disappearance of alcohol from the blood is 100 mg/kg/hr. A 70-kg man loses about 7 gm (9 ml) of alcohol per hr. This is roughly equivalent to the amount of alcohol in a small whiskey or a half-pint of beer. Chronic poisoning is characterized by weight loss, gastroenteritis, polyneuritis, optic atrophy, mental deterioration and often psychosis (Korsakoff's syndrome), delirium tremens and cirrhosis of the liver.

The drunkometer in current use is a portable apparatus for the estimation of the blood ethyl alcohol level by analysis of mixed

---

*1. Below 0.05%, prima facie evidence not under the influence.
2. Between 0.05% and 0.15%, evidence not prima facie, but admissable, with prosecution, if the symptoms warrant.
3. Above 0.15%, prima facie evidence of under the influence.

TABLE 59

CHART OF APPROXIMATE BLOOD ALCOHOL PERCENTAGE

| Drinks | Body Weight in Pounds | | | | | | | | Influenced |
|---|---|---|---|---|---|---|---|---|---|
| | 100 | 120 | 140 | 160 | 180 | 200 | 220 | 240 | |
| 1 | .04 | .03 | .03 | .02 | .02 | .02 | .02 | .02 | Rarely |
| 2 | .08 | .06 | .05 | .05 | .04 | .04 | .03 | .03 | |
| 3 | .11 | .09 | .08 | .07 | .06 | .06 | .05 | .05 | Possibly |
| 4 | .15 | .12 | .11 | .09 | .08 | .08 | .07 | .06 | |
| 5 | .19 | .16 | .13 | .12 | .11 | .09 | .09 | .08 | |
| 6 | .23 | .19 | .16 | .14 | .13 | .11 | .10 | .09 | |
| 7 | .26 | .22 | .19 | .16 | .15 | .13 | .12 | .11 | Definitely |
| 8 | .30 | .25 | .21 | .19 | .17 | .15 | .14 | .13 | |
| 9 | .34 | .28 | .24 | .21 | .19 | .17 | .15 | .14 | |
| 10 | .38 | .31 | .27 | .23 | .21 | .19 | .17 | .16 | |

One drink is 1 oz. of 100 proof liquor or 12 oz. of beer. Subtract .01 for each 40 minutes of drinking. EXAMPLE: A 160 pound person having consumed 4 drinks in less than 40 minutes will have an approximate blood alcohol percentage of .09.

Reprinted by permission of the Medical Letter, Inc., 56 Harrison Street, New Rochelle, New York, 10801.

expired air. The basic procedure involves calculating the weight of alcohol which accompanies 190 mg of carbon dioxide ($CO_2$) in the subject's breath. This is converted to blood alcohol concentration using the observations that (1) alveolar air normally contains close to 5.5 vol.% $CO_2$, i.e. 190 mg of $CO_2$ in 2100 ml of alveolar air at 34°C; and (2) the weight of alcohol present in 1 ml of blood is equal to that present in 2100 ml of alveolar air. The reliability of a breath-alcohol apparatus (drunkometer) depends on observing the correct testing technique and maintaining the entire system under adequate qualified professional personnel and supervision.

Cushingoid symptoms have also been reported from chronic alcohol abuse. Recent evidence suggests that disorders of the liver, heart and bone marrow, although aggravated and accelerated by nutritional deficiencies, are probably caused by cytoxic actions of alcohol, and possibly its metabolite, acetaldehyde, a known potent cytoxin.

*Treatment.* The patient should be put to bed and protected from doing himself harm. Body temperature should be restored to normal. The unabsorbed alcohol should be removed by gastric lavage or emesis, but apomorphine because of its depressant effect should not be used for this purpose. Adequate airway and oxygenation should be maintained. Sodium bicarbonate (1 tsp. to 1 pt. of water) should be offered by mouth every hour to prevent acidosis. If acidosis has already occurred, a 3% to 5% solution of sodium bicarbonate should be administered intravenously until plasma bicarbonate is restored. Intravenous fructose (10%) use in therapy is controversial. Excessive fluids and depressant drugs should be avoided. Barbiturates interfere with the enzymatic action of alcohol dehydrogenase and hinder the body's ability to dispose of alcohol. Because of this interference, the combined depressant effects of moderate amounts of barbiturates and alcohol can be fatal.

Caffeine should be given a prominent place in the treatment because of its excellent pharmacological antagonism to alcohol. Combined with sodium benzoate, it can be given in doses of 0.5 gm (7½ gr) IM. If caffeine is not available, strong coffee by mouth is a good substitute. Excessive use of potent respiratory stimulants is contraindicated. The increase in intracranial pressure which often occurs can be treated with hypertonic intravenous glucose. Urea or mannitol therapy may also prove effective.

In the same eleven years that 45,000 United States servicemen were killed in Vietnam, nearly 300,000 Americans died as the result of alcoholism. The American Hospital Association reported that 25 to 30 per cent of all adult medical-surgical patients in metropolitan hospitals were found to be alcoholics, regardless of the diagnosis. An estimated 9 million persons are alcoholics and account for 50 per cent of our highway and home accidents.

The victims of chronic alcoholism require psychotherapy by a competent, interested physician. Alcoholics Anonymous (*see* listing in local phone directory) will help those patients who genuinely desire help. Disulfiram (Antabuse) therapy over a period of a year may be helpful in overcoming alcohol addiction by inducing sensitivity to alcohol. Reversible drug-induced hepatitis and optic and peripheral neuritis are rare side-effects from this method of therapy.

Management of withdrawal symptoms is

important in treatment of the alcoholic patient. Therapy is directed toward sedation, correction of fluid imbalance and vitamin, mineral and protein replacement.

When ethanol becomes a major source of fuel, as in the excessive drinker, protein, vitamin and mineral deficiencies appear. The patient becomes dehydrated, restless, tense, agitated, depressed, guilty and anxious. Abrupt cessation of drinking results in progressive symptoms, with severity roughly proportional to duration and amount of drinking. Central nervous system involvement is characterized by agitation, confusion, tremulousness, vertigo, ataxia, and occasionally, hallucinations, delirium and convulsions. Cardiovascular manifestations include tachycardia and arrhythmias. Gastrointestinal symptoms are common and include anorexia, nausea, vomiting and diarrhea. Thrombocytopenia commonly occurs in severely alcoholic patients, often unaccompanied by other hematologic abnormalities or folate deficiency and appears to be a direct effect of alcohol. Thiamine deficiency is common and parenteral thiamine should precede glucose administration for the hypoglycemia frequently associated with chronic alcoholism to prevent blocking of the glucose metabolism and pyruvate accumulation. Suicidal tendencies are frequent.

Chlordiazepoxide hydrochloride (Librium®) is a useful drug because it produces greater muscular relaxation than other tranquilizing agents, less drowsiness and less hypotension. The drug also has an anticonvulsant effect. Significant relief occurs within thirty-six hours, even with severe symptoms. Chloral hydrate is used for bedtime sedation. Metronidazole (Flagyl) has recently been found to be an excellent alcohol detoxicant; 500 to 750 mg in divided doses produced marked aversion in two weeks. Fluids and a nourishing diet are effective in correcting fluid imbalance. Vitamin replacement is essential and antispasmodic agents are frequently used.

Table 60 lists documented examples of interactions of drugs with alcohol. Additional effects are discussed in Hansten, P.D.: *Drug Interactions.* Philadelphia, Lea & Febiger, 1975; and Seixas, F.A.: *Ann Intern Med, 83*:86,1975.

## *Alcoholic Liquors*

All alcoholic beverages are chiefly alcohol and water with small amounts of other agents added. Vodka, for example, is simply water and alcohol. Gin is similar to vodka with the addition of flavoring material extracted from juniper berries and orange peel. With other alcoholic liquors, the materials besides water and alcohol are congeners, which signifies simultaneous formulation and are mainly fusel oil, acetaldehyde, organic acids and esters. Fusel oil is a mixture of propyl, butyl and amyl alcohols. The amount of fusel oil present in alcoholic products is so small that its consumption through this vehicle has never been reported to produce any serious toxic effects. Brandy and wine contain traces of methyl alcohol from the breakdown of methoxy groups in the pectin of grape. Brandy and aged whiskey have tannins and other extractives from the charred wood barrel. Ale and beer contain almost as much dextrins as alcohol. Activated charcoal, used in *in vitro* experiments, adsorbs significant amounts of whiskey congeners and appears to be a useful agent for reducing the congeneric material from whiskey. In contrast to other alcoholic drinks, beer causes a diminution in the fibrinolytic activity of the blood. Though no clinical significance is attached to this phenomenon, abnormal clotting times are frequently noted in habitual beer drinkers, and water intoxication with hyponatremia has been documented. Certain essential oils are added to liqueurs and various amounts of sugar to some wines.

| *Common Alcoholic Beverages* | *% Alcohol/Volume* |
|---|---|
| Beer | 4–6 |
| Ale | 5–8 |
| Wine | 10–22 |
| Whiskey<br>Brandy<br>Gin<br>Vodka | 40–55 |

With distilled beverages, the alcohol content is expressed by the term *proof.* In the United States, 100-proof signifies 50 per cent alcohol by volume, with proportional numbers for other concentrations. The British corresponding term is simply *proof,* which means 57 per cent alcohol by volume; and the particular concentration is designated by per cent over or under proof. The British gallon, quart and pint are one-fifth larger than the corresponding United States measures and therefore have 1.37 times as much alcohol as the United States 100 proof liquor.

### *Alcohol, Methyl (Methanol)*

This alcohol, which is obtained from the destructive distillation of wood, is often called "wood alcohol." It is used industrially in chemical synthesis, antifreeze, solvent in shellac and varnish, paint remover and as a denaturant in denatured alcohol. The lethal dose varies between 60 to 250 ml (2 to 8 oz.). The MAC in air is 200 ppm and symptoms can develop from inhalation of fumes while cleaning machinery with the solvent in a closed or poorly ventilated room. Methyl alcohol is much more slowly oxidized in the body than ethyl alcohol. Even after two days, one third of it still remains in the body. Furthermore, it is incompletely burned in the tissues and is oxidized to formic acid, whereas ethyl alcohol is converted into carbon dioxide and water. Severe acidosis is produced by the metabolic products, formaldehyde and formic acid; the pH of the urine may reach 5.0 from the large amounts of formate excreted. The methanol metabolites, formic acid and formaldehyde, are respectively six and sixty times more toxic than methanol. In fatal cases, parenchymatous changes are found in the eyes, liver, kidneys and heart. Edema and petechial hemorrhages occur in the brain, lungs and gastrointestinal tract.

Methyl alcohol intoxication is similar to that seen with ethyl alcohol except that coma intervenes more readily and central depression is more prolonged. Severe gastrointestinal cramps and vomiting are quite characteristic due to the irritant action of methyl alcohol. Vision is often disturbed and blurred early in the course of poisoning and these symptoms occurring after a bout of drinking should immediately arouse suspicion of methanol. The pupils are dilated and do not respond to light; the optic disks are hyperemic and pink. Acidosis, which is characteristic and may be severe, results from the formic acid produced in the body by the oxidation of methyl alcohol. Cyanosis and dyspnea are common. Cardiac depression is frequent with this drug, which itself and through formic acid formation acts as a cardiotoxin. Respiratory and circulatory failure finally develop after many hours or several days of delirium or coma and result in death. If recovery occurs, it is usually slow, and blindness (optic atrophy) may be permanent. Irreversible CNS effects with rigidity, spasticity and hypokinesis have been reported. This prolonged and serious course of poisoning is quite in contrast to that seen from ethyl alcohol.

*Treatment.* Keep the patient warm and in bed. Protect the eyes from light. Control severe acidosis quickly by injecting slowly intravenously 3% to 5% sodium bicarbonate solution (350 to 400 mEq) in 1000 ml of 5% glucose or physiologic saline. Depending on the severity of the poisoning, 150 gm of sodium bicarbonate may be necessary. Check the pH and the carbon dioxide combining power of the blood, or administer alkali until the urine is alkaline. Improvement in the patient's respiration is a good clinical guide. He must be watched closely as patients thus treated with alkali soon become acidotic again. If the patient's respiration is rapidly failing or he is in shock, oxygen should be administered at once. Nikethamide (3 ml of a 25% solution) may be given intravenously slowly. For cerebral edema or hypoglycemia the administration of hypertonic glucose solution is indicated. Valium or sodium pentobarbital may be necessary for controlling the delirium or convulsions which often follow.

The hepatic enzyme alcohol dehydrogenase oxidizes methanol to form formaldehyde but

TABLE 60
SOME DRUG INTERACTIONS WITH ALCOHOL

| *Drug* | *Effect* | *Probable Mechanism* |
|---|---|---|
| Antabuse (disulfiram) | Flushing, diaphoresis, hyperventilation, vomiting, confusion, drowsiness | Inhibits intermediary metabolism of alcohol |
| Anticoagulants, oral | Increased anticoagulant effect with acute intoxication | Reduced metabolism |
| | Decreased anticoagulant effect after chronic alcohol abuse | Enhanced microsomal enzyme activity |
| Antihistamines | Increased CNS depression | Additive |
| Antimicrobials | | |
| Chloramphenicol (Chloromycetin; and others) | Minor Antabuse-like reaction | Inhibits intermediary metabolism of alcohol |
| Furazolidone (Furoxone) | Minor Antabuse-like reaction | Inhibits intermediary metabolism of alcohol |
| Griseofulvin (Fulvicin-U/F; and others) | Minor Antabuse-like reaction | Inhibits intermediary metabolism of alcohol |
| Isoniazid (many mfrs.) | Decreased effect after chronic alcohol abuse | Undetermined |
| Metronidazole (Flagyl) | Minor Antabuse-like reaction | Possible CNS effect |
| Quinacrine (Atabrine) | Minor Antabuse-like reaction | Inhibits intermediary metabolism of alcohol |
| Hypoglycemics | | |
| Chlorpropamide (Diabinese) | Minor Antabuse-like reaction | Inhibits intermediary metabolism of alcohol |
| Phenformin (DBI; Meltrol) | Lactic acidosis | Additive |
| Tolbutamide (Orinase) | Decreased hypoglycemic effect after chronic alcohol abuse | Enhanced microsomal enzyme activity |
| | Increased hypoglycemic effect with ingestion of alcohol, particularly in fasting patients | Suppression of gluconeogenesis |
| | Minor Antabuse-like reaction | Inhibits intermediary metabolism of alcohol |
| Narcotics | Increased CNS depression with acute intoxication | Additive |
| Salicylates | Gastrointestinal bleeding | Additive |
| Sedatives and Tranquilizers | | |
| Barbiturates | Increased CNS depression with acute intoxication | Additive; reduced metabolism |
| | Decreased sedative effect after chronic alcohol abuse | Enhanced microsomal enzyme activity; decreased CNS sensitivity |
| Chloral hydrate (Noctec; and others) | Prolonged hypnotic effect | Mutual potentiation |
| Chlordiazepoxide (Librium; and others) | Increased CNS depression | Additive |
| Chlorpromazine (Thorazine; Chlor-PZ) | Increased CNS depression | Additive; inhibits oxidation of alcohol |
| Clorazepate (Azene; Tranxene) | Increased CNS depression | Additive |
| Diazepam (Valium) | Increased CNS depression | Additive; possible increased absorption |

| | | |
|---|---|---|
| Meprobamate (Miltown; and others) | Increased CNS depression with acute intoxication | Additive; reduced metabolism |
| | Decreased sedative effect after chronic alcohol abuse | Enhanced microsomal enzyme activity |
| Oxazepam (Serax) | Increased CNS depression | Additive |
| Other* | | |
| Phentolamine (Regitine) | Minor Antabuse-like reaction | Inhibits intermediary metabolism of alcohol |
| Phenytoin (Dilantin; and others) | Increased anticonvulsant effect with acute intoxication | Reduced metabolism |
| | Decreased anticonvulsant effect after chronic alcohol abuse | Enhanced microsomal enzyme activity |

*Many alcoholic beverages contain tyramine, which can cause reactions with MAO inhibitors.

From *Medical Letter, 19*:5, 1977. Reprinted by permission of the Medical Letter, Inc., 56 Harrison Street, New Rochelle, New York, 10801.

has more affinity for ethanol than for methanol. If the two are administered jointly, ethanol is oxidized preferentially and methanol is not broken down before it is excreted. The use of ethyl alcohol to inhibit or diminish the toxic effects of methanol was first found effective in rhesus monkeys and is now being used successfully in humans. To prevent the formation of formic acid, a concentration of at least 100 mg of ethanol per 100 ml of blood should be maintained for a 70 kg man (10 ml/hr is considered the minimum dose necessary to suppress the metabolism of methyl alcohol completely). Depending on the severity of intoxication, 3 to 4 oz. of whiskey (45% alcohol) can be given orally every four hours for one to three days. In serious poisoning, ethyl alcohol should be given intravenously as a dilute solution (5%) in bicarbonate or saline. About 3 to 5 per cent of methanol is excreted unchanged through the kidney and the lungs, a slow process and hardly a practical alternative for more effective measures, if available.

Recent studies have shown the feasibility of artificial dialysis in the treatment. It has been demonstrated in laboratory animals that methyl alcohol and its metabolic by-products, formic acid and formaldehyde, can be removed by hemodialysis. A single treatment usually suffices to bring serum methanol levels below 75 mg%, which is considered the toxic threshold. Peritoneal dialysis, although effective, allows longer exposure to methanol and its toxic metabolites. Folic acid has been shown to accelerate methanol elimination in dogs and should be tried in humans.

## *Alcohol, Denatured*

Denatured alcohol is ethyl alcohol which has been adulterated with methyl alcohol (rarely used now for this purpose) and a small quantity of benzine or the pyridine bases. Denaturation or contamination with small amounts of methanol does not necessarily constitute a special problem since ethanol is selectively metabolized while the oxidation of methanol is inhibited in such circumstances. The most common denaturant used now, particularly in cosmetic preparations, is SD-40, which has the following formulation: 3 oz. of brucine (alkaloid) or brucine sulfate, N.F. IX and 500 ml of tert-butyl alcohol. The quantities of brucine present do not create any great hazard, unless an unusually large quantity is ingested.

*Treatment* is similar to that for ethyl alcohol intoxication.

## *Alcohol, Isopropyl (Alcohol, Rubbing)*

Isopropyl alcohol is an isomer of propyl and a homologue of ethyl alcohol. It is similar to the latter in its properties when employed externally but more toxic when taken internally. It is an important industrial solvent and also used as an ingredient of various cosmetics and for medicinal preparations for external use ("rubbing alcohol," etc.). Severe intoxication has occurred from the imbibing of an alcoholic beverage called "scrap-iron" prepared in galvanized drums by fermenting a mixture of yeast, cracked corn or corn meal and sugar with the addition of isopropyl alcohol and naphthalene.

All preparations coming under the classification of *rubbing alcohols* must be manufactured in accordance with the requirements of the Internal Revenue Service. The official formula now in use specifies 8 parts by volume of acetone, 1.5 parts by volume of methyl isobutyl ketone, not less than 68.5 per cent and not more than 71.5 per cent by volume of isopropyl alcohol, the remainder consisting of water and the denaturants, with or without coal-tar colors and perfume oils. Alcohol rubbing compound contains in each 100 ml not less than 355 mg of sucrose octaacetate.

Acetone taken by mouth in doses of 15 to 20 gm daily for several days usually poduces no ill effects other than slight drowsiness, but when inhaled it has more serious consequences. No specific data are available on the acute oral toxicity of methyl-isobutyl ketone in man, but peripheral neuropathy in spray painters has been attributed to this solvent. The probable acute lethal dose is between 0.5 and 5 gm/kg of body weight. The major effective denaturant in the rubbing alcohol is sucrose octaacetate, which is of very low toxicity but has a very bitter taste. A concentration of 0.06% renders even sugar inedible, and this substance would be expected to produce gastric irritation and vomiting long before a toxic dose of the rubbing alcohol could be ingested. The ethanol alone is as toxic as the denaturants used here. In children, 100 to 200 ml of 50% ethanol is often fatal.

Isopropyl alcohol has been reported as producing a wide variety of clinical manifestations, most of them common to ethyl alcohol intoxication. However, certain features may serve to differentiate the two. Isopropyl alcohol is more toxic, probably because of its greater molecular weight, and this is felt to result in an intensified and prolonged course. The presence of acetone in the breath, urine, serum and gastric washing, in the absence of glycosuria or hyperglycemia, may prove an invaluable clue to diagnosis, since 15 per cent of isopropyl alcohol is metabolized to acetone.

The central nervous system is especially vulnerable to isopropyl alcohol and the patient is more likely to show deep refractory narcosis, areflexia and depressed respiration.

Isopropyl alcohol is much more irritating to the gastrointestinal tract and more likely to produce nausea, vomiting, and abdominal pain than ethyl alcohol. Hematemesis and melena may appear early and they are related to ulceration of the gastric mucosa. The secretion of isopropyl alcohol by the salivary glands and the gastric mucosa tends to prolong the action of the alcohol. This physiologic fact is of importance in therapy, since early and repeated gastric lavage may have considerable value.

Extensive hemorrhagic tracheobronchitis, bronchopneumonia and hemorrhagic pulmonary edema have been found at postmortem examination. The mechanism of these changes is not clear but may be related to exhalation of isopropyl alcohol by the lungs. *Treatment* is similar to that for ethyl alcohol. In addition, hemodialysis to reduce blood and tissue levels of isopropyl alcohol should be used if indicated.

### *Alcohol, Amyl (Fusel Oil, Iso-amyl Alcohol)*

This compound is about four times as toxic as ethyl alcohol and causes more severe and prolonged symptoms. The amount of "fusel oil" present in alcoholic beverages is so small that its consumption through this vehicle has never been demonstrated to produce any toxic action. It rarely causes poisoning from its industrial use but has produced severe poisoning from its oral ingestion. The symptoms are headache, vertigo, nausea and vomiting, diarrhea, stupor or delirium and coma. Methemoglobinemia, methemoglobinuria and glycosuria have been reported. Sometimes death may follow. Recovery may be delayed and its aftereffects pronounced. *Treatment* is similar to that for ethyl alcohol. Methylene blue should be used for methemoglobinemia.

### *Alcohol, Allyl (Propenol)*

Allyl alcohol is readily absorbed through the intact skin in toxic and even lethal concentration. Dermatitis of variable types and degrees results, in addition to first- and second-degree burns with vesiculation. The vapors are especially irritating to the eyes and nose, and one hour's exposure to 1000 ppm is fatal to laboratory animals, while a saturated atmosphere can produce death in a few minutes. Ingestion of this material is most toxic, and severe symptoms can occur from contamination of food, cigarettes, etc. The estimated fatal dose is 10 gm.

*Treatment* consists of immediate gastric lavage or emesis if allyl alcohol is swallowed. Activated charcoal in the lavage solution and a residual amount left in the stomach is an effectively absorbent agent. In case of inhalation, remove the individual to fresh air. Give oxygen and apply artificial respiration if necessary. For eye and skin contact, flush thoroughly with water for fifteen minutes, after removing clothing.

### *Alcohol, Cetyl (Hexadecanol)*

This compound is a straight-chain 16-carbon alcohol used to reduce the loss of water by evaporation from large bodies of water such as reservoirs, lakes, ponds, etc. The water is covered with a monomolecular film of this alcohol. Studies show that aquatic life is not affected by this agent.

*Treatment* is unnecessary in case of accidental ingestion since its toxicity is negligible.

### *Glycol (Ethylene, Diethylene, Hexylene, Propylene)*

These agents are heavy liquids with a sweet, acrid taste and are excellent solvents for many water-insoluble substances, including drugs. In animals the toxic dose for ethylene glycol is 4.5 gm/kg, 0.5 gm for diethylene glycol and 20 to 30 gm for propylene glycol.

Many are familiar with the mass poisoning incident in 1938 with an elixir of sulfanilamide compound (72% diethylene glycol, 8% sulfanilamide and 20% flavors, saccharin, caramel and water) in which 105 fatalities were recorded. Fatal minimum total doses in these patients ranged from 5 to 20 ml for all ages. Information from the National Office of Vital Statistics shows that there were twenty-one accidental and two suicidal deaths from ethylene glycol in 1959. These figures indicate that the imbibing of this chemical in antifreeze agents for its alcohol effects, as well as its accidental ingestion by children, is increasing each year. Glycol's warm and sweet taste is similar to glycerin and easily consumed by children and adults. Some consideration should be given by manufacturers to the addition of a bitter additive.

The glycols are successfully converted to glycolaldehyde, glycolic acid and glyoxylic acid (intermediaries) and metabolized in the body to oxalic acid, which damages the brain and causes impairment of renal function and anemia. The central nervous system depression is as severe as and similar to that produced by ethyl alcohol. For diagnosis, chemical reaction tests, boiling point determination and ultrared spectroscopic and paper chromatographic examinations should be done to identify the chemical in container residue or gastric contents. Calcium oxalate crystals in urine sediment and positive results of quantitative determination of oxalates in the urine are strong diagnostic signs.

Oxalate toxicity is not the sole catalyst of clinical manifestation. Recent studies have supported aldehyde production, cofactor utilization and lactic acid accumulation as contributors to morbidity and mortality of ethylene glycol poisoning. The initial symptoms in severe poisoning are those of alcoholic intoxication, with vomiting (occasionally hematemesis), extreme weakness, ataxia, stupor, prostration, cyanosis, anemia, unconsciousness and convulsions. Death may occur early from respiratory failure or later from pulmonary edema or renal failure. Chronic poisoning from inhalation may produce any of the above symptoms in lesser degree.

*Treatment* consists of removing the ingested glycols by gastric lavage or emesis followed by a saline cathartic. A good antidote is 10 ml. of 10% calcium gluconate given slowly intravenously because it precipitates the metabolic product, oxalic acid. Since the hepatic enzyme alcohol dehydrogenase is responsible for the breakdown of ethylene glycol into toxic oxalates which produce the metabolic acidosis and ultimately the renal failure (deposition of oxalate crystals in the renal tubules provokes cytotoxicity as well as obstruction), ethyl alcohol as an antidote in competing for this enzyme has been suggested and used successfully in humans. To be effective, intravenous 100% ethanol as a 5% solution in dextrose and water at a rate of 0.1 ml/kg/hour to maintain blood levels at 1 to 2 mg/ml should be given as early as possible once the diagnosis has been established. Treatment should be continued for three to four days if necessary. Blocking the oxidation of ethylene glycol permits it to be excreted harmlessly. When possible, institute rapid and sustained diuresis with hypertonic mannitol. Early acidosis should be corrected with parenteral bicarbonate or molar lactate solutions.

For depressed respiration, artificial respiration with oxygen may be necessary. In the absence of renal impairment, fluids up to 4 liters should be forced to increase the excretion of glycol. Complete renal failure may respond to the artificial kidney or peritoneal dialysis. Improvement can take place even in the presence of severe uremia. In chronic poisoning it is imperative that the individual be removed from the source of exposure or the environment be changed.

## ALDEHYDES, KETONES, ETHERS AND ESTERS

### *Dimethyl Sulfate*

This agent hydrolyzes in the presence of water to methyl alcohol and sulfuric acid and is used for methylation in the chemical industry. The toxic dose is 1 to 5 gm (15 to 75 gr) and the MAC in air is 1 ppm. Since dimethyl sulfate is caustic to mucous membrances of the eyes, nose, throat and lungs, the following symptoms are characteristic: lacrimation, conjunctivitis, chemosis, photophobia and impairment of vision and color sensation. Direct contact with the skin can cause burns of first and second degree. Hoarseness, cough, edema of the lips, tongue and pharynx, bronchitis, pneumonia and pulmonary edema follow later. In protracted cases there may be injury of the liver and kidneys.

*Treatment.* The patient should be moved to fresh air; skin and mucous membranes should be washed with copious amounts of water (*see* page 46, Chemical Burns of the Eye). Skin corrosions should be treated with weak alkaline wet dressings or by other burn therapy. Cough and bronchospasm may respond to 1% nebulized epinephrine. Prophylactic antibiotics to prevent secondary pneumonia are indicated in severe poisoning. Depressants such as morphine or barbiturates should be used with caution. In contaminated areas, dimethyl sulfate should be deactivated by spraying with water or a 5% sodium hydroxide solution.

### *Tri-Ortho-Cresyl-Phosphate ("Machine Oil")*

This compound is a colorless or pale yellow liquid which is slightly soluble in water and fumes appreciably at 100°C. The meta and para isomeric forms of tri-cresyl-phosphate have negligible toxicological importance.

Tri-ortho-cresyl-phosphate is used as a plasticizer in plastic coatings, in fireproofers and in lubricants. It has occurred as an adulterant in certain pharmaceutical preparations as the fluid extract of ginger (Jamaica ginger, Jake) and of Apiol in Germany. Fatty foods stored in plastics containing this agent may become contaminated and cause symptoms of poisoning.

The lethal dose by ingestion has been estimated to vary between 1 to 10 gm, and the chief pathological lesion is the degeneration of the myelin sheaths of the motor nerve fibers as well as involvement of the affected muscles.

Symptoms of poisoning begin from one to thirty days after exposure, depending on the type (ingestion, inhalation or skin absorption). There is weakness of the distal muscles progressing to wrist and foot drop and flaccid paralysis of the lower extremities with paresthesia. In severe cases the flaccid paralysis may be generalized, affecting even the ocular, laryngeal and respiratory muscles with subsequent death due to respiratory paralysis. Recently 10,000 inhabitants of Morocco were tragically poisoned by the purchase and use of vegetable oil adulterated by "machine oil" containing tri-ortho-cresyl-phosphate. Practically all of these unfortunates suffered severe neurotoxic effects and have been left with more or less paralysis of various muscle groups that will require years of rehabilitation.

*Treatment* consists of immediate gastric lavage or emesis if poison is ingested. After

TABLE 61

ALCOHOL AND TOXIC SUBSTITUTES

| | *Methanol (Methyl Alcohol)* | *Ethanol (Ethyl Alcohol)* | *Isopropanol (Isopropyl Alcohol)* | *Paraldehyde* | *Ethylene Glycol* |
|---|---|---|---|---|---|
| *Use* | Antifreeze<br>Solvent<br>Denaturant | Solvent<br>Beverage | Rubbing alcohol<br>Solvent<br>Lacquer | Hypnotic | Antifreeze |
| Formula | $CH_3OH$ | $CH_3CH_2OH$ | $CH_3CHOH\ CH_3$ | $CH_3CH$ (–O–) $CH$-$CH_3$; O, O; CH; $CH_3$ | $HOCH_2$-$CH_2OH$ |
| Important Metabolites | Formaldehyde<br>Formic acid | Acetaldehyde<br>Acetic acid | Acetone | Acetaldehyde<br>Acetic acid | Oxalic acid |
| Toxicity of alcohol (Narcotic lethal effects) | 0.8 | 1.0 | 2.0 | | |
| Alcohol dehydrogenase used in metabolism | + | + | | | + |
| Lethal dose (Approximate) | 1-4 ml/kg | 300-400 gm | 250 gm | >50 mg/100 ml | 100 gm |
| *Signs and Symptoms* | | | | | |
| 1. CNS depression | + | + | ++ | + | + |
| 2. Acidosis | ++ | + | – | + | ++ |
| 3. Ketosis | – | + | + | – | – |
| 4. Fundi | ++<br>Pink edematous<br>Optic disk | – | – | – | + |
| 5. Respiratory toxicity | + | – | ++ Hemorrhagic tracheo-bronchitis | + | + |
| 6. Gastro-intestinal toxicity | + | + | + | + | + |
| 7. Renal | + | – | + | + | Renal failure<br>Calcium oxalate and hippurate crystals<br>++ |
| 8. Cardiovascular | + | + | – | + | + |
| 9. Hematologic | – | + | + | + | |
| 10. Standard therapy plus (1) Intravenous and oral ethanol | + | – | – | – | + |
| (2) Peritoneal dialysis or hemodialysis | + | + | + | ?+ | + |

Reprinted with permission from Lewis Goldfrank, *Hospital Physician, 11 (10):*14, 1975. Courtesy of F & F Publications, Inc. © 1975.

symptoms of paralysis have developed, the patient should be treated as if he had paralytic poliomyelitis. If weakness of respiratory muscles and depression occur, artificial respiration and oxygen should be given. A respirator or rocking bed may be necessary for several weeks until sufficient recovery occurs. As in poliomyelitis, hydrotherapy, massage and orthopedic care should be given for the paralyzed muscles.

### *Acetaldehyde, Paraldehyde, Metaldehyde and Acrylaldehyde (Acrolein)*

Acetaldehyde is a highly volatile colorless irritating liquid which is used in silver coating and in the chemical industry. Metaldehyde and paraldehyde are polymers of acetaldehyde, and in the presence of acids, decompose to this compound. Paraldehyde is used as a basal anesthetic, metaldehyde for snail bait and acrylaldehyde as a herbicide.

The MAC in air for acetaldehyde is 200 ppm. MAC levels and lethal doses for paraldehyde and metaldehyde have not been established. Acetaldehyde acts as an irritant and depresses all cells. Metaldehyde's action is due to the fact that it is changed to acetaldehyde. Paraldehyde produces depression of the central nervous system as well as the respiratory center.

Poisoning with these agents can produce irritation of all mucous membranes and coma. With exposure to vapors of acetaldehyde, there is lacrimation, photophobia, conjunctivitis, rhinitis, coughing, bronchitis and drowsiness. Ingestion causes nausea, vomiting, diarrhea, narcosis and respiratory failure. Paraldehyde intoxication ordinarily produces sleep without great depression of respiration unless lethal or near lethal amounts are taken. The continued use of large doses of paraldehyde (although its odor is intolerable for most patients) may result in chronic poisoning with visual and acoustic hallucinations, delusions, impairment of memory, intellect, speech, unsteady gait, tremors, anorexia and loss of weight, and its intravenous use can be hazardous and even fatal. In metaldehyde poisoning, in addition to severe gastrointestinal symptoms, there may be marked temperature elevation, muscular rigidity, convulsions, coma and respiratory death.

Acrylaldehyde (acrolein) is a colorless liquid with a sharp penetrating odor detectable at 1 ppm in air; 5.5 ppm causes mucous membrane irritation and 10 ppm can be fatal in a few minutes. Skin contact is the chief occupational hazard, since it can produce severe chemical burns. This compound is highly reactive chemically and readily forms polymers. In closed systems, this polymerization can proceed with explosive violence in the presence of alkaline materials and strong acid.

*Treatment* requires gastric lavage or emesis if these agents have been ingested. The patient should be removed from the source of inhalation exposure, and oxygen and artificial respiration administered if necessary. Contaminated clothing should be removed and the skin thoroughly washed. The remainder of the treatment should be supportive and symptomatic.

### *Acetone*

Acetone is a colorless volatile fluid of aromatic odor and pungent taste with narcotic and solvent properties. Acetone has many industrial uses besides its familiar role as a nail polish remover. The inhalation of the vapors can produce cough, bronchial irritation, headache and fatigue. The American Conference on Governmental Industrial Hygienists has recommended a threshold limit of 1000 ppm. Concentrations should not exceed this value for workers exposed eight hours a day. Ingested acetone causes gastrointestinal symptoms, and in severe cases of poisoning when large amounts are taken, there may be drowsiness followed by coma.

*Treatment* consists of moving the patient from the source of inhalation to fresh air, applying artificial respiration and giving oxygen if required. If acetone is swallowed in any quantity, the stomach should be lavaged or an emetic given. Analeptics and respiratory stimulants should be administered only if necessary.

*Dioxane*

Dioxane is an ether derivative which is used as a solvent for ethylcellulose, oils, resins and waxes. It has both irritant and narcotic effects similar to acetone. The symptomatology and *treatment* are as above for acetone.

*Amyl Acetate (Pear, Banana Oil)*

Amyl acetate is a colorless ester with a sweet pear-like taste and odor. It is employed as a solvent in industry and in cosmetics and perfumes. The inhalation of vapors of this agent may cause irritation of the mucous membranes of the respiratory tract and eye, anorexia, fatigue, headache, vertigo, tinnitus, drowsiness, and in severe poisoning, unconsciousness and coma. Studies of the blood may show severe anemia and eosinophilia.

For *treatment, see* Acetone.

## HYDROCARBONS

*Petroleum Distillates (Kerosene, Gasoline, etc.)*

Kerosene, together with other petroleum products and solvents, accounted for more than 50 deaths, one seventh of all fatal poisonings among children under five in the United States, in 1966. Of 252 children admitted over a ten-year period for kerosene poisoning, the most common cause of poisoning among admissions at the Charity Hospital in New Orleans, 9 died. The incidence from poisoning with petroleum products, principally kerosene, in twelve southern states is four times greater than that in other areas. In the South, kerosene is extensively used for curing tobacco, heating, cooking, and in more remote rural areas, for lighting. This substance is often removed from its original container and put into an empty cola bottle, which is often carelessly left about where thirsty, hungry toddlers do not hesitate to sample it.

Benzene, petroleum spirit, refined solvent naphtha and gasoline are hydrocarbons with more toxic potential. Additives also alter the overall toxicity of gasoline. Stored gasoline presents other serious hazards of combustion and explosion. Gasoline vapors expand to fill the available space. This expansion can split the seams of an unvented can or plastic container and can cause vapor leakage that can ignite or explode from sparks from an electrical unit or appliance. The explosive power of one gallon of gasoline has been compared to the explosive force of fourteen sticks of dynamite. Prolonged immersion in gasoline produces thermal burns, and this, with added vapor inhalation, can cause serious effects and death.

Hydrocarbon ingestion causes symptoms in two organ systems, the central nervous system and the lungs. In addition, there is the direct irritative action on the pharynx, esophagus, stomach and small intestine with edema and mucosal ulceration and the occasional myocardial injury with arrhythmias and electrocardiographic changes. The central nervous system depression occurs soon after ingestion, followed by severe pneumonitis within a few minutes to several hours. Death, when it occurs, is from pulmonary insufficiency, not the central nervous system depression with drowsiness, tremors and occasionally convulsions which, though alarming at times, rarely produce a fatality. Pathological examination of the lungs shows primarily a severe necrotizing pneumonia. If the patient recovers, no later sequelae are seen. The great seriousness of kerosene poisoning, therefore, is due to pulmonary damage. How this damage comes about as a result of swallowing the liquid, especially when a small amount is involved, has been controversial.

One explanation is that the child can easily aspirate some kerosene because of its low surface tension, either directly or in the course of vomiting or during gastric lavage. This may not be observed by the casual observer, for symptoms of choking and coughing may be insignificant or even missing (the material, because of its spreadability, can seep silently down the tracheobronchial tree).

The opposite idea is that kerosene is absorbed from the gut and excreted by way of the lung. In laboratory experiments, however, kerosene placed in the stomachs of experimental animals failed to produce any striking pulmonary injury. Richardson has shown in rabbits that 0.25 ml of kerosene per kg of body weight could cause a fatal pneumonia when injected directly into the trachea; 35 ml/kg was necessary to produce the same degree of fatal pneumonia when instilled by nasogastric tube into the stomach, and since the rabbit does not vomit, it was assumed that the hydrocarbon must reach the lung via the bloodstream. If these values can be applied to children, a child weighing 10 kg would have to ingest 12 ozs. of these hydrocarbons to produce a fatal pneumonia if no aspiration occurred, whereas only 2.5 ml could cause such a fatal pneumonia if aspiration did occur. Recent well-defined animal experiments using for the first time vervet monkeys, determining lung weight/body weight ratios as well as the pathological results, have clearly demonstrated the fact that the pulmonary effects following kerosene ingestion are not due to absorption via the bloodstream or lymphatics from the stomach, but are due to aspiration into the tracheobronchial tree alone (Wolfsdorf, J. and Kundig, H.: *International Pediatric Congress,* Vienna, August, 1971, Department of Clinical and Experimental Pharmacology, University of the Witwatersrand, Johannesburg). These same investigators, again working with primates, were unable to demonstrate CNS effects when kerosene was given via various routes (except carotid artery and left ventricle). Their conclusion was that CNS signs following ingestion of kerosene are probably not due to direct CNS toxicity and that hypoxia secondary to the pneumonitis and other pulmonary effects is the most likely cause of the CNS manifestations.

On these and numerous other experimental data (Huxtable, K.A. et al.), as well as on clinical evidence and many reports of a more severe pneumonia in patients who have had spontaneous or induced vomiting in this type of poisoning, it would appear conclusively that *treatment* without lavage or emesis is not only preferable, but actually the only logical course to follow. Lavage, if used (for concomitant insecticides, etc.), should be done with extreme care. The head and chest should be lowered, copious amounts of water or 3% sodium bicarbonate solution or normal saline can be used and the tube pinched off and quickly withdrawn. The use of syrup of ipecac to produce forcible vomiting in an alert sitting child should be an easier and a safer procedure to use in such a situation when toxic chemicals or insecticides are involved.

The clinical picture produced by kerosene is quite variable. Symptoms appear early and consist predominantly of either mild cerebral depressive effects or respiratory manifestations or, in some children, both at once.

The child may be found coughing and choking with the odor of kerosene on the breath or clothing. If some time has elapsed following ingestion, he may be drowsy or stuporous. In one series, 6 of 101 patients were found unconscious; about 50 of these children had vomited. Most developed fever (sometimes high), tachycardia and tachypnea. Signs of pulmonary involvement include dyspnea and cyanosis with rales, rhonchi, dullness and diminished breath sounds at one or both bases. Following massive aspiration, pulmonary edema may be marked and is usually the cause of death. Most patients are acutely ill, but those with slight pulmonary manifestations often recover in twenty-four to forty-eight hours. Those with combined cerebral and pulmonary involvement are more acutely ill, and it is among these that cardiac dilatation, transient hepatosplenomegaly and abnormal urinary findings are detected. Electrocardiographic abnormalities with arrhythmias may be evidence of primary myocardial injury.

Roentgenographic changes can be seen within an hour or two of ingestion. At first there are multiple, small, patchy densities with ill-defined margins; in more advanced cases the lesions become larger and tend to coalesce. A double gastric fluid level seen on an upright frontal chest x-ray often gives a reliable estimate (as little as 5 ml) of the amount of kerosene ingested by a child. Emphysema may develop. Pneumothorax occasionally occurs. The maximum changes are noted in two to eight hours after ingestion. Among patients who survive, resolution is gradual, the lungs clearing in three to five days, with radiologic signs lagging behind the clinical improvement. Pneumatoceles are occasionally seen in the latent period and usually disappear without treatment. Pulmonary function and chest radiographs have been reported normal up to ten years later in one series.

*Treatment* in kerosene poisoning is nonspecific and symptomatic. Olive or vegetable oil by mouth, 1 or 2 oz. (if not forced) tends to prevent the absorption of kerosene as well as hurry it through the intestinal tract. In the presence of pulmonary signs, oxygen is the most valuable agent to relieve respiratory distress and anoxia. Antibiotics should be administered in severe and symptomatic lung involvement to forestall secondary pulmonary invaders, which can produce additional serious clinical signs and symptoms. Antibiotics, however, should not be used routinely, nor for asymptomatic patients.

Although the use of steroid therapy for the pulmonary edema, as an anti-inflammatory agent and to prevent aggregation of platelets and leukocytes that block the microcirculation in the treatment of the necrotizing pneumonitis has proven to be effective at times, recent experiments with primates (vervet monkeys) have failed to show any demonstrable positive pulmonary effects with the use of steroids as compared with control animals not receiving therapy. Nevetheless, when confronted with severe pulmonary edema and the shock lung syndrome, methylprednisolone over a four- to eight-hour period may be a boost for survival. Systemic effects from the short period of steroid use are unlikely. Appropriate therapy is indicated for fluid and electrolyte imbalance. Thorough washing of contaminated skin and hair is an important part of therapy.

### *Mineral Seal Oil*

This petroleum oil is obtained as a fraction of distillate from crude petroleum in the range of 500° to 700°F. The relative composition of a particular mineral seal oil varies with the source of the crude petroleum. This refined petroleum hydrocarbon contains unsaturated and saturated aliphatic and aromatic hydrocarbons. The unsaturated aliphatic hydrocarbons are largely removed by acid washings. The resulting product is composed principally of saturated aliphatic hydrocarbons of a higher molecular weight than those characteristic of gasoline and kerosene. It also contains some cyclic and branched-chain compounds.

Since mineral seal oil is a heavier "cut" than the gasoline-kerosene fraction, it is more nearly similar to a light lubricating oil and is used especially in furniture and polishing agents. Variable products of red furniture polish may contain from 20 to 99 per cent mineral seal oil. To this hydrocarbon base, less than 1 per cent by volume of various odorizing and coloring agents are added such as oil of cedarwood, cedarleaf, turpentine, camphor, lemon, wintergreen (methyl salicylate) and traces of aniline dye. Kerosene is added to the products with less mineral seal oil.

The morbidity and mortality from poisoning with this compound are of far greater severity than usually seen in the more commonly observed kerosene intoxication. The systemic symptoms are more severe, with drowsiness, lethargy, high spiking temperatures of two or three weeks duration and rather pronounced extensive pneumonitis demonstrated both by physical examination and by x-rays. Resolution may require three to six weeks, but x-ray changes may persist for months. Emphysema is not uncommon as part of the pneumonic picture and pneumothorax has occasionally been reported.

Several possibilities exist which may in whole or in part be the factors involved in producing this more critical clinical course. Since mineral seal oil is a light lubricating oil, it might act both as a pulmonary irritant and as a foreign body in the lung, thus giving signs and symptoms similar in some respects to both kerosene (chemical) pneumonitis and lipoid pneumonia. Thus the pulmonary irritation is compounded. Another factor undoubtedly is that larger amounts of this product are ingested. Red furniture polish is put up in an attractive container, is brightly colored and slightly flavored and though flat, is not unpleasant to the taste. Kerosene, on the other hand, because of its viscosity, pungent odor and acrid taste is seldom taken in any great quantities. A third factor which may contribute to the severity of the pneumonia is the presence of the small quantities of coloring and odorizing agents in most of these products.

*Treatment* is similar to that for petroleum distillates. However, because of the greater potential for pulmonary complications from aspiration, the stomach should *never* be emptied by gagging or by giving an emetic. Gastric lavage should be done (with a cuffed endotracheal tube if available), if at all, only when unusually large amounts are ingested and the risk of producing vomiting during the procedure would be minimal (older child, adult, etc.). The use of a corticosteroid as an anti-inflammatory agent in addition to the antibiotics and other supportive therapy (Croupette®, Isolette®, etc.) is often effective clinically, though not always supported by results obtained in animal experimentation.

### *Stoddard Solvent (Varsol®)*

Varsol is a trademark name for mineral spirits, also known as Stoddard solvent. The Varsols have viscosities below 32 SUS (0.91 to 0.95 centipoises at 25°C) and thus do present an aspiration hazard. Their toxicity is very similar to that of kerosene. Aspiration of as little as a few milliliters may cause chemical pneumonia and pulmonary edema. Although the Varsols vary somewhat in their composition, they all meet the specifications of the Department of Commerce of Stoddard solvent. They are mixtures of various hydrocarbons, including straight– and branched-chain paraffins (aliphatic hydrocarbons), cycloparaffins (naphthenes) and alkyl derivatives of benzene. They contain 30 to 70 per cent paraffins, e.g. heptane, octane; 20 to 50 per cent cycloparaffins; and 10 to 20 per cent aromatics, e.g. xylol. They are used for paint and varnish thinners, for dry cleaning and for general plant machinery cleaning and degreasing. The MAC in air is 500 ppm.

### *Benzene (Toluene)*

Benzene (benzol) occurs in coal tar distillates and is widely used as a commercial solvent. Some motor fuels contain 25 per cent or more of benzene. The MAC is 35 to 50 ppm. Most cases of poisoning are due to the inhalation of vapors in poorly ventilated rooms or from skin contact. A number of deaths have been reported in workmen cleaning out tank cars. The symptoms are due to gastric irritation and to depression of the central nervous system and bone marrow. Mild symptoms consist of irritation of the upper respiratory tract with cough, conjunctivitis, euphoria, dizziness, headache, nausea, vomiting, weakness, constriction in the chest, pallor and burning epigastric pain. More severe symptoms progress to visual blurring, tremors, excitement, delirium, unconsciousness, coma and convulsions. In chronic poisoning from inhalation, there is weakness, drowsiness, anorexia and anemia with abnormal bleeding, which may progress to complete aplasia of the bone marrow. Intentional toluene sniffing can produce renal tubular defects with metabolic acidosis, electrolyte abnormalities and potassium loss. Irreversible brain atrophy with CNS deficits has been documented in toluene-sniffing addicts.

Toluene diisocyanate (TDI) used as a polymerizing agent in the plastics industry has resulted in thrombocytopenic purpura and various upper respiratory tract syndromes. This compound is a highly reactive substance with great sensitizing potential. An initial exposure tends to sensitize the individual, with more severe symptoms occurring after subsequent exposures. Appropriate protective measures for workers with TDI present a major difficulty, since concentrations of the chemical as low as 0.1 ppm are apparently too high for safety.

In the *treatment* it is essential to prevent further absorption by removing the patient from contaminated air and administering artificial respiration and oxygen. If ingested, gastric lavage should be done with care (*see* Kerosene) to avoid aspiration. Follow with mineral oil to prevent further absorption. Emetics should not be given. In skin contamination, the skin should be thoroughly washed with soap and water. Epinephrine, ephedrine or related drugs should not be given since they may induce fatal ventricular fibrillation. In case of aplastic anemia, the advice of a competent hematologist should be sought for use of transfusion, steroids and antibiotics.

*Naphthalene (See page 191)*

*Turpentine*

Turpentine is a colorless oil with characteristic odor and taste obtained from the distillation of pine wood and used as a solvent in paints, polishes and varnishes. The MAC is 100 ppm. As little as 1 tbsp. has caused death in children, while 4 to 6 fl. oz. have produced fatal poisoning in adults.

Hexol, a pine oil distillate related to turpentine and commonly used as a household disinfectant, can also cause symptoms as noted below.

Severe gastrointestinal symptoms arise from the irritant action of the oil. Nausea, vomiting, pain and diarrhea are prominent early effects when turpentine is taken orally. Nervous system stimulation results in excitement and delirium, and these are followed by central nervous system depression and respiratory arrest. The pulse is weak and rapid. The kidneys are irritated and albumin, casts, hemoglobin and red cells appear in the urine; irreversible renal failure, however, rarely occurs. The presence of turpentine bound with glycuronate in the urine imparts to the latter a characteristic odor of violets. Intoxication from prolonged inhalation of the vapors causes conjunctivitis, rhinitis, bronchitis, pneumonia, rapid heart action, nephritis, dizziness and tachypnea.

*Treatment* consists of removing the ingested turpentine by gastric lavage. This should be followed with milk, mineral or vegetable oil or other demulcents to allay gastric irritation. If respiration is depressed, artificial respiration and oxygen should be administered. After the pulmonary edema stage has passed, and if renal function is not impaired, fluids should be forced up to 4 liters daily to maintain urinary output. Those having symptoms from inhalation should be moved from their environment to fresh air and artificial respiration and oxygen used if necessary. The urine and blood should be examined frequently for evidence of complications.

## CORROSIVES

### Acids

*Hydrochloric, Sulfuric, Nitric and Miscellaneous Acids*

These agents are used for cleaning metals and other products as well as in a variety of chemical reactions. Poisoning by mineral acids is usually severe and runs a rapid course. The fatal amount for an adult is between 1 tsp. and ½ oz. of the concentrated chemical, but even a few drops may be lethal if the acid gains access to the trachea. The corrosive effects produced are evident wherever the acid comes in contact with tissue—the skin, mucous membranes, tongue, pharynx, esophagus, stomach and small intestine. The severity of the damage depends on the concentration of the chemical and the duration of exposure. In general, sulfuric acid is the most and hydrochloric acid the least corrosive of the three. Concentrated nitric acid and hydrochloric acid give off fumes which are extremely irritating to the respiratory tract and cause marked inflammation and edema of the pulmonary alveoli. Nitric acid colors tissues a deep yellow. Those coming in contact with any of these acids are severely burned and the skin may be completely charred. If recovery occurs, healing is by scar tissue replacement.

The symptoms of poisoning by these acids are corrosion of the skin and mucosa. Even if the acid is swallowed, so great is the pain that reflex spasm of the glottis prevents some of it from passing down the esophagus and the remainder escapes from the mouth to burn the face. The tongue and mouth are raw and swollen. Also, the posterior pharynx and often larynx are involved, and the resulting edema and inflammation may dangerously impair the patency of the airway. Swallowing and speech are painful and sometimes impossible. The stomach and esophagus (often escapes) are badly burned, as well as the first part of the small intestine. The entire mucosa may eventually slough and disappear. Bloody vomitus containing large shreds of gastric mucosa, severe local and abdominal pain, marked thirst, evidences of severe shock and imminent danger of perforation of the stomach are the outstanding features of ingestion of these acids. Death from shock and collapse may occur from an hour to a day or two later or may intervene suddenly from suffocation if the acid enters the trachea. Coma and convulsions are sometimes terminal events. Death may also ensue from perforation and peritonitis, severe nephritis or pneumonia after a few days' latent period.

Due to the rapidity with which these acids act, any local or general therapy must be carried out quickly and efficiently in order to do any good. Local *treatment* consists of abundant washing of the skin and mucosa with water. If weak alkalis such as sodium bicarbonate or limewater are handy, these may be used but no time should be lost if they are not immediately available. Special care should be given to the eyes; these should be kept open under running water. After all traces of acid are removed, the remainder of local treatment consists of alleviation of pain, prevention of shock and infection and therapy for burns. This latter differs in no way from the treatment of burns due to other agents. Brooke's formula of 1.5 ml of electrolyte and 0.5 ml of colloid per kg of body weight times 50 is useful immediate supportive therapy.

The systematic therapy has first to do with removal of the poison from the stomach. If the patient is seen some time after swallowing the acid, there is danger of perforation from attempts to pass a stomach tube. If the patient is seen early (within an hour), it may be safe to pass, gently, a small well-oiled nasal tube. Copious washing with water or saline solution should then be done. Milk, raw eggs or soap solution can be used as a substitute.

Morphine without stint should be given for alleviation of the severe pain. The respiration should be watched for signs of embarrassment as a result of inhalation of the fumes or acid. The passage of an endotracheal airway may be necessary if laryngeal edema develops. Supportive therapy for shock should be instituted as soon as the antidotal treatment is performed. If the diagnosis of second- or third-degree esophageal or gastric burns is established either by x-ray or by endoscopy, any peritoneal signs or deterioration in the patient's condition is presumptive evidence of gastric necrosis and perforation, and exploratory laparotomy should be done. If the gastric wall is black or ecchymotic, the involved stomach must be resected, along with whatever adjacent organs have been damaged. If the patient recovers, residual gastric ulceration or stenosis of the esophagus or pylorus (a more frequent occurrence in the author's experience) due to scar tissue may require treatment. Hydrochloric acid, being less corrosive, is more likely to cause stenosis than perforation. Steroid therapy has been used for the prevention of esophageal and gastric strictures (*see* Alkalis), but there are some reports of increased incidence of perforation from its use.

### *Hydrofluoric Acid*

Hydrofluoric acid (more toxic than sodium fluoride) is an aqueous solution of hydrogen fluoride in a concentration of 47 per cent and 53 per cent, with a specific gravity of 1.150 and 1.180 respectively. It is used in glass etching and as a corrosive agent in various industries and trades. Contact of hydrofluoric acid with the skin, though it may not cause an immediate reaction, nevertheless can produce severe injury and even death. Low concentrations cause only erythema, but more concentrated solutions cause severe pain and give the skin a blanched and edematous appearance. This is followed by vesication and extensive necrosis of the tissue, which has a tendency to heal slowly. If the nail bed becomes inflamed, the nail may be destroyed or lost, and the destruction may even extend to the bone. The inhalation of high concentrations of hydrofluoric acid may result immediately in vomiting and fatal collapse. With exposure to lower concentrations, the conjunctiva and the mucous membranes of the nose, mouth, larynx, trachea and bronchi show severe inflammation and often ulceration. There may be anosmia, so that the presence of the irritant gas is not noted. With short exposure to low concentrations, cough and lacrimation may be the only symptoms, and they may disappear upon discontinuance of the exposure. When ingested, hydrofluoric acid acts as a violent corrosive poison. Small doses may cause burning pain and constriction in the pharynx, severe gastritis, retching, vomiting and great debility; while larger doses can cause extensive necrosis with perforation of the stomach, shock and death.

*Treatment* consists of immediate gastric lavage with copious amounts of tap water or limewater until the returning fluid is clear. This should be followed by demulcents. In case hydrofluoric vapors are inhaled, the patient should be transferred to fresh air and treated by inhalation of a mist of a 1% solution of calcium chloride. Steroids may be effective for pulmonary edema. Acid burns of the skin are treated with wet dressings of a mixture of magnesium oxide and magnesium sulfate. Areas of severe inflammation and possible necrosis should be infiltrated with a 5% to 10% calcium gluconate solution. If the eye is affected, it can be covered with a 20% magnesium oxide dressing and further treated as outlined in the section for chemical burns. Because of the severe pain, analgesics and sedatives are usually required.

### *Oxalic Acid (Oxalates)*

Oxalic acid and oxalates are used as bleaches and metal cleaners in industry (process engraving, photography, calico printing and dyeing, indigo dyeing, purification of methanol, manufacture of dyes, celluloid, rubber, ceramics, pigments) and in household products (bleaches, metal polishes, anti-rust solutions, paint and varnish removers, ink eradicators). The presence of these compounds about the home has led to numerous accidental ingestions because of the similarity between oxalic acid and Epsom salts and between potassium hydrogen oxalate and cream of tartar. The oxalates present in certain vegetables (rhubarb leaves, beets, etc.) and citrus fruits rarely produce any ill effects, and claims of poisoning from these sources are often greatly exaggerated.

The median adult lethal dose has been reported to be between 15 and 30 gm with death occurring in a few hours. However, as little as 5 gm has caused death.

Corrosive action to mucous membranes is more pronounced with oxalic acid than with its salts and is not due to acidity alone. Severe gastroenteritis and the secondary shock that often results may produce a fatality before specific therapy can be started.

Oxalates combine with serum calcium to form nonionized insoluble calcium oxalate.

The resultant hypocalcemia leads to violent muscular stimulation with convulsions and collapse. The oxaluria which results from the renal excretion of oxalates may cause renal colic and hematuria. Pathologically, the kidney shows cloudy swelling, sclerosis of tubules and hyaline degeneration. Cerebral edema is a frequent finding, along with the corrosive lesions in the mouth, pharynx, esophagus and stomach.

The first manifestations of oxalate poisoning are a burning sensation in mouth and pharynx which may be associated with difficulties in swallowing, edema and ulceration of the oral and pharyngeal cavities. Often the patient experiences pain in the epigastric and lumbar regions followed by hematemesis because of hemorrhagic gastritis and corrosion of the stomach. The patient may suffer from dryness in the mouth and thirst. In spite of the severe inflammatory reactions and corrosions, perforation of the stomach is rare. The intestine may show inflammatory reactions and hemorrhages, resulting in diarrhea with bloody stools. The pulse is usually slow, weak, soft and irregular; the blood pressure may be lowered, the heart may be dilated and the patient may pass into collapse. The respiration is slow and often depressed. There is severe injury of the kidneys, resulting in oliguria, anuria and uremia. Frequently patients suffer from headache, trismus and twitchings of the musculature, especially of the face (tetany), and they may suffer from paresthesia and polyneuritic pain in the limbs. The reflexes may be exaggerated and there may be patellar and ankle clonus. In severe cases, the patient becomes rapidly unconscious and stuporous and develops convulsions, the latter being frequently of uremic origin. The pupils are dilated and react sluggishly, and there may be visual disturbance. The urine may contain albumin, red and white blood cells, hematin and oxalate crystals. Prolonged contact with solutions of oxalic acid has resulted in paresthesia, cyanosis of the fingers, pale yellow discoloration of the fingernails and even gangrene. The inhalation of steam carrying oxalic acid has been reported to cause nosebleeds, excruciating headaches, repeated spells of vomiting, and later backache, loss of weight, nervousness, anemia, albuminuria and prostration.

*Treatment* consists of gastric lavage with limewater (calcium hydroxide), chalk or other calcium salts and the administration of magnesium sulfate as a cathartic. It is essential to stimulate and maintain diuresis, if the renal function remains normal, by the administration of copious amounts of fluids (up to 4 liters daily) to prevent the deposition of calcium oxalate crystals in the renal tubules. Vomiting may be attenuated by the administration of demulcents. The hypocalcemia and some of the systemic effects may be alleviated by the parenteral administration of calcium salts. Otherwise, the treatment has to be symptomatic and supportive. Treatment is designed to precipitate the oxalate in an insoluble form in the stomach; therefore, magnesium sulfate or carbonate or calcium chloride, carbonate or lactate are added to the lavage fluid. Alkalis cannot be used as antidotes against oxalic acid because the salts which are formed in this way are even more soluble than the acid itself and about as poisonous. Magnesium and calcium salts can be used because they precipitate magnesium oxalate and calcium oxalate, which are insoluble. Calcium gluconate 10 ml of a 10% solution should be given intravenously or intramuscularly and repeated if symptoms persist.

In severe cases, parathyroid extract (100 U.S.P. units) should be given IM. Morphine may be necessary for the control of pain.

## Alkalis

Caustic alkali poisoning may result from the ingestion of many household products. Treatment for this type of poisoning varies to a certain extent with the agent ingested, its concentration and whether it is in the liquid or crystalline state. Lye in concentrated solution creates rapid transmural gastric and esophageal necrosis that spreads insidiously to the contiguous organs. Thus, while some alkalis require vigorous and immediate attention, others, such as chlorinated alkalis, are far less dangerous.

Sodium and potassium hydroxide (caustic soda or potash), sodium and potassium carbonates, sodium phosphates, peroxides and oxides are used in the manufacture of soap, chemical synthesis, washing powders, household drainpipe cleaning agents (lye, Drano® [liquid form only contains 9.5 per cent of sodium hydroxide], Pronto®, etc.) and in glycosuria testing tablets (Clinitest® tablets). Liquid Plum'r® has been reformulated to reduce the amount of hydroxide (2.5%) plus potassium silicate (5%) and sodium hypochlorite (4.6%). Several other chemicals have been added which do not affect its toxicity. These compounds combine with protein to form proteinates and with fats to form soap, thus producing, related to the alkali concentration, deep caustic and penetrating burns on contact with tissues. Eight of eleven ingestions of Clinitest tablets resulted in esophageal strictures, some after the ingestion of only one tablet. When swallowed, usually without water, the sodium hydroxide in the tablet acts with saliva to create enough heat to cause a full-thickness esophageal burn.

Symptoms of alkali ingestion are burning pain from mouth to stomach. Swallowing is difficult at first and then impossible. Mucous membranes are soapy and white but become brown, edematous and ulcerated; vomitus is bloody and may contain shreds of mucous membrane. The pulse is feeble and rapid; respiration is increased and collapse may ensue. Death due to shock, asphyxia from glottic edema, or intercurrent infection, pneumonia or mediastinitis may occur in forty-eight to seventy-two hours in severe poisoning. Within weeks or months, or sometimes years, esophageal stricture develops. It is a paradox that corrosive acid ingestion produces fewer permanent effects on the esophagus than do the alkalis, and it is not unusual for individuals suffering from corrosive acid poisoning to develop gastric injury and pyloric stenosis instead of esophageal strictures. However, the ingestion of large amounts of alkali (especially in liquid form) in suicidal attempts can also produce severe and serious caustic lesions in the stomach, and gastroscopy and surgery should not be neglected in these situations if indicated (*see* Acids).

Alkali coming into contact with the skin may produce first–, second–, or even third-degree chemical and exothermic burns depending on concentration of alkali and duration of contact. Eye involvement may cause severe conjunctivitis as well as corneal destruction. The white, thick liquid or paste in the core of some old golf balls may contain sodium hydroxide, and the accidental splashing of this material into the eye may cause serious injury.

In the *treatment,* milk, water or tea (cold preferably) should be given immediately. Since swallowing is painful, difficult and almost impossible at times, flushing or irrigation of the mouth with water is often the only and best immediate therapy. The damage to the esophagus in animal experiments from caustic alkali ingestion occurs within the first minute, and the value of first aid measures thereafter (neutralizing solutions, water, milk or whatever) is of questionable value (Kiviranta, U.: Corrosion of the esophagus and stomach. *Acta Otolaryngol [Suppl],* 81, 1949). Strong acidic antidotes are contraindicated because of the release of heat. Under no circumstances should a gas-releasing carbonated beverage be given. Do *not* use gastric lavage or emetics since the small amount of alkali that usually reaches the stomach is rapidly neutralized by the acid gastric juice. Olive oil or other demulcents ease pain. Esophagoscopy should be done within forty-eight hours by an experienced endoscopist to determine future management of such patients. To avoid perforations, the endoscope should not pass the first site of burn. The absence of oral burns should never preclude this examination as esophageal injury may be present with little or no mouth involvement.

Steroids are effective in diminishing fibroelastic acitivity and act as anti-inflammatory agents in preventing esophageal stenosis in rabbits after the ingestion of lye. These effects suggested the use of steroids for the prevention of stenosis in children who have swallowed a caustic alkali. Recently, similar favorable results were observed in cats, whose esophagi more closely resemble those of children. Clinical reports in humans, though often favorable, have occasionally given equivocal results with this type of therapy. Nevertheless, the use of corticosteroids is rational therapy in that it is less painful, less time-consuming, less expensive and probably more effective in preventing strictures than the older procedure of bougienage as developed by Bokay and Salzer. For children one to four years old, divided doses of 60 mg/day of prednisolone are given for the first four days; 40 mg/day is given for the next four days, and finally 20 mg/day is given until the esophagus is healed, usually in three weeks. Alternate dosage regimen of 2 mg/kg/day of prednisolone or equivalents for three weeks or longer can be used. The standard dose for older children and adults is 60 to 100 mg/day with corresponding decreases in dosage during the treatment program. A broad-spectrum antibiotic suspension is given orally as long as steroids are continued. Large doses of penicillin are administered parenterally for mediastinal or pulmonary complications. BAPN (beta-aminopropionitrile), a lysyl oxidase inhibitor, is a powerful known osteolathyrogen. Lathyrogens specifically inhibit intermolecular covalent bonding in newly synthesized collagen. It has been recently shown that BAPN can prevent stenosis in dogs exposed to esophageal lye burns (Madden, J. W., Davis, W. M., Butler, C., and Peacock, E. E.: Experimental Esophageal Lye Burns: Corrective Established Strictures with Beta-aminopropionitrile and Bougienage. *Ann Surg, 178*:277, 1973). The hypothesis is that wound healing under the influence of BAPN resulted in weakened collagen bonds. This weakness allowed subsequent mechanical dilatation to be more effective. Hopefully, research on BAPN and other similar molecules will provide another and more effective modality of treatment. Penicillamine especially should be explored for similar activity. Insertion of a nasogastric tube for feeding can also help maintain a patent esophageal lumen by preventing adhesions and can aid in future dilatation if necessary.

As an alternate, an older (Salzer) method of treatment, bougienage, may be used. On the third or fourth day, after the inflammation and edema of the esophageal mucosa have subsided, and daily for two weeks, a rubber eyeless catheter filled with mercury or small lead or steel shot should be passed into the stomach. The catheter size should be gradually increased until a No. 32 or 34 enters easily. Dilatation should be continued for four weeks. If the dilator passes with difficulty and partial stricture is suspected or demonstrated by barium swallow or esophagoscopy, dilatation should be continued periodically for at least one year. This method can prevent 75 per cent of esophageal strictures, but cooperation is usually so poor that this figure is seldom attained. Combined therapy of steroids and bougienage is used in some centers.

Formerly, acute and aggressive surgical therapy generally was not considered for severe injuries caused by crystalline lye ingestion. Initial management was conservative. The late complications of esophageal or, more rarely, gastric strictures afforded the surgeon time for a contemplative approach to elective bypass of the obstruction.

In contrast, the natural history of concentrated liquid lye ingestion indicates the need for an aggressive surgical approach, including (1) exploratory laparotomy after roentgenographic confirmation of injury, (2) total gastrectomy for gastric necrosis, (3) right-sided thoracotomy when the distal part of the intra-abdominal esophagus is questionably viable, (4) esophagectomy for esophageal necrosis and (5) delayed restoration of gastrointestinal tract continuity with colon interposition. Failure to remove the esophagus may result in coagulation necrosis spreading to the membranous trachea or aorta adjacent to the esophagus. Recently, the insertion of a silastic intraluminal esophageal splint for three weeks on several patients with full-thickness esophageal burns successfully prevented strictures. Compression of the granulation tissues by the splint left a clean base for complete epithelialization, which established a patent esophageal lumen.

Areas of the skin that come in contact with alkali should be thoroughly cleansed with running water until skin is free of alkali as indicated by disappearance of soapiness. Flowing water from a shower stall equipped with a chair for twelve to twenty-four hours has been used successfully for this purpose when skin area involved has been extensive. In second– or third-degree burns, 2% acetic acid wet dressings should be used for a day or two to complete neutralization of the alkali in deeper tissues since cauterization continues otherwise. Mafenide acetate (Sulfamylon®), which is bacteriostatic and also combines with any remaining active lye to form harmless sodium acetate and mafenide radicals, is an alternate and probably preferable therapy for this purpose.

Alkalis produce some of the most severe chemical eye injuries. The increase in hydroxyl ion concentration beyond the limits of tissue protein stability results in the formation of gel-like alkaline proteinates. In addition, the reaction with fats to form soaps produces considerable damage to the structure of the cell membranes and thus allows the alkali to penetrate rapidly into the tissues. The speed of penetration is responsible for the capacity of alkalis to cause great ocular damage. Treatment consists of the quick, thorough irrigation of the eye with water at the nearest source of supply for five minutes. After installation of a local anesthetic, irrigation with water or normal saline is continued for half an hour. Any attempt to treat a chemical eye injury with a specific neutralizing agent is now considered detrimental. An ophthalmologist should be consulted for degree of damage and specific therapy.

*Treatment of strictures.* In general, single or short strictures, as determined by esophagoscopy or esophagogram, often can be treated by antegrade dilatation (cerebral abscess has rarely been reported to occur with this procedure). Multiple strictures usually require retrograde dilatation through a gastrostomy. Gastrostomy, when necessary, should be placed in the fundus of the stomach directed toward the cardia and should avoid the proximity of the ribs. For chronic strictures, various surgical procedures utilizing colon or intestinal loops or portions of stomach can replace the esophagus in part or preferably totally.

Steriod injections directly into chronic esophageal stenotic lesions have been reported to dramatically and quickly reverse the course of the cicatricial lesion, eliminating the need of further dilatation or instrumentation or making further dilatation more responsive (Waggoner, L. G.: In Bockus, H. L. IEd.I: *Gastroenterology,* 3rd ed. Philadelphia, Saunders, 1976, pp. 289-294).

### *Chlorinated Alkalis (Hypochlorite, Clorox®, Etc.)*

Bleaches are among the most common compounds (household agent or drug) ingested by children. As a matter of fact, ingestion of bleaches represents approximately 5 per cent of all poisonings in children under five years of age reported to the poison control centers, ahead now of aspirin (*see* Table 62 for contents of household bleaches).

These agents are chlorinated alkalis or hypochlorites (Clorox and bleaches of many varieties) that are corrosive with resulting caustic actions depending not only on their variable degrees of alkalinity, but also on their potent oxidizing effects producing "available chlorine." Systemic effects rarely occur, and though harsh to mucous membranes with occasional alarming irritation and edema of the pharynx and larynx, local effects are usually insignificant.

In a survey of two separate reports of 339 and 129 cases of Clorox ingestion, only two patients showed any evidence of esophageal injury. These were mild and of such a nature as to exclude the possibility of the late development of stricture. However, esophageal strictures do occur rarely and have been documented. Routine esophagoscopy for

TABLE 62
CONTENTS OF COMMON HOUSEHOLD BLEACHES

| *Bleach* | *Contents* |
|---|---|
| Sodium hypochlorite solutions | Liquid bleaches commonly referred to as chlorine bleach generally contain about 5% sodium hypochlorite. Packets sold in vending machines may be more concentrated (about 10%). They contain small amounts of free alkali. |
| Sodium perborate bleaches | Generally dry products containing sodium perborate (tetrahydrate) or sodium perborate monohydrate in the range of 15–85%. Other ingredients present may include sodium carbonate, sodium tripolyphosphate, sodium sulfate, sodium silicate, or other common laundry detergent ingredients. These products, therefore, can be strongly alkaline in addition to their borate toxicity. |
| Dichloroisocyanurates and trichloroisocyanurates | Generally dry bleach powders or tablets containing 20–30% of the chloroisocyanurate with phosphates, carbonates, or other ingredients listed above under sodium perborate bleaches. These products may be strongly irritating and their toxicity is due to their corrosive action rather than to any systemic effects. |
| Optical bleaches | These are additives present in some laundry products as fabric brighteners in amounts up to 0.2%. They vary in toxicity from around 2–20 gm/kg. |
| Hair bleaches | These include hydrogen peroxide 6% (20 volume), ammonium hydroxide 1%, vinegar and lemon rinses. |
| Hair neutralizers | Cold wave neutralizers are oxidizing agents and include hydrogen peroxide 6%, sodium perborate about 80–90%, and in some cases sodium bromate about 12–15%. |

evaluation is apparently not indicated unless considerable corrosion of the oropharynx is noted or if unusually large amounts of undiluted solution have been ingested.

There have been incidents documented in which housewives have mixed acid-type toilet bowl cleaners with sodium hypochlorite bleaches that resulted in toxic fumes. The mixture produces chlorine gas which, when inhaled, may cause respiratory irritation (rarely pulmonary edema) with coughing and labored breathing, along with inflammation of the eyes and other mucous membranes (*see* Table 63).

*Treatment* is symptomatic. Sips of milk or other demulcents to allay the burning sensation of the oral mucous membranes are usually all that is necessary. Although these preparations are alkaline, on contact with acid gastric juice or acid solutions they release hypochlorous acid, which is extremely irritating. Buffering the acid by administration of alkali, paradoxic as it may seem, reduces the irritative effect. Vigorous antialkali therapy, however, is rarely indicated. Magnesium hydroxide in milk of magnesia (1 oz.) is a useful antacid, absorbent and demulcent for this purpose. Sodium bicarbonate should be avoided because it releases carbon dioxide which may produce considerable gas and gastric distention.

## *Monopersulfate, Potassium*

This is one of the more recent types of potent oxidizing agents used in bleaching and germicidal preparations for home laundry and bathroom. It has the capacity of oxidizing chloride ion to chlorine, so that the combination of monopersulfate and sodium chloride provides both oxygen and chlorine in an "activated" bleach that can be made almost odorless. Other ingredients which may be formulated with monopersulfate for special purposes are alkyl aryl sulfonates, certain nonionic detergents, some polyphosphate, carboxymethylcellulose, etc. Since monoper-

TABLE 63
EFFECTS OF BLEACH AND HOUSEHOLD PRODUCT MIXTURES

| *Bleach* | *Added agents* | *Chemical reaction* | *Effects* | *Symptoms* |
|---|---|---|---|---|
| Na hypochlorite (Clorox) | Strong acid (toilet bowl cleaners) | $NaOCl + H^+ \rightarrow Cl_2 + H_2O$ & $NaCl$ & $HCO_3$ | Chlorine gas | Extremely irritating fumes; 10–20 mg/cu m causes stinging & burning of eyes, nose & throat. 40–60 mg/cu m fatal |
| Oxidizes as pH becomes neutral | Ammonia ($NH_3$) 16% ammonium hydroxide | $NH_3 + NaOCl \rightarrow NH_2Cl + NaOH$ | Chloramine fumes; acrid, unstable | Watering of eyes, irritation of nose & throat, nausea, "temporarily overcome" |
| Active bleaching pH 4–10 | Lye Strong alkali Na hydroxide | Increase pH and stabilize hypochlorite | No fumes produced, only those attributable to lye itself | Only lye burns |
| pH 11–13, stable | Weak acid (vinegar) | HOCl and OCl | None; slight lowering of pH would enhance bleaching | None |
| No pH change | Laundry detergents | None | None | Only those of constituents |

sulfate forms acidic solutions, an alkaline filler such as sodium carbonate (or soda ash) sufficient to provide a solution pH of 9 to 10 is necessary. The approximate oral lethal dose in male albino rats is 2.25 gm/kg. Aqueous solutions of 2.5% to 3.0% are not irritating on skin of the human forearm or guinea pig; 25% solutions, however, are strong primary irritants on guinea pigs.

*Treatment* is similar to that outlined for alkalis, albeit less vigorous.

## *Ammonia, Ammonium Hydroxide, Picrate and Sulfide*

Ammonia is a gas at ordinary temperatures, while ammonium hydroxide is a liquid containing from 10% to 35% ammonia. Ammonia is used as a refrigerant, fertilizer and in organic synthesis. Ammonium hydroxide is used mainly as a cleaning agent, while the picrate is extensively employed in the munition and fireworks industry. The sulfide salt is used in metallurgy, photographic developers, textiles and in certain "cold wave sets." These compounds injure cells by their direct caustic and necrotizing action, while inhalation can cause pulmonary irritation, edema and pneumonia. Skin contact may cause dermatitis of various types. The MAC of ammonia is 100 ppm, and the lethal dose of ammonium hydroxide is 30 ml (1 oz.) of the 25% concentration.

*Symptoms and Treatment* (*see* Alkalis). Ammonia fumes may cause irritation of the eyes and the upper respiratory tract with cough, vomiting, conjunctivitis and inflammation of the mucous membranes of lips, mouth and pharynx. With high concentration, there is pulmonary irritation with edema, cyanosis, bronchitis and pneumonia. These symptoms require removing the patient from the contaminated area and applying artificial respiration, oxygen and other supportive therapy.

## Gases

Parts per million indicates units of volume of the toxic gas in one million volumes. Since the volume occupied by a gas is dependent on the molecular weight, the following formula must be used to convert from ppm to mg/cu. m.

$$\frac{ppm \times molecular\ weight}{22.4}$$

For example the MAC of carbon tetrachloride 10 ppm represents a concentration of 68 mg/cu. m (1 cu. m = 35.3 cu. ft.). Detectors for many gases are available from the Matheson Company, P.O. Box 85, East Rutherford, New Jersey.

### *Fluorine and Derivatives*

Fluorine and hydrogen fluoride are gases at normal temperature, the former being used in organic synthesis while the latter is used in etching glass and in the petroleum industry. Skin or mucous membrane contact with hydrogen fluoride produces caustic necrotic ulcerations, since it is corrosive to tissue on direct contact. The most prominent findings in fatalities from the inhalation of these compounds are pulmonary edema and pneumonia. The MAC in air for fluorine is 0.1 ppm and 3 ppm for hydrogen fluoride.

The symptoms from these gases are due to inhalation and/or skin contact causing inflammation or corrosion, the severity of which depends on the degree of exposure or contact. Cough, fever, chills, cyanosis, chest pain and constriction, burns and ulcerations of the skin and mucous membranes are the principal manifestations.

*Treatment* is directed toward preventing pulmonary edema and severe burns of the skin and mucous membranes. The patient should be moved from his exposed environment to fresh air and artificial respiration and oxygen given if indicated. The skin should be thoroughly washed under a stream of water for fifteen minutes, and a burn paste of magnesium oxide with 20% glycerine should be applied and allowed to remain long enough to neutralize the caustic effect to the deeper tissues (for sodium [neutral] fluoride poisoning, *see* Chap 2).

### *Cyanide (*Also see *Hydrocyanic Acid)*

This is one of the most rapidly acting of all poisons. In the form of the extremely volatile hydrocyanic acid (prussic acid), its inhalation causes severe toxic effects which lead to death in a very few minutes. The chemist Karl Wilhelm Scheele, discoverer of this acid, was killed by its vapors.

Hydrogen cyanide and its derivatives (acrylonitrile, cyanamide, cyanogen chloride, cyanides, nitroprussides) are used in fumigants, metal cleaners, refining of ores, production of synthetic rubber and in chemical synthesis. In the home, cyanides are present in silver polish, rodenticides and in the seeds of the apple, peach, plum, apricot, cherry and almond. Sodium nitroprusside is used in the treatment of hypertensive crises and to produce a bloodless surgical field for intracranial surgery. Cyanide toxicity and metabolic acidosis have been reported from its excessive use.

Other amygdalin-containing (cyanogenetic glycoside) fruit seeds less frequently or inadvertently consumed are jet beads, choke cherries, cassava beans and bitter almonds. It has been demonstrated that the cyanide content of 100 gm moist peach seed is 88 mg, cultivated apricot 8.9 mg and wild apricot 217 mg. Apricot kernels, widely available in health food stores and promoted as nutritional and medicinal products, have been associated with cyanide poisoning in California. The inadvertent ingestion of 1 to 5 tablets (500 mg) of amygdalin (Laetrile®) caused the death of an eleven-month-old girl, whose father was taking the oral drug for a malignant neoplasm (*JAMA, 238*:482, 1977). Due to the increased interest and changing legislation, amygdalin is becoming more accessible. Its use is controversial, its potential toxic effects are not well known and, unfortunately, many users consider it a harmless vitamin ($B_{17}$).

Amygdalin present in seeds is harmless as such. However, when the seed is crushed and the pulp moistened, the enzyme emulsin, which is also present, produces the following response:

$$\underset{\text{(amygdalin)}}{C_{20}H_{27}NO_{11}} + 2H_2O \longrightarrow \underset{\text{(glucose)}}{2C_6H_{12}O_6} + \underset{\text{(benzaldehyde)}}{C_6H_5CHO} + \underset{\text{(cyanide)}}{HCN}$$

This reaction takes place very slowly in the presence of an acid pH, but in an alkaline medium it occurs quickly, hydrolysis being completed in ten minutes at 20°C. This fact perhaps explains why symptoms of intoxication occur after some delay, since there is an interval for transit from the stomach to the alkaline medium of the duodenum. Calcium cyanamide and ferri– or ferrocyanides do not liberate cyanide when acidified, nor are they metabolized to cyanide *in vivo.* They have a comparatively low order of toxicity with an estimated lethal oral dose of 50 gm for an adult.

Pigmented forms of *Pseudomonas aeruginosa* are capable of producing detectable quantities of cyanide both *in vitro* and *in vivo.* Viscera and eschar from five fatally infected burn patients contained varying amounts of cyanide.

The MAC of hydrogen cyanide is 10 ppm, and the fatal dose is approximately 50 mg (¾ gr). Cyanide compounds, which are capable of releasing hydrocyanic acid, are generally protoplasmic poisons. They paralyze respiration of all cells of the body by interfering with the enzymes controlling the oxidative processes of cell respiration. For this reason, cyanide action has been described as "internal asphyxia." The respiratory center of the medulla ceases to function because its nerve cells can no longer obtain oxygen for their respiration. The venous blood of a patient dying of cyanide is bright red and resembles arterial blood because the tissues have not been able to utilize the oxygen brought to them.

While it is true that some cyanide combines with hemoglobin to form a stable non-oxygen-bearing compound, cyanhemoglobin, this substance is formed only slowly and in a small amount. Death is not due to cyanhemoglobin but to inhibition of tissue cell respiration.

Cyanide is detectable by its bitter almond odor and by specific chemical tests. After oral ingestion of cyanide salts, absorption of some of the material occurs so rapidly and produces death so quickly that the remainder is often found unabsorbed in the gastric contents and should be sought there. The spectroscope also aids in the identification of cyanhemoglobin.

Symptoms may appear with dramatic suddenness when large doses are taken or may be delayed several minutes. Death usually occurs within an hour. Mortality from cyanide is reported as high as 95 per cent. The longer the patient is kept alive, the better his chances are for recovery, because the body detoxifies cyanide by combining it with sulfur compounds to form stable and inactive sulfocyanates. Cardiac manifestations such as atrial fibrillation, ectopic ventricular beats and abnormal QRS with the T wave originating high on the R wave can be detected early by electrocardiographic studies. In addition, there is the naturally occurring enzyme rhodanese which converts the cyanide ion to thiocyanate, a relatively non-toxic compound excreted in the urine, a reaction markedly potentiated in the presence of sodium thiosulfate.

The symptoms which occur in quick succession are giddiness, headache, palpitation, dyspnea and then unconsciousness. There may be some evidences of local irritation from the salts, and this may result in nausea and vomiting. As a rule, depression is already marked before this can occur. Central stimulation is very fleeting, and what are usually called cyanide convulsions are in reality terminal asphyxial convulsions. The breath, as well as the tissues of the body after death, reveals the telltale musty (almonds or macaroons) odor of cyanide. However, it is estimated that 20 to 40 per cent of all people are unable to detect cyanide by odor and are therefore insensitive to this pathognomonic sign.

*Treatment* must be rapid and efficient. The first treatment consists of removing the unabsorbed poison by lavaging the stomach with copious amounts of water through a gastric tube. This should be continued until all odor of cyanide is gone from the lavage fluid. Lavage is best performed even though the patient has survived the ingestion for some time, because a large amount of cyanide, especially if it is in a crude form, may still be unabsorbed. Potassium permanganate solution, 1:5000, or hydrogen peroxide, 1% of the official preparation, may be given as a chemical antidote if handy. No time should be wasted in obtaining them, however, because their value is not great.

The toxicity of cyanide may be reduced by combination with methemoglobin, produced by giving 0.5 gm of sodium nitrite intravenously or inhalations of amyl nitrite. The rationale of this treatment is that nitrite converts hemoglobin to methemoglobin and the resulting ferric iron effectively competes with cytochrome oxidase for the cyanide. Also, cyanide can be converted into relatively nontoxic thiocyanate by giving sodium thiosulfate, 10 to 25 gm of a 25% solution IV.

Amyl or sodium nitrite and sodium thiosulfate have a potentiating action in detoxifying cyanides. The mechanism depends on (1) the successful competition for cyanide ions by methemoglobin with the respiratory enzyme ferricytochrome oxidase and (2) the conversion of the cyanide to thiocyanate. Treatment then should be as follows.

1. Break pearls of amyl nitrite, one at a time, in a handkerchief. Hold the latter over the patient's nose.
2. Fill a syringe with 10 ml of 3% solution of sodium nitrite (0.3 gm) and another with 50 ml of a 25% solution of sodium thiosulfate (12.5 gm).
3. Inject the solution of sodium nitrite and the solution of sodium thiosulfate through the same needle and vein. Discontinue amyl nitrite inhalation.
4. If the poison was taken by mouth, gastric lavage must be done.
5. If poisoning signs reappear or recovery is slow, repeat sodium nitrite and sodum thiosulfate in full doses.
6. In cases of mercuric cyanide poisoning, injection of BAL may be necessary.
7. The dose of sodium nitrite for children with a hemoglobin of 12 gm/100 ml is 10 mg/kg immediately and 5 mg/kg repeated within thirty minutes if necessary.

TABLE 64
VARIATION OF CHILD'S SODIUM NITRITE DOSE WITH HEMOGLOBIN CONCENTRATION*

| *Hemoglobin (gm/100 ml)* | *Initial Dose $NaNO_2$ mg/kg* | *Initial Dose 3% $NaNO_2$ Solution ml/kg* | *Initial Dose 25% Sodium Thiosulfate ml/kg* |
|---|---|---|---|
| 7.0 | 5.8 | 0.19 | 0.95 |
| 8.0 | 6.6 | 0.22 | 1.10 |
| 9.0 | 7.5 | 0.25 | 1.25 |
| 10.0 | 8.3 | 0.27 | 1.35 |
| 11.0 | 9.1 | 0.30 | 1.50 |
| 12.0 | 10.0 | 0.33 | 1.65 |
| 13.0 | 10.8 | 0.36 | 1.80 |
| 14.0 | 11.6 | 0.39 | 1.95 |

* The initial dose of sodium nitrite will produce 26.8% methemoglobinemia. The sodium thiosulfate dose is based on the adult ratio; 5 ml 25% sodium thiosulfate to 1 ml 3% sodium nitrite. Determination of Hb in the presence of excess nitrite ion will be erroneous unless the red cells are washed twice with isotonic saline before the test.

Two antidotes, aminophenols which generate methemoglobin more rapidly than nitrites and cobalt ethylene diamine tetra acetate (Kelocyanor), an effective cyanide-chelating agent, are not yet approved in the United States. In European studies, these antidotes have been found to be more rapid, more efficacious and less toxic than nitrites, which always present the risk of fatal methemoglobinemia. Oxygen 100% plus nonspecific supportive measures for deficits such as lactic acidosis, pulmonary edema and arrhythmias is absolutely essential in the overall management of cyanide poisoning.

### *Sulfides and Derivatives (Carbon Disulfide, Mercaptans, Hydrogen, Sodium and Ammonium Sulfide, Calcium Polysulfide)*

Hydrogen sulfide is a very toxic gas which approaches hydrocyanic acid in the speed and severity of the poisoning it produces. It is a colorless, inflammable gas that is heavier than air and easily recognized by its odor, which resembles that of spoiled eggs. It is perceptible at concentrations as low as 1 ppm. However, even after a short exposure the sense of smell is quickly dulled and this property becomes unreliable when it is most urgently needed.

Hydrogen sulfide is an irritant and irrespirable gas but also causes poisoning by its systemic actions. It is released spontaneously by the decomposition of sulfides and sulfur compounds (sewer gas) and is found in petroleum refineries, tunnels, mines and rayon factories. Carbon disulfide is a liquid which boils at 46°C and is used as an industrial solvent. The mercaptans are gases released in the course of petroleum refining.

Sulfur in doses of 10 to 20 gm causes symptoms of hydrogen sulfide intoxication. The soluble sulfides, upon contact with gastric acid and elemental sulfur by action of colonic bacteria, may produce significant amounts of hydrogen sulfide. The alkaline-soluble sulfides (ammonium, potassium, sodium) are similar in action to alkalis. They cause irritation and corrosion of the skin, and if ingested, they release free alkali in addition to hydrogen sulfide and are strong irritants. Heavy metal sulfides are generally insoluble and have a lower toxic potential (lead sulfide has an oral MLD of 10 gm/kg in guinea pigs). Carbon disulfide has an estimated mean lethal adult dose of 30 to 60 ml and a MAC of 20 ppm. Concentrations over 500 ppm produce systemic symptoms and the estimated lethal exposure is 4000 ppm for one hour.

The MAC in air for hydrogen sulfide is 20 ppm. The fatal dose of soluble sulfides (ammonium sulfide, calcium polysulfide, potassium sulfide, sodium sulfide, thioacetamide) by ingestion has been reported to be as little as 10 gm (⅓ oz.). In low concentrations there is an irritant action, while in high concentrations the depressant effects on the central nervous system are predominant. The irritant action manifests itself on all mucous membranes causing conjunctivitis, palpebral edema, keratitis, photophobia and defects of the cornea resulting in foggy vision and the perception of color rings around lights. It causes irritation of the respiratory tract characterized by rhinitis, tracheitis, bronchitis, pneumonia, pulmonary edema and greenish cyanosis. Exposure to high concentrations results in sudden collapse, convulsions and death from respiratory paralysis. With less severe exposure, there may be nausea and vomiting and the respiration becomes depressed. These reactions may be associated with, or followed by, somnolence, amnesia, unconsciousness, delirium and hallucinations. The patient may have dysphagia, tachycardia and hypotension, and the urine may contain albumin, casts and a few red blood cells. The pupils are nonreactive, and there may be strabismus, diplopia and exophthalmos. The acute poisoning may be followed by bronchitis or pneumonia, bradycardia, myocarditis, cardiac dilatation, periphral neuritis and gastrointestinal disturbances. Chronic exposure to low concentrations may cause headache, irritability, insomnia, bradycardia, loss of appetite, nausea and vomiting. Skin contact with carbon disulfide causes inflammation and caustic burn of the skin, while ingestion may produce cyanosis, respiratory depression, hypotension, drowsiness, tremors, convulsions and death. At autopsy the blood and viscera may have a peculiar greenish cast.

*Treatment* should consist of inducing emesis or doing a careful gastric lavage, unless tissue corrosion is evident. Artificial respiration, if indicated, and oxygen aid tissue oxygenation of sulfides to innocuous sulfates. Administer gastric antacids, milk and demulcents to slow formation of hydrogen sulfide. Sulfides, like cyanide, inhibit oxidative enzymes and thus produce tissue anoxia. Amyl nitrite, by inhalation, and sodium nitrite, 10 ml of a 3% solution slowly IV (as for cyanide therapy), form methemoglobin that in turn inactivates the sulfide to sulfmethemoglobin. This has been effective therapy in experimental sulfide poisoning, but human use has not yet been documented. Atropine may contribute some symptomatic relief but should not be used if severe cyanosis is present. Prophylactic antibiotics for pulmonary edema and topical application of olive oil, epinephrine and local anesthetics are recommended for conjunctivitis and ocular pain. Contaminated clothing should be removed and the skin thoroughly washed with soap and water, and milk of magnesia or bicarbonate paste should be applied to any eroded areas.

Workers (those producing or working with pesticides, dry cleaning substances, paint, paint removers, rayon, rocket fuel, vacuum tubes, wax, optical glass, lacquer, iodine, glue, cellophane, explosives, cement, rubber, certain textiles and various preservatives) who are exposed daily to carbon disulfide may be aided by a new pretoxicosis test based on the reaction of urine with iodine-azide as a simple, rapid, inexpensive measure of response to daily $CS_2$ exposure. The degree of exposure can be easily followed by observing the rate of change of color when urine is treated with the reagent if a worker is given the test at two different times.

The test is based on the fact that a urinary metabolite of $CS_2$ catalyzes the sodium azide-iodine reaction. The time required for the disappearance of the iodine color depends on the degree of exposure of the subject to $CS_2$.

An important asset of the test is that it is sensitive enough to detect exposure to concentrations just below the hygienic standard for workroom air, 50 mg/cu. m. The threshold limit for maximum permissible exposure is 60 mg/cu. m.

Overexposure can be determined easily if two tests are given the same day. If normal color or urinary metabolite values are determined before and after the work period, the individual probably has not been exposed in excess of the hygienic standard. On the other hand, an abnormally rapid color change seen at the end of the day indicates exposure has exceeded threshold values.

The oral administration of antabuse (TETD) in the job replacement examination appears promising by detecting those workers who are not hypersusceptible to the effects of $CS_2$ exposure. This is based on the demonstrated differences in the capacity of the individual to metabolize the sulfur compound TETD and thus provide an index of the capacity of an individual to metabolize $CS_2$. A reduced metabolic capacity for TETD is taken as an indication of hypersusceptibility to $CS_2$ exposure.

### *Carbon Monoxide (CO)*

The menace of carbon monoxide (CO) is due to its enormous affinity for hemoglobin, more than two hundred times that of oxygen, and its simultaneous interference with the release of oxygen from such oxyhemoglobin as is present in the blood. The symptoms of CO poisoning are due to the tissue anoxia that rapidly and ominously ensues and to the fact that carbon monoxide combines with hemoglobin to form carboxyhemoglobin, which is incapable of carrying oxygen. So little a concentration of inspired CO as 1/50 of the normal (20.9%) oxygen content of air is fatal within an hour.

Carbon monoxide is not a direct chemical poison in the sense that chlorine and mustard gas are. It is toxic only because it deprives the tissues of the oxygen they need. It cripples by hypoxia and kills by asphyxiation.

CO itself is colorless, odorless and commonplace. It is present or formed wherever carbon-containing material is incompletely oxidized, as in furnaces with insufficient draft and the exhaust from automobiles.

Exposures to carbon monoxide in the United States may occur in industry around coke ovens and steel-processing plants. The automobile produces large amounts and has been responsible for deaths and chronic exposures of garage mechanics. Increased blood carbon monoxide hemoglobin levels have been measured in drives on congested highways and in traffic policemen at busy intersections during periods of heavy traffic. Exposures can be particularly dangerous if the intake of a car is in the forward part of the hood and low down so that it is in close proximity to the exhaust pipe of the car ahead.

Car exhaust contains 1 to 7 per cent carbon monoxide. This is well into the highly toxic range, and toxic levels can occur within the passenger compartment. Concern over possible poisoning has influenced the ventilation requirements of automotive tunnels. Adequate ventilation becomes more necessary in tunnels at high altitude.

City dwellers are exposed to fairly high concentrations of carbon monoxide from automobile exhausts and power plants. Air along a crowded thoroughfare can contain more than 20 ppm, which does not take long to displace a significant amount of oxygen in the body's hemoglobin. The situation is aggravated on a completely calm day or in temperature inversion. Cigarette smoking increases the amount inhaled by 3 to 10 per cent over the course of a day. Guards in tunnels and workers in kilns or blast furnaces accumulate even more carbon monoxide from smoking.

Charcoal briquettes are intended for use in charcoal grills and hibachis for outdoor cooking. This use does not present a hazard. In enclosed areas, however, where there is little or no ventilation, the large quantities of carbon monoxide gas released by burning charcoal can result in severe poisoning or death. Hibachis should never be used as a source of heat in sleeping quarters. Fatalities (at least forty) have occurred in recent years because of indoor use of charcoal in tents, trailers, campers, automobiles, boats, apartments, houses and other similar unventilated areas.

Illuminating gas is a rather common source for carbon monoxide, although natural gas contains little if any CO (if incompletely burned, however, it produces CO like any other fuel), while coal gas and water gas contain quite large quantities.

It is erroneously thought that a fire in a closed space is dangerous because it exhausts the supply of oxygen, replacing it with carbon dioxide. However, a fire flickers out at an oxygen concentration in which humans can still breathe and function. A fire is dangerous not because it exhausts oxygen but because it emits carbon monoxide. Carbon monoxide is odorless, but unusual odors resulting from poor ventilation and incomplete combustion may signal a dangerous level of carbon monoxide. Hemoglobin combines with carbon monoxide (forming carboxyhemoglobin) 200 to 300 times as readily as it does with oxygen and dissociates from it some 250 times as slowly. Hemoglobin becomes half saturated with oxygen at a partial pressure of 30 mm of mercury and with carbon monoxide at a partial pressure of only 0.12 mm. Furthermore, in the presence of carboxyhemoglobin, oxyhemoglobin can unload its oxygen only when the tissue tension is dangerously low. This may mean that tissue respiratory enzymes have a higher affinity for carbon monoxide than for oxygen. It has been shown that this is true in yeast cells, but it has not been established in cells of animals. In any case, a normally robust man is near collapse if half his 16 gm of hemoglobin is combined with carbon monoxide, whereas an anemic man with only 8 gm of hemoglobin, but with no carbon monoxide, can function reasonably well.

The maximum allowable concentration permitted in industrial installations used to be 100 ppm and was recently reduced to 50 ppm, but even this relatively low figure is too high for prolonged exposure. A useful rule of thumb to determine the factor of safety is to multiply hours of exposure by parts per 10,000 (ppm/100). If the answer is 3, there should be no perceptible effect; if 6, mild symptoms can be anticipated; if 9, symptoms will be pronounced; if 15, death may not be far off. For example, 1 part per 10,000 (100 ppm) breathed for three hours (multiply 1 by 3) is not very dangerous, but it might be so if the time were protracted. In actual fact, the rule does not apply to long periods, as an equilibrium is reached when carbon monoxide concentration is relatively low.

The symptoms produced by the anoxia of acute CO poisoning range from headache and dizziness to syncope and death. Progression in severity is in accordance with the increase in percentage saturation of hemoglobin with CO, and this depends on the concentration of

CO in the atmosphere and the duration of exposure as indicated above An anemic person is of course more susceptible; increased metabolic rate (with greater oxygen demand), as in children, is also deleterious; respiratory volume and cardiac output at time of exposure are factors of importance.

Carbon monoxide levels considered physiologically safe may reduce worker efficiency by impairing psychological function. Psychomotor and judgment inefficiencies are detectable at carboxyhemoglobin blood levels of less than 5 per cent, although physical manifestations usually do not occur until the level reaches 10 to 20 per cent. Judgment errors and the length of time taken to make a judgment increase as the concentration increases. The ultimate consequences of exposure depend on the severity of anoxia produced. Anoxic necrosis may occur in any organ; skin lesions resembling frostbite can vary in degree from areas of erythema and edema to marked vesicle and bulla formation leading to eschar formation. Scalp lesions may evolve into patchy alopecia. Liver damage, heart, brain and kidney lesions, bleeding tendency, leukocytosis, albuminuria and glycosuria occur in a fairly large percentage of patients. What is more, they may first become manifest a week after the acute exposure.

Carbon monoxide poisoning can be a serious threat to the central nervous system and myocardium. These tissues are most sensitive to oxygen deprivation and can show symptoms of hypoxia either promptly or several days after the acute intoxication. Significant electrocardiographic changes occur, including S-T segment and T wave abnormalities, atrial fibrillation and intraventricular block. After massive carbon monoxide exposure and extensive myocardial damage, the serum transaminase may be elevated. Peripheral neuropathy is rare and usually reversible. Roentgenologic abnormalities are noted in approximately 25 per cent of patients, presenting as a soft, veil-like, homogenous density (ground glass) occurring predominantly in the peripheral portions of the lung, probably due to parenchymal interstitial edema. Perihilar haze and peribronchial and perivascular haze (interstitial pulmonary edema usually of cardiac origin) are less common findings. Myonecrosis with marked increase of serum CPK is a rare complication, perhaps from prolonged immobility, in which the patient's own weight compresses the fascia-bound muscle.

Diagnosis is commonly made by the circumstances under which the victim is found. When carboxyhemoglobin is present at 30 vol% saturation or more, a characteristic and diagnostic cherry-red color is imparted to skin, mucous membranes and fingernails. Retinal hemorrhages often occurs and can be helpful in making the correct diagnosis when other signs and symptoms are obscure.

*Treatment* is straightforward, removal of the patient from the poisonous atmosphere and administration of oxygen. Artificial respiration may be necessary, and pure oxygen inhalation should be instituted as rapidly as it is available by means of a face mask, if accessible, preferably under pressure (up to 2.5 atmospheres). It takes 250 minutes of breathing ordinary air to bring carboxyhemoglobin in the blood down to half its value, whereas pure oxygen reduces this time to about 40 minutes. Theoretically, adding 5 to 10 per cent $CO_2$ to oxygen would cause hyperventilation and speed the elimination of CO even more; but, practically, no such effect is observed. Patients with severe CO poisoning suffer from critical metabolic acidosis, and the superimposition of respiratory acidosis with exogenous $CO_2$ is unsound. If respiration is depressed, intubation or manual ventilation may be used, or a respirator may be employed. When revival is necessary, it has been demonstrated that the use of high partial pressures of oxygen in the treatment of carbon monoxide poisoning is of considerable benefit. Ideally, the patient should receive the highest partial pressure of oxygen that can be administered short of producing actual oxygen toxicity (2 to 2.5 atmospheres, as pressure of 3 atmospheres, except by hyperbaric oxygenation, can cause convulsions in the presence of carbon monoxide). A suggested treatment schedule for a patient with severe carbon monoxide poisoning is administration of 100% oxygen in a pressure chamber of (1) 25 lb./sq. in. for twenty minutes; (2) 15 lb./sq. in. for twenty minutes; and (3) 5 lb./sq. in. for ninety minutes, followed by six hours or more of treatment with 100% oxygen at normal atmospheric pressure. This regimen should supply the patient with a plasma-oxygen level sufficiently high for all tissue needs for the two-hour period when about 75 to 80 per cent of the carbon monoxide is eliminated. It is important to remember that an increase in either the partial pressures or the time exposures beyond this suggested schedule may cause the patient to have severe convulsions due to oxygen toxicity. This can be reversed by removing the supply of 100% oxygen and substituting atmospheric air for breathing.

The patient should be kept cool and absolutely quiet to maintain his metabolic rate at a minimum. Recent animal experimentation has shown striking beneficial effects of hypothermia on hypoxia from carbon monoxide, and at least one remarkable recovery in a human has been reported with this type of therapy. However, carbon monoxide has a greater affinity for hemoglobin at reduced temperature and there is a greater than normal oxygen requirement between 28° and 34°C, so hypothermic therapy is still questionable. Blood transfusion or washed RBCs are of value if given early, before myocardial damage occurs, but dangerous when used late. Injection of methylene blue, as was once advocated, is now recognized as useless and perhaps damaging because the oxygen-carrying power of the blood may be further reduced. Intravenous procaine therapy has been found to be an effective therapeutic measure. Stimulants should be avoided. If myonecrosis develops, monitoring of pulses and pressures is necessary to determine the need for early fasciotomy.

Because of the possibility of delayed aftereffects, prognosis after serious poisoning is guarded and hospitalization is advisable. Serial ECGs and LDH, SGOT and CPK determinations are indicated for several days to screen for immediate and/or delayed evidence of myocardial toxicity. Even mild cases of carbon monoxide poisoning require an ECG, as myocardial toxicity does not correlate well with COHb level. Chronic carbon monoxide poisoning is questionable because it does not accumulate in the body after intermittent exposure in the same way that lead, arsenic and many other chemicals do. However, repeated anoxia from carbon monoxide absorption causes gradually in-

TABLE 65
CARBON MONOXIDE POISONING

| *CO in Atmosphere* | *Duration of Exposure* | *Saturation of blood* | *Symptoms* |
|---|---|---|---|
| up to 0.01% | indefinite | 0–10% | None. |
| 0.01–0.02% | indefinite | 10–20% | Tightness across forehead; slight headache; dilatation of cutaneous vessels. |
| 0.02–0.03% | 5–6 hrs. | 20–30% | Headache; throbbing in temples. |
| 0.04–0.06% | 4–5 hrs. | 30–40% | Severe headache; weakness and dizziness; dimness of vision; nausea and vomiting; collapse. Pathognomonic cherry-red color to lips, mucous membranes and skin. |
| 0.07–0.10% | 3–4 hrs. | 40–50% | As above, plus: increased tendency to collapse and syncope; increased pulse and respiratory rate. |
| 0.11–0.15% | 1½–3 hrs. | 50–60% | Increased pulse and respiratory rate; syncope; Cheyne-Stokes respiration; coma with intermittent convulsions. |
| 0.16–0.30% | 1–1½ hrs. | 60–70% | Coma with intermittent convulsions; depressed heart action and respiration; death possible. |
| 0.50–1.00% | 1–2 mins. | 70–80% | Weak pulse, depressed respiration; respiratory failure and death. |

creasing central nervous system damage with sensory loss in the fingers, poor memory and possible mental deterioration.

### *Carbon Dioxide (Carbonic Acid Gas, Anhydride)*

Carbon dioxide is a colorless gas, slightly acid in taste and heavier than air, and therefore has a tendency to accumulate in deep enclosures such as mine pits, silos, tanks and holds of ships. This gas, after absorption, acts as a strong medullary stimulant until high concentrations are reached; then it produces depression with unconsciousness and convulsions.

The symptoms of poisoning depend on the concentration and the period of exposure. As a rule no symptoms of note are experienced until the concentration in the air reaches 3%, at which time dyspnea, headache, vertigo and nausea appear. Toxic concentrations are not reached until 10 vol% of the gas are present. At this level there are visual disturbances, tinnitus, tremors, hyperpnea, profuse perspiration, elevated blood pressure and loss of consciousness. With higher concentration (above 25 vol%), stimulation gives way to depression, leading to stupor, coma, convulsions and death.

Moving the patient to fresh air is paramount in *treatment.* If respiration is depressed, artificial respiration and oxygen should be administered. The use of respiratory and blood pressure stimulants may be necessary if a satisfactory response is not prompt; otherwise the treatment is symptomatic and supportive.

### *Sulfur Dioxide*

Sulfur dioxide is a pungent, irritating, colorless, nonflammable gas, which is used in various chemical industries as an insecticide, antiseptic and bleaching agent and in the manufacturing of paper. Since it can be condensed at $-10°C$ under atmospheric pressure to a colorless liquid, it has also been used as a refrigerant.

Acute poisoning from sulfur dioxide is rare because the gas is easily detected. It is so irritating that contact with it cannot long be tolerated. The chemical is very irritating to the eyes, nose, throat and the upper respiratory tract and to the stomach if swallowed. In contact with the moisture of the mucous membranes, the gas forms sulfurous acid. Reflex spasm of the glottis occurs when the gas concentration is too high and the lungs are protected in this manner. The MAC is 5 ppm.

Symptoms are mainly those of irritant surface effects and consist of coughing, hoarseness, sneezing, lacrimation and dyspnea, and with high concentrations of sulfur dioxide, ulceration of the cornea may occur. Severe inflammation of the bronchial tree and alveolar membrane also results. This can lead to marked pulmonary edema and pneumonitis. Death, however, is infrequent from sulfur dioxide, mainly because the person readily seeks escape from this irritating and irrespirable gas.

*Treatment* consists of moving the patient to fresh air. Gastric lavage with mild alkalis is indicated if the liquid form has been swallowed. Inhalation of mist from a 2% to 5% solution of sodium bicarbonate is beneficial for the irritated upper respiratory tract. The use of a steam vaporizer or "moisture" inhalation is contraindicated since the water vapor may convert sulfur dioxide into the more irritant sulfuric acid. Care of the eyes and symptomatic treatment for pulmonary edema should be used.

### *Formaldehyde (Formalin)*

Formaldehyde is a colorless, irritating gas of pungent odor which is ordinarily available as a 40% solution of formalin and is used as a disinfectant, antiseptic, deodorant, tissue fixative and embalming fluid. Recently employees in some establishments handling women's clothes complained of burning, stinging eyes and headaches. These symptoms were intensified in spring and early summer when new stocks of summer clothes were received.

Formaldehyde-type resins are used to wrinkleproof fabrics, and a fully crease-resistant fabric may retain an amount of this resin equal to one fifth the fabric's weight. If such a fabric is not processed in the heat chamber long enough or at insufficient temperatures, the inadequately polymerized resin leaves a residue of formaldehyde in the fabric. Rayon fabrics in one dress shop contained 5 to 8 mg/10 gm sample of fabric. It is thought that generally the amounts of formaldehyde in dress shops are a severe irritant, but not a hazard to the health of the employees. But one reported exception was a clothes storage facility with formaldehyde in the air five times the amount considered injurious to health. The one remedy at present is adequate ventilation of the shops, with a ventilation rate equivalent to fifteen air changes/hour during critical times. The lowest level at which free formaldehyde in clothes produces symptoms in a formaldehyde-allergic patient is unknown. However, one study indicates that dermatitis occurs when clothing contains more than 0.075 per cent or 750 ppm of formaldehyde.

Occupants of mobile homes have had problems with irritation of the eyes, nose and throat and with headaches, nausea and drowsiness from excess formaldehyde emitted from building materials such as plywood, particle board and chipboard commonly found in such homes. Some have felt chronically ill with difficult breathing. All patients improved when they left their mobile homes for weekends or vacations. Urea-formaldehyde foam, used as insulation in conventional homes, can also be a troublemaker.

Formaldehyde is changed by oxidation in the body to formic acid and harmless methenamine by combination with ammonia. Paraformaldehyde, the polymerized form, can be changed by heat to formaldehyde for fumigating purposes. The lethal dose of formalin is between 60 and 90 ml, causing degenerative changes in the liver, kidney, heart and brain and inflammation and necrosis of the mucous membranes.

If formaldehyde is swallowed, severe abdominal pain is immediately noted. Diarrhea, vomiting and pain in the throat and abdomen occur. Corrosive gastritis can follow with diffuse ulceration, fibrosis and contracture of the stomach, resembling linitis plastica, which may be severe enough to require gastrectomy. Unconsciousness and collapse may intervene in a few minutes. The urine is scanty and contains red blood cells and casts. Death may result from shock in a few hours but is often delayed one or two days. If recovery occurs, it may be rapid and complete.

When the gas is inhaled, symptoms are mainly those of local irritation to the eyes, nose and respiratory tract with conjunctivitis, pharyngitis, tracheitis, etc.

Direct contact of formaldehyde solutions with the skin causes a brown discoloration, tanning dermatitis, with pustulovesicular lesions and occasionally sloughing. Allergic contact dermatitis from formaldehyde (used to give cloth and paper fibers more strength and increase color retention and stability) in clothing textiles and wearing apparel occurs frequently.

*Treatment* consists of immediate gastric lavage with copious amounts of water. If available, a very dilute 0.2% ammonia solution (1 tsp. of strong ammonia water diluted with 1 pt. of water) or a 1% ammonium carbonate solution should be used for the last lavage. Spirits of ammonia diluted with water to 8 ml can be given by mouth. This should be followed by a saline cathartic. The skin, if involved, should be washed thoroughly with soap and water, otherwise the treatment is supportive and symptomatic for shock or anuria if they occur. Immediate gastrectomy may be necessary when there is caustic perforation or gastric necrosis with massive hematemesis.

## *Gasoline Vapor (See Petroleum Distillates)*

Mild poisoning from fumes of gasoline is not rare. It occurs in industry where gasoline is used as a solvent, in dry cleaning establishments and in garages where mechanics are exposed to the vapors. Gasoline sniffing by children and juveniles is not unusual.

Inhalation of high concentrations of gasoline may cause sudden loss of consciousness, coma or even death. Lower concentrations may produce euphoria and flushing of the face, followed by staggering gait, mental confusion, disorientation, ataxia, blurred speech and difficulties in swallowing. After continued or repeated exposure to fairly high concentrations (chronic gasoline poisoning), the patient may develop anorexia and weight loss. He may look pale and suffer from nausea, headache, nervousness, neurasthenic manifestations, muscular weakness and cramps. He may become dull and listless, lose his memory, become confused, suffer from analgesia, paresthesia and myalgia and also develop polyneuritis and anemia. Increased lead absorption has been reported in gasoline sniffing children.

Persons vary greatly in their susceptibility to petroleum vapors not containing other poisonous components. About 0.3% of gasoline vapor in air makes a man dizzy in about fifteen minutes. A man accustomed to breathing the vapors can endure large percentages, but 1% to 2% of gasoline vapor makes most men dizzy in three to five minutes, and this percentage endangers life if exposure is continued for one hour or more.

In the *treatment,* the patient should be moved from his environment to fresh air, and symptomatic measures, particularly artificial respiration and oxygen, should be used if indicated.

### *Chlorine*

Chlorine is used as a bleaching agent, water purificator and in industry. It is a green-yellow gas with a pungent odor. Chlorine water dissolves about twice its volume of chlorine gas, forming a mixture of hydrochloric and hypochlorous acids. It is corrosive because of its acidity and oxidizing potential.

Since chlorine is an extremely active oxidizing agent, it is capable of causing rapid and extensive destruction of organic tissue. This capability is enhanced by the ease of solubility of the gas in water and body fluids and the convertibility of chlorine to an acid.

Low concentrations of chlorine (1 to 2 ppm) usually can be tolerated without undue discomfort. As the airborne level increases to 3 to 6 ppm, the mucous membranes of the eyes, nose and throat become irritated; corrosion of the teeth may follow if exposure is prolonged or chronic. Victims generally respond by sneezing, coughing and tearing, with hemoptysis and headache occurring occasionally. Much of the pathophysiological effect is confined to the nasopharyngeal area, where the gas is absorbed and trapped by moisture in the mucus.

If the amount of chlorine inhaled is sufficient to reach the pulmonary alveoli, the initial symptom is anoxia, with subsequent heart failure likely. Lung tissue reaction is initially congestion and edema. The pathological lesions finally resulting from the reaction to this gas are essentially similar to those of the less-soluble irritant gases: patchy acute and chronic bronchiolar distortion and obliteration, with associated scattered areas of minute scarring, atelectasis and lobular emphysema.

Although there is relatively little substantive data on which to base a safe level for occupational exposure, the American Conference of Governmental Industrial Hygienists believes that a threshold limit value (TLV) of 1 ppm of chlorine in air (with exposure eight hours per day and five days per week) minimizes the danger of chronic changes in the lungs, accelerated aging and erosion of the teeth.

Exposure to chlorine gas produces varying responses depending upon the severity of exposure. Cases may be classified as follows.

1. *Mild.* Minimal sensation of burning of mucous membranes of nose, mouth, throat and perhaps of the eyes is present. There may be slight cough. No *treatment* is necessary and the symptoms clear within a few minutes to an hour.
2. *Moderate.* Immediate, severe irritation of the mucous membranes of the nose, throat

and eyes is accompanied by a distressing, sometimes paroxysmal, cough. Anxiety is usually present. Except for a few rales, physical examination is otherwise normal. X-ray of the lungs is negative. *Treatment* consists of having the patient lie down with the head and shoulders elevated. Oxygen should be administered in periods of a few minutes at a time until the cough and anxiety are relieved. A sedative cough syrup is useful. Often a bronchodilator administered by nebulizer aborts the paroxysmal cough. Inhalation of a spray solution of an aqueous solution of sodium hyposulfite (2%) and sodium carbonate (0.5%) has also proven effective. Most of these patients can be up within a few hours and may return to full activity the following day.

3. *Severe.* Severe productive cough, difficulty in breathing and frequently cyanosis are present. Vomiting may be prolonged. Restlessness and apprehensiveness are often marked. Rales may be heard throughout the lungs. X-ray of the lungs is negative, but the expirogram may show considerable expiratory reduction. *Treatment* consists of rest with the head and shoulders elevated, warmth and reassurance. Inhalation of humidified oxygen for periods of fifteen minutes or longer is effective in alleviating the symptoms and should be repeated as necessary. Oxygen administered with intermittent positive pressure is even more effective. Sedative cough syrups are indicated. Productive cough, bronchial rales and an abnormal expirogram may persist for a day or two. Residual pulmonary damage rarely occurs and recovery is complete. Most patients are able to return to work on the following day.

If a person has been trapped in an area of high concentration of chlorine gas, the physician is confronted with a medical emergency. Shock, coma and respiratory arrest may be present. *Treatment* is supportive and the physician must rely upon his clinical judgment to meet the conditions at hand. Resuscitation measures, including inhalation of 100% oxygen and methods to combat shock, may be required. Corticosteroids may be helpful for pulmonary edema and should be used without hesitation. Complications such as pneumonia, either of infectious or aspiration origin, should be anticipated.

### *Oxygen*

Medicine's increasing use of hyperbaric oxygenation chambers, as well as 100% oxygen in space capsules, has given new importance to the old problem of oxygen toxicity. There are four general manifestations of oxygen toxicity: systemic effects of hyperbaric oxygen; local pulmonary toxicity to oxygen; absorption atelectasis; and the metabolic effects of oxygen at ambient pressure, including retrolental fibroplasia and hematologic changes. In addition to oxygen toxicity, too high a concentration of inspired oxygen can also cause respiratory depression in patients with carbon dioxide retention.

Danger from the inhalation of pure oxygen is considerably increased when it is inhaled under pressure. Pure oxygen at 3 atmospheres pressure can be breathed usually for three hours without distressing symptoms. During the fourth hour, a progressive contraction of the visual field with dilatation of the pupils and some impairment of the central vision are the most consistent phenomena, often associated with peripheral vasoconstriction, increase of pulse rate and extreme pallor of the face. At this stage, dizziness and the feeling of impending collapse, some stupefaction and slowing of the mental processes, fasciculation of the lips and face, some facial perspiration, salivation, nausea, vertigo, malaise, apprehension and choking sensations may occur. With longer exposure patients may show signs of depression or euphoria, anxiety of varying intensity, indifference passing into near-stupor and signs of incoordination. Later they may suffer from visual and auditory hallucinations and may develop rapid panting, or asthma-like attacks, and in severe cases, apnea in inspiratory position.

TABLE 66
MAXIMUM ALLOWABLE CONCENTRATIONS
FOR GASES AND VAPORS*

| *Gas or vapor* | *Concentration ppm* | *Gas or Vapor* | *Concentration ppm* |
|---|---|---|---|
| Acetic acid | 10.0 | Hydrogen sulfide | 20.0 |
| Acetone | 500.0 | Isopropyl alcohol | 400.0 |
| Acrolein | 0.5 | Methanol | 200.0 |
| Allyl alcohol | 5.0 | Methyl bromide | 20.0 |
| Ammonia | 100.0 | Methyl chloride | 100.0 |
| Amyl acetate | 150.0 | Methyl ethyl ketone | 300.0 |
| Aniline | 5.0 | Methylal | 1000.0 |
| Arsine | 0.05 | Methylene chloride | 250.0 |
| Benzene | 25.0 | Methyl chloroform | 250.0 |
| Bromine | 0.5 | Methyl isobutyl ketone | 100.0 |
| Butanol | 50.0 | Monochlorobenzene | 75.0 |
| Butyl acetate | 200.0 | Naphtha, coal tar | 150.0 |
| Carbon disulfide | 20.0 | Naphtha, petroleum† | 500.0 |
| Carbon dioxide | 5000.0 | Nitrobenzene | 1.0 |
| Carbon monoxide | 75.0 | Nitrogen dioxide | 5.0 |
| Carbon tetrachloride | 15.0 | Nitropropane | 25.0 |
| Chlorine | 1.0 | Ozone | 0.2 |
| Chloroform | 50.0 | Phosphine | 0.5 |
| Cyclohexane | 400.0 | Propylene dichloride | 75.0 |
| Dichlorobenzene | 50.0 | Styrene monomer | 100.0 |
| Ether | 400.0 | Sulfur dioxide | 5.0 |
| Ethyl acetate | 400.0 | Tetrachloroethane | 5.0 |
| Ethyl alcohol | 1000.0 | Tetrachloroethylene | 100.0 |
| Ethylene dichloride | 50.0 | Toluene | 200.0 |
| Formaldehyde | 5.0 | Toluene di-isocyanate | 0.01 |
| Hydrazine | 1.0 | Trichloroethylene | 100.0 |
| Hydrogen chloride | 5.0 | Turpentine | 100.0 |
| Hydrogen cyanide | 10.0 | Xylene | 150.0 |
| Hydrogen fluoride | 2.0 | | |

*Expressed in parts per 1,000,000 parts of air.
†Benzene concentration rather than that of total hydrocarbons may be limiting factor.

Such persons may develop convulsions similar to those of idiopathic epilepsy. Hemolytic anemia is often an associated manifestation. Rarely, a person may have attacks of syncope. Some may show confusion and disorientation and suffer from headache, nausea and vomiting, ataxia and occasionally photophobia; some symptoms are aggravated after return to breathing air.

Added to this complex problem is the greatest limiting factor, the Lorrain Smith effect. This is the direct effect of oxygen on alveolar cells, leading to the slow development of pulmonary edema, atelectasis, loss of pulmonary function and death (a total of nine hours at 3 atmospheres hyperbaric oxygen therapy can initiate this chain of events).

*Treatment.* The only available therapy for oxygen toxicity is reduction of the inspired oxygen concentration to as low a level as compatible with an acceptable arterial oxygen saturation. In addition, utilization of ventilatory support, frequent deep breaths to reexpand areas of atelectasis and positive end-expired pressure are indicated when necessary.

Duke investigators support the hypothesis that lipid peroxidation is responsible for hemolytic anemia and convulsions in animals that are exposed to high-pressure oxygen. In addition, they have found that the administration of vitamin E (a well-known antioxidant) can eliminate these toxic effects almost entirely.

It is well established that chronic oxygen toxicity can be prevented by limiting the partial pressure of oxygen to 350 mm of mercury.

The increasing popularity of scuba diving as

a sport may bring the everyday clinician face-to-face with the dangers of decompression sickness, the "bends," particularly in locales where water sports are popular.

Characteristic clinical manifestations of decompression sickness range from relatively minor musculoskeletal pain to serious central nervous system lesions, paraplegia and collapse.

Divers often have to be transported long distances from dive sites to compression chambers; also, symptoms may not appear for hours, or even when they do start, the patient may not be sufficiently aware of them to seek early treatment. In these cases, for example, pure oxygen delivered by mask may help. Pure oxygen tends to hasten inert gas elimination from the body. (The use of nitrous oxide-oxygen mixtures, however, is contraindicated because the properties of nitrous oxide tend to increase bubble size and would thus tend to worsen manifestations.) Heparin has also been shown to be of use in some cases, probably because of its antilipemic (rather than anticoagulant) properties, but should be given in doses as small as 2000 U. q.6h. because it may also cause further damage to vestibular end-organs already damaged by bubbles or hemorrhage. Hypothermia, sympathomimetic amines and other drugs have been proposed, and there is a theoretical basis for the use of agents which affect platelets. Adrenocortical steroids can be used for shock and cerebral edema prevention. Intravenous plasma or substitutes have been useful in the hypovolemia treatment.

Soroche (acute mountain sickness) is noted in some persons at 8000 feet and in almost all persons at 15,000 feet. For most persons affected, soroche is relatively minor and may only force rest or require a few whiffs of oxygen or minor medication. The symptoms, which are of varying severity, are headache, fast heart rate, rapid respiration, dizziness, tingling of fingers, loss of appetite and weakness or intermittent claudication. The person often suffers from insomnia, perhaps with bad dreams. Much more serious effects are angina and acute myocardial infarction, usually seen when someone has preexisting coronary artery disease.

Pulmonary edema can occur within six to thirty-six hours after exposure to high altitudes and can lead rapidly to death. The dryness of high-altitude air, plus the fluid loss from hyperventilation, can result in rapid dehydration while pulmonary edema can occur at the same time. Lowered oxygen tension in arterial blood increases the permeability of the cell membranes, allowing fluid to enter the alveoli and increasing the hypoxia in a self-perpetuating fashion. Further hypoxia results in fluid retention by causing an inappropriate release of an antidiuretic hormone. Rapid respiration, forced out of an open mouth, drops the intraalveolar pressure, increasing fluid transportation over this decreasing pressure gradient.

A dry cough in an individual not having other cold symptoms often signals the onset of pulmonary edema. This is rapidly followed by shortness of breath, wheezing and substernal discomfort. The classic picture of tachycardia, frothy bloody respiration, severe prostration and coma ensues. Diuretics and digitalis show little effect, but the situation can be quickly returned to normal by providing oxygen via a mask. Many hotels and trains in high-altitude areas keep oxygen readily available.

When possible, though, slow acclimatization should be carried out. Best estimates are that it takes about five days to be properly acclimatized to 12,000 or 33,000 feet. A staged ascent is preferable.

As a first response to hypoxia, there is an increased rate and depth of respiration causing a greater blowoff of carbon dioxide. To balance this respiratory alkalosis, the kidneys go into action excreting a larger amount of base. Some investigators report that the respiratory alkalosis of acute altitude exposure can be balanced by pretreatment with small doses of Diamox® (acetazolamide). Although the mechanism of its action is not clearly understood, it is known to lower the conversion of carbon dioxide to bicarbonates by inhibiting the enzyme carbonic anhydrase, which promotes that conversion. In this way it provides more available carbon dioxide for blowoff, causing the body to overbreathe. In addition, it appears to reduce cerebrospinal fluid formation, which lowers its pressure and lessens symptoms. The generally accepted advice is to begin with 250 mg Diamox b.i.d. for two days before and continue two to three days after arrival at high altitudes.

When a trip to high altitudes is anticipated, it is prudent to decrease the total food intake and increase the carbohydrate proportion. Appetite is decreased in high altitudes because lack of oxygen reduces the tone and motility of the stomach. Overloading the stomach may account for the nausea and vomiting often reported. According to James A. Wilkerson's *Medicine for Mountaineering* (Seattle, Mountaineers), a high-carbohydrate diet lowers the effective altitude between 1200 and 1300 feet. It is often helpful to carry hard candy as a dietary supplement.

A reasonable explanation for the first bad nights and severe morning headaches may be that there is a decrease in oxygen saturation during sleep that is equivalent to going up another 1000 feet. A barbiturate taken for one or two nights before and the first few nights after the traveler's arrival minimizes insomnia. Codeine and a salicylate effectively treat the headache. Obviously alcoholic beverages and smoking are interdicted.

The hyperventilation of hypoxia results in dehydration and increased fluid needs. In addition, the water of many mountainous areas is a problem, not only because of the bacterial and parasitic pathogens but because the nonpathogenic bacterial mix is different. Plastic flasks that can hold boiled water for drinking or brushing teeth should be carried. Water boiled for twenty minutes effectively destroys all infectious organisms.

A novel method of combating the drop in intraalveolar pressure noted when open-mouthed hyperventilation occurs is to make use of the principle of PEEP (positive-end expiratory pressure). This is easily done by forcing all expirations out through an empty cigarette holder. This simple trick often prevents the onset of the cycle of hypoxia leading to pulmonary edema.

### *Nitrogen Oxides (Dioxides)*

Inhalation of low concentration of the oxides of nitrogen may cause little or no discomfort of the upper respiratory tract but may result in death hours later due to pulmonary edema. A brief exposure to 200 ppm can be fatal.

"Silo-filler's disease," silage gas poisoning or bronchiolitis fibrosa obliterans due to inhalation of nitrogen dioxide, is especially hazardous for agricultural workers. Nitrogen dioxide is formed when nitric oxide in fresh silage comes in contact with oxygen in the air. Gas production is greatest in alfalfa silage, reaching a peak in twenty-four hours and apparently ending in two or three days. Nitrogen dioxide usually is seen as a yellowish-brown haze if any amount of it has been formed. Though it is an invisible gas in smaller concentrations, it is still dangerous. This gas has an irritating odor similar to laundry bleach. It is heavier than air and therefore remains in the silo below the upper edge of the last door or settles down through the chute to the silo room and into the barn. Inhalation of nitrogen dioxide can produce serious respiratory symptoms with feeling of oppression in the chest, dyspnea, cyanosis, syncope, pulmonary edema and death. Nitrogen dioxide dissolves in water to form a mixture of nitric and nitrous acids, both of which are very irritating and corrosive to the mucous membranes. Due to its relatively low solubility in water, the transient passage of nitrogen dioxide through the upper respiratory tract may not cause significant symptoms but may result in considerable damage to the lower respiratory tract, where the duration of contact and the amount of moisture are greater. The clinical manifestations vary according to the intensity of exposure and the period of inhalation. (The clinical features and chest x-rays of this condition closely resemble sarcoidosis, miliary tuberculosis, histoplasmosis, etc.) This hazard of farming can be avoided simply by not entering a silo during filling and for a week or ten days after completion thereof.

Oxides of nitrogen play a very important role in air pollution because in urban areas, large quantities of these oxides are constantly being generated from such sources as automobiles, diesel engines, thermal power plants, boilers, industrial gaseous wastes, etc.

Combustion of x-ray films results in the production of nitrogen dioxide. Plastic artificial plants also have the potential of giving off this gas. Exposure to nitrogen tetroxide in the missile industry can produce symptoms identical to those from nitrogen dioxide and should be treated in a similar fashion.

*Treatment* consists of immediate administration of oxygen and artificial respiration if necessary. Corticosteroids have been found very effective in relieving the pulmonary edema and symptoms. In addition, antibiotics should be given to prevent secondary bacterial pneumonitis. Education of the farmer to the dangers of toxic silo gas, as well as the safety measures that should be carried out in preventing undue exposure and inhalation, is paramount in the elimination of this serious type of poisoning.

### *Mace (Antiriot Gas)*

Mace contains recrystallized 2-chloroacetophenone, 0.9% 1,1,1 trichloroethane; solvents and propellants; Freon, kerosene, methylchloroform, 4.0%. It produces transient eye irritation which can be severe enough to immobilize the patient.

TOXICITY. In rabbit conjunctival sac, 0.1 ml of the product causes erythema for seventy-two hours. Fluorescein examinations are negative after seventy-two hours.

Monkey eyes sprayed for five seconds at six feet had negative fluorescein examination.

*Treatment* for severe exposure is copious flushing of the eyes, fluorescein examination and anti-inflammatory eye drops. Avoid salves, creams or ointments until 2-chloroacetophenone has dissipated.

### *Phosgene (Carbonyl Chloride)*

Phosgene was first synthesized in 1812 from carbon monoxide, chlorine and activated charcoal in the presence of sunlight. In 1915 the Germans began to use it in chemical warfare, and it is estimated that more than 80 per cent of the deaths due to gas during World War I were due to phosgene. Though now it has several industrial uses, morbidity and mortality are seldom encountered.

Phosgene is a colorless gas that is heavier than air and has a boiling point of 8.2° C. Its formula is $COCl_2$ and, when inhaled, it is slowly hydrolyzed to hydrochloric acid and carbon dioxide in two to twenty-four hours. Phosgene in dilute concentrations has the odor of green corn or new-mown hay but may be pungent in high concentrations. It is only a mild irritant to the eyes and upper airways and, therefore, may be inhaled deeply into the lungs with little discomfort. Smokers note a flat, metallic taste when smoking in the presence of even low concentrations of phosgene. It may be detected in the atmosphere at concentrations of 1 ppm by chemically impregnated strips of paper. The primary disturbance in phosgene poisoning is increased capillary permeability resulting in large shifts of body fluid with resultant decrease in plasma volume. Animal experimentation shows that phosgene acts directly on the lungs, producing severe pulmonary edema (neuroparalytic type mediated by reflex action with resultant sympathetic paralysis and pulmonary vasoconstriction) and marked bronchiolar and bronchial necrosis. It has been postulated that perhaps an enzymatic defect develops which leads to capillary leakage.

*Treatment.* Oxygen administered by nasal catheter and by intermittent positive pressure breathing (IPPB) should be given to decrease

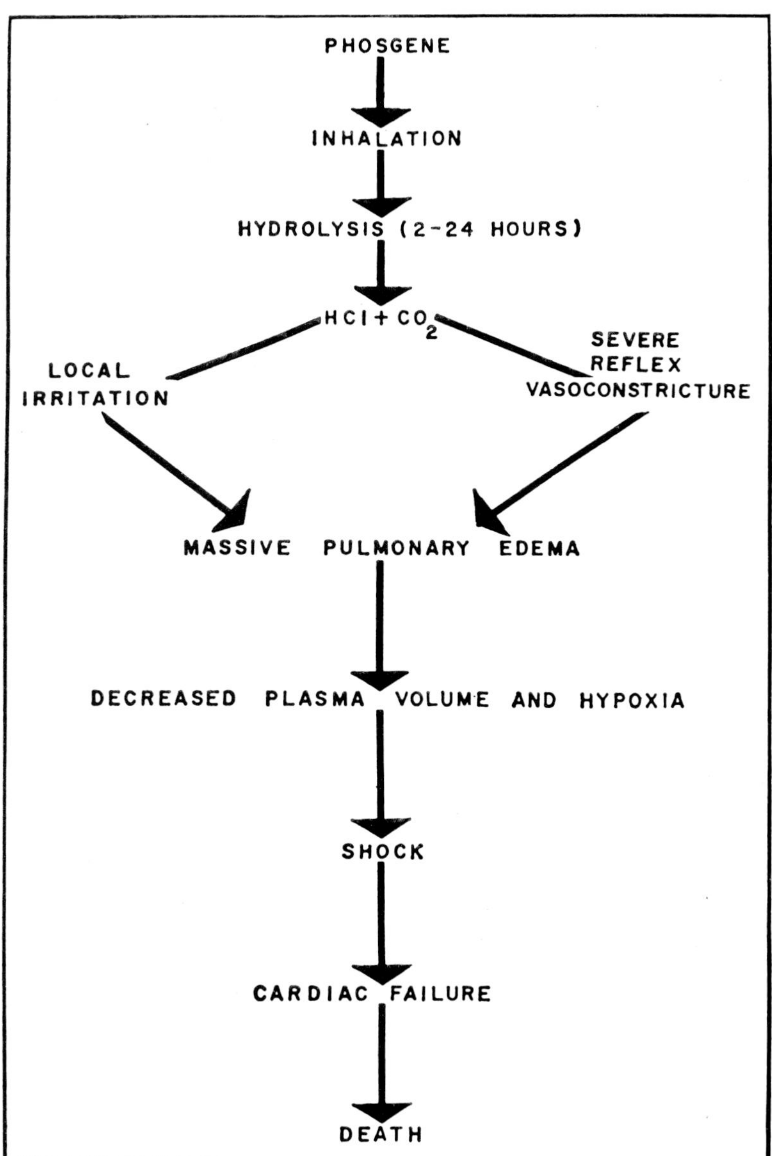


Figure 9. Proposed mechanism of action of phosgene. (Everett, E.D., and Overhold, E.L.: Phosgene poisoning. *JAMA, 205*:243-245, July 22, 1968.)

the hypoxia. Adequate respiratory support should be ascertained by repeated arterial oxygen saturation determinations. If the patient is comatose or cannot handle his secretions, a tracheostomy should be performed. If there is hypotension, it is likely to be due to hypovolemia. A central venous catheter should be employed and the blood volume restored to normal. Morphine is contraindicated since it tends to reduce the hypoxic respiratory drive. Although advocated, digitalization and phlebotomy appear to be of little value in treating the pulmonary edema of phosgene poisoning. Aminophylline should be one of the drugs of choice. It (1) alleviates bronchoconstriction, (2) acts directly on vascular smooth muscle to relieve vasoconstriction, and (3) stimulates the respiratory center. In addition, steroids may be beneficial due to their anti-inflammatory properties. Hexamethylenetetramine (HMT) given intravenously (20 ml of 20% solution) is effective in combatting and preventing progressive lung damage. Prophylactic antibiotics are used on the assumption that the profuse edema fluid would provide an excellent medium for bacterial growth.

## METALLIC POISONS

Many metals present only in minute quantities are essential for the life processes. Some activate enzymes, others facilitate exchange and utilization of oxygen and carbon dioxide. While knowledge is increasing, exact roles are subtle and still all too obscure. Metal poisoning, on the other hand, though understood, is often unrecognized, poorly treated, and attended with severe sequelae and serious prognosis.

TABLE 67
FUNCTION OF METALS IN MAN

| Metal | Function |
|---|---|
| calcium | • body support<br>• blood clotting |
| cadmium | • unknown |
| cobalt | • blood cell formation<br>• spinal cord function |
| copper | • blood cell formation<br>• nerve myelinization<br>• pigmentation |
| iron | • oxygen transport<br>• cellular oxidation |
| magnesium | • activates enzymes |
| manganese | • activates enzyme arginase |
| molybdenum | • nucleic acid metabolism |
| potassium | • vital to cellular life<br>• nerve conduction<br>• muscle contraction<br>• sugar metabolism |
| sodium | • forms external cellular environment |
| zinc | • carbon dioxide exchange<br>• acid secretion |

### *Beryllium*

Beryllium is a light metal which forms the oxide and several soluble and insoluble solutions, all of which are toxic. It is employed in the manufacture of alloys for electrical equipment and ceramics and is also present in some fluorophors used in cathode ray tubes and fluorescent lights. However, these fluorophors have been discontinued by most manufacturers of fluorescent lamps.

Beryllium-copper alloys have been implicated in chronic berylliosis even though some statements in the literature declare that they are nontoxic.

Soluble beryllium salts are easily hydrolyzed with the formation of the free acid, causing severe irritations of the skin with papulovesicular eczematoid, weeping and itchy lesions. When particles penetrate the skin, ulcers and necrosis may occur. Renal lithiasis has been reported in approximately 10 per cent of all cases; the basis for this is not well established, since it occurs with or without hypercalcemia or hypercalcuria. Beryllium is a member of the alkaline-metal group to which calcium, magnesium and strontium belong, and it is presumed that beryllium replaces calcium in the bone and hypercalcemia and hypercalcuria occur. The increased bone density as demonstrated by x-rays in some cases seems to substantiate this hypothesis. The inhalation of the dust of these salts may cause rhinitis, nasopharyngitis, tracheobronchitis and chemical pneumonitis. The acute form of the disease is now rarely seen, but diagnosis of the chronic form remains a problem, which is probably a delayed hypersensitivity reaction with increased blast cell transformation. This theory is supported by the insidious nature of the disease, the latent period between exposure and onset, skin tests and histopathology. There may be a delay of as long as twenty-five years between exposure to toxic beryllium compounds and any sign of disease. Pulmonary involvement causes the syndrome usually present; hence, differential diagnosis of beryllium disease from miliary tuberculosis and Boeck's sarcoid is often difficult. Symptoms range from slight dyspnea on effort to severe orthopnea requiring oxygen, with subsequent right-sided heart failure. Miliary changes may appear on x-ray without symptoms of illness or laboratory evidence of disease. In such cases, a careful occupational history may be helpful. Toxic beryllium compounds may also affect the liver, spleen, lymph nodes, myocardium and kidneys. Disturbance of calcium metabolism in many cases produces a large number of renal calculi. Calcospherite deposits in the lungs compound the pulmonary fibrosis and aggravate the disability. Susceptible individuals are people in occupations using (or formerly using) beryllium (extraction processes, fluorescent light or powder industries, atomic energy development, etc.); persons living or working close to beryllium-using operations; and even persons washing clothes of beryllium-using workers.

*Treatment* is concerned mainly with the handling of those with the chronic manifestations. Skin granulomas and ulcers should be excised surgically. Beryllium dermatitis should be treated with wet dressings and parenteral or oral antibiotics to prevent infections. Steroid therapy (ACTH or cortisone) not only is helpful in decreasing the hypersensitive reaction to beryllium but also useful as an anti-inflammatory agent in the treatment of the chemical pneumonitis. Recently it has been shown that trisodium and calcium edetate induced a definite increase in the total daily excretion of beryllium as well as the concentration of beryllium per liter of urine. The suggested course of treatment as well as the dosage would be similar to that used for lead. It is hopeful that long-term intermittent therapy with a chelating agent such as EDTA may so deplete the body stores of beryllium ion that the clinical course or progress of the disease may be favorably affected. The use of aurintricarboxylic acid (ATA) was reported recently to be effective in protecting monkeys exposed to lethal dosages of beryllium, if given within an hour. Unfortunately, treatment was not successful when experimental dogs were used.

### *Cadmium*

Cadmium is a light metal used for plating metals and in various metallurgic processes. Since it is soluble in an acid medium, the storage of acid food or citrus juices in cadmium-plated (particularly war surplus) containers has in the past caused poisoning. Sales of containers plated with cadmium are banned in many states in order to prevent chemical poisoning from this source. The lethal dose is unknown, but as little as 10 mg (1/6 gr) has caused serious symptoms which are mainly gastrointestinal. Ingestion causes severe nausea, salivation, vomiting, diarrhea, abdominal pain and myalgia. The Japanese *itai-itai* disease or "ouch-ouch" disease in English, so called because of its victim's cries provoked by sudden pains that can occur in various parts of the body, has been found to be due to cadmium pollution of water. Renal and liver damage may follow or accompany the acute symptoms. The inhalation of the practically odorless fumes of cadmium oxide (improper use of silver solder and other sources) as well as other light metals such as zinc, copper, magnesium, etc. ("metal fume fever") causes a different train of symptoms mainly characterized by inflammation of the respiratory tract and pulmonary edema. The MAC in air is 0.1 mg/cu. m. There is a metallic taste with dryness in the mouth, cough, dyspnea, substernal pain, fever, weakness and prostration, bronchitis and pneumonitis. If the symptoms are severe and last over twenty-four hours with chest pain and the patient is a welder, suspect cadmium fume poisoning instead of "metal fume fever." In chronic poisoning from inhalation, there is hyposmia and anosmia, cough, dyspnea, anorexia, weight loss, yellow-stained teeth and irritability. The liver, kidneys and hemopoietic system may be involved.

At present there does not seem to be any acute risk of chronic cadmium poisoning in the population. But what still makes cadmium an important pollutant is its marked tendency to be retained in the body. The organism disposes of only a small percentage of the cadmium it takes in, and the metal is more effectively absorbed by the lungs than by the intestinal tract.

At birth, there is about 1 μg of cadmium in the body. At age fifty, the normal cadmium load is estimated at 30 mg in the United States and 60 mg in Japan. One assumes that the critical level in the kidneys of 200 μg/gm is reached with a total body content of 120 mg. Cadmium, together with lead, mercury and other heavy metals, belongs to a group of pollutants of which we should be especially aware now and in the future. We do not know what cadmium load during the past fifty years has led to the values registered today. It is also uncertain if the kidney level of 200 μg/gm is anything more than a limit beyond which our screening methods cannot discern injury (Tidsskrift for Den Norske Laekeforening, *J Norwegian Med Assoc, 91*:34, 1971). The normal value for cadmium in blood and urine is zero. Harmful exposure limit in urine is 0.05 to 0.1 mg cadmium per liter, or 0.05 to 0.1 μg cadmium per ml.

*Treatment* consists of gastric lavage for ingested cadmium, followed by demulcents. A chelating agent such as calcium edetate 0.5 gm every six hours for one to two weeks has been found to be effective. In serious intoxication it should be given intravenously. In inhalation exposure, the patient should be removed from further exposure and given supportive therapy for pulmonary edema, and calcium edetate should be started as detailed above. BAL is contraindicated. It produces nephrotoxic cadmium compounds. Parenteral cortisone therapy should be administered for severe pulmonary edema.

### *Chromium*

Chromic acid and its salts, the chromates and bichromates, are used in electroplating, steel making, leather tanning, photography, dyeing and in chemical synthesis. Subtle systemic poisoning in addition to well-known surface lesions may be a definite hazard for employees in industries using chromium. In the electroplating process, the metal to be plated is immersed in a solution of chromic acid through which is passed an electric current. Owing to the liberation of oxygen and hydrogen gases at the electrodes, a fine spray of chromic acid arises over the bath, carrying toxic chromium trioxide into the air. The MAC in air for chromic oxide is 0.1 mg/cu. m. The lethal dose of the soluble potassium chromate salt is approximately 5 gm. Contact of chromate solutions with the skin may lead to eczematous dermatitis characterized by a sudden onset, marked edema and ulcer formation. The chromate ulcers have a characteristic punched-out appearance and a tendency to heal slowly. Allergic reaction is not uncommon and is due to sensitization. Exposure to chromate dust or mist may cause conjunctivitis with lacrimation, dark red band of the cornea and ulceration of the cartilaginous part of the nasal septum. The area first turns pale, becomes atrophic, later turns gray and then sloughs, with frequent epistaxis and rhinorrhea. With a short exposure, signs and symptoms from the gastrointestinal tract are rare. Prolonged exposure, however, may result in gastrointestinal disturbances characterized by spasms, gastritis and ulcers of the stomach and intestine. These may be associated with fatigue, lassitude and rheumatic pain. Hepatitis with or without jaundice has been reported in chromate workers and is a serious and incapacitating complication. Long-continued exposure to certain chromates may increase the incidence of cancer of the lungs fifteen times (the incidence is even greater in blacks) and is seen chiefly in the age-group over fifty.

*Treatment.* If ingested, the chromate should

be removed promptly with gastric lavage, and this should be followed by demulcents to alleviate the gastritis. For oliguria or anuria, careful fluid and electrolyte balance should be maintained. In skin contamination the immediate application of a 1% aluminum acetate wet dressing may prevent further irritation and ulceration. Chromate skin ulcers have responded to the use of a 10% edetate ointment. In chronic poisoning, it is imperative that the patient be removed from his source of exposure whether it be from inhalation or skin contact. BAL may be of value in severe systemic intoxication.

### *Lead (Carbonate, Oxide, etc.)*

While lead poisoning ordinarily suggests a slowly developing occupational disease of adults, in children there can be acute manifestations characterized by stupor, convulsions and coma—the features of an encephalopathy—going on to sudden death.

Lead poisoning in children is still too frequent. The reforms that were adopted with awareness of the toxicity of lead, such as avoiding its use for interior paints, did not, unfortunately, remove older buildings from the scene. Furthermore, outdoor house paints may still contain lead. Titanium is gradually replacing lead in paints and those with only 1 per cent lead are unlikely to be very dangerous. The policy of not using lead paint on toys or lead in "lead" soldiers does not protect children from imported playthings or older paraphernalia that may be as hazardous as ever. Plastic beads, necklaces, ceramic glaze (lead oxide), spent lead shot (hazard to poultry and wildlife also), putty and jewelry coated with lead to simulate a pearl appearance are other sources often unnoticed. Chronic use of earthenware containers (particularly for storage of acidic solutions) with lead oxide glaze can release lead in the range of 7 to 20 ppm and produce poisoning. Pottery fired below 2200°F can be assumed to be lead glazed (unless stated otherwise); if fired above 2200° F it can be reasonably certain to be lead-free. The decals used to decorate ceramic dinnerware can be a source of leachable lead (and cadmium) that may be absorbed by foods and beverages, especially if they are acidic. Pewter is an alloy, with tin as the principal constituent. The finest pewter is hardened with a little antimony, copper and bismuth. Inferior pewter may contain varying quantities of lead. Only acidic foods, such as fruit juices, could leach lead from pewter containing lead. The ingestion over a period of time of acidic foods stored or cooked in leaded pewter pots could lead to lead poisoning.

Besides the normal curiosity typical of small children, there is often a craving for unusual things to eat (pica), including flakes of old paint. The colored comic pages of newspapers and color inserts in magazines mouthed and chewed by children are other unsuspected sources for lead poisoning. The yellow coloring of some inserts contain as much as 29,000 ppm of lead (legal limit of lead in house paints is 5000 ppm). The red coloring has 4100 ppm, while black print has 275 ppm of lead.

Lead poisoning is most frequent in children one to five years of age and occurs more often during the sunny months, possibly because vitamin D may enhance the absorption of lead in the same way as it does with calcium. Lead is thus absorbed chiefly from the digestive tract and is distributed throughout the viscera, especially in the liver and kidney, until it is taken up and stored in the skeleton as an insoluble, biologically inert, tertiary lead phosphate. Like calcium, it can be mobilized from the skeleton in metabolic states such as acidosis, or conversely, it can be deposited from the circulation during alkalosis. In addition, poisoning can be caused by the absorption of lead through the skin and by inhalation. Since the use of lead-containing ointments and wet dressings has been discarded by dermatologists, intoxication by absorption is rarely encountered. However, when lead enters the body through the respiratory tract, signs of intoxication develop more quickly than when a tenfold amount of lead is ingested. Epidemics of severe poisoning, with tragic central nervous system involvement, from the inhalation of lead fumes from the burning of storage battery boxes for fuel have been reported in Baltimore, Philadelphia, Detroit and other cities.

Although industrial precautions have generally reduced lead poisoning to a minimum as an industrial hazard, it still occurs occasionally in battery plants and in silver miners who work surface pockets at abandoned sites where soluble lead carbonates exist. It is seldom a hazard, however, to deep miners, where they face nonsoluble lead sulfide rather than lead carbonate. Automobile exhaust and tobacco smoke (persistence of lead arsenate insecticides on tobacco) are sources of lead in the atmosphere, of some concern as an increasing environmental hazard. Spent lead shot, not reaching its target but eaten, can produce lead poisoning and death of some wildlife.

In this country, galvanized iron, copper and plastic pipe are generally used to convey potable water supplies; however, the use of lead pipe is still permitted by many plumbing codes. Under certain conditions, naturally soft waters that are slightly acidic and low in mineral content possess sufficient plumbosolvency to result in appreciable concentrations of lead in water that has been standing in lead pipe overnight. Some cases of lead poisoning from domestic cold water supplies have been reported in Great Britain. In a further study of the lead content of water in Glasgow, Scotland, where many older homes have lead plumbing, a significant correlation was found between the length of lead pipe, the water lead content and the blood lead level of individuals residing in properties with plumbing that is made of lead.

The hazard of lead exposure from domestic water supplies, though small in most areas, is of some concern. The United States Public Health Service drinking water standards (1962) and the Environmental Protection Agency interim primary drinking water standards (1975) impose a limit of lead concentration of 0.05 mg/liter of water. At this level, a consumption of 2 liters of water per day would add a maximum of 0.1 mg/day of lead to the daily intake and contribute about 17 per cent of the total allowable daily intake of 0.2 to 0.6 mg.

There is considerable experimental and clinical evidence in maternal lead poisoning that the fetus is most susceptible to lead toxicity during the stage of most active growth, suggesting that the early pregnancy is most endangered and that the fetus is possibly more sensitive than the young child. Lead in umbilical cord blood correlates with the blood lead of the mother in areas with low, medium or high atmospheric pollution (*Acta Paediatr Scand, 66*:169-175, 1977).

TABLE 68
CALCULATION OF TOLERABLE LEVELS OF LEAD INTAKE TO REFLECT BODY SIZE OF YOUNG CHILDREN

| *Age* | *Body Weight** (*kg*) | *Height** (*cm*) | *Surface Area** (*sq.m*) | *Caloric Requirement** | *Tolerable Lead Intake*† (μ*g/Day*) *Calculated on Basis of* | | | |
|---|---|---|---|---|---|---|---|---|
| | | | | | *kg* | *cm* | *sq.m* | *kcal* |
| Birth | 3.40 | 51.3 | 0.218 | 408 | 68 | 160 | 108 | 87 |
| 6 mo. | 7.15 | 65.8 | 0.250 | 715 | 148 | 205 | 174 | 153 |
| 12 mo. | 9.95 | 78.7 | 0.414 | 995 | 206 | 233 | 205 | 213 |
| 2 yr. | 12.45 | 87.0 | 0.521 | 1250 | 258 | 271 | 258 | 268 |
| 3 yr. | 14.50 | 95.9 | 0.605 | 1400 | 300 | 300 | 300 | 300 |

*Body size of children showing 50th percentile position on growth norms.
†Recalculation of 300 μg/day. Mahaffey has suggested *maximal* intakes from all sources of 100 μg/Pb/day for infants under six months and under 150 μg/day for children over six months of age.
From K. R. Mahaffey, *Pediatrics, 59*:448, 1977. Courtesy of publisher.

Pathophysiologic Effects. Lead poisoning can be difficult to diagnose and is often unrecognized because the symptoms are protean and nonspecific. The chronic form of lead ingestion can simulate any encephalopathy and, in older children, porphyria.

At the cellular level, lead interacts with sulfhydryl groups and interferes with the action of enzymes necessary for heme syntheses for hemoglobin and cytochrome production. Specifically, lead prevents the conversion of delta-aminolevulinic acid to porphobilinogen and the conversion of coproporphyrinogen to protoporphyrin by blocking the action of ALA dehydratase and coproporphyrinogen decarboxylase. This in turn causes ALA and coproporphyrin to accumulate in the urine where they become "markers" for lead poisoning. Lead also blocks ALA synthetase and ferrochelatase (which causes protoporphyrin to accumulate in the red blood cells).

Lead interferes with the sodium potassium ATPase pump mechanism and attaches to RBC membranes causing increased fragility and decreased survival. In addition, lead has an affinity for hemoglobin, and the vast majority of lead bound to the RBC is associated with the hemoglobin moiety. The most clear-cut functional defect caused by lead is the anemia due to decreased heme syntheses. To compensate, the marrow increases RBC production, releasing immature RBCs. Reticulocytes and basophilic stippled cells appear in the blood. The presence of an elevated reticulocyte count in a child with a suspected ingestion can be used to distinguish the anemia of lead poisoning from iron deficiency which results in lowered reticulocyte count. However, children who are malnourished and therefore at greatest risk of lead intoxication often also have iron deficiency anemia.

Acute lead intoxification also affects the kidneys causing a Fanconi-like syndrome, whereas a chronic nephritis is noted with prolonged exposure. In the heart, lead causes swelling of the myocardial fibers which results in myocarditis and eventual fibrosis. The effect of lead on the nervous system is poorly understood. In the CNS, lead causes edema and has a direct cytoxic effect, while the peripheral neuropathy is due to its effect on the myelin sheath. The effects on the CNS are often irreversible, and of those patients who present with encephalopathy, about 85 per cent go on to show signs of permanent brain damage. There is much debate about the effects of chronic exposure to subclinical doses of lead. Evidence is accumulating that even below 60 μg%, the level at which intervention is indicated, lead can have a deleterious effect. Decreased nerve conduction, lower IQs, increased psychomotor activity and learning disorders have all been reported in children whose blood lead is below the "toxic" level (children with subclinical yet excessive lead absorption levels should receive prompt therapeutic and prophylactic treatment to prevent subsequent cerebral dysfunction).

Diagnostic Criteria*

I. Clinical and laboratory criteria
  A. Gastrointestinal manifestations
     One or more of the following:
     1. Anorexia
     2. Intermittent vomiting
     3. Abdominal pain
     4. Constipation
  B. Central nervous system manifestations
     One or more of the following:
     1. Irritability
     2. Drowsiness
     3. Persistent vomiting
     4. Incoordination
     5. Convulsions
     6. Coma
     7. Weakness or paralysis (Neuropathy rare in children. Foot drop and generalized weakness characteristic when seen, whereas the most common manifestation in adults is wrist drop.)
     8. Hypertension

---

* National Clearinghouse for Poison Control Centers.

9. Papilledema and/or optic atrophy
10. Retinal pigmentation (stippling)
11. Paralysis of one or more cranial nerves
12. Elevated cerebrospinal fluid protein content
13. Cerebrospinal fluid pleocytosis
14. Elevated cerebrospinal fluid pressure

C. Hematologic manifestations

One or more of the following:

1. Hypochromic microcytic anemia
2. A significant degree of basophilic stippling of the red blood cells
3. 75 to 100 per cent red fluorescence in erythrocytes examined under ultraviolet light
4. Children with glucose 6-phosphate dehydrogenase (G-6-PD) deficiencies have an increase of whole blood lead levels of 12 per cent when intimately exposed.

D. Excessive coproporphyrinuria

E. Urinary findings

One or both of the following:

1. Glycosuria
2. Aminoaciduria

F. The demonstration of increased radiologic density at the metaphyses of long bones. Lead lines are thicker and heavier than normal growth lines. They may be as much as 5 mm wide and appear often first at the anterior ends of ribs and iliac crests rather than the long bones. Fast-growing bones and deposition of lead and calcium salts are essential to production of these lines in patients with lead poisoning. Appearance time in children depends on quantity ingested and metabolic activity of bone. Lead lines may not be demonstrable until three months after ingestion, when damage has already occurred. Dense transverse bands sometimes result from bismuth deposits, aminopteroylglutamate sodium (aminopterin) administration, healing rickets, vitamin A deficiency and metallic phosphorus.

II. Criteria for lead absorption

The following findings present evidence of absorption of lead in quantities that are known to be capable of inducing intoxication.

A. The finding of a concentration of lead in the blood, as determined by a method of known high sensitivity and precision, of 0.08 mg/100 gm of whole blood or greater. Values of 0.06 to 0.08 mg/100 gm of whole blood are indicative of abnormal absorption of lead but often not a degree of absorption which is capable of inducing symptoms of intoxication. Repeat determinations are preferred.

B. The findings of urinary excretion of lead, as determined by a method of analysis of known high sensitivity and precision, in amounts of 0.08 mg or more per twenty-four hours in patients not receiving treatment to increase lead excretion. Repeat determinations are preferred. A new simplified measuring test of urinary concentration of delta-aminolevulinic acid (ALA) instead of lead itself, using piggyback disposable chromatographic columns, may be the answer in mass screening of children and exposed industrial workers. Prepacked disposable kits for performing this test are available from the Bio-Rad Laboratory, 32nd and Griffin Avenue, Richmond, California. A recently developed ALA dipstick procedure apparently is accurate enough to be used easily and rapidly for screening purposes, but a free erythrocyte porphyrin (FEP) test with one drop of blood (finger prick) is a simple, inexpensive, and an even more reliable plumbism screening test.

III. Exposure to a lead source

A confirmed history, by chemical

identification of the source, of exposure to lead of such a severity and of such duration as to be indicative of a dangerous degree of absorption.

The child who is poisoned by lead has taken in and absorbed dangerous amounts of lead. The presence of clinical and laboratory manifestations in such a child enables a diagnosis of lead poisoning to be made.

CLINICAL AND LABORATORY CRITERIA. Manifestations included under clinical and laboratory criteria are nonspecific, since any of these can be found in other illnesses. Even the increased radiopaque areas or lines at the metaphyses of the long bones are not specific indications of lead absorption, for these are seen with other diseases, e.g. abnormal absorption and storage of other heavy metals and healing rickets. Such lines are not indicative of intoxication but are so frequent in their occurrence in small children who are absorbing abnormal amounts of lead as to serve as a warning. A child exhibiting this manifestation should be investigated carefully with respect to the extent of his absorption of lead.

When any two of the criteria listed under clinical and laboratory criteria for lead occur together with one of the criteria for lead absorption, a diagnosis of lead poisoning may be made with assurance. Two or more of the clinical and laboratory criteria listed may be used to make a presumptive diagnosis of plumbism in children with early manifestations of increased intracranial pressure; such children require removal from the source of lead and emergency treatment. A delay in treatment while a blood or urine analysis for lead is being performed may be hazardous. Edetate calcium disodium (EDTA or versenate) therapy can be instituted while blood or urine determinations are being performed. Treatment can be stopped if repeated lead analyses show the provisional diagnosis to be in error.

The central nervous system is frequently involved in children with lead poisoning, as evidenced by diffuse cortical injury producing generalized convulsions and residual mental retardation. When involvement is associated with abnormal cerebrospinal fluid findings such as increased pressure, elevated protein and variable cell count up to 100, almost all of which are lymphocytes, the diagnosis of lead poisoning with encephalopathy may be made. Spinal puncture (necessary to rule out other CNS disease as well as to clarify the diagnosis), however, must be done with caution since high intracranial pressure and edema of the brain predispose to herniation of the medulla through the foramen magnum. A diagnostic tap should be done with the needle connected to the manometer in a closed system, the pressure recorded, and about 1 ml of fluid withdrawn for chemical analysis, cell count and culture. Repeated determinations of spinal fluid pressure are not recommended.

Excessive coproporphyrinuria is a constant finding in acute episodes; the urinary porphyrin test is a simple and quick screening test to rule in or rule out lead intoxication. It is based on the fact that a normal constituent of urine, porphyrin (principally coproporphyrin type III), is increased in lead poisoning. Theories differ as to its origin, some investigators believing that it is the product of faulty synthesis of hemoglobin, others believing that it represents the result of a breakdown of hemoglobin.

A new technique developed by Bell Laboratories using a portable fluorometer to detect the fluorescence of protoporphyrin requires only a few drops of blood in a capillary tube and is a simple and inexpensive method for large-scale screening. Reactors can then be identified more positively with blood determinations or by the more elaborate atomic absorption spectroscopy (AAS).

*Method:* (1) Pipette 10 ml of a "random" sample of urine into a screw-top tube; (2) add 2 drops of glacial acetic acid, 2 drops of hydrogen peroxide and 2 ml of ether; (3) mix gently in screw-top tube; (4) let stand thirty minutes; (5) view in darkroom using an ultraviolet lamp; (6) record any pink fluorescence of the surface ring as positive.

There is no correlation between the quantitative amount of lead in the urine and the presence of a positive porphyrin reaction. The test may vary from positive to negative in the course of a few months time, or it may stay positive long after cessation of exposure to lead when damage supposedly exists.

The measurement of free erythrocyte porphyrins is a stable and easily measured parameter of lead toxicity. The relationship between blood lead and FEP with time suggests that the combination of blood lead and FEP accurately predicts a degree of risk screened for lead poisoning. The use of FEP alone as a primary screening tool is also easily defensible, as those children with slight elevation of blood lead and normal FEP can be expected in virtually all cases to have normal or falling blood lead at next contact. In addition, children with abnormal FEP and normal blood lead may be at significant risk of lead toxicity or suffering from iron deficiency and deserve further medical attention. Measurement of FEP should, therefore, be a primary tool in screening and diagnosis of lead poisoning. Normal range is 20 to 75 μg/dl of red cells.

Criteria for Lead Absorption. Once the suspicion of lead poisoning is aroused, the most important single consideration in the differential diagnosis is whether or not lead has been absorbed in quantities sufficient to induce illness. This can best be demonstrated by determining the lead content of the blood. The threshold value cited above, 0.08 mg of lead per 100 gm of whole blood, is a critical one. Lead concentrations between 0.06 and 0.08 mg/100 gm of whole blood are indicative of abnormal absorption of lead but often not of a degree which is capable of inducing symptoms of intoxication.

Extensive studies have been made on the variability of the concentrations of lead in the blood and urine of adults and children, both under ordinary circumstances and under conditions of abnormal exposure to lead. In a group of children between the ages of six months and four years, in whom there was no evidence of abnormal intake and absorption of lead, the average blood lead concentration was 0.027 mg/100 gm of blood. In a recent report, the upper normal limit of blood lead concentration in young children is stated to be 0.05 mg/100 gm of blood.

The appraisal of the significance of lead absorption by means of analysis of the urine (ALA test excepted) is more difficult and less effective than that of analysis of the blood, especially with children in whom there is a wide physiologic variation in twenty-four-hour urinary volume. Factors such as dehydration and acidosis, often accompanying the acute episode of lead poisoning in children, can alter urinary lead output in the untreated patient, so that the amount excreted may fall within the normal range. The collection of an uncontaminated sample of urine from a child for the purpose of lead analysis is usually difficult, extreme precautions being required to prevent contamination of the urine with lead.

Administration of calcium disodium EDTA to patients who have abnormal amounts of lead in their tissues is followed by a rise in urinary excretion of lead. This increased lead excretion following edetate administration has been suggested as the basis for a diagnostic test. Patients receiving edetate therapy should excrete 1.5 mg or more of lead in the urine on any one of the first three days of treatment. This test, while by no means as satisfactory as that of the determination of the level of the urinary excretion of lead prior to any therapy, may be more practical than the collection and analysis of a twenty-four-hour urine specimen from an untreated patient where a delay in therapy is hazardous.

Currently, the most reliable method in general use for detecting lead poisoning is atomic absorption spectroscopy (AAS). This laboratory technique requires a large sample of blood drawn from a venous puncture. Because of the size and complexity of the instrument, AAS must be performed in a laboratory by trained personnel. Interpretation of the data requires considerable expertise. The large blood sample is objectionable both to the children and their parents and must be drawn by qualified medical personnel. Simpler and less expensive screening techniques are described elsewhere and should be used first to eliminate nonreactors.

The stippling of red cells in the blood smear is often a better guide to lead damage than the blood or urine lead level. Stippling may be absent in the rare cases of sudden massive ingestions of lead with a rapid onset of symptoms, but usually more than 20 stippled cells per 50 oil immersion fields are present in lead poisoning, and serial determinations show an increase of stippled cells as poisoning becomes manifest. Recently it has been reported that observation of red fluorescence in erythrocytes examined under ultraviolet light is a simple, reliable means of detecting lead poisoning. From 75 to 100 per cent of the erythrocytes were fluorescent in thin wet-drop preparations of heparinized blood in a group of children with untreated lead poisoning. Less than 51 per cent fluorescence occurred in erthrocytes from healthy subjects and patients with various diseases.

Sixteen children with chronic lead intoxication had a mean value of 282 μg/gm of lead in scalp hair. (SD was 22 and range 42 to 975 μg of Pb per gram of hair.) The determination of lead was done in serial segments of hair beginning at the scalp and each measuring 5 to 10 mm in length. In most patients, a twofold to threefold increase in lead was found in the segments of hair proximal to the scalp. In some patients with a record of previous hospitalization for lead intoxication, the entire length of hair accumulated an equal and highly elevated concentration of lead. In contrast, the concentration of lead in hair of forty-one apparently healthy children was 24 μg/gm. (SD was 24.6 and range 2 to 95 μg Pb per gram of hair.) Lead was determined by atomic absorption spectroscopy (*N Engl J Med, 276*:949-952, 1967).

Fecal excretion of lead is a more sensitive index of recent ingestion than blood levels, which may remain elevated for long periods after ingestion has stopped. The upper limit of normal is 123 μg/single stool (mean + 2 SD). Return to normal occurs rapidly after removal of lead.

Glassware and other equipment used in the collection and analysis of blood and urine samples can and should be rendered free of any possible contaminating lead by rinsing with warm 20% nitric acid, followed by thorough rinsing in "lead-free" distilled water. Other special precautions must be taken in the laboratory to prevent contamination of the samples from lead-containing airborne sources during washing and analysis.

Exposure to a Lead Source. Childhood lead poisoning is, in general, a disease of poverty, almost always found in areas of old, run-down housing. The source of lead is usually lead pigment paint applied and reapplied early in this century to walls and fixtures which more recently have been neglected and allowed to fall into disrepair. These coats may be buried beneath other coats of paint covered with wallpaper or they may cover wallpaper or plaster. With neglect, the paint and painted wallpaper peel, and the painted plaster crumbles. Particles may then be picked up and ingested by young children. Lead paint in good condition has also been chewed off surfaces. An adequately safe substitute indoor paint was not made available until about 1940. Lead paint applied to outside surfaces has also been known to be the source of lead in cases of childhood plumbism.

Children's toys and furniture are not significant sources of lead unless repainted with lead pigment paint. Since 1955, the American Standards Association has recommended that only paint with a lead content of 1 per cent or less may be considered safe for use on children's toys, furniture and in housing interiors.

Other sources of lead should be kept in mind (*see* page 255). Numerous cases of poisoning have occurred in both children and adults from inhalation of lead fumes and exposure to ashes resulting from the burning of lead storage battery casings for fuel, a practice sometimes resorted to by destitute families.

Illicit alcohol ("bootleg whiskey," "white lightning," "moonshine") is made in ground stills in which barrels, soldered pipes, automobile radiators, copper tube units sealed with lead solder, etc. are customarily used as condensers. Due to the large quantity of lead that gets into the distillate directly, as well as the additional lead ions which are released wherever the acetic acid distillate from the "mash" comes in contact with solder, illicit alcohol can and often does contain toxic quantities of lead. The drinking of this type of whiskey has produced numerous severe, chronic and fatal cases of lead intoxication usually with encephalopathy in adults, most of whom were chronic alcoholics. Gout is also often seen in chronic imbibers of "moonshine" liquor as a result of lead contamination.

In most cases of childhood lead poisoning, pica, the abnormal appetite for nonedible substances, is responsible for lead ingestion. Children, usually between the ages of one and five years, most often exhibit this abnormal appetite, which may result from an emotional disorder or nutritional deficiency. It has been shown that lead is retained in small amounts in the tissues of an adult with a daily intake of 1 mg of soluble lead in addition to the normal daily dietary intake (0.2 to 0.6 mg of lead). Since lead-pigment-containing paint peelings (a single chip of paint the size of a thumbnail) may contain 100 mg or more of lead, the repeated ingestion of small amounts of these peelings is compatible with absorption and retention of dangerous quantities of lead in the tissues. This eventually results in clinical manifestations of poisoning if the exposure is not interrupted.

An easily performed, inexpensive test allows identification of potentially dangerous lead-containing surfaces and thereby may avert, or help identify, lead poisoning in children. The test is based on the precipitation of lead to an insoluble black lead sulfide.

A chip from the surface of the painted area is removed, or a deep cut made through the paint layers, and a solution of sodium sulfide applied to the chip or the cut surface. *All* old paint layers must be exposed, because the older layers are those most likely to contain lead. Application of a 5% to 8% solution of sodium sulfide causes, in the presence of lead, a color change to black, the intensity of which is directly proportional to the amount of lead present in the paint. A black color develops if the specimen contains between 10 and 25 per cent lead. Although other metals—iron, nickel, mercury, molybdenum—form black sulfides, these metals are not present in house paints in amounts sufficient to cause confusion in interpreting the color change. The test's advantages are that the paint can be tested on the premises, the solution can be carried in one's pocket in a polyethylene squeeze dropper bottle and little training is needed to interpret the color change.

A positive history of pica for paint and a roentgenogram of the abdomen demonstrating radiopaque material in the intestinal tract are valuable clues to the ingestion of lead. A history of ingesting paint chips or chewing on walls or woodwork may or may not be obtained. Often such activity goes unnoticed or the amount ingested is considered insignificant by the parents. The history may be obscure, incomplete or fragmentary. The possibility of the existence of lead poisoning, therefore, must occur to the physician from the nature of the illness itself, and he must be prepared to make a presumptive diagnosis in an acutely ill child without an elicited history of lead ingestion. Diagnosis and therapy must not be delayed because a source of lead is not readily demonstrable. The explanation of the origin of the disease, if it turns out to be lead poisoning, is often found after the fact.

"Symptomatic lead poisoning," when lead levels are below toxic values, can be due to the effects of cadmium, which is much more toxic than lead, present in trace or even contaminated amounts in old paint. Determining cadmium blood levels along with lead may help solve some of these puzzling situations.

In making a final diagnosis involving a child exposed to lead, the following classification for diagnosis is recommended:

A. Asymptomatic increased lead absorption
   This diagnosis refers to the child who shows evidence of presence in the tissues of, and absorption of, abnormally large amounts of lead but who is asymptomatic. A source of lead, evidence of lead absorp-

tion and increased radiologic metaphyseal density of long bones may be demonstrated.

B. Lead intoxication
   1. Lead intoxication without encephalopathy
      Two or more of the clinical and laboratory criteria (excluding central nervous system manifestations accompanied by abnormal cerebrospinal fluid findings) are evidence for absorption of lead in dangerous quantities and demonstration of a lead source enables this diagnosis to be made.
   2. Lead intoxication with encephalopathy
      Two or more of the clinical and laboratory criteria including central nervous system manifestations accompanied by abnormal cerebrospinal fluid findings, evidence for absorption of lead in dangerous quantities and demonstration of lead source make this diagnosis. This category may be subdivided, on the basis of the severity of encephalopathy, into lead poisoning with mild encephalopathy and lead poisoning with severe encephalopathy. The latter group should include those patients who convulse and/or who are comatose for twenty-four hours or longer.
   3. The association of chronic lead poisoning, especially in adults, with hypertension, renal failure and gout also occurs.

The long-term prognosis of childhood plumbism with reference to mental and neurological function may depend upon the severity of the acute symptomatic episode. Therefore this classification should be of prognostic value.

This diagnostic classification is also suggested in order that children who are ingesting abnormally large quantities of lead and children with lead poisoning without encephalopathy are not overlooked. Early diagnosis is essential for a good prognosis in this disease. Removal from lead exposure and therapy with calcium EDTA more often results in a favorable outcome if instituted early. Therapy with calcium EDTA is not as effective once acute lead encephalopathy has occurred. This very effective drug has not significantly reduced the 10 to 15 per cent mortality rate from lead poisoning in children because more often than not therapy is delayed.

*Treatment.* If the poison has been recently ingested, lavage the stomach with warm water or a 1% sodium sulfate solution. A saline cathartic, such as 30 gm (1 oz.) of magnesium sulfate, should be given to flush the lead from the intestinal tract and reduce absorption. Egg white, milk or other demulcents are useful for soothing the irritated gastric mucosa.

To control colic, calcium gluconate 1 gm (15 gr) is given intravenously as a 10% solution and repeated as necessary to obtain relief. Morphine sulfate 15 to 30 mg (¼ to ½ gr) can be given hypodermically for control of severe pain. The maximum dose for children is 1 mg/10 lb. of body weight.

The most effective method of removing lead is the administration of a solution of calcium disodium edetate or versenate (not the sodium salt, edetate disodium, which would chelate calcium as well as lead), which is superior over BAL as a deleading agent because it has a higher therapeutic-to-toxic ratio and a high coefficient of chelation for lead. This drug should be given preferably by intravenous infusion and the concentration should not exceed 3%. One ampule, 5 ml of a 20% solution, must be diluted to at least 33 ml. The following procedure is recommended.

Dilute the 5 ml (1 gm) from an ampule with 250 to 500 ml of isotonic sodium chloride U.S.P. or sterile 5% dextrose solution suitable for intravenous injection. Administer this diluted solution by intravenous drip over a period of one hour. This dose may be administered twice daily for periods up to five days. If additional treatment is indicated, a two-day rest is recommended, to be followed by another five-day course. There is some recent evidence to prove that the stored body lead can be eliminated best by weekly intravenous injections of versenate for several weeks, rather than the daily infusions. The dose for children should not exceed 0.5 gm/30 lb. of body weight, administered as above. Intermittent intramuscular injections of a 20% solution containing 0.5% procaine in a total daily dosage range of 50 to 75 mg/kg of body weight for five to seven days, though painful, is also effective.

Versenate makes available, for the first time, reasonably safe, effective treatment in heavy metal poisoning without organ injury during excretion. A solution of calcium disodium versenate is the calcium chelate of ethylenediaminetetraacetic acid (EDTA). (In the body, calcium is displaced by lead, forming the lead chelate which is nonionized, nontoxic, water-soluble, nonmetabolized and excreted intact.) It cannot produce exacerbation of symptoms during the period of therapy. This compound is potentially nephrotoxic and overdosage or prolonged treatment can cause nephrosis, which usually but not always clears promptly after therapy is discontinued.

Caution should also be used in patients who may have clinical or subclinical potassium deficiency states, since a marked increase in urinary potassium excretion may follow its parenteral use and produce severe hypokalemia. Other side-effects that have been reported include the following: malaise, fatigue, excessive thirst, numbness, tingling, fever, chills, myalgia, arthralgia, headache, nausea, vomiting and histamine-like reactions such as sneezing, rhinorrhea and lacrimation. Skin and mucous membrane manifestations occur with unusual prolonged treatment. Thrombophlebitis proximal to the site of injection occurs frequently if concentrations above 0.5% are used.

Oral administration of EDTA is not as satisfactory (less than 1% absorbed) as parenteral administration and may even be harmful. If excessive quantities of lead are present in the gastrointestinal tract, the resultant chelated lead is well absorbed, and while most of this lead may be excreted in the urine, there is always the possibility that total body lead stores may be increased. The prophylactic oral use of this drug in lead workers should never replace proven preventive and protective measures.

A structural analogue of EDTA, diethylenetriaminepentaacetic acid (DTPA), offers more promise than $CaNa_2EDTA$ in promoting the excretion of lead, iron, cobalt, zinc, chromium, manganese and a number of radioelements, and therefore, it may be the drug of choice for most metal poisons. Calcium trisodium pentetate (DTPA) can be given intramuscularly without serious side-effects at intervals of two weeks with a dosage of 2 to 4 ml (0.5 to 1.0 gm) of a 25% solution. Its use on an ambulatory basis in the management of workers exposed to lead or with mild intoxication seems to be warranted.

The introduction of combined corticosteroid and hypothermia to the therapeutic regimen has not produced any appreciable effect on the survival rate.

Penicillamine (Cuprimine), another chelating agent that can be given orally (preferably on an empty stomach) (20 to 40 mg/kg/day), has been used with encouraging results and deserves further trial in the treatment of lead intoxication as an alternative or an addition to calcium disodium edetate and BAL. It is effective, well tolerated and nontoxic for short-term use. However it is an investigational drug for the treatment of lead and FDA permission for specific use must be obtained.

Chisholm has recently shown that the simultaneous use of BAL and EDTA is far more effective in the treatment of lead encephalitis than EDTA alone. With the drug combination, the blood lead concentrations decreased by 50 per cent per twenty-four hours as a result of enhanced urinary excretion, in contrast to a 20 per cent decrease with EDTA use. In the patients studied, there were no evidences of kidney injury demonstrated in spite of the increased renal lead load. Elevated plasma levels of the enzyme delta-aminolevulinic acid were found to be further increased when EDTA therapy was used, but the concentration was sharply reduced by the addition of BAL. This undoubtedly accounts for the favorable response when both drugs are utilized. The doses used were 4 mg/kg of BAL given alone initially and every four hours thereafter with EDTA (12.5 mg/kg) IM at separate sites for five days. The use of extracorporeal hemodialysis in conjunction with the above treatment has not been of great value.

In lead encephalopathy, with status epilepticus or coma, restricted parenteral fluids and parenteral EDTA and BAL are the mainstays of treatment along with anticonvulsants and intensive supportive care including drugs for diminishing the increased intracranial pressure. Intravenous infusion of urea appears to be a safe and effective drug available for this purpose (mannitol and/or adrenal corticosteroids are often preferred; *see* discussion on Cranial Hypertension). In contrast to other hypertonic solutions, urea is a relatively long-lasting diuretic agent. If not given too rapidly, even large doses are relatively nontoxic. Urea may be administered as a 4% solution in 5% dextrose in water in dosages of 1 gm/kg of body weight per twenty-four hours. Mixture of urea in 10% invert sugar in distilled water or physiologic saline solution can also be given. In severe cases, a 30% solution of urea may be used. The rate of intravenous drip should not exceed 60 to 80 drops per minute. Treatment usually results in active diuresis over a period of eight hours, and the course may be repeated every eight to twelve hours. To prevent extreme dehydration, adequate fluid replacement must accompany urea administration. Electrolyte losses must be replaced. Adequacy of urine excretion must be assured before beginning therapy. The blood urea nitrogen should be determined at intervals; values in excess of 75 mg/100 ml are undesirable. Results from hemodialysis reported so far have been either ineffective or equivocal, although at least one report has shown that the use of edetate calcium disodium followed by peritoneal dialysis measurably increased the amount of lead recovered in the dialysate. This combined treatment should be of value in selected cases, especially where there is renal function impairment or azotemia. Extensive craniectomy with opening of the dura appears to have saved lives and to have prevented, in some instances, irreversible brain damage. In a report of twenty-five surgically treated cases, there were sixteen deaths. The high mortality is a reflection of the desperate status of these patients. Although no conclusion as to the place of surgery in the treatment of plumbic encephalopathy was possible in this article, it was the consensus of the authors that, in selected critical cases, surgery in combination with judicious medical management might save lives.

### *Lead Arsenate and Arsenite*

These compounds are white, heavy powders which are extensively used as insecticides. Intoxication may arise from inhalation of the powder during spraying operations and from the ingestion of contaminated drinking water or food. Because of their low solubility, these salts may be less acutely toxic than expected. Arsenite, however, is more toxic and corrosive than arsenate. The clinical picture of lead arsenate poisoning closely resembles that of lead instead of arsenic, although certain symptoms occasionally are similar to those produced by arsenic. Nevertheless, toxicity is mainly due to the lead component and *treatment* is essentially the same as that for lead poisoning. BAL, however, might be more useful than EDTA in some instances when both lead and arsenic may be responsible for the presenting symptoms. This would be true if a single large dose were ingested for suicidal purposes since arsenic is a more powerful poison than lead, in which case both BAL and EDTA should be used.

### *Lead, Tetraethyl*

This highly toxic compound, introduced in 1923, is an oily liquid which is added in small amounts (1:1000) to gasoline to lessen "knock" by preventing premature combustion. Poisoning arises directly from contact with tetraethyl lead itself, which is absorbed both from the intact skin and lungs. The toxic effect is due to the triethyl lead formed during the breakdown of the tetraethyl compound which causes inflammatory and degenerative lesions in the brain and other tissues. Acute central nervous system excitement results with delirium and mania. The main risk of this type of poisoning exists in industrial workers, but present precautions and prophylactic measures are adequate in eliminating these dangers. The small tetraethyl content in gasoline is not of toxic significance in acute exposures by ingestion or inhalation, but those who were careless about repeated and massive skin contact have developed lead poisoning.

### *Manganese*

This compound in the form of manganese dioxide is used in the manufacture of steel and dry cell batteries. The effects of long-continued ingestion of manganese have not been reported or investigated. The principal manifestations of poisoning are limited to the respiratory tract and the central nervous system. The symptoms consist of cough, nasopharyngitis, bronchitis, pneumonia, headache, lethargy progressing to marked weakness of muscle groups, especially of the lower extremities, spastic gait, tremors of the parkinsonian type, slurred speech, masked facies, sexual impotence and mental deterioration. Chronic manganese poisoning is found chiefly in ore grinders and miners where the inhalation of dust may give rise to respiratory and neuropsychiatric symptoms. The MAC in air is 6 mg/cu. m.

*Treatment.* The patient should be immediately removed from further exposure. Therapy for the respiratory symptoms is mainly symptomatic. Antibiotics and steroids may be beneficial for the chemical pneumonitis. A course of calcium edetate, if given early in treatment, may prevent some of the central nervous system sequelae. BAL also has been effective in reported cases. The parkinsonian symptoms can be controlled to a degree by Artane and other antiparkinsonian drugs. The successful use of L-dopa* (L-dihydroxyphenylalanine) to relieve dystonia and other symptoms of chronic managanese poisoning has produced dramatic improvement of signs and symptoms.

### *Nickel*

This compound and its salts may cause hypersensitization and irritation of the skin with itching papulovesicular lesions, which may become weeping, infected and even necrotic. The skin manifestations may last several weeks or months, and in addition, there is an associated stomatitis and gingivitis. *Treatment* consists of removing the patient from the source of contact and giving appropriate care and therapy to the involved skin.

### *Nickel Carbonyl*

Nickel carbonyl is a colorless liquid formed by passing carbon monoxide over finely divided nickel. It is used in petroleum refining as well as in the Mond process for refining nickel. The lethal concentration of nickel carbonyl is in approximately the same range as hydrogen cyanide. The greatest allowable air concentration is 1 ppm. Though toxic effects are supposedly not cumulative and tolerance is said to develop after repeated exposure to sublethal concentrations, recent reports have incriminated the chronic inhalation of nickel vapors as being carcinogenic. Because the burning cigarette has all the reactants and reaction conditions present which lead to the formation of nickel carbonyl, cigarette smoking, which thus provides ready transport of an active form of nickel into the respiratory system, is now being seriously investigated from this new aspect. (Recent investigations have also implicated an alpha-particle-emitting radioactive element, polonium [$Po^{210}$], a naturally occurring daughter isotope of radium$^{226}$.)

There are two distinct states in the development of symptoms in patients exposed to toxic levels of nickel carbonyl, the initial and the delayed. Initial symptoms include mild frontal

---

* Although there is no firm evidence that levodopa is involved in the genesis of melanoma, there are some individuals with an abnormal susceptibility of melanocytes to levodopa. The possibility of melanoma stimulation by this drug exists and should be kept in mind when used.

headaches, dizziness, nausea, vomiting, soreness and tightness of chest, hacking cough, cold sweats, clammy skin and dyspnea on exertion. These initial symptoms may be quite mild even though the symptoms are more apt to be encountered with exposure to nickel carbonyl as the sole toxic agent rather than with the admixture of nickel carbonyl and carbon monoxide. The initial symptoms frequently pass off gradually with adequate symptomatic treatment. The patient may also remain symptom-free from a few hours to as long as a week after exposure.

In cases of severe exposure, the initial symptoms may merge gradually into the more severe delayed type of reaction. The delayed symptoms include a return of dyspnea, hacking cough and a sense of constriction over the chest and in the midepigastrium. Nausea, vomiting, cyanosis, lethargy and delirium may develop. Death is usually due to pulmonary and cerebral edema. Pathologic changes include hemorrhage into the lungs, brain and adrenal glands, edema of the brain and the lungs and hepatic degeneration.

The pulmonary parenchyma is extremely susceptible to nickel carbonyl. The primary injury occurs in the pulmonary alveoli with maximum severity from the fourth to the sixth days after exposure. Capillary congestion, focal hemorrhages, interstitial edema, interstitial cellular proliferation, fibrinous intraalveolar exudate and hypertrophy of the alveolar lining cells are seen. Lung changes diminish within several days and the tissues return to normal by three weeks except for occasional interstitial fibrosis. The pulmonary parenchyma has a special attraction for nickel. Analysis of nickel in tissue from previously healthy subjects and from a subject dying of nickel carbonyl poisoning shows the highest concentration of nickel in the lungs. Injection of nickel carbonyl labeled with radioactive nickel ($^{63}$Ni) intravenously into rats was followed by detection of 38 per cent of the injected dose in expired air after six hours. This implies that the lungs are a principal route of excretion of nickel carbonyl.

With severe poisoning, the respiratory rate is increased out of proportion to the pulse rate. Thus, a pulse-respiratory ratio of 3:1 or less during the initial stage suggests that a patient may have delayed reactions. Convulsions in a critically ill patient may be a poor prognostic sign.

The liver in nickel poisoning shows moderate central congestion. Nickel carbonyl inhibits synthesis of hepatic ribonucleic acid. Mild pathologic changes also occur in the kidneys with vacuolization of the proximal convoluted tubules but no tubular necrosis.

Urinary excretion of nickel is high for at least twenty-four hours after exposure. The amount of nickel detected in the urine is helpful in judging the severity of the exposure. If the concentration of nickel in the urine collected during an eight-hour interval immediately after exposure is less than 25 μg/100 ml, the exposure may be classified as mild. In such a case, it is anticipated that the delayed symptoms would either not appear or be relatively mild. These patients usually are able to continue their work. When the eight-hour urine is between 25 and 50 μg/100 ml, the delayed symptoms can be expected. If the concentration is above 50 μg/100 ml, the delayed symptoms are likely to be severe and immediate therapy is advised. Treatment with diethyldithiocarbamate is continued until the concentration of nickel in the urine is less than 10 μg/100 ml. Diarrhea and abdominal distension occur in some cases, indicating that nickel is also excreted by the intestines.

Pathologic changes occur mainly in the lungs, liver and brain. Damage of pulmonary tissue is the primary cause of death in fatal cases.

In the *treatment,* 100% oxygen therapy for the pulmonary edema, cyanosis and dyspnea should be given. BAL is a specific antidote in that it increases the urinary excretion of nickel and lowers the concentration in the blood. Sodium diethyldithiocarbamate trihydrate (dithiocarb) as a metal-binding reagent has also proven effective in the treatment of acute nickel carbonyl poisoning. Other measures should include bedrest, antibiotics and steroid therapy for chemical pneumonitis if it occurs.

*Zinc*

Zinc is a soft metal of bluish-white luster with crystalline fraction used for galvanizing containers. Its soluble salts are often incorporated in astringent, escharotic, deodorant and disinfectant agents. Acid food prepared or stored in galvanized zinc cans or utensils may dissolve sufficient zinc metal, which is converted to zinc salts and subsequently ingested with food and liquids in sufficient amounts (225 to 450 mg of zinc sulfate is an emetic dose) to cause severe vomiting with or without nausea.

Mass food poisoning attributable to zinc salts occurs frequently enough that the public needs to be well educated to the dangers of galvanized containers for the preparation and storage of acid food or liquids. The ingestion of solutions of zinc salts can cause intense gastric and substernal pain with violent vomiting and diarrhea, shock and collapse and possibly death. Those who survive may have residual nephritis and strictures of the esophagus and pyloric end of the stomach. Skin contact causes papulovesicular lesions with exfoliation. Inhalation of zinc fumes or other metal fumes (oxides of Al, Sb, Cd, Fe, Mn, Ni, Se, Ag, Cu, Sn) produced in welding, metal cutting and smelting, zinc alloys or galvanized iron can cause "metal fume fever" ("galvo," brass-founder's ague and Brasiere disease) with fever, chills, vomiting, myalgia, tracheobronchitis and often fatal pneumonia.

*Treatment* consists of gastric lavage and the administration of demulcents. In skin contact, the skin should be thoroughly washed with soap and water. A full course of calcium edetate should be given unless one is reasonably certain that poisoning is minimal. Antibiotics and steroid therapy as an anti-inflammatory agent may be useful in the treatment of the chemical pneumonitis that often complicates "metal fume fever."

ZINC CYANIDE. This compound is a white powder which, though tasteless, has an odor of bitter almonds. It has been used as an insecticide, and when accidental ingestion with food has occurred, severe vomiting, diarrhea, dyspnea, cyanosis, convulsions and even death from pulmonary edema have resulted.

ZINC DICHROMATE. This agent is used as a pigment in primers because it is a brilliant orange-yellow powder which is readily soluble. Skin contact, especially from chronic exposure, may cause severe dermatitis.

ZINC OXIDE. This powder is formed when metallic zinc is melted or heated in the presence of air. The ingestion of this compound produces intense gastroenteritis, since severe irritation and even corrosion of the mucosa of the stomach follow the formation of zinc chloride in the stomach by the interaction of zinc oxide and the hydrochloric acid of the gastric juice.

ZINC PHOSPHIDE. (*See* Chap. 2, Phosphine.)

ZINC STEARATE. This soft, bulky powder is a mixture of the zinc salts of stearic and palmitic acids and zinc oxide. Prolonged occupational exposure to the dust may result in diffuse fibrosis of the lung. Infants may aspirate zinc stearate present in commercial talcum powders. A severe irritation of the respiratory mucous membranes is produced with resulting congestion, hyperemia, edema and obstruction of bronchioles with mucus. Bronchopneumonia is common in infants who survive the first day or two. Choking, coughing, cyanosis and signs of suffocation tend to develop immediately. *Treatment* consisting of aspiration of the powder and accumulated secretions by bronchoscopy is worth a trial but is not apt to be effective, because of the marked adhesive quality of the powder. Administration of oxygen is important, and antibiotics along with steroid therapy may be beneficial in combatting the chemical pneumonitis. The use of a Croupette in small children is invaluable.

ZINC SULFATE. This white, odorless astringent powder is efflorescent in dry air and very soluble in water. Its precipitating effect on proteins forms the basis for its astringent and antiseptic properties. As little as 30 gm (1 oz.) has caused fatalities. Symptoms produced from ingestion are burning pain in the mouth and throat, vomiting, watery or bloody diarrhea, tenesmus, retching, anuria, collapse and convulsions. Hyperglycemia has been reported and hepatic and renal damage may be severe.

Zinc deficiency syndrome in Iranian men characterized by iron deficiency anemia, hepatosplenomegaly, hypogonadism, hyperpigmentation and dwarfism has resulted from excessive consumption of wheat containing large amounts of phosphate, which inhibits iron and zinc absorption. Geophagia was also a factor since it contributes additional quantities of phosphate and possibly chelating agents. *Treatment* with zinc salts alone was able to reverse all of the signs and symptoms except for the anemia, which required specific iron therapy.

## *Trace Metals*

Man is constantly exposed to elements that accumulate innocuously in the body. The tin content of canned foods, particularly tomatoes that have been stored for some time, may be alarmingly high, but most of it is insoluble, poorly absorbed and rapidly eliminated. Foods that are properly canned are not dangerous. Aluminum ingested from water, food, cooking ware or antacids may decrease absorption of other substances but is not inherently toxic. Progressive accumulation of titanium has no known harmful or beneficial effects. Acid foods or liquids stored or prepared in galvanized zinc utensils have produced mass food poisoning.

A number of elements are capable of doing harm by usurping the function of essential ones—beryllium substituting for magnesium, silver and gold for copper, rubidium and cesium for potassium, lithium for sodium, arsenic for phosphorus, tellurium and selenium for sulfur, barium and strontium for calcium, tungsten for molybdenum, cadmium and mercury for zinc. Cadmium is one of the worst offenders, disturbing kidney function and increasing reabsorption of sodium. The cadmium level is high in hypertension and is lowered by antihypertensive treatment. Cadmium is also toxic to the testes. Testicular injury in rats produced by cadmium can be prevented by giving zinc simultaneously. Others have found selenium more effective than zinc, because selenium has the capacity for combining with cadmium, as with other metals.

Industrial poisoning occurs with antimony, arsenic, beryllium, cadmium, lead, mercury, strontium, tellurium and thorium. Strontium has had much attention because of its radioactive form in fallout. Fortunately, it is not well absorbed and its concentration in bone rises and falls in response to serum levels. Strontium laid down in teeth, however, is a permanent and undesirable acquisition. It has been found that sodium alginate binds and eliminates strontium without inhibiting absorption of calcium.

Lead poisoning used to be frequent in industry but is now largely limited to pica in children. We all carry lead in our bodies and accumulate it until late middle age, after which we excrete more than we absorb.

Medicinal metal poisoning is still frequent, some of it occurring as a result of the calculated risk of justifiable treatment with toxic substances. Antimony, arsenic, barium, bismuth, boron, gold and mercury have all been involved.

Most of us get enough of the essential trace metals to meet physiologic needs, and few of us are exposed to them in toxic amounts. In deficiency states, supplementation with certain minerals (and vitamins) is advisable, if not mandatory, but in restricted amounts in order to guard against upsetting the delicate balance in their relationship.

Deficiency of copper is rare, and hypercupremia is as undesirable as hypocupremia; but many authorities recommend adding this highly essential element when the diet requires fortifying. The same considerations apply to cobalt, manganese and molybdenum. Recent findings indicate that zinc should be added in areas where natural sources are inadequate. Molybdenum and other metals can be relied upon to counter any tendency zinc may have to aggravate caries. Up to the present, vanadium has not figured in vitamin-mineral preparations. Since it is deficient in many localities, it should perhaps be included for its benefits to the circulation and to the teeth.

### *Tin (Stannic Chloride)*

Tin is an almost silver-white, lustrous, soft, readily malleable metal used in plating and for the impregnation of stockings. Acute tin poisoning is very rare. It has been reported from the ingestion of acid-canned herring and asparagus. The toxic symptoms started after a latent period of five to six hours and were characterized by vomiting, severe colic, meteorism, oppression in the chest and diarrhea, and later by metallic taste and constipation. In a few instances the continued absorption of small quantities of tin has been followed by abdominal pain, nausea, constipation and loss of weight. Some patients have complained about sore throat, mild fever, chilliness, myalgias and arthralgias, and some have shown moderate anemia.

The continued inhalation of small quantities of tin oxide may lead to pneumoconiosis which usually does not show significant fibrosis, the tin particles being deposited in the perivascular and peribronchial regions and along the subpleura lymphatics, producing a sharp shadow in the roentgenogram. Patients suffering from this condition may have shortness of breath, especially upon exertion, slight cough and a reduction of the vital and maximal breathing capacity.

*Treatment* consists essentially in discontinuance of the exposure. The elimination of tin from the organism may be enhanced by the administration of potassium iodide.

### *Titanium Tetrachloride*

This compound is an important intermediate in the production of titanium metal and certain pigments. It is a colorless liquid that fumes strongly in moist air. From a clinical point of view, its most important characteristic is that it reacts violently with water to liberate heat and produce hydrochloric acid. Serious injuries have resulted when workers were sprayed with water after being splashed with the chemical. It should be removed from the body by dry wiping before any washing with water. Burns resulting from its action are deep and slow to heal. A splash of the liquid in an eye may lead to permanent damage. Immediate wiping of the eyelids and adjacent facial structures with a dry cloth, followed by copious washing of the eye with water, is necessary to avoid severe injury. The effect of

TABLE 69
AVERAGE LEVELS OF TRACE METALS*
(gm/70-kg man)

| | | | | | |
|---|---|---|---|---|---|
| Iron | 4 | Antimony | <.09 | Cobalt | <.003 |
| Zinc | 2.3 | Lanthanum | <.05 | Beryllium | <.002 |
| Rubidium | 1.2 | Niobium | <.05 | Gold | <.001 |
| Strontium | 0.14 | Titanium | <.015 | Silver | <.001 |
| Copper | 0.1 | Nickel | <.01 | Lithium | <.0009 |
| Aluminum | 0.1 | Boron | <.01 | Bismuth | <.0003 |
| Lead | .08 | Chromium | <.006 | Vanadium | <.0001 |
| Tin | .03 | Ruthenium | <.006 | Uranium | .00002 |
| Cadmium | .02 | Thallium | <.006 | Cesium | <.00001 |
| Manganese | .02 | Zirconium | <.006 | Gallium | <.000002 |
| Barium | .016 | Molybdenum | <.005 | Radium | .0000000001 |
| Arsenic | <.01 | | | | |

*The table includes nonmetallic elements such as boron, whose chemical behavior is similar to that of true metals.

—After W. H. Strain, AAAS Symposium on geochemical evolution, Denver, 1961, Table 1.

titanium tetrachloride fumes on the lungs is a corrosive one, resulting in chemical bronchitis or pneumonia, which should be treated with corticosteroids and antibiotics. The prevention of fume exposures is important, and all workers who may be subjected to a sudden release of fumes should wear airline masks. Anyone who has been exposed to fumes should be given prophylactic oxygen treatment to minimize the possibility of the development of pulmonary edema.

*Titanium oxide,* on the other hand, is a fairly innocuous substance used as an ingredient in cosmetics and in dentistry to give a natural yellowish tint to artificial teeth.

A four-year study at the National Institute of Nutrition in Tokyo showed that toxic heavy metals are discharged from the body more rapidly by perspiration than by excretion in the urine.

Copper was excreted in the urine at 30 to 60 μg/day, while almost the same amount was removed by only 1 hour of perspiration.

Only 0.9 μg of cadmium was excreted in the urine per day, while an average of 4.4 μg was removed by 1 hour of perspiration. For lead, the respective figures were 17 μg and 11 μg, and for zinc, 100 and 500 μg.

Conversely, the study confirmed that lighter metals—for example, sodium, calcium, barium and magnesium—are removed in smaller amounts by a heavy amount of perspiration than they are by excretion in the urine.

TABLE 70
MAXIMUM BIOLOGICAL ALLOWABLE CONCENTRATIONS

| *Substance* | *Estimated as* | *Maximum allowable concentration (MAC)* | *Biological material* |
|---|---|---|---|
| Lead | Lead | 0.15 mg/liter | Urine |
| Lead | Lead | 0.08 mg/liter | Blood |
| Lead | Coproporphyrin | 0.10 mg/liter | Urine |
| Tetraethyl lead | Lead | 0.12 mg/liter | Urine |
| Tetraethyl lead | Lead | 0.07 mg/liter | Blood |
| Mercury | Mercury | 0.10 mg/liter | Urine |
| Chromium | Chromium | 0.04 mg/liter | Urine |
| Arsenic | Arsenic | 0.10 mg/liter | Urine |
| Arsenic | Arsenic | 3 μg/gm | Hair |
| Benzol | Conjugated sulphates | 70% | Urine |
| Trichloroethylene | Trichloroacetic acid | 50 mg/liter | Urine |
| Acetone | Acetone | 50 mg/liter | Blood |
| Acetone | Acetone | 100 mg/liter | Urine |
| Acetone | Acetone | 0.12 mg/liter | Expired air |
| Alcohol, ethyl | Alcohol | 0.05–0.15% | Blood |
| Toluol | Hippuric acid | 2.4 gm/24 hours | Urine |
| Parathion (organic phosphates) | Cholinesterase activity | reduced by 5% | Blood |
| CO | COHb | 14% | Blood |
| CO | CO | 3 ml% | Blood |
| CO | CO | 0.014% | Expired air |
| HF | Fluoride | 2 mg/liter | Urine |

From E. C. Vigliani: *Med d Lavoro, 50* (No. 5): 323–327, 1959.

TABLE 71
BLOOD, URINE AND TISSUE LEVELS OF METALS
(MICROGRAMS PER 100 ML OR 100 GM)

| | *Blood* | *Urine* | *Liver* | *Kidney* | *Brain* | *Hair and Nails* |
|---|---|---|---|---|---|---|
| *Arsenic* | | | | | | |
| Normal | 0-2.0 | 0-20 | 1-10 | 1-10 | 0-2 | 25-100 |
| Toxic | 100 | 68-350 | | | | 400-9700 |
| Lethal | 100-150 | | 1000-50,000 | 500-15,000 | 50-2000 | |
| *Lead* | | | | | | |
| Normal | 0-30 | <8 | 90-460 | 70-370 | 20-70 | |
| Toxic | 70 | 8 | | | | |
| Lethal | 330 | | | | | |
| *Mercury* | | | | | | |
| Normal | 0-8 | .6-1.6 | 500 | 8-7930 | 120-1520 | 3-600 |
| Toxic | 100 | 5-100 | 2500 | 27,500 | | 6000 |
| Lethal | | | 5000 | | 1000 | |
| *Nickel* | | | | | | |
| Normal | 0.3-6.0 | 0-6 | .5-1.3 | .8-2.4 (Lung) | | 22 |
| Toxic | | | | 7-21 (Lung) | | |
| *Cadmium* | | | | | | |
| Normal | | <.5 | 40-390 | 350-3000 | | .04-.35 |
| Toxic | 4.1 to 28 | 10-50 | | | | 0.4-2.8 μg/gm |
| Lethal | | >100 | | | | |
| *Tin* | | | | | | |
| Normal | 12-14 | 1.1 | 60 | 20 | | |
| *Lithium* | | | | | | |
| Lethal | | | 9.4 | 14.4 | 9.8 | 109 (Bile) |

From Charles L. Winek, Injury by Chemical Agents. In C.G. Tedeschi, L.G. Tedeschi and W.G. Eckert (Eds.), *Forensic Medicine,* © 1977 by W. B. Saunders Company, Philadelphia, Pennsylvania.

## *Chapter 5*

# OCCUPATIONAL HAZARDS

In 1975 the Occupational Safety and Health Administration found that more than three quarters of the industries it inspected had failed to meet established safety standards. Two thirds of the adult population—some 85 million men and women—are in America's labor force, and what many of them do each day to earn a living may be killing them.

Each year occupational hazards kill more than 14,000 people and disable, either temporarily or permanently, more that 2.2 million others. An estimated 500,000 workers develop work-related diseases each year. As many as 100,000 deaths each year may be associated with these diseases. Yet 90 per cent of work-related conditions may never even be suspected nor reported.

Almost every week previously unrecognized health hazards are discovered, new chemicals, new products, new methods of manufacture. But occupational hazards are not confined to the workplace. They extend to the worker's family, to his community and to the environment we all share. Some congenital malformations and diseases, for example, have been linked directly to parental exposure to toxic agents in the workplace. New potentially carcinogenic occupational chemicals are being uncovered and recognized continually, but progress in eliminating these hazards is always a slow process, unless some dire catastrophe occurs.

The Workmen's Compensation Act, which protects over 80 per cent of the work force, almost totally ignores the importance and need for prevention. The main purpose of this law is to protect workers from undue financial burdens created by occupational diseases or injuries. Operating on the premise that disability can be compensated for in dollars alone, the act does very little to prevent hazardous situations leading to disabilities.

Two federal laws aimed at preventing occupational deaths and disabilities are the Federal Coal Mine Health and Safety Act of 1969 and the Occupational Safety and Health Act of 1970. While these acts provide excellent potential for reducing health hazards in the workplace, their implementation has been slow. However, the recent Toxic Substances Control Act (1976), which requires tests for potential harmfulness in new chemicals (and for new uses of existing chemicals), because of the complexities involved, may be most difficult to implement. The "Ames test" is a relatively new procedure for checking the potential mutagenicity and carcinogenicity of chemical substances by monitoring a chemical's effect on bacteria instead of on a group of laboratory animals. The test is a quick and inexpensive screening test, but definitive answers still require animal bioassays, and positive correlation has not been fully achieved. Nevertheless, many scientists believe that the Ames test will have many positive applications, for example, the direct screening of humans for cancer by testing their urine.

Physicians and health professionals involved and interested in occupational health must go beyond "band-aid" solutions and attempt to balance the equation between safety of the work force and industrial productivity.

TABLE 72

OCCUPATIONAL HAZARDS

| *Occupation* | *Hazard* | *Diagnosis* |
|---|---|---|
| Acetaldehyde workers | Acetaldehyde; mercury and its compounds | History; mercury in urine |
| Acetanilid workers | Aniline and other amino compounds of benzol and its homologs | History |
| Acetic-acid makers | Hydrochloric acid; mercury and its compounds | History; mercury in urine |
| Acetone workers | Acetone; mercury and its compounds | History |
| Acetylene workers | Inorganic dust (acetone; ammonia; arsine; carbon disulfide; carbon monoxide; chloride of lime; chromium compounds) | History; chest x-ray; temperature chart; arsenic in urine |
| Acid dippers | Dampness; arsine; cyanogen compounds; hydrochloric acid; nitrous fumes and nitric acid; sulfuric acid | History; arsenic in urine |
| Acid finishers (glass) | Hydrochloric and sulfuric acid; lead and its compounds | History; lead in urine and blood |
| Acridine workers | Acridine | History |
| Acrolein workers | Acrolein | History |
| Agricultural workers | Farmer's lung (inhalation of dust from moldy forage) | History; chest x-ray; circulating antibodies |
| Airplane-dope makers | Acetone; amyl acetate; benzol (benzene) and its homologs (toluol and xylol); carbon tetrachloride; formic acid; methyl Cellosolve® (ethylene glycol; monomethyl ether); tetrachloroethane (acetylene tetrachloride) | History |
| Airplane-hanger employees | Benzine (naphtha-gasoline); benzol (benzene) and its homologs (toluol and xylol); carbon tetrachloride | History |
| Airplane pilots (crop dusting) | Inhalation of various insecticides | History |
| Alcohol-distillery workers | Amyl acetate; amyl alcohol; benzol (benzene) and its homologs (toluol and xylol); mercury and its compounds; methanol (methyl alcohol) | History; mercury in urine |
| Aldehyde pumpmen | Acetaldehyde; methanol (methyl alcohol) | History |
| Alkali-salt makers | Dampness; carbon dioxide; chlorine; hydrochloric acid; sulfur dioxide; sulfuretted hydrogen (hydrogen sulfide) | History |
| Alloy makers | Heat; beryllium; carbon monoxide; cobalt; magnesium; manganese; nickel; selenium compounds; vanadium | History |
| Aluminum extractors | Hydrofluoric acid; manganese | History |
| Alum workers | Sulfuric acid | History |
| Amalgam makers | Mercury and its compounds | History; mercury in urine |
| Amber workers | Lead and its compounds | History; lead in urine |

*Compiled from *U.S. Department of Labor,* Bulletin No. 41.

TABLE 72—*Continued*

| *Occupation* | *Hazard* | *Diagnosis* |
|---|---|---|
| Ammonia workers | Ammonia; calcium cyanamide (cyanamide); carbon monoxide | History |
| Ammonium-salt makers | Heat; ammonia; carbon disulfide; cyanogen compounds; hydrochloric acid; sulfuric acid | History |
| Ammonium-sulfate makers | Sulfuric acid | History |
| Amyl-acetate workers | Amyl acetate; amyl alcohol | History |
| Amyl-nitrite workers | Amyl alcohol | History |
| Aniline-dye makers | (See Dye makers) | History |
| Aniline workers | Aniline and other amino compounds of benzol and its homologs; arsine; benzol (benzene) and its homologs (toluol and xylol); chromium compounds; hydrochloric acid; nitrobenzol and other nitro compounds of benzol and its homologs; nitrous fumes and nitric acid | History; arsenic in urine; methemoglobinemia |
| Animal handlers | Anthrax; fungus infections; septic infections | History |
| Annealers | Heat; ammonia | History |
| Antifreeze makers | Methanol (methyl alcohol); ethylene glycol | History |
| Antimony extractors (refiners) | Heat; antimony and its compounds; pneumoconiosis | History; chest x-ray |
| Antimony-fluoride extractors | Hydrofluoric acid | History |
| Antipyrine makers | Phenylhydrazine | History; hemogram |
| Apple packers | Gentian violet in salvaged newsprint used for packing of boxes, producing epistaxis | History |
| Arc welders | Siderosis; silicosis | History; chest x-ray |
| Arsenic roasters | Heat; arsenic and its compounds (except arsine) | History; arsenic in urine |
| Art-glass workers | Amyl acetate; benzine (naphtha-gasoline); hydrofluoric acid; lead and its compounds; methanol (methyl alcohol); turpentine | History; lead in urine |
| Artificial-amber makers | Formaldehyde | History |
| Artificial-flower makers | Repeated motion, pressure, shock; arsenic and its compounds (except arsine); chromium compounds; lead and its compounds; mercury and its compounds; methanol (methyl alcohol) | History; arsenic in urine; lead and mercury in urine; hemogram |
| Artificial-gem makers | Thallium | History |
| Artificial-ice makers | Sudden variations in temperature; dampness; ammonia; sulfur dioxide | History |
| Artificial-leather workers | Heat; acetone; amyl acetate; aniline and other amino compounds of benzol and its homologs; arsenic and its compounds (except arsine); benzol (benzene) and its homologs (toluol and xylol); butanone (methyl ethyl ketone); butyl alcohol; methanol (methyl alcohol); nitrous fumes and nitric acid; sulfuric acid | History; arsenic in urine; hemogram |
| Artificial-pearl makers | Acetone; amyl acetate; lead and its compounds; nitrous fumes and nitric acid; tetrachloroethane (acetylene tetrachloride) | History; lead in urine |
| Artificial-stone makers | Tar and pitch | History |

TABLE 72—*Continued*

| *Occupation* | *Hazard* | *Diagnosis* |
|---|---|---|
| Asbestos miners* | Asbestos; neoplasia (cancer of the lungs, stomach, colon and mesotheliomas). (See also Miners.) | History; chest x-ray; temperature chart |
| Asbestos-products workers* | Heat; asbestos; benzol (benzene) and its homologs (toluol and xylol); formaldehyde; tar and pitch | History; chest x-ray; temperature chart; hemogram |
| Ashmen | Organic dust; inorganic dust (except asbestos) containing no free silica | History; chest x-ray; temperature chart |
| Asphalt workers | Heat; tar and pitch | History |
| Automobile painters | Dampness; benzol (benzene) and its homologs (toluol and xylol); methanol (methyl alcohol). (See also Painters) | History; hemogram |
| Automobile-radiator cleaners | Oxalic acid | History |
| Babbitters | Antimony and its compounds; lead and its compounds | History; antimony and lead in urine |
| Babbitt-metal workers | Antimony and its compounds; lead and its compounds | History; antimony and lead in urine |
| Bakers | Sudden variations of temperature; organic dust; ultraviolet and infrared rays; carbon dioxide; carbon monoxide | History |
| Baking-powder makers | Carbon dioxide | History |
| Balloon (hydrogen) workers | Arsine | History; arsenic in urine |
| Balloon inflators | Carbon monoxide | History |
| Barbers | Infection; repeated motion, pressure, shock | History |
| Barium-carbonate makers | Barium; sulfuretted hydrogen (hydrogen sulfide) | History |
| Bar-mill workers (iron and steel) | Heat | History |
| Barometer makers | Mercury and its compounds | History; mercury in urine |
| Basic-slag (artificial manure) workers | Inorganic dust (except asbestos) containing no free silica | History; chest x-ray; temperature chart |
| Baters (tannery) | Anthrax | History |
| Beamers (textiles) | Organic dust | History; chest x-ray; temperature chart |
| Beamhouse workers (tannery) | Dampness; anthrax | History |
| Beaterman (paper and pulp) | Dampness; chlorine | History |
| Bed rubbers (stone) | Inorganic dust containing free silica; inorganic dust (except asbestos) containing no free silica | History; chest x-ray |
| Benzine workers | Benzine (naphtha-gasoline) | History; hemogram |
| Benzol purifiers | Benzol (benzene) and its homologs (toluol and xylol); sulfuric acid | History; hemogram |
| Benzol-stillmen | Heat; benzol (benzene) and toluol and xylol | History |
| Beryllium-alloy workers | Beryllium | History |
| Beryllium extractors | Hydrofluoric acid | History |
| Bessemer-converter workers (iron and steel) | Heat; carbon monoxide | History |

*New evidence suggests that the risk of asbestos-induced cancer is greater than previously suspected (over 50% in 600 cases of asbestosis).

TABLE 72—*Continued*

| *Occupation* | *Hazard* | *Diagnosis* |
|---|---|---|
| Beta-still operators (beta-naphthol) | Heat; sulfuric acid | History |
| Bevelers | Inorganic dust (except asbestos) containing no free silica | History; chest x-ray |
| Billet-mill workers (iron and steel) | Heat | History |
| Bisque-kiln workers | Heat; inorganic dust containing free silica; inorganic dust (except asbestos) containing no free silica; carbon monoxide | History; chest x-ray; temperature chart |
| Blacksmiths | Heat; ultraviolet and infrared rays; repeated motion, pressure, shock; carbon dioxide and monoxide; cyanogen compounds; lead and its compounds | History; lead in urine |
| Blasters | Inorganic dust containing free silica; inorganic dust (except asbestos) containing no free silica; carbon monoxide; nitrous fumes and nitric acid; sulfuretted hydrogen (hydrogen sulfide) | History; chest x-ray |
| Blast-furnace workers | Heat; carbon dioxide; carbon monoxide; cyanogen compounds; phosphuretted hydrogen (phosphine); sulfur dioxide; sulfuretted hydrogen (hydrogen sulfide) | History |
| Bleachers | Heat; sudden variations in temperature; chloride of lime; chlorine; chromium compounds; hydrochloric acid; hydrofluoric acid; nitrous fumes and nitric acid; oxalic acid; ozone; phosgene; potassium hydroxide; sodium hydroxide; sulfur dioxide | History |
| Bleachery driers | Heat | History |
| Bleaching-powder makers | Arsine; chloride of lime; chlorine; manganese | History; arsenic in urine |
| Blockers (felt hats) | Heat; carbon monoxide | History |
| Blooders (tannery) | Lead and its compounds | History; lead in urine |
| Blooming-mill workers (iron and steel) | Heat | History |
| Blowers (felt hats) | Organic dust; mercury and its compounds | History; mercury in urine |
| Blowers-out (zinc smelting) | Heat; zinc | History |
| Blue-print makers | Chromium compounds | History |
| Blue-print paper makers | Aniline and other amino compounds of benzol and its homologs; oxalic acid | History |
| Boiler cleaners and washers | Dampness; carbon monoxide | History |
| Boiler-room workers | Heat; carbon dioxide; carbon monoxide | History |
| Boneblack makers | Ammonia; phosphorus | History |
| Bone renders, extractors, etc. | Organic dust; anthrax; acrolein; cyanogen compounds; sulfur dioxide | History |
| Bookbinders | Acrolein; amyl acetate; arsenic and its compounds (except arsine); lead and its compounds; methanol (methyl alcohol); oxalic acid | History; arsenic and lead in urine |
| Bottle-cap makers | Lead and its compounds | History; lead in urine |
| Bottlers (mineral waters) | Carbon dioxide; sulfuretted hydrogen (hydrogen sulfide) | History |
| Brake-lining makers | Asbestos; benzol (benzene) and its homologs (toluol and xylol) | History; chest x-ray; temperature chart |

TABLE 72—*Continued*

| *Occupation* | *Hazard* | *Diagnosis* |
|---|---|---|
| Brass founders | Heat; antimony and arsenic compounds (except arsine); carbon dioxide; carbon monoxide; copper, lead and its compounds; phosphorus; sulfur dioxide | History; lead in urine |
| Brass polishers | Lead and its compounds. (See also Polishers and cleaners [metal].) | History; lead in urine |
| Braziers | Heat; ultraviolet and infrared rays; lead and its compounds; zinc | History; lead in urine |
| Brewers | Heat; sudden variation in temperatures; fungus infections; amyl alcohol; carbon dioxide; carbon monoxide; formaldehyde; hydrofluoric acid; phenol; sulfuric acid | History |
| Brick burners | Heat; carbon dioxide; carbon monoxide; lead and its compounds | History; lead in urine |
| Brick makers | Heat; dampness; inorganic dust containing free silica; inorganic dust (except asbestos) containing no free silica; hydrofluoric acid; lead and its compounds; magnesium; manganese; sulfur dioxide | History; chest x-ray |
| Briquet makers | Arsenic and its compounds (except arsine); tar and pitch | History; arsenic in urine |
| Bromine makers | Aniline and other compounds of benzol and its homologs; bromine; chlorine | History; bromine in urine |
| Bronze-powder makers | Acetone; zinc | History |
| Bronzers | Inorganic dust (except asbestos) containing no free silica; ammonia; amyl acetate; arsenic and its compounds (except arsine); benzine (naphtha-gasoline); benzol (benzene) and its homologs (toluol and xylol); cyanogen compounds; hydrochloric acid; lead and its compounds; manganese; mercury and its compounds; methanol (methyl alcohol); sulfuretted hydrogen (hydrogen sulfide); zinc | History; arsenic and lead in urine; hemogram |
| Broom makers | Organic dust; anthrax; chlorine; formaldehyde; sulfur dioxide | History |
| Browners (gun barrels) | Cyanogen compounds; lead and its compounds; mercury and its compounds; petroleum. (See also Benzine workers.) | History; lead and mercury in urine |
| Brushers (felt hats) | Organic dust; mercury and its compounds | History; mercury in urine |
| Brush makers | Organic dust; anthrax; formaldehyde; lead and its compounds; methanol (methyl alcohol); tar and pitch | History; lead in urine |
| Buffers | Defective illumination; organic dust; inorganic dust containing free silica; inorganic dust (except asbestos) containing no free silica | History; chest x-ray; temperature chart |
| Buffers (rubber) | Amyl acetate; benzine (naphtha-gasoline); lead and its compounds | History; lead in urine |
| Bulb (mercury) makers | Mercury and its compounds | History; mercury in urine |
| Buoy makers | Phosphuretted hydrogen (phosphine) | History |
| Burners (enameling) | Heat; lead and its compounds | History; lead in urine |
| Burnishers (metals) | Defective illumination; antimony and its compounds; benzine (naphtha-gasoline); carbon tetrachloride; sulfuric acid; trichloroethylene | History; antimony in urine; hemogram |

TABLE 72—*Continued*

| *Occupation* | *Hazard* | *Diagnosis* |
|---|---|---|
| Burrers (needles) | Inorganic dust containing free silica; inorganic dust (except absestos) containing no free silica | History; chest x-ray |
| Burr filers | Inorganic dust containing free silica; inorganic dust (except asbestos) containing no free silica | History; chest x-ray |
| Button makers | Organic dust; inorganic dust (except asbestos) containing no free silica; infections; acetone; chloride of lime; formaldehyde | History; chest x-ray |
| Butyl-acetate makers | Butyl alcohol | History |
| Butyl-alcohol makers | Butyl alcohol | History |
| Butyl-cellosolve makers | Ethylene oxide | History |
| Cable makers | Lead and its compounds | History; lead in urine |
| Cable splicers | Dampness; carbon monoxide; lead and its compounds; sulfuretted hydrogen (hydrogen sulfide); turpentine | History; lead in urine |
| Cadmium-alloy makers | Cadmium | History |
| Cadmium and cadmium-compound makers | Arsine, cadmium | History; arsenic in urine |
| Cadmium platers | Cadmium. (See also Electroplaters.) | History |
| Cadmium-vapor-lamp workers | Cadmium | History |
| Caisson workers | Abnormalities of air pressure (compressed air-increased atmospheric pressure); sudden variations in temperature; dampness; defective illumination; carbon dioxide; carbon monoxide; sulfuretted hydrogen (hydrogen sulfide) | History |
| Calcium-cyanamide makers | Heat; inorganic dust (except asbestos) containing no free silica; calcium cyanamide (cyanamide) | History; chest x-ray |
| Calenderers (rubber) | Sudden variations in temperature; inorganic dust (except asbestos) containing no free silica | History; chest x-ray |
| Camphor makers | Amyl acetate; aniline and other amino compounds of benzol and its homologs; hydrochloric acid; zinc | History |
| Candle makers | Acrolein; aniline and other amino compounds of benzol and its homologs; arsenic and its compounds; chromium compounds; sulfuric acid | History; arsenic in urine |
| Canners | Heat; sudden variations in temperature; dampness; septic infections; arsenic and its compounds (except arseniureted hydrogen); carbon dioxide; lead and its compounds | History; arsenic in urine |
| Can sealers | Benzol (benzene) and its homologs (toluol and xylol) | History; hemogram |
| Cap loaders | Mercury and its compounds | History; mercury in urine |
| Carbanilide makers | Carbon disulfide | History |
| Carbide makers | Heat; organic dust; inorganic dust (except asbestos) containing no free silica; ammonia; carbon monoxide | History; chest x-ray |
| Carbolic-acid makers | Benzol (benzene) and its homologs (toluol and xylol); phenol; sulfur dioxide; sulfuric acid | History; routine urine examination; hemogram |
| Carbon-black workers | Heat; organic dust | History; chest x-ray |

TABLE 72—*Continued*

| *Occupation* | *Hazard* | *Diagnosis* |
|---|---|---|
| Carbon-brush makers | Organic dust; inorganic dust (except asbestos) containing no free silica | History; chest x-ray |
| Carbon-dioxide-ice workers | Carbon dioxide | History |
| Carbon dioxide makers | Carbon dioxide | History |
| Carbon-disulfide makers | Carbon disulfide; hydrogen sulfide | History |
| Carbonic-acid makers | Carbon dioxide | History |
| Carbonizers (shoddy) | Organic dust; arseniureted hydrogen (arsine); hydrochloric acid; sulfuric acid | History; chest x-ray; arsenic in urine |
| Carbon-paper makers | Organic dust | History |
| Carbon printers (photography) | Chromium compounds | History |
| Carbon-tetrachloride workers | Carbon disulfide; carbon tetrachloride; phosgene; sulfur chloride | History |
| Carders (asbestos) | Asbestos | History; chest x-ray |
| Carders (textiles) | Organic dust | History; chest x-ray |
| Card grinders (textiles) | Organic dust; inorganic dust (except asbestos) containing no free silica | History; chest x-ray |
| Carpet makers | Organic dust; anthrax; arsenic and its compounds (except arsine) | History; chest x-ray; arsenic in urine |
| Carroters (felt hats) | Arsenic and its compounds; mercury and its compounds; nitrous fumes and nitric acid | History; arsenic and mercury in urine |
| Cartridge makers | Lead and its compounds; mercury and its compounds | History; lead and mercury in urine |
| Case hardeners | Heat; cyanogen compounds | History |
| Casters (metal) | (See Foundry workers; and also particular metal) | History |
| Casting cleaners (foundry) | Inorganic dust containing free silica; inorganic dust (except asbestos) containing no free silica. (See also Acid dippers) | History; chest x-ray |
| Cast scrubbers (electroplaters) | Benzine (naphtha-gasoline); benzol (benzene) and its homologs (toluol and xylol) | History; hemogram |
| Cellulose-formate makers | Formic acid | History |
| Cellulose makers | Dampness; sodium hydroxide; sufur dioxide; sulfuretted hydrogen; sulfuric acid | History |
| Cellulose-products makers | (See Rayon makers; Pyroxylin-plastics workers; Lacquer makers.) | History |
| Cementers (rubber) | Benzine (naphtha-gasoline); benzol (benzene) and its homologs (toluol and xylol); butyl alcohol; carbon disulfide; carbon tetrachloride; dichloroethylene; methanol (methyl alcohol); tetrachloroethane (acetylene tetrachloride); trichloroethylene; turpentine | History; hemogram |
| Cement (Portland) workers | Heat; inorganic dust containing free silica; inorganic dust (except asbestos) containing no free silica; arsenic and its compounds (except arseniureted hydrogen); carbon monoxide; selenium compounds | History; chest x-ray; arsenic in urine |
| Cement (rubber, plastic, etc.) mixers | Acetone; ammonia; amyl acetate; benzine (naphtha-gasoline); benzol (benzene) and its homologs; carbon disulfide; carbon tetrachloride; dioxane (diethylene dioxide); lead and its compounds; pyridine; sulfur chloride; tar and pitch; tetrachloroethylene (perchloroethylene) | History; lead in urine; hemogram |

TABLE 72—*Continued*

| *Occupation* | *Hazard* | *Diagnosis* |
|---|---|---|
| Ceramic workers | (See Pottery workers) | History |
| Chambermen (sulfuric acid) | Sulfur dioxide; sulfuric acid | History |
| Charcoal burners | Carbon dioxide; carbon monoxide | History; chest x-ray |
| Charcoal workers | Organic dust; carbon monoxide | History; chest x-ray |
| Chargers (furnace) | Heat; inorganic dust (except asbestos) containing no free silica; carbon monoxide. (See also particular metal) | History; chest x-ray |
| Chargers (smelting and refining) | Heat; inorganic dust (except asbestos) containing no free silica; carbon monoxide | History; chest x-ray |
| Chasers (steel) | Inorganic dust (except asbestos) containing no free silica | History; chest x-ray |
| Chemists (radium research) | Roentgen rays, radium and other radioactive substances | History; hemogram |
| Chimney masons | Carbon monoxide | History |
| Chimney sweepers | Inorganic dust (except asbestos) containing no free silica; arsenic and its compounds (except arsine); carbon monoxide; tar and pitch | History; chest x-ray; arsenic in urine |
| Chippers | Inorganic dust containing free silica; inorganic dust (except asbestos) containing no free silica; lead and its compounds | History; chest x-ray; lead in urine |
| Chloride-of-lime makers | Chloride of lime; chlorine | History; chest x-ray |
| Chlorinated-diphenyl makers | Chlorinated diphenyls | History |
| Chlorinated-naphthalene workers | Chlorinated naphthalenes | History |
| Chlorinated-rubber makers | Carbon tetrachloride | History |
| Chlorine makers | Chlorine; hydrochloric acid; manganese; mercury and its compounds | History; mercury in urine |
| Chlorine compound makers | Hydrochloric acid | History |
| Chlorodiphenyl makers | Benzol (benzene) and its homologs (toluol and xylol) | History |
| Chloroform makers | Inorganic dust (except asbestos) containing no free silica | History; chest x-ray |
| Chrome workers | Chromium compounds | History; temperature record |
| Chromium platers | Chromium compounds. (See also Electroplaters) | History; temperature record |
| Cigar makers | Organic dust; fungus infections; lead and its compounds; nicotine | History; chest x-ray; temperature record |
| Clay and bisque makers (pottery) | Sudden variations in temperature; dampness; inorganic dust containing free silica; inorganic dust (except asbestos) containing no free silica | History; chest x-ray |
| Clay-plug makers (pottery) | Dampness; inorganic dust (except asbestos) containing no free silica | History; chest x-ray |
| Clay-products workers | (See Pottery workers) | History; chest x-ray |
| Cleaners (metal) | (See Polishers and cleaners [metal]) | History |
| Clothes pressers | Carbon dioxide | History |
| Cloth preparers | Heat; dampness. (See also Bleachers.) | History |
| Cloth singers | Carbon monoxide | History |

TABLE 72—*Continued*

| *Occupation* | *Hazard* | *Diagnosis* |
|---|---|---|
| Clutch-disk impregnators | Benzol (benzene) and its homologs (toluol and xylol) | History; hemogram |
| Coal carbonizers | Sulfuretted hydrogen (hydrogen sulfide) | History; chest x-ray |
| Coal miners | (See Miners) | History |
| Coal passers | Organic dust; inorganic dust (except asbestos) containing no free silica | History; chest x-ray |
| Coal-tar workers | Heat; aniline and other amino compounds of benzol and its homologs (toluol and xylol); carbon monoxide; cresol (cresylic acid); cyanogen compounds; phenol; tar and pitch. (See also Coke-oven workers.) | History; hemogram |
| Cobblers | Organic dust; anthrax; repeated motion, pressure, shock; benzol (benzene) and its homologs (tuluol and xylol); carbon tetrachloride | History; chest x-ray |
| Cobblers (asbestos) | Asbestos | History; chest x-ray |
| Coin makers | Nickel; silver | History; hemogram |
| Coke-oven workers | Heat; ammonia; benzol (benzene) and its homologs; carbon monoxide; sulfur dioxide; sulfuretted hydrogen (hydrogen sulfide); tar and pitch. (See also Coal-tar workers.) | History; hemogram |
| Cold-storage-plant workers | (See Refrigerating-plant workers) | History |
| Collar (fused) makers | Acetone; methanol (methyl alcohol); methyl cellosolve (ethylene glycol, monomethyl ether) | History |
| Collodion makers | Nitrous fumes and nitric acid | History |
| Colored-paper workers | Arsenic and its compounds | History; arsenic in urine |
| Colorers (marble) | Lead and its compounds | History |
| Colorers (white) of shoes | Chromium compounds | History |
| Color makers | Inorganic dust (except asbestos) containing no free silica; ammonia; aniline and other amino compounds of benzol and its homologs; antimony and its compounds; arsenic and its compounds; benzine; benzol and its homologs; bromine; cadmium; chlorine; chromium compounds; cobalt; dimethyl sulfate; lead and its compounds; manganese; mercury and its compounds; methyl bromide; methyl chloride; naphthols; selenium compounds; sulfuric acid; tetrachloroethane; thallium | History; chest x-ray; temperature chart; arsenic, lead, and mercury in urine; hemogram |
| Comb makers | Organic dust; acetone | History |
| Compositors | Inorganic dust (except asbestos) containing no free silica; repeated motion, pressure, shock; aniline and other amino compounds of benzol and its homologs; antimony and its compounds; benzine (naphtha-gasoline); lead and its compounds; turpentine | History; chest x-ray; hemogram |
| Compounders (rubber) | Inorganic dust (except asbestos) containing no free silica; aniline and other amino compounds of benzol and its homologs; antimony and its compounds; arsenic and its compounds (except arsine); benzine; benzol and its homologs; chromium compounds; lead and its compounds | History; chest x-ray; arsenic in urine; hemogram |
| Compressed-air (caisson) workers | (See Caisson workers) | History |

TABLE 72—*Continued*

| *Occupation* | *Hazard* | *Diagnosis* |
|---|---|---|
| Compressed-air (pneumatic tool) workers | (See Pneumatic-tool workers) | History |
| Concentrating mill-workers | Dampness; inorganic dust containing free silica; inorganic dust (except asbestos) containing no free silica; lead and its compounds; manganese; selenium compounds. (See also Oil—flotation-plant workers) | History; lead in urine |
| Coners (felt hats) | Organic dust; mercury and its compounds | History; mercury in urine |
| Construction workers | Dampness; inorganic dust containing free silica; inorganic dust (except asbestos) containing no free silica | History; chest x-ray |
| Copper founders | Arsenic and its compounds; copper | History; arsenic in urine |
| Copper miners | (See Miners) | History |
| Copper refiners and smelters | Heat; antimony and its compounds; arsenic and its compounds; carbon monoxide; copper; hydrofluoric acid; lead and its compounds; manganese; selenium compounds. (See also Oil—flotation-plant workers) | History; arsenic and lead in urine; hemogram |
| Coppersmiths | Arsenic and its compounds; copper | History; arsenic in urine |
| Copper (strip) roller mill workers | Acrolein | History |
| Cordage-factory workers | Anthrax; tar and pitch | History |
| Core makers | Heat; inorganic dust containing free silica; inorganic dust (except asbestos) containing no free silica; carbon monoxide; carbon tetrachloride; zinc | History; chest x-ray |
| Cork workers | Organic dust | History; chest x-ray |
| Cosmetic workers | Arsenic and its compounds; mercury and its compounds; methyl cellosolve; nitrobenzol and other nitro-compounds of benzol and its homologs; aniline compounds | History; arsenic and mercury in urine; hemogram |
| Crayon (colored) makers | Chromium compounds; aniline; lead and its compounds | History; chest x-ray |
| Creosoting plant workers | Dampness; tar and pitch | History; chest x-ray |
| Cresol-soap makers | Cresol (phenol) | History |
| Cresylic-acid makers | Cresol (phenol) | History |
| Crucible mixers | Organic dust; inorganic dust (except asbestos) containing no free silica | History; chest x-ray |
| Crushermen (clay and stone) | Inorganic dust containing free silica; inorganic dust (except asbestos) containing no free silica | History; chest x-ray |
| Crushers (asbestos) | Asbestos | History; chest x-ray |
| Cupola men (foundries) | Heat; carbon dioxide; carbon monoxide | History; chest x-ray |
| Curers, vapor (rubber) | (See Vulcanizers) | History |
| Curriers (tannery) | Organic dust; anthrax; arsenic and its compounds; benzine (naphtha-gasoline) | History; chest x-ray |
| Cut-glass workers | Inorganic dust (except asbestos) containing no free silica; arsenic and its compounds; lead and its compounds | History; chest x-ray; arsenic and lead in urine |

TABLE 72—*Continued*

| *Occupation* | *Hazard* | *Diagnosis* |
|---|---|---|
| Cutlery makers | Inorganic dust containing free silica; inorganic dust (except asbestos) containing no free silica; amyl acetate; lead and its compounds | History; chest x-ray; lead in urine |
| Cutters (oxyacetylene and other gases) | (See Welders) | History |
| Cyanamide makers | Heat; inorganic dust (except asbestos) containing no free silica; calcium cyanamide | History; chest x-ray |
| Cyanogen makers | Cyanogen and its compounds; mercury and its compounds; hydrogen sulfide | History; chest x-ray; mercury in urine |
| Dairy workers | Anthrax; undulant fever (brucellosis) | History; chest x-ray; tuberculin reaction; skin tests for brucellergin |
| Damascening workers | Nitrous fumes and nitric acid | History |
| De-brassers | Nitrous fumes and nitric acid | History |
| Decorators (pottery) | Arsenic and its compounds; benzine; benzol and its homologs (toluol and xylol); lead and its compounds; mercury and its compounds; turpentine | History; arsenic and mercury in urine; hemogram |
| Degreasers | Benzine; benzol and its homologs; carbon disulfide; carbon tetrachloride; chlorinated naphthalenes; dichloroethyl ether; dioxane; ethylene dichloride; methylene chloride; tetrachloroethane; tetrachloroethylene; trichloroethylene | History; hemogram |
| Denatured-alcohol workers | (See particular denaturant) | History |
| Dental workers | Lead and its compounds; mercury and its compounds | History; lead and mercury in urine |
| Depilatory makers | Barium, thallium | History; hemogram |
| Detinning workers | Chlorine | History |
| Detonator cleaners | Mercury and its compounds | History; mercury in urine |
| Detonator filers | Mercury and its compounds | History; mercury in urine |
| Detonator packers | Mercury and its compounds | History; mercury in urine |
| Devil operators (felt hats) | Organic dust; mercury and its compounds | History; mercury in urine; chest x-ray |
| Diamond cutters | Organic dust; inorganic dust (except asbestos) containing no free silica; repeated motion, pressure, shock | History; chest x-ray |
| Diamond polishers | Lead and its compounds | History; chest x-ray |
| Diatomaceous-earth workers | Inorganic dust containing free silica; cristobalite | History; chest x-ray |
| Dichloroethylene workers | Dichloroethylene | History; hemogram |
| Digester-house workers (paper and pulp) | Heat; sudden variations of temperature; sulfur dioxide; sulfuretted hydrogen | History; chest x-ray |
| Dimethylsulfate workers | Arsine; dimethyl sulfate; methanol; nitric and sulfuric acid | History; arsenic in urine; chest x-ray |
| Dinitrobenzol workers | Nitrobenzol and other nitro compounds of benzol and its homologs | History; hemogram |
| Dinitrophenol workers | Dinitrophenol | History; temperature chart; examination of eyegrounds and lens |

TABLE 72—*Continued*

| *Occupation* | *Hazard* | *Diagnosis* |
|---|---|---|
| Dioxane makers | Dioxane | History |
| Dippers | (See Acid dippers) | History |
| Dippers (gun cotton) | Nitrous fumes and nitric acid | History |
| Dippers (rubber) | Benzine; benzol and its homologs; carbon tetrachloride | History; hemogram |
| Dishwashers | Fungus infections | History |
| Disinfectant makers | Acetaldehyde; aniline and other amino compounds of benzol and its homologs; arsenic and its compounds; benzol and its homologs; bromine; carbon dioxide; chloride of lime; chlorine; cresol; cyanogen compounds; formaldehyde; mercury and its compounds; ozone; phenol; picric acid; sulfur dioxide | History; arsenic and mercury in urine; hemogram |
| Divers | Compressed air (increased atmospheric pressure); carbon dioxide; carbon monoxide | History |
| Doffers (textile) | Heat; dampness; organic dust | History; chest x-ray |
| Dope workers | (See Airplane-dope makers) | History |
| Dressers (glass) | Heat | History |
| Dresser tenders (textile) | Heat; sudden variations in temperature; dampness | History; chest x-ray |
| Driers | Sudden variations in temperature; carbon dioxide; carbon monoxide | History; chest x-ray |
| Driers (felt hats) | Sudden variations in temperature; methanol (methyl alcohol) | History |
| Driers (lacquer) | Ultraviolet and infrared rays | History; hemogram |
| Driers (rubber) | Benzine; benzol and its other homologs; carbon disulfide | History; hemogram |
| Drier workers (foundries) | Carbon monoxide | History |
| Dry-cleaners | Amyl acetate; benzine; benzol; carbon disulfide; carbon tetrachloride; dichloroethylene; ethylene dichloride; methanol; oxalic acid; tetrachloroethane; tetrachloroethylene; trichloroethylene; turpentine | History; chest x-ray |
| Drying-room workers (miscellaneous) | Sudden variations in temperature; carbon dioxide; carbon monoxide | History; chest x-ray |
| Dye makers | Acetaldehyde; acetone; acridine; ammonia; aniline and other amino compounds of benzol and its homologs; antimony and arsenic compounds; arsine; barium; benzol; bromine; butyl alcohol; carbon dioxide; carbon tetrachloride; chloride of lime; chlorine; chromium compounds; cresol; cyanogen compounds; dimethyl sulfate; dinitrophenol; dioxane; ethyl bromide and chloride; formaldehyde; formic acid; furfural; hydrochloric acid; lead and its compounds; manganese; mercury and its compounds; methanol; methyl bromide; methyl cellosolve; methyl chloride; methylene chloride; naphthols; nitrobenzol; nitrous fumes and nitric acid; oxalic acid; phenol; phenyl hydrazine; phosgene; picric acid; pyridine; sodium hydroxide; sulfur dioxide; sulfuretted hydrogen; sulfuric acid; thallium; trichloroethylene; turpentine; uranium; vanadium (See Phenylenediamine.) | History; hemogram; temperature chart; examination of lens and fundus; examination of urine for arsenic, lead and mercury |
| Dyers | Acetone; ammonia; amyl acetate; aniline and other amino compounds of benzol and its homologs; antimony and lead; arsenic and its compounds; benzine; chromium compounds; ethylene dichloride; hydrochloric acid; manganese; methanol; nitrous fumes and nitric acid; oxalic acid; phenol; picric acid; pyridine; sulfur chloride; titanium oxide; uranium; vanadium | History; hemogram; chest x-ray; urine for arsenic and lead |

TABLE 72—*Continued*

| *Occupation* | *Hazard* | *Diagnosis* |
|---|---|---|
| Electrical-transformer makers | Chlorinated diphenyls; chlorinated naphthalenes | History |
| Electric-condenser makers | Chlorinated diphenyls; chlorinated naphthalenes | History |
| Electric-induction furnace workers | Mercury and its compounds | History; mercury in urine |
| Electrode makers | Organic dust; tar and pitch | History; chest x-ray |
| Electrolytic process (copper) workers | Arsine | History; arsenic in urine |
| Electroplaters | Antimony and arsenic compounds; benzine; benzol; cadmium; carbon disulfide; carbon tetrachloride; chlorinated naphthalenes; chromium and cyanogen compounds; formic acid; hydrochloric acid; hydrofluoric acid; lead and mercury compounds; nickel; nitrous fumes and nitric acid; potassium hydroxide; sulfuric acid; tetrachloroethane; trichloroethylene | History; hemogram; temperature chart; arsenic, lead and mercury in urine |
| Electrotypers | Sudden variations in temperature; organic dust; inorganic dust (except asbestos) containing no free silica; ammonia; antimony and its compounds; lead and its compounds | History; chest x-ray; lead in urine |
| Embalmers | Formaldehyde; mercury and its compounds | History; mercury in urine |
| Embalming-fluid makers | Mercury and its compounds | History; mercury in urine |
| Embossers | Mercury and its compounds | History; mercury in urine |
| Embroidery workers | Lead and its compounds | History; lead in urine |
| Emery-wheel makers | Inorganic dust (except asbestos) containing no free silica; lead and its compounds | History; chest x-ray; lead in urine |
| Enamelers | Inorganic dust containing free silica; amyl acetate; antimony; arsenic and its compounds; benzine; benzol; carbon disulfide; carbon monoxide; chromium; lead; manganese; nickel; tetrachloroethane; turpentine | History; chest x-ray; hemogram; arsenic and lead in urine |
| Enamel makers | Amyl acetate; antimony and arsenic compounds; barium; benzine; benzol; carbon disulfide; carbon monoxide; chromium compounds; hydrochloric acid; hydrofluoric acid; lead and its compounds; manganese; methyl cellosolve; nitrous fumes and nitric acid; tetrachloroethane; turpentine | History; hemogram; arsenic and lead in urine |
| Engravers | Inorganic dust (except asbestos) containing no free silica; benzol; copper; hydrochloric acid; lead and mercury and their compounds; nitrous fumes and nitric acid; oxalic acid; sodium hydroxide; sulfuric acid | History; hemogram; refraction; chest x-ray; urine for lead and mercury |
| Etchers | Arsine; hydrochloric acid; hydrofluoric acid; nitrous fumes and nitric acid; phenol; sulfuric acid | History; arsenic in urine |
| Ether makers | Sulfuric acid | History |
| Ethyl-benzene makers | Ethyl benzene | History; hemogram |
| Ethyl-bromide makers | Ethyl bromide and ethyl chloride | History; bromine in urine |
| Ethyl-chloride makers | Ethyl bromide and ethyl chloride | History; bromine in urine |
| Ethylene-dibromide makers | Bromine; ethylene dibromide | History; bromine in urine |

TABLE 72—*Continued*

| *Occupation* | *Hazard* | *Diagnosis* |
|---|---|---|
| Ethylene-dichloride makers | Ethylene dichloride | History |
| Ethylene-oxide makers | Ethylene oxide | History |
| Examiners using fluoroscope or roentgen ray | Roentgen rays; radium and other radioactive substances | History; hemogram |
| Excavation workers | Fungus infections | History |
| Explosives workers | Acetaldehyde; acetone; ammonia; amyl acetate; amyl alcohol; aniline and other amino compounds of benzol and its homologs; antimony and its compounds; benzol; bromine; carbon dioxide; carbon disulfide; chromium compounds; cresol; dinitrophenol; formaldehyde; lead and its compounds; mercury and its compounds; methanol; nitrobenzol and other nitro compounds of benzol and its homologs; nitroglycerin; nitrous fumes and nitric acid; phenol; phosphorus; picric acid; pyridine; sulfuric acid | History; chest x-ray; hemogram; urine for bromine, lead, mercury; examination of lens and fundus |
| Extractors (gold and silver) | (See Gold and silver refiners and extractors) | History |
| Extractors (oils and fats) | Acetone; benzine; benzol and its homologs; carbon disulfide; ethylene dichloride; tetrachloroethane; trichloroethylene | History; hemogram |
| Fat renderers | Sudden variations in temperature; anthrax; acrolein; magnesium; ozone; sulfuretted hydrogen; sulfuric acid | History |
| Feather curers | Organic dust; arsenic and its compounds | History; chest x-ray; arsenic in urine |
| Feather workers | Organic dust; aniline and other amino compounds of benzol and its homologs; arsenic and its compounds; benzine; benzol and its homologs; methanol; sulfur dioxide; turpentine | History; chest x-ray; arsenic in urine |
| Felt-hat makers | Organic dust; carbon monoxide; mercury and its compounds; methanol; nitrous fumes and nitric acid; sulfuric acid | History; chest x-ray; mercury in urine |
| Felt makers | Heat; anthrax; sulfuretted hydrogen | History; chest x-ray |
| Ferrosilicon workers | Arsenic and its compounds; arsine; phosphuretted hydrogen | History; arsenic in urine |
| Fertilizer makers | Organic dust; inorganic dust containing free silica; inorganic dust (except asbestos) containing no free silica; anthrax; acrolein; ammonia; arsenic and its compounds; arsine; benzol; calcium cyanamide; carbon dioxide; cyanogen compounds; hydrochloric acid; hydrofluoric acid; magnesium; manganese; nicotine; nitrous fumes and nitric acid; sulfur dioxide; sulfuretted hydrogen; sulfuric acid | History; chest x-ray; arsenic in urine |
| Fiberizers (asbestos) | Asbestos | History; chest x-ray |
| Fiber workers | Organic dust | History; chest x-ray |
| Filament makers and finishers (incandescent lamps) | Amyl acetate; carbon monoxide; methanol; thallium | History; hemogram |
| File cutters | Inorganic dust (except asbestos) containing no free silica; lead and its compounds | History; chest x-ray; lead in urine |
| Filers | Inorganic dust (except asbestos) containing no free silica; lead and its compounds | History; hemogram; chest x-ray; lead in urine |
| Filling-station workers | Benzine; carbon monoxide; lead and its compounds; tetraethyl lead | History; hemogram; lead in urine |

TABLE 72—*Continued*

| *Occupation* | *Hazard* | *Diagnosis* |
|---|---|---|
| Finishers (leather) | Organic dust | History; chest x-ray |
| Fire-extinguisher makers | Carbon dioxide; carbon tetrachloride; ethyl bromide and ethyl chloride; ethylene dibromide; methyl bromide | History; hemogram |
| Fireworks makers | Antimony and its compounds; arsenic and its compounds; barium; manganese; mercury and its compounds; phosphorus; picric acid; thallium. (See also Explosives workers) | History; arsenic and mercury in urine; hemogram |
| Flangers (felt hats) | Carbon monoxide | History; chest x-ray |
| Flavoring-extract makers | Amyl acetate; amyl alcohol; benzol; butyl alcohol; nitrobenzol and other nitro compounds of benzol and its homologs | History; hemogram |
| Flax-rettery workers | Sulfuretted hydrogen | History |
| Flax spinners | Heat; organic dust | History; chest x-ray |
| Flint workers | Inorganic dust containing free silica; inorganic dust (except asbestos) containing no free silica | History; chest x-ray |
| Floor-polish makers | (See Polish makers) | History |
| Flour-mill workers | Organic dust; fungus infections | History; chest x-ray |
| Flue cleaners | Inorganic dust (except asbestos) containing no free silica; carbon monoxide; sulfur dioxide; tar and pitch | History; chest x-ray |
| Flue-dust recoverers (sulfuric-acid mfr.) | Thallium | History; hemogram |
| Fly-paper makers | Arsenic and its compounds; organic phosphate | History; arsenic in urine |
| Food irradiators | Ultraviolet and infrared rays | History; hemogram |
| Formaldehyde workers | Formaldehyde | History |
| Formers (felt hats) | Organic dust; mercury and its compounds | History; chest x-ray; mercury in urine |
| Formic-acid workers | Formic acid; oxalic acid | History |
| Foundry workers | Inorganic dust containing free silica; inorganic dust (except asbestos) containing no free silica; ultraviolet and infrared rays; carbon dioxide; carbon monoxide. (See also particular metal) | History; chest x-ray; hemogram |
| Frosters (glass and pottery) | Chromium compounds | History |
| Fruit preservers | Sulfur dioxide | History |
| Fullers (textiles) | Benzol, and its homologs; carbon tetrachloride; dichloroethyl ether; tetrachloroethane | History; hemogram |
| Fur carders | Organic dust; anthrax | History; chest x-ray |
| Fur handlers<br>clippers<br>cutters | Organic dust; anthrax; mercury and its compounds; sulfuretted hydrogen | History; chest x-ray; temperature chart; arsenic and mercury in urine |
| Furnace workers | Heat; inorganic dust (except asbestos) containing no free silica; ultraviolet and infrared rays; carbon monoxide. (See also particular metal) | History; chest x-ray; hemogram |
| Furniture polishers | Organic dust; repeated movement, pressure, shock; amyl acetate; benzine (naphtha-gasoline); chromium compounds; methanol; petroleum; turpentine | History; chest x-ray |
| Fur preparers | Organic dust; anthrax; formaldehyde; mercury and its compounds; nitrous fumes and nitric acid | History; chest x-ray; mercury in urine |

TABLE 72—*Continued*

| *Occupation* | *Hazard* | *Diagnosis* |
|---|---|---|
| Fur pullers | Organic dust; anthrax | History; chest x-ray |
| Fused-quartz workers | Inorganic dust containing free silica | History; chest x-ray |
| Fusel-oil workers | Amyl alcohol | History |
| Galvanizers | Acrolein; ammonia; arsenic and its compounds; arseniureted hydrogen; benzine; hydrochloric acid; lead and its compounds; nitrous fumes and nitric acid; sulfur dioxide; sulfuric acid; trichloroethylene; zinc | History; chest x-ray; arsenic and lead in urine; hemogram |
| Garage workers | Acrolein; benzine; carbon monoxide; lead and its compounds; tetraethyl lead | History; chest x-ray; lead in urine |
| Gardeners | Undulant fever (brucellosis); arsenic, lead and compounds; calcium cyanamide; nicotine and other insecticide poisoning | History; skin test for brucellergin; arsenic and lead in urine |
| Gas (illuminating) workers | Ammonia; arsine; benzol and its homologs; carbon monoxide; cyanogen compounds; hydrofluoric acid; phenol; sulfuretted hydrogen; tar and pitch; trichloroethylene | History; hemogram; arsenic in urine |
| Gasoline blenders | Aniline and other amino compounds of benzol and its homologs; benzine; benzol and its homologs; ethyl benzene; ethylene dibromide; lead and its compounds; nitrobenzol and other nitro compounds of benzol and its homologs; tetraethyl lead | History; hemogram; lead in urine |
| Gasoline-engine workers | Acrolein; benzine; carbon monoxide | History; hemogram |
| Gas purifiers | Ammonia; cyanogen compounds; phenol; sulfuretted hydrogen | History; hemogram |
| Gassers (textile) | Carbon monoxide | History |
| Gelatin makers | Anthrax; acrolein; sulfur dioxide | History |
| Gilders | Amyl acetate; benzine; benzol; cyanogen compounds; mercury and its compounds; methanol; nitrous fumes and nitric acid; pyridine | History; hemogram; mercury in urine; temperature chart |
| Glass blowers | Heat; inorganic dust; ultraviolet and infrared rays | History; chest x-ray; hemogram |
| Glass colorers | Cadmium; chromium compounds; cobalt; selenium and tellurium compounds | History; chest x-ray |
| Glass cutters | Inorganic dust (except asbestos) containing no free silica | History; chest x-ray |
| Glass finishers | Inorganic dust (except asbestos) containing no free silica; hydrochloric acid; hydrofluoric acid; lead and its compounds; sulfuric acid | History; chest x-ray; hemogram; lead in urine |
| Glass-furnace workers | Heat; inorganic dust containing free silica; inorganic dust (except asbestos) containing no free silica; ultraviolet and infrared rays; carbon monoxide. (See also Glass mixers.) | History; chest x-ray |
| Glass mixers | Inorganic dust containing free silica; inorganic dust (except asbestos) containing no free silica; ultraviolet and infrared rays; antimony and arsenic compounds; barium; hydrochloric acid; lead and its compounds; magnesium; manganese; selenium compounds; sodium hydroxide; thallium; uranium; vanadium | History; chest x-ray; arsenic and lead in urine; hemogram |
| Glass polishers | Lead and its compounds | History; lead in urine |
| Glass (safety) makers | Butyl alcohol; methanol; tetrachloroethane | History; hemogram |

TABLE 72—*Continued*

| *Occupation* | *Hazard* | *Diagnosis* |
|---|---|---|
| Glaze dippers (pottery) | Antimony; arsenic and its compounds; chromium compounds; hydrochloric acid; lead and its compounds; manganese | History; chest x-ray; arsenic and lead in urine |
| Glaze mixers (pottery) | Inorganic dust containing free silica; inorganic dust (except asbestos) containing no free silica; antimony, lead and arsenic and their compounds; hydrochloric acid; manganese | History; chest x-ray; arsenic and lead in urine; hemogram |
| Gloss-kiln workers | Carbon monoxide; lead and its compounds | History; hemogram; lead in urine |
| Glove makers (leather preparers) | Dampness; organic dust. (See also Tannery workers) | History; hemogram |
| Glue workers | Organic dust; anthrax; septic infections; acrolein; ammonia; benzine; carbon dioxide; carbon disulfide; carbon tetrachloride; cresol; hydrochloric acid; nitrobenzol; sulfur dioxide; sulfuretted hydrogen; sulfuric acid; trichloroethylene | History; chest x-ray; hemogram |
| Glycerin refiners | Oxalic acid | History |
| Gold and silver refiners and extractors | Inorganic dust (except asbestos) containing no free silica; arsenic and its compounds; arsine; bromine; chlorine; cyanogen compounds; formaldehyde; hydrofluoric acid; lead and mercury compounds; sulfur chloride | History; chest x-ray; arsenic, bromine, lead and mercury in urine; hemogram |
| Gold beaters | Inorganic dust (except asbestos) containing no free silica | History; chest x-ray |
| Grain-elevator workers | Organic dust; fungus infections; carbon dioxide | History; chest x-ray |
| Granite workers | (See Stonecutters) | History |
| Graphite workers | Heat; organic dust; inorganic dust (except asbestos) containing no free silica | History; chest x-ray |
| Grinders (colors) | (See Color makers) | History |
| Grinders (metals) | Inorganic dust containing free silica; inorganic dust (except asbestos) containing no free silica; antimony and lead compounds | History; lead in urine |
| Grinding-wheel makers | Inorganic dust containing free silica; inorganic dust (except asbestos) containing no free silica | History; chest x-ray |
| Guncotton dippers | Nitrous fumes and nitric acid; sulfuric acid | History; chest x-ray |
| Guncotton pickers | Organic dust | History; chest x-ray |
| Gypsum workers | Inorganic dust (except asbestos) containing no free silica; sulfuretted hydrogen | History; chest x-ray |
| Hair workers | Dampness; organic dust; anthrax; septic infections; mercury and its compounds | History; chest x-ray; mercury in urine |
| Hardeners | (See Temperers) | History |
| Hardeners (felt hats) | Mercury and its compounds; methanol | History; mercury in urine |
| Harness makers | Organic dust | History; chest x-ray |
| Heel makers (shoe) | Organic dust | History; chest x-ray |
| Hemp workers | Organic dust | History; chest x-ray |
| Hide workers | Fungus infections | History; chest x-ray |
| Horn workers | Organic dust | History; chest x-ray |
| Hot-rod rollers (iron and steel) | Heat | History |

TABLE 72—*Continued*

| *Occupation* | *Hazard* | *Diagnosis* |
|---|---|---|
| Hydraulic-construction workers | Dampness | History; chest x-ray |
| Hydraulic miners | Dampness | History; chest x-ray |
| Hydrochloric-acid makers | Arsine; hydrochloric acid; sulfuretted hydrogen; sulfuric acid | History; chest x-ray |
| Hydrocyanic-acid makers | Cyanogen compounds; sulfuric acid | History; chest x-ray |
| Hydrofluoric-acid makers | Hydrofluoric acid | History; chest x-ray |
| Ice (artificial) makers | (See Artificial-ice makers) | History |
| Ice-cream makers | Dampness; ammonia; carbon dioxide | History; chest x-ray |
| Incandescent-lamp makers | Amyl acetate; carbon monoxide; lead and mercury and their compounds; methanol; thallium | History; lead and mercury in urine; hemogram |
| Ink makers | Ammonia; arsenic and its compounds; barium; benzine; benzol; bromine; carbon monoxide; carbon tetrachloride; chlorine; chromium compounds; cresol; formaldehyde; hydrochloric acid; lead and its compounds; mercury and its compounds; methyl cellosolve; nitrobenzol and other nitro compounds of benzol and its homologs; oxalic acid; potassium hydroxide; silver; turpentine; vanadium | History; hemogram; arsenic, lead and mercury in urine |
| Insecticide makers | (See specific insecticide) | History; hemogram; urinalysis. |
| Inspectors using fluoroscope or roentgen ray | Roentgen rays, radium and other radioactive substances | History; hemogram |
| Instrument-dial (luminous) painters | Roentgen rays, radium and other radioactive substances | History; hemogram |
| Insulation (sound) (heat) workers | Inorganic dust containing free silica; inorganic dust (except asbestos) containing no free silica | History; chest x-ray |
| Insulators (wire) | Antimony and arsenic compounds; benzol; carbon tetrachloride; chlorinated diphenyls; chlorinated naphthalenes; ethylene dichloride; tar and pitch | History; hemogram; arsenic in urine |
| Iodine makers | Chlorine | History |
| Iron and steel workers (all departments) | Heat; inorganic dust (except asbestos) containing no free silica; ultraviolet and infrared rays; arsenic and its compounds; carbon monoxide; titanium oxide. (See also particular occupation and Alloy makers) | History; chest x-ray; arsenic in urine; hemogram |
| Irradiators (food) | Ultraviolet and infrared rays | History; hemogram |
| Japan makers | Arsenic and lead and their compounds; benzine; methanol; turpentine | History; chest x-ray; arsenic and lead in urine |
| Japanners | Arsenic and lead and their compounds; benzine; methanol; turpentine | History; arsenic and lead in urine; hemogram |
| Jewelers | Inorganic dust (except asbestos) containing no free silica; amyl acetate; arsine; cyanogen compounds; hydrochloric acid; lead and mercury and their compounds; nitrous fumes and nitric acid; sulfuric acid | History; refraction; chest x-ray; arsenic, lead and mercury in urine |
| Junk (metal) refiners | Heat; inorganic dust (except asbestos) containing no free silica; lead and its compounds; zinc | History; chest x-ray; lead in urine |
| Jute workers | Organic dust; inorganic dust containing free silica; inorganic dust (except asbestos) containing no free silica | History; chest x-ray |

TABLE 72—*Continued*

| Occupation | Hazard | Diagnosis |
|---|---|---|
| Kiln tenders | Heat; carbon monoxide | History; chest x-ray |
| Knitting-mill workers | Organic dust | History; chest x-ray |
| Labelers (paint cans) | Lead and its compounds | History; lead in urine |
| Lace makers | Organic dust | History; chest x-ray |
| Lacquerers | Acetone; amyl acetate; amyl alcohol; arsenic and its compounds; benzine; benzol; carbon tetrachloride; ethyl benzene; ethylene dichloride; formic acid; lead and its compounds; methanol; methylene chloride; pyridine; tetrachloroethane; trichloroethylene; triorthocresyl phosphate; turpentine | History; hemogram; arsenic and lead in urine |
| Lacquer makers | Acetaldehyde; acetone; ammonia; amyl acetate; amyl alcohol; arsenic and its compounds; barium; benzine; benzol; butanone; butyl alcohol; carbon tetrachloride; cellosolve; chlorinated diphenyls; chlorinated naphthalenes; dioxane; ethylene dichloride; formaldehyde; formic acid; hexanone; hexone; lead and its compounds; methanol; methyl cellosolve; methylene chloride; nitrous fumes and nitric acid; pentane; pyridine; tetrachloroethane; trichloroethylene; triorthocresyl phosphate; turpentine | History; hemogram; arsenic and lead in urine |
| Lampblack makers | Organic dust; petroleum; phenol | History; chest x-ray |
| Lamps (electric) | (See Incandescent-lamp makers) | History |
| Lapidaries | Inorganic dust (except asbestos) containing no free silica | History; chest x-ray |
| Lard makers | Acrolein | History; chest x-ray |
| Lasters (shoe) | Organic dust; methanol | History; chest x-ray |
| Laundry workers | Heat; dampness; carbon monoxide; chloride of lime; chlorine; ozone; formaldehyde | History; chest x-ray |
| Lead-arsenate makers | Arsenic and lead and their compounds | History; arsenic and lead in urine |
| Lead burners | Arsine; lead and its compounds | History; arsenic and lead in urine |
| Lead-foil makers | Heat; lead and its compounds | History; lead in urine |
| Lead miners | Lead and its compounds. (See also Miners) | History; chest x-ray |
| Lead-pipe makers | Lead and its compounds | History; lead in urine |
| Lead platers (on iron) | Mercury and lead compounds | History; lead and mercury in urine |
| Lead-salts makers | Lead and its compounds | History; lead in urine |
| Lead smelters | Heat; antimony; lead; selenium; tellurium; arsenic and its compounds; cadmium; carbon monoxide; sulfur dioxide | History; chest x-ray; arsenic and lead in urine; hemogram |
| Leather workers | Organic dust; anthrax; amyl acetate; barium; carbon tetrachloride; hydrochloric acid; methanol; trichloroethylene. (See also Tannery workers) | History; chest x-ray |
| Lime burners | Heat; arsenic; inorganic dust (except asbestos) containing no free silica; carbon dioxide; carbon monoxide | History; chest x-ray; arsenic in urine |
| Lime-kiln charges | Inorganic dust (except asbestos) containing no free silica; carbon dioxide; carbon monoxide | History; chest x-ray |
| Lime pullers (tannery) | Dampness; anthrax | History; chest x-ray |

TABLE 72—*Continued*

| *Occupation* | *Hazard* | *Diagnosis* |
|---|---|---|
| Lime workers | Inorganic dust (except asbestos) containing no free silica | History; chest x-ray |
| Linen workers | Organic dust | History |
| Linoleum makers | Heat; organic dust; inorganic dust (except asbestos) containing no free silica; acrolein; amyl acetate; arsenic and its compounds; barium; benzine; benzol; carbon tetrachloride; chromium compounds; lead and its compounds; manganese; methanol; sulfuric acid; turpentine | History; chest x-ray; hemogram; arsenic and lead in urine |
| Linotypers | Antimony; lead and its compounds; carbon monoxide | History; lead in urine |
| Linseed-oil boilers | Acrolein; carbon dioxide; lead and its compounds | History; lead in urine; chest x-ray |
| Litharge workers | Lead and its compounds | History; lead in urine |
| Lithographers | Inorganic dust (except asbestos) containing no free silica; repeated motion, pressure, shock; aniline and other amino compounds of benzol and its homologs; arsenic and its compounds; benzine; benzol and its homologs; chromium compounds; hydrochloric acid; lead; mercury; methanol; nitrous fumes and nitric acid; oxalic acid; sulfuric acid; tetrachloroethane; turpentine | History; lead and mercury in urine; chest x-ray; hemogram |
| Lithopone makers | Barium; cadmium | History; temperature chart |
| Lithotransfer workers | Lead and its compounds | History; lead in urine |
| Longshoremen | Infections (anthrax); manganese | History; temperature chart |
| Luminous-dial-factory workers | Roentgen rays, radium and other radioactive substances | History; hemogram |
| Luters (zinc smelting) | Heat; zinc | History |
| Lye makers | Potassium hydroxide; sodium hydroxide | History |
| Manganese-dioxide workers | Manganese | History |
| Manganese grinders | Manganese | History; chest x-ray |
| Manganese-ore separators | Manganese | History; chest x-ray |
| Manganese-steel makers | Manganese | History; chest x-ray |
| Manometer makers | Mercury and its compounds | History; mercury in urine |
| Maple bark peelers | Pneumonitis with diffuse nodular infiltrate (cryptostroma corticale spores) | History; chest x-ray |
| Marble cutters | Inorganic dust (except asbestos) containing no free silica | History; chest x-ray |
| Marblers (glass) | Heat | History; chest x-ray |
| Match-factory workers | Dampness; organic dust; inorganic dust (except asbestos) containing no free silica; antimony and its compounds; carbon disulfide; chromium compounds; lead and its compounds; manganese; phosphorus; potassium hydroxide; sulfuretted hydrogen | History; chest x-ray; lead in urine |
| Mattress makers | Organic dust; anthrax | History; chest x-ray |
| Mechanics (gas engines) | Carbon monoxide; petroleum | History |
| Melters (foundry, glass) | Heat | History; chest x-ray |

TABLE 72—*Continued*

| *Occupation* | *Hazard* | *Diagnosis* |
|---|---|---|
| Mercerizers | Hydrochloric acid; sodium hydroxide; sulfuric acid | History; chest x-ray |
| Mercury-alloy makers | Mercury and its compounds | History; mercury in urine |
| Mercury bronzers | Mercury and its compounds | History; mercury in urine |
| Mercury miners | Mercury and its compounds (See also Miners) | History; mercury in urine |
| Mercury-pump workers | Mercury and its compounds | History; mercury in urine |
| Mercury-salt workers | Mercury and its compounds | History; mercury in urine |
| Mercury smelters | Heat; carbon monoxide; mercury and its compounds; sulfur dioxide | History; mercury in urine |
| Mercury-solder workers | Mercury and its compounds | History; mercury in urine |
| Mercury-vapor lamp makers | Mercury and its compounds | History; mercury in urine |
| Metalizers | Cadmium; lead; selenium; zinc | History; lead in urine |
| Metal polishers and cleaners | (See Polishers and cleaners [metal]) | History |
| Metal-polish makers | (See Polish makers) | History |
| Metal turners | Inorganic dust (except asbestos) containing no free silica | History; chest x-ray |
| Metal washers | Benzine (naphtha-gasoline) | History; hemogram |
| Metal workers | (See particular occupation) | History |
| Methane (synthetic) makers | Carbon monoxide | History |
| Methyl-alcohol workers | Acetone; carbon monoxide; methanol | History |
| Methyl-bromide makers | Bromine; methanol; methyl bromide | History; bromine in urine |
| Methyl-chloride makers | Hydrochloric acid; methanol; methyl chloride | History |
| Methyl-compounds makers | Methanol | History |
| Methylene chloride workers | Methylene chloride | History |
| Mica strippers or splitters | Inorganic dust (except asbestos) containing no free silica | History; chest x-ray |
| Mica workers | Inorganic dust (except asbestos) containing no free silica | History; chest x-ray |
| Microscopists | Repeated pressure, motion, shock | History; refraction |
| Millers | Fungus infections | History; chest x-ray |
| Millinery workers | Aniline and other amino compounds of benzol and its homologs; benzine; benzol and its homologs; methanol; turpentine | History; hemogram |
| Mineral-earth workers | Inorganic dust (except asbestos) containing no free silica | History; chest x-ray |
| Miners | Heat; dampness, defective illumination; inorganic dust containing free silica; inorganic dust (except asbestos) containing no free silica; asbestos; repeated motion, pressure, shock; carbon dioxide; carbon monoxide; manganese; nitrous fumes and nitric acid; silver; sulfuretted hydrogen | History; chest x-ray; sputum examination; tuberculin reaction |

TABLE 72—*Continued*

| *Occupation* | *Hazard* | *Diagnosis* |
|---|---|---|
| Minkery workers | Anthrax | History; temperature chart |
| Mirror silverers | Acetaldehyde; ammonia; benzol; cyanogen compounds; formaldehyde; formic acid; lead and its compounds; mercury and its compounds; silver | History; chest x-ray; hemogram; lead and mercury in urine |
| Mixers (felt hats) | Organic dust; mercury and its compounds | History; chest x-ray |
| Mixers (rubber) | Inorganic dust (except asbestos) containing no free silica; benzol; aniline and other amino compounds of benzol; formaldehyde; formic acid; lead and its compounds | History; chest x-ray; hemogram; lead in urine |
| Mixing-room workers (miscellaneous) | Organic dust; inorganic dust (except asbestos) containing no free silica | History; chest x-ray |
| Mold breakers (foundry) | Inorganic dust containing free silica; inorganic dust (except asbestos) containing no free silica | History; chest x-ray |
| Molders (asbestos) | Asbestos | History; chest x-ray |
| Molders (pottery) | Carbon monoxide | History; chest x-ray |
| Monotypers | Antimony and its compounds; carbon monoxide; lead and its compounds | History; lead in urine |
| Mordanters | Amyl alcohol; antimony and its compounds; arsenic and its compounds; benzine; benzol and its homologs; chloride of lime; chromium compounds; cyanogen compounds; formic acid; nitrous fumes and nitric acid; vanadium | History; hemogram; arsenic in urine |
| Mottlers (leather) | Amyl acetate; methanol | History |
| Muriatic-acid makers | (See Hydrochloric-acid makers) | History |
| Mushroom workers | Nitrogen dioxide and organic dust | History; diffuse pulmonary infiltration with fever, cough, malaise, chest and abdominal pain, yellow, green or bloody sputum. X-ray appearance of diffuse pneumonitis; Puerto Rican migrants mainly involved |
| Musical-instrument makers | Lead and its compounds | History; lead in urine |
| Naphthylamine workers | Aniline and other amino compounds of benzol and its homologs | History; hemogram |
| Neon-lights lettermakers | Carbon monoxide | History |
| Nickel extractors | Nickel | History; temperature chart |
| Nickel platers | Dampness. (See also Electroplaters) | History; temperature chart |
| Nickel-purification workers (Mond process) | Nickel; nickel carbonyl | History; temperature chart |
| Nitraniline workers | Aniline and other amino compounds of benzol and its homologs | History; hemogram |
| Nitrators | Nitrobenzol and other nitro compounds; nitrous fumes and nitric acid; sulfuric acid | History; hemogram; temperature chart |
| Nitric-acid workers | Ammonia; lead and its compounds; nitrous fumes and nitric acid; sulfuric acid | History; temperature chart; chest x-ray; lead in urine |

TABLE 72—*Continued*

| *Occupation* | *Hazard* | *Diagnosis* |
|---|---|---|
| Nitrobenzol workers | Benzol and its homologs; nitrobenzol and other nitro compounds of benzol and its homologs; nitrous fumes and nitric acid; sulfuric acid | History; temperature chart; hemogram |
| Nitrocellulose workers | Acetone; amyl acetate; amyl alcohol; arseniureted hydrogen; benzol; methyl cellosolve; nitrous fumes and nitric acid; sulfuric acid. (See also Pyroxylin-plastics workers) | History; hemogram; temperature chart; arsenic in urine |
| Nitroglycerin makers | Arsine; lead and its compounds; nitroglycerin; nitrous fumes and nitric acid; sulfuric acid | History; temperature chart; arsenic and lead in urine |
| Nitrous-oxide workers | Nitrous fumes and nitric acid | History; temperature chart |
| Oilcloth makers | (See Linoleum makers) | History |
| Oilers | Petroleum | History |
| Oil extractors | (See Extractors [oils and fats]) | History |
| Oil-flotation-plant workers | Petroleum; sulfur dioxide; sulfuretted hydrogen. (See also Concentrating-mill workers) | History |
| Oil purifiers | Sulfuric acid | History |
| Oil refiners | (See Petroleum refiners) | History |
| Oil-well workers | Petroleum; sulfuretted hydrogen | History |
| Open-hearth-department workers (iron and steel) | Heat; carbon monoxide | History; chest x-ray; temperature chart |
| Ore-concentrating-mill workers | (See Concentrating-mill workers) | History |
| Oxalic-acid makers | Cyanogen compounds; nitrous fumes and nitric acid; oxalic acid; potassium hydroxide | History; temperature chart |
| Oxy-acetylene cutters | (See Welders) | History |
| Ozonators | Ozone | History |
| Painters | Acetone; amyl acetate; amyl alcohol; aniline and other compounds of benzol and its homologs; antimony and its compounds; arsenic and its compounds; barium; benzine; benzol; carbon disulfide; carbon tetrachloride; chromium compounds; lead and its compounds; manganese; mercury and its compounds; methanol; nitrous fumes and nitric acid; trichloroethylene; turpentine | History; chest x-ray; temperature chart; hemogram; arsenic, lead and mercury in urine |
| Painters (luminous watch and instrument dials) | Roentgen rays; radium and other radioactive substances | History; hemogram |
| Painters (tar) | Tar and pitch | History; chest x-ray; temperature chart |
| Paint makers | Acetone; amyl acetate; amyl alcohol; aniline and other amino compounds of benzol and its homologs; antimony and mercury compounds; arsenic and its compounds; barium; benzine; benzol; cadmium; carbon disulfide; carbon tetrachloride; chlorinated diphenyls; chlorinated naphthalenes; chromium compounds; hydrochloric acid; lead and its compounds; methanol; phenol; pyridine; selenium compounds; sodium hydroxide; sulfuric acid; tar and pitch; titanium oxide; trichloroethylene; turpentine; uranium | History; hemogram; lead, arsenic and mercury in urine |
| Paint-remover makers | Benzine; benzol; butanone; carbon tetrachloride; cresol; dichloroethyl ether; dioxane; furfural; methanol; methylene chloride; phenol tetrachloroethane; trichloroethylene; sodium and potassium hydroxide | History; hemogram |

TABLE 72—*Continued*

| *Occupation* | *Hazard* | *Diagnosis* |
|---|---|---|
| Paint removers | Inorganic dust (except asbestos) containing no free silica; acetone; amyl acetate; benzine; benzol and its homologs; butanone; carbon tetrachloride; cresol; dichloroethyl ether; lead and its compounds; methylene chloride; phenol; tetrachloroethane; trichloroethylene | History; chest x-ray; hemogram; lead in urine |
| Paper glazers | Arsenic and its compounds | History; arsenic in urine |
| Paperhangers | Inorganic dust (except asbestos) containing no free silica; arsenic and its compounds; chromium compounds; formaldehyde; lead and its compounds | History; chest x-ray; temperature chart; arsenic and lead in urine |
| Paper makers | Sudden variations in temperature; fungus infection; ammonia; amyl acetate; arseniureted hydrogen; chlorine; chromium compounds; formaldehyde; hydrochloric acid; hydrofluoric acid; lead and its compounds; magnesium; potassium hydroxide; sodium hydroxide; sulfur dioxide; sulfuretted hydrogen; sulfuric acid; titanium oxide. (See also particular occupation) | History; chest x-ray; temperature chart; arsenic and lead in urine |
| Paper-money makers | Chromium compounds | History; temperature chart |
| Paraffin workers | Acetone; benzol (benzene) and its homologs; carbon disulfide; carbon tetrachloride; ethylene dichloride; petroleum | History; hemogram |
| Parakeet handlers | Psittacosis | History; serologic reaction; temperature chart |
| Paris-green workers | Arsenic and its compounds | History; arsenic in urine |
| Parrot handlers | Psittacosis | History; serologic test; temperature chart |
| Patent-leather makers | Amyl acetate; carbon monoxide; lead and its compounds; methanol; oxalic acid; ozone; sulfuric acid; turpentine | History; lead in urine |
| Pencil makers | Acetone; aniline and other amino compounds of benzol and its homologs; arsenic and its compounds; benzol; chromium compounds; pyridine | History; hemogram; arsenic in urine |
| Perfume makers | Acetone; ammonia; amyl acetate; aniline and other amino compounds of benzol and its homologs; benzine; benzol and its homologs; butyl alcohol; carbon tetrachloride; cresol; dichloroethylene; dimethyl sulfate; ethyl bromide and ethyl chloride; formic acid; hydrochloric acid; methanol; methyl chloride; methylene chloride; naphthols; nitrobenzol and other nitro compounds of benzol and its homologs; phenol; potassium hydroxide; sulfuric acid; trichloroethylene | History; hemogram; urinalysis |
| Petroleum refiners | Acetone; acrolein; ammonia; aniline and other amino compounds of benzol and its homologs; benzine; benzol; carbon monoxide; dichloroethyl ether; hydrochloric acid; lead and its compounds; methylene chloride; nitrobenzol and other nitro compounds of benzol and its homologs; petroleum; sodium hydroxide; sulfur dioxide; sulfuretted hydrogen; sulfuric acid; trichloroethylene; turpentine | History; chest x-ray; hemogram; lead in urine |
| Pewter makers | Antimony and its compounds; tin with lead, brass or copper | History; chest x-ray; temperature chart |

TABLE 72—*Continued*

| *Occupation* | *Hazard* | *Diagnosis* |
|---|---|---|
| Pharmaceutical workers | Organic dust; acetone; acrolein; aniline and other amino compounds of benzol and its homologs; antimony and its compounds; arsenic and its compounds; benzol and its homologs; bromine; calcium cyanamide; carbon dioxide; carbon tetrachloride; chloride of lime; dinitrophenol; dioxane; ethyl bromide and ethyl chloride; ethylene dibromide; ethylene dichloride; formic acid; magnesium; manganese; mercury and its compounds; methyl bromide; methyl chloride; methylene chloride; naphthols; nitroglycerin; nitrous fumes; nitric acid; phenol; phenylhydrazine; phosgene; phosphorus; picric acid; potassium hydroxide; sodium hydroxide; sulfuric acid; tellurium compounds; tetrachloroethane; tetrachloroethylene; trichloroethylene; turpentine; uranium | History; chest x-ray; temperature chart; hemogram; arsenic, bromine, mercury and lead in urine; examination of lens and fundus |
| Phenol makers | Benzol (benzene) and its homologs; phenol; sulfuric acid | History; hemogram |
| Phenylhydrazine workers | Phenylhydrazine | History; hemogram |
| Phosgene makers | Carbon monoxide; chlorine; phosgene | History |
| Phosphate extractors | Hydrochloric acid | History |
| Phosphate-mill workers | Inorganic dust (except asbestos) containing no free silica; hydrofluoric acid; phosphorus. (See also Fertilizer makers) | History; chest x-ray; temperature chart |
| Phosphine workers | Carbon monoxide; phosphuretted hydrogen | History |
| Phosphor-bronze workers | Phosphorus | History; chest x-ray; temperature record |
| Phosphoric-acid makers | Cyanogen compounds; nitrous fumes and nitric acid; sulfuric acid | History; temperature record; chest x-ray |
| Phosphorus-compound makers | Phosphorus-sulfuretted hydrogen | History |
| Phosphorus-evaporating machine operators | Phosphorus; sulfuric acid | History; chest x-ray |
| Phosphorus extractors | Hydrofluoric acid; phosphorus; phosphuretted hydrogen | History; chest x-ray |
| Phosphorus (red) makers | Phosphorus; phosphuretted hydrogen | History; chest x-ray |
| Phosphuretted-hydrogen workers | Phosphuretted hydrogen | History |
| Photoengravers | Ammonia; amyl acetate; benzol; chromium compounds; methanol; nitrous fumes and nitric acid; potassium hydroxide | History; hemogram; temperature chart; chest x-ray |
| Photographers | Defective illumination; ultraviolet and infrared rays; methanol | History; refraction; temperature chart; chest x-ray |
| Photographic-film makers | Defective illumination; amyl acetate; bromine; butyl alcohol; nitrous fumes and nitric acid; silver. (See also Pyroxylin-plastics workers) | History; refraction; temperature chart; chest x-ray |
| Photographic-material workers | Acetaldehyde; acetone; ammonia; aniline and other amino compounds of benzol and its homologs; barium; benzol; chlorine; chromium compounds; cresol; cyanogen compounds; formaldehyde; hydrochloric acid; mercury and its compounds; phenol; picric acid; sulfuric acid; tellurium compounds; trichloroethylene; turpentine; uranium; vanadium. (See also Photographic film makers) | History; hemogram; temperature chart; mercury in urine |

TABLE 72—*Continued*

| *Occupation* | *Hazard* | *Diagnosis* |
|---|---|---|
| Photograph retouchers | Lead and its compounds | History; lead in urine |
| Photogravure workers | Chromium compounds; nitrous fumes and nitric acid | History; temperature chart; chest x-ray |
| Picklers | Arseniureted hydrogen; cyanogen compounds; hydrochloric acid; hydrofluoric acid; nitrous fumes and nitric acid; sulfuric acid | History; chest x-ray; arsenic in urine |
| Picric-acid makers | Benzol (benzene) and its homologs; nitrous fumes and nitric acid; phenol; picric acid; sulfuric acid | History; temperature chart; hemogram |
| Pigeon fatteners (breeders) | Anthrax; interstitial pneumonitis | History; temperature chart; chest x-ray |
| Pigment makers | (See Color makers) | History |
| Pipe fitters | Lead and its compounds. (See also particular liquid piped) | History; lead in urine |
| Pitch workers | Heat; arsenic and its compounds; cresol; tar and pitch | History; chest x-ray; temperature chart; arsenic in urine |
| Planer men (stone) | Inorganic dust containing free silica; inorganic dust (except asbestos) containing no free silica | History; chest x-ray; temperature record |
| Plasterers | Dampness; inorganic dust (except asbestos) containing no free silica; anthrax | History; chest x-ray; temperature chart |
| Plaster-of-paris workers | Inorganic dust (except asbestos) containing no free silica | History; chest x-ray; temperature chart |
| Platers | (See Electroplaters; Metalizers) | History |
| Platinum extractors | Bromine | History; bromine in urine |
| Plumbers | Arsine; carbon monoxide; lead and its compounds. (See particular substance piped) | History; arsenic and lead in urine; hemogram |
| Pneumatic-tool workers | Inorganic dust (except asbestos) containing no free silica; repeated motion, pressure, shock | History; chest x-ray; temperature chart |
| Polishers and cleaners (metal) | Organic dust; inorganic dust containing free silica; inorganic dust (except asbestos) containing no free silica; repeated motion, pressure, shock; benzine; benzol; cyanogen compounds; hydrochloric acid; methanol; oxalic acid; pyridine; silver; trichloroethylene; turpentine | History; chest x-ray; temperature chart; hemogram |
| Polish makers | Inorganic dust (except asbestos) containing no free silica; amyl acetate; aniline and other amino compounds of benzol and its homologs; benzine; benzol; carbon tetrachloride; cyanogen; dioxane; methanol; nitrobenzol and other nitro compounds of benzol and its homologs; oxalic acid; trichloroethylene; turpentine | History; chest x-ray; temperature chart; hemogram |
| Polyvinyl chloride workers | (See Vinyl-chloride workers) | |
| Porcelain makers | (See Pottery workers) | History |
| Potassium hydroxide makers | Potassium hydroxide | History |
| Pottery workers | Heat; dampness; inorganic dust containing free silica; inorganic dust (except asbestos) containing no free silica; arsenic and its compounds; carbon dioxide; carbon monoxide; chromium compounds; cobalt; hydrochloric acid; hydrofluoric acid; lead and its compounds; manganese; mercury and its compounds; selenium compounds; sulfur dioxide. (See also particular occupation) | History; chest x-ray; temperature chart; arsenic and mercury in urine |

TABLE 72—*Continued*

| *Occupation* | *Hazard* | *Diagnosis* |
|---|---|---|
| Pouncers (felt hats) | Organic dust; inorganic dust containing free silica; inorganic dust containing no free silica | History; chest x-ray; temperature chart |
| Pourers (foundry) | Heat | History; chest x-ray; temperature chart |
| Powder makers | (See Smokeless-powder makers) | History |
| Preparers (tannery) | Anthrax; septic infections | History; chest x-ray |
| Preservative makers and handlers | Formaldehyde | History; chest x-ray |
| Pressmen (oil refining) | Dampness; petroleum | History; chest x-ray |
| Pressmen (printers) | (See Printers) | History |
| Pressroom workers (rubber) | Aniline and other amino compounds of benzol and its homologs; antimony and its compounds; arsenic and its compounds; benzine; benzol | History; chest x-ray; hemogram; arsenic in urine |
| Primers (explosives) | Mercury and its compounds | History; mercury in urine |
| Printers | Inorganic dust (except asbestos) containing no free silica; aniline and other amino compounds of benzol and its homologs; antimony and its compounds; arsenic and its compounds; benzine; benzol; carbon monoxide; carbon tetrachloride; cyanogen compounds; lead and its compounds; mercury and its compounds; methanol; tetrachloroethylene; turpentine | History; chest x-ray; hemogram; arsenic, mercury and lead in urine |
| Printers, textile | (See Textile printers) | History |
| Puddlers (iron and steel) | Heat; carbon monoxide; manganese | History; chest x-ray |
| Pullers-out (felt hats) | Heat | History; chest x-ray |
| Pulp-mill workers | Heat; dampness. (See also Paper makers) | History; chest x-ray |
| Putty makers | Inorganic dust (except asbestos) containing no free silica; benzine; carbon disulfide; lead and its compounds | History; chest x-ray; temperature chart; hemogram |
| Putty polishers (glass) | Inorganic dust (except asbestos) containing no free silica; lead and its compounds | History; chest x-ray; lead in urine |
| Pyridine makers | Pyridine | History; hemogram |
| Pyrites burners | Heat; inorganic dust (except asbestos) containing no free silica; arsenic and selenium compounds; sulfur dioxide; sulfuretted hydrogen | History; chest x-ray; hemogram; arsenic in urine |
| Pyroxylin-plastics workers | Organic dust; acetaldehyde; acetone; acrolein; amyl acetate; amyl alcohol; aniline and other amino compounds of benzol and its homologs; benzine arseniureted hydrogen; benzol; butyl alcohol; carbon monoxide; carbon tetrachloride; cyanogen compounds; dichloroethylene; dioxane; ethylene dibromide; lead and its compounds; methanol; methyl cellosolve; nitrous fumes and nitric acid; sulfuretted hydrogen; sulfuric acid; tetrachloroethane; triorthocresyl phosphate | History; chest x-ray; hemogram; arsenic and lead in urine |
| Quarrymen | Inorganic dust containing free silica; inorganic dust (except asbestos) containing no free silica | History; chest x-ray |
| Quartz workers | Inorganic dust containing free silica | History; chest x-ray |
| Radioactive-paint makers | Roentgen rays, radium and other radioactive substances | History; hemogram |

TABLE 72—*Continued*

| *Occupation* | *Hazard* | *Diagnosis* |
|---|---|---|
| Radioactive-water makers | Roentgen rays, radium and other radioactive substances | History; hemogram |
| Radiologists | Roentgen rays, radium and other radioactive substances | History; hemogram |
| Radio-tube makers | Mercury and its compounds | History; mercury in urine |
| Radium miners | Roentgen rays, radium and other radioactive substances | History; hemogram |
| Radium-ore-reduction workers | Roentgen rays, radium and other radioactive substances | History; hemogram |
| Radium specialists | Roentgen rays, radium and other radioactive substances | History; hemogram |
| Rag workers | Organic dust; anthrax; septic infections | History; chest x-ray |
| Rayon makers | Ammonia; amyl acetate; benzine; butyl alcohol; carbon disulfide; chlorinated diphenyls; chlorine; cyanogen compounds; dioxane; formaldehyde; hydrochloric acid; methanol; methylene chloride; nitrous fumes and nitric acid; oxalic acid; sodium hydroxide; sulfuretted hydrogen; sulfuric acid; tetrachloroethane | History; hemogram; chest x-ray |
| Reclaimers (rubber) | Aniline and other amino compounds of benzol and its homologs; benzol; carbon disulfide; hydrochloric acid; lead and its compounds; mercury and its compounds; nitrous fumes and nitric acid; sulfuric acid | History; hemogram; lead and mercury in urine; temperature chart |
| Red-lead workers | Lead and its compounds | History; lead in urine |
| Refiners (metals) | Arsenic and its compounds; arseniureted hydrogen; carbon monoxide; hydrochloric acid; lead and its compounds; mercury and its compounds; nitrous fumes and nitric acid; sulfur dioxide, sulfuric acid. (See also particular occupation) | History; chest x-ray; arsenic, lead and mercury in urine |
| Refrigerating-plant workers | Sudden variations in temperature; dampness; ammonia; carbon dioxide; carbon monoxide; ozone | History; chest x-ray |
| Refrigerator (mechanical) makers and repairmen | Acrolein; ethyl bromide and ethyl chloride; methyl bromide; methyl chloride; methyl formate; sulfur dioxide | History; chest x-ray |
| Resins (synthetic) makers | Organic dust; acetaldehyde; acetone; chlorinated diphenyls; chlorinated naphthalenes; cresol; dichloroethyl ether; formaldehyde; furfural; methanol; methyl cellosolve; oxalic acid; phenol; selenium compounds; trichloroethylene; vinyl chloride | History; chest x-ray |
| Roller coverers (cotton mill) | Heat; organic dust | History; chest x-ray |
| Rollers (metals) | Heat | History; chest x-ray |
| Roll setters (iron and steel) | Heat | History; chest x-ray |
| Roll wrenchers (iron and steel) | Heat | History; chest x-ray |
| Roofers | Lead and its compounds; tar and pitch | History; chest x-ray; lead in urine |
| Roofing-material workers | Heat; inorganic dust (except asbestos) containing no free silica; asbestos; tar and pitch | History; chest x-ray |
| Rope makers | Organic dust; tar and pitch | History; chest x-ray |
| Rotogravure workers | Benzol (benzene) and its homologs | History; hemogram |
| Roughers (iron and steel) | Heat | History; chest x-ray |

TABLE 72—*Continued*

| *Occupation* | *Hazard* | *Diagnosis* |
|---|---|---|
| Rubber-cement makers | (See Cement [rubber] mixers) | History |
| Rubber-glove makers | Benzine (naphtha-gasoline) | History; hemogram |
| Rubberized-asbestos-board makers | Benzine (naphtha-gasoline) | History; hemogram |
| Rubber (synthetic) makers | Acetaldehyde; amyl alcohol; aniline and other amino compounds of benzol and its homologs; chlorine; chloroprene; cresol; nitrous fumes and nitric acid; sulfur chloride | History; hemogram; temperature chart; chest x-ray |
| Rubber-tire builders | Benzine; benzol and its homologs | History; hemogram |
| Rubber workers | Organic dust; inorganic dust containing free silica; inorganic dust (except asbestos) containing no free silica; acetone; aniline and other amino compounds of benzol and its homologs; antimony and its compounds; arsenic and its compounds; barium; benzine; benzol; carbon disulfide; carbon tetrachloride; chromium compounds; ethylene dichloride; formaldehyde; formic acid; lead and its compounds; magnesium; methanol; nitrous fumes and nitric acid; phenol; pyridine; sodium hydroxide; tellurium compounds; tetrachloroethane; trichloroethylene; turpentine. (See also particular occupation) | History; chest x-ray; temperature chart; arsenic and lead in urine |
| Sagger makers | Dampness; inorganic dust (except asbestos) containing no free silica; lead and its compounds | History; chest x-ray |
| Salt extractors (coke-oven by-products) | Ammonia; sulfuric acid | History |
| Salt preparers | Heat; sudden variations in temperature; inorganic dust (except asbestos) containing no free silica | History; chest x-ray |
| Sand blasters | Inorganic dust containing free silica; inorganic dust (except asbestos) containing no free silica | History; chest x-ray |
| Sand cutters | Inorganic dust containing free silica | History; chest x-ray |
| Sanders | Inorganic dust containing free silica; inorganic dust (except asbestos) containing no free silica | History; chest x-ray |
| Sanding-machine operators | Inorganic dust containing free silica; inorganic dust (except asbestos) containing no free silica | History; chest x-ray |
| Sandpaperers (enameling and painting auto bodies, etc.) | Inorganic dust (except asbestos) containing no free silica; lead and its compounds | History; chest x-ray; lead in urine |
| Sandpaper makers | Inorganic dust containing free silica; inorganic dust (except asbestos) containing no free silica | History; chest x-ray |
| Sand pulverizers | Inorganic dust (except asbestos) containing no free silica | History; chest x-ray |
| Saw filers | Inorganic dust (except asbestos) containing no free silica | History; chest x-ray |
| Sawyers (stone) | Inorganic dust containing free silica; inorganic dust (except asbestos) containing no free silica | History; chest x-ray |
| Scourers (belts) | Benzol (benzene) and its homologs | History; hemogram |
| Scourers (metals) | Benzine (naphtha-gasoline); carbon tetrachloride; nitrous fumes and nitric acid; sulfuric acid; trichloroethylene | History; hemogram |
| Scourers (wood lasts, shoes) | Organic dust | History; chest x-ray |
| Scouring-powder makers | Inorganic dust containing free silica; inorganic dust (except asbestos) containing no free silica | History; chest x-ray |

TABLE 72—*Continued*

| *Occupation* | *Hazard* | *Diagnosis* |
|---|---|---|
| Scrapers (foundry) | Inorganic dust containing free silica; inorganic dust (except asbestos) containing no free silica | History; chest x-ray |
| Screen tenders (pulp mill) | Dampness | History; chest x-ray |
| Screen workers (lead and zinc smelting) | Inorganic dust (except asbestos) containing no free silica; lead and its compounds | History; chest x-ray; lead in urine |
| Sealers (incandescent lamps) | Carbon monoxide | History |
| Sealing-wax makers | Arsenic and its compounds; turpentine | History; arsenic in urine |
| Selenium refiners | Selenium compounds | History |
| Sewage-purification workers | Chlorine | History; hemogram |
| Sewage workers | Dampness; ammonia; benzine; carbon dioxide; carbon monoxide; sulfuretted hydrogen | History; chest x-ray; hemogram |
| Shade-cloth makers | Benzine; benzol and its homologs | History; hemogram |
| Shale-oil workers | (See Petroleum refiners) | History |
| Shavers (felt hats; fur; tannery) | Dampness; organic dust; anthrax; septic infections | History; chest x-ray |
| Shearers | Infection; undulant fever (brucellosis) | History; skin test for brucellergin |
| Sheep-dip makers | Arsenic and its compounds | History; arsenic in urine |
| Sheet-metal workers | Lead and its compounds | History; lead in urine |
| Shellackers | Amyl acetate; benzine; benzol; butyl alcohol; lead and its compounds; methanol; turpentine | History; hemogram |
| Shellac makers | Ammonium; amyl acetate; benzine; benzol; butyl alcohol; lead and its compounds; methanol; turpentine | History; hemogram; lead in urine |
| Shell fillers | Dinitrophenol; nitrobenzol and other nitro compounds of benzol and its homologs; nitroglycerin; picric acid | History; hemogram; examination of lens and fundus |
| Sherardizers | Zinc | History |
| Shifters | Organic dust; inorganic dust (except asbestos) containing no free silica | History; chest x-ray |
| Shingle stainers | Benzine (naphtha-gasoline) | History; hemogram |
| Shipyard workers | Tar and pitch | History |
| Shoddy workers | Organic dust; anthrax; septic infections; arseniureted hydrogen; chlorine; hydrochloric acid; sulfuric acid | History; hemogram; arsenic in urine |
| Shoe dyers | Lead and its compounds; nitrobenzol and other nitro compounds of benzol and its homologs | History; hemogram; lead in urine |
| Shoe-factory operatives | Organic dust; anthrax; acetone; amyl acetate; benzine; benzol; carbon tetrachloride; methanol; tetrachloroethane; trichloroethylene; turpentine | History; chest x-ray; hemogram |
| Shoe finishers | Sudden variations in temperature; ammonia; amyl acetate; amyl alcohol; benzine; benzol; methanol | History; chest x-ray; hemogram |
| Shoe-heel (wood) coverers | Acetone; amyl acetate; benzine; benzol and its homologs; methanol | History; hemogram |
| Shooting-gallery workers | Mercury and its compounds | History; mercury in urine |

TABLE 72—*Continued*

| *Occupation* | *Hazard* | *Diagnosis* |
|---|---|---|
| Shot makers | Antimony and its compounds; arsenic and its compounds; lead and its compounds | History; arsenic and lead in urine |
| Silicon-alloy makers | Inorganic dust containing free silica | History; chest x-ray |
| Silk weighters | Lead and its compounds; tin | History; lead in urine |
| Silk workers | Organic dust; septic infections | History; chest x-ray |
| Silo workers | Carbon dioxide; nitrous gases (Also see Farmer's lung disease.) | History; chest x-ray |
| Silverers (mirror) | See Mirror silverers | History |
| Silver-foil makers | Silver; argyria | History |
| Silver melters | Carbon monoxide; cyanogen compounds; silver | History; chest x-ray |
| Silver miners | Arsenic and its compounds; lead; silver; argyria | History; arsenic in urine; chest x-ray |
| Silver-nitrate makers | Silver; argyria | History |
| Silver platers | Silver. (See also Electroplaters) | History |
| Silversmiths | Silver; argyria | History |
| Singers (cloth) | Carbon monoxide | History |
| Sintering-plant workers | Inorganic dust (except asbestos) containing no free silica | History; chest x-ray |
| Sizers (felt hats) | Heat; mercury and its compounds | History; chest x-ray; mercury in urine |
| Skimmers (glass) | Heat; ultraviolet and infrared rays | History; hemogram |
| Slag workers | Inorganic dust containing free silica; inorganic dust (except asbestos) containing no free silica | History; chest x-ray |
| Slate workers | Inorganic dust containing free silica; inorganic dust (except asbestos) containing no free silica | History; chest x-ray |
| Slaughterhouse workers | Dampness; infections; anthrax; septic and intestinal infections; undulant fever (brucellosis) | History; skin test for brucellergin; chest x-ray; hemogram; ova and parasites |
| Slip makers (pottery) | Dampness; inorganic dust (except asbestos) containing no free silica; lead and its compounds | History; chest x-ray |
| Slushers (porcelain enameling) | Lead and its compounds | History; lead in urine |
| Smelters | Lead; inorganic dust containing free silica; inorganic dust (except asbestos) containing no free silica; sulfur dioxide. (See also particular metal) | History; chest x-ray |
| Smokeless-powder makers | Acetone; amyl acetate; amyl alcohol; benzol; carbon disulfide; nitrobenzol and other nitro compounds of benzol and its homologs; nitroglycerin; nitrous fumes and nitric acid; phenol; picric acid | History; hemogram |
| Smoothers (glass) | Dampness; inorganic dust (except asbestos) containing no free silica | History; chest x-ray |
| Soap (abrasive) workers | Inorganic dust containing free silica; inorganic dust (except asbestos) containing no free silica | History; chest x-ray |
| Soap makers | Organic dust; septic infections; acrolein; amyl acetate; arsenic and its compounds; benzine; benzol; carbon tetrachloride; dichloroethyl ether; ethylene dichloride; formaldehyde; formic acid; hydrochloric acid; manganese; methanol; nitrobenzol and other nitro compounds; potassium and sodium hydroxide; sulfuretted hydrogen; sulfuric acid; tar and pitch; tetrachloroethane; tetrachloroethylene; trichloroethylene | History; chest x-ray; temperature chart; hemogram; arsenic in urine |

TABLE 72—*Continued*

| *Occupation* | *Hazard* | *Diagnosis* |
|---|---|---|
| Soda makers | Ammonia; arseniureted hydrogen; carbon dioxide; carbon monoxide; chlorine; nitrous fumes and nitric acid; sulfuretted hydrogen; sulfuric acid | History; chest x-ray; arsenic in urine |
| Sodium-hydroxide makers | Dampness; chlorine; sodium hydroxide | History; chest x-ray; temperature record |
| Sodium-silicate makers | Inorganic dust containing free silica | History; chest x-ray |
| Sodium-sulfide makers | Sulfuretted hydrogen | History |
| Softeners (tannery) | Organic dust | History; chest x-ray |
| Solderers | Ultraviolet and infrared rays; arsine; cadmium; carbon monoxide; cyanogen compounds; hydrochloric acid; lead and its compounds | History; hemogram; arsenic and lead in urine |
| Solder makers | Antimony and its compounds; cadmium; lead and its compounds | History; lead in urine |
| Sole stitchers (Blake machine) | Mercury and its compounds | History; mercury in urine |
| Soot packers | Organic dust; arsenic and its compounds | History; arsenic in urine; chest x-ray |
| Spice makers | Organic dust | History; chest x-ray |
| Spinners (asbestos) | Asbestos | History; chest x-ray |
| Spinners (textiles) | Organic dust; repeated motion, pressure, shock, etc. | History; chest x-ray |
| Sprayers (metals) | (See Metalizers) | History |
| Sprayers (trees) | Arsenic and its compounds; cyanogen compounds; lead and its compounds | History; arsenic and lead in urine |
| Spreaders (rubber works) | Carbon tetrachloride | History; temperature chart; chest x-ray |
| Stamp-mill workers | Heat; dampness; inorganic dust containing free silica; inorganic dust (except asbestos) containing no free silica | History; chest x-ray |
| Starch makers | Organic dust; carbon dioxide; sulfuretted hydrogen | History; chest x-ray |
| Starters (felt hats) | Heat; mercury and its compounds | History; mercury in urine |
| Statuary workers | Inorganic dust containing free silica; inorganic dust (except asbestos) containing no free silica | History; chest x-ray |
| Stearic-acid makers | Acrolein | History; chest x-ray |
| Steel (chrome) makers | Chromium compounds | History; temperature chart |
| Stereotypers | Antimony and its compounds; lead and its compounds | History; lead in urine; chest x-ray |
| Stiffeners (felt hats) | Mercury and its compounds; methanol | History; mercury in urine |
| Still (coal tar) cleaners | Heat; benzol and its homologs; tar and pitch | History; chest x-ray |
| Stillmen (carbolic acid) | Heat; phenol | History; chest x-ray |
| Stillmen, operating | Heat. (See also particular chemical) | History |
| Stitchers (shoes) | Methanol | History |
| Stokers | Heat; inorganic dust (except asbestos) containing no free silica; ultraviolet and infrared rays; carbon monoxide | History; chest x-ray |

TABLE 72—*Continued*

| *Occupation* | *Hazard* | *Diagnosis* |
|---|---|---|
| Stone (artificial) makers | Inorganic dust (except asbestos) containing no free silica; inorganic dust containing free silica | History; chest x-ray |
| Stone cutters | Inorganic dust containing free silica; inorganic dust (except asbestos) containing no free silica | History; chest x-ray |
| Stone masons | Inorganic dust containing free silica; inorganic dust (except asbestos) containing no free silica | History; chest x-ray |
| Storage-battery makers | Amyl acetate; antimony and its compounds; arsine; cadmium; carbon monoxide; lead and its compounds; mercury and its compounds; nickel; sulfur dioxide; sulfuric acid | History; chest x-ray; lead and mercury in urine |
| Straw cutters | Fungus infections | History; chest x-ray |
| Straw-hat makers | Organic dust; acrolein; amyl acetate; chloride of lime; formaldehyde; methanol; tetrachloroethane | History; chest x-ray |
| Sugar cane workers | Inhalation of dust from dried sugar cane or bagasse (bagassosis) | History; pneumonitis or bronchiolitis; chest x-ray |
| Sugar refiners | Heat; dampness; organic dust; inorganic dust (except asbestos) containing no free silica; ammonia; barium; carbon dioxide; chlorine; hydrochloric acid; sulfur dioxide; sulfuretted hydrogen; sulfuric acid | History; chest x-ray |
| Sulfates makers | Sulfuric acid | History |
| Sulfides makers | Sulfuretted hydrogen | History |
| Sulfite cooks (pulp mill) | Heat; sulfur dioxide | History; chest x-ray |
| Sulfur burners | Heat; inorganic dust (except asbestos) containing no free silica; arsenic and its compounds; sulfur dioxide | History; chest x-ray; arsenic in urine |
| Sulfur-chloride makers | Chlorine; hydrochloric acid; sulfur chloride; sulfuric acid | History |
| Sulfur-dioxide makers | Carbon monoxide; sulfur dioxide | History |
| Sulfurers (malt and hops) | Sulfur dioxide | History |
| Sulfur extractors | Carbon disulfide | History |
| Sulfuric acid workers | Ammonia; arsenic and its compounds; arsine; lead and its compounds; nitrous fumes and nitric acid; selenium compounds; sulfur dioxide; sulfuretted hydrogen; sulfuric acid; vanadium | History; arsenic and lead in urine; chest x-ray |
| Sulfur miners | Sulfur dioxide; sulfuretted hydrogen | History; chest x-ray |
| Sumackers (tannery) | Dampness; anthrax | History; chest x-ray |
| Takers-down (glass) | Heat | History; chest x-ray |
| Talc workers | Inorganic dust (except asbestos) containing no free silica. Exposure to fibrous talc dust is more hazardous than to granular talc, although prolonged exposure to both can produce talcosis of the lung with impairment of pulmonary function. | History; chest x-ray |
| Tallow refiners | Inorganic dust (except asbestos) containing no free silica; acrolein; carbon disulfide; sulfuric acid | History; chest x-ray |
| Tank cleaners | Arsine; benzine; benzol; hydrofluoric acid; tar and pitch; tetraethyl lead. (See also particular chemical) | History; chest x-ray; arsenic in urine |

TABLE 72—*Continued*

| *Occupation* | *Hazard* | *Diagnosis* |
|---|---|---|
| Tannery workers | Dampness; infection; ammonia; amyl acetate; aniline and other amino compounds of benzol and its homologs; arsenic and its compounds; benzine (naphtha-gasoline); carbon dioxide; chloride of lime; chromium compounds; cyanogen compounds; formaldehyde; formic acid; hydrochloric acid; lead and its compounds; mercury and its compounds; oxalic acid; picric acid; sodium hydroxide; sulfur dioxide; sulfuretted hydrogen; sulfuric acid | History; chest x-ray; hemogram; lead and mercury in urine |
| Tapers (airplanes) | Tetrachloroethane | History; hemogram |
| Tappers (smelting) | Heat. (See also particular metal) | History |
| Tar (distillery) workers | Heat; arsenic and its compounds; cresol; tar and pitch. (See also Coal-tar workers) | History; chest x-ray; temperature chart; arsenic in urine |
| Taxidermists | Organic dust; anthrax; septic infections; arsenic and its compounds; mercury and its compounds | History; chest x-ray; mercury and arsenic in urine |
| Tear-gas makers | (See War-gas makers and Mace.) | History |
| Teazers (glass) | Heat; carbon monoxide | History |
| Temperers | Heat; calcium cyanamide; carbon monoxide; cyanogen compounds; lead and its compounds; mercury and its compounds; petroleum; sulfuric acid | History; lead and mercury in urine |
| Tetraethyl-lead makers | Bromine; lead and its compounds; tetraethyl lead | History; lead and bromine in urine |
| Textile (asbestos) workers | Asbestos | History; chest x-ray |
| Textile-comb makers | Inorganic dust (except asbestos) containing no free silica | History; chest x-ray |
| Textile printers | Heat; amyl acetate; aniline and other amino compounds of benzol and its homologs; antimony and its compounds; arsenic and its compounds; cadmium; carbon monoxide; chlorine; chromium and lead compounds; cyanogen compounds; manganese; mercury and its compounds; methanol; nitrous fumes and nitric acid; phenol; sulfuric acid; turpentine; vanadium | History; chest x-ray; hemogram; lead and mercury in urine |
| Thallium workers | Thallium | History |
| Thermometer makers | Mercury and its compounds; methyl chloride; thallium | History; mercury in urine |
| Tile makers | Heat; sudden variations in temperature; inorganic dust containing free silica; inorganic dust (except asbestos) containing no free silica; lead and its compounds; uranium. (See also Pottery workers) | History; chest x-ray; lead in urine |
| Tin-foil makers | Heat; lead and its compounds | History; chest x-ray; lead in urine |
| Tinners | Heat; dampness; acrolein; ammonia; arsenic and its compounds; arseniureted hydrogen; hydrochloric acid; lead and its compounds | History; chest x-ray |
| Tin-plate-mill workers | (See Iron and steel workers) | History |
| Tin-recovery workers | Chlorine | History |
| Tire builders | (See Rubber-tire builders) | History |
| Tobacco denicotinizers | Ethylene dichloride; trichloroethylene | History |
| Tobacco moisteners | Dampness; carbon dioxide | History |

TABLE 72—*Continued*

| *Occupation* | *Hazard* | *Diagnosis* |
|---|---|---|
| Tobacco seedling treaters | Benzol (benzene) and its homologs | History |
| Tobacco workers | Organic dust; nicotine | History; chest x-ray |
| Toolmakers | Inorganic dust (except asbestos) containing no free silica | History; chest x-ray |
| Top fillers (foundry) | Heat; inorganic dust (except asbestos) containing no free silica | History; chest x-ray |
| Towermen (sulfuric acid) | Arsine; nitrous fumes and nitric acid; sulfur dioxide; sulfuric acid. (See also Sulfuric-acid workers) | History; arsenic in urine |
| Toy makers | Amyl acetate; arsenic and its compounds; lead and its compounds | History; lead and arsenic in urine |
| Transfer workers (pottery) | Lead and its compounds; turpentine | History; lead in urine |
| Transparent wrapping materials workers | Acetone; carbon disulfide; hydrochloric acid; sodium hydroxide; sulfuretted hydrogen; sulfuric acid | History; chest x-ray |
| Treaders (rubber) | Benzine (naphtha-gasoline); benzol (benzene) and its homologs | History; hemogram |
| Trichloroethylene workers | Trichloroethylene | History |
| Trinitrotoluol makers | Benzol (benzene) and its homologs; nitrobenzol and other nitro compounds of benzol and its homologs | History; hemogram |
| Tube makers (glass) | Heat | History; chest x-ray |
| Tubulators (incandescent lamps) | Carbon monoxide | History |
| Tumbling-barrel workers | Inorganic dust containing free silica; inorganic dust (except asbestos) containing no free silica | History; chest x-ray |
| Tunnel workers | Compressed air (increased atmospheric pressure); inorganic dust containing free silica; inorganic dust (except asbestos) containing no free silica; carbon dioxide; nitrous fumes and nitric acid; sulfuretted hydrogen | History; chest x-ray |
| Turners-out (glass) | Heat | History; chest x-ray |
| Turpentine extractors | Heat; turpentine | History; chest x-ray |
| Type cleaners | Benzine (naphtha-gasoline); methanol | History; hemogram |
| Type founders | Antimony and lead and their compounds | History; lead in urine |
| Type melters | Acrolein; lead and its compounds | History; lead in urine |
| Typesetters | (See Compositors) | History |
| Ultramarine-blue makers | Sulfur dioxide | History |
| Upholsterers | Organic dust; anthrax; methanol | History; chest x-ray |
| Uranium miners | Roentgen rays, radium and other radioactive substances; uranium; rates of lung cancer are excessive only in those working underground for five or more years. | History; hemogram |
| Uranium workers | Roentgen rays, radium and other radioactive substances; uranium | History; hemogram |
| Vanadium-steel workers | Heat; vanadium | History; chest x-ray |
| Vapor curers | (See Vulcanizers) | History |
| Varnishers | Acetaldehyde; acetone; amyl alcohol; aniline and other amino compounds of benzol and its homologs; benzine; benzol; butyl alcohol; carbon disulfide; carbon tetrachloride; dichloroethylene; ethylene dichloride; formic acid; lead and its compounds; manganese; methanol; tetrachloroethane; trichloroethylene; turpentine | History; hemogram; chest x-ray; temperature chart |

TABLE 72—*Continued*

| *Occupation* | *Hazard* | *Diagnosis* |
|---|---|---|
| Varnish makers | Acetaldehyde; acetone; acrolein; ammonia; amyl acetate; amyl alcohol; aniline and other amino compounds of benzol and its homologs; arsenic and its compounds; barium; benzine (naphtha-gasoline); benzol (benzene) and its homologs; butyl alcohol; carbon disulfide; carbon tetrachloride; chlorinated diphenyls; chlorinated naphthalenes; dioxane; ethylene dichloride; formic acid; furfural; hexone; lead and its compounds; manganese; methanol; methyl cellosolve; ozone; phenol; sodium hydroxide; sulfur chloride; tretrachloroethane; trichloroethylene; turpentine | History; hemogram; chest x-ray; arsenic and lead in urine |
| Varnish-remover makers | Benzine; benzol; dichloroethyl ether; hexanone; pentanone; tetrachloroethane | History; hemogram |
| Vatmen | Heat; dampness; carbon dioxide | History; chest x-ray |
| Vat varnishers | (See Varnishers) | History |
| Vault workers | Carbon dioxide | History |
| Velvet makers | Heat; arsenic and its compounds | History; chest x-ray; arsenic in urine |
| Vignetters | Hydrochloric acid | History |
| Vinegar workers | Acetaldehyde; carbon dioxide | History |
| Vinters | Carbon dioxide | History |
| Vinyl-chloride makers | Vinyl chloride; acroosteolysis of fingers (associated with the hand cleaning of polymerizers) | History |
| Vulcanizers | Ammonia; aniline and other amino compounds of benzol and its homologs; antimony and its compounds; benzine; benzol; carbon dioxide; carbon disulfide; chromium compounds; methanol; selenium compounds; sulfur chloride; sulfur dioxide; sulfuretted hydrogen | History; chest x-ray; hemogram |
| Vulcanizers (steam) | Heat; dampness | History; chest x-ray |
| Wallpaper printers | Heat; sudden variations in temperature; arsenic and its compounds; chromium, lead and their compounds | History; chest x-ray; arsenic and lead in urine |
| Warehouse workers | Anthrax | History; temperature chart; chest x-ray |
| War-gas makers | Arsine; benzol; bromine; chlorine; cyanogen compounds; dimethyl sulfate; phosgene; picric acid; sulfur chloride | History; chest x-ray; hemogram; temperature chart |
| Washers (metal) | Benzine (naphtha-gasoline). (See also Degreasers) | History |
| Watch-dial (luminous) painters | Roentgen rays, radium and other radioactive substances | History; hemogram |
| Water gilders | Mercury and its compounds | History; mercury in urine |
| Waterproofers (paper and textiles) | Benzine; benzol; carbon tetrachloride; chromium compounds; formaldehyde; tar and pitch | History; hemogram; temperature chart |
| Water purifiers | Barium; chloride of lime; chlorine; ozone | History |
| Wax makers | Benzol; chlorinated diphenyls; chlorinated naphthalenes; ozone; sulfuric acid; trichloroethane; turpentine | History; hemogram |
| Wax-ornament makers | Acrolein; arsenic and chromium and their compounds | History; arsenic in urine |
| Weavers (asbestos) | Asbestos | History; chest x-ray |
| Weighers | Organic dust; inorganic dust (except asbestos) containing no free silica | History; chest x-ray |

TABLE 72—*Continued*

| *Occupation* | *Hazard* | *Diagnosis* |
|---|---|---|
| Welders | Ultraviolet and infrared rays; arsenic and its compounds; benzol; cadmium; carbon monoxide; chromium and its compounds; copper; hydrofluoric acid; lead and its compounds; manganese; mercury and its compounds; nitrous fumes and nitric acid; ozone; phosphorus; phosphuretted hydrogen; selenium compounds; zinc | History; chest x-ray; hemogram; arsenic and mercury in urine |
| Well workers | Carbon dioxide | History |
| White-lead workers | Carbon dioxide; lead and its compounds | History; lead in urine |
| Window-shade makers | Benzine; benzol | History; hemogram |
| Wire drawers | Arsenic and its compounds; hydrochloric acid; sulfuric acid | History; arsenic in urine |
| Wirers (incandescent lamps) | Amyl acetate | History |
| Wood-alcohol distillers | Acetone; carbon monoxide; methanol | History |
| Wooden-heel workers | Anthrax | History |
| Wood-last scourers (shoes) | Organic dust | History; chest x-ray |
| Wood polishers | (See Furniture polishers) | History |
| Wood preservers | Arsenic and its compounds; dinitrophenol; mercury and its compounds; phenol; sulfuric acid; tar and pitch | History; arsenic and mercury in urine; examination of lens and fundus |
| Wood stainers | Chromium compounds; lead and its compounds | History; lead in urine |
| Woodworkers | Organic dust; benzine (naphtha-gasoline); methanol | History; hemogram; chest x-ray |
| Wool carders | Organic dust; anthrax | History; hemogram |
| Wool scourers | Dampness; anthrax; acetone; ammonia | History; hemogram; chest x-ray |
| Wool spinners | Organic dust; anthrax | History; hemogram |
| Wool workers | Organic dust; anthrax | History; hemogram |
| Wringers (guncotton) | Nitrous fumes and nitric acid | History |
| Writers of books | Mogigraphia; "Amarbleosis"; anorexia; insomnia; scotomata. | History; characteristic physical findings |
| Yeast makers | Acetaldehyde; carbon dioxide; hydrofluoric acid; sulfuric acid | History |
| Zinc-chloride makers | Benzol and its homologs; chlorine; hydrochloric acid | History; hemogram |
| Zinc-electrode makers | Mercury and its compounds | History; mercury in urine |
| Zincers | Cyanogen and its compounds | History |
| Zinc miners | Arsenic and its compounds; lead and its compounds; manganese. (See also Miners) | History; chest x-ray; lead and arsenic in urine |
| Zinc smelters and refiners | Inorganic dust containing free silica; inorganic dust (except asbestos) containing no free silica; antimony, lead, arsenic and their compounds; cadmium; carbon monoxide; manganese; selenium compounds; sulfur dioxide; tellurium compounds; zinc. | History; chest x-ray; lead and arsenic in urine |
| Zoological technicians | Undulant fever (brucellosis) | History; temperature chart; skin test with brucellergin |

## THE FORGOTTEN CASUALTY

Of all persons exposed to hazardous substances, the victim of dermatitis is the forgotten casualty. All too often "skin rashes" are overlooked or dismissed as minor injuries by those looking for more dramatic evidence of poisoning. In terms of home poisoning, this attitude is probably justified; however, in industry, dermatitis is the leading occupational disease. Unfortunately, the threat of occupational dermatitis is too often overlooked in accident prevention activities.

Occupational acne (chloracne) occurs among workers exposed to insoluble cutting oils, crude petroleum, coal tar, heavy tar distillates, coal tar pitch, chlorinated hydrocarbons and weed killers such as 2,4-dichlorophenol and 2,4,5-trichlorophenol. The most potent of all these chemicals, as far as their acne-forming properties are concerned, are the chloronaphthalenes, chlorodiphenyls and chlorodiphenyloxides. Nearly all workers exposed to these three substances for several months or more develop acne-like lesions on the exposed parts unless the most stringent rules of cleanliness for clothes and body are observed. The inorganic compounds of chlorine do not cause occupational acne either by external contact or by internal administration. Nor do the acneiform lesions occur among workers with the solvent chlorinated hydrocarbons, although all the solvents can injure the skin by direct contact, and these substances may even cause systemic poisoning when absorption occurs. Individuals with dry, fair skin are less commonly affected than those with oily and/or dark skin. Those with acne vulgaris or a history thereof should not be

TABLE 73
MAXIMUM ALLOWABLE CONCENTRATIONS
FOR TOXIC FUMES AND DUSTS*

| *Fume or Dust* | *Concentration mg/cu m* |
|---|---|
| Arsenic | 0.25 |
| Beryllium | 0.002 |
| Cadmium | 0.1 |
| Chlordane | 2.0 |
| Chlorodiphenyls | 1.0 |
| Chloronaphthalenes | 1.0–5.0 |
| Chromic acid and chromates | 0.1 |
| Cyanide (alkaline) as CN | 5.0 |
| DDT | 2.0 |
| Dieldrin | 0.25 |
| o-Dinitrocresol | 0.2 |
| Fluoride dusts, smokes | 2.0 |
| Iron oxide | 15.0 |
| Lead (chromate & sulfide) | 0.5 |
| Lead tetraethyl | 0.1 |
| Lead (other inorganic) | 0.2 |
| Lindane | 0.5 |
| Manganese | 5.0 |
| Mercury | 0.1 |
| Parathion | 0.1 |
| Pentachlorophenol | 0.5 |
| Selenium | 0.1 |
| Sulfuric acid | 1.0 |
| Tetraethyl pyrophosphate | 0.1 |
| Tetryl | 1.5 |
| Thallium | 0.1 |
| Thiram | 5.0 |
| Titanium dioxide (chemical pneumonitis) | 15.0 |
| Trinitrotoluene | 1.5 |
| Zinc chromate | 0.2 |
| Zinc oxide fume | 15.0 |

*Expressed in mg/cu m of air.

TABLE 74
MAXIMUM ALLOWABLE CONCENTRATIONS
FOR MINERAL AND INERT DUSTS*

| *Mineral or Dust* | *Concentration† $X10^6$/cu ft (M.P.P.C.F.)* |
|---|---|
| Aluminum oxide | 25.0 |
| Asbestos | 5.0 |
| Glass | 30.0 |
| Granite | 10.0 |
| Inert—insoluble | 30.0 |
| Inert—soluble | 35.0 |
| Limestone | 35.0 |
| Mica | 20.0 |
| Silica, amorphous | 5.0 |
| Silica, quartz | 2.5 |
| Silica mixtures—approximately inversely proportional to free silica content | |
| Silicon carbide | 25.0 |
| Talc | 20.0 |

*All values in millions of particles/cu ft of air by standard light-field count (M.P.P.C.F.).

†In cases in which dust is generated from materials with high quartz content, measures should be taken to subtract any "background" or inert dust from actual dust counts obtained.

employed in the manufacturing of these compounds. The coexistence of chloracne and porphyria cutanea tarda (PCT) occurs frequently in these workers and should not be overlooked.

## Acne Eruptions Induced by Drugs and Chemicals

A. Hormones
   1. Corticotropin
   2. Corticosteroids
   3. Testosterone
   4. Estrogen and Progestogen

B. Halogens
   1. Iodine
   2. Bromine
   3. Chlorine
   4. Fluorine

C. Oils and Tars
   1. Industrial chloracne (*see above*)

D. Miscellaneous
   1. Quinine
   2. Disulfiram (Tetraethylthiuram disulfide)
   3. Cod liver oil
   4. Thiouracil
   5. Thiourea
   6. Trimethadione
   7. Chloral

Today, as on every working day throughout the United States, one quarter of all workers are exposed to skin irritants and sensitizing chemicals in the performance of their jobs. Of these, 10 per cent lose time from work because of skin diseases directly traceable to chemicals and other substances they are required to handle. Each case of dermatitis costs over $200, but the overall cost to industry and its workers is still a matter of conjecture. Many firms do not know the extent of their dermatitis problem nor the amount of lost time it incurs. However, fifteen years ago, the United States Public Health Service estimated the annual loss from industrial dermatitis to be over $100 million. The cost of ignoring the forgotten casualties comes rather high!

Safety techniques to protect against the dermatitis hazard have been worked out and strictly applied in larger plants. They are not reaching the 2½ million smaller establishments which employ more than half the workers and in which 70 per cent of all industrial accidents occur.

The most effective method of combatting industrial dermatitis is educating workers on how to recognize its causes and how to prevent skin disease before it happens. Warnings on the labels and identification of hazardous ingredients which act as skin irritants and strong sensitizers are frequently the only informational media to educate most workers about the risks of dermatitis from commercial and industrial chemicals.

Occupational acro-osteolysis has been found in some workmen who clean by hand the vats in which vinyl chloride polymer plastics are made. The disease consists of Raynaud's phenomenon, scleroderma-like changes on the hands and forearms and dissolution of terminal phalanges of the hands. The incidence of the disease among workers in the plastics industry, specifically those engaged in the production of polyvinyl chloride from vinyl chloride, is approximately 3 per cent.

Two men also had delayed emptying of the stomach. The disease process was reversed when the men were removed from their jobs, but shortening of the terminal phalanges persisted.

Asthmatic symptoms may result from exposure to chemicals encountered in rubber, lacquer, shellac and beauty culture industries. The specific chemical may be antigenic, causing immediate hypersensitivity. Patients often have other allergies.

In the rubber industry, the accelerator ethylenediamine is usually the causative agent. Monoethanolamine, ammonium thioglycolate, ethylenediamine and hexamethylenamine in hair-set and cold-wave lotions or in nail polish may cause allergic reactions in beauty operators and patrons and their husbands. In lacquer and shellac industries, wheezing, heaviness in the chest, severe

TABLE 75
A. MATERIALS AND INDUSTRIAL EXPOSURES ASSOCIATED WITH OCCUPATIONAL DERMATITIS AND/OR ASTHMA

| | |
|---|---|
| Aliphatic polyamines | Epoxy resin users |
| Castor beans | Castor oil extractors, fertilizer workers, farmers |
| Chloramine-T | Pharmaceutical workers |
| Cobalt dust | Cobalt refinery workers, cobalt alloy makers |
| Complex platinum salts | Platinum refiners |
| Flour | Millers and bakers |
| Formaldehyde | Phenolic and amino resin workers, fumigators, laboratory workers |
| Hexavalent chromium compounds | Chromate workers |
| Hops | Brewers and farmers |
| Karaya gum | Hair dressers |
| Paraphenylenediamine | Fur dyers |
| Penicillin | Pharmaceutical workers, nurses |
| Phthalic anhydride | Chemists, epoxy resin users |
| Pink-rot fungus of celery (Sclerotinia sclerotiorum) | Celery pickers |
| Pyrethrins | Insecticide makers and users |
| Ragweed pollen | Farmers, highway workers, grain handlers |
| Spices | Spice workers, bakers, sausage makers |
| Tobacco | Cigarette factories and employees |
| Toluene diisocyanate | Polyurethane foam makers |
| Wood dust | Sawmill workers, woodworkers |
| Wool | Wool handlers |

B. MATERIALS AND INDUSTRIAL EXPOSURES ASSOCIATED WITH URTICARIA

| | |
|---|---|
| Aliphatic polyamines | Epoxy resin users |
| Aminothiazole | Pharmaceutical workers |
| Ammonia | Ammonia workers |
| Castor bean pomace | Castor oil extractors, fertilizer workers, farmers |
| Complex platinum salts | Platinum refiners |
| Formaldehyde | Phenolic and amino resin workers, fumigators, laboratory workers |
| Lindane | Insecticide workers, cotton dusters |
| Penicillin | Pharmaceutical workers, nurses |
| Sodium sulfide | Photographers |
| Spices | Spice workers, bakers, sausage makers |
| Sulfur dioxide | Paper mill workers |
| Tobacco stems (plants) | Tobacco warehouses, workers, and farmers |

asthma, allergic coryza or skin manifestations occur with exposure to ethylenediamine and hexamethylenamine used as solvents and paint thinners. Intradermal skin tests with the chemical agents result in an immediate wheal reaction, and inhalation of the specific chemical causes recurrence of symptoms.

## OCCUPATIONAL HAZARDS OF PAINTERS AND SCULPTORS

Media are indispensable to the visual arts, contemporary or traditional, and though unobtrusive and subordinate to the artist's message, they have always been apparent to the observer and their dangers known to the physician. Bernardino Ramazinni commented over 250 years ago on the ill health of painters, which he attributed to the materials they handled. Contaminating the air, these materials were thought to penetrate the seat of the "animal spirits," "enter the abode of the blood" and disturb the economy of the "natural functions."

Concepts of pathogenesis have changed,

but the traditional media-fresco, tempera, oil, encaustic and water color employed two and one-half centuries ago are still in common use. Their toxic contents of lead, arsenic and cadmium are still likely to cause harm to the unwary. The newer materials add substantially to the list of hazards. Synthetic products such as fiberglass, ethyl silicate, vinyl acetate and vinyl chloride may have an adverse effect on the skin and eyes by direct irritation or allergenic action. More serious systemic illness may be caused by diluents and solvents such as carbon tetrachloride or benzine, which are best replaced by less toxic substances. Newer materials used by sculptors also present serious occupational hazards. The well-known risks of silicosis in stone grinding and clay modeling are now overshadowed by dangers associated with the increasing use of metals. Welding, soldering, brazing, shell molding and casting carry a potential for lead and carbon monoxide poisoning, cadmium or ozone pneumonitis, as well as other diseases ("metal fume fever").

None of these injuries to health need occur if the artist takes precautions. Good personal hygiene, as well as specific preventive measures appropriate to the material used, forestalls damage. Unfortunately, unlike the industrial worker trained in prophylaxis under supervision of industrial management, the lone, individualistic, independent artist often knows little about the potentially noxious nature of his materials and lacks guidance in avoiding occupational dangers. It is important that public health authorities as well as practicing physicians provide the much needed information and counsel.

## PNEUMOCONIOSES

The consequences of early uncontrolled dust exposures are revealed today in high social benefits paid out for pneumoconiosis. Some 27,000 claims for pneumoconioses, amounting to $132 million, have been settled by workmen's compensation agencies in eighteen states since 1950. The Social Security Administration estimates that 15,000 workers under sixty-five years of age are in current payment status for disability due to pneumoconioses and that they and their dependents are receiving $18 million a year in benefits.

The term "pneumoconiosis" literally means dust retained in the lung, with no implication as to whether disease is present. No single classification of the pneumoconioses has been widely accepted, since its development depends upon a number of factors related to the worker and to the dust. Worker factors include duration of exposure to the dust and susceptibility; factors related to the dust comprise its chemical composition, particle size and concentration. The following are pneumoconioses which are best understood, most commonly seen and more widely accepted as definite clinical entities.

1. Silicosis
2. Coal workers' pneumoconiosis
3. Asbestosis
4. Diatomite pneumoconiosis
5. Shaver's Disease
6. Talcosis
7. Pulmonary siderosis
8. Byssinosis
9. Bagassosis
10. Farmer's lung
11. "Mainliner's lung" (Drug addicts)
12. Miscellaneous (Mica, Kaolin, Feldspar, Cement, Gypsum, Fluorspar, Sepiolite, Sulfur, Jute, Moura seed, Grain)

### *Silicosis (Grinders' Rot, Miners' Consumption, Miners' Phthisis, Potters' Asthma, Stonemasons' Phthisis)*

Silicosis is a pneumoconiosis caused by the inhalation of finely divided silicon dioxide (silica) in the free state, which may be in a crystalline form such as in quartz, cristobalite and tridymite, or in a noncrystalline or amorphous form such as in opal. Silica in the nonfree or combined state, namely a silicate, refers to silica in chemical combination. Thus, the feldspars are aluminum silicates with potassium, sodium, calcium or barium. Other silicates include kaolin, mica, serpentine, shale, slate and talc. A pneumoconiosis associated with the inhalation of the dust of a silicate is termed a "silicatosis." Silica and silicates, composing almost the entire crust of the earth, constitute the major portion of all rocks and their products such as soils, sands and clays.

Silicosis may be either of an acute or a chronic nature. The former is referred to as rapidly developing silicosis rather than as acute silicosis.

The etiology, symptomatology and pathology of rapidly developing silicosis are not well understood. The disease has been most often reported in manufacturers and packers of abrasive soap powders, in sandblasters working in enclosed tanks and in high-power drillers of tunnel rock. Suspected factors are exposure to very finely divided crystalline silica dust; exposure to massive amounts of free crystalline silica; synergistic action of other ions; differences in individual susceptibility; and presence of concomitant infection, especially tuberculosis.

The time of exposure to silica dust is relatively short in the reported cases of rapidly developing silicosis, varying from eight to eighteen months from the first exposure to the time of the onset of symptoms. After development of symptoms, the survival time is likely to be very short. The clinical picture of this type of silicosis is characterized by pulmonary insufficiency, with dyspnea, tachypnea and cyanosis leading to the development of cor pulmonale. Many cases have been complicated by pulmonary tuberculosis. The chest roentgenogram in rapidly developing silicosis shows diffuse fibrosis with no visible typical nodulation. Roentgenographic evidence of pulmonary tuberculosis is often present.

Chronic pulmonary silicosis, the type usually encountered in industry, is produced, as a rule, only after years of silica dust inhalation. The disease is reported to occur most commonly in the mining industries but is also seen in numerous other industries such as potteries, foundries, stonecutting and stone finishing, tile and clay producing and glass manufacturing.

Clinically, silicosis may follow one of several courses. The simple, uncomplicated form, frequently called simple discrete nodular silicosis, often does not progress beyond the stage where the nodules comprise a relatively small amount of the total lung tissue. This form of silicosis may present itself symptomatically only as a slowly increasing, nondisabling, exertional dyspnea, and the chest roentgenogram usually reveals uniformly distributed, discrete densities up to 10 mm in diameter. Very often, there is also seen enlargement of the shadows cast by the tracheobronchial lymph nodes.

In some silicotic patients, there is seen to develop in the upper portions of both lungs large irregular masses of dense fibrous tissue. When these conglomerate masses appear on the x-ray, the disease may be categorized as conglomerate silicosis. In this form of the disease, the presence of advanced fibrosis and diffuse obstructive emphysema may lead to severe respiratory crippling due to a decrease in the maximum breathing capacity and an increase in the residual lung volume. At this stage, the clinical symptoms, in addition to dyspnea on exertion, may include a productive cough, chest pain and marked weakness. Cor pulmonale, probably caused by the increase in pressure required to force blood through a damaged pulmonary capillary bed, is a late and frequently fatal complication.

Tuberculosis is considered a common complication of silicosis. This combination is frequently manifested by the appearance of coalescent or conglomerate shadows on a chest roentgenogram which previously had demonstrated only shadows suggestive of simple discrete nodular silicosis.

### *Coal Workers' Pneumoconiosis*

One out of every ten miners working in the Appalachian soft-coal fields is afflicted with job-related pneumoconiosis, associated with the chronic inhalation of coal dust, according to a two-and-one-half-year U.S. Public Health Service study. In about 3 per cent of active miners, the disease has progressed from simple pneumoconiosis to the irreversible and ultimately fatal pulmonary massive fibrosis, characterized by massive destruction of lung tissue and often severe emphysema. The Federal Coal Mine Health and Safety Act of 1969 attacks pneumoconiosis from four directions: detection, control, prevention and compensation.

The dust to which a coal worker may be exposed is complex in nature. Besides the dust arising from the disintegration of coal, which itself is always intimately associated with other minerals, silicious dust of various types is derived from the rock strata above and below the coal seam. In the simple or uncomplicated form of coal workers' pneumoconiosis, the lungs contain a large quantity of coal dust which is aggregated into foci surrounding the respiratory bronchioles, frequently causing them to dilate (focal emphysema). The fibrosis produced is strikingly sparse, the coal dust being held in a fine mesh of reticulin fibrils, stellate in appearance, and contrasting markedly with the rounded, whorled nodule of silicosis. The advanced or complicated form starts within a few coal foci as a collagen fibrosis and subsequently enlarges and coalesces to form a dense mass of fibrous tissue. This fibrosis may occupy much of a lobe or even a whole lung and is thought usually to be due to tuberculosis superimposed upon a lung heavily laden with coal dust. Because of the nature of this condition, it is often referred to as progressive massive fibrosis (PMF) and carries with it the implications of a grave prognosis, with death frequently resulting from tuberculosis or pulmonary insufficiency or from cor pulmonale secondary to obliteration of the pulmonary vascular bed by fibrous tissue invasion.

The roentgenographic characteristics of simple coal workers' pneumoconiosis include discrete opacities up to 10 mm in diameter, which may be arranged in groups or spread diffusely throughout the lung fields. In the complicated form of the disease, the earliest roentgenographic evidence of PMF is the presence, usually on a background of simple pneumoconiosis, of larger, less well defined opacities, often resembling reinfection-type tuberculosis in both position and appearance. These large shadows tend to increase in size and to coalesce. They later may contract, with resultant severe distortion of the lung architecture.

### *Asbestosis*

Asbestos is a general term used to describe several indestructible fibrous mineral silicates which differ in their chemical composition and physical properties. About 95 per cent of the world's asbestos production is derived from chrysotile. Deposits of this mineral are found in many countries, but the largest mines are located in Canada. In 1920, world production of asbestos was about 300,000 tons; in 1930, it had increased to about 500,000 tons. At present, it is over 4 million tons/year, with the United States consuming about 40 per cent of the world production. Because asbestos does not burn or conduct heat or electricity well, it is widely used to make insulation, brake linings and many other products.

Exposure to asbestos is a potential industrial hazard. Related diseases include pulmonary fibrosis and carcinoma, bronchiogenic cancer, malignant pleural mesothelioma and abdominal tumors. Malignancy after asbestosis is particularly common in dockyard employees, asbestos textile workers and miners and processors of the mineral. Of men with asbestosis, 50 per cent die of pulmonary malignancy. For those who smoke, the incidence is greater. Use of the agent is increasing, and it is never destroyed. Asbestosis is virtually ubiquitous, and it has an estimated 3000 uses. The Occupational Safety and Health Administration (OSHA) of the U.S. Department of Labor mandated, beginning in 1976, a new and much lower level of on-the-job pollution by this fibrous, metallic silicate. In places of employment, the level must not exceed 2 fibers/ml, as a time-weighted average for an eight-hour day, with peaks not to exceed 10 fibers. The previous standard was 5 fibers/ml, again with peaks not to exceed 10.

As regards floor tile, shingles and similar products, there is little possibility of dangerous asbestos exposure from the normal use or wear of such products. The asbestos in these products is "locked in" with cement, plastic and other binding materials, and they release measurable levels of asbestos dust only through the on-job sawing or cutting necessary for installation. Its utilization in brake linings may represent some danger. Effect of exposure is often delayed and occupational cause of the disease overlooked, though at present it is thought to be inconsequential from these exposures.

Asbestos may act as a cocarcinogen in conjunction with iron, chromium and nickel. Metal complexes acting with other chemical carcinogens may cause the malignant effect. Naturally occurring oils, jute oil from sacks or emulsions added for processing may be responsible. Another possible mechanism is the ability of asbestos fibers to migrate within tissues. It has been documented that lung cancer deaths are much higher in asbestos workers who smoke than among nonsmokers. Air pollution is an additional factor. Exposure is also a nonoccupational hazard. Men in eastern Finland, where asbestos is mined, have six times as much lung cancer as residents of other parts of that country and Norway.

Prolonged inhalation of asbestos fibers (the most important types are chrysotile, a simple magnesium silicate, which constitutes 95 per cent of the asbestos used in the United States; amosite and anthophyllite, which are complex magnesium iron silicates; and crocidolite, a complex sodium iron silicate) between 20 and 50 μ long may result in the production of a typical pulmonary fibrosis with severe respiratory disability. Asbestos fibers smaller than 20 μ in length are believed to be incapable of initiating a fibrogenic response. On the basis of experimental studies, it was found that this fibrosis is due to the mechanical action of the asbestos fiber. The fibers, upon being deposited in the terminal bronchioles, initiate a tissue response that appears to be a defense mechanism resulting in the coating of the fiber with the ultimate production of what is known as the asbestos or asbestosis body. If large quantities of the fibers are inhaled over a prolonged period of time (10 to 20 years), the tissue reaction progresses until a generalized, diffuse fibrosis becomes evident. This fibrosis is seen first in the lower lobes of the lungs but eventually, if exposure continues, appears in the other lobes as well. Respiratory insufficiency and cardiac failure may occur.

The roentgenogram of the chest with pulmonary fibrosis resulting from prolonged inhalation of asbestos fibers shows a typical pattern. In the early or first stages of the disease, the shadows are fine, diffuse and homogeneous and appear characteristically at the bases of both lungs. The typical nodular pattern of silicosis is not seen in asbestosis; rather, the affected lung fields present a ground-glass appearance. In moderately advanced or second-stage asbestosis, the infiltration is more evident but remains generally confined to the lower lobes. The heart borders may become indistinct or shaggy, a condition which has been referred to as "porcupine" heart. In far advanced or third-stage asbestosis, the infiltrate can be seen throughout the middle and upper lung fields; however, the apices generally remain clear. There is almost complete obliteration of the cardiac outline, the domes of the diaphragm and the costophrenic sulci.

There is no typical clinical picture for asbestosis. The disease is insidious in its onset and is slowly progressive so long as inhalation of the fiber continues. There is a gradual increase in cough and expectoration, anorexia and weight loss, all combined with slowly increasing dyspnea. Cyanosis and clubbing of the fingers are rare findings. When an acute pneumonitis develops in the presence of established asbestosis with fibrosis, recovery is often delayed because healing is slow and relapses are frequent. As to the relationship between asbestosis and tuberculosis, it is fairly well established that asbestosis does not predispose to the development of tuberculosis, nor does it aggravate an apparently healed lesion. However, asbestosis and lung cancer are known hazards for workers in the asbestos insulation industry; so, perhaps, is malignancy of the stomach and colon. Recently, a rare neoplasm derived from the living cells of the pleura and peritoneum, "mesothelioma," has been found to be on the increase in this group. A typical clinical symptom of pleural mesothelioma is the characteristic stoop caused by retractions in this fibrous tumor.

Asbestos in substantial amounts has been found in a number of industrial cities' water supply. There is at present no firm basis for recommending a change in water supply because of potential carcinogens such as asbestos or chemical pollutants.

### *Diatomite Pneumoconiosis*

There are three forms of diatomaceous earth: crude, calcined and flux-calcined. The crude contains no crystalline form of free silica, and the flux-calcined has 30 per cent cristobalite. The particle size of finished diatomite powder products is usually under 10 μ.

As with most pneumoconiosis-causing dusts, the longer the exposure to diatomite dust, the more is the chance of developing demonstrable lung changes; however, it has been shown that exposure to this dust for as little as one to three years may produce definite roentgenographic evidence of pneumoconiosis. In addition, the extent and severity of diatomite pneumoconiosis correlate with the cristobalite content of the dust involved.

Radiographic changes resulting from exposure to diatomite dust can roughly be divided into two groups: (1) changes of a linear-nodular type and (2) changes resulting in the production of coalescent opacities, usually superimposed on definite linear-nodular changes. In this type of pneumoconiosis, pulmonary signs and respiratory symptoms correlate poorly with roentgenographic changes, except where massive confluent lesions are present, in which case pulmonary disability may be extreme.

When tuberculosis is superimposed on diatomaceous earth pneumoconiosis, the infection often pursues a benign course until cavitation supervenes. The course then is frequently one of slow deterioration despite modern treatment including collapse procedures and chemotherapy.

### *Shaver's Disease (Corundum Fume Fibrosis, Bauxite Fume Fibrosis)*

Shaver's disease is a pneumoconiosis of occupational origin resulting from the inhalation of the fume emitted by electric furnaces used in the production of corundum. This fume is rich in alumina and silica, both of which are in the free state and are largely amorphous in structure. The fume is further characterized by its small particle size, generally smaller than 0.5 μ and extending down to about 0.02 μ. Although the noxious agent or agents within this fume have not been identified, both silica fume and finely divided aluminum are believed to be capable of causing lung damage if inhaled in significant amounts.

In contrast to classical silicosis, Shaver's disease may develop in a relatively short time, often the period between first exposure and onset of symptoms being as brief as twenty-four months. The most outstanding symptom of this disease is shortness of breath, usually mild in the early stages of illness but worsening as it progresses. Sudden attacks of extreme breathlessness are not uncommon and may indicate the occurrence of spontaneous pneumothorax, a condition seen with disturbing frequency among those afflicted with this disease. Additional signs and symptoms include cough productive of frothy white sputum, chest tightness and pain, weakness and fatigue. There is no evidence to suggest that this disease predisposes to pulmonary tuberculosis.

The chest roentgenogram characteristically reveals bilateral granular haziness, widened mediastinum, heavy fibrotic strands, distortion and elevation of the diaphragm and radiographic evidence suggestive of emphysematous bullae.

### *Talcosis*

Pure talc is a hydrated magnesium silicate, similar in chemical composition to asbestos. It is a flaky mineral, but also occurs in a fibrous state. When crushed, it forms a smooth bland powder which is used for a wide variety of purposes. Commercial talc varies markedly in its composition, and the mineral talc itself is usually only a minor component present in combination with other minerals such as dolomite, tremolite, magnetite, serpentine, mica and anthophyllite. Varying amounts of free silica may also be present.

Numerous investigators have shown that prolonged inhalation of mixed talc results in the production of significant lung damage even though there is little or no free silica present. Histopathologic examination of lung sections usually reveals the presence of mild to moderate peribronchial and perivascular fibrosis with dilatation of many small bronchi and bronchioles. In more advanced cases the fibrosis may be extensive. Roentgenographic evidence of emphysematous bullae and fibrosis is usually demonstrable. A striking feature very frequently noted upon histologic examination of affected lung tissue sections is the presence of many brilliantly birefringent, needle-shaped particles in the areas of fibrosis. X-ray diffraction studies have indicated that these particles are talc. Another commonly reported finding is the presence of asbestos-like bodies embedded in the fibrous tissue. These structures have been most frequently seen in specimens of lungs which have been found to contain appreciable quantities of tremolite, considered to be the main pathogenic mineral. They are less commonly seen in specimens which contain only small amounts of this mineral. When the characteristic talc lesion is modified by significant amounts of free crystalline silica in the inhaled dust, the entire clinical, pathologic and roentgenographic picture may be greatly changed. There may be a greater tendency toward the formation of massive lesions; fibrosis may be more intense, and damage to the pulmonary vascular bed may be extreme. True classical silicotic nodules are uncommon in such cases.

Potential occupational exposures include cosmetic workers, paint makers, paper makers, pottery makers, rubber cable coaters, rubber tire makers, talc millers, talc miners and talcum powder makers.

### *Pulmonary Siderosis*

Siderosis is a benign pneumoconiosis resulting from the deposition of inert iron dust in the lung. Neither fibrosis nor emphysema is usually associated with this condition unless, as often happens, there is concomitant exposure to silica dust. Siderosis does not usually result in the production of disability, nor does it show any predisposition to pulmonary tuberculosis or lung cancer.

The chest roentgenogram in siderosis closely resembles the picture seen in uncomplicated silicosis. There may be, in both conditions, discrete nodular densities evenly distributed throughout the lung fields. Emphysema is rare, and the formation of the conglomerate masses which are often seen in silicosis rarely occur in siderosis.

The differential diagnosis between siderosis and silicosis is difficult, especially since they may occur together. The diagnosis can usually be made, however, on the basis of medical and occupational histories, physical examination, chest roentgenograms, pulmonary function studies and an appraisal of the work environment.

### *Byssinosis*

Byssinosis, the result of chronic irritation of the lung by flax, hemp and cotton dust, is a disabling disease occurring among textile workers throughout the world; current protective measures, such as ventilation systems, do not provide adequate protection. There is evidence that respiratory symptoms consistent with byssinosis occurred in the hand-picked cotton era, but an increase in incidence appears to have followed the change to machine-picked cotton in the 1950s. Cotton now used is generally lower in grade because of the presence of more trash (particles of dried boll, stem and leaves) gathered by the mechanical picker which cannot be completely removed in ginning, and in milling is reduced to respirable-sized particles. Exposure to this very fine dust is thought to be responsible for the bronchial release of histamine and the symptoms of byssinosis. The disease can be acquired in all processes of the cotton industry, from ginning to spinning. The characteristic clinical symptom is a sensation of tightness in the chest on Mondays or the first day after an absence from work. Ventilatory capacity, as measured by forced expiratory volume (FEV) is reduced. A significant drop in FEV on Mondays can be used for spot-testing workers at risk of byssinosis. As the disease progresses, the worker is affected every working day by chest tightness, dyspnea and effort intolerance. Chronic bronchitis and emphysema may develop, and death from cor pulmonale may be the eventual outcome. There is no characteristic pattern identifiable on the chest roentgenogram.

Recent evidence indicates that the causative agents are in the pericarp and bracts of the cotton plant rather than in the fibers and seeds. A method is thus required to separate the cotton fibers from the plant material before ginning to provide absolute protection. Although industrial hygiene practices have been improved in plants, the raw cotton is dirtier due to increased mechancial picking and contains more of the harmful bracts. The American Conference of Governmental Industrial Hygienists has proposed that the safe level of lint-free cotton dust be set at 0.2 mg/cu. m.

### *Bagassosis*

Bagassosis is an occupational disease resulting from the inhalation of dust from dried sugar cane fiber or bagasse, which has become an important industrial material. It is used in insulating and acoustic materials as well as in the manufacture of paper, fertilizer, explosives, animal feed and refractory brick. Chemically, bagasse consists of approximately 4 per cent ash and 2 per cent protein, the rest being cellulose, resins and complex plant carbohydrates. The fresh fiber is apparently innocuous, and illness follows contact only with old bagasse which has been baled and allowed to dry. This fact evidently accounts for peculiarities of the distribution of the disorder. The disease has been absent from most of the great cane-growing areas of the world but has recently appeared at a newly established paper mill in Puerto Rico where approximately eighty cases have been observed. There have been four deaths among the reported cases and many cases probably go undetected. Typically, bagassosis presents as an acute pneumonitis or bronchiolitis, often with roentgenographic features of miliary tuberculosis. Some findings appear to be compatible with alveolar hypoventilation secondary to bronchiolitis, but more study is needed to clarify the physiological defect in this disease. One patient with a severe, fulminating form of bagassosis deteriorated rapidly while miliary tuberculosis, bronchiolitis of bacterial or viral origin, or the Hamman-Rich syndrome were considered, and he received multiple antibiotics and antituberculosis drugs. When he was given cortisone and ACTH as a lifesaving measure, he had immediate and dramatic relief. He was asymptomatic at the end of six weeks; his lungs cleared in four months; and almost three years later he remains well.

Roentgenograms of the chest often disclose the presence of miliary shadows symmetrically distributed throughout both lungs, which appear very similar to the shadows seen in typical miliary tuberculosis. Patchy areas of increased densities suggesting bronchopneumonic infiltration are also seen. Lesions are usually more in evidence in the hilar areas and at the lung bases, while the apices are often spared. The cardiac shadow may be enlarged and the pulmonary artery segment may be very prominent.

The great majority of patients suffering from bagassosis tend to improve spontaneously when they are removed from contact with the offending agent. Symptoms gradually abate over a period of several weeks, and recovery usually takes place in one to six months. However, some impairment of pulmonary function may be detected for longer periods, and the question of whether there occurs permanent functional lung damage has not yet been answered.

### *Farmer's Lung (Hypersensitivity Pneumonitis)*

*Thermopolyspora polyspora* and another thermophilic organism *(Micromonospora vulgaris)* were isolated from the lungs of patients with clinically, histologically and immunologically proven farmer's lung. The organism was found to react in identity experiments with known cultures of *T. polyspora.* It also reacted with identity in double diffusion experiments with other patients with farmer's lung who had recent or active disease. Spores from thermophilic actinomycetes, mainly *Micropolyspora faeni,* also produce offending antigen in moldy material. Another discovery is that the serum of patients with this disease reacts in a highly specific way with an antigen extracted from moldy hay. Simplified hemagglutination tests for detection of antibodies to thermophilic actinomycetes are available for the diagnosis of farmer's lung. Pigeon and budgerigar breeders or fanciers, maple bark strippers and mushroom pickers are other occupational hazards reported to produce acute febrile interstitial pulmonary disease which resembles farmer's lung and affects the peripheral gas-exchanging tissues. The disease is caused by inhalation of the antigens in the environment or in the avian excreta. Workers in the furrier's trade can also develop this condition from the inhalation of hair shafts and dust. It has been recently documented that one does not always have to implicate an occupational exposure, for thermophilic organisms can be found in home humidifiers and air conditioning systems. Fever, shivering, malaise and loss of weight are accompained by cough and dyspnea, crepitant rales, evidence of impaired carbon monoxide transfer and decreased lung compliance. The most consistent radiologic pattern is a combination of coarsening of bronchovascular markings, fine sharp nodulations and reticulation or honey-combing throughout the lung parenchyma consistent with an interstitial process. In seven affected pigeon fanciers and five affected budgerigar fanciers, precipitins were present against antigens in the avian excreta and serum proteins. In the pigeon fanciers, the attacks tended to come on five to six hours or more after the exposure; in the budgerigar fanciers* the onset tended to be insidious and the patients presented with advanced lung damage. Inhalation tests provoked a febrile response after six to seven hours, together with the other symptoms and signs. Skin tests gave, in all except two cases, dual reactions consisting of an immediate wheal followed after three to four hours by an extensive, edematous reaction, regarded as being of the Arthus type. A strong immunological response, consisting of the appearance of precipitins, results from the entry of the organic avian antigens through the respiratory tract, and the evidence suggests that the clinical manifestations are the result of a precipitin-mediated hypersensitivity reaction. Immediate improvement is induced by steroids, but there is no evidence that their benefits are long-term. Industrial, agricultural and specific antigen exposures should be limited or avoided if at all possible. Prevention is accomplished by avoiding moldy material, wearing masks, ensiling a crop after drying or wilting and spraying bales with 2% propionic acid, a fungicide. Efforts should be made to

*Parakeet breeder or owner.

TABLE 76
ANTIGENS CAUSING HYPERSENSITIVITY PNEUMONITIS

| *Agent* | *Typical Exposure* |
|---|---|
| *Molds* | |
| Thermophilic actinomycetes | |
| *Micropolyspora faeni* | Dairy farming |
| *Micromonospora vulgaris* | Sugar cane processing, mushroom growing, air conditioners |
| Alternaria | Paper mill |
| Maple bark *(Cryptostroma corticale)* | Paper making |
| Cork dust (Suberosis) | Cork making |
| Redwood sawdust | Saw mills |
| *Penicillium casei* | Cheese washing |
| *Aspergillus clavatus* and *fumigatus* | Malt processing |
| *Mucor stolonifer** | Paprika processing |
| *Lycoperdon pyriformis** | Treatment of epistaxis |
| *Other Plant Antigens* | |
| Wood dust | Carpentering |
| Coffee bean dust | Coffee roasting |
| Sisal dust* | Sisal processing |
| Legumes (especially lentils)* | Aspiration pneumonitis |
| Roof thatch* | New Guinea native huts |
| "Blackfat" tobacco* | Smoking moldy tobacco |
| Castor bean pomace | Fertilizer |
| *Antigens from Animal Sources* | |
| Bird droppings (avian) | Pigeon breeding; breeding of parakeets, budgerigars |
| Fur dust | Sewing furs |
| Pituitary snuff (pigorox protein) | Diabetes insipidus |
| Smallpox virus | Nursing |
| Grain weevil *(Sitophilus granarius)* | Laboratory exposure |
| *Bacterial Antigens* | |
| Tuberculin* | Laboratory exposure |
| Bacillus subtilis enzymes* | Detergent manufacture |

*Suspected but not proven.

clean out central humidifiers and air conditioning systems regularly.

Screening for malabsorption (gluten enteropathy) should be carried out in all patients with allergic alveolar disease, since a number of these patients have been found to have celiac disease.

### *"Mainliner's Lung" (Drug Addicts)*

This condition occurs frequently and is being recognized more often by clinicians and radiologists. It is the result of septic or particle-laden narcotic or drug doses being injected intravenously. The first capillary bed that the junk reaches is the lung, and that is where the first clear pathologic effect can sometimes be seen. The possibilities for lung damage among "pushers" are not limited to abscesses. Pieces of cotton or other particulate foreign matter also end up in the lung, blocking pulmonary arterioles or capillaries.

## ENVIRONMENTAL HAZARDS

### *Air Pollution*

Air pollutants are substances that either are not normally present in the atmosphere or, if they are, their natural concentration is so increased by man's activities that they, or compounds which they form, become annoying or a health hazard. Besides particulate matter, such as smoke and fly ash, pollutants include oxides of nitrogen, sulfuric acid,

TABLE 77
OCCUPATIONS POTENTIALLY ASSOCIATED WITH PNEUMOCONIOSES

*Aluminum Pneumoconiosis*
- Fireworks maker
- Ammunition maker

*Asbestosis*
- Asbestos weaver
- Auto mechanic
- Brake manufacturer
- Carpenter
- Clutch manufacturer
- Filter maker
- Floor tilemaker
- Insulator
- Logger
- Mill worker
- Miner
- Roofer
- Shingle maker
- Shipbuilder
- Steam fitter

*Baritosis*
- Barite miner
- Barite miller
- Ceramics worker
- Glassmaker
- Paint maker
- Rubber worker
- Well driller

*Bagassosis*
- Cane worker
- Insulation maker
- Papermaker
- Wallboard worker

*Beryllium Disease*
- Alloy maker
- Bronze maker
- Ceramics worker
- Electronic tube maker
- Extraction worker
- Fluorescent lamp maker
- Metallurgist
- Missile worker
- Neon sign maker
- Nuclear energy worker
- Phosphor maker
- Propellent maker
- Toxicologist
- X-ray tube maker

*Coal Miners' Pneumoconiosis*
- Coal miner
- Motorman
- Roof bolter
- Tipple worker
- Trimmer

*"Hard Metal" Pneumoconiosis*
- Abrasives maker
- Cutting tool worker
- Drill maker

*Kaolinosis*
- Brick maker
- Ceramics worker
- China maker
- Miner
- Papermaker
- Potter

*Shaver's Disease*
- Abrasives maker

*Siderosis*
- Demolition man
- Fettler
- Flame cutter
- Foundryman
- Grinder
- Metal worker
- Metalizer
- Polisher
- Scarfer
- Shipbreaker
- Welder

*Silicosis*
- Abrasives worker
- Bricklayer
- Brickmaker
- Ceramics worker
- Coal miner
- Diatomite worker
- Enameller
- Fettler
- Filter maker
- Foundryman
- Glassmaker
- Insulation worker
- Miner
- Motorman
- Polisher
- Quarry man
- Sandblaster
- Shot blaster
- Stonecutter
- Stonedresser
- Stonedriller
- Tunnel driver

*Talcosis*
- Cable maker
- Ceramics worker
- Cosmetic worker
- Miner
- Papermaker
- Plastics worker
- Rubber worker

Lloyd B. Tepper, M.D., University of Cincinnati. The work history in industrial dust disease. *Semin Roentgenol* 2:235–243, 1967.

hydrocarbons, hydrogen sulfide, carbon monoxide, pollens (allergens), beryllium and lead. Inhaled air pollutants primarily affect the respiratory system. Diseases most likely influenced by air pollution include chronic bronchitis, emphysema, bronchiectasis, cor pulmonale and bronchogenic carcinoma. Yet a mountain of studies by sophisticated clinicians and biochemists has failed to link a single specific pollutant or group of pollutants in a causal relationship to any of these diseases. Nevertheless, it is estimated that over 150 million tons of pollutants spew forth into our air each year in the form of dangerous gases, dusts and fumes. The 15,000 quarts of air that each citizen breathes daily bring into the fragile tissues of bronchial pathways and lungs a portion of these contaminants, and it is assuredly not far-fetched to assume that the delicate mucous membrances are sooner or later affected. The vulnerability of patients with lung disease on sudden exposure to highly polluted air has been clearly recorded. In Donora,

Pennsylvania, in 1948, 20 people died during a four-day episode of severe pollution, and 22 died in Poza Rica, Mexico, in 1950 in a period of an hour or so. Mortality studies suggest that 4,000 persons died within a period of five weeks as a result of a very dense "fog" that struck London in 1952.

In general, air pollution seems to be more of a problem as the size of communities increase, with their growing population and expanding industrialization. Moreover, what seems to be a factor in one situation is not necessarily a factor in another. A major source of air pollution in the United States, for example, is automobile exhaust, emitting large quantities of unsaturated hydrocarbons, nitrogen oxides, carbon monoxide and carbon dioxide. Irradiated by sunlight, these emission compounds produce the photo chemical smog characteristic of Los Angeles and other urban complexes with heavy automobile congestion. However, in England, the major source of air pollution is not the automobile but soft coal, the basic domestic fuel. Sulfur dioxide escaping from burning coal mixes with air and produces sulfur trioxide, which is changed into sulfuric acid when moistened. In the presence of fog,

TABLE 78
POLLUTANTS

| *Pollutants* | *Where They Come From* | *What They Do* |
|---|---|---|
| Aldehydes | Thermal decomposition of fats, oil, or glycerol. | Irritate nasal and respiratory tracts. |
| Ammonias | Chemical processes—dye-making, explosives, lacquer, fertilizer. | Inflame upper respiratory passages. |
| Arsines | Processes involving metals or acids containing arsenic, soldering. | Break down red cells in blood; damage kidneys; cause jaundice. |
| Carbon Monoxides | Gasoline motor exhausts. | Reduce oxygen-carrying capacity of blood. |
| Chlorines | Bleaching cotton and flour, and many other chemical processes. | Attack entire respiratory tract and mucous membranes of eyes; cause pulmonary edema. |
| Hydrogen cyanides | Fumigation, blast furnaces, chemical manufacturing, metal plating. | Interfere with nerve cells; produce dry throat, indistinct vision, headache. |
| Hydrogen fluorides | Petroleum refining, glass etching, aluminum and fertilizer production. | Irritate and corrode all body passages. |
| Hydrogen sulfides | Refineries and chemical industries, bituminous fuels. | Smell like rotten eggs; cause nausea; irritate eyes and throat. |
| Nitrogen oxides | Motor vehicle exhausts, soft coal. | Inhibit cilia action so that soot and dust penetrate far into the lungs. |
| Phosgenes (carbonyl chloride) | Chemical and dye manufacturing | Induce coughing, irritation, and sometimes, fatal pulmonary edema. |
| Sulfur dioxides | Coal and oil combustion.* | Cause chest constriction, headache, vomiting, and death from respiratory ailments. |
| Suspended particles (ash, soot, smoke) | Incinerators, almost any manufacturing. | Cause emphysema, eye irritations, and possibly cancer. |

From *Medical World News*, February 3, 1967.

* Sulfur dioxide is also widely used as a preservative in certain common foodstuffs, i.e., dried fruits. The recent practice of packaging these foods in hermetically sealed plastic containers has tended to retain the $SO_2$ content. The ingestion of such foods without adequate prior aeration or cooking has been observed to produce coughing, laryngeal irritation, and a sense of constriction of the chest in normal individuals.

carbon particles in London chimneys mix with sulfur dioxide to contaminate the air. Dust storms and forest and grass fires add a vast share of their own pollutants to the atmosphere.

Perhaps the most significant human activity to produce air pollutants is combustion, whether in industrial or home furnaces, the engines of motor vehicles and jet planes or incinerators.

Home heating, in the total scheme of things a minor source of air pollution in most places, is a good example of how much contamination combustion can cause—and how it can be controlled by switching to other energy sources. If 100,000 homes all burned an average grade of bituminous coal during 40°F weather, they would produce some 307,000 lb. of air pollutants daily. If the same 100,000 homes burned oil, 42,000 lb. of pollutants would result. But if natural gas heated the 100,000 homes, only 10 lb. of pollutants would be produced every day. And the pollution would fall to zero if the homes were heated by electricity.

Pollutants resulting from processes such as attrition, vaporization and combustion fall into two broad categories: particulates (solid matter and liquid droplets) and gases.

Particulates larger than 10 $\mu$ in diameter, such as coarse dust particles or the fly ash impurities remaining after coal is burned, settle out of the air quickly and so are significant pollutants only near their source. Those between 1 and 10 $\mu$ in diameter travel further, the distance they cover depending on their size. Ordinary soot often falls in this category.

The most troublesome particulates are those less than 1 $\mu$ in diameter; they are usually referred to as aerosols because they are small enough to remain suspended in air and travel with it. Aerosols can absorb radiant energy and conduct heat quickly to the surrounding gases of the atmosphere, gases that are incapable of absorbing radiant energy by themselves. As a result, the air in contact with the aerosols becomes much warmer.

The principal chemicals to compose air pollutants follow.

NITROGEN OXIDES. While nitrogen itself constitutes 78 per cent of the atmosphere and is generally benign, some of its oxides are not. Nitric oxide, a colorless, somewhat toxic gas, is formed when combustion takes place at a high enough temperature to cause a reaction between the air's nitrogen and oxygen. Such temperatures are reached only in efficient combustion processes or when combustion occurs at high pressure, as in automobile cylinders or electric power plants. In most urban areas the car is the single largest producer of nitric oxide, which moves so rapidly from the engine cylinder to the cooler exhaust pipe that it is prevented from decomposing to nitrogen and oxygen, as it would if cooling were slower.

Varying amounts of nitric oxide are converted to the much more damaging nitrogen dioxide. The greater the presence of hydrocarbons and sunlight in the atmosphere, the more nitric oxide is converted. Nitrogen dioxide is the only major pollutant gas that is colored, yellow-brown, so it can significantly affect visibility. It also has a pungent, sweetish odor that is detectable at 1 to 3 ppm, a level sometimes reached in downtown areas or traffic jams.

SULFUR AND ITS COMPOUNDS. The prevalence of sulfur as a pollutant lies in the fact that it is almost invariably present as an impurity in coal and fuel oil, which accounts for the recent shift from those energy sources to natural gas and electricity in many localities.

The major oxide of sulfur that is produced in combustion is sulfur dioxide, a heavy, pungent, colorless gas that combines easily with water vapor to become sulfurous acid, a colorless liquid. The acid, mildly corrosive, is harmful in itself because it can yellow paint, but as a pollutant it is perhaps more important for its ability to combine with atmospheric oxygen to form sulfuric acid, which is even more corrosive and can take the form of an irritating mist.

Not only can sulfur compounds irritate the upper respiratory tract, cut down visibility on highways and over cities and corrode material surfaces, they can also produce distinctly unpleasant odors. Smelliness is particularly characteristic of hydrogen sulfide gas and the mercaptans, even at low concentrations.

CARBON AND ITS OXIDES. The most noticeable carbon pollutant, particularly to the housewife, is soot, a product of incomplete combustion. It is composed of finely divided carbon particles clustered together in long chains. Because the particles are so fine, their surfaces are exceptionally broad in relation to their weight, allowing them to attract a variety of chemicals from the surrounding air.

Carbon monoxide is a gas found at relatively high concentrations in the urban atmosphere, yet its effects, particularly in the realm of health, are uncertain. Controlled laboratory experiments have shown that 100 ppm can cause dizziness, headache and other toxic symptoms, but studies of persons in traffic accidents have failed to show that their driving ability was imparied by carbon monoxide in the air at the time.

Carbon dioxide is not normally considered a pollutant, but in the presence of atmospheric moisture it converts to carbonic acid, which corrodes many materials. Some scientists believe that the huge amounts of it entering the atmosphere daily are slowly warming the earth's air envelope, a process that will result in the partial melting of the polar ice caps.

HYDROCARBONS. Of the hundreds of solid, liquid and gaseous hydrocarbons found in nature, only a few are harmful to man. The major hydrocarbon pollutants are in the olefin and aromatic series, which are primarily discharged from incomplete combustion. The olefins participate in the formation of photochemical pollution, while a number of aromatic compounds are believed to be carcinogenic.

OZONE. The allotropic form of oxygen, an early and continuing product of photochemical pollution formation, assures the continued oxidation of other pollutant chemicals and so is constantly measured by air pollution control specialists to determine the oxidant level of the atmosphere at any given time. In itself it can cause coughing, headache and severe fatigue, as well as damage to plant life and materials. Although long-term effects in the human of exposure to ozone have not been reported in the literature, animal studies indicate that repeated daily exposures to ozone at 1 ppm concentration lead to emphysematous and fibrotic changes in the lungs, cellular effects manifested by decreased oxygen consumption and chromosomal changes.

Ozone does occur naturally in the environment. In rural areas, a normal concentration of 0.05 ppm of total oxidants has reached levels occasionally approximating 1.0 ppm.

The odor threshold of ozone is 0.02 to 0.05 ppm, although hypersensitive individuals may detect a concentration of 0.001 ppm. Some individuals find the characteristic pungent odor pleasant, but to most people the odor is disagreeable.

Some scientists warn that the earth's protective sunscreen of ozone is threatened by several atmospheric pollutants, particularly aerosol propellants (chlorofluoromethanes) and bromine compounds, which can be dissociated by the very short wave lengths present only in the stratosphere to release free chlorine atoms, which break down ozone. They claim that depletion of the stratosphere ozone layer, which filters out the sun's harmful ultraviolet radiation, could increase the incidence of skin cancer, cause serious damage to crops and affect climate.

According to the Federal Aviation Administration, many of the adverse effects of air travel previously attributed to jet lag and other causes may in fact be caused by ozone. At concentrations of 0.2 to 0.5 ppm, ozone can cause fatigue and reduce ability to concentrate. It can also reduce visual acuity, especially at night, both through direct eye irritation and by reducing oxygen supply to the retina. Since such effects could impair a pilot's performance and thus endanger lives of passengers, the FAA is now studying effects of ozone on lung function, vision, and task performance of volunteers and is preparing to issue regulations defining allowable concentrations of ozone in the aircraft.

Until more is known, pilots are advised to

don oxygen masks. The aircraft industry is installing filters on certain aircraft, and the passengers and stewardesses can ward off the effects of ozone by remedies that include vitamins A and E and orange juice.

PEROXYACETYL NITRATE. Peroxyacetyl nitrate (often called PAN) and the aldehydes are also products of photochemistry and affect the eyes, skin and respiratory tract.

These are the most common atmospheric pollutants, but not the only ones. Many others can contaminate the air just as dangerously but generally do so in more circumscribed areas, such as the environs of factories or farm fields.

Besides causing adverse health effects, air pollution is responsible for physical damage ranging from disintegration of nylon stockings to the crumbling of marble in buildings. It has even been held responsible for white house paint turning black almost overnight. Severe smog has reduced visibility to such an extent that airplane service has been suspended, ferryboats have collided and traffic accidents increased. Agriculture is affected, too. Vegetation is stunted, and damage to crops may be so great that the entire farm enterprise may be lost.

The solution to this hazard to our environment is varied and complex, yet two important conclusions can be clearly ascertained.

1. The technical know-how, as well as the actual control devices, is now available for the control of almost any air pollution problem existing from stationary sources and soon will be available for the control of vehicular sources (efficient crankcase and tail pipe devices are now being tested to greatly eliminate automobile emissions).
2. Each community must determine for itself the degree of clean air it desires and the price it is willing to pay for this eventuality.

The primary interest of the medical profession in air pollution is to realize adequate health standards. This can be achieved only through research, engineering and legislation. Adequate control has been possible only in those areas where clear and enforceable standards have provided both the compulsion and the common goal to meet them.

The American Medical Association, recognizing the hazards of air pollution, has created a Department of Environmental Health. The department is (1) seeking legislation which will provide for research, technical assistance and interstate enforcement on the federal level (Air Quality Act of 1967); (2) providing liaison necessary to stimulate medical participation through local medical societies; and (3) bringing to bear its influence on any aspect of air pollution that requires attention.

## *Polluted Air In The Home*

The air inside most houses is probably as polluted as the air outside them. Contaminated air does not stop at the doors of a building. In summer, when the windows are open, the outside air can circulate freely; even in winter some outside air continues to enter. Not so obvious is the pollution caused by common household activities and contributed to by poor planning and construction of many dwellings. In the kitchen, gas appliances consume large amounts of oxygen and produce smoke, charged with potentially harmful matter. Chlorine from the water escapes in steam, along with fats and oils used in cooking. These substances mixed with the emanations from gas stoves are probably only slightly irritating, but daily exposure over a number of years may be harmful.

Chemicals in cleaners, solvents, abrasives, bleaches, pesticides and air fresheners have invaded the household. None of these chemicals are harmful provided that all safety measures are followed. The labels of the products carry such warnings as the following: Keep windows open when spraying; wear rubber gloves when dusting; keep children and pets out of the room; do not inhale fumes. Unfortunately very few users read or follow these rules when embarking on a cleaning spree. Repeatedly it has been stressed that a mixture of two or more such compounds can be toxic, but these warnings have had little effect.

**AIR POLLUTION**

| SOURCE | TONS/YEAR | % OF TOTAL |
|---|---|---|
| INDUSTRY | 23,000,000 | 16.7 |
| POWER PLANTS | 20,000,000 | 14.0 |
| MOTOR VEHICLES | 86,000,000 | 60.5 |
| SPACE HEATING | 8,000,000 | 5.5 |
| REFUSE DISPOSAL | 5,000,000 | 3.4 |
| TOTAL | 142,000,000 | |

| | TONS/YEAR |
|---|---|
| Carbon monoxide | 66,000,000 |
| Oxides of nitrogen | 6,000,000 |
| Hydrocarbons | 12,000,000 |
| Sulfur oxides | 1,000,000 |
| Lead compounds (as lead) | 190,000 |
| Particulates | 1,000,000 |

**VEHICLE EXHAUST EMISSIONS AND STANDARDS**

| POLLUTANT | UNCONTROLLED VEHICLE | CALIFORNIA STANDARDS 1966* | CALIFORNIA STANDARDS 1970 |
|---|---|---|---|
| HYDROCARBONS | 900 PPM** | 275 PPM | 180 PPM |
| CARBON MONOXIDE | 3.5 % | 1.5 % | 1.0 % |
| OXIDES OF NITROGEN | 1500 PPM | 350 PPM | 350 PPM |

* National standards for hydrocarbons and carbon monoxide beginning with 1968 model vehicles.
** Parts Per Million.

*Despite the staggering tonnages of industrial waste released into the atmosphere annually, the automobile is responsible for some two thirds of the total amount. Detroit seems certain to meet Federal standards, but planners stress that emission levels must be lowered still further if the air is to remain breathable.*

**PRESENT AND FUTURE AUTOMOBILE EMISSION CONTROL LEVELS**

| | UNCONTROLLED AUTOMOBILE, 1963 | | NATIONAL STANDARDS, 1968 | | COMMERCIALLY FEASIBLE, 1970 | | COMMERCIALLY FEASIBLE, 1975 | | EXPECTED ULTIMATE, AFTER 1980 | |
|---|---|---|---|---|---|---|---|---|---|---|
| | TYPICAL EMISSION LEVELS | ESTIMATED POLLUTION PER CAR/YEAR | | | | | | | Less than | Less than |
| EXHAUST | | | | | | | | | | |
| HYDROCARBONS | 900 ppm | 300 lbs. | 275 ppm | 90 lbs. | 1800 ppm | 60 lbs. | 50 ppm | 20 lbs. | 25 ppm | 10 lbs. |
| CARBON MONOXIDE | 3.5 % | 1700 lbs. | 1.5 % | 750 lbs. | 1.0 % | 500 lbs. | 0.5 % | 250 lbs. | .25 % | 120 lbs. |
| NITROGEN OXIDES | 1500 ppm | 90 lbs. | 1500 ppm | 90 lbs. | 600-800 ppm | 40 lbs. | 250 ppm | 15 lbs. | 100 ppm | 10 lbs. |
| CRANKCASE BLOWBY (hydrocarbons) | | 130 lbs. | | none | | none | | none | | none |
| EVAPORATION (hydrocarbons) | | 90 lbs. | | 90 lbs. | | none | | none | | none |
| TOTAL | | 2310 lbs. | | 1200 lbs. | | 600 lbs. | | 285 lbs. | | 140 lbs. |

Figure 10.

TABLE 79
AIR POLLUTANTS

| *Pollutant* | *Health Effects* |
|---|---|
| Sulfur dioxide ($SO_2$)<br>Sulfuric acid ($H_2SO_4$)<br>Sulfate-salt particles<br>Lead alkyls | Sulfuric acid irritates the nose and throat at concentrations of about 15 parts per million. In the bronchi, erosion of the lining epithelium, submucosal edema, and thrombosis of the smaller arteries and veins occur. Lead alkyls, if increased, have serious potential. |
| Carbon monoxide (CO) | Acute carbon monoxide poisoning results in signs and symptoms of anoxia. |
| Ozone ($O_3$) | Air passages are irritated, causing pain in the chest, cough, dyspnea, and nausea, at concentrations above 0.2 parts per million. Known effects include pulmonary edema (later fibrosis), stimulation of cellular healing, and reaction with various proteins to produce antigens. |
| Nitrogen dioxide ($NO_2$) | Exposure to high concentrations can result in acute airway obstruction, bronchiolitis obliterans, and death. |
| 3,4-Benzpyrene and other polycyclic hydrocarbons | Suspected as carcinogenic. Benzpyrene results mainly from burning or distilling of furnace fuels and is known to cause cancer in animals. |
| Olefinic hydrocarbons | Precursors of compounds, such as acrolein and formaldehyde, which cause eye irritation. |

Another nuisance and source of potential distress is the basement garage. The ceiling above the garage is not airtight and may permit carbon monoxide fumes to invade the living quarters above.

How many cases of migraine and other types of headaches, rashes, premature skin aging, allergies, respiratory disturbances and irritability are the consequences of exposure to such an unusual chemical milieu can only be surmised.

Some of these indoor pollution problems have relatively simple solutions. Properly sized exhaust fans or protective hoods connected to flues can eliminate most combustion and cooking pollutants from the kitchen. Better building codes can prevent leakage of carbon monoxide fumes from basement garages to living quarters.

## *Radioactive Air Pollution (Fallout)*

Now that man is contaminating the general atmosphere with products of nuclear fusion and fission, the significance of such pollutants is a matter of grave concern which is being carefully and extensively investigated. The effects from occupational and industrial exposures have long been suspected and well documented. Workers in the pitchblende mines in Czechoslovakia developed a relatively high incidence of pulmonary carcinoma that is apparently related to exposure to radon gas. The increased risk of leukemia in radiologists also seems well established. The former use of irradiation of the thymus in infants is highly suspected of producing an increased rate of thyroid cancer. The broad study carried out by the Atomic Bomb Casualty Commission in Hiroshima and Nagasaki has provided valuable preliminary information about the hazards of direct wholebody irradiation, but the effects of fallout (radioactive dust) remain to be determined.

Fallout is small pieces of dust and debris which are made radioactive by nuclear explosions. When a hydrogen bomb is exploded close to the ground, thousands of tons of these tiny particles of dust and debris are sucked upward high into the air. They help form the mushroom cloud which is always seen with one of these explosions. Some of the radioactive matter spills out of the cloud near the explosion. Most of it is carried by the wind, and it can settle to earth anywhere, continuing to give off radioactivity until it decays.

The long-range interrelation of preventive medicine and geopolitics is defined forcefully and clearly by Breslow (*Am J Public Health, 48*:913, 1958).

When considering latent effects of contaminating the atmosphere with ionizing radiation, it becomes necessary to recognize that fall-out from a single explosion will persist for decades and its effects will extend over generations. Geneticists agree that the number of mutations—and most of these are harmful—is strictly proportional to the amount of radiation received. There is no "safe" or harmless dose. Some evidence also implies that even small doses of radiation may cause leukemia and bone cancer in a small proportion of exposed persons, but this small proportion must be applied to the entire world population. Thus, nuclear explosions of the past twelve years may indeed be causing an unknown number of cases. Taking into account the exposure of the entire world population this number may not be inconsiderable.

There are four basic principles to be always considered in any discussion of fallout.

1. Fallout is dangerous and its potential is unlimited.
2. There are effective available protective measures against it.
3. The best protection comes from individual or community shelters built to specifications.
4. The optimum protection is planned and prepared in advance.

## *Water Pollution*

Prior to 1960, daily dependable supplies of fresh water were more than adequate to meet daily water demands. Industrial growth, increased population and higher standards of

TABLE 80
WATER POLLUTANTS

| *Type* | *Description* | *Effects* |
|---|---|---|
| Sewage and other oxygen-demanding wastes | Putrescible organic substances | Reduction of oxygen dissolved in water which is injurious to fish life; further reduction of dissolved oxygen to zero results in a septic condition |
| Infectious agents | Organisms which may cause typhoid fever, virus infections, and intestinal disorders | Potential danger to persons who drink this water and to participants of aquatic sports |
| Plant nutrients | Dissolved mineral substances used as food by aquatic plants | Enhanced growth of algae; intensified taste and odor |
| Synthetic organic chemicals | Household detergents, insecticides, pesticides, and weed killers | Injurious to aquatic life; possible injurious effects from long-term ingestion |
| Other chemicals (inorganic and mineral substances) | Salt,* acids, and other manufactured chemicals from mining, petroleum, agricultural, etc. industries | Increased cost of water treatment, reduction of recreational value; injurious to aquatic life |
| Sediments | Soil and mineral particles which are washed from land | Erosion of machinery, such as water pumping equipment; reduction of fish and shellfish population; plugging of water filters |
| Radioactive substances | Waste products from mining and refining of radioactive minerals and from use of refined radioactive substances | Cumulative effects of exposure to radiation |
| Heat | Water used for cooling purposes | Injurious to fish and other aquatic life |

*Toxic chromium compounds mixed with highway salt to prevent deterioration of cars not properly undercoated for winter season.

living have resulted in increased consumption of water during the past several decades, so that daily need for fresh water now exceeds daily supply. Estimates are that by 1980, we shall be using almost 600 billion gallons daily of fresh water, but only 515 billion gallons will be available. The long-range problem of supply and demand is giving state and national officials grave concern.

Pollution in rivers, streams and lakes increased almost sixfold in the past sixty years and is continuing to increase. In the past, pollution problems were local in origin and were controlled locally. Serious pollution problems could be avoided for the most part by dilution provided by streams. Today, water pollution is a complex national problem. Among the factors which have been responsible for growth of the pollution problem are increased population, urbanization and industrial growth. Certain synthetic detergents present a special and serious problem because they are not removed by conventional waste treatment methods and pass through processes for purifying water.

In small communities, the detergent waste from homes seeps through the soil into well water. In fact, so much detergent waste now seeps through the soil that the "runoff" water in the watersheds of big city reservoir systems is also being polluted. Normally, waste matter in soil is broken down by bacterial action. Detergents, however, are man-made synthetics, unaffected by bacteria. Those using the inorganic base alkyl-benzene sulfonate (ABS) pass intact through sewage treatment, and passing through home faucets with built-in aerators, the detergents may foam again.

TABLE 81
SOME LEADING OCCUPATIONAL CARCINOGENS

| *Carcinogen* | *Cancer type* | *Industry* | *Population at Risk* |
|---|---|---|---|
| Inorganic arsenic | Lung, lymphatic | Copper smelting | 1.5 million |
| Asbestos | Lung, bladder | Mining, insulation, brake linings | 1 million |
| Bis(chloromethyl)-ether (a contaminate of chloromethyl-methyl ether [CMME]) | Lung (small cell) | Water conditioners; possibly textiles, shoemaking | Several thousand; total unknown (most potent carcinogen tested in nineteen years by Institute of Environmental Medicine) |
| Benzene and 4-aminobiphenyl | Leukemia, bladder | Rubber | 2 million |
| Benzidine, beta-naphthylamine | Bladder | Dyestuffs | Unknown |
| Cadmium oxide | Prostate | Welding, metal processing | 100,000 |
| Chromic acid | Lung | Chrome plating | 15,000 |
| Coke-oven emissions, coal tar pitch | Lung, scrotal | Steelmaking, aluminum | At least 10,000 |
| Vinyl chloride* | Liver | Plastics | At least 10,000 |
| Plutonium | Lung | Mining, nuclear energy | Unknown |

*There have been no significant vinyl chloride related diseases at plants where operations have been maintained at relatively low levels of exposure. The hazard of either liver angiosarcoma or skin disease in most plants in the United States is minimal under present working conditions. Noncirrhotic portal fibrosis with associated portal hypertension is more frequently observed in workers in Wales exposed to vinyl chloride than is angiosarcoma.

Sources: National Institute of Occupational Safety and Health; International Agency for Research on Cancer, World Health Organization; Health Research Group.

# Chapter 6

# DRUGS

The drug bill of the American people amounts to over \$8½ billion a year. In 1972, the public spent about \$5½ billion on prescriptions and \$3½ billion on packaged medication, of which over \$600 million went for aspirin (more than 20 million lbs. consumed) and analgesics. This means that practically every household has some type of pill or medicine around. Too frequently adults assume that these drugs are harmless and leave them where young children can easily reach them.

Some of the drug poisoning in small children is due to overdosing, but a great deal of it is like any other household poisoning, the child simply swallows something he has found. Since flavored aspirin tablets were first marketed for children in 1949, the incidence of poisoning has increased to an alarming degree. The flavor is so palatable that children search every nook and corner for this candy aspirin. Often parents themselves are at fault for referring to this and other flavored medications as candy instead of clearly stating that these preparations are medicines given only for illnesses. The 1976 report from the National Clearinghouse for Poison Control Centers covering 473 centers in forty-four states showed that 71,495 cases of poisoning (over 50%) were caused by medicines. Of this number, aspirin ingestions had dropped to 4.1 per cent from the 18.5 per cent high in 1970.* This remarkable drop in incidence, morbidity and mortality can be attributed to the effectiveness of safety closures.

*Treatment* for drug intoxication should be carefully planned. Unless a basic plan is established, panic, confusion and inappropriate treatment may impede resuscitation.

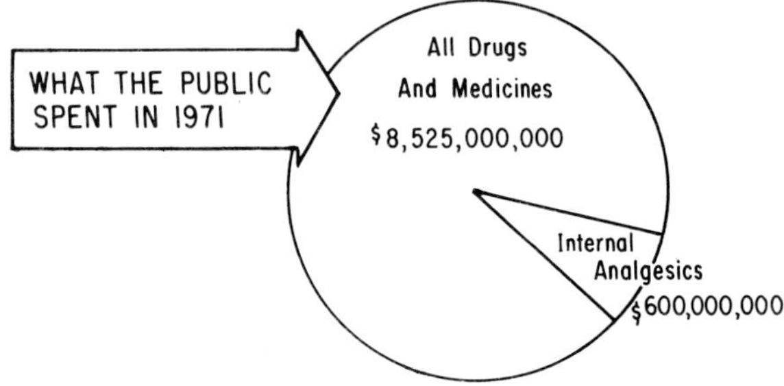


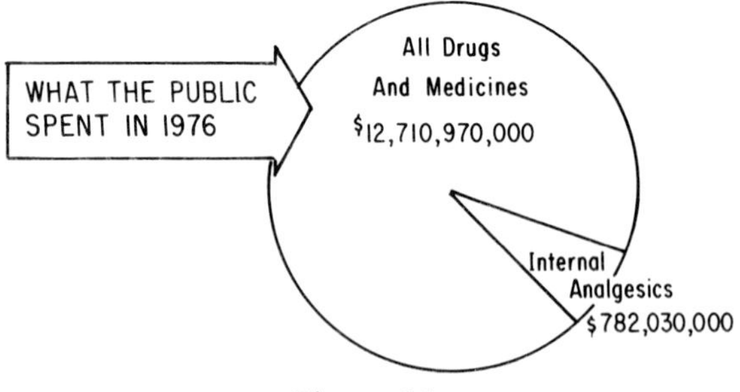


Figure 11.

Establishing respiratory exchange is most important. The airway is cleared of secretions, and an oropharyngeal or endotracheal airway may be inserted. Often, however, extension of the head and forward displacement of the mandible are sufficient. Mechanical respirators may be needed to maintain adequate oxygen exchange. Mouth-to-mouth breathing may be necessary pending the arrival of mechanical respirator equipment. Physiologic improvement of the patient's condition is often notable when tissues receive adequate oxygen.

*In children under 5 years of age.

A large nasogastric tube is used to empty the stomach, and a sample of gastric contents is analyzed. The patient's general condition is assessed, and pertinent information is obtained.

Generally, legs are elevated above the level of the right auricle to allow venous drainage of the lower extremities. The usual shock position promotes circulatory pooling in the head and thorax. Cardiac failure may necessitate alterations in position.

Elastic bandaging of the legs prevents venous stasis. Passive leg exercises are advisable if depression is extreme. The patient is turned from side to side every two hours to reduce atelectasis and promote pulmonary drainage.

Homeostasis is maintained by parenteral fluid. Amount is based on blood electrolyte concentrations and urine output. An indwelling urethral catheter is placed in the bladder to permit accurate hourly measurement of output. When the kidney is not damaged, fluid therapy is aided by hourly measurement of urine specific gravity.

If oliguria is associated, electrocardiographic examination and frequent measurement of serum potassium are required.

Vital signs are recorded every fifteen minutes or more frequently if values are labile or if vasopressors are administered.

Drugs should be given only when specifically required. In only a few cases, such as cyanide poisoning, is therapy with an antidote urgent. Intensive supportive therapy reduces the need for medication.

Central nervous system stimulants should not be used to improve respiration. The drugs impact a false sense of security, and harmful reactions such as rebound depression or convulsions may occur. If the myocardium is hypoxic, epinephrine may induce fatal ventricular fibrillation.

Intravenous vasopressors such as phenylephrine, methoxamine or methamphetamine may be required if the patient has tachycardia above 110 pulse beats per minute, prolonged capillary filling time, pallor or diaphoresis. Moderate hypotension as low as 80 mm Hg does not necessitate vigorous therapy with vasopressors unless urinary output is depressed. Extremely potent agents, such as levarterenol bitartrate, are rarely used; potent vasoconstrictors may significantly depress urinary output.

## FOOD-DRUG INTERACTIONS

Several years ago, a major antidepressant had to be withdrawn from the market when unusually severe side-effects were noted in patients taking it. Research into the cause of these reactions turned up the fact that cheeses with a high tyramine content were the culprit.

Armed with that knowledge, the product's manufacturer was once again able to market it, along with suitable precautionary material. And the food-drug interaction field came into its own.

Since that time, a host of interactions of this nature have filled the literature. Unfortunately, there has been no ongoing effort to screen out the rare interactions from the more common ones.

In the following Table 82, many of the interactions, both rare and prevalent, are listed. In most instances, the information presented is not intended to be an absolute in forbidding the intake of these foods (full disclosures should be consulted for absolute prohibitions). Patients on reaction-prone drugs should avoid excessive intake of those foods which may have a deleterious effect on the action of the medications they are taking (the interaction potential of broad beans may be lessened by thorough cooking).

TABLE 82
A SAMPLING OF POSSIBLE FOOD-DRUG REACTIONS

| Drug | Food reaction possibility | Drug | Food reaction possibility |
|---|---|---|---|
| aminophylline | vitamin B complex | griseofulvin | fatty foods |
| anticoagulants | cabbage, cauliflower, carrots, corn, fish and fish oils, liver, mineral oil, mushrooms, oats, papain, peas, potatoes, pork, soybeans, spinach, strawberries, tomatoes, wheat, wheat germ, wheat bran, wine, vitamins C & K. | iron salts | cereals, eggs, milk and milk products, vitamins C & E, |
| | | l-dopa | broad beans, vitamin B complex |
| | | lincomycin | vitamin B complex |
| | | MAO inhibitors (ex: phenelzine, tranylcypromine) | aged cheddar cheeses and others, alcohol, yogart, yeast, amino acids, bananas, beer, broad beans, canned figs, chicken liver, chocolate, cola drinks, coffee, licorice, milk and milk products, pickled herring, tea |
| bisacodyl | milk and milk products | | |
| catecholamines (ex: isoproterenol, epinephrin) | bananas, coffee, cocoa, riboflavin, tea, vitamine B complex | | |
| chlortetracycline | milk and milk products | methacycline | milk and milk products |
| chloramphenicol | riboflavin, vitamin B complex | oral contraceptives | mineral oil |
| corticosteroids | vitamin A | penicillin | certain cheeses |
| digitalis-glycosides | dextrose, licorice | procarbazine | bananas |
| erythromycin (oral) | acid drinks like cranberry, orange and lemon juices, | reserpine | vitamin B complex |
| | | sulfonamides | mineral oil |
| furazolidone | beef, broad beans, certain cheeses, chicken liver, pickled herring, wine | tetracyclines | milk and milk products, riboflavin, vitamin B complex |
| | | thiazides | licorice |

## ROLE OF DRUGS IN SUICIDE

Drugs play an important role in the problem of suicide. In 1963, according to the Office of Vital Statistics, there were 20,819 suicides (22,060 in 1969). Of these, 2666, or more than 12 per cent, resulted from intentional ingestion of overdoses of analgesics and soporifics (Table 85). Other methods of committing suicide, such as firearms or hanging, were used more frequently than drugs. Carbon monoxide for suicidal purposes is employed as often as are drugs.

The number of suicides due to ingestion of excessive doses of various drugs is shown in Table 86. Barbiturates (Class E970 B) are still the most frequently used drug for suicide at the present time, with an increase in morbidity in the past ten years. The advent of tranquilizers has not decreased the use of barbiturates for suicidal purposes. About 75 per cent of all suicidal deaths by drugs were due to barbiturates in 1963. There were 321 documented barbiturate deaths in 1968.

TABLE 83
UNITED STATES SUICIDE RATES

Source: U.S. Public Health Service

| | *1972* | | *1968* | | *1967* | | *1965* | |
|---|---|---|---|---|---|---|---|---|
| | Male | Female | Male | Female | Male | Female | Male | Female |
| Poisoning | 3,242 | 3,208 | 2,960 | 2,724 | 2,949 | 2,746 | 3,179 | 2,816 |
| Hanging and strangulation | 2,510 | 790 | 2,265 | 834 | 2,112 | 666 | 2,453 | 744 |
| Firearms and explosives | 10,852 | 2,496 | 9,078 | 1,833 | 8,766 | 1,784 | 8,457 | 1,441 |
| Other | 1,164 | 742 | 1,076 | 602 | 1,360 | 942 | 1,401 | 1,016 |
| Totals | 17,768 | 7,236 | 15,379 | 5,993 | 15,187 | 6,138 | 15,490 | 6,017 |

TABLE 84
INTERNATIONAL SUICIDE RATES

Source: World Health Organization
The following table gives death rates per 100,000 population for suicide in various countries and localities. The figures are for 1970, the latest year for which data are available.

| *Country or Locality* | *Rate* | *Country or Locality* | *Rate* |
|---|---|---|---|
| Hungary | 34.8 | Australia | 12.4 |
| Czechoslovakia | 25.3 | Bulgaria | 11.9 |
| Austria | 24.2 | United States | 11.6 |
| Sweden | 22.3 | Canada | 11.3 |
| Denmark | 21.5 | Poland | 11.3 |
| West Germany | 21.5 | New Zealand | 9.6 |
| Finland | 21.3 | Norway | 8.4 |
| Switzerland | 18.6 | Netherlands | 8.1 |
| Belgium | 16.5 | Scotland | 7.6 |
| France | 15.4 | | |

TABLE 85
NUMBER OF SUICIDAL DEATHS BY SPECIFIC CAUSES ACCORDING TO INTERNATIONAL CLASSIFICATION

| *Class* | *Name* | *1963* | *1960* | *1957* | *1954* |
|---|---|---|---|---|---|
| E 970 | Analgesics and soporifics | 2,666 | 1,616 | 993 | 856 |
| E 971 | Other liquids and solids† | 733 | 741 | 651 | 811 |
| E 972 | Domestic gas | 175 | 186 | 204 | 366 |
| E 973 | Other gas‡ | 2,211 | 1,787 | 1,499 | 1,483 |
| E 974 | Hanging | 3,057 | 3,366 | 3,559 | 3,370 |
| E 975 | Submersion | 576 | 616 | 641 | 621 |
| E 976 | Firearms | 9,595 | 9,017 | 7,841 | 7,539 |
| E 977 | Cutting | 417 | 488 | 449 | 466 |
| E 978 | Jumping | 791 | 697 | 518 | 521 |
| E 979 | Other | 598 | 517 | 274 | 315 |
| *Totals* | | 20,819 | 19,031 | 16,629 | 16,348 |

*Data from U.S. Department of Health, Education and Welfare, Office of Vital Statistics.
†Strychnine, phenol, and cresol compounds; lye and potash; mercury; arsenic; and fluorides.
‡Motor vehicle exhaust gas and carbon monoxide.

It is likely that some of the suicides due to ingestion of barbiturates were unintentional since many patients experience a state of mental confusion after a dose of barbiturates; they are unable to remember that they have already taken the drug. These states, also known as "automatism," can occur after ingestion of low to moderate, relatively "non-

TABLE 86
NUMBER OF SUICIDAL DEATHS BY SPECIFIC CAUSE IN INTERNATIONAL CLASSIFICATION E 970 (SUICIDE AND SELF-INFLICTED POISONING BY ANALGESIC AND SOPORIFIC SUBSTANCES)*

| *Class* | *Drugs* | *1963* | *1960* | *1957* | *1954* |
|---|---|---|---|---|---|
| A | Morphine and other opium derivatives | 7 | 12 | 12 | 16 |
| B | Barbituric acid and derivatives | 1,997 | 1,290 | 817 | 721 |
| C–G | Salicylates, antipyretics, and bromides | 76 | 57 | 29 | 23 |
| H | Other analgesic and soporific substances | 488 | 226 | 123 | 87 |
| M | Unspecified drugs | 98 | 31 | 12 | 9 |
| *Total* | | 2,666 | 1,616 | 993 | 856 |
| *Total suicides* | | 20,819 | 19,031 | 16,629 | 16,348 |

*Data from U.S. Department of Health, Education, and Welfare, Office of Vital Statistics.

lethal" amounts of barbiturates. Unintentional ingestion of excessive additional doses may take place during these confused periods.

The incidence of suicide owing to ingestion of barbiturates, other analgesic and soporific substances and the tranquilizer meprobamate is given in Table 87. The striking difference in the incidence of suicide between barbiturates and meprobamate becomes particularly impressive when it is realized that the use of meprobamate, at least in the United States, is of a similar order of magnitude as the use of barbiturates.

The remarkable difference between the number of deaths produced by barbiturates and meprobamate is probably due to two factors. The first is the observation that meprobamate does not cause confusional states and the second is the much lower toxicity of the tranquilizer. With barbiturates, the ingestion of five to fifteen hypnotic doses may be fatal. With meprobamate and other tranquilizers of this type, ingestion of fifty or more therapeutic doses is usually survived.

TABLE 87
NUMBER OF SUICIDES DUE TO BARBITURATES (CLASS E 970 B), OTHER ANALGESIC AND SOPORIFIC SUBSTANCES (CLASS E 970 H), AND MEPROBAMATE DURING 1954-1963*

| *Year* | *Suicide by Barbiturates* | *Suicide by Other Analgesic and Soporific Substances* | *Suicide by Meprobamate* |
|---|---|---|---|
| 1954 | 721 | 86 | — |
| 1955 | 781 | 94 | 1 |
| 1956 | 765 | 95 | 3 |
| 1957 | 817 | 122 | 1 |
| 1958 | 912 | 167 | 1 |
| 1959 | 1,073 | 178 | 1 |
| 1960 | 1,290 | 226 | 0 |
| 1961 | 1,341 | 250 | 2 |
| 1962 | 1,738 | 360 | 2 |
| 1963 | 1,997 | 484 | 1 |
| Total | 11,435 | 2,062 | 12 |

*Data for barbiturates and other analgesic and soporific substances from U.S. Department of Health, Education, and Welfare, Office of Vital Statistics. Data for meprobamate from published literature and records of the medical department of Wallace Laboratories.

## DRUG-INDUCED HEMOLYTIC ANEMIA AND ALTERED THERAPEUTIC RESPONSES (INBORN ERRORS OF METABOLISM)

Human genetics, through the advances of biochemical genetics, has important implications for the practitioner, with regard to both diagnosis of disease and its drug treatment. Table 88 list examples of genetic polymorphisms in man in which enzyme defects lead to drug sensitivity or to an alteration of therapeutic responses. When primaquine was first found to be effective in eradicating vivax malaria, it was given to our troops returning

## Methods of Suicide Used By Americans

| | 1964 | | 1972 |
|---|---|---|---|
| Firearm and explosive | | 9,806 | 11,348 |
| Poisoning | | 5,541 | 6,450 |
| By analgesic and soporific substances | 2,543 | | 3,972 (combined) |
| By other solid and liquid substances | 685 | | |
| By gases | 2,313 | | 2,478 |
| Hanging and strangulation | | 3,005 | 3,300 |
| Jumping from high places | | 752 | * |
| Submersion (drowning) | | 541 | * |
| Cutting and piercing instruments | | 382 | * |
| Other and unspecified means | | 556 | 1,906 |

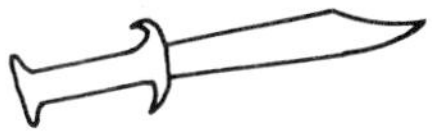

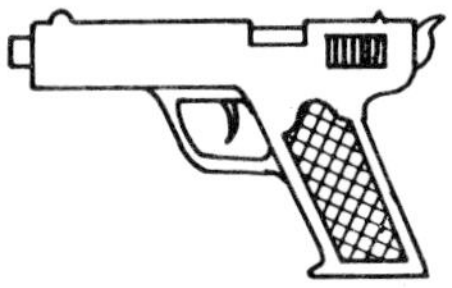

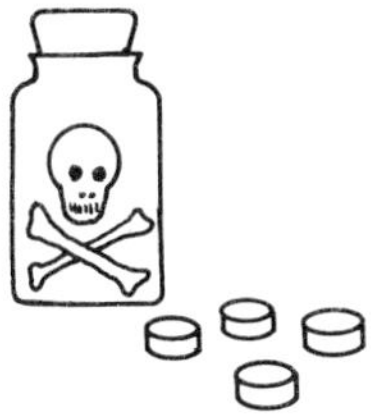

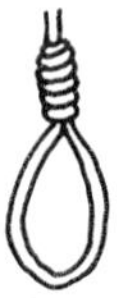

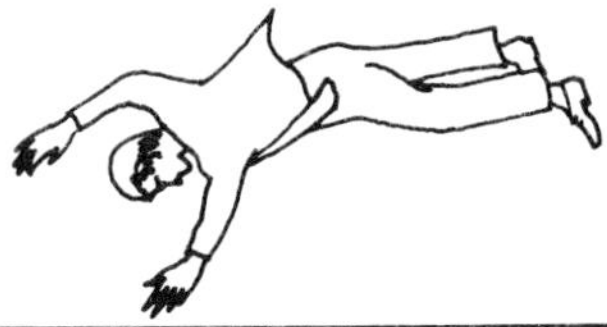

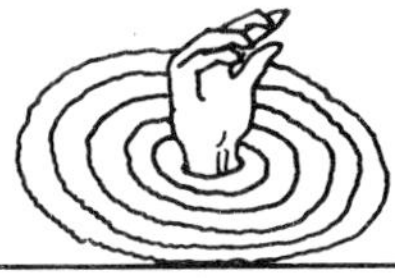

* Included in "Other and unspecified means."

Figure 12.

from Korea. It was soon learned that although it is nontoxic for whites, it produces hemolysis in a significant number of blacks. Alving and his co-workers showed that the red cells of a person sensitive to the drug are deficient in glucose-6-phosphate dehydrogenase or zwischen ferment, an enzyme in the so-called pentose shunt, one of the main pathways by which glucose is metabolized in all cells. This enzyme catalyzes the removal of hydrogen from glucose-6-phosphatase to form 6-phospho-gluconate. The hydrogen is attached to triphosphopyridine nucleotide (TPN) to form reduced triphosphopyridine nucleotide (TPNH). Later studies showed that the primaquine-sensitive red cells have low levels of reduced glutathione, which is necessary for maintenance of the integrity of the red cell membrane. The glutathione is kept reduced by an enzyme, glutathione reductase, but the hydrogen must be supplied by the reduced triphosphopyridine nucleotide formed in the first reaction. This defect in glucose-6-phosphate dehydrogenase (G-6-PD) has been found in 10 to 15 per cent of healthy black American males and in about 1 per cent of healthy whites (most of these whites inhabiting or having originated from the Mediterranean basin). The defect occurs in a more severe form in Sephardic Jews, Sardinians, Arabs, Greeks and many other southern European, Middle Eastern and Oriental population groups. G-6-PD deficiency is inherited as a sex-linked recessive characteristic.

There is another, much rarer form of G-6-PD deficiency which results in a chronic hemolytic anemia of the congenital, non-spherocytic type, even in the absence of drug exposure.

Other factors influencing primaquine-type hemolysis are the nature and dose of the drug ingested. Compared to primaquine, an 8-amino-quinoline, other antimalarial 8-amino-quinolines such as pamaquine (plasmochin) or quinocide cause an even more severe hemolysis. A dose of 15 mg primaquine per day administered to healthy G-6-PD-deficient individuals induces only a moderate hemolysis with mild anemia. Chloroquine (Aralen®), 0.3 gm/day, or quinacrine, 0.1 gm/day, causes even less hemolysis and no anemia.

In the treatment of vivax malaria, primaquine eliminates the tissue stages of malaria parasites and is curative. Chloroquine and quinacrine, however, are not curative but suppress clinical attacks. Thus, in the treatment of vivax malaria, neither chloroquine nor quinacrine can substitute for primaquine. Moreover, when used in combination with primaquine, quinacrine increases the hemolytic effect. Accordingly, one method of treatment of vivax malaria, which can safely be given to G-6-PD-deficient individuals, consists of 45 mg primaquine combined with 0.3 gm of chloroquine administered one time/week for eight weeks. Hydroxychloroquine may be substituted for chloroquine.

It has been learned that another disease, favism, can be ascribed to the same defect. Favism is a disease characterized by hemolysis that occurs when certain persons, especially Italians and Greeks, eat the fava bean or inhale the pollen from the fava plant. This disorder apparently does not occur in blacks with this enzymic deficiency. Moreover, it has been shown that naphthalene (moth balls), sulfonamides (particularly the long-acting ones such as Kynex®, Azulfidine®, etc.),

TABLE 88
GENETIC POLYMORPHISMS PRODUCING DRUG-INDUCED HEMOLYTIC ANEMIA OR ALTERED THERAPEUTIC RESPONSE

A. Drug sensitivities
  Glucose-6-phosphate dehydrogenase
    a. Primaquine hemolysis
    b. Favism
    c. Effect of sulfonamides, naphthalene, nitrofurantoin (Furadantin®), para-aminosalicylic acid, sulfoxone (Diasone®), BAL, methylene blue, chloroquine, vitamin K analogues, antipyretics, etc.
B. Influence of environment, illness, pregnancy, periods of "stress and strain"
C. Acetylating of isonicotinic acid hydrazide (INH)
  1. Rapid—1 hour
  2. Slow—6 hours—neuropathy
D. Pseudocholinesterase apnea
  (due to a defect or altered activity of pseudocholinesterase)
  1. Succinylcholine (Anectine®)
  2. Decamethonium
E. Influence of barbiturates on porphyria

| DRUG REACTIONS | Fixed eruptions | Erythema multiforme | Exfoliative dermatitis | Periarteritis nodosa | Serum sickness | Shock | Granulocytopenia | Hemolytic anemia | Thrombocytopenic purpura | Aplastic anemia | Hepatitis |
|---|---|---|---|---|---|---|---|---|---|---|---|
| **Drugs** | | | | | | | | | | | |
| Acetanilid | X | | | | | | | | | | |
| Acetazolamide | | | | | | | | | X | X | |
| Aminopyrine | | | | | | | X | | | X | |
| Aminosalicylic acid | X | | X | | | X | | | X | X | X |
| Anesthetics | | | | | | X | | | | | |
| Antihistamines | | X | | | | | X | | | | |
| Antimony salts | X | | | | | | | | | | |
| Antipyrine | X | X | | | | | | | | | |
| Arsenicals | X | X | X | | X | | X | | X | X | X |
| Aspirin | | | | | | X | | X | | | |
| Barbiturates | X | X | X | | X | | X | | | | X |
| Belladonna | | | X | | | | | | | | |
| Bromides | | X | | | | | | | | | |
| Carbarsone | | | X | | | | | | | | |
| Chloramphenicol | | X | | | | | X | X | X | X | |
| Chlordiazepoxide | | | | | | | X | | | X | |
| Chlorothiazide | | | | | | | | | X | X | |
| Chlorpropamide | | | | | | | | | X | X | X |
| Corticotropin | | | | | X | X | | | | | |
| Cortisone | | X | | | | X | | | | | |
| Dehydrocholic acid | | | | | | X | | | | | |
| Diethylstilbestrol* | | | X | | | | | | | | |
| Digitalis | | | | | X | | | | | | |
| Digitoxin | | | | | | | | | X | | |
| Dinitrophenol | | | X | | | | | | | | |
| Diphenhydramine | | | | | | X | | | | | |
| Diphenylhydantoin | | | | | | | X | | X | | |
| Dipyrone | | | | | | | X | | | | |
| Erythromycin estolate | | | | | | | | | | | X |
| Estradiol | | | | | | | | | | X | |
| Estrogens | | | | | | | | | X | | X |
| Folic Acid | | | | | | X | | | | | |
| Gamma benzene hexachloride | | | | | | | X | | | X | |
| Gold salts | X | X | X | | | | X | | X | X | X |
| Heparin | | | | | X | | | | | | |
| Hydantoins | | X | X | X | X | | | | | | X |
| Hydralazine | | | | | X | | | | | X | |
| Insulin | | | | | X | | | | | | |
| Iodides | X | | X | X | X | X | | | | | |
| Isoniazid | | | | | X | | X | | | | X |
| Liver extract | | | | | X | | | | | | |
| Meperidine | | | | | | X | X | | | | |
| Mephenytoin | | | | | | | X | | | X | |
| Meprobamate | | | | | | | X | | X | | |
| Mercupurin | | | | | | | | | | | X |
| Mercurials | X | | X | X | X | X | | | | X | |

* Maternal ingestion of diethylstilbestrol during pregnancy appears to increase the risk of vaginal adenocarcinoma developing years later in the offspring exposed.

| DRUG REACTIONS | Fixed eruptions | Erythema multiforme | Exfoliative dermatitis | Periarteritis nodosa | Serum sickness | Shock | Granulocytopenia | Hemolytic anemia | Thrombocytopenic purpura | Aplastic anemia | Hepatitis |
|---|---|---|---|---|---|---|---|---|---|---|---|
| Methantheline | | | X | | | | | | | | |
| Methimazole | | | | | | | X | | | | |
| Monoamine oxidase inhibitors | | | | | | | | | | | X |
| Naphthalene | | | | | | | | X | | | |
| Nitrofurantoin | | | | | | | | X | | | |
| Novobiocin | | | | | | | | | | | X |
| Opium alkaloids | | | | | | X | | | | | |
| Penicillin | X | X | X | | X | X | X | X | X | X | X |
| Phenacemide | | | | | | | X | | X | X | X |
| Phenacetin | X | X | | | | | | X | | | |
| Phenindione | | | | | | | X | | | | X |
| Phenolphthalein | X | X | | | | | | | | | |
| Phenothiazines | | | X | | X | X | X | X | X | X | X |
| Phenylbutazone | | X | X | | X | | X | | X | X | X |
| Pollen extracts | | | | | | X | | | | | |
| Potassium perchlorate | | | | | | | | | | X | |
| Procaine | | | | | | X | | | X | | |
| Procainamide | | | | | | | X | | | | X |
| Quinacrine | X | | X | | | | | | | X | X |
| Quinidine | X | | | | X | | | X | X | | |
| Quinine | X | | X | | X | | | | X | | |
| Ristocetin | | | | | | | X | | X | X | |
| Salicylates | X | X | | | X | | X | | | | |
| Salicylazosulfapyridine | | | | | | | | X | | | |
| Serums | | | | X | X | | | | | | |
| Streptomycin | | X | X | | X | X | X | X | X | X | X |
| Sulfadiazine | | | | | | X | | | | | |
| Sulfadimethoxine | | | | | | | | | | X | |
| Sulfamethoxypyridazine | | | | | | | | | X | X | |
| Sulfisoxazole | | | | | | | | | | X | |
| Sulfobromophthalein | | | | | | X | | | | | |
| Sulfocyanates | | | | | X | | | | | | |
| Sulfonamides | X | X | X | X | X | | X | X | X | X | X |
| Testosterone | | | | | | | | | | | X |
| Tetracycline | X | X | | | X | | X | X | | X | |
| Thiamine | | | | | | X | | | | | |
| Thiazides | X | | X | | | | | | | | X |
| Thiosemicarbazone | | | | | | | X | | | | |
| Thiouracils | | | | X | | | X | | X | | |
| Thorium dioxide | | | | | | X | | | | | |
| Tolbutamide | | | | | | | X | | X | X | |
| Triacetyloleandomycin | | | | | | | | | | | X |
| Tripelennamine | | | | | X | | | | | | |
| Vaccines | | X | | | X | | | | | | |
| Viomycin | | | | | X | | | | | | |

Figure 13. Reprinted with permission from Dr. Dale Friend and the *Journal of the American Pharmaceutical Association.*

nitrofurantoin (Furadantin®), BAL, methylene blue, quinidine, vitamin K analogues and a number of other drugs and agents can produce this reaction in persons who possess this enzyme defect. Thus we now have a logical explanation of a number of diverse diseases or drug sensitivities previously totally unexplained. Many are due to a common genetic defect inherited as a sex-linked recessive and intermediate trait.

A third point is inherent in these observations. It shows that certain genetic defects would have remained unexpressed were it not for changed environmental circumstances. As one geneticist remarked about favism: It would not have occurred if the fava bean grew in the Far North, since Eskimos do not possess the defect. As he expressed it, it was necessary for the gene flow and the bean flow to come together for the defect to become apparent. In this day and age, with the tremendous development and widespread intake of new drugs, we must expect and be on the lookout for other instances of this phenomenon. In addition, many industrial physicians are now determining G-6-PD abnormalities in preplacement job examinations to screen persons who may be hypersusceptible to specific chemicals in their work and environment.

Another instance is the discovery that all persons fall into two categories in regard to the way in which they metabolize isonicotinic acid hydrazide, or INH, the antituberculosis drug. There are rapid inactivators and slow inactivators, depending on an acetylating enzyme. One hour after a dose of isonicotinic acid hydrazide, the rapid inactivator achieves the same blood level that the slow inactivator requires six hours to achieve. Obviously one might suspect that this may affect the response to treatment in a tuberculous patient. Perhaps treatment might not be so effective in a rapid inactivator. Actually, studies performed thus far show that this is not the case. That is, therapeutic failures to isonicotinic acid hydrazide occur almost equally among rapid and slow inactivators, and the development of drug-resistant organisms does not appear to be affected by this genetic polymorphism. However, there is suggestive evidence that there is higher incidence among the slow inactivators of the peripheral neuropathy, which is the chief toxic manifestation of isonicotinic acid hydrazide. This is a phenomenon that affects many other drugs (sulfapyridine, sulfamethazine, hydralazine, dapsone, phenelzine) and that illustrates how genetic constitution may influence therapeutic response and even the development of toxicity.

The development of apnea in persons given succinylcholine and decamethonium drugs, used as muscle relaxants, is another example. This has been shown to be due to a defect or at least to altered activity of pseudocholinesterase. There is even one report of successful treatment of apnea by the injection of pseudocholinesterase.

The deleterious effect of barbiturates in persons possessing the inborn error of metabolism of acute intermittent porphyria has been well documented. Barbiturates can induce or aggravate an acute attack, perhaps causing permanent neurologic damage or even death. There is much evidence to suggest that many persons possessing this genetic metabolic defect of porphyrin metabolism might well live a normal life span without having an acute attack if they are not given a barbiturate.

During severe illness such as diabetic acidosis or bacterial or viral infections, the susceptibility to hemolysis in G-6-PD-deficient individuals may be greatly increased. Even acetylsalicylic acid, which at high doses of 4 to 12 gm/day ordinarily causes no more hemolysis than chloroquine or quinacrine, may cause a severe hemolysis at lower doses during such illnesses. In the presence of complicating illness, during pregnancy and during periods of severe stress and strain, physicians should be especially cautious in the administration of medicines of any kind to G-6-PD-deficient patients. Lead blood levels are increased as much as 12 per cent in those children exposed to lead who have this deficiency.

A recent study by Oski has shown that another enzyme system is abnormal in white but not in black patients with glucose-6-phosphate dehydrogenase deficiency. All of five white patients studied had markedly reduced erythrocytic acid phosphatase activity; none of five black patients had this deficiency. Like glucose-6-phosphate dehydrogenase deficiency, the erythrocytic acid phosphatase deficiency was related in some as yet undefined way to glucose metabolism. Normal erythrocytes incubated with glucose at 37°C for twenty-four hours showed no fall in acid-phosphatase activity; however, incubation without glucose caused a fall of 75 per cent in acid-phosphatase activity. Large doses of analgesics containing acetophenetidin (phenacetin) can produce serious hemolytic anemia without glucose-6-phosphate dehydrogenase deficiency or autoimmune mechanism. Recognition of Heinz bodies in the red blood cells often is the clue to diagnosis. Since many patients are reluctant to admit to taking analgesics, Heinz bodies should be sought in all cases of hemolytic anemia negative to the Coombs' test.

All studies in Germany so far indicate that only about 20 per cent of mothers taking thalidomide at the period of fetal organogenesis actually gave birth to deformed infants. This would indicate that if thalidomide is to do its damage, another predisposing factor must be present.

There is an apparent parallel between the effects of thalidomide and those of diseases known to be genetically transmitted, especially panmyelopathy (Fanconi's aplastic anemia) which is capable of producing phocomelia. It is known, of course, that panmyelopathy is caused by the blocking of an enzymatic reaction. This is probably true of thalidomide as well. More specifically, the thalidomide may in some way interfere with the metabolic pathways connected with the so-called generator of the limbs. Recent animal experiments have shown that thalidomide (or its metabolites) decreases cellular oxygen consumption by interfering with intermediary energy metabolism, and this could lead to developmental anomalies of the organism.

Drug-induced hemolytic anemia has also been described in individuals with a relatively rare hemoglobinopathy, hemoglobin Zurich. The same drugs which cause hemolysis of G-6-PD-deficient red cells cause hemolysis of cells from patients with this hemoglobinopathy. This hemoglobin is apparently unusually susceptible to oxidation, possibly because the abnormality in amino acid sequence occurs near the point of attachment of heme to globin.

In rare cases, drug-induced hemolysis may result from the development of antibodies which, in the presence of the drug, agglutinate red cells. Stibophen (Fuadin), penicillin, quinine, quinidine and phenacetin have all been implicated in such hemolytic anemias.

Drug-induced hemolytic anemia may also occur in some individuals who have neither G-6-PD deficiency, hemoglobin Zurich nor demonstrable antibodies. Some such cases appear to be related to impaired renal function resulting in unusually high drug levels in the blood. In other cases, the cause of sensitivity has not yet been determined. Sometimes the onset of drug-induced hemolysis is explosive; the patient complains of the symptoms of anemia—weakness, palpitation and pallor—and in addition there may be back pain, jaundice, abdominal cramps and the passage of dark urine. In other instances, hemolysis is less acute, and the routine determination of hematocrit or hemoglobin levels may give the first indication that the patient has become anemic during drug therapy. It also is possible that the anemia may pass unnoticed by both physician and patient with the hemoglobin concentration spontaneously returning to normal after drug therapy is discontinued.

The diagnosis of drug-induced hemolytic anemia is generally not difficult. When the administration of a drug known to be capable of inducing hemolysis is accompanied by a fall in the hemoglobin level of several grams per 100 ml over a period of a few days, and the hemoglobin returns to normal after withdrawal of the drug, a diagnosis of drug-induced hemolysis is clearly suggested.

In the early phase of hemolysis, Heinz bodies may often be seen in the red blood cells

TABLE 89
SOME OXIDANTS AND DRUGS THAT MAY CAUSE HEMOLYSIS IN G-6-PD DEFICIENCY

| | | | |
|---|---|---|---|
| Analgesics | Acetylsalicylic acid (aspirin) [1]<br>Acetophenetidin (phenacetin) [1]<br>Acetanilid<br>Phenazone<br>Aminopyrine, Antipyrine | Antimalarials | Pamaquin<br>Primaquine<br>Chloroquine[1]<br>Mepacrine<br>Quinine |
| Sulfonamides | Sulfanilamide,<br>$N^2$-acetylsulfanilamide<br>Sulfapyridine<br>Sulfacetamide<br>Sulfafurazole[1]<br>Sulfamethoxypyridazine<br>Salicylazosulfapyridine<br>Septrin, Bactrim[1,2] | Miscellaneous | Quinidine<br>Probenecid[1]<br>Procainamide[1]<br>Antazoline[1]<br>Diphenhydramine[1]<br>Ascorbic acid[1]<br>Vitamin $K_1$[1]<br>Piperazine |
| Sulfones | Dapsone<br>Thiazolsulfone | | Nalidixic acid<br>Isoniazid |
| Other Antimicrobials | Nitrofurantoin<br>Furazolidone<br>Nitrofurazone<br>Chloramphenicol[1]<br>*p*-Aminosalicylic acid[1] | | Tolbutamide<br>Methyldopa<br>Methylene blue<br>Naphthalene<br>Fava pollen and beans<br>Dimercaprol-BAL<br>Mestranol |

1. Reported as hemolytic agents but cause hemolysis only in conjunction with other factors such as infection or high drug doses.
2. The only reported hemolytic episodes were during infections, making the role of the drug unclear, but it should be avoided whenever possible.

Reprinted, by permission, from *The New England Journal of Medicine, 287*:994, 1972.

in appropriately stained preparations. When hemolysis is rapid, hyperbilirubinemia and the urinary excretion of heme compounds may be noted. In addition, reticulocytosis usually occurs several days after the decline of the hemoglobin level, although this may occasionally be masked by the disorder for which the drug was administered. Several simple, accurate methods for the detection of glucose-6-phosphate dehydrogenase (G-6-PD) deficiency, the most common cause of sensitivity to drug-induced hemolysis, are listed below. However, blood levels of this enzyme in individuals with G-6-PD deficiency may be transiently normal immediately after hemolysis occurs.

The G-6-PD defect can be identified by various tests of the blood.

1. By the findings of a record level of glutathione (GSH).
2. By the GSH stability test in which blood is incubated with acetyl phenylhydrazine.
3. By direct spectrophotometric measurement of the enzyme G-6-PD.
4. By the discovery of Heinz bodies in red blood cells.
5. By the methemoglobin reduction test which involves the oxidation of hemoglobin to methemoglobin by sodium nitrite and its subsequent enzymatic reconversion to hemoglobin in the presence of methylene blue. This redox dye affects the pentose phosphate pathway and activities, reduces triphosphopyridine nucleotide and methemoglobin reductase in normal, but not in G-6-PD-deficient erythrocytes. This simple rapid test can identify individuals who will experience hemolysis of clinical significance during the administration or ingestion of many drugs, chemicals and plants.
6. A recent simplified method to detect G-6-PD deficiency in erythrocytes is based on the reduction of the tetrazolium dye,

MTT, by reduced triphosphopyridine nucleotide. First, 5 ml of blood is mixed with 1 ml of ACD solution in heparinized capillary tubes. To correct for hematocrit variations, blood is sedimented overnight or centrifuged. The sedimented or packed erythrocytes are removed from the tube and applied to both sides of treated paper. The paper is placed in distilled water at room temperature for about twenty minutes, then blotted with filter paper; this performance is repeated once or twice to remove all traces of hemoglobin. As much water as possible is blotted from the paper, and the spot test reagent solution is applied. A strong purple color develops in two minutes with healthy erythrocytes, but little or no color develops when erythrocytes are deficient in G-6-PD. The paper may be flooded with distilled water to stop the reaction, dried and kept as a semipermanent record in a dark envelope.

7. A one-stage simple screening procedure. In the presence of cyanide as a catalase inhibitor, G-6-PD-deficient red cells are rapidly oxidized by the $H_2O_2$ generated by the coupling oxidation of ascorbate and oxyhemoglobin. The resulting brown hemoglobin pigment appearing in deficient blood suspension is readily perceived by the naked eye.

The *treatment* of drug-induced hemolytic anemia consists primarily of the recognition that drug-induced hemolysis is occurring and the withdrawal of the responsible medication. Hematinics, such as iron, liver or vitamins, are of no benefit and are not indicated. Transfusion is to be avoided whenever possible because of its inherent risks. In blacks with drug induced hemolysis due to G-6-PD deficiency, hemolysis due to most drugs is self-limited and usually subsides even if drug administration is continued. In whites, this may not be the case, but hemolysis ceases within a few days of withdrawal of drug. A good reticulocyte response suggests that recovery will be prompt. It is often suggested that a fluid intake and administration of alkali may be helpful in preventing renal complications of acute blood destruction, although the clinical benefits of such a regimen have not been clearly documented. However, anuria from drug-induced hemolysis is very rare, and recovery from drug-induced hemolysis is the rule.*

Human cytogenetics is for the first time providing explanations for many drug side-effects, which up to now have been obscure. In order to avoid mishaps or to institute early and effective treatment of abnormal chemical or drug reactions, biochemical determinations of activity of specific enzymes are required.

*Since methylene blue is known to cause hemolysis in a G-6-PD deficient individual, ascorbic acid is the treatment of choice for methoglobinemia.

## KNOWN RETINOTOXIC DRUGS

A. Digitalis glycosides (25%)
B. Phenothiazine derivatives
C. Indomethacin
D. Chlorpropamide (Diabinese)
E. Corticosteroids
F. Oxygen
G. Chloramphenicol
H. Quinoline
   1. Optochin
   2. Chloroquine (Aralen)
   3. Hydroxy-chloroquin (Plaquenil®)
   4. Plasmochin®

Systemically administered drugs can have a significant effect on ocular structures. With autonomic agents, the effect can be predicted and occurs shortly after drug administration. Other drugs produce ocular injury only after long-term administration and could not have been anticipated on the basis of information available from animal experimentation (human effects cannot always be produced) or short-term clinical investigation. The chelating agent D-penicillamine given over a period of several months was unsuccessful in reversing ocular pigmentation produced by long-

TABLE 90
GASTRODUODENAL ULCERS—ROLE OF DRUGS

| *Pathogenesis* | *Drugs* |
|---|---|
| Inciting localized damage to the vulnerable mucosa | Cinchophen<br>Aspirin (Salicylates)<br>Phenylbutazone |
| Excessively stimulating hydrochloric acid, providing aggravation and a chronicity factor | Histamine<br>Caffeine<br>Reserpine |
| Reducing mucosal resistance which yields to aggressive action of acid and pepsin | Cinchophen<br>Corticotropin and adrenal steroids<br>Phenylbutazone<br>Aspirin (Salicylates) |
| Interference with the reparative processes and the resultant delay in healing | Corticotropin<br>Antimetabolites (5-fluorouracil) |

TABLE 91
DRUG-INDUCED SYSTEMIC LUPUS ERYTHEMATOSUS

| | |
|---|---|
| Hydralazine hydrochloride (Apresoline®) | Diphenylhydantoin sodium (Dilantin®) |
| Penicillin | Mephenytoin (Mesantoin®) |
| Phenylbutazone | Trimethadione (Tridione®) |
| Sulfadiazine (Sulfonamides) | Primidone (Mysoline®) |
| Procainamide hydrochloride (Pronestyl®) | Ethosuximide (Zarontin®) and possibly other succinamides (Celontin® and Milontin®) |
| Isoniazid | Oral contraceptives |
| Heavy metals | Para-aminosalicylic acid |
| Thiourea derivatives | Hydralazine |
| Thiazides | Griseofulvin |
| Iodides | Tetracycline |
| Phenothiazines (Chlorpromazine, etc.) | |
| Quinidine | |

TABLE 92
DRUG REACTIONS IN THE AGED

| *Medication* | *Possible Side Effects* |
|---|---|
| Anesthesia and Analgesia | |
| Anesthetic gases or vapors | Dangerous stress |
| Ether | Sudden circulatory collapse |
| Cyclopropane | Inciting cardiac irritability |
| Local anesthetics | Hypothermia |
| Curare-like compounds | Respiratory embarrassment |
| Premedication | Effect more pronounced |
| Opiates | Respiratory depression (use 2/3 dose) |
| Meperidine | Bronchodilation |
| Phenylbutazone | Toxicity potential increased |
| Hypnotics and Tranquilizers | |
| Barbiturates | Increased sensitivity and bizarre response |
| Bromides | Increased bromism and impaired renal function |
| Phenothiazines | Extrapyramidal reactions |
| Hormones | |
| Corticosteroids | Electrolyte disturbances, edema, hypertension |
| Methandrostenolone | Increased BSP retention |
| Cardiovascular Drugs | |
| Anticoagulants | Intensification of action due to impaired renal function |
| Antihypertensives—Reserpine, Thiazides | Emotional distress<br>More frequent potassium loss |
| Cardiac glycosides | Possibility of toxic reactions |
| Vasopressors | Increased therapeutic action |
| Anti-infective Agents | Tendency toward accumulation, especially with long-acting sulfonamides |

term phenothiazine administration. Table 92 is a partial list of the drugs with which side-effects may occur in the geriatric patient and where reduction in dose seems indicated.

Dosage schedules in the young differ from those used in adult patients. It is not, however, always realized that the elderly patient may require special consideration where the dose of drugs is concerned. However, until the causes of altered drug pharmacology are better understood and clarified in the older age-groups, functional or biologic age is a more important guide than chronologic age as a factor in the modification of drug activity in human subjects.

## ACETAMINOPHEN (PARACETAMOL)

There is a general lack of knowledge in the United States, as compared to the European (especially the British) experience, concerning the toxicity of acetaminophen. This may be

TABLE 93
DRUGS CAPABLE OF CAUSING FIXED ERUPTIONS

Acetanilid
Aconite
Acriflavine
Aminopyrine
Amphetamine
Anthralin
Antihistaminic drugs
Antimony compounds
Antipyrine
Arsenicals
Barbiturates
Belladonna alkaloids
Chloral hydrate
Chloroquine phosphate
Cinchophen
Codeine
Copaiba
Diethylstilbestrol
Digitalis
Disulfiram
Emetine hydrochloride
Eosin
Ephedrine
Ergot
Formaldehyde solution
Hydantoins
Hydralazine
Iodine
Ipecac
Karaya gum
(legumes)
Meprobamate
Mercurials
Methenamine
Morphine
Opium
Oxyphenisatin acetate
Penicillin
Pentaerythritol tetranitrate
Phenacetin
Phenolphthalein
Phenothiazines
Potassium chlorate
Quinacrine hydrochloride
Quinine
Rauwolfia alkaloids
Reserpine
Saccharin
Salicylates
Streptomycin
Sulfonamides
Tartar emetic
Tetracyclines
Tetraiodofluorescein
Thiram
(vermouth)
(wormseed)

*Disseminated skin eruptions produced by drugs are common and usually easily recognized, but those that appear only in one or very few areas, the so called fixed eruptions, occur relatively infrequently and are often puzzling diagnostic problems. If the drug responsible for the "fixed eruption" is repeated at sufficiently long intervals, the lesion will heal either completely or partially and reappear in the same place with each renewed exposure to the offending medication. Thus the term "fixed" has an anatomic and not a temporal connotation.

TABLE 94
DRUGS AND STEVENS-JOHNSON SYNDROME (ERYTHEMA MULTIFORME)

| | |
|---|---|
| Sulfonamides | Aminosalicylic acid |
| (sulfamethoxypyridazine, | Penicillin |
| sulfamethoxine, | Chloramphenicol |
| sulfadiazine, | Chlorpropamide |
| sulfamerazine, | Measles vaccine |
| sulfathiazole) | Phensuximide |
| Hydralazine | Smallpox vaccine |
| Diphenylhydantoin | Phenobarbital |
| Trimethadione | Tetracycline |
| Phenylbutazone | Thiazide derivatives |
| Antipyrine | Clindamycin |

TABLE 95
DRUGS AND EXFOLIATIVE DERMATITIS

| | |
|---|---|
| Phenylbutazone | Allopurinol |
| Diphenylhydantoin | Actinomycin D |
| Sulfonamides | Barbiturates |
| Penicillin | Iodides |
| Gold salts | Mesantoin |
| Arsenicals | Phenacemide |
| Antimony compounds | Quinacrine |
| Mercurials | Quinidine |
| Aminosalicylic acid | Tetracycline |
| Chlorpropamide | Vitamin A |
| Phenothiazines | |

TABLE 96
DRUGS AND TOXIC EPIDERMAL NECROLYSIS

| | |
|---|---|
| Dapsone | Diphtheria inoculations |
| Phenylbutazone | Gold salts |
| Acetazolamide | Penicillin |
| Aminopyrine | Phenolphthalein |
| Sulfonamides | Polio vaccine |
| Diphenylhydantoin | Tetanus antitoxin |
| Nitrofurantoin | Tetracycline |
| Barbiturates | Tolbutamide |
| Brompheniramine | Allopurinol |

TABLE 97
DRUG-INDUCED MALABSORPTION

| *Drug* | *Nutrient Affected* |
|---|---|
| Biguanides, colchicine, digoxin, ethacrynic acid, 5-fluorouracil, indomethacin, L-dopa, neomycin, phenobarbital, salicylate, sulfonylureas | Glucose, xylose |
| Aminopterin, biguanides, colchicine, fenfluramine, kanamycin, neomycin | Triglycerides |
| Cholestyramine, colchicine, colestipol, neomycin | Fat-soluble vitamins |
| Biguanides, cortisone, neomycin, tetracyclines | Calcium |
| Allopurinol, cholestyramine, magnesium trisilicate, neomycin | Iron |
| Biguanides, colchicine, neomycin, para-aminobenzoic acid | Vitamin $B_{12}$ |
| Aminopterin, cholestyramine, diphenylhydantoin, neomycin, phenobarbital, salicylazosulfapyradine | Folic acid |
| Biguanides, cathartics, chlorothiazide, colchicine, ethacrynic acid | Water and electrolytes |

TABLE 98
DRUGS PRODUCING HYPERGLYCEMIA

| | |
|---|---|
| Nalidixic acid | Estrogens |
| Diphenylhydantoin | Corticosteroids |
| Lysergic acid diethylamide | Indomethacin |
| Isoniazid | Thiazides |
| Nicotinic acid | Caffeine |
| Oral contraceptives | Chlorpromazine |
| Epinephrine (and conegers) | Marihuana |
| Glucagon | Ethacrynic acid |
| Diazoxide | Salicylates |
| Thyroid | Nicotine |
| Androgens | |

due to the fact that serious acetaminophen poisoning is truly lacking in this country because these preparations are packaged in small volumes and low concentrations. The half-life of acetaminophen is short, one to two hours. This compound does not produce the gastrointestinal, hemorrhagic or the acid-base disturbances of aspirin, but it has a more subtle form of toxicity which can be serious and fatal with massive ingestion.

Patients ingesting toxic quantities of acetaminophen demonstrate three phases in their course. The *first* phase begins within hours after ingestion and consists mainly of anorexia, nausea, vomiting and diaphoresis. Patients are generally pale and feel quite ill. Coma or

TABLE 99
DRUGS PRODUCING GYNECOMASTIA*

| | |
|---|---|
| Estrogens | Amphetamines |
| Androgens | Radioiodine |
| Desoxycorticosterone | Oleandomycin |
| Digitalis | Tetracycline |
| Isoniazid | Vincristine |
| Griseofulvin | Phenothiazines |
| Reserpine | Heroin |
| Spironolactone | Marihuana |
| Progesterone | Clonidine |
| Gonadotropins | (Often sign of |
| Ant. pituitary extract | hyperthyroidism) |

*Gynecomastia has been reported in a number of patients receiving maintenance hemodialysis and the H2 receptor blocker, cimetidine.

CNS depression is not a feature unless they have ingested other drugs. In the *second* phase, these symptoms abate in severity but continue for a period of forty-eight hours. Meanwhile, hepatic enzymes, bilirubin and prothrombin time rise into the abnormal range as hepatonecrosis ensues. Clinically there is pain in the right hypochondrium as the liver becomes enlarged and tender. Urinary output may be reduced due to dehydration, renal damage and the antidiuretic effect of the drug. Rarely, anuria may develop in association with hepatic failure, but the BUN may be disproportionately low as the liver damage prevents formation of some urea. The *third* phase follows at three to five days and is marked by hepatic necrotic sequelae including jaundice, coagulation defects, hypoglycemia and encephalopathy as well as renal failure and myocardiopathy. Death is primarily due to hepatic failure and is dependent upon the degree of hepatic necrosis. Although acetaminophen is a metabolite of phenacetin, studies have not demonstrated the methemoglobin formation seen in chronic phenacetin abusers.

Acetaminophen is rapidly absorbed from the GI tract, with a peak plasma concentration reached within 70 to 160 minutes of ingestion. Once absorbed, a small portion is metabolized by the hepatic cytochrome[450] P oxidase system to an active intermediate metabolite which is thought to produce hepatotoxicity. It is normally detoxified by conjugation with glutathione and excreted via the urine. In the overdose situation, when glutathione is rapidly utilized and the stores drop to less than 30 per cent of normal, the unconjugated metabolite can bind to various hepatocellular constituents and produce necrosis, Liver damage may occur in adults who ingest more than 10 to 15 gm of acetaminophen (200 to 250 mg/kg, about thirty-five tablets). However, the degree of liver damage does not seem to correlate well with the amount of the ingested dose. A dose of 25 gm (approximately seventy-five tablets) or more in an adult is thought to be potentially fatal. Plasma half-life ($\tau$½) is the most consistently accurate method of predicting which patients will develop hepatic damage. If the $\tau$½ exceeds four hours, it may be assumed that liver damage has occurred. If the $\tau$½ exceeds twelve hours, hepatic coma is a possibility.

Single plasma levels are not as reliable in predicting outcome as multiple levels. British studies show that plasma levels greater than 300 mg/ml at four hours, or 120 mg/ml at twelve hours, were uniformly associated with hepatic injury, in contrast to the lack of toxicity at levels less than 120 mg/ml at four hours, or 50 mg/ml at twelve hours. It has therefore been suggested that patients with plasma levels between 120 mg/ml and 300 mg/ml at four hours, or 50 mg/ml and 120 mg/ml at twelve hours, should have repeat determinations so that $\tau$½ may be calculated.† It must be borne in mind, however, that it is usually very difficult to obtain the precise time of ingestion.

Fatalities have been reported with ingestion of 6 gm of acetaminophen. All patients who have ingested 5 gm or more should be hospitalized for monitoring and symptomatic and supportive therapy as needed in spite of the fact that patients have survived without toxicity having ingested three to four times that amount.

It is recommended that the use of antiemetics, aspirin and especially acetaminophen in children whose signs and symptoms (sudden onset of vomiting with CNS disturbance)

†Plot patients' plasma acetaminophen concentration against a line joining 200 μg/ml at 4 hours and 60 μg/ml at 12 hours on a semilog graph of concentration vs. time. If concentration is below this line, liver damage should be clinically insignificant, and treatment can be stopped.

suggest Reye's syndrome (RS) be discouraged for the following reasons. (1) The possibility exists, although unproven, that these drugs adversely affect the course of the disease. (2) The extrapyramidal signs caused by antiemetics may be confused with the CNS involvement in RS, which is now considered to be among the ten major causes of death in children aged one to ten years.

*Treatment.* Assessment and management of an acetaminophen overdose should proceed along two simultaneous paths. One involves a specific approach to the overdose itself, while the other involves a more general evaluation of encephalopathy and altered mental status.

Despite the rapid gastrointestinal absorption of acetaminophen, prevention of further absorption should be attempted up to twenty-four hours following ingestion. This should include induction of emesis or copious gastric lavage (depending in the patient's level of consciousness) and administration of a cathartic and activated charcoal (although of limited value with this agent). Forced diuresis may be beneficial in hastening the excretion of acetaminophen. However, as the drug's metabolites (glucuronide and sulfate conjugates) are rapidly excreted in the urine under normal circumstance, and since there is a possibility of renal tubular damage and antidiuresis, forcing fluids may be dangerous. If initiated, it must be instituted cautiously, with close monitoring of BUN and electrolytes. Hemodialysis reduces the $\tau$ ½ of acetaminophen, but there is no good evidence that it alters the clinical course, as hepatic injury is an early event. Peritoneal dialysis is ineffective because of the strong protein-binding properties of acetaminophen. Hemadsorption of acetaminophen over activated charcoal is still experimental. At present, the only hope of preventing hepatic injury appears to be administration of an agent that inactivates the toxic metabolites of acetaminophen, and at present, no such approved antidote exists. Therapeutic administration of glutathione has been attempted without success. The British literature reports successful treatment of acetaminophen overdosage with apparent protection from significant hepatic necrosis using parenterally administered cysteine and cysteamine (glutathione precursors capable of crossing cell membranes). It is theorized that these precursors, like glutathione, can inactivate the toxic intermediate metabolite via preferential conjugation. These agents, however, have not been approved and are still considered experimental in the United States.

Oral methionine (Pedameth®), 2.5 gm every four hours up to 10 gm, has recently been found effective in reducing the frequency and severity of acetaminophen-induced liver damage. Although this compound has few side-effects and is of low toxicity, it does have the potential to aggravate a preexisting hepatic disease, and therefore should only be given early (before ten hours) after ingestion, before the likely acetaminophen hepatic effects take place (Goulding, R. et al.: Oral Methionine in the Treatment of Severe Paracetamol [Acetaminophen] Overdose. *Lancet, 2, 7990*:829-830, 1976).

N-Acetylcysteine (Mucomyst®), based on preliminary evaluation, appears to act as a glutathione substitute and to directly combine with the toxic acetaminophen metabolite. It is presently being recommended as the oral drug of choice (loading dose of 140 mg/kg followed by 70 mg/kg every four hours for a total of eighteen doses), if given within twelve hours after ingestion. Acetylcysteine must be given early to be effective in blocking the covalent binding of the toxic metabolite that produces hepatic necrosis.

Once severe hepatic toxicity has occurred, treatment is supportive, with the hope that hepatic function will return. Administration of high-dose steroids, exchange transfusion, cross-circulation with laboratory animals and liver transplantation have all been performed with varying degrees of success. Anthihistamines, high- and low-dose steroids and ethacrynic acid may enhance acetaminophen toxicity and should be avoided.

## ACONITINE (ACONITE)

Aconitine is an almost obsolete drug formerly used widely for its antipyretic action and depressant effects on the heart. It is obtained from a plant often cultivated in gardens and known as wolfsbane or monkshood. The active substance is the alkaloid aconitine. The lethal dose is 2 to 4 mg of aconitine or 15 to 30 ml of the tincture. The stimulation of the medullary centers caused by aconite results in slowing of the heart and reduction of blood pressure. The drug also stimulates the peripheral sensory system, and tingling of the skin and mucosa is prominent after both local and systemic use. Overdose causes nausea, vomiting, cardiovascular collapse, dyspnea, chest pain, restlessness, diplopia and shock. Death usually occurs from direct paralysis of the heart.

*Treatment* is purely symptomatic. Aconite is not employed any more in modern therapeutics for its systemic actions, due to its toxicity and because therapeutic doses border on the dangerous. However, poisoning still occurs from confusion of aconite with other plants such as horseradish. Inasmuch as cutaneous absorption can occur and cause serious poisoning, aconite is seldom used for its local counterirritant and anodyne effects.

## ALUMINUM COMPOUNDS

Aluminum is a bluish-white, malleable, radiopaque metal that is handled in the form of ingots, sheets, leaves and powder, only the latter being of toxicological importance. Aluminum acetate is a white powder of slightly acidic odor used as a mordant, siccative, astringent and deodorant. Aluminum chloride is another soluble salt used for its astringent and antiseptic effects. Aluminum ammonium sulfate (alum) is used as a styptic agent, for the purification of water, in baking powder and in various industries. Concentrated solutions used as a mouthwash can cause severe stomatitis and gingivitis with necrosis. The ingestion of such solutions produces hemorrhagic gastritis. Insoluble aluminum hydroxide, on the other hand, is used primarily for its demulcent and absorbent actions as in antacid agents. It exerts its antacid effect by a chemical reaction with HCl, which results in the formation of $AlCl_3$. In the intestinal tract, the aluminum chloride reacts with the alkaline secretions to form basic aluminum salts which are not absorbed and therefore do not affect the acid-base balance nor impair renal function. Aluminum hydroxide, which has been widely used in dialysis therapy to lower serum phosphate levels by decreasing phosphorus absorption from the gut through the formation of insoluble aluminum phosphate, has been incriminated as the probable causative agent for dialysis dementia (encephalopathy). Discontinuing its use has largely eliminated this complication.

Aluminum hydroxide is essentially a nontoxic compound. Long-term administration to animals of doses many times greater than those employed in patients has not caused untoward effects. Some individuals are intolerant to the astringent action of the drug and experience nausea and vomiting. Constipation as a result of the astringent action can be circumvented by combined therapy with a mildly cathartic antacid such as magnesium oxide or trisilicate.

The soluble salts as aluminum acetate and chloride may occasionally cause dermatitis of various types and degrees that necessitate discontinuance of therapy. However, serious manifestations of toxicity are not usually seen. The ingestion of traces of aluminum through the use of cooking utensils is harmless.

## AMPHETAMINES (*See* SYMPATHOMIMETIC AMINES)

## ANESTHETICS, GENERAL

The compounds most commonly used for general anesthesia are ether, halothane, chloroform, nitrous oxide, methoxyflurane (Penthrane®), ethyl chloride cyclopropane and ethylene. Ketamine hydrochloride (Ketaject®, Ketalar®) is a noninhalation general anesthetic (IM, IV) used mainly for brief surgical and diagnostic procedures (adverse effects are distinct and recognizable). The symptoms of toxicity and the treatment are approximately the same for all (*also see* Ether).

Symptoms include deepened unconsciousness, rapid heart, loss of reflexes and cardiac and respiratory failure. A toxic nephropathy associated with methoxyflurane anesthesia has been documented with marked diuresis instead of diminished urine volume as the predominate clinical finding.

*Treatment* consists of discontinuing the anesthetic, oxygen inhalations under slightly positive pressure, caffeine and sodium benzoate 0.5 gm (7½ gr) subcutaneously, pentylenetetrazol (Metrazol) 0.2 gm (3 gr) IV. If complete cardiac arrest occurs, not over five minutes are available to reestablish the heartbeat. Every physician who performs any surgical procedures should have a routine laid out in advance for this possible reaction.

The most effective measures follow.

1. Indirect cardiac massage.
2. Striking the precordium forcibly with the fist.
3. Epinephrine (Adrenalin®) hydrochloride (1:1000 solution) 15 minims (1 ml) intracardially may be tried using a long lumbar puncture needle inserted next to the sternum in the third or fourth left interspace and directed medially and downward. To be of any possible benefit this injection must be made into the cavity of either ventricle; if the ventricular muscle is injected there is a tendency to cause fibrillation. Intravenous procaine is of little, if any, value.
4. Direct cardiac massage. If the chest is opened, the importance of ensuring adequate oxygenation of the cardiac muscle through massage of the heart or adjacent large vessels should not be overlooked. This applies even in the presence of fibrillation.

Drug interactions in anesthesia are common and often catastrophic. Before a patient undergoes anesthesia, his past and present drug therapy history for side-effects should be thoroughly discussed, and the anesthesiologist should be familiar with the relevant standard effects of the drugs used and the possibilities of interactions that exist among them, as well as with the anesthetic agents to be used (for extensive listing and discussion of interactions, *see Drug Therapy,* January 1976).

## ANESTHETICS, LOCAL

Systemic toxic symptoms are usually due to inadvertent injection of the local anesthetic intravascularly, injection into highly vascular tissue or rapid absorption of topically applied drugs from inflamed mucous membranes (*also see* Procaine). The major toxic effects are convulsions, circulatory depression (shock) and respiratory depression. Vasovagal reaction is the most common cause of fainting with dental anesthesia. Shock is usually due to myocardial depression and peripheral vasodilatation. Most instances of sudden cardiovascular collapse occur with topical application of a local anesthetic to the respiratory tract.

Systemic sympathomimetic symptoms such as nervousness, tachycardia, increased blood pressure and angina pectoris occur chiefly when a local anesthetic containing a vasoconstrictor is injected directly into a vein. Injection of a vasoconstrictor into a vein can also cause serious drug interactions if the patient has been taking a monoamine oxidase inhibiting drug as an antidepressant or as an antihypertensive. The hazard of an adverse effect on the normal or diseased cardiovascular system from the small amount of epinephrine in dental local anesthetics has been somewhat exaggerated. The main hazard of vasoconstrictors is their use where circulation is easily compromised; they can cause necrosis in tight tissue compartments such as the digits, nose, ears and penis.

Allergic reactions to local anesthetics are rare; skin reactions may occur in dentists and in persons who use preparations containing local anesthetics for the relief of sunburn and other minor burns, wound pain, itching or hemorrhoids. Methylparaben and other parabens used as preservatives in some local anesthetic preparations are capable of causing allergic reactions when administered topically.

Hypersensitivity to a local anesthetic cannot be determined reliably by skin testing or by instillation into the conjunctivae. Therefore, a careful history of allergic reactions to a particular drug should be obtained from the patient before administering a local anesthetic.

Neonatal asphyxia has been reported with cyanosis, apnea, bradycardia and convulsions from faulty maternal caudal anesthesia (mepivacaine, Carbocaine®) where the drug has been introduced directly into the fetus. In addition, placentral transfer and biologic transformation possibilities need further study. Prilocaine, though less toxic to the cardiovascular and central nervous system, can cause reversible methemoglobinemia which may progress to cyanosis. Like other local anesthetics, it does cross the placental barrier to produce methemoglobinemia and cyanosis in the fetus. A benzocaine-containing teething gel produced methemoglobinemia (severe cyanosis) twenty to thirty minutes after topical application in a fourteen-month-old infant without abnormal hemoglobins.

*Treatment* is different for the early convulsive stage and for the later shock stage. The administration of oxygen with a manually operated ventilation device is usually sufficient to control anoxia in the convulsive stage and it avoids the need to administer a central nervous system depressant such as a barbiturate. With the respiratory depression that frequently accompanies shock caused by local anesthetics, the indication for assisted respira-

TABLE 100
LOCAL ANESTHETICS

| *Local Anesthetic* | *Indications* | *Action** |
|---|---|---|
| *Para-aminobenzoic acid esters* | | |
| Procaine (Novocain and other brands) | Infiltration; nerve block | Short |
| Chloroprocaine (Nesacaine and other brands) | Infiltration; nerve block | Short |
| Tetracaine (Pontocaine) | Topical, respiratory tract; infiltration; spinal; nerve block | Long |
| *Benzoic acid esters* | | |
| Cocaine | Topical, respiratory tract | Medium |
| *Amides* | | |
| Lidocaine (Xylocaine and other brands) | Topical, respiratory tract; infiltration; spinal; nerve block | Medium |
| Mepivacaine (Carbocaine) | Infiltration; nerve block | Medium |
| Prilocaine (Citanest) | Infiltration; nerve block | Medium |

*Duration depends not only on intrinsic pharmacological properties, but also on volume and concentration of the solution and whether it is combined with a vasoconstrictor. For infiltration, most local anesthetics are effective in a 0.25% to 1% concentration; for nerve and epidural block, in a 1% to 2% concentration; for topical application to the respiratory tract, in a 1% to 5% concentration.

tion along with other measures is more urgent than with other causes of shock. Because of reduced cardiac output and peripheral vasodilatation in local anesthetic shock, the use of a vasopressor agent which has both vasoconstrictive and heart stimulating (inotropic) effects, such as levarterenol bitartrate (norepinephrine, Levophed) is indicated. Initial doses range from 5 to 50 μg, with smaller doses used for maintenance. Plasma volume expanders should be used if necessary and precede the administration of vasopressor agents (*see* Chap. 1 for treatment of methemoglobinemia if it occurs).

## ANTHELMINTICS

A primary consideration in the choice of an anthelmintic is its ease of administration, therapeutic index and a minimum of side-effects. Many of the compounds still being employed are therapeutic relics and moreover are highly toxic. New synthetic drugs are rapidly displacing the older empirical agents. They are safe and clinically more effective and are the anthelmintics of choice. Table 101 includes most of the old and more recent anthelmintics now being used and their potential toxicity.

TABLE 101
ANTHELMINTICS

| *Drug* | *Helminth* | *Side-Effects* | *Treatment* |
|---|---|---|---|
| Aspidium Oleoresin (Male Fern) | Tapeworm | Gastroenteritis, xanthopsia, amblyopia, jaundice, vertigo, myalgia, trismus, coma and convulsions | Symptomatic. Saline cathartic to remove the drug from the intestinal tract. Control convulsions with short-acting barbiturates. |
| Thiabendazole (Mintezol®) | Oxyuris<br>Ascaris<br>Strongyloides<br>Hookworm<br>Trichinosis<br>Larva migrans | Nausea, vomiting, vertigo, headache, marked weakness, leukopenia and crystalluria | Discontinue use or reduce dosage. |
| Kousso (Cusso) | Tapeworm | Chemically related to aspidium, but less active and less toxic | Symptomatic and supportive. |
| Pelletierine Tannate | Tapeworm (*Taenia solium*) | Gastroenteritis, dizziness, mydriasis, muscle weakness, paralysis and respiratory depression | Saline cathartic. Symptomatic. Support respiration and use respirator if indicated. |
| Chenopodium Oil | Ascaris | Gastroenteritis, tinnitus, amblyopia, hepatic and renal injury; profound depression followed by coma | Saline cathartic. Supportive for circulatory and central nervous system depression. |
| Santonin | Ascaris | Xanthopsia, headache, vomiting, confusion, diarrhea, convulsions, respiratory and circulatory failure | Saline cathartic. Symptomatic and supportive for convulsions, circulatory and respiratory depression. |
| Thymol | Hookworm | *See* Phenol. The systemic effects, however, are not as severe unless unusually large amounts are ingested | (*See* Phenol.) |
| Betanaphthol | Hookworm | Gastroenteritis, hepatic and renal damage, hemolytic anemia and convulsions | Gastric lavage followed by 2 to 3 oz. of vegetable oil, blood transfusions and symptomatic. |
| Carbon Tetrachloride | Hookworm | *See* Chapter 3. Has been replaced by tetrachloroethylene | |
| Tetrachloroethylene | Hookworm<br>Ascaris<br>Whipworm | Similar to carbon tetrachloride, except far less toxic | *See* Chapter 3. |

TABLE 101—*Continued*
ANTHELMINTICS

| *Drug* | *Helminth* | *Side-effects* | *Treatment* |
|---|---|---|---|
| Methylrosaniline Chloride (Gentian Violet) | Strongyloides<br>Oxyuris | Nausea, vomiting, diarrhea and abdominal cramps | Discontinue use or reduce dosage. |
| Hexylresorcinol | Hookworm<br>Ascaris<br>Oxyuris<br>Dwarf Tapeworm<br>Whipworm | Local irritant when applied in high concentration. Oral administration can cause gastroenteritis and irritation of the mouth. Systemic toxicity of the drug is low | Discontinue use. |
| Diethylcarbamazine (Hetrazan®) | Filarial nematodes | Fever, leukocytosis, lymphadenitis, joint pains, headache, malaise, nausea, vomiting and skin rashes | Discontinue use or reduce dosage. |
| Pyrvinium Pamoate (Povan) | Oxyuris | Nausea, vomiting and diarrhea. Stools are colored bright red (spilled material will stain) | Discontinue use or reduce dosage. |
| Piperazine | Oxyuris<br>Ascaris | Nausea, vomiting, diarrhea, methemoglobinemia, blurred vision and general muscle weakness with ataxia and loss of reflexes which are reversible. EEG abnormalities are common. Precipitated petit mal seizures have been reported | Discontinue use or reduce dosage. |
| Phenothiazine N.F. | Veterinary preparations for helminthic infestations in domestic animals. | Hemolytic anemia, drug fever and skin rashes | Discontinue use. Alkalinize urine. Blood transfusion if indicated. |
| Miracil D (Nilodin®) | Schistosoma (flukes) | Nausea, vomiting, vertigo, tremors, headache, sweating, hepatic and renal damage and convulsions | Discontinue use. Symptomatic and supportive. |
| Thiabendazole (Mintezol®) | Toxocariasis<br>Trichinosis | Nausea, vomiting, crystalluria (odor to urine), Steven-Johnson syndrome | Discontinue use. |
| Mebendazole (Vermox®) | Oxyuris<br>Ascaris<br>Whipworm | Nausea, abdominal pain and diarrhea. Contraindicated in pregnancy | Symptomatic and supportive. |
| Antimony Compounds (Fuadin®, Tartrates) | Schistosoma (flukes) | *See* Chapter 3. | |
| Chloroquine (Aralen) | Giardia<br>Tapeworm | *See* Chapter 6. | |
| Quinacrine (Atabrine®) | Giardia<br>Tapeworm | *See* Chapter 6. | |
| Bephenium Hydroxynaphthoate (Alcopara®) | Hookworm<br>Ascaris | Nausea, vomiting, diarrhea and abdominal pain | Discontinue use or reduce dosage. |
| Pyrantel Pamoate | Ascaris<br>Oxyuris | Nausea, vomiting, abdominal cramps, anorexia and transient elevation of SGOT levels | Use only for ascaris and oxyuris. Do not use concomitantly with piperazine or if liver dysfunction exists. |

## ANTIBIOTICS AND CHEMOTHERAPEUTICS

The discovery, development and production of antibiotics and chemotherapeutic agents for the treatment of infectious diseases and infections constitutes one of the greatest advances of all time in medical therapeutics. However, in the choice of any anti-infective

| | | |
|---|---|---|
| *Metabolic or Endocrine Effects* | | |
| Weight gain* | Hypothalamic effect | Small rations |
| Edema | Increased antidiuretic hormone secretion | Wait |
| Lactation, gynecomastia, menstrual irregularities | Estrogenic effect | Reassurance |
| False pregnancy test | Urinary metabolite (?) | Use immunologic tests |
| Impotency in men, increased libido in women | Estrogenic effect | Reassurance |
| *Miscellaneous* | | |
| Unexpected deaths | Dose; previous brain damage or seizures | Completely unpredictable; watch doses in known seizure patients |
| Hypostatic pneumonia; trophic ulcers | Age; neglect | Adequate nursing care |
| Anesthetic complications | Blocked pressor reflexes | Stop drug prior to elective surgery |
| Local inflammation, gangrene | At injection site or perivenous leakage | Avoid parenteral drug when possible |
| Electrocardiographic abnormalities | Vagolytic, quinidine-like effects | Uncertain |
| Potentiation of other drugs, alcohol | Dose | Avoid polypharmacy; warn patient |
| Teratogenic effects | Phocomelia with trifluoperazine; not established | Avoid drugs in fertile or pregnant women as much as possible |
| Pigmentary retinopathy | Toxic doses | Keep dose under 800 mg daily of thioridazine |
| Melanin pigmentation; corneal and lens deposits | Chlorpromazine 2 years or more; high dose | Switch to "low-dose" piperazine derivative |

*Thioxanthine, amitriptyline and lithium carbonate are other drugs that can produce weight gain.
Hollister, L. E.: *JAMA, 189*:311, 1964.

2 mg/kg and biperiden hydrochloride (Akineton®) have been even more effective in the treatment of these complications. As a matter of fact, the marked response to diphenhydramine often aids diagnosis. Recent reports, however, indicate that intravenous diazepam is the agent of choice for the management of drug-induced dystonia.

In summary, the following are the important points in management.

1. Ingestions are frequently multiple.
2. Recurrence is frequent.
3. If short-acting barbiturates are required to manage convulsions secondary to neuroleptic overdosage, the dosage should be reduced because of the potentiation of CNS depression.
4. Severe dystonias secondary to neuroleptic overdose should be managed with non-atropinizing antiparkinsonism agents, especially if tricyclic antidepressants are also taken, since neuroleptic-tricyclic antidepressant combination can give an atropine psychosis.
5. Phenothiazine overdose may block effects of emetics.
6. Dialysis and forced diuresis are not effective for phenothiazine and tricyclic antidepressant overdose.
7. Tricyclic antidepressant overdose (*see* page 472) has significant atropine-like central nervous system effects and peripheral effects; the latter are particularly grave in relation to the cardiovascular system. Physostigmine salicylate (Antilirium) 1 to 3 mg IV has been effective in managing both central and peripheral effects. Physostigmine has also been reported to reverse phenothiazine-induced coma in a child. Neostigmine (Prostigmin®) and pyridostigmine (Mestinon®) have been useful in managing the peripheral atropine-like effects.
8. There may be a "rebound" of symptoms of tricyclic antidepressant overdose seventy-two hours or more after initial satisfactory response to treatment. This includes cardiac effects.
9. Extreme caution is necessary when using sympathomimetics, stimulants or sedatives in the management of monoamine oxidase inhibitor overdose.
10. Effects of phenothiazine overdose are maximum within four to six hours; with monoamine oxidase inhibitors, more than twenty-four hours may be required.

## ATROPINE (BELLADONNA, STRAMONIUM)

It is a rare home that does not have at least one preparation containing atropine or some other belladonna derivative in the medicine cabinet. These alkaloids are widely used for ophthalmic, cutaneous, rectal and gastrointestinal conditions, and overdosage is often not readily recognized.

Although infants appear to tolerate unusually large therapeutic doses in gastrointestinal colic, they (and retarded children in particular) are ordinarily quite sensitive to atropine. Thus intoxication may follow if, through error, eye drops are instilled in the nose. Severe toxic symptoms may also occur when atropine or scopolamine is substituted for the weaker drug, homatropine. Finally, accidental ingestion and eating berries or seeds containing belladonna alkaloids, as in the jimsonweed, may cause poisoning. While all parts of this plant are poisonous, the seeds are especially toxic since they contain scopolamine and hyoscyamine as well as atropine. Attempts at suicide, or rarely hypersensitivity, have produced their share of acutely ill patients, but only a few deaths. Asthmador® is a proprietary drug sold in powder form to be ignited and the vapors inhaled for the relief of asthma.* It contains two solanaceous herbs, *Atropa belladonna* and *Datura stramonium,* and has produced severe psychotic state (agitation, confusion, hallucinations, ataxia and slurred speech) and physical signs of atropinization in students who have ingested this preparation "for kicks." Asthmador and other asthma

*Asthmador has recently been discontinued in the United States as an over-the-counter asthma remedy.

powders are popular with the younger set because of their availability and lack of legal restrictions. They may also be incorporated into various hallucinogenic drugs to potentiate their effect or for economic deception to stretch the supply of a true hallucinogen. Hallucinations occur in about 50 per cent of the users; delirium and serious toxic symptoms are seen in only 25 per cent. Five deaths are known to have occurred due to impairment of judgment and physical coordination from the effects of stramonium-containing asthma powders.

The fatal dose of atropine is not known, although 10 to 20 mg in children and about 100 mg in adults have been estimated as lethal. Wide variation in tolerance is known to exist, however, and patients have survived ingestion of as much as 1 gm of the drug.

Signs and symptoms of atropine poisoning develop quickly and have vividly been described as "Hot as a hare, blind as a bat, dry as a bone, red as a beet, and mad as a wet hen." The first manifestation is an almost immediate sensation of dryness and burning of the mouth. Talking and swallowing become difficult or impossible. There is intense thirst. Blurred vision and marked photophobia reflect the pupillary dilatation and loss of accommodation. The skin becomes flushed, hot and dry. Tachycardia and fever develop, the temperature sometimes rising to the alarming height of 42.8°C (109°F) in infants. The heart rate, however, may not rise unduly in infants and old people. The desire to void urine is present, but there is difficulty in doing so.

These signs and symptoms are often accompanied by marked confusion and muscular incoordination. Mania, delirium and frankly psychotic behavior may develop and continue for hours or days. A rash may appear, followed by desquamation, especially in the region of the face, neck and upper trunk. Circulatory and respiratory collapse occur with more severe overdosage.

The diagnosis of atropine poisoning is not always easy because the victim is frequently mistaken for a psychotic. In children, the marked skin flush and high temperature suggest the onset of an exanthematous infection. Diagnosis is usually made on the history of drug ingestion plus the confirmatory signs and symptoms. Injection of 10 to 30 mg of methacholine may be used as a pharmacologic test of intoxication. Failure to produce moistening of the mucous membrances of the mouth, lacrimation, sweating and gastrointestinal hyperactivity help to confirm the impression of an overdose of atropine or a belladonna alkaloid. A useful biologic test is to place one drop of the patient's urine in a cat's eye. If atropine is being excreted, mydriasis promptly occurs.

The *treatment* of atropine poisoning is mainly symptomatic; no specific antidote is available. If a patient is seen almost immediately after ingestion of the drug, the stomach should be lavaged, preferably with a 4% tannic acid solution. This must be done at once if it is to accomplish anything, because atropine is rapidly absorbed from the gastrointestinal tract.

The patient should be placed in a darkened room to avoid irritation of the eyes or a miotic may be instilled. Small doses of pilocarpine are useful for its parasympathomimetic effect and for improving the visual disturbance and dry mouth. The serious features of intoxication produced by the central action of atropine are, however, uninfluenced by oral pilocarpine nitrate, which now is available only in bulk powder form in the United States. The increased body temperature, which may be a severe problem in children, is treated with ice packs and sponging. Oxygen is indicated if respiration is inadequate, and a respirator may be required. For the manic patient or the occasional patient in convulsions, small doses of barbiturates, chloral hydrate or paraldehyde are recommended; large doses are contraindicated because they depress respiratory action. Occasionally an indwelling catheter is necessary if the patient has difficulty in initiating micturition. Pilocarpine in 10 to 15 mg doses or methacholine in 10 to 30 mg doses (although not effective against the serious central symptoms) can alleviate the dryness of the mouth and mydriasis which may often be the most annoying symptoms.

Anticholinesterase agents reverse the action of atropine, but most of these drugs, e.g. pyridostigmine and neostigmine (Prostigmine), have quaternary ammonium groups which do not cross the blood-brain barrier and therefore are ineffective against the central action of atropine and atropine-like compounds; physostigmine, on the other hand, is a tertiary amine and readily enters the brain. When a diagnosis of delirium or coma due to atropine-like drugs is made, 2 mg physostigmine should be given IM or IV and repeated every fifteen to thirty minutes if necessary, since this drug has a very short half-life. Phenothiazine has a central atropine-like action and is contraindicated in the treatment.

A rabbit serum enzyme (azolesterase) has been found effective in the treatment of atropine, homatropine and benzoylcholine chloride poisoning. It has little or no effect on other alkaloids and apparently increases the toxicity of amprotropine phosphate. Until the enzyme-containing fraction is isolated and further clinical studies made, the therapeutic value of this preparation is still undetermined.

Scopolamine intoxication is of importance because it is contained in commonly used proprietary preparations (Sominex®, etc.). The toxic dose of scopolamine is 3 to 5 mg (12 to 20 Sominex tablets) and the fatal dose of atropine is about 100 mg. Specific side-effects include widely dilated pupils, delirium and hyperirritability (psychosis), tachycardia, dry mouth, warm skin and coma.

Scopolamine differs from atropine in that tachycardia and hyperirritability are less likely, and loss of consciousness may occur sooner. The following diagnostic test has been suggested in questionable cases.

Inject 10 to 30 mg methacholine (Mecholyl®) SC. Absence of resulting salivation, lacrimation, sweating, or hyperactivity of the intestinal tract is good evidence of atropine or scopolamine poisoning.

Specific *treatment* is as outlined above for atropine with particular emphasis on the use of physostigmine salicylate as the antidote of choice.

## BARBITURATES*

Acute barbiturate intoxication is a potentially fatal form of poisoning in which the eventual clinical outcome is often solely related to the level of supervision and care that is provided by attending physicians and nurses. In contrast to many other forms of poisoning, acute barbiturate intoxication is more often purposeful than accidental, more common in adults than children and especially frequent among members of the medical profession and its allied disciplines. A past history of one or more suicidal attempts can often be elicited and the importance of follow-up psychiatric care cannot be emphasized too strongly. It also represents a form of intoxication in which an elemental knowledge of the clinical pharmacology of barbiturates is an absolute prerequisite to optimum and intelligent management.

### *Clinical Pharmacology of Barbiturates*

All barbiturates are chemical derivatives of barbituric acid (Fig. 15). The pharmacologic characteristics of each drug are largely determined by the chemical nature of the side chains at $R_1$ and $R_2$. In general, those agents with long side chains possess a short duration of action and a high degree of potency, and hepatic degradation contributes importantly to their inactivation. In contrast, those agents with shorter side chains exhibit a longer duration of action and less potency, and

*Robinson, R.R. (Professor of Medicine and Chief, Division of Nephrology, Dept. of Medicine, Duke University Med. Center, Durham, N.C.); Treatment of Acute Barbiturate Intoxication. In Arena, Jay (Ed): Symposium on advances in the treatment of poisoning *Mod Treat 8*:561, 1971.

excretion by the kidneys provides a more important means for their elimination from the body. Pharmacologic characteristics of greatest importance to therapy have been listed in Table 110 for each of the common barbiturates.

### *pK*

The pK is equivalent to the pH at which the ionized and non-ionized forms of an acid or base are equal in concentration. All barbiturates are weak organic acids whose pK values range between 7.2 and 8.0 (Table 110). From the shape of the titration curve of a weak acid against a base (Fig. 16), it can be seen that a weak acid whose pK is close to the physiologic pH is less ionized in biologic fluids than one whose pK is considerably higher. For example, about 5 per cent of the total concentration of phenobarbital (pK 7.2) is non-ionized at pH 7.4, whereas 98 per cent of secobarbital (pK 7.9) is non-ionized at the same pH. Obviously, minor pH alterations can effect large changes in per cent ionization if the pK of the drug is close to the physiologic pH. Phenobarbital is 50 per cent nonionized at pH 7.2 but less than 4 per cent non-ionized at pH 7.5. Conversely, the degree of ionization is affected very little by pH changes of a similar nature when the pK is relatively high (secobarbital is 99% non-ionized at pH 7.2 and 98% non-ionized at pH 7.5).

This physicochemical characteristic of weak acids is of great importance because it is generally held that lipid-containing biologic membranes are freely permeable to the non-ionized species but relatively impermeable to the ionized form. Consequently, the passive diffusion and eventual distribution of total barbiturate across a given cellular surface (gastric mucosa, blood-brain barrier, adipose tissue, etc.) are greatly influenced by the pH gradient across that particular cell wall. Non-ionized barbiturates diffuse passively across cellular membranes from an area of high concentration (the relatively acid side of the membrane) to an area of lower concentration (the relatively alkaline side of the membrane) until diffusion equilibrium is achieved.

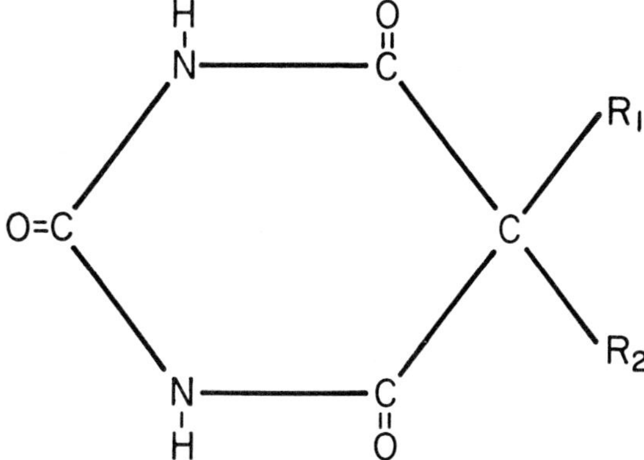


Figure 15. Chemical structure for derivatives of barbituric acid.

TABLE 110
PHYSICOCHEMICAL PROPERTIES OF COMMON BARBITURATES

| *Generic name* | *Proprietary name* | *pK* | *Lipid partition coefficient** | *Plasma protein binding (%)* | *Fatal dose (gm)* | *Fatal plasma conc. (mg/100 ml)* |
|---|---|---|---|---|---|---|
| *Long-acting* (>6 hours) | | | | | | |
| Barbital | Veronal | 7.74 | 1 | 5 | 10 | 15 |
| Phenobarbital | Luminal | 7.24 | 3 | 20 | 5 | 8 |
| *Intermediate-acting* (3–6 hours) | | | | | | |
| Amobarbital | Amytal | 7.75 | | | | |
| Butabarbital | Butisol | 7.74 | | | | |
| *Short-acting* (<3 hours) | | | | | | |
| Pentobarbital | Nembutal | 7.96 | 39 | 35 | 3 | 3.5 |
| Secobarbital | Seconal | 7.90 | 52 | 44 | 3 | 3.5 |

*Between methyl chloride and an aqueous buffer. Higher coefficients reflect greater solubility in lipid.

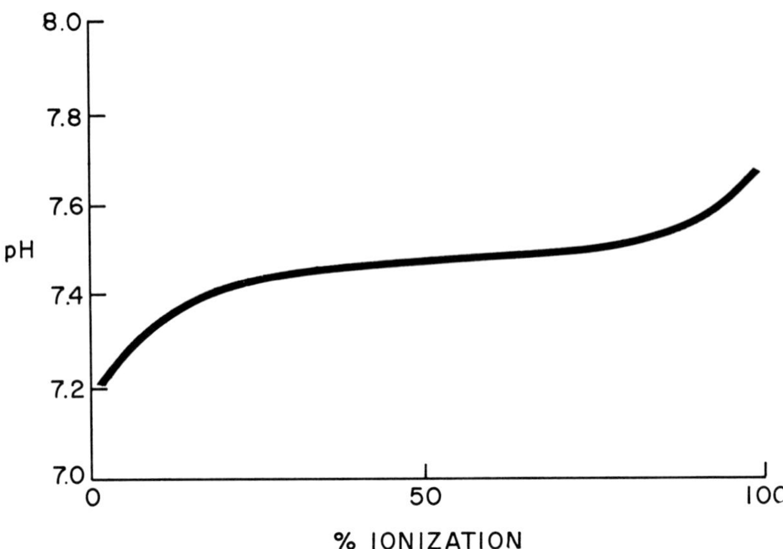


Figure 16. Titration curve for a weak organic acid (pK 7.5) against a base. Curve is similarly shaped for most barbiturates although its relationship to the vertical pH scale will vary according to specific pK value of each drug (pH = pK = 50% ionization.)

At equilibrium, the transmembrane concentrations of non-ionized barbiturate are equal, but the concentration of total barbiturate (non-ionized plus ionized forms) is always higher on the more alkaline side because the per cent contribution of non-ionized to total acid is lower at the higher pH. This is an important reason barbiturates are so rapidly absorbed from the acid gastric contents (where all barbiturates are almost 100% non-ionized and therefore freely diffusible) into the relatively alkaline blood. Of course, barbiturates such as phenobarbital which are ionized more completely within the physiologic range of blood pH are much less lipid-soluble and therefore enter peripheral tissues much less completely than agents such as secobarbital which are almost completely non-ionized at any physiologic blood pH (*see above*). This circumstance contributes to the fact that phenobarbital administration is accompanied by higher plasma concentrations of total barbiturate (but lower tissue concentrations) than those observed after equivalent doses of secobarbital. Agents such as secobarbital are so highly soluble in lipid that their rate of transfer across biologic membranes is mainly limited by their rate of delivery to the membrane itself. Although much less lipid-soluble throughout the usual range of blood pH, the tissue penetrance of agents such as phenobarbital can still vary considerably because their degree of ionization is so responsive to minor changes of blood pH; their tissue solubility may be enhanced during systemic acidosis and diminished during systemic alkalosis.

### *Duration of Action*

The duration of action of any barbiturate is determined by a complex interrelationship between many variables: dose, rate of absorption, rate of metabolic degradation or excretion of the active drug, drug tolerance and rate of removal of nonmetabolized and active drug from the central nervous system. There is good correlation between duration of action and the mechanism by which active drug is eliminated from the body. Short-acting agents are principally eliminated via hepatic degradation with the subsequent excretion of inactive metabolites in urine. Hepatic degradation plays a lesser role in the elimination of long– and intermediate-acting agents. The renal excretion of unaltered and therefore active drug provides a much more important route of disposal for these agents.

*Hepatic Degradation*

All barbiturates undergo metabolic degradation by the liver to some degree. Metabolic disposal by this organ is a relatively rapid process as compared to the rate at which barbiturates are excreted in the urine. After ingestion, the short-acting drugs are initially and rapidly sequestered in the tissues so that their effect on the central nervous system is terminated rapidly. These agents are then mobilized slowly and immediately degraded by the liver, and their inactive metabolites are then excreted in urine. Longer-acting drugs such as phenobarbital rely more heavily on the slower process of urinary excretion.

*Renal Excretion*

Unaltered drug is first filtered at the glomerulus, after which it undergoes net renal tubular reabsorption via a pH-dependent process of passive diffusion. The passive renal tubular reabsorption of these weak organic acids can be diminished (and excretion thereby increased) by reducing the concentration of the diffusible or non-ionized form of the drug at the reabsorptive site via an increase in either the volume or pH of tubular fluid. Osmotic diuresis increases the excretion of most barbiturates by increasing the volume of fluid at the reabsorptive site. In contrast, urinary alkalinization does not increase urinary excretion greatly except in the case of agents such as phenobarbital whose pK values are well below 8.0, which is the maximum urine pH. Variations in tubular fluid pH exert much less effect on the urinary excretion of drugs such as pentobarbital or secobarbital whose pK values are close to 8.0. In the case of secobarbital (pK 7.9, the tubular fluid concentration of its freely diffusible (and therefore readily reabsorbed) non-ionized form can be reduced to no less than 50 per cent of the total concentration—even assuming that a pH of 7.9 could be maintained throughout the nephron for a sufficiently long period to be of practical benefit.

*Plasma Protein Binding*

All barbiturates are bound by plasma proteins to varying degrees (*see* Table 110). This factor is important because the extent of protein binding greatly influences filterability at the glomerulus (and thereby the rapidity of renal excretion) and the ease with which the drug can be removed from the body via procedures such as hemodialysis or peritoneal dialysis. In general, long-acting barbiturates are much less bound to the plasma proteins, and hence more dialyzable, than are the short-acting compounds.

*Initial Evaluation of Patient*

Acute barbiturate intoxication must always be differentiated from other forms of coma or central nervous system injury. Information regarding occupation, possible trauma, and previous psychiatric illnesses, attempts at suicide and drug usage should be obtained. Particular attention should be directed toward obtaining an accurate history regarding the type, amount and time of drug ingestion, the duration of coma and the associated ingestion of alcohol. The depth of coma is often greater than might be expected from the plasma barbiturate concentration alone if alcohol and barbiturate ingestion have occurred concomitantly. Empty medicine bottles may provide a clue to the type of ingested barbiturate.

The patient who is admitted to the hospital with clinical signs of shock after barbiturate intoxication is characteristically in a state of deep coma. Corneal and deep tendon reflexes are absent and pupillary response to light is minimal. The rectal temperature is reduced to levels averaging only 95°F (35°C), and the skin is cool with the temperature in the ventrum of the great toes averaging only 79°F (26°C). The skin of the earlobes, nose or fingers is often cyanotic, reflecting the marked impairment in ventilation. Bullous lesions on the skin, although not specific, are sufficiently characteristic to be strongly suggestive of the diagnosis. A modest increase in heart rate is usually observed, but rates in excess of 130 beats/minute are uncommon. The systolic blood pressure is typically reduced to levels of less than 80 mm Hg. However, the values obtained with the sphygmomanometer are usually 10 to 20 mm Hg less than those obtained on direct measurement after insertion of a catheter into an artery. Moist rales are unusual, but rhonchi and wheezes indicative of atelectasis or pneumonia are often detected, particularly when the patient has aspirated oral or gastric contents.

The initial physical examination should include an assessment of the vital signs, the extent of respiratory depression, the depth of coma and a search for evidence of trauma and neurologic abnormalities. Evidence of preexisting diseases such as hypertension, cirrhosis and diabetes mellitus must be sought. The odor of the breath may indicate the presence of associated alcohol ingestion or diabetic ketoacidosis. Special attention should be paid to the status of the corneal and deep tendon reflexes, the pupillary light reflex, the bowel sounds and the response to verbal commands and deep painful stimuli.

The depth and severity of coma can be used to reflect the severity of intoxication. The following classification of coma has proved useful.

Grade I. Patient is comatose, deep tendon reflexes are intact and the patient withdraws from painful stimuli.

Grade II. Patient is comatose and fails to respond to painful stimuli but the reflexes are intact and vital signs are stable.

Grade III. Patient is comatose with no response to painful stimuli, deep tendon reflexes are absent or markedly depressed, and vital signs are stable.

Grade IV. Patient is comatose with no response to painful stimuli, deep tendon reflexes are absent, and there is respiratory depression and/or circulatory instability.

Regardless of the status of the neurologic examination, patients should be classified as Grade IV if cyanosis or sustained hypotension is present. On occasion, some patients promptly revert to a lesser grade of coma when such conditions as dehydration, anoxia and hypotension have been corrected. Patients whose coma is no more than Grade I or II should always recover with little more than good supportive care. Frequent and serial observations of the severity of coma provide the single most useful guide to the adequacy of subsequent therapy. An appropriate flow sheet is always desirable.

Minimum laboratory evaluation at the time of the first examination should include roentgenographic examination of the chest and skull, routine urinalysis, and estimates of the hematocrit, white blood cell and differential counts. Blood should be obtained for typing and crossmatching, and an aliquot should be saved for future drug analysis if necessary. When available, measurements of the blood urea nitrogen concentration and pH and the plasma concentrations of electrolytes, total barbiturate and creatinine should be obtained.

Measurements of plasma barbiturate concentration by most clinical laboratories do not distinguish between the type of barbiturate ingested or between the parent active compound and its inactive metabolites. A single isolated meaurement is often of little value except to confirm the presence of barbiturate in plasma. Furthermore, it should be remembered that the depth and duration of coma are related more closely to the barbiturate concentration in the brain than the concentration in plasma. The results of an initial measurement of the plasma barbiturate concentration must always be related to the clinical setting in which it was obtained if it is to be of real prognostic value. For example, patients who have acquired tolerance through habitual drug use can be expected to exhibit higher plasma barbiturate concentrations for any grade of coma, and patients who have simultaneously ingested other sedatives or tranquilizers may appear in deeper coma than would be expected from the plasma barbiturate concentration alone. Similarly, because of the smaller distribution space for phenobarbital, the associated ingestion of a small amount of this agent may raise the plasma barbiturate concentration inordinately when the concurrent ingestion of shortacting agents actually provides the major means of intoxication. Under these circumstances, the actual prognosis may not be as ominous as suggested by the plasma barbiturate concentration.

Although there are notable exceptions such as those outlined above, an initial plasma concentration of 3.5 mg/100 ml for short-acting drugs and 8.0 mg/100 ml for long-acting drugs should be regarded as potentially fatal. These plasma concentrations are apt to be encountered after the ingestion of total doses of 3.0 gm for short-acting drugs or 5.0 gm for long-acting drugs. Serial measurements of the plasma barbiturate concentration can often provide a valuable guide to the adequacy of therapy.

### *Treatment*

Regardless of the exact diagnosis, *treatment* should be instituted immediately if acute barbiturate intoxication is suspected. For practical purposes, acute intoxication with intermediate-acting agents resembles that produced by long-acting agents. In both of these groups there is a longer interval between ingestion and the onset of coma, shock or respiratory depression. Coma is apt to be prolonged and long-term provision of general supportive care may be required. In contrast, shock and anoxia may appear much more quickly after the ingestion of short-acting drugs. Coma is more often severe and death can occur rapidly. In this situation, the management of circulatory and respiratory collapse represents the immediate therapeutic problem.

TABLE 111
BARBITURATE BLOOD LEVELS AT CONSCIOUS RETURN

| *Long-acting barbiturates (lethal 10–12 mg % or greater)* | *mg/100 ml* |
|---|---|
| Barbital (Veronal) | |
| Phenobarbital (Luminal) | 5–9 mg |
| Mephobarbital (Mebaral®) | |
| Diallylbarbituric Acid (Dial) | |
| *Intermediate-acting barbiturates (lethal 4 mg % or greater)* | |
| Amobarbital (Amytal) | |
| Aprobarbital (Alurate®) | |
| Butabarbital (Butisol) | 2–4 mg |
| Butethal (Neonal®) | |
| Hexethal (Ortal®) | |
| Vinbarbital (Delvinal®) | |
| *Short-acting barbiturates (lethal 2 mg % or greater)* | |
| Cyclobarbital (Phanodorn®) | |
| Pentobarbital (Nembutal) | |
| Secobarbital (Seconal) | |
| Hexobarbital, sodium (Evipal) | 1–2 mg |
| Thiamylal, sodium (Surital®) | |
| Thiopental, sodium (Pentothal) | |

*Note:* These figures are approximate and from limited studies. Wide variations are possible and the clinical class of the barbiturate must be known if the quantitative assay is to be of value. Variable factors are the age of the patient, previously established drug tolerance, and coexisting unrelated illnesses. Relatively low levels may be associated with a fatal outcome in elderly or debilitated patients and much higher levels can be tolerated by individuals who are chronic users of these compounds. In the final analysis the depth of anesthesia depends on concentration of the drug in the brain, not in the blood, and serum levels therefore are unreliable as *absolute* guides to therapy.

The importance of close observation and quality nursing care cannot be stressed too strongly. The caloric intake must be maintained with parenteral fluids, water and electrolyte losses must be replaced and sites of infection must be detected and treated promptly. The eyes may be patched to prevent corneal damage, the patient should be placed on an alternating-pressure-type mattress and turned frequently (every two hours) and good oral hygiene must be observed.

*Ventilation*

An adequate airway must be assured at once if respiratory depression is present. Its importance to the maintenance of adequate ventilation is obvious; in addition, the passage of barbiturates across the blood-brain barrier into the central nervous system may be facilitated during hypoventilation and respiratory acidosis. An oropharyngeal airway may prove adequate if respiratory depression is not severe. On the other hand, if respiration is not spontaneous, endotracheal intubation with a cuffed tube should be carried out immediately. This maneuver greatly facilitates the regular removal of bronchial secretions in patients who are severely comatose. Nevertheless, bronchoscopy may still be required on occasion. A tracheostomy should be considered if assisted ventilation via an endotracheal tube is required for more than forty-eight to seventy-two hours.

Patients who require assisted ventilation can best be maintained with positive-pressure breathing on room air at a rate of 10 to 12 cycles/minute. High concentrations of oxygen should not be used since hypoxia sometimes provides the major stimulus to respiration in these patients, and its overcorrection may be followed by prolonged apnea when assisted ventilation is discontinued. The depth (volume) and rate of assisted respiration should be adjusted periodically to maintain the arterial blood $pCO_2$ at approximately 40 mm Hg. Serial measurements of the $pCO_2$ and pH in arterial blood are desirable to minimize the occurrence of either hyperventilation or hypoventilation.

*Circulatory Depression*

The blood pressure may return to normal in many patients after dehydration has been corrected and adequate ventilation has been restored. A slow intravenous infusion of 0.85% saline should be started immediately in all patients if for no other reason than the maintenance of ready access to the circulatory system should it be required for any reason. Many patients exhibit clinical evidence of dehydration (elevated hematocrit, increased plasma protein concentration, decreased skin turgor over the forehead, etc.). Salt and water deficits, if present, must be replaced with appropriate intravenous fluid therapy. In many patients, neither the blood pressure nor the urine output can be restored to normal until these deficits have been replaced. Although a completely reliable rule of thumb does not exist, if hyponatremia coexists with dehydration, initial replacement therapy can safely consist of 0.85% saline alone; if hypernatremia is present, initial replacement therapy can consist mainly of 5.0% dextrose in water or perhaps 0.45% saline in 2.5% dextrose in water (prepared by mixing 0.85% saline with 5.0% dextrose in water in equal volumes). If the serum sodium concentration is normal in the presence of dehydration, replacement therapy can be initiated with 0.6% saline solution (prepared by mixing 700 ml of 0.85% saline with 300 ml of 5% dextrose in water). In any event, once dehydration has been corrected, aggressive fluid therapy must not be continued until the adequacy of urine flow and renal function has been established.

Additional measures are required if hypotension does not respond to the correction of dehydration, hypovolemia or hypoxia. Some patients still exhibit severe hypotension in the presence of apparently normal hydration. Under these circumstances, it has been our policy to initiate therapy with a rapid (one to four hours) intravenous infusion of 1 to 2 liters of 0.85% saline and 500 ml of a plasma expander such as 6.0% dextran (dextran 6.0% in saline or Gentran® in Travert® or an artificial plasma preparation [Plasmanate®]). Plasma volume expanders can be administered safely to adults at rates of 10 to 20 ml/min (or even faster in some instances) and a total dose of 500 ml generally serves to increase plasma volume by 5 to 8 per cent. Total pediatric doses can be estimated at 10 to 15 ml/kg. Subsequent doses and rates of administration must be determined by the clinical response of the patient. Large volumes of isotonic saline (5 to 6 liters) over a relatively short period (eight to twelve hours) may be tolerated well if renal function is adequate. Nevertheless, overhydration and an inordinate expansion of plasma volume with the subsequent appearance of heart failure are potential hazards. Serial monitoring of the central venous pressure may sometimes serve to warn the physician of undue plasma volume expansion and impending congestive heart failure.

Vasopressor drugs have proved satisfactory in patients whose blood pressure is unresponsive to adequate hydration and plasma volume expansion. An intravenous infusion of metaraminol (Aramine® 1.0% injection) or levarterenol (Levophed 0.2%) has been lifesaving in many patients. Metaraminol, 50 to 150 mg in 250 to 500 ml of 0.85% saline, can be administered at a rate sufficient to maintain the mean arterial pressure between 80 to 85 mm Hg. Levarterenol, one 4 ml ampule in 400 to 500 ml of 0.85% saline, can be used in similar fashion. Regardless of which vasopressor agent is used, the mean arterial pressure should not be sustained above 90 mm Hg, since there is evidence in intoxicated patients that a greater increase in mean arterial pressure may be accompanied by an undesirable fall in cardiac output and a sharp rise in peripheral vascular resistance.

Although it is required rarely and its real value has not yet been established with certainty, a rapid intravenous injection of 100 mg of hydrocortisone (Solu-Cortef®) over a one-minute period may be tried if shock and/or hypotension are refractory to usual forms of therapy. Similar doses may be repeated every hour to six hours.

### *Gastric Lavage*

Gastric lavage has been advocated for many years in patients with acute barbiturate intoxication. However, in view of the rapidity of barbiturate absorption from the gastrointestinal tract, it is thought that this procedure is of little or no value unless the patient is seen within the first few hours after ingestion. Even so, an extremely low drug yield is obtained all too often. One group of investigators was able to remove over 100 mg of barbiturate in only ten of seventy-two patients (Harstad, E., Meiler, K.O. and Simeson, M.H.: Uber den Wert der Magenspulung bei der Behandlung von Akuten Vergiftungen. *Acta Med Scand, 112*:478,1942).

Recently recommended has been the use of activated charcoal with a saline lavage solution. This adsorbs varying but considerable amounts of drugs. Wash the stomach with 250 to 500 ml of the charcoal-saline slurry and continue the lavage with normal saline until the return is clear. Follow this with 500 to 1000 ml of castor oil in 50 ml aliquots using a Toomey syringe for instillation and withdrawal. The solubility of sedatives makes castor oil quite effective. In addition, concretions, if present, can be dissolved. Some oil enters the intestine if bowel sounds are still present and initiates diarrhea to remove some of the drug. If lavage is carried out in a comatose patient, a cuffed endotracheal tube should be inserted to minimize the danger of pulmonary aspiration. Emetics should never be used because of the same potential hazard.

Regardless of whether or not gastric lavage is carried out, it is wise to empty the stomach of its contents after an endotracheal tube has been inserted and its cuff has been inflated. Gentle nasogastric suction can be carried out intermittently during the period of coma to minimize the risk of spontaneous vomiting and subsequent aspiration.

### *Analeptic Drugs*

Central nervous system stimulants have been used extensively. Nevertheless, there is little evidence that the use of these agents either lowers the mortality rate or shortens the duration of coma. At the present time, it is generally felt that these drugs contribute little or nothing to the management of acute barbiturate intoxication. Many of the patients who appear to respond to these agents have such a light degree of coma that eventual recovery would have been expected without their use. In addition, their administration may so confuse the clinical picture that accurate assessment of the patient's true response to therapy becomes impossible. Furthermore, their use is sometimes associated with the appearance of such adverse side-effects as seizures, cardiac arrhythmias, vomiting and hyperpyrexia.

Nevertheless, if the clinical status of the patient is deteriorating rapidly, it may be advisable to administer either an amphetamine, bemegride or the newer agent ethamivan (Emivan®). If ethamivan is used, its dosage and route of administration depend upon the depth of coma and respiratory depression. Initially, ethamivan can be given intravenously to adults as a single slow injection (two to five minutes) in doses of 1 to 2 mg/kg. Subsequent doses can be administered as often as every ten minutes until easy arousal is achieved. Sneezing, coughing, laryngospasm and muscle twitching may occur if the administered dose is excessive.

### *Diuretics*

It has been recognized for some time that the rate of urinary barbiturate excretion is directly related to increasing urine flow. This observation is consistent with the hypothesis that filtered barbiturate is subsequently and partially reabsorbed via passive diffusion. Although the renal clearance of all barbiturates is increased at high rates of urine flow, this relationship is more apparent for long-acting drugs such as phenobarbital than for short-acting drugs such as pentobarbital or secobarbital. Perhaps as much as 10 per cent of the filtered load of certain short-acting agents may be excreted during marked diuresis, whereas 20 per cent of the filtered load of phenobarbital may be excreted at similar rates of urine flow. However, some investigators have failed to distinguish between the urinary excretion of active drug and its inactive metabolites so that the actual excretory rates (and perhaps the clearances) of unaltered drug may be somewhat lower than those indicated above. Bloomer has suggested that diuresis increases the excretion of active pentobarbital only slightly whereas the clearance of its inactive metabolites rises more rapidly (Bloomer, H.A.: Limited Usefulness of Alkaline Diuresis and Peritoneal Dialysis in Pentobarbital Intoxication *N Engl J Med, 272*:1309, 1965). For these reasons, it is probable that forced diuresis is more effective in patients who have been poisoned with long-acting barbiturates. Nevertheless, clinical observations suggest that forced diuresis has shortened the duration of coma in all types of barbiturate intoxication, and plasma barbiturate concentrations have been observed to fall more rapidly, even in patients who have been intoxicated with short-acting compounds. It is our present opinion that a trial of diuretic therapy is indicated in all patients whose degree of coma is Grade II or greater.

As long as a satisfactory urine flow is obtained, the method of achieving sustained diuresis is relatively unimportant except for differences in adverse side-effects that may be associated with a particular form of therapy. However, it may be impossible to secure an adequate water diuresis with fluids such as 2.5% to 5.0% dextrose in water because of an increased release or activity of antidiuretic hormone either due to hypovolemia and/or a direct stimulatory effect of the barbiturates themselves. For this reason, the use of osmotic diuretics is generally required to secure an adequate and sustained diuresis. Organomercurials, thiazides, ethacrynic acid, furosemide, sodium bicarbonate or lactate, glucose, Tham buffer, urea and mannitol have all been used with varying success.

Several authors have emphasized that an average daily urine volume of 8 to 14 liters (6 to 10 ml/min.) must be obtained to achieve maximum results. Electrolyte and fluid losses must be replaced on an hour-by-hour basis during diuresis of this magnitude. This can only be accomplished by hourly measurements of the sodium and potassium concentration in urine. Despite the potential hazard of urinary tract infection, the required hourly assessment of fluid balance is greatly facilitated by the insertion of an indwelling bladder catheter. Overhydration can occur rapidly, especially in the presence of underlying acute or chronic renal disease. Similarly, severe dehydration with hypernatremia can develop with remarkable rapidity if losses of electrolytes and water are not replaced regularly. An intravenous infusion of either 0.45% sodium chloride in 2.5% dextrose in water or 0.85% saline alone generally provides adequate replacement therapy until measurements of urinary electrolyte concentrations are available. At that time, potassium chloride may be added to the intravenous infusion in an amount equivalent to the measured urinary losses of this cation.

Mannitol or urea have proved to be the most useful osmotic diuretics in our own experience. Mannitol (Osmitrol®) is perhaps preferable because an infusion of urea precludes the use of BUN measurements as an index of renal function, dehydration, etc. Mannitol is administered initially as a single intravenous injection, 0.5 gm/kg or approximately 100 to 150 ml of 25% mannitol in an average-sized adult. If the urine flow rises above 180 ml (3 ml/min.) during the first hour after its injection, a constant intravenous infusion of 5% to 10% mannitol is begun at a rate sufficient to achieve and maintain the desired urine flow. Since mannitol is confined mainly to the extracellular space, plasma volume expansion can occur with an associated reduction in the plasma bicarbonate concentration and the appearance of mild systemic acidosis. Although both of these potential side-effects are undesirable, they are relatively insignificant when compared to the gain that is obtained from forced diuresis itself.

Recently, the use of newer and potent diuretic drugs such as ethacrynic acid (Edecrin®) or furosemide (Lasix®) has been suggested. Although experience with these agents is limited, urine flows as high as 16 ml/min. have been observed after the administration of ethacrynic acid. Similar results can be attained with furosemide if renal function is adequate. If furosemide is used, the intravenous administration of 40 mg in single doses every four to six hours provides an adequate dosage schedule in many adults. Permanent sensorineural hearing loss has been reported with furosemide administration.

### *Alkalinization*

Urinary alkalinization is a more effective form of therapy in patients with phenobarbital intoxication than in those who have ingested short-acting agents. For reasons that have been outlined above, the urinary excretion of barbiturates with higher pK values is little affected by urinary alkalinization. In experimental animals, phenobarbital excretion can be increased tenfold by urinary alkalinization (pH 7.8 to 8.0), although this effect is less apparent at high rates of urine flow. The excretion of secobarbital and pentobarbital is much less affected. If an alkalinizing agent such as sodium bicarbonate is used, the associated appearance of systemic alkalosis possesses the added advantage of facilitating barbiturate removal from peripheral tissues by creating a more favorable pH gradient between intracellular fluid and blood.

Sodium bicarbonate, sodium lactate and Tham buffer have all been used successfully as alkalinizing agents. We prefer the use of sodium bicarbonate for several reasons, one of which includes the fact that the bicarbonate anion penetrates cell walls very poorly so that a favorably high pH gradient between cell and

TABLE 112
TREATMENT OF BARBITURATE INTOXICATION

| *Condition* | *Treatment* | *Guides* |
|---|---|---|
| Respiratory insufficiency | Airway, suction; endotracheal intubation, cuffed tube, lavage; Humidified oxygen; Mechanical ventilation, pressure- or volume controlled ventilator | Arterial $Po_2$, $O_2$ saturation, $Pco_2$, pH, minute ventilation; x-ray film of chest; airway pressure |
| Hypovolemia | Albumin, 5% solution, 1 liter, then dextrose, 10% in sodium chloride 0.9 solution; potassium chloride supplement, 40–120 mEq | Central venous pressure, arterial pressure, urine output and osmolality |
| Low urinary output | Fluid infusion furosemide, 40 mg IV or ethacrynic acid, 25 mg IV | Urinary output and osmolality |
| Heart failure | Digoxin, 0.5 mg IV, followed by 1–4 doses of 0.25 mg digoxin at 1–2 hr intervals | Central venous pressure, ECG |
| Pneumonia | Ampicillin sodium, 1 gm every 4 hours IV; methicillin sodium, 1 gm every 6 hours IV; chloramphenicol sodium succinate, 500 mg every 6 hr IV; gentamicin sulfate, 0.75 mg/kg every 6 hr IM | Sputum and blood culture, with antibiotic sensitivity; chloramphenicol after aspiration of gastric contents; gentamicin for gram-negative bacteria resistant to other antibiotics |
| Dialysis | Peritoneal<br>Lipid<br>Hemodialysis (preferred) | Barbiturate levels of 3.5 mg/100 ml for short acting drugs and 8–10 mg/100 ml for long acting agents; impaired hepatic and renal function |

blood is perhaps established more easily. The intravenous administration of a single dose of sodium bicarbonate (45 mEq or one 50 ml ampul of 7.5% sodium bicarbonate) followed by a constant intravenous infusion of 0.75% sodium bicarbonate is usually sufficient. Its rate of infusion must be adjusted according to the results of serial measurements of urine pH in order to insure the occurrence of maximum urinary alkalinization. Similar results can be achieved by the infusion of equivalent amounts of sodium lactate.

It has been shown recently that maximum urinary alkalinization can be attained more predictaby if sodium bicarbonate administration is followed by the administration of acetazolamide (Diamox). This is particularly true when maximum urinary alkalinization may be limited by filtration rate depression, tissue hypoxia or intense osmotic diuresis. Acetazolamide is administered as a single intravenous injection of 250 mg every six hours. Its administration should always be accompanied by an infusion of sodium bicarbonate as outlined above, since urinary alkalinization with acetazolamide alone is also accompanied by the appearance of systemic hyperchloremic acidosis, an event which might tend to minimize the egress of barbiturate from peripheral tissues.

### *Hemodialysis*

An increased rate of removal of barbiturate from the body is the primary objective of either hemodialysis or peritoneal dialysis. Hemodialysis has now been used extensively in the treatment of barbiturate intoxication. *In vitro,* using a four-layer Kiil dialyzer at a blood flow rate of 400 ml/min., the dialysances of phenobarbital, amobarbital, pentobarbital and secobarbital are 110, 95, 85 and 65 ml per minute respectively. Estimates of removal rates or dialysances during actual dialyses *in vivo* have almost always been lower. In general, it has been suggested that a single six-hour hemodialysis can effect the removal of an amount of barbiturate which is comparable to that removed during twenty-four hours of sustained diuresis or peritoneal dialysis. Of course, even greater amounts of drug can be removed if hemodialysis is prolonged or its use is accompanied by the maintenance of sustained diuresis. Unfortunately, it is often difficult to maintain an adequate diuresis during the period of hemodialysis.

Long-acting drugs such as phenobarbital can be extracted in greater quantity than short-acting drugs such as secobarbital or pentobarbital which are better removed by a newer technique of lipid dialysis. This observation can be attributed, at least in part, to the fact that short-acting agents exhibit a greater degree of binding to plasma proteins and, hence, are less dialyzable, as well as to the fact that the plasma concentrations of short-acting drugs are usually lower than those of long-acting drugs so that their diffusion gradient from plasma to dialysate fluid is also less.

The actual value of hemodialysis in acute barbiturate intoxication has been difficult to assess. Mortality figures have indicated thus far that conservative measures alone represent the most successful form of therapy for all types of barbiturate poisoning. In at least one center, the mortality rate has been less than 1 per cent when no measures other than general supportive care and/or diuretic therapy were used. Of course, these results were achieved at a large center where the physicians and nurses are highly skilled and experienced. In contrast to these results, mortality figures have been highest in those centers where hemodialysis has been applied most extensively (Henderson, L.W. and Merrill, J.P.: Treatment of Barbiturate Intoxication *Ann Intern Med, 64*:876, 1966. Setter, J.G., Maher, J.F. and Schreiner, G.E.: Barbiturate Intoxication: Evaluation of Therapy Including Dialysis in a Large Series Selectively Referred Because of Severity. *Arch Intern Med, 117*:224, 1966). However, factors such as a higher referral of desperately ill patients for dialysis may well have contributed to these results. Despite disconcerting figures such as these, it is our own clinical impression that hemodialysis can be lifesaving in many patients.

At present, the use of hemodialysis is considered in patients who have ingested a potentially fatal dose of drug (Table 110), who exhibit a plasma barbiturate concentration above 3.5 mg/100 ml for short-acting drugs or 8 mg/100 ml for long-acting drugs or who demonstrate Grade III or IV coma that does not appear responsive to more conservative measures. In addition, it is often indicated in patients with underlying renal or hepatic disease where the normal routes of drug disposal are impaired and in patients who have also ingested other sedatives or tranquilizers that may be dialyzable. Prompt and immediate referral to a dialysis center is imperative as soon as the need for hemodialysis is contemplated. A recently developed resin column hemoperfusion system (*see* page 66) appears to be more effective than hemodialysis.

### *Peritoneal Dialysis*

This procedure has not yet been applied extensively to the management of barbiturate intoxication despite the fact that several observers have reported the occurrence of clinical improvement during its use. It possesses the distinct advantage of being applicable in any community hospital, and several authors have described the technique of intermittent peritoneal dialysis in full detail. However, because it is less efficient than hemodialysis, it can be anticipated that less drug will be removed per unit period of time. Removal of short-acting drugs is more limited because of lower plasma concentrations and greater binding to plasma proteins. Some investigators have reported increased extraction via the addition of plasma albumin (5 gm/100 ml of Albumisol) or tromethamine (Tham buffer) to commercially available dialysate fluid (Inpersol®, Dianeal®, Peridial®). The addition of Tham (150 mol/liter) has effected a twentyfold rise in phenobarbital extraction in experimental animals by maintaining an alkaline pH in the dialysate fluid so that drug removal is thereby enhanced. Nevertheless, sustained peritoneal dialysis with Tham-containing fluids does not appear advisable until wider clinical experience has been acquired regarding the possible adverse systemic effects of Tham absorbed from the peritoneal cavity. At present, the combined use of osmotic diuresis and conventional peritoneal dialysis with standard commercial fluids seems most appropriate for general use.

### *Complications*

Pulmonary complications (infection, atelectasis, aspiration, etc.), urinary tract infection (consequent to the use of an indwelling bladder catheter), acute pulmonary edema, acute tubular necrosis subsequent to hypotension and/or hypovolemia, and several bullous lesions of the skin are some of the most important complications of acute barbiturate intoxication. Of these, infection (pulmonary and urinary tract) is most frequent. Although the prophylactic use of antibiotics is sometimes recommended, it has been our own policy to reserve the use of antibiotics for the treatment of a specific infection. This policy requires that the physician must be constantly aware of the hazards of infection in a comatose patient, and that he must search for its possible presence each day.

Acute pulmonary edema may be a direct consequence of barbiturate intoxication itself rather than related to such factors as iatrogenic plasma volume expansion. Its recognition may be difficult in the presence of severe respiratory depression, and it may occur when the central venous return and pressure are relatively low. In addition to rapid digitalization, the administration of vasopressor agents may be particularly helpful if systemic hypotension is present. Phlebotomy should be avoided if hypovolemia is present, and morphine and its analogues are definitely contraindicated.

### *Tests*

A simple and rapid screening test (five minutes) for the presence or absence of barbiturates in 2 ml of blood has been reported in the *British Medical Journal* volume 2, page 1040, October 26, 1963. The extraction of the barbiturate from the blood into chloroform, the reaction with mercuric ions and color tests with diphenylthiocarbazone (dithizon) for any mercury barbiturate in the chloroform are all performed in a 100 ml beaker. The other important feature of the method is that extraction of the barbiturate from the buffered blood is performed by magnetic stirring, using only 10 ml of chloroform. If a water-operated magnetic stirrer is used, the apparatus can be made portable, dependent only on a water supply and a suction device. The glass suction tube is 3/16 in. (0.5 cm) in diameter and is taped onto a supporting stand so that it dips into the beaker, thus enabling an aqueous phase in the beaker to be drawn off, leaving 10 ml of the lower chloroform layer *in situ.* The technique works equally well on whole blood, serum, urine and stomach washes. Salicylate, even in the highest toxic levels in blood or urine, does not interfere with detection.

Until recently, the cobaltamine test was the only one of any value in the investigation of barbiturate toxicology. Today, purification using chromatography and countercurrent techniques, followed by identification using x-ray diffraction or infrared spectrophotometry and assay by means of ultraviolet spectrophotometry are routine methods of analysis.

### *Prognosis and Follow-up Care*

The overall mortality from acute barbiturate intoxication is generally less than 5 to 7 per cent. The incidence of subsequent suicide attempts, often with the same drug, is high. For this reason, follow-up psychiatric care is of great importance. Arrangements for such care should be made during the period of acute intoxication since it is at this time that a great deal of valuable psychiatric history can be obtained from patients and their relatives.

The idea that the combination of an emetic substance with a sedative drug would prevent overdosage of the latter because the large dose of emetic would cause vomiting and thus empty the stomach receives some practical support from past experience with powdered ipecac and opium (Dover's powder), which is an extremely safe preparation for this very reason. When a large dose is taken, vomiting is produced by the ipecac. In this instance, however, the emetic action is produced by local gastric irritation.

With a centrally acting emetic like apomorphine, the situation is more difficult. The emetic drug would have to be absorbed at least as readily and preferably better than the sedative, and, unfortunately, the absorption of apomorphine (a parenterally used drug) from the stomach is somewhat erratic. The emetic dose of apomorphine when given orally is also extremely variable, and it would be difficult to find an amount which could be guaranteed not to produce emesis when incorporated along with a therapeutic dose of a barbiturate and at the same time would be certain to cause emesis if an overdose were taken.

A further and more serious difficulty arises in that apomorphine, in addition to its emetic action, retains most of the central depressant activity of morphine. It may cause serious depression and even collapse, which is particularly liable to happen when the patient is already depressed by another sedative drug such as a barbiturate. In these circumstances, vomiting may not occur, and the existing depression may become much more profound. For these reasons it is unlikely that any attempt to prevent barbiturate poisoning in which apomorphine was combined with the barbiturate would be uniformly successful, and clearly such a preparation would be potentially dangerous.

## BISMUTH COMPOUNDS

These preparations are used both for their local and systemic effects. Bismuth subsalicylate (soluble in oil), bismuth sodium triglycollamate and thioglycolate (soluble in water) are given parenterally in the treatment of infectious diseases and warts. On the other hand, the insoluble salts (bismuth subcarbonate, subnitrate, glycobiarsol) are employed in the treatment of diarrhea and intestinal diseases. Oral bismuth subgallate is used to control odor and consistency of the stool in patients with colostomy or ileostomy.

Acute bismuth poisoning rarely occurs. The use of bismuth subnitrate in the treatment of diarrhea has led to acute and often severe or fatal intoxication, but this is not due to the action of bismuth. The nitrate is changed by bacteria in the colon to nitrite, and the absorption of the latter in larger amounts can cause severe nitrite poisoning, with methemoglobinemia, cyanosis, dyspnea, hypotension and death from respiratory arrest. Bismuth subcarbonate should always be used instead of the nitrate since it is entirely safe and just as effective.

Chronic bismuth intoxication has many of the characteristics of chronic lead and arsenic poisoning. The gastrointestinal symptoms are colic, diarrhea, nausea and vomiting and anorexia. The intestinal symptoms are largely due to the precipitation in the mesenteric capillaries of bismuth sulfide with resulting embolization. The stools are black, due to the presence of bismuth sulfide. The mouth shows evidence of bismuth deposition in the endothelial and fibrous cells in the summits of the papillae and in the mucosal surfaces of the palate, cheeks and gums. This is manifested in a blue-gray bismuth line and a diffuse or patchy bluish color of the mucosa. It may persist for years and resist attempts at removal. Stomatitis also characterizes more severe grades of bismuth poisoning.

Various skin lesions may appear, followed by an exfoliative dermatitis. Severe headache and puzzling grippe-like attacks may usher in bismuth poisoning. Peripheral neuritis and liver damage are occasionally seen and juandice may accompany the latter.

Bismuth has a nephrotoxic as well as a

hepatotoxic action, chiefly on the proximal convoluted tubules. Changes in the medulla and spinal cord may produce signs and symptoms related to the central nervous system. Blood dyscrasias including agranulocytosis, aplastic anemia and purpura have been reported. In childhood poisoning, roentgenograms of growing bone, like lead and other heavy metals, give the appearance of healed rickets. Intracytoplasmic and intranuclear eosinophilic inclusions are found in 85 per cent of the patients. These refractile spherical bodies are readily stained by the PAS reagent.

The prolonged use of oral bismuth subgallate in colostomy patients has produced a neurological syndrome characterized by malaise, lassitude and dysesthesia, progressing to loss of memory, tremor and impaired coordination. Signs and symptoms were reversible when therapy was discontinued.

In the *treatment,* recovery is likely if dimercaprol (BAL) is given early. Administer an emetic or remove stomach contents with gastric lavage followed by a saline cathartic. General measures should include atropine and meperidine (Demerol) to relieve the gastrointestinal discomfort. For the stomatitis, any good mouthwash and attention to oral hygiene is necessary. Fluid, 2 to 4 liters daily, should be given if kidney function is not impaired. In case of cyanosis due to methemoglobinemia use methylene blue.

## BROMIDE

Though bromides no longer enjoy very great popularity in therapeutics, intoxication is still relatively common. Doses that would be sufficient to cause acute poisoning are so irritating to the stomach that nausea and vomiting occur almost immediately. Acute, severe intoxication is therefore rare, although it may occur following administration in the face of impaired renal function. The twelve-day plasma half-life of bromide is another factor in producing toxic symptoms, if taken daily over a period of time.

Bromide poisoning is almost always chronic and insidious and most commonly due to self-medication with numerous proprietary "nerve tonics," sedatives, hypnotics and remedies for headaches. For example, Bromo-Seltzer® has 250 mg potassium bromide per dose, while Sleep-eze® has 0.125 mg scopolamine hydrobromide per dose. Although free of bromides in the United States, Sominex is a bromide preparation in Canada. From 2 to 10 per cent of patients admitted to mental hospitals formerly suffered from some degree of bromism, the tabulated incidence depending greatly on how often serum bromide tests were done. Bromide intoxication mimics many psychotic states and should be considered whenever a clinical diagnosis is uncertain.

Sodium, potassium and ammonium bromides are water-soluble and absorbed rapidly from the intestine and are distributed throughout the extracellular fluid in much the same fashion as chlorides. They displace chlorides while the total body halide level remains constant. Excretion is extremely slow and takes place chiefly through the kidneys, and with continued intake of bromides there is a steady accumulation in the body fluid. The toxic concentration of bromides is quite variable. Generally, blood levels above 125 mg/100 ml are considered in the toxic range, though higher levels (150 to 200 mg) are sometimes well tolerated and severe intoxication is sometimes seen with much less.

Symptoms of bromism most commonly and seriously involve the central nervous system. Nerve cells, it is supposed, are particularly sensitive to the replacement of chloride by bromide in the extracellular fluid; it is possible that some bromide ions pass the cell membrane and exert their effect intracellularly. Skin, glandular secretions and the gastrointestinal tract are also affected.

The mental and neurologic effects are

TABLE 113
MANIFESTATIONS OF CHRONIC BROMIDE INTOXICATION

| | |
|---|---|
| *Psychiatric* | Confusion<br>Impaired memory<br>Hallucinations<br>Drowsiness<br>Extreme excitement<br>Paranoia |
| *Neurologic* | Ocular bobbing<br>Weakness<br>Coma<br>Tremors<br>Incoordination<br>Positive Babinski<br>Hyperactive or hypoactive deep tendon reflexes<br>Papilledema |
| *Dermatologic* | Pigmentation<br>Acneiform rash<br>Nodular lesions on the legs<br>Pustular lesions |
| *Gastrointestinal* | Anorexia<br>Furred tongue<br>Constipation<br>Foul breath |

extremely variable, ranging from mere accentuation of the sedative effects of the drug to overt mania, delirium, hallucinations and coma. Transitory schizophrenia has been reported during bromide intoxication. Frequently the patient continues to use bromides for the very nervous symptoms that are produced by them. These disturbances may develop suddenly and may stimulate almost any functional or organic mental and neurologic disorder. Usually, however, the pattern is bizarre, and this suggests a possible drug intoxication. The neurologic features consist of weakness, fatigability, coarse tremors of the hands, tongue and lips, and sluggishness, incoordination, headache, a staggering gait, thickened speech, drowsiness and disturbed reflexes.

About 25 per cent of patients with bromism have some form of dermatitis, usually an acneiform rash, but the eruption may be nodular or varied and mimics many other patterns. As some bromide is excreted through the tears and respiratory tract, it may cause mild conjunctivitis, lacrimation, rhinitis and bronchial irritation. Similarly, the gastric secretion of bromide may irritate and cause anorexia, furred tongue, foul breath and constipation.

Diagnosis is usually considered if a history of prolonged ingestion is elicited, but such a history may be unobtainable. In any event, the diagnosis is confirmed by determination of the serum bromide level. Acute bromide intoxication may manifest itself by an abnormal SMA-6, as there is a transient elevation of total serum chloride and bromide both measured as chloride by analyser. Electroencephalographic records are frequently abnormal, and the cerebrospinal fluid protein is elevated. Evidence of CNS depression in newborns of neurotic or psychotic mothers and neonatal bromide intoxication, among others, should be ruled out.

In severe cases when the rapid removal of bromides may be essential, hemodialysis with the artificial kidney or peritoneal dialysis is a very rapid effective procedure. *Treatment* otherwise usually takes one to four weeks and consists primarily of stopping all sources of bromides and supplying sodium chloride to displace and hasten the elimination of the bromides.

Sodium chloride, 6 to 12 gm daily, should be given orally in divided doses, together with a fluid intake of at least 4 liters. If required, isotonic salt solution may be given intravenously. Ammonium chloride may be used instead, with the possible advantage of more rapid excretion of bromides due to its diuretic effect; in cardiac patients it may be especially desirable. Mercurial and thiazide diuretics are also valuable in facilitating the elimination of bromides and reportedly shorten the duration of the poisoning. Gastric and salivary glands secrete bromides preferentially to chloride. Continuous gastric aspiration with concomitant repeated gastric secretory stimulation with betazole (Histalog®), to remove bromide, has been used successfully in the treatment of bromism and actually is more effective quantitatively than renal excretion.

## CAFFEINE

Caffeine is the most powerful of the xanthine derivatives as a central nervous system stimulant. It is also valuable for its effect on the myocardium, smooth muscle and kidney.

All cola beverages contain caffeine. The Federal Food and Drug Administration permits the use of caffeine in these beverages to 1.2 gr (72 mg)/12 oz. bottle (6 mg/oz.). Low-calorie drinks are allowed only half (3 mg/oz.) as much caffeine.

The amount of caffeine found in the following beverages, on a per-fluid-ounce basis, is as follows: Coca-Cola,®, 4.6 mg; Pepsi-Cola®, 3 mg; and Royal Crown Cola®, 3.5 mg.

The caffeine content of an average cup of coffee*, prepared from 15 to 17 gm of coffee and averaging 5 fl. oz., is approximately 18 mg/fl. oz. Strong tea* contains the same amount of caffeine, although average tea approximates 12 to 15 mg/fl. oz. Cocoa contains about 6 mg/oz. Popular pain-relieving drugs often contain 20 mg or more of caffeine per dose.

*The caffeine content in coffee and tea varies widely by brand and blend.

The fatal overdose of caffeine has been estimated to be approximately 10 gm. Untoward reactions, however, can occur after the ingestion of 1 or more gm. These are mainly referrable to the central nervous system and circulatory system. Insomnia, restlessness and excitement are the earliest symptoms and may progress to mild delirium. Sensory disturbances such as tinnitus and flashes of light are common. The muscles twitch and become tense. Hematemesis has been reported. Respiration increases and tachycardia and extrasystoles are frequent. The diuretic action of the drug may be prominent. In the most severe cases, strychnine-like convulsions may appear. Chronic caffeinism can produce low-grade fever.

In the *treatment,* gastric lavage should be employed if large amounts have been ingested. The central nervous system symptoms of caffeine poisoning may be readily controlled by the administration of depressant drugs. The short-acting barbiturates are effective for this purpose. Adequate amounts of oral or parenteral fluids should also be given to maintain hydration (*see* Xanthines).

## CALCIUM

Calcium salts are specific in the immediate treatment of low-calcium tetany regardless of etiology. They are also employed for their antispasmodic, diuretic, antacid and circulatory actions.

### *Calcium Chloride (27% calcium)*

Contact with concentrated solutions causes erythema, exfoliation, ulceration and scarring of the skin. The salt can be given by mouth or intravenously. It should never be injected into tissues, and perivenous infiltration should be avoided or necrosis may occur. Orally it should be administered with a demulcent vehicle or irritation and ulceration of the gastrointestinal tract may occur, and for the same reason it should never be given by gavage to infants.

### *Calcium Gluconate (9% calcium)*

This salt can be given orally, intravenously or intramuscularly, and though the calcium content is low, it has the marked advantage of being nonirritating to subcutaneous tissue or gastrointestinal tract. Nevertheless, it should not be used in a 10% solution IM in infants, as abscess formation at the site of injection may result. Repeated intravenous injections can produce sensation of heat, fever, nausea, vomiting and oppression in the chest.

### *Calcium Lactate (13% calcium)*

This salt has the physical properties of calcium gluconate, is administered by the oral route, and has practically no side-effects.

### *Calcium carbonate (40% calcium)*

This is a safe, insoluble salt, taken orally and converted to available soluble calcium salts in the bowel.

### *Dibasic and Tribasic Calcium Phosphate*

These are innocuous, insoluble, tasteless salts used as gastric antacids and are particularly valuable when both calcium and phosphorus are needed.

### *Calcium Levulinate (13% calcium)*

This salt has a bitter, saline taste and can be given orally in powder form or parenterally as a 10% solution.

Calcium intoxication (hypercalcemia) causes anorexia, nausea, vomiting, dehydration, weakness, lethargy, coma and death. It is a medical emergency which requires prompt treatment regardless of its diverse etiologies (hyperparathyroidism, sarcoidosis, malignancy, hypervitaminosis D, etc.). Unless the serum calcium level is reduced below 16 mg/100 ml, there is danger of sudden death.

*Treatment.* Once the hypercalcemic syndrome is recognized, effort should be made to hydrate the patient and to correct any electrolyte deficits which may be present. If a daily urine volume exceeding 2500 ml can be maintained, the serum calcium level often falls by 2 to 4 mg/100 ml. This usually results in considerable improvement in the clinical status of the patient. If adequate hydration fails to provide a safe serum calcium level, an attempt should be made to correct the hypercalcemia by means of drug therapy. The most dependable and rapidly acting agent for this purpose is the chelating agent, sodium ethylenediaminetetraacetic acid (EDTA). Unfortunately, chelation is a temporary measure and renal damage may at times be inflicted by large amounts of EDTA administered for prolonged periods.

The intravenous and oral administration of sodium or magnesium sulfate is effective in reducing serum calcium levels. Calcium forms an ion-pair association with sulfate on an electrostatic, rather than a covalent, basis. Apparently, the binding forces are strong enough to prevent reabsorption of calcium ions without altering the usual rapid clearance of sulfate by the kidney. This cannot be recommended as a proved therapeutic approach, but it appears worthy of trial.

Inorganic phosphate, orally as the disodium or dipotassium salt or intravenously as 1 liter of 0.1 M solution of disodium phosphate and monopotassium phosphate (0.081 mol $Na_2HPO_4$ plus 0.019 mol $KH_2PO_4$, to provide solution of pH 7.4), has recently been found effective.

The response to the administration of adrenal corticosteroids may be both therapeutically beneficial and diagnostically significant. It is well known that the adrenal steroids have a hypocalcemic effect in certain clinical situations. Tetany can be precipitated by the administration of hydrocortisone to patients with hypoparathyroidism. Hydrocortisone, 300 mg daily, or the equivalent dosage of any one of the active compounds should be used in attempting to control hypercalcemia.

Artificial dialysis, if available, is an expedient temporary measure to permit time for some other modality to become effective. $Na_2HPO_4$, by mouth and intravenously, also has been used with some success.

## CANCER CHEMOTHERAPEUTIC AGENTS

The chemotherapeutic agents in cancer are given, in many instances, to the maximum tolerated dose in an attempt to elicit a therapeutic response. Severe and sometimes prolonged host toxicity may occur with some drugs, and their toxic manifestations as well as

TABLE 114
TOXICITY OF CANCER CHEMOTHERAPEUTIC AGENTS

| *Drug* | *Dosage and Route of Administration* | *Acute Side-effects* | *Toxicity* | *Precautions** | *Major Indications* |
|---|---|---|---|---|---|
| *Alkylating Agents* | | | | | |
| Mechlorethamine (nitrogen mustard, Mustargen) | 0.4 mg/kg as a single dose IV or in 2 divided doses | Nausea and vomiting, local phlebitis | Bone-marrow depression | Strong local irritant; administer through a running IV infusion | Hodgkin's disease and other lymphomas, carcinoma of the lung |
| Cyclophosphamide (Cytoxan) | 500-1500 mg/m² as a single dose IV; or 60-120 mg/m² per day PO; dose decreased if severe leukopenia develops | Nausea and vomiting; hyponatremia and water intoxication | Bone-marrow depression, alopecia, cystitis | Maintain adequate fluid intake to avoid cystitis | Hodgkin's disease and other lymphomas, multiple myeloma, neuroblastoma, carcinomas of the breast, ovary, lung |
| Chlorambucil (Leukeran) | 0.1-0.2 mg/kg per day; PO dose decreased if severe bone-marrow depression develops; only 2-4 mg daily may be necessary in chronic lymphocytic leukemia | Nausea, vomiting (with high doses) | Bone-marrow depression | None | Chronic lymphocytic leukemia, Hodgkin's disease and other lymphomas, carcinomas of the breast and ovary |
| Busulfan (Myleran) | 2-10 mg/day PO for 2-3 weeks; maintenance with 1-3 mg daily | None | Bone-marrow depression, pulmonary fibrosis, hyperpigmentation of skin, gynecomastia | None | Chronic myelocytic leukemia, polycythemia vera |
| Melphalan (Alkeran) | 0.2 mg/kg per day PO × 4 q-6 weeks (myeloma); or 0.1 mg/kg per day PO for 2-3 weeks; maintenance with 2-4 mg/day when bone marrow has recovered | Nausea and vomiting (with high doses) | Bone-marrow depression | None | Multiple myeloma, carcinoma of the ovary |

*All alkylating agents and many other antineoplastic drugs should be used only if absolutely necessary in pregnant women, since they are abortifacient or teratogenic.

| | | | | | |
|---|---|---|---|---|---|
| Triethylene-thiophosphoramide (Thiotepa) | 0.2 mg/kg per day IV × 5 | None | Bone-marrow depression | None | Hodgkin's disease and other lymphomas, carcinomas of the breast and ovary |
| *Cycle-dependent Antimetabolites* | | | | | |
| 5-Fluorouracil (5-FU, Fluorouracil) | 12 mg/kg per day IV × 4, then alternate days at 6 mg/kg × 4 or until toxicity; repeat course monthly or give weekly IV dose of 12-15 mg/kg; maximum dose 1 gm for either regimen | Occasional nausea and vomiting | Bone-marrow depression, diarrhea, stomatitis, alopecia, neurotoxicity | Decrease dose in patients with diminished liver, renal or bone-marrow function, or after adrenalectomy | Carcinoma of stomach, colon, pancreas, liver, ovary, breast |
| Floxuridine (FUDR) | 24 mg/kg per day IV × 4, then alternate days at 6 mg/kg × 4 or until toxicity; repeat course monthly or give weekly IV dose of 24-30 mg/kg; or 0.1-0.6 mg/kg daily as continuous intra-arterial infusion | Same as 5-FU | Same as 5-FU | Same as 5-FU | Same as 5-FU |
| Cytarabine (cytosine arabinoside, ara-C, Cytosar) | *Leukemia:* 3 mg/kg per day IV for 1-3 weeks; or 2.5 mg/kg q.12h.IV for 1-3 weeks (with 6-thioguanine); or intrathecally, 20-30 mg/m² *Head and neck cancer:* 1 mg/kg q12h SC for 5-7 days | Nausea, vomiting (with high doses), headache | Bone-marrow depression, megaloblastic anemia, occasional hepatic toxicity | Contraindicated in nonleukemic patients with poor bone-marrow function; use with caution in liver disease | Acute myeloblastic leukemia, lymphomas, carcinoma of the head and neck |
| Methotrexate (MTX, amethopterin, Methotrexate) | *Choriocarcinoma:* 10-30 mg/day PO or IM × 5 *Acute leukemia, maintenance:* child, 1.25-5 mg/day PO; adult, 5-10 mg/day PO; or both, 30 mg/m² IM or PO twice weekly | None | Bone-marrow depression, megaloblastic anemia, diarrhea, stomatitis, vomiting; alopecia less common, occasional hepatic fibrosis, vasculitis, pulmonary fibrosis | Adequate renal function must be present, and urine output must be maintained. Salicylates have a synergistic toxic effect and should be used cautiously, if at all | Choriocarcinoma, acute leukemia, carcinoma of the head and neck, breast and testicular tumors; adjuvant for osteosarcoma |

TABLE 114—*Continued*
TOXICITY OF CANCER CHEMOTHERAPEUTIC AGENTS

| *Drug* | *Dosage and Route of Administration* | *Acute Side-effects* | *Toxicity* | *Precautions* | *Major Indications* |
|---|---|---|---|---|---|
| | *Meningeal leukemia:* 0.2-0.4 mg/kg intrathecally *Head and neck tumor:* 50 mg/day intra-arterially with concomitant or sequential systemic antidote, leucovorin | | | | |
| 6-Mercaptopurine (6-MP, Purinethol) | 2.5 mg/kg per day PO | Occasional nausea, vomiting, anorexia | Bone-marrow depression, hepatotoxicity associated with bile stasis and necrosis | Hyperuricemia can occur with breakdown of large numbers of tumor cells; allopurinol sometimes prevents this, but 6-MP dose should then be reduced to at most ⅓ of usual dose | Acute leukemias |
| 6-Thioguanine (6-TG, Tabloid) | 100 mg/m² PO q.12h. for 8 days, often in combination with cytarabine | Rare gastrointestinal intolerance | Bone-marrow depression | None | Acute myeloblastic leukemia |
| *Antibiotics* | | | | | |
| Dactinomycin (actinomycin D, Cosmegen) | 15-40 μg/kg per week IV for 3-5 weeks in adults; 15 μg/kg per day IV × 5 in children | Pain on local infiltration with skin necrosis; nausea and vomiting in many patients 2 h. after dose; occasional cramps and diarrhea | Bone-marrow depression stomatitis, diarrhea, erythema, hyperpigmentation with occasional desquamation in areas of previous irradiation | Administer through running IV infusion; use with care in liver disease and in presence of inadequate marrow function; prophylactic antiemetics are helpful | Wilms' tumor, neuroblastoma, embryonal rhabdomyosarcoma, Ewing's sarcoma, choriocarcinoma, testicular and carcinoid tumors |
| Mithramycin (Mithracin) | 25-50 μg/kg IV on alternate days for 3-8 doses or until toxicity develops | Anorexia, nausea | Bone-marrow depression, hepatic damage with decreased production of clotting factors, stomatitis, azotemia | Very toxic drug; its use on alternate days with strict adherence to monitoring of LDH, BUN, prothrombin time, and platelet count before each dose can increase therapeutic index by de- | Embryonal cell carcinoma of the testis |

| | | | | | |
|---|---|---|---|---|---|
| | | | | creasing toxicity; contraindicated in liver or kidney dysfunction and in patients with coagulation disorders or thrombocytopenia | |
| Mitomycin C (Mutamycin) | 0.05 mg/kg IV per day × 6, then alternate days until 50 mg total dose | Nausea, vomiting; local inflammation and ulceration if extravasated | Neutropenia, thrombocytopenia, oral ulceration, nausea, vomiting, diarrhea | Administer through running IV infusion or inject with great care to prevent extravasation | Lymphomas, gastrointestinal carcinomas, carcinomas of the breast, cervix, lung, head, neck |
| Bleomycin (Blenoxane) | 10-20 mg/m² IV or IM 1-2 ×/week; start with 5 mg for first 2 doses in lymphoma | Fever, chills, nausea, vomiting; local pain or phlebitis less frequent | *Skin:* hyperpigmentation, thickening, nail changes, ulceration, rash, peeling, alopecia<br><br>*Pulmonary:* pneumonitis with dyspnea, rales, infiltrate can progress to fibrosis; more common in patients over 70, and with more than 400 mg total dose, but unpredictable | Watch for hypersensitivity in lymphoma with first 1-2 doses; use with exreme caution in presence of renal or pulmonary disease; start in hospital under observation do not exceed total dose of 400 mg | Lymphomas, testicular tumors, squamous cell carcinomas of skin, penis, vulva, head, neck |
| Doxorubicin (Adriamycin) | 60-100 mg/m² IV q.3 weeks | Nausea, vomiting, fever, local phlebitis, necrosis if extravasated, red urine (not blood) | Bone-marrow depression, alopecia, cardiac toxicity related to cumulative dose, stomatitis | Administer through running IV infusion; avoid giving to patients with significant heart disease, follow for EKG abnormalities and signs of heart failure | Acute lymphoblastic leukemia, sarcomas, neuroblastoma, lymphoma, Ewing's sarcoma, carcinoma of the bladder, breast, thyroid, lung. Does not cross the blood-brain barrier and not useful for brain tumors |
| *Plant Alkaloids* | | | | | |
| Vinblastine (Velban) | 0.10-0.15 mg/kg per week IV | Severe, prolonged inflammation if extravasated; occasional nausea, vomiting, headache, and paresthesias | Bone-marrow depression, particularly neutropenia; alopecia, muscle weakness, occasional mild peripheral neuropathy, mental depression | Administer through running IV infuson or inject with great care to prevent extravasation; decrease dose in liver disease | Hodgkin's disease and other lymphomas, choriocarcinoma, carcinoma of the breast, testicular tumors |

TABLE 114—*Continued*
TOXICITY OF CANCER CHEMOTHERAPEUTIC AGENTS

| *Drug* | *Dosage and Route of Administration* | *Acute Side-effects* | *Toxicity* | *Precautions* | *Major Indications* |
|---|---|---|---|---|---|
| | | | 2-3 days after treatment, rarely stomatitis | | |
| Vincristine (Oncovin) | 0.4-1.4 $mg/m^2$ IV weekly in adults; 2 $mg/m^2$ weekly in children | Local inflammation if extravasated; hyponatremia and water intoxication | Paresthesias, weakness, loss of reflexes, constipation; abdominal, chest, and jaw pain; hoarseness, footdrop, mental depression; marrow toxicity generally mild, anemia and reticulocytopenia most prominent; alopecia | Administer through running IV infusion or inject with great care to prevent extravasation; decrease dose in liver disease; patients with underlying neurologic problems may be more susceptible to neurotoxicity; alopecia may be prevented by use of scalp tourniquet for 5 minutes during and after administration | Acute lymphoblastic leukemia, lymphomas, Wilms' tumor, neuroblastoma, testicular tumors, carcinoma of the breast |
| *Nitrosoureas* | | | | | |
| Carmustine (BCNU) | 75-100 $mg/m^2$ per day IV ×2; repeat course in 6-8 weeks | Burning pain along vein, facial flushing, nausea and vomiting 4-6 h. later | Bone-marrow depression 3-6 weeks after administration; occasional renal and hepatic toxicity | Slow infusion rate to prevent local pain; use antiemetics; patients with impaired bone-marrow function should have a lower dose or not receive drug | Hodgkin's disease and other lymphomas, brain tumors, myeloma, melanoma |
| Lomustine (CCNU) | 130 $mg/m^2$ PO; repeat in 6-8 weeks | Occasional nausea and vomiting | Same as BCNU | Use antiemetics; reduce dose for patients with impaired marrow function | Same as BCNU |
| Dacarbazine (DTIC-Dome) | 150-250 $mg/m^2$ per day IV ×5; or 950-1200 $mg/m^2$ IV once | Nausea and vomiting diminishing with continued dose; occasional flu-like syndrome | Bone-marrow depression | Use lower dose in patients with impaired marrow or renal function | Melanoma, Hodgkin's disease |
| *Miscellaneous* | | | | | |
| Procarbazine (Matulane) | 50-300 mg/day PO with slow buildup in dose | Nausea and vomiting especially if high doses are used too rapidly; improves after first few days | Bone-marrow depression after 3-4 weeks, lethargy, drowsiness; fever, myalgia, arthralgia | Decrease dose in patients with hepatic, renal, or marrow dysfunction; synergism with CNS de- | Hodgkin's disease and other lymphomas |

| | | | | | |
|---|---|---|---|---|---|
| | | | | pressants (phenothiazines, barbiturates) may be seen as well as an Antabuse-like reaction with ethanol; monoamine oxidase inhibitory activity sometimes occurs and sympathomimetic drugs, cheese, bananas should be avoided | |
| Hydroxyurea (Hydrea) | 80 mg/kg q.3 days PO; or 20-30 mg/kg per day | Anorexia and nausea | Bone-marrow depression, megaloblastic anemia; stomatitis, diarrhea, and alopecia are less common | Decrease dose in patients with marrow and renal dysfunction | Chronic myelocytic leukemia, melanoma |
| Mitotane (*o,p'*-DDD, Lysodren) | 8-10 gm/day PO in 3-4 divided doses; tolerated dose varies from 2 to 16 gm/day | Nausea and vomiting which limits the dose | Somnolence, lethargy, visual disturbances, dermatitis | Low dose should be used initially, with gradual buildup to maximum tolerated dose (usually 8-10 gm/day) | Carcinoma of the adrenal cortex |
| *Steroids* | | | | | |
| Glucocorticoids | 40-100 mg daily PO of prednisone or equivalent; maintain at lower doses, if possible | Epigastric distress | Weight gain, truncal obesity striae, skin fragility, moon facies, euphoria and psychosis, peptic ulcers, osteoporosis; enhanced risk of infection, diabetes, hypertension | Consider prophylaxis of tuberculosis in patient with history of or exposure to tuberculosis or with lymphoma; use antacids for gastric distress | Acute and chronic lymphocytic leukemia, Hodgkin's disease and other lymphomas, myeloma, carcinoma of the breast |
| Estrogens | *Diethylstilbestrol Prostate cancer:* up to 1 mg/day PO *Breast Cancer:* up to 15 mg/day PO in divided doses<br><br>*Chlorotrianisene (TACE) Prosate cancer:* 12-25 mg/day PO | Nausea and vomiting with large doses | Gynecomastia in men, breast tenderness in women; high doses have been implicated in increased cardiovascular deaths in men with cancer of the prostate | Use at low doses in men with prostate cancer; use in postmenopausal breast cancer patients only, since estrogens can exacerbate the disease in premenopausal women; serum calcium can rise rapidly in breast cancer patients shortly after therapy is started, espe- | Carcinoma of the prostate and breast |

TABLE 114—*Continued*
TOXICITY OF CANCER CHEMOTHERAPEUTIC AGENTS

| *Drug* | *Dosage and Route of Administration* | *Acute Side-effects* | *Toxicity* | *Precautions* | *Major Indications* |
|---|---|---|---|---|---|
| | | | | cially with bony disease; edema may occur with poor cardiac function | |
| Androgens | *Testosterone propionate:* 50-100 mg 3×/week IM<br><br>*Fluoxymesterone (Halotestin, Ora-Testryl):* 20-30 mg/day PO | Occasional nausea and vomiting occur more frequently at higher doses | Fluid retention, virilization, (increased facial hair, acne, deepening of voice, clitoral hypertrophy), hypercalcemia, liver function abnormalities with rare jaundice, increased red cell mass | Use with care in elderly patients with cardiac, liver, or renal disease with nephrotic syndrome (edema), and in immobilized patients, especially likely to develop hypercalcemia | Carcinoma of the breast |
| Progestational agents | *Medroxy-progesterone acetate:* 400-800 mg/week IM or PO<br><br>*Hydroxyprogesterone caproate:* 1000 mg IM twice weekly<br><br>*Megestrol acetate (Megace)* 20 mg b.i.d. PO | None | Occasional liver function abnormalities; occasional alopecia and hypersensitivity reactions | Use with care in presence of liver dysfunction | Carcinoma of the kidney, breast, endometrium |
| L-Asparaginase | 10-500 IU/kg per day IV ×2-20; or 100-500 IU/kg 3×/week | Allergic reactions, fever, anorexia, nausea, vomiting | Liver dysfunction (albumin, cholesterol, and clotting factors), which improves with continued dose; hyperglycemia, sometimes with nonketotic coma; pancreatitis, rarely renal failure; anaphylactic shock | Serum should be monitored for antibody to the drug prior to each dose; epinephrine should be available; rise in BUN and ammonia is due to action of the enzyme and is not evidence for toxicity | Acute lymphoblastic leukemia |
| Daunorubicin (daunomycin, rubidomycin) | 1 mg/kg per day IV ×5; or 30-60 mg/m$^2$ per day IV ×3; or 30-60 mg/m$^2$ per week IV | Nausea, vomiting, fever, local phlebitis, necrosis if extravasated, red urine (not blood) | Bone-marrow depression, alopecia, cardiac toxicity related to cumulative dose, stomatitis | Administer through running IV infusion; avoid giving to patients with significant heart disease, follow for EKG | Acute myeloblastic and lymphoblastic leukemia |

| | | | | | |
|---|---|---|---|---|---|
| | | | | abnormalities and signs of heart failure | |
| Streptozotocin | 1 g/m² per week IV for 5-6 weeks | Nausea, vomiting, abdominal cramps, diarrhea | Renal failure, renal tubular acidosis | Slow infusion rate to prevent local pain, contraindicated in renal disease | Malignant insulinoma, carcinoid |
| 5-Azacytidine | 150-300 mg/m² per day IV ×5; or 150-200 mg/m² 2×/week for 2-8 weeks | Fever, nausea, vomiting, diarrhea, hypotension | Bone-marrow hypoplasia | Rapid administration may lead to hypotension or fever | Acute myeloblastic leukemia; possibly melanoma, carcinoma of the breast and colon |
| Estramustine phosphate (Estracyt) | 600-1000 mg PO daily; or 300-450 mg IV daily | Nausea, vomiting, phlebitis, urticaria | Thrombocytopenia (rare); gynecomastia (rare) or breast tenderness | Early nausea and vomiting are controllable with phenothiazines. | Carcinoma of the prostate |
| Hexamethylmelamine | 4-15 mg/kg per day PO for 21-90 days; usually limited by gastrointestinal toxicity | Nausea, vomiting | Mild marrow suppression; agitation, confusion, depression; dermatitis, cystitis | None | Carcinomas of the lung, ovary, breast, cervix, bladder; lymphoma |
| Semustine (methyl-CCNU) | 175-200 mg/m² PO; repeat in 6-8 weeks | Nausea, vomiting 4-6 h. after administration | Bone-marrow depression, occasional renal and hepatic toxicity | Use antiemetics; reduce dose in face of impaired marrow function | Melanoma, gastrointestinal carcinoma, Hodgkin's disease and other lymphomas |

From Marsh and Mitchell, Chemotherapy of Cancer, II, *Drug Therapy*, p. 44, October, 1976. Courtesy of Biomedical Information Corporation, Publisher, New York, New York.

their pharmacological benefits must be clearly understood for their safe and yet adequate administration. Table 114 will be helpful in this regard.

Leucovorin (citrovorum factor) is a potent agent for neutralizing the immediate toxic effects of methotrexate on the hematopoietic system. Where large doses or overdoses have been given, calcium leucovorin may be administered by intravenous infusion in doses up to 75 mg within twelve hours, followed by 12 mg intramuscularly every six hours for four doses. Where average doses of methotrexate appear to have had an adverse effect, 2 to 4 ml (6 to 12 mg) of calcium leucovorin may be given intramuscularly every six hours for four doses. In general, where overdosage is suspected, the dose of leucovorin should be equal to or higher than the offending dose of methotrexate and should best be administered within the first hour. Use of calcium leucovorin after an hour delay is much less effective. Because of the current use of methotrexate in the treatment of skin disorders (psoriasis, etc.), this drug is now more available for accidental ingestion by children. Prompt administration of leucovorin (folinic acid) is important if severe toxicity is to be avoided.

Of great interest to many physicians is L-asparaginase, which is prepared from *E. coli* and is effective in acute lymphoblastic leukemia and in lymphosarcoma. It is now being studied for possible use in a number of other malignant diseases. As new drugs are added, they replace the less effective older ones. Cortisone is now rarely used, being replaced by more satisfactory adrenal steroid derivatives, and phenylalanine mustard instead of urethane is the drug of choice for multiple myeloma.

In children receiving mercaptopurine (Purinethol®) for leukemia, the concomitant administration of allopurinol (Zyloprim®), which is a xanthine oxidase inhibitor, calls for a reduction of up to 75 per cent in the therapeutic dose requirement of mercaptopurine. In intensive chemotherapy or in radiation therapy for leukemia, lymphomas or other malignancies, allopurinol controls ensuing hyperuricemia and hyperuricosuria and helps prevent uric acid nephropathy. Allopurinol is not a uricosuric drug *per se;* it reduces both serum and urinary uric acid levels by inhibiting the formation of uric acid.

## CAMPHOR AND CAMPHORATED OIL

Camphor is present in some moth-repellent cakes and balls as well as in camphorated oil used as a rubefacient. Camphorated oil is a 20% solution of camphor in oil, and as little as one teaspoonful has caused death in a child. Camphor is a cyclic ketone for the hydroaromatic terpene group. Its absorption through mucous membranes occurs rapidly; toxic levels may be achieved within a few minutes after ingestion. Most of the camphor is promptly removed from the bloodstream by entering either the liver, where it is conjugated to glucuronic acid after being oxidized to campherol, or the lipid deposits, where it is highly soluble. Ultimately the conjugated form is excreted by the lungs and can be detected on the breath.

Early symptoms are headache, a sensation of warmth, excitement, nausea, vomiting and delirium. Camphor odor of the breath and urine is characteristic. The skin becomes clammy, and the face is alternately flushed and pale. The pulse is weak and rapid. Twitching of facial muscles and muscular spasms may be followed by generalized convulsions and circulatory collapse.

*Treatment* is largely symptomatic, as for other central stimulants. Gastric lavage and emetics are indicated if the patient is seen before the onset of severe symptoms, followed by activated charcoal. A short-acting barbiturate, i.e. sodium pentobarbital, 0.3 gm IV, ether inhalations or chloral hydrate should be employed in controlling convulsions. Injectable diazepam (Valium) is a useful adjunct in status epilepticus and severe recurrent seizures. Lipid dialysis can remove great quantities of camphor and be a lifesaving procedure.

Artificial respiration and oxygen may be necessary in case of respiratory failure. Opiates, digestible oils and alcohol must be avoided. Intravenous fluid and plasma may be required to combat shock and maintain electrolyte balance.

## CANTHARIDIN (SPANISH FLY)

This preparation is used as a skin irritant or vesicant. It also has an intense irritant action on mucous membranes. It is excreted by the kidney and irritates the urinary tract. Irritation of the bladder causes urgency of urination, and irritation of the urethra results in priapism, thereby giving cantharidin an undeserved popular reputation as an aphrodisiac.

Spanish fly, or cantharides, is a powder derived from certain crushed beetles belonging to the order Coleoptera, family Meloidae, which contain less than 0.6 per cent of the active ingredient, cantharidin. Cantharidin is the anhydride of a simple aromatic acid, cantharidic acid, which forms biologically active soluble salts with alkali. The acid itself is soluble only in fats, ether and alcohol.

The lethal dose has been reported as small as 10 mg (1/6 gr); however, two cases of survival following ingestion of more than 75 mg are on record. Necrosis of the esophageal and gastric mucosa and intense congestion of the genitourinary tract with hemorrhage in the renal pelvis, ureters and bladder may be found pathologically.

The principal manifestation of poisoning are burning pain in throat and stomach, swelling and blistering of tongue, dysphagia, severe gastroenteritis, salivation, nausea, vomiting, bloody diarrhea, severe colic, tenesmus, burning pain in back, bladder and urethra, hematuria, strangury and thirst. Heart and respiration are briefly stimulated and then greatly depressed. There may be delirium, syncope and tetanic convulsions, collapse and finally coma.

*Treatment.* Because of the dysphagia, gastric lavage should be used cautiously in removing the ingested drug. Demulcents may allay the local pain in the mouth and upper gastrointestinal tract. In face of severe respiratory depression, morphine should not be used. The cardiovascular collapse and shock may require blood transfusions, parenteral fluids or levarterenol. Short-acting barbiturates are necessary if convulsions occur. Adequate fluids should be maintained to promote diuresis. Alcohol, fats and oils promote absorption and should be avoided. Alkali produces soluble salts which remain biologically active and should not be used in treatment.

## CATHARTICS

Drugs have been used since time immemorial for the purpose of promoting defecation. Since many agents are widely self-administered by lay persons, a knowledge of their use and possible reactions (Table 115) is desirable for the treatment of overdosage or when these compounds are accidentally ingested. Inorganic phosphate salts (sodium phosphate and biphosphate) have produced hyperphosphatemia, hypocalcemia and tetany in infants. Special precaution should be taken when administered as enemas to children with Hirschsprung's disease. Podophyllum interferes with cellular mitosis and has been shown to be embryocidal and growth-retarding in mouse fetuses and is not considered a safe cathartic, especially since much safer laxatives are available.

TABLE 115
CATHARTICS

| Compound | Time of Action | Cramping | Time Taken | Site of Action | Possible Reactions |
|---|---|---|---|---|---|
| *Emodin* | | | | | |
| Cascara | 8 hr. | None | h.s. | Colon | Pigmented rectal mucosa. |
| Senna | 6 hr. | 4 plus | h.s. | Colon | Nausea and vomiting. Hypokalemia. |
| Rhubarb | 4-8hr. | 1 plus | day | Colon | Constipation. Nausea, vomiting and headache. Skin: Macular, vesicular and hemorrhagic lesions. |
| Aloe | 8-12 hr. | 3 plus | h.s. | Colon | May cause nephritis. |
| *Resins* | | | | | |
| Jalap | 3-4 hr. | 1 plus | day | Small intestine | |
| Colocynth | 2-3 hr. | 4 plus | day | Small intestine | Overdose causes severe prostation. |
| Elaterin | | | | | |
| Gamboge | | | | | |
| Podophyllum (not considered a safe cathartic due to its potential toxicity in man and embryotoxicity in animals) | 12-24 hr. | Varies with individual | h.s. | Small intestine | Contact dermatitis and conjunctivitis. Podophyllum resin is cytotoxic, arresting epidermal mitosis, and is used in the treatment of condylomata acuminata and verruca vulgaris. It is very toxic and the lethal dose is 0.3 to 0.6 gm. Symptoms consist of vomiting, diarrhea, ataxia and coma. Treatment is symptomatic, supportive and washing off after use. |
| *Irritant Oils* | | | | | |
| Castor Oil | 2-6 hr. | + or − | day | Small intestine | No specific. |
| Croton Oil | 1-3 hr. | 4 plus | day | Small intestine | Nausea, vomiting and hemorrhagic gastroenteritis which may lead to shock and death. |
| Phenolphthalein | 4-8 hr. | None | day or night | Colon and less in small intestine | Hypersensitivity with colic, palpitation and decreased respiration. Skin: macular plaques, pruritis, burning and occasional vesiculation and ulceration. |
| Phosphates (Phospho-Soda) | 1-8 hr. | + or − | day or night | Small and large intestine | Hypocalcemia. Inorganic phosphate (Fleet) enemas should be used cautiously in children with Hirschsprung's disease. |
| Calomel (Mercurous Chloride) | 12 hr. | None | h.s. | Small intestine | Diuresis. Mercury poisoning and toxic nephritis. Acrodynia. |
| Saline Cathartics | 2-6 hr. | None | day | Small and large intestine, via peristalsis | Magnesium poisoning. Dehydration. Diuresis and toxic nephritis. |
| Bulk Cathartics | 4-20 hr. | None | anytime | ———— | Rare hypersensitivity. Rare obstruction. |
| Petrolatum | 10-18 hr. | None | h.s. | GI lubricant | Chronic mesenteric adenitis. |

| | | | | | |
|---|---|---|---|---|---|
| | | | | | Decreased vitamin A and D absorption. Lipoid pneumonia. |
| Dioctyl Sodium Sulfosuccinate* | 12-24 hr. | None | anytime | Increases wetting efficiency of intestinal water and promotes formation of oil-water emulsions to keep stools soft | None |
| Dihydroxyanthraquinone (Dorbane®) | 8-12 hr. | 1 plus | day | Peristaltic stimulant, colon | May produce a brick reddish or orange discoloration of the urine. This is of no clinical significance. |

*Dialose® Plus has produced reversible hepatic dysfunction (chronic, active and lupoid hepatitis) in some habitual users because of the incorporated drug oxyphenisatin. This compound is present in various other cathartic preparations.

General measures for *treatment* are to delay absorption by giving tap water, milk or liquid petrolatum and then removal by gastric lavage or emesis, followed by milk or demulcents to relieve gastrointestinal irritation. Atropine, 1 mg every four hours, reduces gastrointestinal secretions, and meperidine (Demerol), 100 mg, is indicated for pain or severe tenesmus. Hydration should be maintained by oral or intravenous fluids. In the case of magnesium salt or inorganic phosphate poisoning, calcium gluconate 10 ml of 10% solution may be needed as a specific antidote.

## CHLORAL HYDRATE

Chloral hydrate is a white solid, but chloral is a colorless caustic liquid of pungent odor. Chloral, although used in the chemical industry, is primarily one of the oldest and best hypnotics. Its usual therapeutic dose is 1 gm, but this depends on the state of excitability of the nervous system, and in mania and delirium, larger amounts can be given. The concomitant use of chloral hydrate and coumarin anticoagulants requires dosage reduction of the latter (reduces the biologic half-life) to avoid excessive hypothrombinemia with risk of bleeding. As little as 5 gm have caused death, but on the other hand, recovery from 30 gm has been reported. Tolerance to this drug develops to a certain extent and allows a larger dose to be taken. Normal liver function is necessary, however, in order for the habituated person to take these increased amounts with impunity because the liver plays an important part in detoxifying chloral hydrate. If the hepatic function is impaired, poisoning may occur more rapidly since chloral hydrate is metabolized to trichloroacetic acid or trichloroethanol. "Knockout drops" are produced when chloral is added to alcohol, and this combination is extremely depressing.

Acute poisoning by chloral hydrate results in deep stupor or coma within thirty minutes to one hour because absorption from the gastrointestinal tract is rapid. Death may occur in a few hours or more promptly from sudden cardiovascular collapse. In addition to the deep narcosis, respiration is slow and shallow, the body temperature is subnormal, the blood pressure is low and the skin is cyanotic and moist. The pupils are contracted and may even show the pinpoint constriction usually associated with acute morphine poisoning. If the heart is diseased, chloral hydrate may exert a direct myocardial action which results in collapse and death. When the heart is normal, death is usually respiratory in character. Cardiac arrhythmias have been documented. Recovery may be characterized by severe hemorrhagic gastritis from the local corrosive irritant action of the drug on the esophagus (esophageal stricture has been reported) and stomach mucosa, jaundice from liver injury and albuminuria from renal irritation. This parenchymatous damage is much milder but basically similar to that characteristic of delayed chloroform poisoning.

*Treatment* is essentially similar to that for barbiturate poisoning. The stomach is lavaged, the patient is kept warm, the shock syndrome is treated if it develops and respiration and blood pressure are supported by the same measures used for barbital poisoning. Intravenous glucose has the triple function of aiding the circulation, supplying glycogen to protect the liver and aiding diuresis to ensure elimination of the poison which as a glycuronide is excreted by the kidneys.

Chronic chloral hydrate intoxication occurs only in chloral habitués, and chloral addiction, though common formerly, is rarely encountered today. The syndrome closely resembles chronic alcoholism. Both have in common nutritional disturbances, skin lesions, severe gastritis and nervous system symptoms. Even delirium tremens has been reported from abrupt withdrawal of chloral hydrate. Death is not infrequent in these unfortunates either from cardiac or hepatic involvement. Treatment consists of the same measures that are used in chronic alcoholics and morphine addicts and is best carried out in a nursing home or institution specializing in this field of work. Psychotherapy and rehabilitation are essential.

Chloral betaine (Beta-Chlor®), a chemical complex of chloral and betaine, has an identical action on the central nervous system as that of chloral hydrate. The virtual elimination of undesirable gastrointestinal effects has made its use more desirable. However, the similarities between the two drugs indicate that the same degree of caution is necessary. Patients with known hepatic or renal impairment should not be given chloral betaine or chloral hydrate.

## CINCHOPHEN (NEOCINCHOPHEN)

These compounds have been used often in the past as analgesics, antipyretics and uricosuric agents, but because of their hepatotoxic effects they are now rarely employed except in patent medicines and proprietary mixtures. The lethal dose varies from 5 to 30 gm, and approximately 1 per cent of those who take the drugs for any length of time will develop liver damage. The principal manifestations are cutaneous, gastrointestinal and hepatic. Skin lesions vary in purpuric and scarlatiniform rashes, urticaria and vesicular eruptions. Minor symptoms from the gastrointestinal tract such as epigastric pain, eructation, loss of appetite and diarrhea may be due to local irritation or may be indicative of systemic poisoning and the beginning of toxic hepatitis, manifestations of which often begin with nausea and vomiting; the liver becomes tender and painful, jaundice develops, and in fatal cases is followed by gradual deterioration, stupor, coma and death from yellow atrophy of the liver. The onset of toxic hepatitis is unpredictable; it may develop after a few doses or after prolonged treatment with the drug. Occasionally it is associated with degenerative changes in the heart muscle. In rare cases agranulocytosis occurs.

In *treatment,* the stomach should be lavaged to remove any ingested poison. This should be followed by saline catharsis. Intravenous fluids should be given for the vomiting and lactated Ringer's or bicarbonate solution given for acidosis if it occurs. The treatment of toxic cirrhosis is symptomatic and supportive and is similar to that for chloroform and carbon tetrachloride injury to the liver.

## CITRIC ACID

Exchange transfusion procedures, recent medical and surgical methods of treating bleeding esophageal varices in patients with portal hypertension and bold techniques in heart and major vessel surgery, have increased the possibilities for the development of citrate toxicity.

High concentrations of serum citrate are likely to occur during multiple transfusions of citrated blood in patients with liver disease or mechanical obstruction to hepatic circulation or during rapid or prolonged infusion of citrated blood or plasma in any individual with or without liver disease.

Depression of serum ionized calcium levels is the main danger of high citric acid levels resulting from multiple transfusions of citrated blood. Reduced calcium concentrations may cause tetany, disturbances in blood coagulation and hypotension leading to vascular collapse and death.

In normal patients, if the rate at which citrate is infused is below 0.5 mg/kg of body weight per minute, the serum citrate ion concentration remains below 9 mg/100 ml, and the calculated ionized calcium level stays above 4.2 mg/100 ml; these levels are within the normal range. However, if the same amounts are given to patients with advanced liver disease, serum citrate levels rise above normal, and ionized calcium drops below normal.

As the rate of infusion is increased to 1 mg/kg/min., or approximately 500 ml of blood in 15 min., the concentration of citrate rises above 9 mg/100 ml in about 50 per cent of normal patients and in almost all subjects with liver disease. The ionized calcium level falls correspondingly.

At the lower rates of infusion, the concentration of serum citrate is roughly proportional to the infusion rate. When infusion rates are above 1 mg/kg/min., the resultant serum citrate level correlates more closely with total dose than with infusion rate.

Use of intravenous calcium salts generally is not satisfactory in the *treatment* of citric acid intoxication because of difficulty in determining correct dosages. The dose of calcium chloride is considerably smaller than that of calcium gluconate since it contains more calcium by weight. Calcium overdosage may be a serious consequence. Myocardial citrate toxicity can be avoided almost completely by giving 1 ml of $CaCl_2$ (which contains three times more ionic calcium per milliliter than calcium gluconate) simultaneously with each 100 ml of rapidly transfused citrated blood.

Decalcified blood collected by passage across a cation-exchange resin is almost ideal for multiple, rapid transfusions. During passage across the resin, serum calcium, as well as potassium and magnesium, is replaced with sodium ion, and clotting is prevented. During multiple transfusions of blood collected in this manner, the calcium ion lacking in the transfusions can be accurately replaced.

Packed or resuspended red blood cells can also be substituted for citrated blood.

## COBALT

Following reports of cobalt as an erythrocyte-stimulating agent, cobaltous chloride enjoyed widespread use as a hematinic. This metal, however, has potential toxic actions, and physicians should familiarize themselves with these as well as accurate dosage levels. The most important toxic effect of cobalt seems to be the production of goiter, with or without clinical or laboratory evidence of thyroid dysfunction. Saikkonen, in his experiments with rats, demonstrated a rise in urinary coproporphyrin after a single dose of cobalt and suggested that the well-documented rise in erythrocyte counts induced by cobalt might well be the result of tissue hypoxia. Profound hyperlipemia with subsequent xanthoma formation has been ascribed to chronic ingestion of cobaltous chloride contained in a hematinic product. Cobalt used as an antifoaming agent has been implicated in producing the "beer drinker's (enlarged) heart."

## COCAINE

Cocaine is obtained from the leaves of *Erythroxylon coca* and other species of Erythroxylon trees which are indigenous to Peru and Bolivia. Synthetic cocaine is an ester of benzoic acid and a nitrogen-containing base.

Cocaine is absorbed rapidly by all mucous membranes and is detoxified in the liver by hydrolysis; orally ingested cocaine is rapidly hydrolyzed in the stomach, making that route of administration much less toxic than inhalation (whether illicit snorting or as part of anesthesia in advance of bronchoscopy) or intravenous injection. The drug's duration of action is 20 to 40 minutes, and the absolute fatal dose by oral administration is generally accepted to be 1200 mg, with the $LD_{50}$ approximately 500 mg. But 200 to 300 mg used before bronchoscopy in the throat of a patient who has not been protected with small amounts of short-acting barbiturates could produce a reaction; amounts as low as 30 mg have been reported to cause fatal cardiac arrhythmias. Because of the great variation in the toxicity of cocaine, the drug is no longer used hypodermically, but it still remains a most effective and favored agent for inducing anesthesia by topical application. Illegal supplies of cocaine have been mixed with boric acid so that cocaine users may be ingesting 150 mg of boric acid daily (10 mg/day recommended limitation), which could produce serious and even fatal intoxication. The effects of cocaine are due to direct stimulation of the cerebral cortex and the centers in the midbrain as well as the sympathomimetic effects.

The symptoms of mild intoxication are exhilaration, easy laughter, tachycardia, sweating, dilated pupils, anorexia, anxiety and confusion. Hallucinations (bugs crawling under the skin; visual) and delusions develop with larger doses, and in extreme cases convulsions and apnea may result in respiratory death. Chronic poisoning from ingestion, injection or absorption produces euphoria, anorexia, weight loss, personality changes and eventually mental deterioration. Addiction to cocaine usually is not as marked as that which develops to morphine, and though psychic dependence is great, the physical dependence is not as clearly demonstrable as in the case of morphine addiction. Thus the abstinence syndrome is less marked and withdrawal less difficult. The treatment is not unlike that described under narcotic addiction.

*Treatment* of acute poisoning consists of removing remaining cocaine from skin or mucous membranes by washing with tap water or normal saline solution. Absorption from an injection site should be limited by tourniquet or ice pack. For ingested drug, delay absorption by giving water, milk or charcoal and then remove by gastric lavage or emesis followed by saline catharsis. To control convulsions, the administration of short-acting barbiturates such as thiopental sodium, 2.5% slowly intravenously, should be started without delay because symptoms progress with great rapidity. If convulsions interfere with respiration, oxygen, artificial respiration and the cautious use of a curare-like drug (succinylcholine, etc.) may be helpful. For shock, the patient should be placed in shock position and intravenous fluids with levarterenol or a blood transfusion given. Propranolol (Inderal®) has been reported to be useful. In the chronic user who is restless, sleepless and paranoid, the benzodiazepines (almost never the phenothiazines) have a beneficial effect.

TABLE 116
THE "CAINE" PHASES

| | *Central Nervous System* | *Circulatory System* | *Respiratory System* |
|---|---|---|---|
| Early stimulative phase | Excitement, apprehension, other symptoms of emotional instability<br>Hallucinations<br>Sudden headache<br>Nausea, vomiting<br>Twitchings of small muscles, particularly of face and fingers | Pulse variations, probably slowing<br>Usual elevation in blood pressure; possible fall<br>Skin pallor | Increased respiratory rate *and* depth |
| Advanced stimulative phase | Convulsions, tonic and clonic—resembles grand mal seizure | Increase in both pulse rate *and* blood pressure | Cyanosis<br>Dyspnea<br>Rapid, gasping or irregular respirations |
| Depressive phase | Muscle paralysis<br>Loss of reflexes<br>Unconsciousness<br>Loss of vital functions<br>Death. | Circulatory failure<br>No palpable pulse<br>Death | Respiratory failure<br>Ashen gray cyanosis<br>Death |

## CODEINE

Codeine resembles morphine pharmacologically, but its actions are milder. Lethal dose is 0.5 to 1.0 gm. It is obtained commercially from morphine by the process of methylation. This masking of the phenolic hydroxy radical with a methyl group results in a product that is less habit-forming and less depressing to respiration. Codeine is also, however, weaker in its narcotic and analgesic effect than morphine, and the central nervous system stimulatory ("convulsant") characteristic is intensified. Its analgesic effect is fleeting and large doses are required to achieve it. Smaller doses may potentiate the effect of other hypnotics and analgesics. Its use in children is limited, in the majority of cases, to conditions that justify its action as an antitussive or an analgesic particularly the former. The recommended dose as an antitussive in children is kept small (4 to 8 mg) because repeated medication may be necessary and because fluid intake may be limited (codeine is excreted 80% in the urine). Large doses may actually increase the irritability of the cough and respiratory mechanisms, with the attendant increase in the secretions of the tracheobronchial tree. Large doses, furthermore, may produce neurologic stimulation that overrides the desired antitussive or analgesic effect. In adults optimal doses produce less sedation, respiratory depression, and gastrointestinal, urinary and pupillary effects than morphine. Nausea, vomiting, constipation and diarrhea occur less frequently, and poisoning is not common. Moderate doses of codeine may occasionally cause restlessness, excitement, vertigo and mydriasis. Larger doses of 0.5 to 0.8 gm or more have caused muscle weakness, tremors, miosis, delirium, coma, convulsions and respiratory and circulatory depression with death. Although codeine is an addicting drug, its addiction potential is less than that of the other opiates. It gives less psychic satisfaction than morphine, and larger doses over a longer period of time are required to produce addiction. *Treatment* should be similar to that for morphine.

Codeine analogues (oxycodone, dihydrocodeine, hydrocodone, dihydrocodeinone) are usually available on the United States market only in combination drugs, and none offer sufficient advantages to offset their greater addiction properties. *Treatment* of overdosage with these compounds is similar to the management of codeine as described above.

## COLCHICINE (COLCHICUM)

These drugs are used as analgesic agents and in the treatment of gout and recently were reported to be effective for periodic peritonitis (recurrent polyserositis, familial Mediterranean fever). Colchicine is the active alkaloid present in all parts of the plant, meadow saffron. It is excreted slowly and converted in the body to oxydicolchicine, which in large doses causes cell destruction.

Symptoms of poisoning are severe abdominal pain, nausea, vomiting and diarrhea. The diarrhea soon becomes profuse, watery and bloody due to a hemorrhagic gastroenteritis. A reversible malabsorption syndrome is often produced. Considerable amounts of fluid, electrolytes and plasma are lost through the bowel, and in this respect the syndrome is similar to acute arsenic poisoning. Even when given by injection, colchicine causes gastrointestinal irritation. Burning of the throat and skin are also prominent symptoms. Because of the extensive vascular damage, shock occurs. The kidney, another site of excretion of colchicine, is also involved, followed by hematuria and oliguria. The pulse is rapid and weak. Muscular weakness is pronounced, with paralysis and death resulting from respiratory arrest usually within a day or two. Consciousness is present to the end, but terminal delirium or convulsions may appear. Chronic administration of colchicine may cause agranulocytosis, aplastic anemia, decrease in absorption of vitamin $B_{12}$, peripheral neuritis and delirium.

The fatal dose varies considerably. As little as 15 ml of colchicum seed tincture, corresponding to 7 mg of colchicine, has proved fatal; but much larger doses have been survived. *Treatment* of acute colchicine poisoning, in addition to gastric lavage, should be directed very early against shock. Shock symptoms should be treated by intravenous saline, glucose or blood. For the muscular weakness with respiratory depression, artificial respiration and oxygen should be administered. Atropine and morphine aid in relieving the intense abdominal pain. The remaining measures are purely symptomatic, supportive ones.

## CONTRACEPTIVES, ORAL

The older oral contraceptives contain both estrogen and progestin, while the drugs are separated in the newer sequential tablets. These drugs should not be used in women with breast or genital cancer, liver disease or thromboembolic disorders. Other precautions include (1) not prescribing for young women in whom epiphyseal closure is not complete (oral contraceptive drugs are sometims used to treat acne and dysmenorrhea in girls); (2) withholding the medication in the immediate postpartum period in the nursing mother because of possible inhibition of lactation as well as the possibility of estrogen-induced changes in the infant; (3) patients with a history of psychic depression should be carefully observed during treatment; (4) the drug should be discontinued if there is a sudden onset of severe headache, dizziness or blurred vision or if examination discloses papilledema, retinal hemorrhages or visual-field defects; and (5) contraceptive hormones can impair glucose tolerance enough to interfere with the control of diabetes.

Accidental ingestion of these popularly used preparations by small children is on the increase and often presents a problem when large numbers are taken. Even though no serious toxicity has so far been reported when this has occurred, emesis or gastric lavage should be carried out in the event of an unknown or large dose ingestion.

## CORTICOSTEROIDS

This vast group of compounds of carbohydrate-regulating hormones of the adrenal cortex is used therapeutically chiefly for substitution therapy in adrenal insufficiency. In addition, they are extensively used for collagen diseases, rheumatic fever, lupus erythematosus, severe allergic manifestations, etc.

The effects of accidental ingestion of a large number of glucocorticoid compound tablets have not been reported (oral doses of 5 gm/kg of prednisolone in mice failed to cause death), but prolonged use of these agents can produce mental symptoms, facial rounding (moon face), abnormal fat deposits, fluid retention (edema), excessive appetite, weight gain, hypertrichosis, acne, striae, ecchymosis, increased sweating, pigmentation, dry scaly skin, thinning scalp hair, increased blood pressure, tachycardia, thrombophlebitis, decreased resistance to infection, negative nitrogen balance with delayed bone and wound healing, headache, weakness, menstrual disorders, accentuated menopausal symptoms, neuropathy (including neuritis and paresthesias), fractures (osteoporosis), peptic ulcer (activation, perforation, hemorrhage), decreased glucose tolerance, hypopotassemia, adrenal insufficiency, polyarteritis nodosa, impaired renal function and lupus-erythema-

TABLE 117

COMPLICATIONS DUE TO INFECTION-PROMOTING AND ANTI-INFLAMMATORY EFFECT IN STEROID TREATMENT

| *Complication* | *Mechanism* | *Prevention* | *Management* | *Prognosis* |
|---|---|---|---|---|
| Active tuberculosis | Inhibition of host defense | Tuberculin test; chest x-ray | Antitubercular drugs; withdraw steroids | Very good |
| Histoplasmosis | Inhibition of host defense | Histoplasmin test; chest x-ray; serologic tests? | Withdraw steroids | Unknown |
| Viral infection | Inhibition of host defense; increased virulence | Withhold steroids if history negative particularly for varicella | Withdraw steroids | Guarded (generally good) |
| Bacterial infection | Inhibition of host defense; increased virulence (shock) | Early recognition of infection: stained smear; early use of antibiotics | Increase steroid dosage; increase and widen antibiotic coverage; hospitalize | Good |
| Gastrointestinal ulcers and complications | Anti-inflammatory; increased acidity; increased pepsinogen | X-ray subjects in advance; antacids; dietary measures | Reduce dosage or eliminate steroids; measures appropriate to complications | Good |
| Periarteritis | Unknown | Unknown | Probably withdraw steroids | Guarded |

TABLE 118

COMPLICATIONS DUE TO HORMONE EXCESS ENCOUNTERED IN TREATMENT WITH STEROIDS

| *Complication* | *Mechanism* | *Prevention* | *Management* | *Prognosis* |
|---|---|---|---|---|
| Cushing's syndrome | Hormone excess | Avoid overdosage | Reduce dosage or eliminate steroids | Excellent |
| Growth arrest | Pituitary inhibition | Avoid overdosage | Reduce dosage | Excellent |
| Diabetes mellitus | Anti-insulin: accelerates gluconeogenesis | Blood sugar tests*: if familial, steroid glucose-tolerance test | Increase insulin; reduce steroid dosage | Excellent (temporary, reversible) |
| Osteoporosis (bone fracture) | Antianabolic | High-protein diet; anabolic hormones; prevent immobilization; Sulkowitch test; periodic spine x-rays | Withdraw steroids; anabolic hormones; high-protein diet | Good |
| Psychosis | Unknown | Withhold from prepsychotic patients | Withdraw steroids; shock therapy if necessary | Good (reversible) |

*Fasting and 2-hr. postprandial blood sugar tests and glucose-tolerance test.

TABLE 119
AVAILABLE CORTICOSTEROIDS AND THEIR RELATIVE POTENCIES
(Amount of synthetic needed to have effect equal to 25 mg of cortisone or 20 mg of hydrocortisone)

| *Generic Name* | *Chemical name* | *Equivalent doses (mg)* |
|---|---|---|
| Cortisone | 11-dehydro-17-hydroxycortisone | 25 |
| Hydrocortisone (cortisol) | 17-hydroxycorticosterone | 20 |
| Prednisone | 1-delta-dehydrocortisone | 5 |
| Prednisolone | 1-delta-1-dehydrohydrocortisone | 5 |
| Methylprednisolone | 6-alpha-methylprednisolone | 4 |
| Triamcinolone | 9-alpha-fluoro-16-alpha-hydroxyprednisolone | 4 |
| Paramethasone | 6-alpha-fluoro-16-alpha-methylprednisolone | 2 |
| Fluprednisolone | 6-alpha-fluoroprednisolone | 1.5 |
| Dexamethasone | 9-alpha-fluoro-16-alpha-methylprednisolone | 0.75 |
| Betamethasone | 9-alpha-fluoro-16-beta-methylprednisolone | 0.6 |

tosus-like changes. Hepatomegaly and abdominal distention have been observed in children. Corticosteroid therapy produces more severe side-effects than treatment with corticotropin. They occur more often in women than in men and at all ages.

*Treatment* of accidental ingestion is immediate gastric lavage or emesis, otherwise in the face of critical indication or severe symptoms, these drugs need be discontinued or the dosage reduced only temporarily and given on alternate days.

## CURARE (CHONDODENDRON TOMENTOSUM EXTRACT, DIMETHYL TUBOCURARINE CHLORIDE, IODIDE, ETC.)

Curare has been used as a generic term that includes all drugs acting in the vicinity of the myoneural junction and often referred to as "muscle relaxants." In therapeutic doses, it blocks myoneural transmission to skeletal muscle and may depress ganglionic impulses in the autonomic nervous system.

Since these compounds are for parenteral use, they should be employed only by those thoroughly familiar with their dosage, effects and dangers. Poisoning from curare is almost always the result of clinical overdosage or injudicious use of drug. Symptoms of intoxication consist of agitation; complete paralysis of voluntary muscles, starting with those of the face and neck, spreading to extremities and finally to the diaphragm and the intercostal muscles; elevated temperature; bradycardia; diuresis; and respiratory depression. Consciousness is not affected and death is by asphyxia. When curare or curarine is swallowed, the action is similar to, but much less severe than, after injection.

*Treatment* includes the prompt early insertion of an endotracheal catheter and the use of a positive-pressure artificial respirator with oxygen until muscle power returns. Both physostigmine and neostigmine are pharmacologic antagonists to the muscle-paralyzing effect of curare, but neostigmine is more effective. Neither is adequate to counteract great overdosage and may increase curarization in large doses. Recently, edrophonium chloride (Tensilon®) and neostigmine (Prostigmin) have been used to combat overdosage of curariform drugs, with effective results. Atropine should be combined with anticurares to counteract the undesirable side-actions, especially the tendency to cause profuse secretion. The excessive use of the anticurares may be detrimental, not only because of their side-actions, but also because these drugs often potentiate rather than antagonize curare activity. Moreover, prompt and adequate artificial respiration is the important factor in the treatment of overdosage with curares; the anticurares are of secondary and limited value.

## DEXTROMETHORPHAN HYDROBROMIDE

Dextromethorphan hydrobromide is related to the synthetic analgesic levorphanol, but possesses little or none of its analgesic activity nor any of its addictive properties. It has become popular as a substitute for codeine in cough preparations. Clinical evidence indicates that this drug is about equal to codeine in action when administered in doses up to 20 mg. Further increase in dosage does not seem to increase its antitussive effectiveness into the range of the morphine-like agents.

The incidence of untoward effects produced by dextromethorphan has been low, with drowsiness and gastrointestinal upset as the principal manifestations seen. Toxic doses in animals produce ataxia, hyperexcitability, convulsions and death from respiratory failure. Symptoms reported following human intoxication include nausea, vomiting, drowsiness, dilated pupils, blurred vision, nystagmus, flushed skin, vertigo, ataxia, shallow respiration, urinary retention, stupor and coma.

In *treatment,* the stomach should be lavaged or an emetic used, followed by a saline cathartic. Otherwise, only supportive and symptomatic measures are required. The antidotal efficacy of the morphine antagonists such as nalorphine, levallorphan or naloxone has not been fully established for dextromethorphan, but the recent use of naloxone immediately reversed ataxia and other symptoms in a two-year-old child.

## DEXTROPROPOXYPHENE HYDROCHLORIDE (DARVON®)

This is a synthetic analgesic drug which is related pharmacologically to codeine. Animals fed toxic doses of dextropropoxyphene have developed varying degrees of central nervous system and respiratory depression. Although addictive qualities of Darvon are apparently slight, potential habituation should be suspected in any case of excessive use of this drug. The following effects have been reported in humans: nausea, vomiting, dizziness, ptosis, convulsions, hypoxia, pulmonary edema, cardiovascular collapse and coma. Neonatal withdrawal symptoms associated with the maternal use of propoxyphene have been reported, and its constant use during pregnancy should be discouraged.

Although propoxyphene is considered a relatively safe drug when used in recommended doses, in combination with alcohol, tranquilizers, sedative-hypnotics and other central nervous system depressants, additive serious depressant effects may occur which can cause severe toxicity and death. Total propoxyphene-related fatalities increased from 196 in 1972 to 315 in 1974, the last year for which complete data were available.

*Treatment.* There is no antidote for dextropropoxyphene poisoning. Animal studies have indicated that nalorphine hydrochloride or levallorphan tartrate may be of value in the treatment of respiratory depression caused by this drug, and recent reports of its use in children indicated that it was of definite value and may have been the most important therapeutic measure used. Naloxone hydrochloride (Narcan), since it is available, is now the narcotic antagonist of choice. Analeptic drugs (amphetamine, caffeine with sodium benzoate, etc.) must not be given because fatal convulsions may be produced. Activated charcoal adsorbs significant amounts of Darvon and should be administered, after which the stomach should be emptied as soon as possible, following the ingestion of larger than therapeutic amounts. Additional charcoal should then be administered. The induction of gastric lavage or emesis is contraindicated, however, if the patient is comatose or is convulsing. Measures designed to ensure adequate pulmonary ventilation by keeping the airway clear, by administration of oxygen and by artificial respiration are necessary if respiratory depression exists. Therapy for pulmonary edema should include vigorous efforts to decrease intravascular volume, decrease venous return, improve arterial oxygenation and combat acidosis. If convulsions occur, efforts to maintain adequate pulmonary ventilation must be intensified. Seizures may be controlled by the administration of parenteral short-acting barbiturates or by deep intramuscular injection of paraldehyde. These drugs must be given cautiously because of their respiratory depressant action. Careful attention must be paid to fluid balance because of the possible occurrence of nephrogenic diabetes insipidus. Although this compound is dialyzable, dialysis has not been greatly effective so far.

## DIAMETHAZOLE (ASTEROL®)

Diamethazole is a practically odorless, colorless, antifungal agent available as 5% ointment, 5% tincture and 5% dusting powder.

This compound has definite neurotoxic effects on infants and there have been several reports of convulsions following its use. The application of excessive doses in its prolonged use for several weeks has been followed by hallucinations, tremors, muscular twitching and weakness, incoordination and ataxia. This preparation should never be used for children under six years of age, and in adults the weekly dose should not exceed 60 gm of the tincture or ointment. Every precaution should be taken to prevent getting Asterol into the mouth, eyes or nose. In the event of irritation or failure to obtain prompt therapeutic relief, use of the drug should be discontinued. (This product was discontinued in the United States [1966] but is still available in Europe.)

## DIGITALIS

In use for hundreds of years, digitalis is still the most effective drug for congestive heart failure of the so-called low-output type. Unfortunately, digitalis, its various preparations and the numerous individual principles in pure form, however derived, are capable of toxic effects when used in little more than the therapeutic dose. Unlike most drugs, it has only a slight margin of safety; less than twice the useful dose is toxic. To employ digitalis with a heavy hand is to invite serious poisoning, and the incidence of such trouble is increasingly alarming. In addition, the complexities of digitalis therapy as to dosage, absorption, half-life and interaction with other drugs is just now being recognized and appreciated.

Digoxin is almost completely metabolized or excreted unchanged in the urine in five days; its peak effect is seen at one to three hours after administration, and the serum half-life is twenty-four hours. On the other hand, digitoxin is almost completely excreted in eighteen days and the peak effect is seen at eight to ten hours and may last as long as seventy-two hours. Digitoxin is almost completely absorbed from the gastrointestinal tract, in contrast to 50 to 90 per cent of digoxin. Absorption is complete by 2 hours after ingestion. More than 80 per cent of digoxin and digitoxin are excreted in the urine, but only 10 per cent of digitoxin is unchanged.

The number of accidental ingestions of cardiac glycosides by children is increasing each year, probably because of the greater number of digitalis compounds prescribed for our aging population and often carelessly left about the home in open handbags, on tables, etc. The slightly sweet taste of glycosides appeals to children, which further increases the possibility of accidental ingestion. The use of special containers with safety closures for these preparations should be encouraged, along with a label, "Keep out of the reach of children," or some similar warning statement.

The functions of the drug are complex, multiple and interrelated, but the major therapeutic usefulness of digitalis is probably due to its direct action on the myocardium, producing a more vigorous systolic contraction. To some degree it seems to stimulate the vagus reflexly; of importance in atrial fibrillation is the drug's effect on the atrioventricular conduction bundle, where it especially increases the refractory period, slows the rate of conduction and thus aids in reducing the ventricular rate. During therapy, the electrocardiogram may demonstrate shortening of the Q-T interval with concave depression of the descending limb of the T wave and "sagging" of the S-T segment; prolongation of the P-R interval can occur early. These changes, while typical (so-called digitalis effect), are neither specific for digitalis nor indicative of the amount given.

Intoxication occurs, primarily and most obviously, with overdosage. It may follow administration of slowly excreted materials at unduly short intervals, inaccurate adjustment of the patient's own requirements and susceptibility (there is no "standard" dose or response) and possible failure to note early toxic signs. Forcing the drug for "intractable failure" is hazardous, and so is the use of it for so-called high-output failure, where the response is ordinarily poor. It is now appreciated also that, while a patient may be doing well under digitalis correctly administered, the addition of drugs causing a loss of potassium (mercurial diuretics, steroids) may precipitate intoxication.

The following (preventable) factors are largely responsible for digitalis intoxication.

1. The drug sometimes is administered for incorrectly diagnosed heart failure or for dyspnea from pulmonary, rather than cardiac, disease.
2. Administration may be premature, without waiting for the effects of rest and nursing or before determining if the patient received the drug shortly before hospital admission.
3. Diuretics given concurrently aggravate digitalis toxicity. Triamterene (Dyrenium®) is a potassium-sparing diuretic which can be used effectively and safely.
4. Potentially dangerous arrhythmias related to digitalis therapy may occur without warning symptoms such as anorexia, nausea, vomiting or visual disturbance—a hazard that increases the importance of electrocardiographic assessment of cardiac condition before digitalization.
5. Belief that an optimum dose always reduces ventricular rate persists, but in patients with sinus rhythm, the drug may reduce the rate only slightly, if at all. In those with atrial fibrillation, rapid ventricular action may be due to ventricular ectopic beats from digitalis intoxication. In those with atrial fibrillation and irregular ventricular action, ventricular rhythm may become regular during digitalization as the result of complete A-V block with regular A-V rhythm or nonparoxysmal A-V tachycardia.
6. Refractory heart failure may be a manifestation of digitalis toxicity, but if not recognized as such, it may be treated by even more digitalis.
7. Treatment continued without adequate clinical control and electrocardiographic assessment may lead to intoxication, as may failure to discontinue administration for an adequate time if signs of overdosage are seen.

## Toxic Manifestations of Digitalis

A. Gastrointestinal
   1. Anorexia
   2. Nausea
   3. Vomiting
   4. Diarrhea
B. Neurologic
   1. Mental depression, personality changes, delirium, psychoses.
   2. Abnormal visual sensations (10% to 25%)
      a. Color (especially yellow and green)
      b. Scotomata

c. Blurred or dimmed vision
3. Cerebral excitation manifested as headache, vertigo, increased irritability
4. Peripheral neuritis

C. Cardiac
1. Changes in rhythm
 a. (1) Ventricular premature contractions, coupled rhythm
  (2) Atrial fibrillation
  (3) Atrial tachycardia with or without block
  (4) Ventricular tachycardia
 b. Heart block
  (1) Prolonged P-R interval
  (2) Dropped beats
2. Heart failure: mesenteric infarction from circulatory failure with low cardiac output and hypotension
3. Electrocardiographic changes
 a. S-T segment depression
 b. T wave changes
 c. Changes in rhythm

D. Other
1. Gynecomastia
2. Anemia-eosinophilia-thrombocytopenia
3. Allergic manifestations such as skin rash, urticaria, etc.
4. Profound fatigue
5. Generalized muscular weakness

Toxicity is perhaps more frequently seen with the potent purified derivatives (especially if slowly excreted) than with the whole leaf, but manifestations are the same no matter what preparation is used. The symptoms of intoxication may be local, central or cardiac in origin. Local irritation of the gastrointestinal tract is more likely to occur with the digitalis leaf, but such symptoms as fatigue, anorexia, nausea and vomiting can be due to the central effects of toxic doses of the glycosides as well as the leaf. Digitalis fatigue is unique in that it does not lessen toward evening, but remains steady and increases with even slight increments of the drug. Other central manifestations include yellow or green visions, halos, scotomata, flickering vision and "snowflake" effects; oculomotor paresis and amblyopia may occur. Headache, drowsiness and convulsions are known to have been caused by digitalis. Gynecomastia is an unusual and rare complication. Psychic effects include depression (a change in personality with increasing depression may be the first sign of digitalis intoxication), confusion, defects in memory and concentration, delirium and frank psychotic episodes. Sometimes the delirium lasts for weeks, even though provoked by a short-acting glycoside. Digitalis delirium frequently is associated with aortic valve lesions and may occur as the earliest and possibly the only sign of intoxication without electrolyte changes, Cheyne-Stokes respiration, anoxia or administration of sedatives. Elderly patients are affected most often.

Of greatest importance, however, are the cardiac manifestations of toxicity. Any conceivable arrhythmia may develop, one of the common early forms being premature beats. Ventricular extrasystoles may arise from one of many foci and appear in couples or groups as bigeminy, trigeminy, etc., or there may be atrial arrhythmias or sinus arrest and various degrees of atrioventricular block; or nodal rhythm, wandering pacemaker or Wenckebach arrhythmia may occur. Bursts of uni– or bidirectional ventricular tachycardia herald severe intoxication, and ventricular fibrillation and death may follow. Atrial arrhythmias are often encountered and include atrial fibrillation, flutter and tachycardia with block. The development of a slow, regular rhythm in a patient previously fibrillating with a rapid ventricular rate should alert the physician to the possible existence of a nodal rhythm or complete AV block due to excessive accumulation of digitalis. It is important to note also that electrocardiographic evidence of intoxication may be only sporadic, and constant clinical observation of the patient on digitalis is required.

There is no specific level of dosage at which toxicity appears. It varies with each patient and is affected by the patient's age, the etiology of his heart disease, associated electrolyte imbalances and perhaps unknown factors. Older patients appear to be more sensitive to digitalis therapy, perhaps because their heart disease is more advanced and the ratio between the effective and toxic dose is for them even further decreased.

Sometimes one cannot decide whether an ill patient has received too much or too little digitalis, although usually the diagnosis can be readily made by history, physical examination and electrocardiogram. If a decision is not possible, it is safer to assume that the patient is overdigitalized. This is the error of choice; the reverse error, treating toxicity with additional digitalis, is more immediately catastrophic. A rapid saliva test using the mean potassium-calcium product (markedly elevated) found in saliva may be helpful in separating the digitalis-toxic patients from the non-digitalis toxic group. This method allows presymptomatic detection of potential digitalis toxicity in patients at risk.

Since the gastrointestinal, nervous and electrocardiographic phenomena of advanced heart failure may be hard to distinguish from those of digitalis intoxication, various digitalis tolerance tests have been devised. Small doses of lanatoside C or ouabain are given intravenously to see whether the patient improves with additional glycoside. Serious toxicity is minimized by the fact that these are short-acting, rapidly excreted drugs. An even shorter-acting glycoside, acetyl strophanthin, may be used in the same way. Such tolerance tests are, of course, also hazardous and must be weighed against expected benefits. They are best used when the likelihood of digitalis overdosage is thought to be less than that of underdosage.

*Treatment.* In massive ingestion, gastric lavage and oral administration of ipecac may result in increased vagal activity, a response to be avoided in the setting of digitalis-induced vagal hyperactivity and the possibility of high degrees of atrioventricular block. Alternative procedures in the management of this problem should include treatment with atropine prior to lavage, the use of a small-diameter nasogastric tube with prewarmed lavage solutions and the avoidance of ipecac and apomorphine hydrochloride.

If the diagnosis of digitalis toxicity is considered, further administration of the drug is stopped immediately. In mild cases a reduction in dosage may be sufficient. The patient is closely observed, and if toxicity persists or is severe, potassium chloride in oral doses of 2 to 10 gm dissolved in fruit juice may be effective within thirty minutes. In severe intoxication, intravenous potassium chloride may be given in doses of 3 gm (40 mEq) in 500 ml of dextrose solution over an hour, under electrocardiographic observation. The infusion is halted immediately upon cessation of signs of toxicity or upon peaking of the T waves. Potassium itself is a potentially toxic drug, but poisoning with oral medication is rare with good urinary output. Potassium therapy is effective in the presence of a normal serum level; it should not be given if the level is elevated.

Magnesium sulfate can be given in a dose of 20 ml of 20% solution. Its action is of very short duration and therefore of questionable clinical value. It has an antiarrhythmic effect on the myocardium and is especially effective in abolishing premature ventricular contractions (bigeminy) and ventricular tachycardia due to digitalis. Diphenylhydantoin (Dilantin), the widely used anticonvulsant drug, has recently been demonstrated in animals and humans to correct digitalis toxicity arrhythmias that have been refractory to usual therapy. The drug is particularly effective in supraventricular and ventricular arrhythmias. It is also of benefit in controlling paroxysmal atrial and ventricular arrhythmias but has had little or no effect on atrial flutter and fibrillation.

Profound depression of the myocardium after IV administration has been reported, and the hemodynamic characteristic of diphenylhydantoin should be familiar to the clinician before use. Measures such as hypothermia, dialysis, extracorporeal circulation and exchange transfusion have not proven effective experimentally because digitalis is rapidly fixed to the cell and does not diffuse quickly.

Some of the antihistamines, particularly antazoline, are effective against ventricular

TABLE 120
DRUG THERAPY FOR DIGITALIS TOXICITY

| *Drugs and other Methods* | *Mild Toxicity* | *Severe Toxicity* | *Contraindications* |
|---|---|---|---|
| Potassium | KCl 1-2 gm q.4h. | 40-60 mEq/liter KCl in 500 ml 5% DW (distilled water) IV injection (1-3 h.period) under EKG monitor and periodic serum $K^+$ determination | Hyperkalemia, uremia, 2nd and 3rd degree A-V block, SA block |
| Dilantin (diphenylhydantoin) | 100 mg t.i.d. or q.i.d. by mouth | 125-250 mg IV injection (2-3 min. period) under EKG monitor. Same dosage may be repeated every 5-10 min. | 2nd and 3rd degree A-V block, SA block, marked sinus bradycardia |
| Xylocaine (lidocaine) | | 1 mg/kg body weight IV injection every 20 min. Maximum dose: 750 mg | (Same as Dilantin) |
| Inderal (propranolol) | 10-30 mg t.i.d. or q.i.d. before meals and at bedtime | 1-3 mg slow IV injection (not to exceed 1 mg/min.) under EKG monitor. Second dose may be repeated after 2 min. Additional medication should not be given within less than 4 h. | Bronchial asthma, allergic rhinitis, marked sinus bradycardia, SA block, 2nd and 3rd degree A-V block, cardiogenic shock, heart failure, pulmonary hypertension |
| Pronestyl (procainamide) | 250-500 mg q.3-4h. by mouth | 50-100 mg every 2-4 min. slow IV injection or 1 gm in 200 ml 5% DW IV drip (30-60 min. period) under EKG monitor. Maximum doses: 2.0 gm | (Same as Dilantin) |
| Quinidine | | 0.6 gm in 200 ml 5% DW IV drip (30-60 min. period) under EKG monitor | (Same as Dilantin) |
| Atropine sulfate | 1-2 mg IV | | |
| Magnesium sulfate | Slow (1 ml/min.) IV infusion (20 ml of 20% solution) under continuous EKG monitoring. | | |
| Artificial pacemaker | Temporary demand pacemaker may be indicated for 3rd degree A-V block and occasionally for 2nd degree A-V block, SA block or marked sinus bradycardia. | | |
| DC countershock | *Not recommended* except as a last resort after all available measures have been exhausted. To prevent postcardioversion arrhythmias, administer Dilantin 125-250 mg IV 5-10 minutes before DC countershock. | | |
| Sodium EDTA | Not recommended for clinical use. | | |

Note: Immediate digitalis withdrawal is *always* the first step!

arrhythmias, and saturated lactones (THFA) are reported to be antagonstic to digitalis effects on the A-V conduction, but sufficient clinical experience is lacking. Beta-adrenergic blocking agents (propranolol and others) have also been found to be successful in reversing the arrhythmias of digitalis intoxication, but side-reactions (nausea, vertigo, paresthesia, hypotension) are common. Atropine is an old standby in the treatment of nodal arrhythmias and is known to increase the minimal lethal dose of cardiac glycosides.

Serious arrhythmias like ventricular tachycardia may be treated with procainamide. It is given orally in doses of 1.0 gm, and doses of 0.5 gm may be repeated every two or four hours. Intravenously, doses of 250 to 1000 mg may be given at a maximum rate of 100 mg/min. Procainamide may, however, cause hypotension and occasionally ventricular tachycardia and is to be administered with caution and under electrocardiographic control. Quinidine has been used for the arrhythmias of digitalis toxicity, but some authorities consider it dangerous. An external cardiac pacemaker should be used for cardiac arrest. In the accidental ingestion of large doses by children or adults for suicidal intent, the administration of an intravenous solution of the chelating agent sodium or dipotassium (not calcium) edetate produces a hypocalcemia that may counteract the toxic symptoms of digitalis. EDTA does not remove the calcium ion; instead it chelates the calcium ion, thus reducing the synergistic action of the calcium present on the activity of digitalis. However this therapy is little used since more effective therapy is now available. The dangerous arrhythmias usually begin to convert to sinus rhythm within a few minutes. In some patients, the effect of sodium edetate is temporary, but slower potassium chloride may be given, if necessary, once the rapid initial improvement has been obtained with the chelating agent.

Intravenous administration of citrate salts (sodium and potassium) has been reported to neutralize the toxic effects of digitalis overdose in experimental animals and correct abnormal heart rhythm without causing serious side-reactions.

Most cases of serious digitalis toxicity may be avoided or treated early if the physician remembers that toxicity occurs at different dosage levels in different patients or even in the same patient at different times. Patients should be told that they are on digitalis and containers should be clearly labeled. The parenteral administration of digitalis is more dangerous and is seldom necessary. The use of divided increments with careful observation permits the physician to approximate most nearly the elusive clinical state of "optimal digitalization." Large daily oral doses of vitamin E (200 to 300 mg) have been recently used successfully in checking digitalis intoxication. Several types of insoluble nonabsorbable bile-acid-binding polymers, which have been shown to interrupt the enterohepatic circulation of bile acids, may prove to be important adjuncts in the treatment of digitalis intoxication. These types of resins include cholestyramine, a quaternary ammonium styrenedivinylbenzene copolymer, and colestipol (U-26597A), an insoluble copolymer of tetraethylenepentamine and epichlorohydrin. A Boston team has recently found specific antibodies to reverse a digitalis overdose and intoxication. Finally, thorough familiarity with the pharmacology, indications and contraindications of one rapidly acting and one slower form of digitalis contributes much to reduce this dangerous iatrogenic condition.

## DIPHENOXYLATE HYDROCHLORIDE (LOMOTIL®)

Lomotil (diphenoxylate hydrochloride 2.5 mg with atropine 0.025 mg/tablet or teaspoonful) is a very popular antidiarrheal agent. A dose of 15 mg diphenoxylate hydrochloride is equal to 45 mg of codeine, while 2.5 mg diphenoxylate equals 4 ml of camphorated tincture of opium in its antidiarrheal action. Its pharmacologic action is closely related to meperidine (Demerol) and strongly inhibits rhythmic contractions of the smooth muscle of the gastrointestinal motility. There is a very narrow range between the therapeutic and toxic doses. Therapeutic dose is 3 to 10 mg/day in a child and 20 mg/day in an adult.

Toxicity in children has resulted from as few as six tablets, and twelve tablets have caused death in a two-year-old child. Because of the narrow range between the therapeutic and toxic doses, many physicians oppose its use in young children, and the FDA package insert guidelines for Lomotil contradict its use in children under two years of age.

The first signs and symptoms are of

atropine toxicity: hyperpyrexia, flushing of the skin and tachypnea. Early convulsions are probably due to the hyperpyrexia. The pupils are miotic and unresponsive to light due to the narcotic effect. There is generalized hypotonia and loss of the deep tendon reflexes. The atropine toxicity signs last two to three hours.

The second phase begins abruptly with a drop in temperature, disappearance of flush and progressive depression of the central nervous system. Respiration becomes slow and shallow and may cease. Major seizures at this time are attributed to hypoxia. Paralytic ileus may also be present.

*Treatment.* Establish an adequate airway with an endotracheal tube, and as soon as the life-support mechanisms are stabilized, perform gastric lavage. Gastric lavage is useful even many hours after ingestion because of the decrease in gastrointestinal motility due to the pharmacologic activity of the drug. Activated charcoal administered in doses five to ten times the estimated weight of the ingested compound (10 to 20 gm minimum) should be followed with a nonabsorbable saline cathartic 250 mg/kg PO every three or four hours until adequate stooling occurs. A respirator should be at the bedside. IV fluids should be given, but not to the extent of precipitating cerebral edema, which is a real possibility. Naloxone HCL (Narcan) IV, SC or IM should be given in doses 0.01 mg/kg at first sign of respiratory depression. Since the duration of action of diphenoxylate is much longer than naloxone, this may have to be repeated if the respiratory depression recurs. It may be necessary at intervals of ten to fifteen minutes to monitor against recurrent respiratory depression. The bladder should be catheterized to avoid reabsorption of atropine and because urinary retention frequently recurs. Hemodialysis, peritoneal dialysis or exchange transfusions are not beneficial.

## ERGOT AND ERGOT ALKALOIDS

Ergot is a parasitic fungus which grows on rye. It is used in various proprietary mixtures as an abortifacient. The derivatives ergotamine and dihydroergotamine are used in the treatment of headaches, while ergonovine and methylergonovine are employed as uterine stimulants. The lethal dose of ergot may be as low as 1 gm, but fatalities from purified derivatives are rare. Ergot and its alkaloids, in addition to being potent adrenergic blocking agents, also stimulate smooth muscles of the arterioles, intestines and uterus, as well as excite and depress the central nervous system.

Symptoms of acute poisoning are referable as a rule to the gastrointestinal, central nervous and peripheral vascular systems. Abdominal pain, nausea and vomiting and diarrhea appear quite early. Constriction in the throat and precordium suggestive of angina pectoris may occur. Disturbances of speech and vision, delirium, paresthesias and motor difficulties of the extremities, epileptiform convulsions and coma follow in more serious cases. Abortion may occur in pregnant women and fatal hemorrhage ensue. Muscle pains and weakness and numbness and tingling of the fingers and toes are forerunners of the gangrene which may occur in severe ergot poisoning. The gangrene is due to endothelial injury and consequent thrombosis and involves the most distal parts of the extremities first. It may then extend up the limbs for varying distances. Gangrene takes several days to develop, and there are usually ample premonitory signs of deficient circulation such as paresthesia, pain, numbness, cyanotic color and skin changes. Gangrene can ocur from the repeated use of therapeutic doses of ergot or its alkaloids. It is more apt to appear in patients with peripheral vascular disease, severe toxemia or hepatitis and jaundice. Patients with infections, arteriosclerosis, peripheral vascular or cardiac, kidney or liver disease should not be given ergot preparations. Pregnancy is another obvious contraindication. Occasionally trismus develops as the main toxic symptom from ergotamine ingestion, resulting from stimulation of the trigeminal motor nucleus in the pons.

Symptoms of chronic poisoning (ergotism) from ingestion, injection or application to mucous membranes can be produced either from contraction of blood vessels and reduced circulation (numbness, tingling and coldness of the extremities, pain in the chest and gangrene of the fingers or toes) or from the central nervous system involvement (tremors and convulsions), which rarely occurs in iatrogenic ergotism (excessive ingestion of ergot compounds).

*Treatment* consists of delaying absorption of ingested compounds by giving water or milk and then removing by gastric lavage or emesis, followed by saline cathartic. The gastrointestinal effects often yield to injections of atropine sulfate in 0.5 mg doses. Muscle pains of the extremities respond in milder cases to intravenous calcium gluconate, 10 ml of a 10% solution. For incipient gangrene, papaverine hydrochloride may be given as a vascular antispasmodic in oral or hypodermic doses of 30 to 60 mg or intravenously in 30 mg amounts. This compound is hepatotoxic, probably on a hypersensitivity basis, and should not be used for any prolonged period.

Mecholyl in doses of 5 to 20 mg or choline esters and nitrates may be used also as a vasodilator. A continuous intravenous infusion of the potent vasodilator sodium nitroprusside has recently been used with complete resolution of signs and symptoms of peripheral ergotamine-induced peripheral ischemia after other therapy had failed. While these agents cannot repair endothelial damage, remove thrombi or recanalize thrombosed vessels, they may improve collateral circulation so that there is adequate blood brought to the extremities to arrest or repair the gangrenous process. Instruments supplying passive vascular exercise or intermittent venous occlusion should also be employed before an extremity is sacrificed by surgery.

Before using the preparations in Table 121 for migraine, the patient should be checked for contraindications: vascular disease, pregnancy, liver and kidney disease, hypertension, sepsis and cachexia. By trial and error, the physician should learn to estimate the total amount of ergot necessary to stop an individual's attacks and should attempt to give this effective total in the first dose early in the attack. This amount should be given one to two hours to work before adding further doses. If the maximum amount of ergot therapy has been used within four to five hours without effect, further ergot for migraine headache is apt to be futile and may only promote prostration and nausea. In general, there should be at least two days of each week in which the patient takes no ergot.

Sansert® (methysergide maleate), which is not an ergot derivative, has been reported to produce retroperitoneal fibrosis in some individuals, with occasional involvement of

TABLE 121
ERGOT DERIVATIVES MAXIMUM DOSAGE IN USE FOR MIGRAINE

| *Commercial Product* | *Composition* | *Usual Initial Dose* | *Maximum Initial Dose* | *Maximum Amount in One Day* |
|---|---|---|---|---|
| | | *Oral ingestion* | | |
| Gynergen® tablets (Sandoz) | Ergotamine tartrate 1 mg | 1 to 3 mg | 5 mg | 10 mg |
| Bellergal® tablets (Sandoz) | Ergotamine tartrate 0.3 mg | 1 to 2 | 3 | for attacks in children 6 |
| | Bellafoline 0.1 mg Phenobarbital 20 mg | 1 to 2 | 4 | for prophylaxis in adults 8 |
| Bellergal® spacetabs (Sandoz) | Ergotamine tartrate 0.6 mg | 1 | 2 | for attacks in children 3 |
| | Bellafoline 0.2 mg Phenobarbital 40 mg | 1 | 2 | for prophylaxis in adults 4 |

TABLE 121—*Continued*
ERGOT DERIVATIVES MAXIMUM DOSAGE IN USE FOR MIGRAINE

| *Commercial Product* | *Composition* | *Usual Initial Dose* | *Maximum Initial Dose* | *Maximum Amount in One Day* |
|---|---|---|---|---|
| Cafergot® P-B tablets (Sandoz) | Ergotamine tartrate 1 mg<br>Caffeine 100 mg<br>Bellafoline 0.125 mg<br>Pentobarbital 30 mg | 1 to 2 | 3 | 6 |
| Wigraine® tablets (Organon) | Ergotamine tartrate 1 mg<br>Caffeine 100 mg<br>Acetophenetidin 130 mg<br>Belladonna alkaloids 0.1 mg | 1 to 2 | 3 | 6 |
| Migral® tablets (Burroughs Wellcome) | Ergotamine tartrate 1 mg<br>Caffeine 50 mg<br>Cyclizine 25 mg | 1 to 2 | 3 | 6 |
| | | *Sublingual administration* | | |
| Ergomar® tablets (Cooper) | Ergotamine tartrate 2 mg | 1 | 2 | 4 |
| | | *Aerosol inhalation* | | |
| Medihaler-Ergotamine® (Riker) | Ergotamine tartrate 0.36 mg/inhalation | 1 to 2 inhalations | 4 inhalations | 6 inhalations |
| | | *Rectal suppositories* | | |
| Cafergot suppositories (Sandoz) | Ergotamine tartrate 2 mg<br>Caffeine 100 mg | ½ to 1 | 1 | 3 |
| Cafergot P-B suppositories (Sandoz) | Ergotamine tartrate 2 mg<br>Caffeine 100 mg<br>Bellafoline 0.25 mg<br>Pentobarbital 60 mg | ½ to 1 | 1 | 3 |
| Wigraine suppositories (Organon) | Ergotamine tartrate 1 mg<br>Caffeine 100 mg<br>Belladonna alkaloids 0.1 mg<br>Acetophenetidin 130 mg | 1 | 2 | 4 |
| | | *Parenteral injection* | | |
| Gynergen (Sandoz) ampules, 0.5 ml and 1 ml | Ergotamine tartrate 0.5 mg/ml | SC and IM<br>0.5 ml | 1 ml | 1.5 ml |
| | | IV (to be used with great caution)<br>0.3 to 0.5 ml | 0.5 ml | 1 ml |
| Dihydroergotamine or DHE 45 (Sandoz) ampules, 1 ml | Dihydroergotamine 1 mg/ml | SC and IM<br>0.7 to 1 ml | 1.5 ml | 3 ml |
| | | IV<br>0.5 ml | 1 ml | 1.5 ml |
| Sansert® (Sandoz) | Methysergide maleate (not an ergot derivative) 2 mg | | 2 mg t.i.d. p.c. | 8 mg |

the pleura, immediate subjacent pulmonary tissues and the cardiac valves (the precipitation of fibrotic changes in patients already predisposed to disorders of collagen is also a distinct possibility). Reversible vasculitis of the iliac vessels with secondary ureteral obstruction, bilateral hydronephrosis and diminution of renal function have also been documented. Arterial insufficiency or shutdowns of major vessels, or both, have occurred with prolonged use; thus therapy with this compound should not exceed six months without reasonable drug-free intervals of two or three weeks.

## ESTROGENS, CONJUGATED U.S.P.

Conjugated estrogens, U.S.P., is a mixture of the sodium salts of the sulfate esters of the estrogenic substances, principally estrone and equilin, that are of the type excreted by pregnant mares. Conjugated estrogens contains 50 to 65 per cent of sodium estrone sulfate and 20 to 35 per cent of sodium equilin sulfate, calculated on the basis of the total conjugated estrogens content.

Poisoning reports reveal no significant acute toxicity in accidental ingestion cases. Symptoms and findings have been insignificant except for minimal nausea and vomiting from large amounts.

*Treatment* is symptomatic, but usually none is necessary. However, if large amounts are ingested, lavage or emesis is advisable.

## ETHER AND OTHER ANESTHETIC AGENTS

Ether, chloroform, trichloroethylene, ethyl chloride, halothane (Fluothane®) and divinyl ether (Vinethene®) are liquid anesthetic agents; while ethylene, cyclopropane and nitrous oxide are gases used to produce general anesthesia. Ether is also used in industry as a solvent.

The administration of halothane to patients with known liver or biliary tract disease is not always recommended since hepatic necrosis and cholestatic jaundice may occasionally occur following its use. However, death has been rarely attributed to the use of this anesthetic agent, and its overall record of safety far outweighs its potential hazard. Halothane is also ill-advised for obstetrical anesthesia, since the uterine relaxation produced responds poorly to oxytocics, and for those with increased intracranial pressure, unless a reduction of pressure is first effected. Plasma bromide levels in patients following halothane anesthesia may remain elevated for prolonged periods (three weeks).

These anesthetics depress all functions of the central nervous system in descending order from the cortex to the medulla. Excessive amounts stop respiration, and if oxygen is diminished and carbon dioxide is increased, irregularities of ventricular contraction, ventricular fibrillation and damage to the heart, liver and kidneys are likely to occur.

The principal manifestations of poisoning with these agents are excitement, stupor, unconsciousness and paralysis of respiration. Convulsions may follow increased carbon dioxide in alveolar air. Chronic industrial exposure may lead to anorexia, weight loss, insomnia, irritability, polycythemia and nephritis.

Most of the signs and symptoms of ether poisoning clear up upon discontinuance of the exposure. It is therefore essential that the patient be transferred to fresh air, the body kept warm and artificial respiration given if necessary. It is imperative in serious cases that an adequate airway be maintained and the secretions removed. The blood pressure should be stabilized with intravenous fluids or blood transfusions. In chlorinated anesthetic poisoning, 10 ml of 10% calcium gluconate solution intravenously is advisable as a nonspecific cellular protectant for the liver.

In treating hypoxia, an arterial $PO_2$ in the range of 60 to 90 mm Hg usually can be obtained with less than 60% oxygen so pulmonary oxygen toxicity can be avoided. When greater than 60% oxygen is required, the physician should aggressively try to improve alveolar gas exchange so that the inspired oxygen concentration can be lowered. The use of continuous positive-pressure breathing in this setting may be helpful.

## GLUTETHIMIDE (DORIDEN)

This drug is a popular oral nonbarbiturate sedative. On the basis of the $LD_{50}$ for mice, it has been estimated that the lethal dose for adults is about 40 gm. However, 10 to 20 gm have caused death and even smaller doses can be lethal if taken concomitantly with other sedatives (barbiturates, alcohol, etc.). Acute intoxication can occur when amounts of 3 gm or more of glutethimide are ingested, and coma has resulted in adults from the ingestion of 5 gm. Rapid, accurate methods for Doriden determination are available, utilizing thin-layer and gas chromatography.

The principal manifestations of poisoning are ataxia, nystagmus, mydriasis, drowsiness, coma and respiratory and central nervous system depression. Although hypothermia is seen early, hyperpyrexia is often associated with coma, which may occur twenty-four hours after ingestion. In addition, tachycardia, hypotension, sluggish or absent deep tendon reflexes, cyanosis and sudden apnea may occur. Respiratory rates are not frequently depressed, yet adequate ventilation is often a problem. In children particularly, fever, flushing of the skin and dryness of mucous membranes closely resemble atropine poisoning. Marked dermographism is common.

In *treatment,* gastric lavage (because of greater solubility in oil than in water, use castor oil emulsion, leaving some in the stomach to hasten elimination) should be done, with an inflatable cuff if necessary, even several hours after ingestion. Large doses of castor oil (up to a pint) have been reported to dramatically cut coma time in patients who had taken overdoses of lipophilic drugs such as ethchlorvynol, methyprylon, methaqualone and glutethimide (the tricyclics and benzodiazepines also have a high affinity for fat). The concept is that by increasing the overall fat content of the body, these drugs are absorbed from the body. By giving additional castor oil, the pool of fats available for solution is constantly changed. Activated charcoal can absorb large amounts of glutethimide and should be given after the stomach has been emptied. Fluids should be restricted to 1500 ml in adults. Overhydration can produce pulmonary and cerebral edema. Since less than 2 per cent of oral glutethimide is excreted by the kidneys, forced diuresis is of little value. While stimulants counteract cardiovascular and respiratory depression, they do not hasten the return of reflexes or consciousness, and they may obscure the natural course of toxicity. A cuff-type endotracheal tube with alternating pressure respirator assures adequate ventilation. In moderate intoxication (blood levels less than 2.5 mg%), central nervous system stimulants, support of blood pressure with vasopressor agents and maintenance of pulmonary ventilation may be required. Megimide (bemegride) competes with, or is metabolized by, the same enzyme as Doriden and is not therapeutically effective. If the patient does not respond or if the blood level of glutethimide is over 3 mg% aqueous or lipid, hemodialysis (removes drugs and its metabolites 100 to 400 times faster than the kidneys) should be considered. The following are the established criteria for hemodialysis: (1) coma plus ingestion of 10 gm or more of glutethimide; (2) coma with a blood level of 3 mg% or more; (3)

progressive deepening of anesthesia or clinical deterioration; (4) widely dilated and unresponsive pupils; (5) shock which is resistant to pressor agents; (6) prolonged central nervous system depression; (7) hypothalamic signs; (8) persistent respiratory difficulties despite a good airway (cyanosis, severe hypoxia, etc.); and (9) development of severe complications (aspiration pneumonia, etc.). At the earliest signs of infection, antibiotic therapy should be started immediately, while endotracheal intubation or tracheotomy, when indicated, should never be delayed.

## GOLD

Gold and its salts (sodium thiosulfate, sodium thiomalate, NF aurothioglucose, aurothioglycanide) are used in the treatment of arthritis, lupus erythematosus and other conditions. Apparently there is very great variation in personal tolerance of these drugs, not only in different individuals, but also in the same person at different times. The chief toxic effects are fever; nausea; vomiting; diarrhea; photosensitivity; metallic taste; proteinuria; hematuria (nephritis and nephrosis); uremia; various skin disorders such as papulovesicular lesions, urticaria and exfoliative dermatitis, all attended with severe pruritis; granulocytopenia; thrombocytopenia; purpura and aplastic anemia.

*Treatment* consists of prompt discontinuation of the medication. Dimercaprol, if given early and before irreversible damage has been done, is a very effective therapeutic agent. Calcium disodium edetate and D-penicillamine have also been reported to be effective in the treatment of gold toxicity. Antihistamine therapy is useful for the allergic reactions, and specific supportive therapy should be given for the renal and hematological complications. Parenteral N-acetylcysteine (NAC), an investigational new drug used for correcting the serum and tissue sulfhydryl (SH) group depletion, has been documented as an effective chelating agent for gold (and other metal) intoxication and deserves further evaluation.

## HYDRALAZINE

Hydralazine (Apresoline) and related synthetic phthalazine derivatives are employed as antihypertensive agents with the dual capacity of reducing blood pressure and at the same time increasing renal blood flow.

Untoward effects from hydralazine therapy include chills, malaise, loss of weight, myalgia, muscle stiffness, arthralgia which is sometimes migratory, hematuria, pleuritic pain, abdominal pain, fatigability, acute glossodynia and nocturnal itching of the knees and ankles.

The physical findings reveal fever which has been reported to reach a temperature of 40°C (105°F). Arthopathy may be generalized with hot, swollen, tender and inflamed joints which resemble rheumatoid arthritis, particularly in the fusiform swelling of the proximal interphalangeal joints. Severe joint effusion may also occur. Among the skin eruptions, a butterfly rash has been seen. Erythema of the hands and severe erythematous reaction to ultraviolet light have been noted, and petechiae and ecchymosis are occasionally found. Also, tender muscles, pericardial friction rub, painful lymphadenopathy, hepatosplenomegaly, subcutaneous nodules, peripheral neuropathy (pyridoxine deficiency) and polyneuritis occur. These symptoms and signs have occurred singly or in varying combinations.

Reports of abnormal laboratory findings in most patients with symptoms of intoxication include positive L.E. cell, false positive serological tests for syphilis, hyperglobulinemia, decrease in serum cholesterol levels, microcytic or normocytic anemia with pancytopenia, increase in sedimentation rate and abnormal cephalin-cholesterol flocculation and thymol turbidity tests.

## HYPOGLYCEMIC AGENTS (ORAL)

At present, there are several hypoglycemic agents available for oral use in the treatment of selected patients with diabetes. Three are sulfonylurea compounds, tolbutamide, tolazamide and chlorpropamide (although classified as sulfonamide derivatives, they have no antibacterial action); biguanide and phenformin differ from the sulfonylureas chemically and in their mode of action (extrapancreatic). Phenylbutazone, oxyphenbutazone, probenecid, salicylates, bacteriostatic sulfonamides and the monoamine oxidase inhibitors may potentiate the hypoglycemic effects of these compounds. Lactic acidosis is known to be associated with phenformin therapy in diabetics; any impairment of renal function increases this risk.

On the basis of both laboratory tests and clinical experience, the toxicity of all oral hypoglycemic agents appears to be relatively low. Cholestatic jaundice has occurred rarely after the use of tolbutamide and more often after large doses of chlorpropamide. Hypoglycemic reactions are a distinct possibility during the transition period between the discontinuance of insulin and the initiation of a sulfonylurea compound. The risk of such a reaction is greatly increased if tolbutamide or chlorpropamide is administered together with insulin or phenformin. Occasionally a prolonged severe hypoglycemic reaction may occur even with conventional doses, especially in elderly diabetics with renal insufficiency. Deep and prolonged coma without persistent hypoglycemia has been reported from the ingestion of a large quantity of acetohexamide (Dymelor®).

Patients who are taking one of these sulfonylurea compounds, particularly chlorpropamide, may also note an intolerance to alcohol. When such a patient drinks an alcoholic beverage, he may experience an unusual flushing of the skin, particularly of the face and neck, similar to that which is noted when disulfiram (Antabuse) is given. This effect may be prevented if the patient is instructed to take an antihistaminic drug orally one hour before he takes the alcoholic drink.

Other untoward reactions to the sulfonylurea compounds have been reported, including gastrointestinal upsets and allergic skin manifestations such as pruritis, erythema, urticaria and morbilliform or maculopapular eruptions. Most of these dermatologic effects are transient; if they persist, the oral agent should be discontinued. Gastrointestinal effects, diarrhea and loss of appetite can be troublesome and occur more frequently when phenformin is administered. The reactions are central in origin and may be controlled by adjusting the dosage or substituting time-disintegration capsules for tablets. If the symptoms persist, the drug should be discontinued temporarily. Reversible hypothyroidism may occur with prolonged therapy.

Hematopoietic reactions such as leukopenia, thrombocytopenia and agranulocytosis have been reported after the use of the sulfonylurea derivatives but not after the use of phenformin. In contrast to the bacteriostatic sulfonamide drugs, the sulfonylurea drugs have not caused hematuria, crystalluria or other signs of renal damage. Hence, alkalinization of the urine or a large fluid intake is not necessary when these agents are employed. Hypernatremia and water intoxication have been reported with chlorpropamide therapy.

*Treatment* of willful or accidental ingestion of overdosage should be immediate gastric lavage or emesis followed by careful observation and therapy for severe hypoglycemic symptoms and/or shock.

## IODINE AND ITS COMPOUNDS

Iodine is a brownish, flaky element which is practically insoluble in water, but readily soluble in alcohol. It is used most often as the official U.S.P. tincture (2% iodine and 2% NaI in 50% alcohol); it is also available as strong iodine tincture (7% iodine and 5% KI in 83% alcohol), Lugol's solution (5% iodine and 10% KI in aqueous solution) and iodine ointment (4% iodine).

Iodoform, iodochlorhydroxyquin and sodium and potassium iodides are all powders or crystals having the same solubility properties. The fatal dose of iodine and iodoform is estimated to be 2 gm; whereas fatalities from iodochlorhydroxyquin and iodide salts rarely occur.

Iodochlorhydroxyquinoline* (Entero-Vioform®), or clioquinol as it is known on the European market, has produced subacute myelo-optic neuropathy (SMON) when used for the treatment of gastroenteritis. An incidence of over 10,000 has occurred in Japan where the drug has been withdrawn from the market. The condition is not always reversible.

Although accidental ingestion of the tincture or of Lugol's solution occurs frequently, such poisoning rarely ends fatally, for while iodine may do damage locally, it is not a severe systemic poison due to its poor absorption, as such, into the circulation.

The corrosive action of iodine on the gastrointestinal mucosa causes severe pain in the mouth, throat and stomach, often accompanied by nausea, vomiting and diarrhea. The vomitus may be blue if starch is present in the stomach. Iodine secreted in the saliva causes a metallic taste in the mouth. Application of iodine or iodoform to the skin may cause vesiculation, weeping and crusting. Iodine compounds given parenterally can cause fatal collapse as a result of hypersensitivity, while prolonged ingestion of these substances can cause iodism with skin erythema, urticaria, acne, conjunctivitis, stomatitis, anorexia, weight loss and nervous symptoms. Rarely fever can be the sole manifestation of iodism.

Finally, the corrosive action of iodine may lead to circulatory collapse, and with aspiration resulting in bronchopneumonia, is the chief cause of death when it occurs. Enlargement of the salivary glands is an unusual toxic reaction that occasionally arises and should be recognized, since it may save a patient considerable expense and his physician embarrassment in not having to go through an extensive differential diagnosis examination. Discontinuing treatment brings rapid decrease in the size of these glands with a return to normal in a few days. Iodide salts (calcium, potassium, etc.) are commonly used in expectorants and cough preparations. Prolonged use may result in iodism, hypothyroidism and goiter.

Recommendations.

1. Iodides should be used as expectorants only in patients with chronic disease who have a reproducible, clear-cut amelioration which cannot be obtained with a less toxic agent. The dosage should be as low as possible, and the drug should be used for the shortest time possible.
2. Iodides should never be used as expectorants during pregnancy and should be discontinued or decreased during breast-feeding.
3. Iodides should not be prescribed as expectorants during adolescence because of their potential to induce acneiform eruptions, exacerbate existing lesions and adversely affect the thyroid.
4. Iodides should never be prescribed as expectorants for patients with goiter.
5. All preparations containing iodides should be clearly labeled as to their iodide content, with the warning that they are contraindicated in pregnancy since they can produce goiter in the newborn.

In the *treatment,* give a suspension of starch or flour (1 tbsp./1 pt. of water) to precipitate the iodine, and administer a dilute solution (1% to 5%) of sodium thiosulfate orally to convert iodine chemically to the relatively inert iodide and tetrathionate. Protein in the form of milk or egg white may also be used. All the reaction products must be removed later by gastric lavage. Intravenous administration of glucose, saline and electrolyte solutions helps to support the circulation and to counteract dehydration. Whole blood and

*and other halogenated hydroxyquinolines

plasma may also be required to combat shock. Morphine for pain and antibiotics against infection are also desirable. Anaphylactic reactions should be treated with epinephrine 0.3 to 1.0 ml of 1:1000 solution IM or IV and repeated as necessary. Diphenhydramine (Benadryl) and steroids may also be used effectively for this purpose.

## IPRONIAZID PHOSPHATE-MARSILID (ISONICOTINOYL-2-ISOPROPYLHYDRAZINE)

This is the isopropyl derivative of isoniazid, which was used for a time as a tuberculostatic agent and as a "psychic energizer." However, the toxic effects of this compound produced numerous central nervous system manifestations, as well as jaundice with hepatitis, and these adverse symptoms have caused the withdrawal of this drug from the market (*see* Monoamine Oxidase Inhibitors).

## IRON COMPOUNDS

The incidence of poisoning by iron salts seems to be related to the status of iron therapy in any given period. Cases of accidental and homicidal poisoning from iron salts were widely reported in the literature of the middle nineteenth century. Reports of accidental iron intoxication did not appear again in print until 1934, and since 1947 they have appeared with sufficient frequency to warrant editorial attention. Approximately 2000 persons are poisoned each year in the United States, with a high fatality rate. For example, from 1969 to 1972 there were 31 deaths and 54.3 known hospitalizations in children under five years of age from ingestion of iron-containing products.

Until the last decade of the nineteenth century, iron therapy was widely employed in the treatment of hypochromic anemias due to body iron deficiencies. At the turn of the century, a definite change in attitudes toward the value of iron therapy occurred as the result of the belief that inorganic iron was not absorbed from the gastrointestinal tract. The small doses of iron salts then used had little therapeutic effect, and the value of iron fell into disrepute of iron therapy previously set forth by Sydenham and Blaud, namely, large doses and the greater potency of ferrous salts, began to be reconfirmed through use.

In recent years, ferrous sulfate has been used extensively for the treatment of iron deficiency anemia, and even some blood banks give the tablets routinely to donors. The more widespread use of this compound has increased the opportunity for accidental poisoning in young children. Coloring and candy-coating of this medication make it more appealing to small children, thereby magnifying the danger. The magnitude of the hazard is evident in the vital statistics on fatal accidental iron poisoning recorded in the United States and Great Britain in recent years.

There are at present over 120 iron preparations on the market. Chelated iron compounds are almost as effective as the others in the treatment of iron deficiency anemia and less toxic. A child would have to take four times as many chelated iron tablets as standard ones to get the same toxic effect. The administration of parenteral iron preparations, iron dextran (Imferon®) and iron sorbitol citric acid complex (Jectofer®) has been associated with fever, lymphadenopathy, nausea and vomiting, arthralgias, animal sarcoma (Imferon), urticaria, severe peripheral vascular collapse and fatal anaphylactoid reactions. Parenteral therapy should be limited to very specific situations in which orally administered iron is ineffective or contraindicated.

The daily diet of the average man contains about 10 to 15 mg of elemental iron, of which 1 to 15 mg is absorbed. The estimated daily loss from all sources is about 0.5 to 1.5 mg. Acute or chronic iron overload does not significantly increase the excretion. Iron is absorbed in the ferrous form; after crossing the mucosal cell it is converted to the ferric form and picked up by transferrin, the iron-binding protein. In this form iron is strongly chelated. Transferrin is usually only one-third saturated. When the quantity of iron in the circulatory system exceeds the iron-binding protein, some of the iron attaches itself to albumin, and the remainder circulates in the free form. Presumably it is this free or unbound iron which produces toxicity. The average human lethal dose is about 200 to 250 mg of iron per kg of body weight. Ambiguous labeling of many iron-containing products often results in misinterpretation of actual elemental iron content. Often the labels contain just the iron salt content. Elemental iron is equivalent to 20 per cent of the salt as ferrous sulfate or 33 per cent as ferrous fumarate and approximately 10 per cent for the gluconate salt. This can be misleading; for example, 2 gm of ferrous sulfate is equivalent to 400 mg of elemental iron, a potentially fatal dose for a young child. In a study of chewable vitamins, it was found that the elemental iron content varied from 400 to 3000 mg/container, the latter equivalent to seven times the lethal dose. None of these products warned of the danger of an excess of ingested iron. As few as ten 0.3 gm tablets of ferrous sulfate have proved fatal in a child. In general, the lethal range is achieved when the serum Fe level exceeds the total iron-binding capacity (TIBC). A serum Fe level of greater than 500 μg/100 ml is in the lethal range.

Serum iron determination is the best test for confirmation of diagnosis and for detecting severity of acute poisoning. Although iron tablets are radiopaque, abdominal roentgenograms are not always a reliable means of confirming iron tablet poisoning or of assessing removal of iron from the gastrointestinal tract. Whole, partially fragmented or powdered tablets can be visualized in the stomach and small bowel but usually cannot be seen if dissolved, in fine suspension or obscured by food bolus.

The mechanism of action in iron poisoning is not known. Pathological findings have failed to give a satisfactory explanation for death. Opinions are divided as to whether the fatal outcome is due to shock secondary to local tissue damage to the gastrointestinal tract, to systemic effects following the passage of large quantities of iron into the bloodstream or to the metabolic effects of absorbed iron resulting in respiratory collapse.

Interference with hepatocellular enzyme activities is undoubtedly an important etiological factor producing toxicity, since in iron overload in animals and man, there is an increase in the activity of a number of oxidative enzymes and glucose-6-phosphate in the parenchymal cells. This is followed by a loss of activity of these same enzymes in the same areas which previously showed the increase.

One of the unique features of iron metabolism is that iron has no organ of excretion. Iron released from the catabolism of iron compounds is not excreted and must be fed back into anabolic iron pathways. Overloading with parenterally administered iron is not compensated for by increased fecal or urinary excretion. Iron found in the feces represents only unabsorbed iron; the intestine has no power to regulate through excretion the amount of iron in the body. Urinary excretion of iron is negligible, and increased ingestion of iron is not accompanied by elevated urinary excretion. Thus, the capacity to regulate the amount of iron in the body lies in the absorption mechanism. However, a significant quantity of urinary feroxamine gives the urine a pink "vin rosé" color and is evidence that the serum iron level is high enough to produce toxicity.

Iron is absorbed by the mucosal cells of the intestinal tract, more readily in the ferrous than in the ferric form. How iron passes through the mucosal cell and into the bloodstream is unknown. The absorption of iron is not a question of simple diffusion across a membrane but involves a metabolic transportation through the intestinal mucosa. Presumably, the mucosal cell regulates the rate of absorption from the gastrointestinal tract and seems to act as a barrier to the rapid entrance of iron into the circulation.

The pathological picture is usually that of hemorrhage and necrosis of the stomach and intestinal mucosa. The liver is frequently involved, showing mild cloudy swelling to small areas of complete necrosis. Among some survivors, fibrosis of the liver and pyloric stenosis have been described. In most cases there has been a marked dilatation of the right side of the heart, with pulmonary congestion and occasional hemorrhage. There have not been any particular abnormal findings in other organs of the body.

There are four known critical phases in iron poisoning with a likely fifth phase that has, as yet, not been clinically documented.

I. Hemorrhagic gastroenteritis occurring one-half to one hour or more after ingestion; this may be accompanied by shock, acidosis, coagulation defects and coma.

II. Delayed profound shock presenting twenty to forty-eight hours after ingestion (serum iron levels usually above 500 mg%).

III. Liver injury and failure not previously implicated as a sole cause of death. A study of the enzyme histochemical changes induced in the livers of acutely iron-overloaded rabbits has shown alterations in several enzymes involved in oxidative metabolism. Electron-microscopic examinations show early and severe mitochondrial injury responsible for this disturbance.

IV. A late phase of gastric scarring and contracture, with pyloric obstruction due to the corrosive action of iron salts, appearing four weeks or longer after ingestion.

V. Theoretical phase of cirrhosis due to subfatal liver injury is possible, but has not yet been reported.

The principal manifestations of poisoning are vomiting and circulatory collapse. Lethargy, vomiting (odor of iron in vomitus and on breath), fast and weak pulse, low blood pressure, pallor, cyanosis, ataxia and coma appear within one-half to one hour after ingestion. These symptoms may disappear after four to six hours, followed by a six– to twenty-four-hour asymptomatic period in which the child seems to improve rapidly. A second crisis occurs with cyanosis, vasomotor collapse, pulmonary edema, coma and death within twelve to forty-eight hours.

Assessing the severity of volume depletion may be difficult; one cannot estimate volume loss based only on hematocrit values. Hemodilution and equilibration necessary to alter hematocrit may take up to twenty-four hours. One of the most helpful and simplest techniques in testing volume depletion is the "tilt" or "orthostatic changes" test. Orthostatic changes are determined by taking a patient's pulse and blood pressure in the horizontal (supine) position and comparing the values to those obtained with the patient seated with the legs hanging over the side of the bed. Rough estimation of volume deficits are correlated with these changes. The response is also dependent upon numerous other factors such as age, autonomic nervous system function (diabetes, tabes dorsalis, postsympathectomy states, etc.) and drug use (antipsychotics such as chlorpromazine, sedatives, antihypertensives, etc.).

In the absence of any of these complicating factors, a volume deficit of 500 ml usually results in an increase of approximately 20 beats/min. in heart rate when a patient moves from the supine to the sitting position. A deficit of 1000 ml results in approximately a 30 beats/min. increase with a possible slight decrease in systolic blood pressure, while with a deficit of 1500 ml, the tachycardia is accompanied by a decrease of approximately 15 mm Hg in the systolic blood pressure.

The *treatment* for severe iron intoxication is directed toward removing the iron and combating shock and has to be immediate, vigorous and sustained, for the mortality is still 30 to 50 per cent. Teamwork is necessary to carry out the following procedures.

1. Clearance with suction and maintenance of an open airway.
2. Control of shock with available intravenous fluids, blood, plasma and oxygen.
3. Gastric lavage, using the largest caliber tube possible, with a concentrated solution of sodium bicarbonate, 5% disodium phosphate duohydrate (one-half-strength Fleet® enema solution can be substituted) or milk until the returning fluid is clear. After lavage, proportional amounts of these solutions should be left in the stomach. Either ferrous carbonate or ferrous phosphate is formed, both of which are poorly absorbed (*see* Apomorphine, which could be especially valuable in removing large particles from the stomach and producing reflux of enteric-coated tablets from the upper intestinal tract).
4. Retention in the stomach of 100 to 300 ml of one of the above solutions. A demulcent, such as egg white, may be added to the bicarbonate or phosphate solution.
5. Rectal lavage with one of the above solutions if there is diarrhea, hyperperistalsis of the intestinal tract or a lapse of three hours or more since ingestion of the iron.
6. In critical cases, oral administration of half the total intravenous dose of edetate (EDTA), 35 to 45 mg/kg/24 hr., may be indicated. The effectiveness of oral edetate in acute iron poisoning, however, remains to be confirmed. The chelating agent diethylenetriamine-penta-acetic acid (DTPA), obtained from Geigy Pharmaceuticals, has a stability constant for iron 1000 times that of EDTA, and up to 109 mg% iron has been excreted in the urine following its administration.
7. Collection of blood for complete blood count, typing, crossmatching, blood pH, serum proteins, iron, sodium, potassium, chloride and carbon dioxide determinations as well as for liver function tests. Faced with the problem of delays of several hours or longer in obtaining SI level results, a rapid screening test (Fischer test) for the detection of iron in the serum in excess of the iron-binding protein has been developed (Fischer, D.S. and Price, D.C.: A Simple Serum Iron Method Using the New Sensitive Chromogen Tripyridyl-S-triazine. *Clin Chem, 10*:21-31, 1964). Mix 0.2 ml of bathophenanthroline and 0.1 ml of the reducing agent hydroxylammonium chloride in an iron-free glass or plastic tube and add 0.5 ml clear serum or plasma. If the test serum turns red, it contains free iron in excess of the serum iron-binding capacity. A positive reaction with the bathophenanthroline reagent represents an SI level that exceeds the TIBC by 50 μg/100 ml or more. The test takes about ten minutes, and the results frequently are available before the completion of gastric lavage. Although experience with this test in the clinical setting is limited, patients with a positive reaction should immediately be given deferoxamine parenterally. If the results of the test are negative, chelate therapy is withheld, but fluids are administered intravenously in order to control dehydration and acidosis. If the results are uncertain, use deferoxamine parenterally, at least until the SI level and TIBC are known.
8. Critically ill patients should receive edetate IV. If none has been given orally, the intravenous dose should be 70 to 80 mg/kg/24 hr. in dextrose or normal saline solution in an 0.5% to 2% concentration. If oral edetate is used (and the rate of its absorption through a gut wall damaged by iron is not known), only half the above dose should be used intravenously, 35 to 40 mg/kg/24 hr.
9. Deferoxamine mesylate (Desferal®) 1 to 2 gm IV or IM, a chelating agent isolated from *Streptomyces pilosus,* has been demonstrated to produce urinary excretion of about 15 mg of iron in patients with

hemochromatosis and 5 mg of iron in normal persons; its effectiveness in the treatment of acute iron poisoning is well documented.

This drug is a sideramine of microbial origin with a molecular weight of 561. As the soluble mesylate salt, it binds 8.5 mg of trivalent iron per 100 mg of chelate with an avidity comparable to that of the plasma iron-binding protein transferrin. Given by mouth, deferoxamine is not absorbed to any significant degree; in the gut, especially at an acid pH, the drug binds inorganic iron and greatly reduces its absorption. An additional advantage is that it does not chelate other metals, such as calcium. Given intravenously, deferoxamine combines with iron to form ferrioxamine, which is to a large extent excreted in the urine, though some is metabolized in the body. Relatively high levels of urinary iron excretion, ease of administration by the intravenous or intramuscular route, lack of clinically significant excretion of other metals and freedom from serious toxic side-effects make the use of deferoxamine in the removal of excess body iron of considerable value.

The rationale for use of deferoxamine mesylate in the treatment of acute iron intoxication is based on the twofold aim of (1) binding iron that is circulating in plasma in excess of transferrin-binding capacity to render it nontoxic while hastening its excretion in the urine (deferoxamine increases urinary excretion of iron by 100 times); and (2) binding iron remaining in the gastrointestinal tract to prevent its absorption. Parenteral administration of the drug is used to effect the first aim; administration orally or by gastric tube is designed to achieve the second goal. As with use of other iron-chelating agents such as EDTA, DTPA and EDDHA, deferoxamine is but an adjunct to various supportive measures designed to combat symptoms of iron toxicity. The dose of Desferal sufficient to chelate the iron may be calculated on the basis of the amount of iron ingested, but since this information may be difficult to obtain, it has been recommended that 5 to 10 gm of Desferal be given by mouth immediately. Most children will not drink this bitter material, so it may have to be given by nasogastric tube.* An additional 1 to 2 gm should be administered slowly intravenously to chelate iron that has been absorbed. Rapid infusion has been reported to produce severe hypotension. A small percentage of patients receiving this drug intravenously have demonstrated flushing of the skin, urticaria, tachycardia, hypotension and a shock-like state. Based upon animal experiments, it has been felt that this phenomenon is due to histamine release. These effects have not as yet been seen in those receiving Desferal intramuscularly. Since blood levels are comparable within fifteen minutes with this route of administration, it would seem preferable to intravenous injections. It is possible that the potential side-effects from deferoxamine and the iron-deferoxamine complex can be minimized by the use of a vasopressor agent (Levophed, etc.) to prevent the blood pressure from reaching or remaining at critically low levels and hemodialysis to augment the excretion of the toxic complex, which is dialyzable. Desferal is contraindicated in patients with severe renal disease or anuria since the drug and the chelate are excreted primarily by the kidney. Cataracts have been observed in three patients who were treated for prolonged periods in chronic iron storage disease. The amount of absorbed iron is difficult to estimate either by history or serum iron values, and since there is no significant reported toxicity to Desferal in the recommended doses and because of the potential danger from iron overdose, it is recommended that all suspected cases of serious iron overdose or poisoning receive oral* and parenteral therapy. Treatment should not await the results of the serum iron determinations. If serum iron values remain high, repeated parenteral Desferal may be necessary. Color changes in the urine can provide both a diagnostic indicator and a guide for subsequent therapy. A reddish discoloration occurs when iron levels exceed 350 μg%, at which point the iron-binding capacity of the serum is usually saturated.

10. Peritoneal dialysis or hemodialysis, even though iron is reported to be nondialyzable, has been used successfully and should be seriously considered if severe first-phase symptoms are present and urine flow is greatly reduced or absent.

    Early exchange transfusion, if facilities and personnel exist for its performance, is an even more effective procedure. It has the additional advantage of permitting precise regulation of blood pressure if it is properly done and may also help to correct or avert the coagulation deficiencies that can be a problem in serious cases. Significant GI bleeding may require fibrinogen.

    Acidosis may become severe and is often relatively refractory; sodium bicarbonate 3 to 5 mEq/kg intravenously as needed should be administered. The occasional hypoglycemia that develops should be taken care of by glucose in the IV fluids. The rare victim with hyperpyrexia can be managed by tepid sponging and adequate hydration. Convulsions can be controlled with either paraldehyde or diazepam (Valium).

11. After these immediate emergency measures have been carried out, roentgenograms of the abdomen should be taken for visualization of radiopaque iron tablets in the gastrointestinal tract.
12. Collection of all urine for early detection of possible oliguria and study of the urine sediment for evidence of renal tubular damage.
13. Administration of prophylactic antibiotics, particularly if aspiration of foreign matter into the airway has occurred, and of multiple vitamins, which should include vitamin B complex.
14. Guided by the clinical picture and the daily iron levels in serum and, if measurements are available, by the urinary output of edetate (EDTA) and iron, intravenous and/or oral* edetate is continued in a total daily dose of no more than 70 to 80 mg/kg. The duration of treatment with this drug should not be and need not be longer than five days.
15. Follow-up liver function tests and study of the gastrointestinal tract with a radiopaque medium for inflammatory and necrotic changes or strictures.

*There are a few reports suggesting that large oral doses of deferoxamine can be absorbed and result in systemic toxicity. Its oral use is now being questioned by some clinical toxicologists.

TABLE 122
RECOMMENDED DOSAGE REGIMENS FOR DEFEROXAMINE

*Oral*

*Dose:* 5 to 10 gm via nasogastric tube following gastric lavage.*

*Intramuscular*

For all patients not in shock or severely intoxicated,

*Dose:* 20 mg/kg IM every 3 to 12 hours, depending upon the clinical picture, degree of intoxication as estimated from amount ingested and serum iron levels, and response to therapy.

*Intravenous*

For severely ill patients and those already in a state of cardiovascular collapse, and for those with a serum iron level of 300 μg/100 ml or more.

*Dose:* 40 mg/kg by *slow* infusion. The rate of infusion should not exceed 15 mg/kg/hr. in order to avoid hypotensive reactions. The dose is lowered to 20 mg/kg and repeated every 4 to 12 hours depending upon the patient's clinical status. With very severe intoxication, therapy may have to be continued 2 to 3 days.

*There are a few reports suggesting that large oral doses of deferoxamine can be absorbed and result in systemic toxity. Its oral use is now being questioned by some clinical toxicologists.

## ISONIAZID (ISONICOTINIC ACID HYDRAZIDE, I.N.H., NYDRAZID, NICONYL)

Isoniazid is used in the treatment of tuberculosis and is supplied in 25, 50 or 100 mg tablets; 10 mg/ml syrup; and 10 or 100 mg/ml intramuscular injection. It is an inhibitor of monoamine oxidase and potentiates the toxic effects of alcohol and barbiturates. It is rapidly absorbed from the gastrointestinal tract with maximum blood levels achieved one to three hours after ingestion, and peak excretion in two to four hours. Within twenty-four hours, over 80 per cent of an ingested dose appears in the urine, mainly as the acetyl derivative, and over 10 per cent in the bile.

Death has resulted from ingestion of 14.4 and 15 gm by adults; 8.3 gm by a two and one-half year-old; 5.3 gm with beer by an adult; 3 gm by a thirteen-year-old; and following mistaken intravenous administration of 4 to 6 gm to two elderly patients. Adults have survived oral doses of 12.5 gm without and 20 gm with hemodialysis. Intramuscular doses of 35 to 40 mg/kg in humans caused tachycardia and convulsions but were not lethal. Toxic symptoms have been caused by a few grams in adults and by 1 to 2 gm in young children. Frequent side-effects of therapy are fever, myalgia, arthralgia, nausea and anorexia.

The predominant symptoms of isoniazid intoxication are tachycardia, muscular twitching and generalized tonic and clonic convul-

TABLE 123
FIRST-LINE ANTITUBERCULOSIS DRUGS*

| *Drug* | *How Supplied* | *Administration and Adult Dosage* | *Adverse Reactions* | *Caution in Use* |
|---|---|---|---|---|
| Aminosalicylic acid (PAS) | Tablets<br>Powder | Oral, with meals; 10-12 gm day in divided doses | Gastrointestinal distress (dyspepsia, diarrhea) | Presence of peptic ulcer or colitis<br>Use of anticoagulants |
| Ethambutol | 100 mg and 400 mg tablets | Oral; 15-25 mg/kg once daily | Diminished visual acuity (optic neuritis)<br>Hepatitis? | Presence of gout (or elevated blood uric acid level) |
| Isoniazid (isonicotinic acid hydrazide; INH) | 100 mg and 300 mg tablets<br>Parenteral solutions | Oral; 300 mg once daily | Hepatitis<br>Peripheral neuritis | Alcoholism |
| Rifampin | 300 mg capsules | Oral; 600 mg once daily | Hepatitis<br>Renal hypersensitivity reactions (related to interruption of treatment)<br>Thrombocytopenia | Use of anticoagulants, oral contraceptives, digitalis?, or steroids? |
| Streptomycin | Powder<br>Solutions | Intramuscular; 1 gm every one to three days | Neurotoxicity, vestibular and auditory branches of eighth cranial nerve | Use of other neurotoxic drugs<br>Presence of renal insufficiency |

*Second-line agents are ethionamide, pyrazinamide, cycloserine, viomycin, kanamycin, capreomycin and thioacetazone.

sions. Exaggerated reflexes, tinnitus, vertigo, weakness, vomiting, electrolyte imbalance (hyperkalemia, metabolic acidosis), hyperglycemia, acetonuria, sudden drop in blood pressure, stupor and psychosis have been reported. Severe cases exhibit coma, convulsions, apnea, cyanosis, arrhythmia and death from respiratory arrest or circulatory failure. Toxic encephalopathy is a rare complication. Transient paresthesias and peripheral neuritis or liver damage may occur, and optic neuritis with atrophy and blindness has been reported. Isoniazid-associated hepatitis is a serious concern and is being investigated. If suspected, SGOT levels should be followed.

*Treatment.* Because of the rapid onset of symptoms, which may begin within thirty minutes after ingestion, induce emesis only if it is possible to do so prior to the onset of central nervous system stimulation. Lavage within the first two or three hours is advised but should not be attempted until convulsions are under control. Maintain respiration. Give intravenous sodium bicarbonate to correct the metabolic acidosis. To control convulsions, give IV short-acting barbiturates. Diazepam IV is helpful in aborting seizures not stopped by other medication (isoniazid-induced seizures do not respond to anticonvulsants unless the serum pH is corrected). In addition, pyridoxine hydrochloride (adult dose, 200 to 400 mg intravenously) may be given, as it has shown an incomplete antagonism against isoniazid convulsions in animals. It has been recommended that the manufacture of isoniazid tablets be restricted to those in combination with pyridoxine (a ratio of 30 to 100 mg). Analeptic drugs are contraindicated. Hemodialysis, peritoneal dialysis and exchange transfusion have all been successfully employed in treating patients who ingested potentially lethal doses. Isoniazid blood levels drop at twice their normal rate during hemodialysis. Osmotic forced diuresis (mannitol, urea, furosemide, ethacrynic acid) also hastens excretion.

## MAGNESIUM

Magnesium salts rarely cause poisoning, for after the oral ingestion, the normal kidney is capable of excreting the magnesium ion with sufficient rapidity to prevent the accumulation of toxic amounts. In impaired renal function, however, the oral administration of large doses of magnesium salts may sometimes lead to toxicity despite the slow rate of absorption. This is likely to occur when magnesium sulfate is employed as a dehydrating cathartic in the treatment of the edema of nephritis. The ensuing symptoms of central depression may be mistaken for uremia. The blood pressure falls and death results from respiratory paralysis. Aluminum hydroxide instead of magnesium antacids should be given to uremic patients with hyperphosphatemia or gastritis. Magnesium ions are toxic to the heart muscle, but direct paralysis of the heart occurs only from the rapid intravenous injections of large amounts of magnesium salts. The respiratory and circulatory failure produced by these drugs can be antagonized promptly by the parenteral administration of calcium chloride or gluconate, by artificial respiration and by the hypodermic injection of 0.5 to 1.0 mg of physostigmine. The administration of large amounts of fluids enhances the urinary excretion of these salts. Because of the depressant effects of magnesium salts, they should not be used for their cathartic action in patients poisoned by orally ingested barbiturates.

The practice of administering large amounts of a hypertonic solution of magnesium sulfate by slow drip per rectum to induce dehydration in the management of increased intracranial pressure and cerebral edema is particularly dangerous. Even in the presence of normal renal function, a significant rise in the level of plasma magnesium can be observed and fatal poisoning has been reported. Death has also resulted from a magnesium sulfate enema in a child with congenital megacolon and in newborns for use in the treatment of hyaline membrane disease.

## MARIHUANA (CANNABIS)

Marihuana is obtained from the flowering tops of hemp, the female plant of *Cannabis sativa,* an herb of the family Moraceae. Tetrahydrocannabinol (THC) is the active synthesized principle. The tops of the flowers are covered with hairs rich in resinous exudate which contains most of the active ingredients. Hemp grows wild in many parts of the world. In the United States, its cultivation is restricted to only four states and is under strict federal regulatory control. However, it grows wild in gardens, backyard lots and along the roadside. In Eastern countries the resinous exudate is employed as a beverage and a sweetmeat and is also smoked, but in America it is commonly dried and smoked in cigarettes called "reefers," "joints" or "sticks" containing "hay," "grass," "pot," "weed" or "tea."

The acute symptoms are exhilaration, giggling, inflamed conjunctivae and dryness of the mouth. The symptoms vary with the individual's personality. Most however, enter a dreamy state, and euphoria, imagination and perceptions are increased and vivid. The response to rhythm allows a more rapid tempo and improvisation becomes easy. Some, on the other hand, in the company of others tend to be restless, talkative and jocose, but when let alone they become quiet, drowsy and sleepy. After a period of drowsiness lasting one to four hours, they awaken feeling let down and experience many of the symptoms seen in an alcoholic hangover.

After repeated administration and high dosage, other effects are noted: lowering of the sensory threshold, especially for optical and acoustical stimuli, thereby resulting in a feeling of intensified appreciation of works of art; hallucinations, illusions and delusions that predispose to antisocial behavior; anxiety and aggressiveness as a possible result of the various intellectual and sensory derangements; and sleep disturbances.

In the psychomotor sphere, hypermotility occurs without impairment of coordination. Among somatic effects, often persistent, are injection of the ciliary vessels and oropharyngitis, chronic bronchitis and asthma. These conditions and hypoglycemia with ensuing bulimia are symptoms of intoxication, not of withdrawal.

There is little difficulty in recognizing the intoxication of a person who has smoked a significant amount of marihuana in the preceding few hours. If the physician has an opportunity to smell the smoke of a "reefer," a characteristic sweet pungent odor somewhat like burning alfalfa or hay is noted. Federal, state and local narcotic enforcement officers and certain clinical laboratories may be helpful in identifying the odor or the dried marihuana preparation, should the latter come into the physician's hands. The chronic effects lead to a progressive mental deterioration, tremors, physical weakness, anorexia, pallor, icterus and decrease of sensation and sexual potency. There is reduction of willpower and concentration. Marihuana does not give rise to biological or physiological addiction. However, scientists report that marihuana remains in the bloodstream for three days, that it takes more than eight days for the body to rid itself of all chemical traces and that the drug and its byproducts accumulate in tissues (especially in fatty tissues such as brain and testicles) with chronic use. Noteworthy abuse reports include lowered sperm counts and testosterone levels to the point of temporary infertility, likely related to the retention of the drug in the testes. Still other investigators have documented effects on body cellular processes with reduction of T-lymphocytes and resultant interference in the immune mechanism, reduction of DNA and RNA synthesis and an increased number of cells with broken chromosomes. In addition, emphysema, pharyngitis and bronchitis have been reported, as well as premalignant lesions in living tissues. A substantial medical literature exists to implicate significant health hazards as a result of marihuana smoking. The most active component of marihuana (THC) is fat soluble and it is likely to appear in breast milk. However the long range effects of this toxin on the nursing infant has not as yet been documented but the potential for ill effects exists. About 60 per cent of U.S. marihuana comes from Mexico and it has recently been discovered that much of it is contaminated with the herbicide, paraquat, which has the potential of producing pulmonary fibrosis among long-term heavy users. Instead of killing off completely the marihuana by spraying with paraquat, large batches of the heavily contaminated substance are being salvaged and brought into the country illegally. Thus far induced lung damage has not been reported in humans.*

*However, the recent report of Dr. Donald C. Zavala (Chest, *74*:418-420, October, 1978) "An Effect of Paraquat on the Lungs of Rabbits" should give genuine concern for individuals who smoke contaminated marihuana cigarettes.

## METHADONE (DOLOPHINE®)

Methadone was synthesized by German chemists in 1941 and came into clinical usage following World War II. The neurophysiologic effects of methadone, with a few exceptions, are indistinguishable from those of morphine. The effects on the cardiovascular system include (1) peripheral vasodilation which may produce orthostatic hypotension; (2) occasional sinus bradycardia; and (3) depression of sensitivity of the respiratory center to $CO_2$, which may lead to elevated $PCO_2$, cerebrovascular dilatation and elevated cerebrospinal fluid pressure. Methadone may cause spasm of the biliary tract and urinary retention. Miosis is less than that seen with morphine.

Methadone is readily absorbed from the gastrointestinal tract and rapidly leaves the bloodstream. Its effects may be prolonged for up to forty-eight hours. The lethal dose of methadone is unknown; 10 to 20 mg/kg causes death from respiratory failure in the rhesus monkey.

The average quantity of methadone prescribed for patients on a methadone maintenance program is 80 to 120 mg/day (higher doses are occasionally prescribed) taken by mouth in 2 to 4 oz. of Tang® or fruit juice or in solutions prepared by dissolving noninjectable tablets in water. When taken by maintenance patients whose special tolerance for narcotics decreases the pharmacological effects of this medication, this dose produces no sedation, no impairment of respiration nor other adverse effects. However, the same dose causes severe respiratory depression if taken by nontolerant subjects not on the methadone program and is likely to be fatal in children. The ingestion of methadone under such circumstances constitutes an acute emergency, requiring immediate diagnosis and treatment with the specific and effective antidotes which are available for the serious respiratory depression which follows.

Methadone is dispensed in prescription-labeled bottles, with the name of the patient, the hospital and the prescribing physician on each bottle. If a child has ingested a dose, an empty container (and in it traces of the orange-juice-like fluid) may be found nearby. The patient responsible for the medication should, of course, be questioned, if available. A child age two to six who takes a full dose of methadone becomes progressively comatose over a period of one-half to three hours and, if untreated, can die of respiratory failure within this time. Respiratory depression in older children or nontolerant adults, albeit less devastating, could be severe enough to warrant vigorous therapy.

In *treatment* artificial respiration is indicated immediately if breathing has stopped or if its rate or depth has become too low to maintain effective ventilation. If equipment is available, an airway tube should be inserted and a respirator mask applied, e.g. an Ambu respirator with bag and nipple for oxygen supply. An endotracheal tube with inflatable cuff is desirable for comatose patients to protect against aspiration of vomitus, but no time should be lost in looking for the special equipment required and a trained anesthetist to insert the tube. Narcan (naloxone hydrochloride), 0.01 mg/kg, given IV, IM or SC, is the antidote of choice. If Narcan is not available, Nalline (nalorphine hyrochloride), dose 0.1 mg/kg, or Lorfan (levallorphan tartrate), dose 0.02 mg/kg, are also effective IV or IM antidotes for narcotic overdose. These latter two agents, however, may augment the degree of respiratory depression if the diagnosis of narcotic poisoning is in error. They can be harmful if the depression of breathing is due to poisoning with barbiturate or to other disease processes. Narcan is free from this danger, producing no respiratory depression, psychotomimetic effects, circulatory changes or miosis and therefore is safe to use when the diagnosis is in doubt.

Briefly, Narcan's advantages over the other antagonists are as follows.

1. Narcan as an essentially pure narcotic antagonist does not possess depressant agonistic properties. Unlike nalorphine and levallorphan, Narcan does not produce respiratory depression, pupillary constriction or psychotomimetic effects. Therefore, it is a safer drug.
2. Narcan is the only specific antidote for treating the narcotic depression, including respiratory depression, induced by pentazocine (Talwin®) overdosage. Nalorphine and levallorphan are ineffective against pentazocine-associated respiratory depression.
3. Narcan is effective in the treatment of any degree of narcotic-induced respiratory depression. Nalorphine and levallorphan have not been shown to be effective in the treatment of mild degrees of depression.
4. In this period of polydrug abuse resulting in mixed overdoses, Narcan is a safe diagnostic agent as well as a therapeutic drug. If respiratory depression is due to non-narcotic drugs, the administration of Narcan can help rule out narcotics as the etiologic agent. If the depression is due to narcotics, Narcan promptly reverses the depression. On the other hand, nalorphine and levallorphan administered to a patient with mild narcotic or non-narcotic depression may augment the depression.

If respiration has improved in response to the first injection of antidote but is not yet adequate, it should be repeated in five minutes and again in ten minutes. If, however, the first injection has had no significant effect, the diagnosis of narcotic overdose may be in error. In case of such doubt, it is safe to repeat the injections of Narcan, but further administration of Nalline or Lorfan should be deferred for at least thirty minutes while adequate ventilation is maintained by artificial respiration and the patient's clinical status carefully reevaluated. Establish a routine of close observation to ensure that the victim is examined carefully every fifteen minutes, or more often, during the first twenty-four hours. If the patient is a young child, the crib should be put beside the nurse's desk in a good light so that respiration can be observed continuously. Narcotic antagonists should not be used to attempt to counteract light coma in adequately breathing patients, but an antidote must be readily available to treat recurring respiratory depression which often follows the primary resuscitation. The antidotal action of narcotic antagonists is only two to three hours, while the depressant effect of methadone may last from twenty-four to forty-eight hours. After successful initial resuscitation, further injections of narcotic antagonists may be given intramuscularly which should be about 50 per cent greater than the intravenous dose. The onset of action of narcotic antagonists is slower (five to ten minutes) after intramuscular than after intravenous injection (one to two minutes). The difference in speed of onset of action is unimportant if the patient is being watched closely and if the narcotic antagonist is given before respiration has become seriously depressed again. In treating comatose infants and small children, it is advisable to maintain a slow intravenous drip of glucose-saline solution (2 parts 5% glucose mixed with 1 part saline solution) for the first twenty-four hours. This ensures adequate hydration and provides a route for intravenous medication, if needed for treatment of circulatory collapse. Emptying the stomach by lavage is indicated if the procedure can be done immediately after ingestion. However, if the victim is not seen after an hour or more, lavage not only interferes with the much more important artificial ventilation but also is potentially dangerous (tracheobronchial aspiration in comatose patients). Gastric lavage in comatose patients should only be performed after ventilatory resuscitation and tracheal intubation with a well-fitting cuffed tube. Dialysis is contraindicated (the amount of methadone in blood is negligible, even after a fatal ingestion). Central nervous system stimulants are ineffective against the depressant actions of methadone and synergistic to the deleterious stimulant effects of this drug and should not be used.

The importance of secure custody of methadone must be emphasized by physicians prescribing this medication. In general, the medication has been responsibly handled by patients being treated by methadone maintenance programs. There have, however, been 3 serious poisonings of children (2 fatal) from approximately 2 million doses dispensed in New York City over a five-year period. These incidents and deaths were due to carelessness and neglect. With the widespread use of methadone on an ambulatory basis, many more, similar tragic events will occur (30 already have) unless some safer container and/or mechanism is developed for the handling of this potentially toxic compound.

## MONOAMINE OXIDASE INHIBITORS (MARPLAN®, NARDIL®, NIAMID®, PARNATE®, ETC.)

These drugs are primarily psychopharmacologic agents used specifically to relieve depressive symptoms. In angina pectoris, they are useful adjuncts in management through reduction in frequency of attacks and pain. Their principal effects are increased psychomotor activity, blocking action on certain parts of the autonomic nervous system and a potentiating action on unrelated drugs (imipramine, amitriptyline, barbiturates, phenothiazine derivatives, etc.). The exclusive reliance on these compounds to prevent suicidal attempts is unwarranted, as there may be a delay in the onset of therapeutic effect or even an increase in anxiety and agitation.

The side-effects from the use of these drugs, even in standard dosages, are multiple and may include the following: restlessness, overstimulation or insomnia, weakness, headaches, dizziness and drowsiness, dry mouth, nausea, abdominal pain, diarrhea or occasionally constipation. Rare symptoms are skin rashes, urinary retention, tachycardia, transitory hypertension (often precipitated by amphetamine and ingestion of cheese protein) with headache, postural hypotension, tinnitis, chills, sweating, edema, blurred vision, paresthesia, cardiac arrhythmias (depressed myocardial contractility), muscle spasm, tremors and impotence. At higher or toxic doses, the symptoms are similar but more severe.

The use of these drugs is not recommended when there is a history of hepatic or renal disease. They have also been shown to have potentiating effects on certain drugs, such as sympathomimetics, central nervous system depressants, hypotensive agents and alcohol. Under no circumstances should they be administered together or in rapid succession with Tofranil (imipramine) or Elavil® (amitriptyline). When monoamine oxidase inhibitors are combined with phenothiazine derivatives or other compounds known to affect blood pressure, elderly patients and those with cardiovascular inadequacies should be observed more closely because of the possibility of additive hypotensive effects.

The ingestion of ripened cheese can induce severe paradoxical hypotension due to the amines (tyramine, beta-phenylethylamine tryptamine) produced from amino acids of casein by bacterial action in the processing of

TABLE 124
ADVERSE EFFECTS WITH CONCURRENT ADMINISTRATION OF OTHER AGENTS AND MAO INHIBITORS

| *Agent* | *Reaction* | *Comments* |
|---|---|---|
| Foods | | |
| Cheese, yogurt, sour cream | Severe headache, hypertension, cardiac arrhythmia | Intracranial bleeding, circulatory failure and death have occurred |
| Beer, Wine | | |
| Yeast products | | |
| Broad Beans | | |
| Coffee, cola beverages, chocolate | Hyperexcitability | |
| Avocados, bananas, canned figs | | |
| Sympathomimetic drugs | | |
| Amphetamine | Severe headache, hypertension, cardiac arrhythmias, chest pain | Intracranial bleeding, circulatory failure and death have occurred |
| Dextroamphetamine | | |
| Methamphetamine | | |
| Ephedrine | | |
| Metaraminol | | |
| Phenylephrine | | |
| Phenylpropanolamine | | |
| Mephentermine | | |
| Antidepressants | | |
| Imipramine | Hypertension, convulsions, hyperpyrexia, cardiotoxicity | Rare but may be fatal EKG monitoring with maximum dosage |
| Amitriptyline | | |
| CNS depressants | | |
| Anesthetics | Hypotension, coma, shock | |
| Meperidine | | |
| Morphine | | |
| Barbiturates | | |
| Codeine | | |
| Alcohol | | |
| Other MAO inhibitors or overdosage | Agitation, tremor, opisthotonus, coma, hyperpyrexia | No antidote available, administration of other drugs hazardous |
| Antihypertensives | | |
| Thiazide diuretics | Potentiates hypotensive effect | |
| Methyldopa | May cause hypertensive reaction | |
| Phenothiazines | Increased extrapyramidal reactions (parkinsonism, dystonias)<br>Hypotension | |
| Insulin | Hypoglycemic reactions | |
| Antiparkinson drugs | Potentiation | |

cheese. Tyramine is the most toxic substance, since it is many times more powerful a pressor agent than are the other amines. (Beer and wine have also been incriminated.)

*Treatment* should consist of general supportive measures, close observation of vital signs and conservative steps to counteract specific symptoms as they occur. In case of accidental or deliberate ingestion of large amounts, gastric lavage or an emetic should be used immediately. The simultaneous use of activated charcoal appears to be logical as an

TABLE 125
TYRAMINE IN FOODS AND BEVERAGES
(μg/gm or μg/ml)

| | |
|---|---|
| *Cheeses:* | |
| Camembert | 86 |
| Emmentaler | 225 |
| N.Y. State Cheddar | 1,416 |
| Gruyère | 516 |
| Processed American | 50 |
| *Pickled herring* | 3,030 |
| *Beverages:* | |
| Chianti | 25 |
| Sherry | 4 |
| Beer | 2–4 |

adsorbent agent. External cooling is recommended if hyperpyrexia occurs. Careful use of barbiturates to relieve myoclonic reactions or convulsions may be necessary; however, extended therapy should be avoided, as effects may be prolonged by these compounds. Parenteral sodium bicarbonate is extremely effective in correcting cardiac arrhythmias, if they occur. When hypotension requires treatment, the standard measures for managing circulatory shock should be initiated. If pressor agents are used, the rate of infusion should be regulated by careful observation of the patient. Monoamine oxidase inhibitors may sometimes increase the pressor response, as has been demonstrated with levarterenol. Phentolamine methane sulfonate given slowly intravenously is the treatment of choice for hypertensive crises and the hypertension that follows the ingestion of cheese. Forced diuresis and dialysis are of questionable value since these compounds are protein-bound and lipophilic and therefore not easily dialyzable.

## MORPHINE (NARCOTICS)

Morphine poisoning may occur from attempts at suicide or accidentally from an inadvertently excessive dose administered therapeutically. Under certain conditions, an otherwise safe dose may become toxic. Very young infants are very susceptible to morphine, and patients with hypothyroidism may be poisoned with therapeutic doses. On the other hand, the individual with heightened reflex excitability of his nervous system may take two, three or more times the ordinary dose and suffer few if any serious effects. For example, a patient with severe pain from renal colic or coronary disease may be given 45 to 60 mg of morphine before he obtains relief of pain, and his respiration is not seriously embarrassed. Naturally, the addict is quite tolerant of large amounts, but even he can die from an overdose. Generally, however, the toxic dose of morphine for a nonaddicted person who is not in pain is somewhere in the neighborhood of 60 mg, and serious symptoms are usually experienced after doses of 100 mg. The outlook becomes less favorable as the amount increases, and doses above 250 mg carry a serious prognosis with death occurring as a result of the marked respiratory depression and consequent anoxia. Of the injected or ingested morphine, 90 per cent is excreted in the urine, either free or conjugated with glucuronic acid. The feces contain from 7 to 10 per cent of the remaining drug.

Acute narcotic poisoning produces a profound depression of the central nervous system from above downward and a stimulation from below upward. Thus it produces sleep, relief of pain and respiratory depression from its action on the cerebral cortex and medulla. Occasionally stimulation of the medulla with excitation of the vomiting center causes severe retching.* The chief action of morphine other than on the nervous system is a stimulatory effect on certain smooth muscles; however, this is not important from the toxicological standpoint. Onset of action is slightly quicker and nausea somewhat less with diacetylmorphine (heroin) than with other narcotics, but not enough to compensate

*Nausea and vomiting in patients given morphine can often be prevented postoperatively by having them drink hot tea. Morphine is secreted in the stomach as the emetic, apomorphine, but the tannic acid in hot tea changes this to tannate, avoiding the reabsorption of the apomorphine.

for its clearly recognized increased hazard of inducing addiction. Certain compounds, especially codeine and thebaine, manifest more pronounced stimulation, and indeed under certain circumstances, thebaine action resembles strychnine.

By the time the physician is called to see the patient, stupor or sleep has already intervened. Soon the patient can no longer be aroused and sinks into a coma. The respiration by this time is quite shallow and slow and may number only two to six per minute. Occasionally, a Cheyne-Stokes type of respiratory rhythm may be observed. As a result of the asphyxia, the patient is cyanotic. The blood pressure is first maintained, but it soon begins to fall gradually because of deleterious effects of anoxia on the capillaries, with a consequent increase in their permeability and loss of blood proteins. This eventually leads to irreversible shock if treatment is not instituted. The pupils are symmetrically constricted, but if anoxia supervenes, they may dilate markedly, which is often noted as death approaches. The trend of pinpoint and symmetrical pupils and marked respiratory depression should strongly suggest a diagnosis of acute morphine poisoning. The musculature of the body is extremely flaccid, and the jaw may relax to such an extent that the tongue may block the pharynx. The Babinski reflex may show dorsal flexion. The skin is cold and moist with perspiration. In some people, skin rashes, urticaria and pruritus are observed. Itching of the nose is a fairly common feature of morphine action. Occasionally, rather atypical features may be present. Excitement which may pass into mania, or delirium can occur, and even convulsions are noted in rare individuals. Excitement is more likely to result from codeine or heroin than from morphine, and convulsions are seldom seen in adults but sometimes occur in children. Nausea and vomiting may be a prominent feature. Death occurs from respiratory failure, and the heart continues to beat for a short while after breathing has ceased.

*Treatment* consists of gastric lavage, which should be done as soon as the patient is seen. There may be morphine left in the stomach even several hours after ingestion due to delay in emptying. The stimulation attendant on the passing of the tube is in itself beneficial. Ipecac and apomorphine as emetics are especially contraindicated here, since most narcotic compounds (particularly heroin) have potent antiemetic effects. They are rarely effective and there is always the possibility of aspiration as well as synergism with depression. Chemical antidotes, if available, such as dilute solutions of potassium permanganate or tincture of iodine to oxidize the morphine may be used for lavage and followed with a slurry of activated charcoal (1 gm of charcoal adsorbs 800 mg of morphine).

Before the stomach tube is completely removed, a saline cathartic solution should be given to hasten the unabsorbed drug through the intestinal tract. If the patient is conscious, attempts should be made to keep him awake by giving strong black coffee by mouth and by physical stimulation. After the onset of definitive symptoms, treatment is directed mainly at maintaining respiratory exchange and giving narcotic antagonists. Comatose patients develop respiratory obstruction due to soft-tissue relaxation in the upper airway and to accumulation of secretions in the pharynx and tracheobronchial tree. The obstruction can be overcome by hyperextension of the head and lifting the mandible forward to clear the airway, by aspiration of obstructing secretions and by the insertion of an artificial airway when needed. If the respiratory effort is satisfactory, an oropharyngeal airway may suffice. In deep coma, however, an endotracheal tube is indicated to ensure patency of the airway, to reduce the respiratory dead space and to facilitate the removal of secretions. These tubes should be changed every twelve hours. Doxapram hydrochloride (Dopram®) 3 to 5 ml intravenously is an extremely safe, nonspecific respiratory stimulant. It usually has an immediate, dramatic effect, but unfortunately it is short lasting—only three to five minutes. The occurrence of pulmonary edema several hours after recovery from coma in heroin overdosage has been well documented. The pathogenesis is unclear but hypoxia may be an important factor. Oxygen given under intermittent positive pressure along with conventional therapy should result in a good clinical response.

Some attempt must be made to estimate the adequacy of respiration. Generally, the tidal volume should exceed 300 ml. Cyanosis does not have to be visible for a diagnosis of respiratory inadequacy to be made. Some estimation of ventilation is offered by the color of the lips, fingernails and mucous membranes. If they are pink, oxygenation is probably satisfactory. However, carbon dioxide levels may be high in spite of good oxygenation. The goal of therapy of narcotic overdosage is to obtain normal blood gas values (pH 7.42, $pCO_2$ 40, $pO_2$ 90) with the patient breathing room air. Therefore, a heparinized sample of arterial blood should be obtained and analyzed for these values. Values for blood gases on victims of narcotic overdosage vary with the clinical situation, as the following examples indicate. If the patient is comatose when first seen, typical values might be pH 7.20, $pCO_2$ 70, $pO_2$ 35. Such values represent a combined metabolic and respiratory acidosis. If treatment has been successful, no respiratory complications are present and the patient is breathing supplemental oxygen, then a typical set of values might be pH 7.40, $pCO_2$ 40, $pO_2$ 120 (depending upon the percent of inspired oxygen). If pulmonary edema is present, however, then the initial respiratory acidosis persists and the arterial blood gas picture might be pH 7.30, $pCO_2$ 60, $pO_2$ 45.

Respiration must be assisted in patients with inadequate pulmonary ventilation as determined above, and artificial respiration must be instituted in the apneic patient. Many types of mechanical respirators are available and are useful under these circumstances. In the absence of mechanical devices, manual artificial ventilation can be used, or manual rhythmic compression of a breathing bag attached to a mask can be resorted to. Any anesthetic machine may be used for artificial ventilation. A respiratory rate of at least 25/min. is desirable. The advice and aid of an anesthesiologist should be sought in these procedures. As soon as adequate ventilation has been provided, the patient should be given naloxone (Narcan) intravenously (*see* pp. 441-442). A favorable response to naloxone administration should be considered diagnostic of narcotic overdosage. Naloxone has been called a "pure narcotic antagonist" and does not possess the agonistic (depressant) properties characteristic of other narcotic antagonists. Therefore, if naloxone is given to a patient who has taken an overdose of barbiturate, for example, no harm has been done. The response to treatment should be carefully noted, since it gives clues to the clinical situation. After treatment with naloxone, the patient may be alert and oriented or he may show persistent lethargy or symptoms of withdrawal. An alert and oriented patient may or may not indicate that treatment is successful. Patients with persistent lethargy should be given special attention. Lethargy may represent the effect of other depressant drugs, or it may represent arterial hypoxemia secondary to pulmonary edema. Patients with symptoms of withdrawal after treatment with naloxone usually are narcotic addicts. Failure of response to narcotic antagonists suggests that the drug producing coma was not a narcotic or that substances (a bag of heroin contains 1 to 5 per cent heroin with quinine, lactose, mannitol, baking soda and other materials used as a "filler") or conditions in addition to narcotics are producing coma.

In severe toxicity, the cardiovascular system is usually depressed and requires supportive measures. In the early phases when hypotension is due to vasodilatation, vasopressors should be given. If the hypotension is accompanied by a slow pulse, ephedrine, 25 mg IV or 50 mg IM, effects a sustained rise in pressure and increase in pulse. If the pulse is rapid, either methoxamine (Vasoxyl®), 3 to 5 mg IV or 10 mg IM, or phenylephrine (Neo-Synephrine), 1 mg IV or 5 mg IM, is preferable because these drugs slow cardiac rate. If there is shock, plasma or plasma expanders should be administered.

Additional measures consist of maintenance of proper fluid and electrolyte balance; maintenance of normal temperature; frequent change in the patient's posture to obviate pulmonary complications; repeated catheterization to avoid distention of the bladder; and symptomatic therapy for itching, nausea, vomiting; and confusion during the recovery period. Usually the narcotic antagonist decreases the severe gastrointestinal symptoms, but if these persist, they may be relieved by administering an antiemetic drug such as Marezine®, Dramamine or Thorazine, in doses of 50 mg IM, repeated every four to six hours if necessary. Care should be exercised to prevent damage to eyes, lips and mouth by taping the eyes shut and by lubricating the lips to prevent dryness and cracking. Attention must be paid to oral hygiene. Antibiotics should be used as a prophylactic measure in the prevention of bacterial pneumonia.

Apneic infants, born of addictive mothers or mothers to whom narcotics have been given during labor, may benefit from the narcotic antagonists. Nalorphine 0.2 to 0.5 mg, 0.04 to 0.1 mg of levallorphan in 2 ml of solution, or preferable naloxone (Narcan) 0.010 to 0.015 mg/kg can be injected into the infant's umbilical vein. The larger doses may be given intramuscularly. Onset of respiration and increased muscle tone should appear within a few minutes following intravenous injection if the depression is due to the narcotics given the mother. In children, the dose of nalorphine is 0.1 mg/kg of body weight, while the dosage for levallorphan is 0.02 mg/kg. However, the administration of naloxone has completely supplanted the use of other narcotic antagonists.

Diazepam (1 to 2 mg intramuscularly every eight hours if necessary) appears to be a safe and effective drug for the treatment of neonatal narcotic withdrawal symptoms. Control may be quickly achieved with a short course of therapy without serious side-effects or the occurrence of rebound symptoms when the drug is discontinued. (For further discussion of this topic, *see* page 448.)

## MORPHINE (NARCOTIC) ADDICTION

It is not within the scope of this book to include a detailed discussion of so complex a problem. A brief review will suffice.

There are over a half-million narcotic addicts now in the United States. Narcotic addiction is characterized by four principal phenomena: tolerance, habituation, physiologic dependence and tendency to relapse after repeated "cures." Diagnosis of addiction is simple if the physician keeps them in mind. The presence of pinpoint pupils and scars or needle marks on the skin should arouse suspicion. An absolute diagnosis can be made by the administration of small doses of nalorphine (2.5 mg), levallorphan (0.5 mg) or preferably naloxone. (0.01mg/kg).

Narcotic addiction is a chronic, relapsing disorder. This, plus the not infrequent criminal activities of addicts, their skill in manipulating those about them in relation to their addiction and the remarkable social stigma associated with addiction, results in many frustrations for physicians who undertake their treatment. For these reasons, many physicians avoid the treatment of addicted persons. Yet, the withdrawal of an addict and the treatment of any underlying personality disorder he may have are certainly medical problems. If addicts are to obtain the medical treatment they need and often seek, it must be given by physicians. It is evident that each physician whose services are sought by an addict with an apparently sincere desire for treatment is obligated either to provide the indicated treatment himself or to refer the patient to a professional colleague skilled in and willing to undertake such treatment.

The management of narcotic addiction is a highly specialized problem requiring a well-integrated program that includes expert medical, psychiatric and nursing care. In some areas the patient may be admitted to a public, local or state institution where treatment programs exist. When local or state facilities are not available, the patient can be referred to the U.S. Public Health Service Hospital at Lexington, Kentucky, or Forth Worth, Texas, for patients residing west of the Mississippi.

The withdrawal *treatment* may be abrupt, rapid or gradual. Of these, the rapid method is preferable except in those with chronic illness such as cardiac and pulmonary disease, in which case the drug is withdrawn gradually. Regardless of the daily amounts the addict consumes, the dose of morphine is reduced to about 32 mg every six hours. This stabilizing dose is usually sufficient to avoid craving and to prevent withdrawal symptoms. This dose is continued for three to four days, then rapidly reduced until the patient is receiving 10 mg/dose. At this time the 10 mg dose of morphine is alternated with 30 mg of codeine for one day. Thereafter, codeine alone is given for two or three days, after which all narcotic medication is discontinued. This schedule of withdrawal involves about one to two weeks.

Supportive therapy, consisting of psychological support, nonaddictive analgesics for muscle pain, non-narcotic drugs for control of diarrhea, tranquilizers or mild sedatives such as chloral hydrate to relieve tension and to assure sleep and adequate food and fluids is essential.

An alternative method is the use of the methadone substitution method. After the stabilization period, methadone is substituted in the ratio of 1 mg to 4 mg for morphine; to 2 mg for heroin; to 1 mg for Dilaudid; and to 20 to 30 mg for Demerol or codeine respectively. Methadone is then continued for one week, after which it is rapidly withdrawn over a period of three days. The abstinence syndrome which follows withdrawal of methadone is considerably less severe than after morphine withdrawal. This medication appears to have two useful effects: (1) relief of narcotic hunger and (2) induction of sufficient tolerance to block the euphoric effect of the average illegal dose.

The single massive oral dose of methadone (Dole-Nyswander) treatment of heroin addiction has not had the extensive use or follow-up to warrant the expectations and permanent results predicted. Cyclazocine has been used as a useful and effective alternative compound to methadone maintenance treatment, and diazepam has been effective in reducing the duration and severity of withdrawal symptoms in a large group of adolescent heroin addicts.

The Narcotic Addict Treatment Act of 1974 (Public Law 93-281, May 1974) placed federal government control of methadone on a firm legal foundation. This additional control was accomplished by giving to the Drug Enforcement Administration (DEA) of the Department of Justice the responsibility for registering all practitioners who use methadone or other narcotic drugs in the treatment of narcotics addiction.

Neonatal narcotic addiction is creating a problem in large metropolitan cities, and experience has indicated that withdrawal symptoms following maternal use of methadone are more severe than those following heroin abuse. While some infants manifest withdrawal symptoms immediately after birth, generally the syndrome does not set in until the third to fifth day (as long as two weeks later with methadone). The symptoms most frequently encountered are unusual irritability; tremors; high-pitched, incessant, shrill, prolonged crying; vomiting; diarrhea; sneezing; hypotonicity; respiratory distress; excessive sweating; excessive mucus secretion; and failure to gain weight. Convulsions occur primarily with methadone withdrawal. Many of the babies are premature. The preferred treatment is chlorpromazine, given in doses ranging from 0.7 mg/kg to 1.2 mg/kg every six hours, depending upon the severity of the case, with reduction of dosage after one to two weeks; average duration of treatment is two to four weeks. However, intramuscular diazepam has been documented as being even more effective than chlorpromazine and may be the treatment of choice. However, there is some concern that sodium benzoate and the benzoic acid/benzoate combination contained in injectable diazepam have been shown *in vitro* to displace bilirubin from its binding site on albumin, and therefore have the potential of producing bilirubinemia and kernicterus. Other drugs used for treatment are phenobarbital and paregoric elixir. Paregoric dosage is 3 to 5 drops before each feeding (up to 20 drops for methadone withdrawal). Phenobarbital dosage is 8 to 10 mg/kg/day in three or four individual doses. The goal of therapy is an infant who is no longer irritable and hyperactive, is able to feed and sleep between feedings and no longer has diarrhea or vomiting. Occasionally, withdrawal is mild and requires no specific therapy other than a neutral thermal environment, swaddling, gentle handling and careful feeding. Supportive therapy such as provision of adequate fluid, electrolytes and calories; treatment of suspected infection; and correction of metabolic problems, particularly hypoglycemia and hypocalcemia, is most important.

In general, 50 per cent of treated infants require therapy for ten to twenty days, with 25 per cent requiring less than ten days and 25 per cent requiring up to forty days of treatment (methadone withdrawal takes longer than heroin withdrawal).

The disposition and long-term care of the infant of an addicted mother represents the greatest overall challenge. Prior to the infant's discharge, the home environment must be investigated to determine whether or not the child's well-being and safety can be assured. Following discharge, there must be continued supervision of the child's care. The supervision requires close collaboration among social workers, public health nurses and physicians.

Neonatal withdrawal syndrome to a variety of transplacentally acquired (maternal) drugs has been recognized since the 1800s. Utilizing methods of gas chromatography, mass spectrometry and computer systems, indentification of a number of drugs or their metabolites producing withdrawal symptoms in the human neonates is now being readily recognized. In addition to the opiates and their derivatives, barbiturates (phenobarbital), hydroxyzine hydrochloride and other ataractics and psychotropic agents, the tricyclics and any number of other drugs taken throughout pregnancy have the potential of producing the withdrawal syndrome. Depending on the half-life of the specific drug, the duration for excretion by the neonate has been reported to be two to eight days.

## MYRISTICIN (NUTMEG, MACE)

Nutmeg or mace intoxication is caused by myristica, a yellowish volatile oil which is the essential oil of nutmeg and of nutmeg flower oil, which has the following toxic volatile principles: eugenol, isoeugenol, geraniol, safrol and bormeol. The usual toxic dose is 5 to 15 gm of powdered nutmeg. The effects which appear in one to six hours are mainly due to central nervous system stimulation and are manifested by excitement, flushing of the skin, tachycardia, absence of salivation, hallucinations (psychedelic), drowsiness, delirium and unconsciousness. The gastrointestinal symptoms of nausea, vomiting and diarrhea occur soon after ingestion. Hepatic necrosis has been reported with severe poisoning. *Treatment* consists of 2 to 4 oz. of mineral or castor oil followed by gastric lavage and a saline cathartic. Milk or other demulcents can be given after lavage to allay gastric irritation. Convulsions should be controlled by administration of ether or a quick-acting barbiturate. Myristicin has been isolated from the smoke of commercial cigarettes and this biologically active compound may be responsible for some of the effects attributed to nicotine.

## NITRITES, NITRATES, GLYCERYL TRINITRATE

Amyl nitrite, ethyl nitrite, sodium nitrite, glyceryl trinitrate (nitroglycerin) and other organic nitrates are used therapeutically to dilate coronary vessels and to reduce blood pressure. Occasionally, nitrates such as bismuth subnitrate or nitrate from well water may be converted to nitrite by the action of intestinal bacteria and cause nitrite poisoning. Public Health Service Drinking Water Standards set the limit of 45 mg/liter of nitrate ion in drinking water to avoid infant methemoglobinemia. The conversion of *nitrates* to *nitrites* constitutes the hazard. Unchanged nitrates ordinarily do not produce methemoglobinemia. This occurs more frequently in infants because of their susceptible fetal hemoglobin and a relative lack of enzymes that reconvert the methemoglobin to hemoglobin.

The spores of *Bacillus subtilis,* which cannot be suppressed during the production of dried milk powder, can also produce this reaction if the formula water happens to be contaminated with nitrates. Dried powdered buttermilk (lactic acid) formula, on the other hand, is safe for artificial feeding because it contains *Streptococcus lactis,* an organism producing nisins, which exert an antibiotic effect preventing the growth of *B. subtilis.* Fresh spinach and beets have relatively high concentrations of nitrates (1000 ppm and over) and on standing after cooking the more highly toxic nitrites are formed. (Methemoglobinemia in fourteen infants ages two to ten months has been reported.) The normal urinary output of nitrate is about 0.5 gm/day derived mainly from green vegetables. Nitrites are also used to preserve the color of meat, in pickling or in other salting processes.

The following lethal doses have been reported: ethyl nitrite in a three-year-old child, 4 gm ("Sweet Spirits of Niter," 3.5 to 4.5 per cent of ethyl nitrite given in the formula of a four-month-old infant produced fatal methemoglobinemia); glyceryl trinitrate, 2 gm; sodium nitrite, 2 gm; nitrates 0.5 to 5.0 gm/kg. The allowable residue of nitrite in food is 0.01 per cent. More than 10 ppm of nitrate in well water may induce methemoglobinemia in infants.

Drug nitrites dilate blood vessels throughout the body by a direct relaxing effect on smooth muscles and they can also cause methemoglobinemia. The pathologic findings are chocolate-colored blood as a result of conversion of hemoglobin to methemoglobin and congestion of all organs.

An offshoot of amyl nitrite, N-butyl nitrite, has become a "street" drug called "poppers" (also "locker-room," "jack," "rush," "aroma" or "bullet"). Because of the resultant rush of blood and oxygen to the brain, a facial flushing and a temporary high occurs a few seconds after sniffing. Its use in the drug subculture is its improvement of dancing and sex.

The principal manifestations of poisoning with these drugs are fall of blood pressure and cyanosis. Acute poisoning from ingestion, injection, inhalation or absorption from skin or mucous membranes produces headache, flushing of the skin, vomiting, dizziness, collapse, marked fall of blood pressure, cyanosis, coma and respiratory paralysis. Repeated administration may lead to chronic poisoning. Nitroglycerin workers show marked tolerance to repeated exposure. This tolerance disappears rapidly, and short absence from exposure may lead to severe poisoning from amounts that were previously safe.

*Treatment* consists of delaying absorption of ingested nitrites or nitrates by giving water, milk or activated charcoal and then removing them by gastric lavage or emesis, followed by catharsis. Keep the patient warm and recumbent in shock position. Administer oxygen and artificial respiration if necessary. Remove completely from the skin by scrubbing with soap and water for all skin contacts, and treat severe methemoglobinemia with dyspnea and cyanosis by methylene blue injection. Transfuse with whole blood or use plasma expanders as indicated. Avoid epinephrine and other vasoconstrictor drugs since spontaneous reflexes usually generate and maintain arteriolar constriction in nitrite poisoning. If reflex bradycardia occurs, atropine can be used as a blocking drug.

## PARA-AMINOPHENOL ANALGESIC COMPOUNDS (ACETANILID, PHENACETIN [ACETOPHENETIDIN], ETC.)

These drugs are used alone or in combination with other drugs in a number of proprietary analgesic compounds. Poisoning nearly always occurs from the medical misuse rather than from attempts at self-destruction. The lethal dose varies from 5 to 20 gm. Considerable individual susceptibility to these drugs is manifested and the toxic dose for one person may be harmless for another. Acetanilid, however, is definitely more toxic than phenacetin (acetophenetidin).

Acetaminophen (N-acetyl-*p*-aminophenol, Liquiprin® and Tempra®) is a major metabolic end product of acetanilid and phenacetin with fewer adverse effects. Rate and degree of temperature reduction, though not significantly greater, is more sustained with acetaminophen-aspirin combination than with either drug alone. (For a more complete discussion, *see* Acetaminophen, p. 346.)

The characteristic feature of poisoning by these drugs (acetaminophen excepted) is cyanosis. This is due to the formation of methemoglobin (probably due to an abnormal metabolic pathway), and if there is much of this altered pigment, the symptoms are those of anemia. The patient may be cyanotic and yet the characteristic absorption bands for methemoglobin may not be seen in the spectroscope either because the concentration of pigment is not sufficiently high or because the cyanosis is due to sulfhemoglobinemia. The presence in the blood of para-aminophenol itself may also account for the skin color. Dyspnea, weakness, anginal pain and circulatory failure also occur and in part are due to the interference with oxygen transport by the blood. Symptoms suggestive of cinchonism may appear but are rare. In severe cases, there is subnormal body temperature, prostration, shallow breathing, confusion and collapse. The pulse is weak and rapid, and the heart is directly affected by para-aminophenol in a manner similar to the toxic action of aniline. Hypoglycemia in children has been reported with overdosage of acetaminophen. Liver and kidney damage result from these drugs, and jaundice, oliguria or anuria may be noted. The urine shows the "indophenol" reaction as a result of the renal elimination of para-aminophenol paired with glycuronic or sulfuric acid. Dark brown urine, with the unusual property of reducing silver nitrate solutions in the cold, may be a useful clue leading to the recognition of unsuspected phenacetin intoxication or abuse. Confirmation may be obtained by the detection of phenacetin metabolites in the urine by simple one-way chromatography after acid hydrolysis. Skin reactions also follow the use of these drugs, especially phenacetin (acetophenetidin), and are erythematous or urticarial in nature. They may be accompanied by a stomatitis. Death may occur after a period of delirium, collapse and coma. Patients with organic disease and especially with cardiac or pulmonary pathology are more susceptible to poisoning with acetanilid. The chronic form of poisoning may be extremely difficult to diagnose unless the drugs are suspected of being the cause. Cyanosis, weakness, shortness of breath, anorexia, loss of weight, insomnia anemia and brownish urine are the outstanding features. The oxygen-carrying capacity of the blood is lower than that indicated by the value of the hemoglobin because some of the latter is rendered incapable of carrying oxygen.

Although long considered a drug of limited toxicity, phenacetin (acetophenetidin) has in recent years come under criticism as a possible source of renal damage (interstitial nephritis, pyelonephritis and papillary necrosis) in patients who consume large amounts of it over long periods. Most of this drug is converted to N-acetyl-*p*-aminophenol, a compound that is also marketed as an analgesic under the generic name acetaminophen. To date, there is only circumstantial evidence that phenacetin or its degradation products cause renal damage. However, the clinical as well as the experimental evidence, when adequate animal dosage is used, is significant enough that phenacetin-containing drugs should be used with caution in patients with known renal disease. In any unexplained serious chronic renal disease, phenacetin addiction should be kept in mind and, if found, treated accordingly. Massive ingestion of acetaminophen for suicidal purposes has produced hepatic necrosis and renal failure. Abnormal electroencephalographic changes have also been reported in chronic and prolonged users of phenacetin.

The combined abuse of aspirin with phenacetin as an analgesic increases the potential of renal injury and disease. Aspirin inhibits the tissues' defenses against oxygen damage by interfering with two enzymes in the hexose monophosphate shunt, thereby laying the tissues open to damage by the metabolic product of phenacetin (acetylparaminophenol).

There is no specific *treatment* for poisoning by these compounds. The medicine should be withdrawn at the earliest possible moment. If a large single dose is the cause of the intoxication, the stomach should be lavaged and a saline cathartic given. If the cyanosis or anemia is severe, transfusion may be needed. This is especially true if a hemolytic crisis has occurred. If there is cardiovascular collapse, warmth, rest and intravenous glucose are helpful. Other symptomatic measures to support the respiration and circulation should be employed as needed. Forced diuresis could be dangerous in the face of possible renal failure and should be used with caution, if at all. With evidence of prolonged half-life and high levels of unconjugated drug, dialysis would appear efficacious.

Cysteamine, an investigational drug which inactivates the toxic metabolite of acetaminophen, showed therapeutic promise in acetaminophen intoxication. A dose of 2 gm intravenously over ten minutes followed by three 400 mg doses at intervals of four to eight hours has been used in adults. Comparatively smaller doses should be used for children. Subsequent documentation has failed to verify any substantial benefits. Histologic evidence of liver damage showed a possible beneficial effect of cysteamine, but this therapy did not prevent renal or pancreatic damage (*see* Acetaminophen, 346).

For methemoglobinemia levels above 40 per cent, methylene blue should be given immediately and repeated in one hour if necessary.

## PARASYMPATHOMIMETIC (CHOLINERGIC) AGENTS

These compounds are chiefly of two types: (1) choline derivatives, which are similar to acetylcholine, and (2) cholinesterase inhibitors, which prevent the destruction of the endogenous acetylcholine. The following are some of these agents with their approximate adult MLD: physostigmine (eserine), 0.06 gm; neostigmine, 0.06 gm; pilocarpine, 0.13 gm; methacholine (Mecholyl), 0.03 gm; and muscarine, 10 mg.

Their principal effects and symptoms are parasympathomimetic stimulation with tremors, miosis, vertigo, marked peristalsis with involuntary defecation and urination, vomiting, cardiac inhibition, bradycardia, dyspnea, convulsions and death due to respiratory failure or cardiac paralysis.

*Treatment* should consist of immediate, thorough emptying of the stomach by either gastric lavage or emetics. Artificial respiration may be required until the specific antidote atropine can be given. The patient should be kept fully atropinized (1 to 2 mg every fifteen to thirty minutes) throughout the entire crisis. It must be remembered, however, that atropine blocks only the muscarine effects, and if tremors are severe or a convulsion is impending or occurring, a short-acting barbiturate should be administered. It may be necessary to maintain an airway with suctioning until the patient has fully recovered. Pro-Banthine® is alternate and drug of choice.

## PAREGORIC (CAMPHORATED TINCTURE OF OPIUM)

Paregoric is a hydroalcoholic solution containing not more than 129.6 mg of powdered opium per 29.573 ml (1 fl. oz.) with anise oil, benzoic acid and camphor. It is a tincture of 0.4% opium (0.04% morphine) and is now the major narcotic used in many cities. Paregoric is an exempt item in most states and can be purchased at pharmacies without prescription. It is estimated that two thirds of all addicts are now using this anodyne for intravenous injection.

The drug is usually concentrated by boiling before intravenous instillation. Users often mix paregoric with amphetamines, secobarbital, glutethimide, other barbiturates or tripelennamine. The talcum filler of tripelennamine has been associated with diffuse pulmonary granuloma and subsequent pulmonary hypertension (*see* "Blue Velvet"). The benzoic acid, camphor and anise of paregoric are irritants and lead to occlusive sclerosis after intravenous instillation. Therefore, the median cubital vein (most often used by heroin addicts) as well as the femoral, popliteal, axillary and saphenous veins are often used. The external jugular vein is, however, the most frequent site of injection because of its large size and ready accessibility. A scar at the base of the neck just above the clavicle is the pathognomonic sign of paregoric addicts. An additional unexplained hazard is the report of penicillin G-resistant staphylococcal infections in addicts, despite the fact that the infections were acquired outside of the hospital.

## PHENOL AND DERIVATIVES (CRESOL, NAPHTHOL, MENTHOL, THYMOL, GUAIACOL, RESORCINOL, ETC.)

Phenol is a white aromatic solid, soluble in water in 1:15 dilution. Creosotes (wood or coal tar) are mixtures of phenolic and other compounds obtained by the destruction and distillation of wood or coal. Despite the fact that phenol is little employed in therapeutics today, the many derivatives are used as antiseptics, disinfectants, caustics, germicides, surface anesthetics and preservatives. An antimildew agent containing pentachlorophenol used in the terminal rinse of diapers and nursery linens has produced "a sweating syndrome" and fever with two deaths and severe intoxication in nine additional infants. The lethal dose of phenol is between 2 and 10 gm.

Phenol is a general protoplasmic poison and enters into a loose combination with protein. It can penetrate tissue very deeply and is readily absorbed from all surfaces of the body. Local gangrene occurs from prolonged contact with tissue, and such accidents were not infrequent in the former widespread use of phenol as an antiseptic or local anesthetic. Irritation is soon replaced by anesthesia due to the death of nerve endings, and tissue necrosis follows. The chemical is also absorbed readily into the bloodstream from the gastrointestinal tract. It causes widespread capillary damage and paralysis and also acts on the cells of the kidney, heart and nervous system. The body detoxifies phenol by oxidizing close to one half of it and conjugating much of the remainder as ethereal sulfates and phenolic glycuronates. Both the conjugated fraction and a smaller unbound portion are excreted through the kidneys. In smaller amounts, it has a salicylate-like stimulating effect on the respiratory center causing a respiratory alkalosis which is later followed by acidosis. Methemoglobinemia may also occur.

The symptoms are both local and systemic. The local effects of phenol on the skin and mucosa are those of tissue destruction. The skin is white and anesthetized, and the ulcers and sloughing which follow heal very slowly by scar formation.

The systemic effects are those produced by the action on the gastrointestinal tract—pain, nausea, vomiting, diarrhea—and those due to the action of the poison on the vital structures of the body. Cardiovascular collapse and shock quickly develop. Central nervous system stimulation is transitory and soon followed by respiratory and central depression. Renal damage is often severe and anuria may result. The little urine that is passed is characteristically smoky and contains albumin, casts and red blood cells. A small fraction of the phenol may be excreted by the lungs and impart an aromatic odor to the breath.

Phenol can be detected in the blood, tissues and urine. A few drops of ferric chloride will turn the urine a blue or violet color if phenolic compounds are present.

In the *treatment* of ingested poison, its absorption should be delayed by giving milk, olive oil or vegetable oil followed by repeated gastric lavage. Mineral oil and alcohol are contraindicated because they increase the gastric absorption of phenol (their use is still suggested in some texts). Castor oil 60 ml (2 oz.), which dissolves phenols, retards their absorption and hastens their removal, should then be given. This in turn can be followed by a saline cathartic. For skin and mucosal lesions, the surfaces should be washed with large amounts of water for fifteen minutes followed by the application of castor oil (as a surface solvent) or 10% ethyl alcohol. Daily dressing may then be applied to the affected parts.

Specific therapy for acidosis, convulsions or shock should be instituted as the need arises.

## PHENOLPHTHALEIN

The accidental ingestion of an overdose of a laxative containing phenolphthalein usually need not cause alarm, because phenolphthalein is not a highly toxic substance. The number of bowel movements seldom exceeds six in the first twenty-four hours. There may be two to three movements after that. As a rule, the bowel action returns to normal not later than the third day. If urine or feces are alkaline, they may acquire a red color. This is not blood.

Aside from laxation, the course is likely to be uneventful. Only rarely has prostration, vertigo, dyspnea or any other systemic effect been observed. Chronic usage may produce a fixed drug eruption.

The tendency to overtreat should be guarded against.

*Treatment.* The following suggestions for the management of phenolphthalein overdosage are recommended.

1. Gastric lavage should be instituted if the patient is seen early enough after ingestion; otherwise, this procedure is not necessary.
2. Vomiting should not be induced in children, as aspiration of particles vomited may cause difficulties.
3. Activated charcoal in teaspoonful doses, suspended in milk, water or non-carbonated beverage (but not in fruit juices) every one or two hours. An excess of charcoal is harmless. If excessive laxation develops, continue charcoal until the laxative action subsides.
4. If a very large quantity of phenolphthalein has been taken, it may be advisable to administer a therapeutic dose of castor oil. This aids in quickly eliminating the major portion of the phenolphthalein ingested. No saline cathartic, alkalis, glycerin, propylene glycol, alcohol or other solvents of phenolphthalein should be given, as they may increase the laxative action.
5. The person should remain quiet, but not confined to bed. Regular diet. No restriction of fluids, except fruit juices.
6. Bismuth, kaolin or other bowel movement restraining drugs, except activated charcoal, are contraindicated. They may prolong the action of the retained portion of the laxative by slowing up evacuation. (Factitious diarrhea induced by phenolphthalein can be confirmed by adding 0.1 N sodium hydroxide to the stools [or urine], which produces a characteristic purple color.)

## PHOSPHATE COMPOUNDS

Sodium phosphate compounds are frequently used as laxatives for both adults and children. Especially popular is a mixture of sodium biphosphate ($NaH_2PO_4$) and sodium monophosphate ($NaHPO_4$) commercially known as Fleet enema or, in the oral preparation, as Phospho-Soda®. This mixture contains 2178 mEq/liter of sodium and 1756 mEq/liter of phosphate. It acts osmotically. The hypertonic solution of sodium biphosphate and sodium monophosphate raises the fluid volume of the colon, distends it and thereby increases the peristalsis. Even though some of the anion is absorbed, if kidney function is normal, no toxic accumulation occurs. However, hypocalcemic tetany following the absorption of inorganic phosphates from enemas has been reported in adults and children, especially those with Hirschsprung's disease. The retention of phosphate ions depresses the serum calcium and tetany may result. *Treatment* is simple and clear-cut with the administration of parenteral elemental calcium.

## PHOTOSENSITIZING COMPOUNDS

Skin eruptions provoked by light and limited to exposed surfaces are being induced more and more by recently introduced drugs and chemicals. This condition has been observed with the following drugs.

1. Sulfonamides
2. Sulfonylurea hypoglycemics (carbutamide, tolbutamide [Orinase] and chlorpropamide [Diabinese])
3. Chlorothiazide and related diuretics
4. Phenothiazines, benzodiazepines and tricyclics
5. Demethylchlortetracycline (Declomycin® and tetracyclines)
6. Griseofulvin
7. Nalidixic acid (NegGram®)
8. Promethazine (Phenergan®)
9. Furocoumarins, psoralens
10. Aminobenzoic acid
11. Gold and silver salts
12. Chlorosalicylamide
13. Halogenated salicylanilides, carbanilides in germicidal soaps) and phenols
14. Barbiturates
15. Trimethadione (Tridione)
16. Salicylates
17. Local anesthetics of procaine group
18. Estrogens, progesterones
19. Cyclamate, calcium
20. Oral contraceptives
21. Thiothixene (Navane®)
22. Miscellaneous group
    a. Acridine, anthracene
    b. Azine
    c. Oxazine, oxazone
    d. Bergamot-Rul (perfumes, flavoring agents)
    e. Pitch
    f. Quinine and other antimalarials
    g. Selenium
    h. Pyridine
    i. Phenanthrene
    j. Phenylbutazone
    k. Arsenicals
    l. Citrus oils (orange, lemon, lime)
    m. Stilbamidine
    n. Benadryl
    o. Triethylene melamine (TEM)
    p. Hexachlorophene
    q. Coal and wood tars
    r. Petroleum products
    s. Dyes
    t. Plants (*see* Table 138)
    u. Pyrazinamide
    v. Sunscreens (PABA, Neo-A-Fil®)
    w. Azathioprine (Imuran®)
    x. Quinidine
    y. Isoniazid
    z. Hexachlorobenzene

Photosensitization, though undesirable and sometimes alarming, is not ordinarily associated with serious or permanent untoward effects. (For photosensitization produced by plants, *see* Chap. 9.)

If exposure to sunlight is unavoidable, topical sunscreening agents (not the popular suntanning agents) should be employed. Ultra-Violet Absorbing Lotion (UVAL®) containing 10% sulisobenzone (2-hydroxy-4-methoxy-benzophenone-5-sulfonic acid) is the most effective preparation available. The next most useful are red veterinary petrolatum (RVP®) and 15% *p*-aminobenzoic acid (PABA). Unlike PABA, the RVP prevents sunburn from exposure to light waves above as well as below 32000 Ångström units. PABA itself occasionally causes photosensitive reactions.

## PICRIC ACID

Picric acid or trinitrophenol is a yellow powder used in the dye industry, manufacture of explosives and occasionally therapeutically as an antiseptic. The lethal dose has been found to be as little as 1 gm, but severe poisoning can also follow chronic exposure to high concentrations of dust of picric acid.

The local irritant properties of this compound can cause severe conjunctivitis, palpebral edema, keratitis and yellow vision. Contact with the skin gives rise to intense pruritic dermatitis with vesicles and weeping lesions. The systemic effects are those of an acute gastroenteritis with severe abdominal pain, nausea and vomiting and diarrhea. The vomitus is yellow in color. The kidneys are often seriously involved, and acute nephritis is not uncommon. The urine is red in color and greatly reduced in volume. Complete anuria may occur and can result in death from uremia. The renal involvement may in part be due to the hemolytic action of picric acid on red blood corpuscles. The liver is also damaged and jaundice ensues, but the yellow color of the skin and mucous membranes is due to staining from the acid itself. In severe acute poisoning, nervous system symptoms are prominent and consist of headache, progressive depression and finally coma and death.

*Treatment* is purely symptomatic. If the poison has been ingested, gastric lavage with a 5% solution of sodium bicarbonate should be used and repeated until all the yellow color has disappeared from the wash water. This should be followed by a saline cathartic. If the kidney is not impaired, large amounts of oral or parenteral fluids should be given. For skin contacts, the skin should be thoroughly washed (about fifteen minutes) with a 5% solution of sodium bicarbonate. The papulovesicular weeping dermatitis that often results can be treated with wet dressings of a weak alkaline solution. If the eyes are involved, *see* page 46 for suggested therapy and management.

### Porphyria-inducing Drugs

Barbiturates
Phenobarbital, sodium
Sulfonethylmethane (Trional®)
Glutethimide (Doriden)
Diphenylhydantoin, sodium (Dilantin)
Bemegride (Megimide)
Phensuximide (Milontin)
Hexachlorobenzene
Diallyl-barbituric acid (Dial®)
Sulfonmethane (Sulfonal®)
Methyprylon (Noludar®)
Mephenytoin (Mesantoin)
Meprobamate (Miltown®)
Methsuximide (Celontin)
Griseofulvin
Alcohol (excessive intake)
Diethylstilbestrol (DES)
Methotrexate
Chloroquine phosphate

These compounds in *in vitro* test system have demonstrated a definite potential for inducing porphyria. Therefore, they should be considered to be contraindicated in patients with known hepatic porphyria and in their families and near relatives.

## PROCAINE (TETRACAINE, DIBUCAINE, PIPEROCAINE, DIMETHISOQUIN [QUOTANE®], ETC.)

The number of synthetic local anesthetics is so large that it is impossible to consider all of them. Procaine, one of the first to be synthesized, is probably the most widely used of all local anesthetics. It is about one-fourth as toxic as cocaine, but in spite of this, it sometimes causes systemic effects in unusually sensitive individuals. Deaths have been reported from the administration of as little as 0.01 to 0.13 gm of procaine. Such reactions are due to sensitization and fortunately are rare. Death is usually characterized by cardiovascular collapse and occurs soon after the administration of procaine.

The principal manifestations of poisoning with these agents are dizziness, cyanosis, fall of blood pressure, twitching, convulsions, coma, bronchial spasm and respiratory failure. *Treatment* is similar to that given for cocaine and for shock (*see* page 69):

## PYRAZOLON ANALGESICS (AMINOPYRINE, DIPYRONE, ANTIPYRINE, PHENYLBUTAZONE, ETC.)

These drugs are used as analgesics for the treatment of rheumatic diseases and other painful disorders. The lethal dose varies from 5 to 30 gm, but deaths from acute poisoning are rare. Practically all of the fatalities are due to agranulocytosis from idiosyncrasy and sensitization to these compounds. The ingestion of as little as 1 gm has caused a fatal agranulocytic reaction. Antipyrine is the only one likely to cause methemoglobinemia, but this rarely occurs. Although they all cause sodium chloride and water retention, phenylbutazone particularly is most potent in this respect.

The principal symptoms of acute poisoning from the pyrazolons are dizziness, nausea, vomiting, mental disturbances, cyanosis, coma and convulsions. In chronic intoxication from phenylbutazone, the manifestations are epigastric pain, vomiting, anorexia, urticaria, edema, oliguria and cyanosis. In 1 per cent of patients therapeutic doses cause, in addition, agranulocytosis with fever, sore throat and membranous exudate; hepatitis with hepatosplenomegaly and jaundice; exfoliative dermatitis; gastric or duodenal erosion with bleeding or perforation; and adrenal necrosis. Aminopyrine also causes agranulocytosis in 1 per cent or more of patients, while antipyrine is more often responsible for exfoliative dermatitis. In preexisting renal disease, anuria and uremia follow if large daily doses (over 600 mg) of these drugs are given. Seven deaths, three of them in children, were attributed to dipyrone in the United States in the mid 1960s. Have this many lives been saved through the use of this drug?

The immediate *treatment* is similar to that outlined for the para-aminophenol analgesics, with gastric lavage and the use of methylene blue for cyanosis and methemoglobinemia. In addition, definitive therapy should be used for the treatment or prevention of uremia, agranulocytosis, hepatitis, gastroduodenal bleeding and exfoliative dermatitis if these problems arise.

## QUININE AND CINCHONA COMPOUNDS

Quinine is the chief alkaloid of cinchona bark, which also contains several closely related drugs, one of which is quinidine. In addition, there are synthesized quinine derivatives such as the hydrocupreines.

Quinine is a general protoplasmic poison. This is presumably the basis for its use in malaria. It also has definite actions on the peripheral and central nervous systems and on muscle, skeletal, cardiac and uterine systems. Under certain circumstances quinine can cause hemolysis of red blood cells.

The outstanding symptoms seen in the course of quinine poisoning constitute a syndrome called cinchonism. This is not only caused by quinine, quinidine and their natural and synthetic congeners, but it is also produced to a certain extent by the salicylates and cinchophen. Cinchonism consists of ringing in the ears, difficulty in hearing and dizziness; blurred vision with scotomata, disturbed color vision, photophobia, diplopia and diminished visual fields; headache, nausea and vomiting, diarrhea and epigastric discomfort; flushing of the skin, sweating, fever and cutaneous rashes. The latter may be papular, urticarial or even scarlatiniform in character, and occasionally inflammatory edema of the face occurs. Cerebral symptoms consist of apprehension, confusion, excitement and syncope. Asthmatic and anginal symptoms may also be noted. It can be emphasized then that the second and the eighth cranial nerves are especially involved, and the remaining symptoms are chiefly referable to the gastrointestinal tract, skin and cerebrum.

In the milder cases of poisoning, only tinnitus, slight visual disturbances, headache and nausea are noted. In the more severe type of intoxication, all the above-mentioned signs and symptoms are fully developed. The pulse becomes weak, breathing shallow, weakness marked, temperature subnormal and the skin cyanotic. Deaths occur from respiratory or circulatory collapse. Delirium, coma or convulsions may appear terminally. If the patient recovers, there may be permanent damage due to the toxic action of quinine on the optic nerve and retinal and auditory ganglion cells. The toxicity for the heart is due to the quinine depression of myocardial contractility and conductivity. At times, quinine may cause intravascular hemolysis of red blood cells with hemoglobinuria, suppression of renal function, anuria and uremia. This is usually associated with aestivoautumnal malaria due to the *Plasmodium falciparum* and has been called blackwater fever. The fatal oral dose of quinine for adults is about 8 gm (1 gm for children), but much larger doses have been taken with recovery. Death may occur in a few hours or be postponed for a day or two. Inasmuch as death is due to respiratory failure which occurs late in the course of poisoning, and since quinine is excreted and destroyed with fair rapidity, if the patient survives several hours, his chances for recovery become progressively better.

The quinine content of the so-called tonic waters is usually no greater than 30 mg/500 ml of water. In hypersensitive individuals, however, this is enough to produce a reaction. Gin-and-tonic purpura is well documented, and the aperitif Dubonnet® (7 mg quinine per 100 ml) has also been reported to produce purpura.

The usual quinine salt taken is the sulfate form; this is fairly insoluble and slowly absorbed. The stomach should therefore be thoroughly washed, and magnesium sulfate given to hasten the passage of the unabsorbed drug through the intestine. There are no specific measures to counteract the systemic action of quinine, but symptomatic and supportive *treatment* must be given. The respiratory depression should be met with stimulants, oxygen and artificial respiration if necessary. The blood pressure should be maintained by injections of levarterenol. Body heat should be conserved. The visual impairment may be treated with amyl nitrite inhalations on the basis of the retinal vascular constriction observed in these cases. Mecholyl might prove as efficacious as it has been in tobacco amblyopia. Atropine should be instilled in the eyes, and an ophthalmologist consulted in treating the visual disturbances in these patients. Hemoglobinuria may necessitate blood transfusion and the use of alkalis.

1. Quinidine is the dextroisomer of quinine and is somewhat more toxic than quinine. This may be due to the fact that this drug is especially used in auricular fibrillation, where accidents can occur based in large part upon the pathological physiology of the disease itself. A patient may manifest milder toxic reactions (which are usually listed as idiosyncrasy) to quinine and not to

quinidine, and the reverse is also true. The side-effects of quinidine are listed below.

*Cardiotoxicity*

- Atrioventricular and intraventricular block
- Ventricular ectopy: premature beats—single or in groups—or ventricular tachycardia and fibrillation
- Excessive depression of myocardial contractility
- Quinidine with digitalis increases the risk of syncope and sudden death due to ventricular fibrillation

*Noncardiotoxic side-effects*

- Nausea, vomiting, and diarrhea
- Cinchonism, signaled by vertigo, tinnitus, deafness, confusion (dementia), headache, fever, allergic reactions, or blurred vision
- Thrombocytopenia—rare, but may be fatal
- May cause hemolysis in glucose-6-phosphate-deficient patients
- Lupus erythematosus and granulomatous hepatitis
- Hepatotoxic effects

The danger signs of quinidine are detailed below. All forms of ectopy or heart block are preceded by a 50 per cent prolongation of the QRS interval above the baseline.

- Immediately stop quinidine when the QRS interval is expanded by 50 per cent or increased 0.12 to 0.14 second, or when the serum level is greater than 9 μg/ml
- Also stop quinidine in the presence of newly induced ventricular premature beats or tachycardia
- Stop quinidine when there are signs of advanced toxicity: severe tinnitus, blurred visions, frequent vomiting, severe diarrhea and cramps, headache, fever, confusion, and delirium

*Treatment.* IV hypertonic sodium chloride solution and lidocaine.

2. The synthetic hydrocupriene compounds (optochin, numoquin) show a specific toxicity to the optic nerve, and blindness has occurred from their former use in human pneumococcal pneumonia. The retinal damage is severe even with small doses; for this reason these compounds are rarely used.
3. Plasmochin is a synthetic quinoline derivative which is not closely related chemically to quinine but is used against malaria as an adjuvant to, rather than a substitute for, quinine. It is especially effective against the sexual forms (gametocytes) of the plasmodia. It does not cause cinchonism but may cause methemoglobinemia, cyanosis, cardiac irregularities, abdominal pain, vomiting, necrosis of the liver, jaundice and collapse. The margin of safety is relatively narrow.
4. Chloroquine is another quinoline derivative, now being employed frequently in the treatment of rheumatoid arthritis and lupus erythematosus. This drug is rapidly and completely absorbed from the gastrointestinal tract, and since its pharmacological action is similar to quinine, it is imperative in the case of poisoning that the stomach be emptied promptly. Induction of emesis should be attempted in the home before bringing the patient to the hospital for gastric lavage. The rapid occurrence of respiratory and cardiac arrest in acute chloroquine poisoning is due to its complete and rapid absorption resulting in high blood concentrations and depression of vasomotor function and respiration. Peripheral neuropathy, myopathy, toxic psychosis, convulsions and severe retinopathy (*see* below) are distressing side-reactions from the prolonged use of this drug. Teratogenic effects have also been documented. Non-enteric-coated ammonium chloride, 1 gm three or four times a day, may hasten the urinary excretion of chloroquine. Hydroxychloroquine in usual doses has been reported to produce severe vertigo in some patients.
5. Quinacrine (Atabrine®) resembles quinine in its therapeutic action in malaria, but it is a synthetic chemical entirely unrelated to the quinine alkaloids. It is a yellow acridine

dye and colors the skin, urine and tissues, including the central nervous system, this same hue. Atabrine does not cause cinchonism but may produce fever, regional and abdominal pain, headache, and occasionally transient psychoses. This preparation is now being used effectively in the treatment of recurrent pleural effusion and ascites associated with certain neoplastic diseases. Convulsions occurred in two individuals, but both were on corticosteroids which are known to lower the seizure threshold. The cerebrocortical stimulant effects of quinacrine also are well documented.

Ocular symptoms often develop in patients taking synthetic antimalarial drugs. Difficulty with close work, halos around lights, poor adjustment to glare, diplopia and inadequate night vision are among the commonest disorders. Keratopathy and retinopathy are common in persons receiving large doses for long periods. Reversible paralysis of the lateral rectus muscle and whitening of hair and lashes are also reported, and antimalarial drugs may cause macular lesions. Potential toxicity should not be overlooked, even though treatment value is undisputed.

Ocular abnormalities result from all commonly used synthetic antimalarial drugs, including chloroquine diphosphate, hydroxychloroquine, amodiaquin and quinacrine hydrochloride. Corneal lesions develop in about 86 per cent of patients taking chloroquine longer than one month and may disappear without permanent ocular damage when medication is stopped. Anesthetic properties of some antimalarial drugs may account for decreased or absent corneal sensitivity. Retinal lesions caused by antimalarial drugs include arteriolar narrowing, abnormal macular pigmentation and depigmentation, optic disk pallor, peripheral retinal pigmentation and scotomas. Although the mechanism of retinal damage is unknown, prolonged chloroquine therapy has a definite role, since it can produce irreversible retinopathy of a serious nature, probably due to direct drug deposition in ocular tissues instead of a hypersensitivity phenomenon. It has been demonstrated that detectable amounts of chloroquine were found in the urine, red blood cells and plasma of patients with chloroquine retinopathy for as long as five years after their last known drug ingestion. The urinary excretion of chloroquine can be increased by acidification of the urine with oral ammonium chloride and parenteral BAL. This type of therapy appears promising and is worth further trials. Asymptomatic, drug-related retinopathy may be reversible. Patients on continuous therapy should consult a competent ophthalmologist every three to six months. Blue-black mucocutaneous hyperpigmentation (ochronosis), not related to alcaptonuria, has been reported with quinacrine and related antimalarial drug therapy.

Children are especially sensitive to the 4-aminoquinoline compounds. A number of fatalities have been reported following the accidental ingestion of chloroquine, sometimes in relatively small doses (for example, 0.75 or 1 gm in a three-year-old child). Patients should be strongly warned to keep these drugs out of the reach of children.

Chloroquine is very rapidly and completely absorbed after ingestion; in accidental overdosage, toxic symptoms may occur within thirty minutes. These consist of headache, nausea and vomiting, drowsiness, visual disturbances, cardiovascular collapse and convulsions, followed by sudden and early respiratory and cardiac arrest. The electrocardiogram may reveal atrial standstill, nodal rhythm, prolonged intraventricular conduction time and progressive bradycardia leading to ventricular fibrillation and/or arrest. *Treatment* is symptomatic and must be prompt, with immediate evacuation of the stomach by emesis (at home before transportation to the hospital) or gastric lavage until the stomach is completely emptied. Convulsions, if present, should be controlled before attempting gastric lavage: If due to cerebral stimulation, cautious administration of an ultra short-acting barbiturate may be tried, but if due to anoxia, convulsions should be corrected by oxygen administration, artificial respiration or, if in shock with hypotension, by vasopressor therapy. Because of the importance of supporting respiration, tracheal intubation or tracheostomy followed by gastric lavage has also been advised.

In vascular collapse, vasopressors should be administered intravenously, because of the more rapid action. Intravenous molar sodium lactate may improve the response to the vasopressor and may help to reverse cardiotoxic effects of quinoline compounds (as shown for quinidine), although sodium lactate tends to reduce urinary excretion of chloroquine. In the event of cardiac arrest, immediate thoracotomy and cardiac massage is required. Peritoneal dialysis and exchange transfusions have also been suggested to reduce the level of the drug in the blood. Hemodialysis has been recently documented as being far more effective than peritoneal dialysis for quinidine intoxication when high blood flow rates through the artificial kidney can be maintained. However, dialysis in dogs did not reduce mortality from chloroquine poisoning, and peritoneal dialysis in a twenty-eight-month-old infant was unsuccessful.

A patient who survives the acute phase and is asymptomatic should be closely observed for at least twenty-four hours. Fluids may be forced and sufficient ammonium chloride may be administered for a few days to acidify the urine to help promote urinary excretion.

## SALICYLAMIDE

Salicylamide, chemically 2-hydroxybenzamide, has an $LD_{50}$ of 1.4 gm/kg in rats, but there are marked species differences in animals which preclude making accurate evaluation of its comparable toxicity with aspirin. Comparison of three antipyretic drugs shows that aspirin and acetaminophen are comparable in effectiveness for reducing temperatures in febrile children, while salicylamide is less effective (*Am J Dis Child, 114*:284-287, 1967). Salicylamide causes depression of the central nervous system as opposed to stimulation produced by acetylsalicylic acid. Hyperpnea, respiratory alkalosis, metabolic acidosis and alteration of the prothrombin time do not occur as they do in salicylate intoxication. Salicylamide is not hydrolized to salicylic acid, and its toxity in humans has not been established. There is no specific antidote and *treatment* is entirely symptomatic.

## SALICYLATE

Aspirin, like other medications, has been deliciously flavored so that it is acceptable to children, but as a result, children readily mistake it for candy. Methyl salicylate (oil of wintergreen) has such a sweetish odor and is so highly attractive that children do not hesitate to drink it. Its application as a dermatological ointment, especially in the treatment of psoriasis, has produced thirteen documented deaths by percutaneous absorption. Assiduous treatment by parents is another serious cause of salicylate poisoning.* Parents know that aspirin is beneficial in a febrile illness, but they are much too inclined to refer to it as candy, and most of them are not aware that there is a rule of safe dosage: For each year up to the age of five, children can be given 65 mg (1 gr) every four to six hours, not more, since these are maximum doses. The toxic dose is considered to be in the range of 75 to 150 mg/lb. The combined use of aspirin and acetaminophen produces a more sustained antipyretic effect than either drug alone, although the rate and degree of temperature reduction is not significantly altered.

Continued administration of salicylates can

*A fatality occurred in a two-week-old infant given a 1¼ grain tablet every four hours for three days for colic and crying.

lead to cumulative toxicity. Administration to an infant who is dehydrated, who takes little fluid or who has reduced urinary output calls for the sort of additional care that is hardly within the comprehension of most parents.

The salicylates (methyl salicylate excepted) are rapidly and well absorbed from the digestive tract, including the stomach, and are found in all tissues afterward. Elimination is largely via the kidney, starting as early as ten to fifteen minutes after a therapeutic dose and continuing for several hours; but traces can appear in the urine for three days or more. About 20 per cent of the salicylate is oxidized in the tissues, and 70 per cent is excreted in the urine. However, this can be less than 50 per cent in dehydration and/or decreased urinary excretion.

Methyl salicylate has other characteristics which are of practical importance. It contains more salicylate than other remedies: one teaspoonful (5 ml) is equivalent to about twenty-one aspirin tablets (325 mg each). The absorption of methyl salicylate (because of its methyl radical) may be delayed for hours; consequently, when oil of wintergreen has been swallowed, gastric lavage is almost always worth the trouble, even several hours later.

The pharmacologic effects of salicylates in large doses are fairly well, though not completely, understood. They consist, in the main, of a marked increased in the metabolic rate and an initial hyperventilation that is followed, in severe cases, by a metabolic acidosis. The first sign noted is the rapid, deep and pauseless ("panting dog") breathing. This hyperventilation is ascribed to some direct stimulating action on metabolism and the respiratory center, as well as to the increased metabolic rate, and it results in removing excessive carbon dioxide. With the loss of $CO_2$ there is primary reduction of serum $CO_2$ level, and the blood pH rises. There is at first, then, a respiratory alkalosis. A compensatory renal retention of chlorides and excretion of sodium alleviate the alkalosis to a measurable degree. In adults and older children, the matter ends there, and (if the drug is withdrawn) recovery ensues within a few days.

In infants and in others receiving disproportionately large doses, there develops next a metabolic acidosis, and the pH falls to normal and then to the acid side of normal. Among the factors producing the acidosis may be included some loss of sodium and potassium (kidney may retain potassium and excrete hydrogen ions in spite of blood pH of over 7.45) via the urine during the initial alkalosis and, to an extent, the ketosis of dehydration, starvation and fever; but these (and accumulation of salicylate ion) are not regarded as an entire explanation. It has been suggested that an effect of salicylate may be a metabolic change at the cellular level so that organic acid metabolites (Krebs cycle) accumulate apart from ketone bodies.

Severe hypoglycemia has been reported in salicylate intoxication, resulting from interference with key enzyme systems. The exact mechanism for this is not clearly understood, since blood insulin concentration apparently is not increased. However, salicylate does influençe carbohydrate metabolism by causing a marked reduction or disappearance of liver glycogen and an interference with adenosine triphosphate formation. These metabolic changes are responsible for a decreased synthesis of carbohydrate, and along with an increased glucose utilization by the patient due to vomiting and inanition, a rather marked reduction in blood sugar may result with or without neurological manifestations. On the other hand, hyperglycemia occurs occasionally, which may be difficult to distinguish from diabetic acidosis. The hyperglycemia may be partially due to activation of hypothalamic sympathetic centers releasing epinephrine or to increased glucose-6-phosphatase activity, with decreased aerobic metabolism.

The development of the metabolic acidosis is indistinguishable by clinical observation alone, for acidosis is now a stimulus to hyperventilation and consequent reduction in serum $CO_2$. As a matter of fact, this reduction serves as a compensatory mechanism to the metabolic acidosis. Hence, the child's breathing and the serum $CO_2$ fail to show which phase of intoxication is present, and as the urine is not necessarily alkaline during alkalosis (paradoxical aciduria seen with systemic alkalosis and associated potassium deficiency), it affords no clarification. Blood pH must be determined for recognition of the state of acidosis. The question is not academic, since therapy is guided by chemical status of the child. In children under three years of age, who have the highest incidence, ketosis develops so rapidly that the preliminary alkalotic phase is rarely seen. Acidemia is often associated with impaired consciousness, which carries a grave prognosis. Noncardiogenic pulmonary edema can occur in severe salicylate intoxication (propoxyphene, heroin and methadone are other drugs reported to produce this effect).

The ferric chloride test is presumptive for salicylate poisoning and is simple and frequently useful. Normally ferric chloride gives a Burgundy red color if aceto acetic acid is present, but the color does not appear if the specimen is acidified and boiled before adding the 10% ferric chloride. If salicylate ion is present, however, the test is positive even after boiling and gives a violet color. The test is of no quantitative value, however, since a strongly positive test may be found in association with relatively low blood levels of salicylate. Neither can the test be used to identify aspirin in gastric contents since the color complex is formed only with free salicylic acid. Phenistix® reagent strip, impregnated at one end with ferric and magnesium salts and cyclohexylsulfamic acid (primarily designed for detection of phenylketonuria), provides a simple, rapid, definitive procedure for detecting salicylate intoxication. The reactive portion of Phenistix gives a gray-green to blue color with phenylketones and a brownish-purple color with salicylate. The latter reaction occurs in two intensities: a "small" reaction corresponding to approximately 25 to 50 mg/100 ml free salicylate and a "large" reaction corresponding to 150 or more mg per 100 ml. These reactions are read against a special color chart available from the manufacturer.

Although urine specimens after single small doses of aspirin may give a positive reaction with the reagent strip, serum tests with the reagent strip are negative in the absence of intoxicating levels. Consequently, a simple,

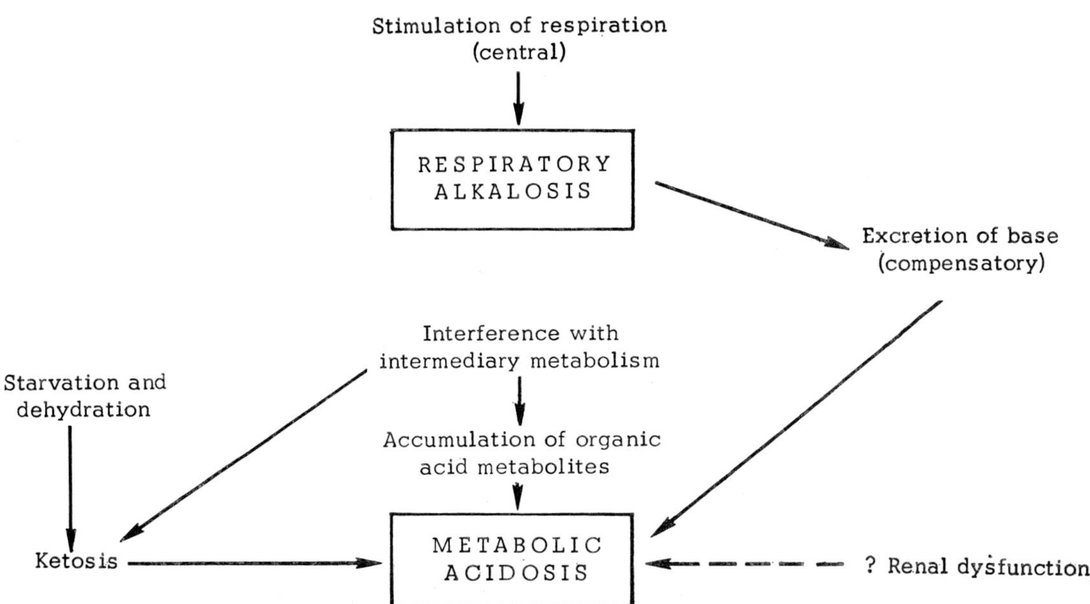


Figure 17. Proposed pathogenesis of the acid-base disturbances of salicylate intoxication in children.

useful screening test for recognition of salicylate intoxication can be accomplished quickly in the following two steps: (1) Test urine with reagent strip. Negative result excludes salicylate intoxication. Positive result requires performance of second step. (2) Test blood serum with reagent strip. Negative result excludes salicylate intoxication. Positive result indicates probable salicylate intoxication. The single known confusion reaction with the procedure occurs when very large quantities of phenothiazine metabolites in urine produce a color similar to that obtained with small quantities of salicylate. Differentiation between the two reactions is simple: Addition of one drop of 20 N sulfuric acid to the reacted strip bleaches out color due to salicylate but intensifies color due to phenothiazine metabolites.

Serum salicylate levels above 35 mg/100 ml can produce symptoms of salicylate intoxication in children. Spuriously high salicylate levels can be obtained in the newborn with hyperbilirubinemia unless methods are used in which potentially interfering substances such as bilirubin are removed either by extraction or precipitation. Trinder's method is a simple, accurate and rapid laboratory test. Possible toxicity cannot be accurately predicted or excluded by a single salicylate level determination when the ingested quantity is unknown. Done's method for estimating degree of toxicity views the serum salicylate level as a function of time. Ingested salicylate is totally absorbed in about four hours; decline in serum salicylate concentration then approaches a first-order reaction. Extrapolation back to time zero yields a theoretical value ($S_0$) for the highest salicylate level attained, which can then be compared with the severity of symptoms. Correlation between magnitude of $S_0$ and extent of symptoms is significantly better than that obtained using observed salicylate values. Done's method aims at accurate selection of patients requiring intensive treatment for salicylate intoxication rather than prediction of symptom development, and his derived cutoff level assuring absence of symptoms is 50 mg/100 ml.

Patients with serum salicylate values or calculated $S_0$ above 40 mg/100 ml require hospitalization or close supervision at home. Patients with values between 30 and 40 mg per 100 ml require hospitalization only if symptoms of salicylate intoxication are noted. Analyses of $S_0$ values help explain apparent discrepancies between a determined serum salicylate value and the patient's actual physical condition. It should be noted that the $S_0$ concept is applicable only to patients who have ingested toxic amounts of salicylate in a single dose, and sufficient time must have elapsed so that the major portion of the salicylate may be assumed to have been absorbed. Otherwise, the regression curve is likely to be distorted. For practical purposes, this period of absorption is considered to be at least six hours. In chronic poisoning—therapeutic overdosing for a period of days—there is little relationship between blood level and severity of poisoning; patients with serious and even fatal toxic reactions may have relatively low levels of salicylate in the blood.

The management of salicylism includes close observation and knowledge of the multiple effects of salicylates on the body such as the increase in body metabolism, lengthened prothrombin time, the blocked enzyme systems which normally aid utilization of ketones, the dehydration (chemical imbalance and salicylate toxicity combining to impair the peripheral circulation), and as an end result, the accumulation of ketone bodies and other acid metabolic products which cannot be handled by the kidney, changing the original resiratory alkalosis into a metabolic acidosis. The role of salicylates as a cause of encephalopathy and hepatic dysfunction has now been fairly well established. These effects have incriminated salicylate intoxication as a possible etiological factor for Reye's syndrome.

*Treament.* If the patient is seen within four hours (six hours for methyl salicylate) of ingestion, the stomach should be emptied by thorough emesis or lavage, followed by maximum dose of activated charcoal by mouth or gastric tube (if lavaged). This absorbs large quantities of salicylates and greatly decreases blood salicylate levels. Fever

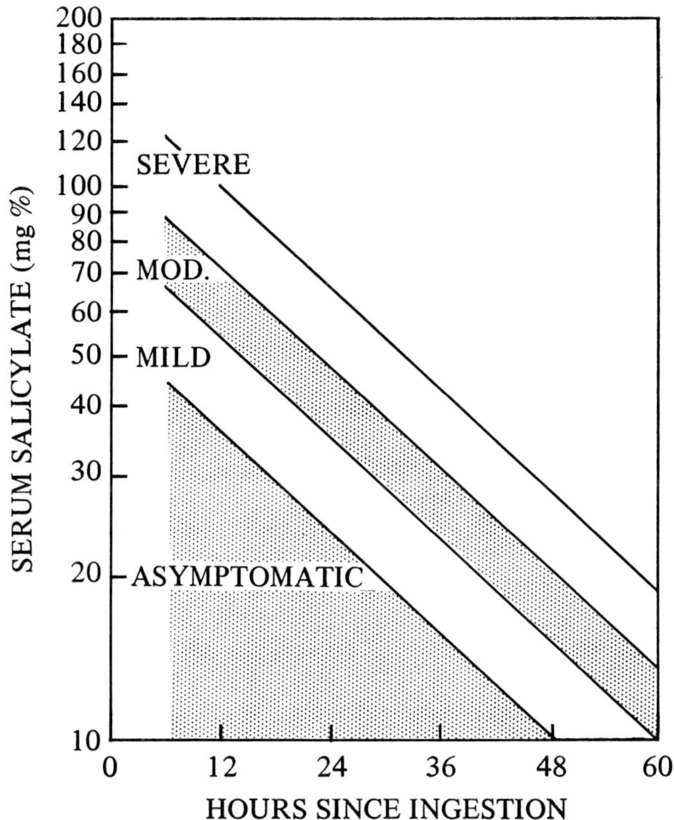


Figure 18. Done's nomogram relating serum salicylate concentration and expected severity of intoxication at varying intervals following the ingestion of a *single* massive dose of salicylate.

is reduced by cold or tepid sponging; in addition there is evidence to suggest that hypothermia may restore the binding capacity of serum albumin for salicylate; large quantities of parenteral fluids are given to offset dehydration and to augment elimination of salicylates by increasing urine flow; vitamin K is administered to combat the bleeding tendency due to hypoprothrombinemia. Under certain circumstances, salicylates depress the synthesis of K-dependent clotting factors in the liver. Quick has demonstrated that aspirin (not sodium salicylate) prolongs the bleeding time by depressing a plasma factor that controls bleeding from small vessels and that it is not the salicylate content but the acetyl linkage that determines this action. Glucose is needed to overcome ketosis and hypoglycemia if present, electrolyte solutions to correct electrolyte imbalance and sodium bicarbonate (contraindicated in the early phase when respiratory alkalosis prevails, although there is some doubt that uncomplicated respiratory alkalosis occurs in the very small infant) to increase the blood pH and also because salicylates are more promptly excreted in an alkaline urine. Alkalinizing the urine by sodium bicarbonate infusion can result in a 50 per cent reduction in plasma salicylate concentration within two to five hours. This type of therapy may obviate the use of the more risky and dangerous exchange transfusion and dialysis. Hypokalemia, potassium cellular deficiency or intracellular sodium intoxication is possible and would require conjunctive potassium administration. There are very few conditions that require as much KCL. These patients are almost always markedly depleted of potassium, and it is most difficult to alkalinize the urine unless a good intake of KCL is maintained.

The dose of parenteral sodium bicarbonate (3.75%, 44.6 mEq/50 ml ampule) necessary to alkalinize the urine is approximately 5 mEq/kg of body weight, which can be given in divided doses over a twelve-hour period. Two of the 5 mEq cations should be given as potassium to prevent alkalosis and to avoid renal tubular potassium depletion with paradoxical aciduria (acid urine despite alkalemia).

In advanced acidosis, the alkalinization of the urine by sodium bicarbonate or other alkalinizing agents is often difficult to obtain, and a serious alkalosis may even be precipitated. Actually, replacement of potassium deficits can be more effective in alkalinizing the urine under these circumstances. In addition, potassium deficiency plays an important role in the pathogenesis of severe salicylate intoxication, particularly in small children, so that the administration of this ion serves a dual purpose. Potassium may be dangerously depleted owing to direct effect of salicylate on potassium excretion by the renal tubules.

Oxygen should be administered to supply the brain, kidneys and other tissues. Hemodialysis with the artificial kidney, peritoneal dialysis and exchange transfusions may be lifesaving procedures for methyl salicylate or severe salicylate poisoning. It has been demonstrated that the efficiency of peritoneal dialysis in removing protein-bound substances such as salicylates can be greatly enhanced when 5% human albumin (Albumisol) is used in the dialysis solution. Combining fluids and bicarbonate with concomitant intermittent peritoneal dialysis produces a salicylate removal rate that is up to three times greater than if only fluids and bicarbonate are used.

When renal function is adequate and in the absence of hypotension, forced alkaline diuresis and oral potassium citrate (K-Lyte®) 200 mEq/sq. m over an eight-hour period is a satisfactory method of therapy. This combined therapy alkalinizes the urine more quickly with smaller amounts of sodium bicarbonate. An intravenous drip of 2% sodium bicarbonate (or M/6 sodium lactate), 0.9% sodium chloride and 5% dextrose, in rotation, is given up to a volume of 2 liters/hour for the first three hours (adults) subject to the maintenance of normal jugular venous pressure and the absence of crepitations at the lung bases. The regimen uniformly producing best results includes intravenous administration of sodium bicarbonate (44 mEq/kg) and potassium citrate (35 mEq/kg) in 5% glucose, plus sodium bicarbonate by push in a dose of 3 mEq/kg followed by 1.5 mEq/kg every fifteen minutes up to three times, and potassium citrate by oral or nasogastric route (200 mEq/sq. m/eight hours). An indwelling catheter is used to empty the bladder hourly. Serum salicylate level is measured on admission and every hour thereafter. Alkali is omitted from the infusion when the patient's urine attains a pH of 8.0. An intake of 6 to 8 liters of fluid is necessary to produce 3 to 4 liters of urine during the first eight hours of treatment. If adequate diuresis is not obtained in three hours, dialysis should then be used.

To help the body metabolize salicylate, acetazolamide (Diamox) has recently been used effectively in therapy. This carbonic anhydrase inhibitor causes the urine to become alkaline within minutes after administration. The fear of worsening a metabolic acidosis is offset by giving sodium bicarbonate at the same time. The organic base, Tham (tris-hydroxy-methyl-amino-methane) solution with a pH of 8.6, has been used to accelerate the rate of renal excretion of salicylates. The tris buffer promptly alkalinizes the urine and has been effective in patients who had not responded satisfactorily to standard sodium bicarbonate therapy. In selected cases with complete and careful monitoring, this could be the treatment of choice. The renal clearance of salicylate is increased with corticosteroid administration resulting in a reduced serum level of free salicylates. This is most likely due to steroid ability to increase glomerular filtration rate and diminish tubular reabsorption of water.

Chronic salicylate intoxication can produce gastrointestinal bleeding and symptoms of confusion, bizarre behavior and hyperventilation. It is often confused with frank hysteria, diabetic coma or other types of organic delirium. Aspirin-induced bleeding from the gastrointestinal tract manifests itself in two forms: the frequent occult loss of blood which reportedly occurs in 70 per cent of patients taking repeated doses of aspirin and the uncommon overt hemorrhage. Two mechanisms have been implicated in the causation of the occult bleeding: local irritation of the gastric mucosa and hemostatic disturbance. The former, evidenced by mucosal congestion and by accumulation of DNA in gastric washings due to excessive epithelial shedding, is unrelated to the presence of hydrochloric acid. The hemostatic abnormality is essentially that of prolonged bleeding time, probably caused by reduction in platelet stickiness. Recent evidence shows that aspirin prevents the release of adenosine diphosphate (ADP) from platelets. This release apparently enhances the stickiness of platelets and accelerates clot formation.

### Salicylate Poisoning Treatment Scheme

I. Immediate (emesis or gastric lavage)
  - A. Evaluation of severity of intoxication (extrapolation method of Done)
  - B. Appraisal of status of dehydration
  - C. Determination of acid-base imbalance. Test urine with Phenistix paper and Nitrazine® paper
  - D. Determination of electrolyte imbalance
  - E. Draw blood for the following laboratory tests:
    1. Salicylate level
    2. $CO_2$ combining power
    3. Plasma $CO_2$ content
    4. pH
    5. Serum electrolytes

II. Pending laboratory report
  - A. Start intravenous fluids (5% glucose in ⅓ physiologic saline)
  - B. If dehydration is severe, hydrating solution should be given at the rate of 8 ml/sq. m body surface per minute for thirty to forty-five minutes
  - C. After that time, slow down hydrating solution to 2 ml/sq. m/min.
  - D. Correct bicarbonate and potassium deficits as indicated (average requirements: 5 mEq $NaHCO_3$ per kg and 2 mEq K per kg for twelve hours)
  - E. In presence of clinical acidosis and acid urine, $NaHCO_3$ should be given in initial hydrating solution

III. In life-threatening intoxication, consider exchange transfusion (in small infants), peritoneal dialysis with 5% albumin solution (Albumisol) or dialysis with artificial kidney

IV. Administer vitamin K and B complex, the route of administration depending on the condition of the patient

V. Maintenance management
  - A. Test each urine voided with Nitrazine paper
  - B. Periodic (frequent) determination of the following.
    1. Blood $CO_2$ combining power
    2. Blood $CO_2$ content
    3. Blood pH

## SILVER SALTS

The salts of silver that most often cause toxic symptoms are acetate and nitrate because they are available in many households. Silver nitrate caustic pencils may be broken up and eaten by children. Less than 2.5 gm is generally harmless, but larger amounts may cause severe symptoms. Ingestion of between 2.5 and 10 gm may be fatal, and over 10 gm almost always causes death.

Symptomatology includes burning of the throat and epigastrium, violent abdominal pain, black vomitus, and in severe cases, convulsions and coma which may be terminal. The continued absorption of small quantities of organic and inorganic silver salts results in argyria or argyrosis, which may be a local or generalized pigmentation wherever silver is deposited in the tissues. It predominantly affects those sections of the body which are exposed to light; but often the conjunctivae, mucous membranes of the nose and the lunulae of the fingernails are the first to be discolored; these changes should caution against further exposure.

*Treatment* includes sodium chloride 15 gm (½ oz.), well diluted, by mouth; gastric lavage with large amounts of warm water; morphine sulfate or Demerol for pain; magnesium sulfate as a purgative by mouth; and caffeine and sodium benzoate 0.5 gm (7.5 gr) subcutaneously. Hospitalization of patient for definitive therapy and observation is advised if more than 2.5 gm have been swallowed.

## SULFONES, ETHYL (SULFONAL, TRIONAL, TETRONAL)

For many years these compounds were widely used as hypnotics, but with the advent of barbiturates, they soon were discarded and are now rarely prescribed in the United States. Slow onset of action and excretion, cumulative toxicity, marked and protracted after-depression and untoward effects on the skin, liver, kidney and blood (hematoporphyrins and methemoglobin) characterize these drugs and contraindicate their use in preference to less toxic and more useful sedative-hypnotic agents.

In acute poisoning the stomach should be emptied by emesis or gastric lavage followed by a saline cathartic since the drug is very insoluble and slowly absorbed. The remainder of the *treatment* should be symptomatic and supportive.

## SULFONAMIDES

Sulfonamide compounds and their acetyl derivatives (sulfapyridine, sulfathiazole, sulfadiazine, etc.) are chemotherapeutic agents used in the treatment of bacterial infections. These drugs frequently precipitate in the kidney tubules or in the ureters, causing renal damage and blocking the excretion of urine. Lethal results have been caused by daily therapeutic doses, but death is usually due to the hematopoietic effects and rarely to hepatic or renal failure. Sulfonamides diffuse freely into all tissues, and secretions of the body, including milk, fetal products and the cerebrospinal fluid, in concentrations approximating those found in the blood. From 90 to 95 per cent of the administered dose is excreted by the kidney. Of this, from 30 to 65 per cent is in the form of an acetyl ester, thought to be synthesized by the liver. In general, all sulfonamides are handled in a similar manner.

Toxic and even fatal effects have been caused by therapeutic doses of 2 to 5 gm daily. Animal experiments, however, indicate a low toxicity. Sulfanilamide is a drug absorbed relatively slowly but completely from the digestive tract or from parenteral injection. Poisoning is almost invariably associated with medicinal use. Severe reactions must be considered to be due to idiosyncrasy. The intensity or type of reaction does not seem related to the size of dose or the blood concentration. The toxic actions of sulfonamides are variable from patient to patient. All the effects can be related to the aniline radical and are largely due to an action on blood or the hematopoietic system. Cyanosis due to sulfanilamide (but not to other sulfonamides) is frequent; in a few cases this is associated with methemoglobinemia and, in rare instances, to sulfhemoglobinemia. Sulfanilamide, but not its derivatives, inhibits carbonic anhydrase and thereby causes diuresis and acidosis.

Many patients exhibit symptoms of cerebral and gastrointestinal effects such as anorexia, colic, nausea, vomiting, dizziness, headache, drowsiness or even unconsciousness. A toxic fever may develop one or more days after the infectious fever has subsided and precedes the development of the more serious manifestations of poisoning, namely acidosis, acute hemolytic anemia, agranulocytic angina, dermatitis or toxic neuritis. Jaundice of hepatic origin occasionally occurs. The dermatitis is generally maculopapular, but it may be manifested by almost any form of rash, including purpura.

The less serious symptoms disappear within a day or two after cessation of sulfonamide administration. The grave symptoms require one to three weeks for remission. When death occurs, it is usually several days after the first dose.

*Treatment* consists of stopping the administration of the drug immediately. If large doses have been swallowed, give an emetic or perform gastric lavage. If kidney function is normal, fluids should be forced up to 4 liters/day to speed the excretion of the drug. To increase renal excretion, the urine should be alkalinized by oral or intravenous sodium bicarbonate. Specific therapy for anuria or agranulocytosis must be employed if these complications develop. Aplastic anemia requires repeated blood transfusions as well as supportive therapy. Methylene blue 1% should be administered for the rare occurrence of methemoglobinemia.

## SULFONAMIDE (THIAZIDE) DIURETICS

Chlorothiazide (Diuril), an oral sulfonamide diuretic and antihypertensive drug, was first used in 1958. Since then a whole series of related compounds have been introduced: (1) bendroflumethiazide (Naturetin®); (2) benzthiazide (Exna®); (3) chlorthalidone (Hygroton®); (4) cyclothiazide (Anhydron®); (5) hydrochlorothiazide U.S.P. (HydroDIURIL®, Esidrix®, Oretic®); (6) hydroflumethiazide (Saluron®); (7) methyclothiazide (Enduron®); (8) polythiazide (Renese®); (9) quinethazone (Hydromox®); and (10) trichlormethiazide (Naqua®, Metahydrin®).

In addition to the sulfonamide side-effects already enumerated, the following additional reactions have been encountered with these agents: hypokalemia, hypochloremic alkalosis, azotemia, nausea, vomiting, diarrhea, glycosuria (diabetogenic), dizziness, paresthesias, skin rash, photosensitivity and blood dyscrasias.

Severe renal or hepatic insufficiency is the only contraindication to therapy with these agents. However, certain cautions in their use are important. Patients receiving prolonged therapy should be observed regularly for signs of electrolyte imbalance (anorexia, nausea, muscle weakness, drowsiness), and sodium, potassium and chloride levels in the serum should be determined periodically. Patients in whom potassium depletion may occur (those with hepatic cirrhosis and those who are also receiving digitalis, corticosteroids, or corticotropin) should take some food daily that is high in potassium content, e.g. orange juice, or a potassium salt may be prescribed. Clinical evidence does not indicate that any of these agents is superior to the others with respect to the possible production of hypokalemia. Reversible hyperparathyroidism may develop with the prolonged use of thiazide diuretics.

Patients with cirrhosis and ascites should be observed for impending hepatic coma, which is presaged by fetor hepaticus, flapping tremor, confusion and drowsiness. These agents should be used cautiously in patients with gout; the concomitant use of an uricosuric agent may be necessary if blood uric acid levels become elevated. The hyperglycemic action of these drugs should not preclude their use in diabetic patients, but only the minimal effective dose should be given. When these diuretics are given in combination with other hypotensive agents, the doses of the latter should be reduced to avoid sudden decreases in blood pressure.

In elderly patients with advanced arteriosclerosis, coronary or cerebral thrombosis may be precipitated by the use of these drugs, especially if the patient is receiving ganglionic blocking agents, e.g. the quaternary ammonium compounds, hexamethonium, and tetraethylammonium chloride, or has undergone a sympathectomy in the past. Since these patients may have a marked hypotensive response, the usual doses should be reduced by one-half.

There is a lack of information concerning definite deleterious effects on the fetus when these diuretics are administered to pregnant women.

## SYMPATHOMIMETIC AMINES

Epinephrine, ephedrine, amphetamine (meth– and dextro–), naphazoline, methylphenidate (Ritalin) and related synthetic agents are widely used in therapeutics. These drugs all have powerful cortical excitant actions in addition to their effects on the autonomic nervous system. Amphetamines especially are used and abused by individuals to overcome sleepiness or provide increased energy and alertness. Their use for this purpose, if not under medical control, should be condemned. The dangers lie in the elimination of the warning signal of fatigue (often responsible for fatal auto or truck accidents), the possibility of habit formation, and with continued use, undesirable circulatory effects. The efficacy of the amphetamines for weight reducing is due primarily to their increased metabolic effect, however, other factors such as diuresis, enhanced muscle tone and activity, restlessness, sleeplessness and diminished appetite are also responsible. Amphetamines are also widely used in pediatrics in the treatment of the minimal brain-damaged hyperactive child. Investigators have found that normalization of the pupillary ability to contract following a test dose is a fairly reliable indicator that amphetamine therapy is likely to work.

Chronic poisoning and addiction are brought about by continued consumption of excessive amounts of sympathomimetic amines (particularly the amphetamines) over long periods. Their effects are similar to those of cocaine but are milder and do not develop as rapidly. Their abuse is common among alcoholics and barbiturate addicts. The symptoms are apprehension, jerky choreiform movements, tachycardia, hypertension, mydriasis, insomnia and anorexia. A toxic psychosis, characterized by the development of hallucinations and delusions of a paranoid character, may appear. Continual chewing or teeth-grinding movements, with rubbing of the tongue along the inside of the lip resulting in trauma and ulcers of the tongue and lip, frequently occur.

Unpleasant symptoms often follow the administration of a therapeutic dose of 0.3 ml of a 0.1% solution of epinephrine. Such a dose, given intravenously, may produce fatal ventricular fibrillation. The subcutaneous lethal dose is about 10 mg. Ephedrine and its salts have not been known to cause death, although a therapeutic dose of 15 to 20 mg may be followed by symptoms of intoxication. Amphetamine (meth– and dextro–, lethal dose for children is 5 mg/kg), naphazoline, tramine, synephrin, phenylephrine, etc. are often taken in large doses without fatalities, although alarming symptoms from idiosyncrasy do occur. These particular compounds resemble epinephrine and ephedrine in a number of respects but differ from them chiefly in possessing greater ability to stimulate the higher nervous centers, particularly the cortex.

Symptoms of toxicity from these drugs are palpitation, fever, tachycardia, chills, sometimes bradycardia, extrasystoles, heart block, nausea, vomiting, cold perspiration, blanching of the skin, elevation of blood pressure and pain in the chest: all are evidences of sympathetic stimulation. Mydriasis may occur.

Central actions result in insomnia, anxiety and tremor. These are more marked with epinephrine, amphetamine, methamphetamine and ephedrine. Delirium and convulsions precede collapse and coma. Collapse may occur from myocardial depression associated with pulmonary edema. These drugs, particularly epinephrine, are especially dangerous in association with chloroform, chloral hydrate, tribromoethanol (Avertin®), carbon tetrachloride or ethyl chloride, since the chlorine and bromine derivatives of methane (and probably all general anesthetics) sensitize the heart muscle to epinephrine and predispose to ventricular fibrillation.

may be administered if hypertension is prominent. Chlorpromazine (Thorazine), 1 to 2 mg/kg intramuscularly repeated as necessary, has been found effective in controlling the marked central nervous system excitation and the concomitant hypertension, and there should be no hesitation in the use of this drug. However, recent investigations have indicated that Haldol® and Inapsine® are more effective in much smaller doses than chlorpromazine and should be given further clinical trial.* If cardiovascular collapse occurs, the blood pressure should be maintained with levarterenol, and oxygen and artificial respiration given for shallow respiration or cyanosis.

SYMPTOMS

| *Mild* | *Moderate* | *Severe* |
|---|---|---|
| Restlessness | Confusion | Convulsions |
| Tremors and tics | Delirium | Circulatory collapse |
| Insomnia | Hallucinations | Hyperpyrexia |
| Talkativeness | Panic states | Chest pain |
| Irritability | Profuse sweating | Subarachnoid hemorrhage (beaded angiographic pictures) |
| Tachycardia | Tachypnea | Coma and death |
| Flushing of skin | Hypertension | |
| Increased sweating | Extrasystoles | |
| Dilatation of pupils | Dyskinesia (similar to those produced by phenothiazines) | |
| Dryness of mouth | | |
| Glycosuria | | |
| Hyperactive reflexes | | |
| Analgesia | | |
| Fever | | |

The use of amphetamines intravenously is a form of drug abuse with an addictive and relapse potential comparable to that of opiates or cocaine and which is favored by many drug abusers over heroin.

*Treatment* of poisoning from this general group should consist of delaying the absorption of the ingested drug by giving tap water or milk and charcoal and then removing them by gastric lavage or emesis followed by saline catharsis. Specific treatment consists of the administration of central nervous system depressants, especially paraldehyde or a barbiturate. If convulsions are imminent, a short-acting barbiturate should be given intravenously.

Alpha-adrenergic blocking agents such as phenoxybenzamine (Dibenzyline) and nitroglycerin (0.5 mg) or sodium nitrite (60 mg) Since the kidneys are the major route of excretion, some 45 per cent of ingested doses appearing unchanged in the urine, ample fluids are an essential part of therapy. Excretion in the urine may be as high as 80 per cent when the urine is acid, and acidification is a good therapeutic effort. Peritoneal dialysis in experimental animals has been a successful form of therapy and should be used in severe poisoning.

*Treatment* of chronic poisoning from the amphetamines consists of sedation, withdrawal of the drugs and a program of psychotherapy similar to that used for the treatment of any drug addiction.

*Intravenous Inapsine® (droperidol) plus acidification of the urine and external measures of reducing body temperature produced rapid improvement in a seriously intoxicated patient.

## TRICYCLIC COMPOUNDS

Drugs in this class include imipramine (Tofranil), desipramine (Norpramin®, Pertofrane®), amitriptyline (Elavil), nortriptyline (Aventyl®), protriptyline (Vivactil®), trimipramine (Surmontil®) and opipramol. Doxepin hydrochloride, a dibenzoxepin compound, is structured similarly to amitriptyline except for the replacement of one carbon atom by an oxygen atom in the tricyclic ring.

Tricyclic antidepressants may be additive with or may potentiate the action of CNS depressants such as alcohol, sedatives or hypnotics. Numerous drugs (barbiturates, ethchlorvynol, MAO inhibitors, phenothiazines, haloperidol, sympathomimetics, levothyroxine, levodopa, phenylbutazone, others) have been reported to affect the response to tricyclic antidepressants or themselves when used concomitantly.

There have been a number of serious cardiac arrhythmias, conduction disturbances and heart blocks associated with intoxication from tricyclic antidepressant tranquilizers. The most commonly seen disturbances of cardiac function from overdoses of these drugs are supraventricular tachycardia, widening of the QRS complexes, depression of the S-T segments and abnormal T waves. Disturbances of rhythm and conduction which have been reported include atrial and ventricular tachycardias, flutters and fibrillations, wandering pacemaker, multifocal extrasystoles (ectopic beats), complete or partial atrioventricular and intraventricular blocks and cardiac arrest.

In addition to the cardiac disturbances, intoxication with tricyclic antidepressants also produces the peripheral signs of atropinism and central nervous system, with symptoms of vomiting, thirst, drowsiness or dizziness, signs of mydriasis, nystagmus, agitation or stupor, bowel and bladder paralysis, muscle rigidity, tremors, hyperreflexia, athetoid or clonic movements, convulsions, hyper– or hypotension, depressed respiration, cyanosis, hyper– or hypothermia and coma. When a patient has convulsions or coma, signs of atropinism and cardiac arrhythmias, one should strongly suspect tricyclic antidepressant poisoning specifically and intoxication by other anticholinergic drugs and chemicals in general.

The most serious phase appears to be the first twelve hours; however, in children the tricyclics are especially treacherous. When a verified ingestion occurs, it probably would be wise to hospitalize the child for monitoring for at least forty-eight or more hours, even though the patient may be asymptomatic at the time of admission. During recovery, a deep lethargy may alternate with tremors, agitation, delirium, hallucinations, mental confusion and persistent insomnia. In some cases sudden relapse and death have occurred after seeming recovery from the effects of tricyclic drugs.*

*Treatment* of intoxication from tricyclic antidepressant tranquilizers is supportive and symptomatic, with particular attention to the correction of cardiac arrhythmias and maintenance of blood pressure and respiration. Vital signs should be monitored continuously. ECG monitoring is advisable, and severely intoxicated cases should be treated in an intensive care unit. A most reliable and valid clinical indication of a severe tricyclic overdose is a QRS duration of 100 msec or greater on a routine ECG within the first twenty-four hours when plasma measurements are unavailable (levels of 1000 mg/ml are considered toxic). Cardiac arrhythmias may progress to cardiac arrest due to ventricular fibrillation or asystole. Death may occur rapidly following a sudden drop of blood pressure and pulse rate. The use of defibrillators and internal or external pacemakers has been advocated. However, in one nonfatal case, an external DC defibrillator produced no alleviation of arrhythmias, and in a fatal case an external pacemaker was tried unsuccessfully.

Since many toxic effects of tricyclic antidepressants are anticholinergic in nature, physostigmine salicylate (Antilirium®) (a centrally

*Tricyclic agents have a half-life in the body of 60 to 80 hours, a factor that may explain sudden relapses and death.

acting anticholinesterase agent, the only commonly used inhibitor that readily penetrates the blood-brain barrier) may be used as an antidote for severe overdosage. Delirium, hallucinations, coma, myoclonic and choreiform movements and cardiac arrhythmias often respond to physostigmine. Frequent administration of physostigmine may be necessary as it is short-acting and patients may suddenly relapse. The drug is usually administered to adults in a dose of 2 mg by *slow* IV injection; it may cause convulsions if given too rapidly. This dose may be repeated in twenty minutes if there is no response. If the drug is effective, additional doses of 1 to 4 mg may be administered every thirty to sixty minutes as necessary. The initial pediatric dose is 500 μg, which may be administered every five minutes until a response is obtained or a maximum of 2 mg is given; thereafter, the lowest effective dose may be repeated as necessary. Physostigmine should not be used routinely, as side-effects may include excess cholinergic activity and seizures. In severe tricyclic antidepressant overdosage resulting in cardiac disturbances or coma, the benefits of physostigmine usually outweigh the risks. Like many antiarrhythmic agents, physostigmine can cause myocardial depression, as do the tricyclics, therefore compounding this effect. Most adverse effects of physostigmine can usually be controlled by administration of a peripherally acting anticholinergic agent such as propantheline bromide (Pro-Banthine) in preference to the centrally acting drug atropine, which could potentiate the CNS effects of the original intoxicant.

As it is not possible to predict which patient will respond, it may be necessary to try more than one antiarrhythmic drug. Intravenous sodium diphenylhydantoin has dramatic antiarrhythmic properties and may also be of value in preventing convulsions, which occur frequently. Congestive heart failure is treated by careful digitalization. However, digitalization should be avoided in a situation where an increase in AV block and multiple ventricular ectopic beats are likely to occur. The administration of sodium bicarbonate and potassium may aid in treating the cardiovascular effects, and in one series, sodium bicarbonate was the most clinically effective method of treatment of arrhythmias in children; experimental studies support this view. Convulsions may cause a dangerous increase in the cardiac workload. Agitation, tremors and convulsions have been successfully treated with parenteral barbiturates. However, use of barbiturates is questionable if drugs that inhibit monoamine oxidase have also been taken by the patient in overdosage or in recent therapy. Also, barbiturates may increase respiratory depression, particularly in children. Diazepam (Valium) has been used as an alternative to barbiturates for controlling convulsions and is considered the drug of choice by some, but its short duration is a disadvantage. Paraldehyde is also effective and has a longer duration of action. It is advisable to have equipment available for artificial ventilation and resuscitation. Hypotension and shock may be treated by intravenous fluids of glucose, saline solution or plasma and cautious administration of vasopressor agents such as levarterenol (l-norepinephrine; Levophed), phenylephrine or metaraminol which increase blood pressure without increasing heart rate. Any of these sympathomimetic drugs may induce cardiac arrhythmias and must therefore be used with caution. Other sympathomimetic drugs such as epinephrine and isoproterenol which stimulate the beta-adrenergic receptor sites of the heart should be avoided, as they cause additional increases in the heart rate and may lead to fatal ventricular fibrillation. Respiration must be maintained. Intratracheal artificial respiration is effective, and the need for it should be anticipated. Patients should be observed for possible recurrence of respiratory distress following resumption of spontaneous breathing.

Various methods have been attempted to hasten excretion of these drugs. They are absorbed quickly from the gastrointestinal tract and are largely bound to plasma proteins. In addition, they are rapidly accumulated in the body tissues so that high serum concentrations do not occur. They are excreted in the urine largely as glucuronides of the demethylated and hydroxylated metabolites.

They are also reportedly secreted into the stomach after absorption. Beneficial effects have been reported from use of exchange transfusion, repeated gastric lavage and osmotic diuresis. Although evidence is equivocal as to the effectiveness of osmotic diuresis in removing significant amounts of these drugs, it is the general belief that diuresis is beneficial. Osmotic diuresis with mannitol has been employed in the treatment of a number of cases of intoxication with tricyclic antidepressant drugs. In one adult, only 5 per cent of the ingested dose of amitriptyline was recovered in the urine (as amitriptyline and its principal metabolites) following a ten-hour period of forced diuresis with mannitol. Since these drugs also promote urinary retention, catheterization should be considered if diuresis is attempted. Care must also be used to prevent overhydration leading to increased cardiac workload. Continuous or repeated gastric lavage has also been recommended to speed excretion. (Since cardiac arrest in patients with arrhythmias may be precipitated by lavage, precaution should be taken to control the arrhythmia first.) While continuous gastric lavage was effectively employed in a child intoxicated with imipramine who exhibited coma, convulsions and cardiac disturbances, it may be unwise to attempt during convulsive stages. Hemodialysis and peritoneal dialysis are not effective in removing significant amounts of these drugs since they bind rapidly and extensively to tissue proteins.

## VANADIUM

Vanadium compounds are used in the television (color picture tubes) and steel industries and are often contaminants of heavy fuel oils, the residue of combustion of which may contain considerable quantities of the oxide. Inhalation of high concentrations of small particles of vanadium phosphors and pentoxide dust has produced skin manifestations and severe irritation of the eyes, nose, throat and lungs with pulmonary edema. Subsequent exposures, even though minimal, produced much more serious effects indicating the possibility of an allergic phenomenon.

Ascorbic acid has a protective and antidotal effect against vanadium poisoning in mice, rats and dogs. When administered in doses as low as 125 mg/kg of body weight to mice twenty minutes before vanadium injection, the vitamin prevented death in thirty-nine of forty animals. When rats were injected with ascorbic acid after the appearance of poisoning symptoms, 70 per cent survived. Fatal doses of vanadium administered to dogs were also made ineffective by antidotal injection of ascorbic acid. *In vitro,* polarographic studies indicate that the reduction of vanadium by ascorbic acid may be responsible for the detoxification. The vanadium-antagonizing action of calcium disodium ethylenediamine tetra-acetate ($CaNa_2EDTA$) is less effective, since signs of toxicity are arrested sooner and recovery is more rapid after ascorbic acid therapy. BAL therapy has been ineffective.

## VERATRUM (VERATRAMINE, VERATRINE, ETC.)

The veratrum alkaloids, the most important being protoveratrine, are a group of chemically related compounds obtained from liliaceous plants belonging to the suborder melanthaceae. They act mainly on the cardiovascular system, respiration, nerve fibers and skeletal muscles. These drugs have been employed in the past for the treatment of hypertension, toxemias of pregnancy and certain nephropathies. However, in modern therapeutics their use is practically obsolete.

The principal signs of intoxication are gastrointestinal symptoms and fall of blood pressure. They consist of nausea, severe vomiting, unpleasant taste, salivation, diarrhea, muscular weakness, epigastric and substernal pain, diplopia, bradycardia and extreme hypotension. However, with very large doses, the blood pressure may be elevated due to the direct effect of the drug on the vasomotor center in the brain.

*Treatment* should consist of removal of the ingested compound or plant by gastric lavage or emesis followed by activated charcoal and saline cathartic. Atropine blocks the reflex fall of blood pressure and can be given in 2 mg doses subcutaneously every hour until symptoms are controlled. Sympathetic blocking agents such as phentolamine hydrochloride (Regitine®) 50 to 100 mg orally or hydralazine 10 to 20 mg IM can be given for hypertension.

## VITAMINS

Americans are buying and consuming large quantities of vitamin supplements, believing that more of a good thing must be better than just a little. Occasionally this quest for health through self-administered vitamins leads to illness and death. The public is spending over $450 million a year on over-the-counter purchases of vitamins. The cost of vitamins incorporated into foods is an unknown added expenditure.

Undoubtedly, most sales are made in behalf of children, who after the second year of life neither require nor derive any great benefit from additional vitamins beyond those contained in the usual American diet. Healthy children fed adequate amounts of properly selected foods need no supplemental vitamins except vitamin D, and this is usually amply supplied by fortified milks and foods. Healthy adults receiving adequate diets also have no need for supplementary vitamins except during pregnancy and lactation. The only supplementary vitamins shown to be useful in the routine management of children are D, C and K in the newborn infant. Vitamin A deficiency is very rarely seen in children in this country and usually only in those in whom there is interference with normal absorption of fat and in children kept for long periods on a hypoallergenic, milk-free diet without animal fat. Whereas the prolonged use of forty to fifty times the usual amount of vitamin A is necessary to produce toxic symptoms, in the case of vitamin D only four to five times the ordinary amount may induce adverse effects. Dietary deficiency is rare in the case of vitamin K; its use is primarily for hemorrhagic conditions due to hypoprothrombinemia. There is little danger of harm from ingesting large quantities of the water-soluble vitamins because the excess is excreted readily. Folic acid, however, presents a special problem. In therapeutic dosage, folic acid may mask the presence of pernicious anemia and permit neurological lesions to develop while supporting a normal erythrocyte count.

The development of flavored chewable polyvitamin preparations has increased the incidence of ingestion of these compounds by children. It has been our experience so far that very little ill effect has resulted from these mishaps. Chewables with fluoride usually contain 1 mg of sodium fluoride per tablet and would not ordinarily produce serious symptoms, even if a full bottle of one hundred were taken by a child two or three years of age (*see* Fluoride). However, acute increased intracranial pressure from vitamin A and the possibility of toxicity in those with poor hepatic or renal function should be considered, and when an unusually large number has been taken, they should be removed by emesis or gastric lavage.

In addition to unavailability of proper foods, the principal cause of vitamin deficiency is intake of alcohol or illicit drugs, which interferes with food intake or its utilization. (In alcoholism, not only is intake of vitamins reduced but there is also an increased need for vitamins for ethanol metabolism.) Other causes are malabsorption disorders; bowel surgery; intestinal, pancreatic and liver disease; malignancy; and chronic heart failure, infection and neurologic disease. In addition, vitamin supplementation is essential during pregnancy and the postnatal period in the infant. Any form of physiologic stress may result in reduced vitamin stores and utilization.

Circulating or urinary levels of vitamins can provide evidence of vitamin deficiency and so allow treatment before symptoms appear. However, patients may have signs and symptoms of hypovitaminosis even though vitamin levels are normal. This may be due to malutilization. Thus, in assessing vitamin nutriture, it is important to measure not only vitamin levels but also the activity of metabolically active products of vitamins, which may be impaired.

TABLE 126
VITAMINS—PHYSIOLOGIC REQUIREMENTS

I. *Thiamine*
Thiamine is necessary to catalyze reactions concerned with carbohydrate metabolism. Studies of volunteers maintained on a thiamine deficiency regimen indicate that acute depletion of this vitamin leads to nausea, vomiting, anxiety and hypotension, all of which are corrected by replacement therapy. Chronic deficiency leads to peripheral neuritis, encephalopathy, and beriberi heart disease.

II. *Electron transport vitamins—riboflavin, nicotinic acid*
Enzymatic forms of riboflavin and nicotinic acid act as hydrogen acceptors and are therefore needed for adaptation to physiologic stress. Riboflavin depletion is characterized by photophobia, vascularization of the cornea, atrophic epidermis, cheilosis, glossitis, and anemia. Nicotinic acid depletion is characterized by dermatitis, glossitis, mental changes, peripheral neuritis, and anemia.

III. *Nucleogenic vitamins—vitamin $B_{12}$, folic acid, vitamin $B_6$ (pyridoxine)*
Vitamin $B_{12}$, folic acid and vitamin $B_6$ directly or indirectly catalyze DNA synthesis. Their depletion leads to glossitis, gastritis, reduced protein synthesis and impaired healing after tissue injury. The biologic half-life of vitamin $B_{12}$ in plasma is 5 to 14 days. In contrast to vitamin $B_{12}$, folate depletion develops rapidly in persons whose diet is devoid of this vitamin for several weeks. Folate deficiency leads to a decrease in serum folate within 3 weeks; hematologic abnormalities appear after 7 weeks; increased formiminoglutamic acid is excreted after 14 weeks; and anemia becomes overt after 4½ months. Vitamin $B_6$ deficiency may occur in a person who maintains an inadequate diet or receives drugs such as isoniazid. Anemia and neuritis are common accompaniments of a deficiency state in adults, whereas irritability, convulsions and behavioral disorders are characteristic in infants.
Folic acid deficiency may result from drug therapy. Diphenylhydantoin (Dilantin) interferes with folic acid absorption, and reciprocally, folic acid therapy may increase the frequency of seizures in epileptic subjects by antagonizing the activity of anticonvulsants, especially diphenylhydantoin. If convulsions become more frequent when epileptic patients receive folic acid prophylactically or therapeutically, either the dose of folic acid should be reduced or the dose of anticonvulsant increased, or both. Patients on chronic dialysis require folic acid supplements because the vitamin, like other water-soluble vitamins, is dialyzable.
Inadequate utilization of the vitamin most commonly results from treatment with a folic acid antagonist such as methotrexate, the diuretic triamterene (Dyrenium) or the antimalarial pyrimethamine (Daraprim). Since these folic acid antagonists block the reduction of folic acid to a metabolically useful form, treatment of folic acid deficiency due to such drugs is not accomplished with folic acid, but with folinic acid (Leucovorin, citrovorum factor), the most stable and only commercially available reduced form of folic acid, in a dose of 5 to 15 mg orally three times daily; it is well absorbed when taken orally.

IV. *Fat-soluble vitamins—vitamins A, D, K and E*
Vitamins A, D, K and E are essential for a variety of key metabolic reactions. Vitamin A deficiency leads to skin changes, night blindness and xerophthalmia; vitamin D depletion is responsible for rickets; and vitamin K deficiency results in hypoprothrombinemia. Marked deficits of vitamin E lead to hemolytic anemia. Excessive quantities of fat-soluble vitamins lead to hypervitaminosis syndromes. Thus, vitamin A and vitamin D intoxication are common in children receiving excess amounts of these vitamins.

V. *Vitamin C*
A deficiency of this vitamin may interfere with adrenal function, vascular tone and cell integrity. Severe deficiency leads to scurvy. Daily use of excessive amount of vitamin C can produce urinary tract oxalate stones.

VI. *Pantothenic acid and biotin*
Pantothenic acid, a ubiquitous substance in nature, is necessary for coenzyme A activity. Its deficiency may lead to fatigue, headache, gastrointestinal disturbances or peripheral neuropathy. Biotin is also ubiquitous. A deficiency is noted only rarely and is characterized by glossitis, dermatitis, lassitude and paresthesia.

TABLE 127
VITAMINS

| | *Food and Drug Administration MDR** | | | *National Research Council RDA*** | | |
|---|---|---|---|---|---|---|
| Age | A (units) | D (units) | C (mg) | A (units) | D (units) | C (mg) |
| Infants 0–1 | 1500 | 400 | 10 | 1500 | 400 | 30 |
| Children 1–3 | 3000 | 400 | 20 | 2000 | 400 | 40 |

*Minimum daily requirements.
**Recommended daily allowance.

Vitamin therapy should provide balanced amounts of vitamins, for deficiency of one vitamin may lead to malabsorption of another. Proteins and minerals must also be given, since vitamins alone are not sufficient in preventing or correcting vitamin deficiency. On the other hand, excessive amounts of fat-soluble vitamins should be avoided (hypervitaminosis A and D are common in such cases). It may be necessary to monitor the response to vitamin therapy, since many preparations do not contain a balanced mixture.

### *Known Drugs Capable of Producing Vitamin Deficiencies*

Anticonvulsants, contraceptive steroids, methotrexate, pyrimethamine and aspirin can produce folic acid deficiency; metformin can increase vitamin $B_{12}$ requirements; INH (isonicotinic hydrazide), thiosemicarbazide, hydralazine, penicillamine and L-dopa can produce vitamin $B_6$ deficiency; INH produces niacin deficiency; boric acid can increase riboflavin requirements (not yet documented in humans); aspirin, indomethacin and contraceptive steroids produce vitamin C deficiency; anticonvulsants (long term therapy) can produce vitamin D deficiency; while coumarin anticoagulants and cholestyramine can increase vitamin K requirements.

### *Hypervitaminosis A*

Vitamin A poisoning or hypervitaminosis A is due to the excessive and indiscriminate use of vitamin A concentrates for daily vitamin requirements, acne and other skin disorders. The toxic factor in vitamin A poisoning is probably the permanently elevated plasma vitamin A level. Clinical hypervitaminosis A develops only after the liver is no longer able to remove from the circulation the excess amount ingested. Hepatic dysfunction may be the basis for the vitamin A poisoning, and faulty or limited excretion may contribute to maintenance of high blood levels. Chronic excessive ingestion of vitamin A may stimulate fibrogenesis and lead to a disorder resembling hepatic cirrhosis. Any patient with chronic liver disease of unknown cause should be checked for possible hypervitaminosis A.

In rats, excess vitamin A has been shown to cause acceleration of periosteal proliferation, rapid consumption of epiphyseal cartilage and remodeling of bone attended by osteoclasis. Hemorrhages due to hypoprothrombinemia are common in vitamin A poisoning in animals but are rare in humans.

The chief symptoms in children are a long latent period, irritability, anorexia, scaly skin eruption, pain along the bones most exposed to trauma, swollen legs and forearms, pruritus, alopecia, cracked and bleeding lips and tender swellings of the skull. Hepatosplenomegaly, hyperpigmentation, hypercalcemia, persistent severe headache, exophthalmos, papilledema and a craving for butter may be present. A massive dose of vitamin A may cause an acute benign hydrocephalus (pseudotumor) from increased intracranial pressure. Roentgenograms have shown hyperostoses of the bones involved, occasional mottling of epiphyses, thinning of the calvarium, decalcification of the skull and vertebrae and calcification of pericapsular structures.

Vitamin A intoxication in adults causes symptoms which are similar to those of hypervitaminosis A in children but are usually milder. Structural bone changes are not likely to occur, and bone and joint pains are not so severe. Menstrual alterations, exophthalmos and pigmentation of the skin have been reported. Transitory increased intracranial pressure has been noted only in severe acute toxicity.

*Treatment* consists merely of withdrawal of the vitamin. Since decreased serum ascorbic acid values have been reported, large doses of vitamin C may be of some therapeutic benefit. Steroid therapy helps alleviate the benign increased intracranial pressure. Most signs and symptoms disappear within a few weeks, but the hyperostoses remain evident for several months after clinical recovery has occurred.

Carotenes of plant origin are readily converted into vitamin A by the liver, where it is stored and from which it is released as needed by the tissues. In the prolonged ingestion of carotene foods (carrots, yellow squash, sweet potatoes, spinach, oranges, yellow corn and beans, egg yolks, butter, kale, apple juice, pumpkins, turnips, parsnips, rutabagas, papaya) and in diabetes mellitus, hypothyroidism and disorders of the liver, the conversion of carotene may be disturbed and it may appear in unusual amounts in the blood, producing carotenemia, an innocuous condition in which the skin (particularly the soles and the palms) shows a yellow discoloration. The sclerae, however, are not involved. The possibility of symptomatic vitamin A intoxication from a diet high in carotenoids would be most unlikely. Lycopenemia, a condition similar to carotenemia except the skin is more highly tinted a deep orange-yellow, is due to high serum and hepatic levels of lycopene from excessive ingestion of tomato juice (rarely from beets, rose "hips," berries left on rose bushes and red-colored foods such as chili). Lycopene differs from the active isomer, beta-carotene, only in that the terminal beta-ionone rings are open and a double bond is substituted at the terminal dimethylated carbon atoms. Both substances, for the most part, travel the same metabolic pathways, but lycopene is physiologically inert and cannot form vitamin A, which accounts for the excessive serum and hepatic storage. Lycopene is neither toxic nor beneficial.

### *Hypervitaminosis D*

When unusual symptoms develop in a patient receiving vitamin D, toxic hypervitaminosis D should be suspected. Usually the intoxication develops only after amounts of the vitamin in excess of 100,000 IU have been taken daily for several months, but lower doses may be toxic. If the vitamin intake is not limited, the condition can be fatal. Excess intake of vitamin D in pregnancy has been implicated in producing infantile hypercalcemia, supravalvular aortic stenosis, mental retardation and a distinctive elfin facies in infants.

Indications of poisoning include nausea and vomiting, diarrhea, fatigue, weight loss, headache, paresthesias, depression, normocytic normochromic anemia (refractory to liver, iron and vitamin $B_{12}$, probably occurs in all patients but is rarely the most prominent symptom), urinary frequency, nocturia, albuminuria, hematuria, progressive loss in urinary concentrating power, rise in blood urea nitrogen, elevated serum calcium and phosphorus with normal alkaline phosphatase and roentgen signs of diffuse demineralization of bones or periarticular calcification. These symptoms and signs can appear in any order or combination.

Although many of these conditions also occur with primary hyperparathyroidism, the serum phosphorus and alkaline phosphatase levels in hypervitaminosis D are normal or but slightly elevated, whereas in the endocrine disorder the serum phosphorus is usually low associated with pronounced elevation of the alkaline phosphatase.

Vitamin D intake of infants and pregnant women should be continuously and carefully supervised with supplements used only when indicated and not routinely.

Hypervitaminosis D should be prevented but, once developed, must not be overlooked. If the vitamin is discontinued, renal failure and irritation usually disappear and the metastatic calcification in the kidneys and soft tissue generally reabsorbs. Inorganic phosphate orally as the disodium or dipotassium salt or intravenously as 1 liter of a 0.1 M solution of disodium phosphate and monopotassium phosphate (0.081 mol of $Na_2HPO_4$ plus 0.019 mol of $KH_2$ $PO_4$ to provide solution of pH. 7.4), and oral sodium or magnesium sulfate are effective in the treatment of the hypercalcemia and in relieving the symptoms of vitamin D intoxication. However, glucocorticoids are more rapid and effective in reducing serum calcium levels. The use of intravenous sodium citrate in lowering the amount of ionized calcium in the blood has little beneficial effect. Peritoneal dialysis, using a calcium-free balanced electrolyte solution to which 4% glucose is added, has recently been found to be very effective in removing vitamin D from the body.

### *Hypervitaminosis K*

The indiscriminate administration of vitamin K and its analogues is made on the assumption that they are harmless and the physician often believes that he is doing something of real value for his patient by giving him such a preparation during a hemorrhagic episode, regardless of etiology. Even in the face of predetermined hypoprothrombinemia, it is the common practice to give vitamin K in greater than adequate doses and to continue the treatment well beyond the time required to correct a true deficiency. Hypoprothrombinemia due to a seriously diseased liver cannot be corrected by vitamin K therapy, and many patients with this disorder can actually be harmed by frantic administration of these compounds. Hypervitaminosis K in animals has produced aplastic anemia, petechial hemorrhages, renal tubular degeneration and focal hemorrhages in many organs. Premature infants given large does of the water-soluble analogue of vitamin K have developed hemolytic anemia and kernicterus. Adults with liver diseases have had depression of prothrombin activity after large doses of vitamin K, and other alterations in liver function have been detected in individuals with previously normal liver function. Therefore, it should be emphasized that vitamin K and its analogues should be prescribed only for hemorrhagic conditions due to hypoprothrombinemia, except in advanced liver disease, and that treatment be given in therapeutic doses no longer than is necessary to restore prothrombin activity to normal.

Phytonadione (fat-soluble) and the variable synthetic name brand types (AquaMEPHYTON®, Mono-Kay®, Konakion®, etc.) of the naturally occurring form of vitamin $K_1$ are the preparations of choice since they are safer, and unlike the analogues, their effectiveness does not depend on the ability of the body to transform it into a utilizable form. These products should only be given subcutaneously (infants) or intramuscularly. Intravaneous administration is rarely indicated and must be done slowly.

## VOLATILE OILS

Volatile or essential oils are colorless liquids which evaporate readily at room temperature and consist of mixtures of saturated or unsaturated cylic hydrocarbons, ethers, alcohols, esters and ketones. These oils or the plants containing them—apiol, nutmeg, pine, absinthe, pennyroyal, juniper, savin, rue, tansy, eucalyptus, turpentine and menthol—are used as skin irritants. Many have undeserved reputations as abortifacients.

Ingestion of 15 ml of a volatile oil has caused fatal poisoning. Volatile oils intensely irritate all tissues and produce congestion and edema in the lungs, brain and gastric mucosa. The kidneys reveal degenerative changes.

The principal manifestations of poisoning with the volatile oils are vomiting and circulatory collapse. Symptoms from ingestion are dysphagia, nausea, vomiting, diarrhea, dysuria, hematuria, unconsciousness, shallow respiration and convulsions. Inhalation causes dizziness, rapid shallow breathing, tachycardia, bronchial irritation and unconsciousness or convulsions. Anuria, pulmonary edema and bronchial pneumonia may complicate recovery after either type of exposure. An amount of volatile oil capable of inducing abortion is likely also to produce irreversible renal damage.

In the *treatment,* give 60 to 120 ml of liquid petrolatum or castor oil, then remove oils by gastric lavage with tap water or emesis, taking extreme care to prevent aspiration. Follow these procedures immediately with a saline cathartic. Administer artificial respiration if necessary. The general measures are as follows.

1. Give milk, 250 ml, or mineral oil, 30 ml, as necessary to allay gastric irritation.
2. Atropine, 1 mg, to decrease bronchial secretions.
3. Fluids to 4 liters daily to maintain maximum urinary output if kidney function is normal and danger from pulmonary edema has passed (after first twenty-four hours).
4. Keep patient warm and quiet.
5. Treat pulmonary edema and anuria if they occur.
6. Control convulsions by cautious administration of short-acting barbiturates.

In prevention, volatile oils must be stored safely. Medications containing turpentine or other volatile oils should be labeled and kept out of children's reach. Masks capable of absorbing organic vapors should be used if atmospheres or environments containing high concentrations of volatile oils must be entered.

## XANTHINES (AMINOPHYLLINE, THEOPHYLLINE, THEOBROMINE, CAFFEINE, ETC.)

The xanthines are widely used in the treatment of bronchial asthma and certain acute cardiovascular conditions. Their effectiveness in asthma is based on their ability to relax the smooth muscle of the tracheobronchial tree and reduce edema of the bronchial mucosa, while their potent diuretic action is also beneficial for cardiac failure.

The clinical manifestation of overdosage of aminophylline may be central nervous system stimulation with unusual restlessness and irritability; this is an early sign and may progress to tremors, epileptiform convulsions, drowsiness and coma. Prolonged increase in gastric secretion may be manifested by nausea, persistent vomiting or even hematemesis. Increased urine output may be associated with reversible albuminuria and dehydration. Cardiovascular collapse or even death may result.

*Treatment* of a full-blown case of poisoning in children is difficult. Gastric lavage is indicated if hyperreflexia is not present. Aluminum hydroxide gel should be given as an antacid and protective agent against gastrointestinal irritation. Oxygen inhalation by mask or in a tent, both with and without intermittent positive pressure, has been employed. Short-acting barbiturates can be injected cautiously to control neuromuscular irritability and convulsions. Intravenous fluids to combat dehydration and antibiotics to prevent complicating infections are also useful and necessary measures, when indicated. Since xanthine is 2,6-dioxypurine and closely related to uric acid (2,6,8-trioxypurine), the uricosuric drug allopurinol (Zyloprim) might be found to be effective in the treatment of acute xanthine intoxication. Allopurinol acts by inhibiting xanthine oxidase, blocking the formation of uric acid from xanthine. Charcoal hemoperfusion is useful.

Theophylline is the most active of the xanthine agents, and the combination with ethylenediamine makes it more soluble and more completely absorbed. The xanthines stimulate the central nervous system, augment gastric secretions, cause diuresis and exert central and peripheral actions on the cardiovascular system. To eliminate preventable iatrogenic intoxication, the following dosages are recommended in the oral and rectal administration of aminophylline for the treatment of bronchial asthma in children: (1) suspension tablets given orally: 5 mg (1/12 gr)/kg of body weight; the dose may be repeated every eight hours, but not oftener than every six hours; (2) rectal suppository or retention enema: 8 mg (1/8 gr)/kg of body weight; the dose may be repeated every eight hours, but not oftener than every six hours, and is to be restricted to patients in whom oral administration is not practical; (3) for severe obstructive dyspnea, 0.25 gm aminophylline in 10 ml of diluent can be given intravenously over a period of eight to ten minutes and repeated in fifteen to twenty minutes if necessary. Rapid administration has been accompanied by intense reactions and in some instances death. More prolonged bronchial relaxation can be accomplished by the infusion of 200 to 500 ml of 5% dextrose in distilled water containing 0.5 gm aminophylline.

TABLE 128
MISCELLANEOUS DRUG COMPOUNDS

| *Drug* | *Use* | *Toxic Effect* | *Treatment* |
|---|---|---|---|
| Absinthe | Stomachic liquor | Optic neuritis; convulsions; mental deterioration | Discontinue use; give anticonvulsive therapy |
| Acacia | Emollient; demulcent;stabilizer for colloids | IV administration has caused fatal pulmonary edema and liver damage | Do not administer IV |
| Acedicon (dihydrocodeinone enolacetate) | Analgesic; sedative; narcotic | Addiction; vascular collapse; constipation | Gastric lavage followed by saline cathartic |
| Acenocoumarol (Sintrom®) | Anticoagulant | Hemorrhage; GI irritation | Discontinue use immediately; give water-soluble vitamin K |
| Acetaminophen (Tempra, Liquiprin) | Analgesic; antipyretic | Drowsiness and CNS depression; hypoglycemia | Gastric lavage or emesis; supportive. *See* Acetaminophen |
| Acetarsone (Acetarsol®) | Dysentery; trichomonal infections | Various skin rashes and exfoliation; fever, malaise and vomiting; renal and hepatic injury; agranulocytosis | Discontinue use; arsenic therapy |
| Acetazolamide (Diamox) | Carbonic anhydrase inhibitor; diuretic; epilepsy; glaucoma; etc. | Drowsiness; paresthesia; thrombocytopenia; agranulocytosis; skin eruptions; ureteral colic; urinary calculi | Discontinue use; do not use in any type of suprarenal gland failure |
| Acetic Acid | Household flavoring agent (essence of vinegar 14% acetic acid, vinegar 4% to 6%, glacial 100%) | Severe pain in mouth and throat followed by grayish-white ulcers; hematemesis; pulmonary edema; subnormal temperature with shock and collapse | Gastric lavage with weak alkali; demulcents, particularly milk; oxygen and caffein as needed |
| Acetohexamide (Dymelor®) | Antidiabetic | Hypoglycemia; GI irritation; skin rash; alcoholic-like effect | Discontinue use or reduce dosage |
| Acetomeroctol (Merbak®) | Antiseptic | Occasional urticaria progressing to weeping dermatitis; rarely, anemia, leukopenia and liver | Discontinue use; BAL therapy |

*Drugs indicated by an asterisk have been removed from the market or are obsolete.

TABLE 128—*Continued*
MISCELLANEOUS DRUG COMPOUNDS

| *Drug* | *Use* | *Toxic Effect* | *Treatment* |
|---|---|---|---|
| | | damage; ingestion may cause symptoms of mercury salt poisoning | |
| Acetone | Solvent | Nausea; vomiting; abdominal pain; characteristic fruit odor on breath; cough with bronchial irritation | Remove from source of exposure; supportive therapy |
| Acetone Cyanohydrin | Solvent | Nausea; vomiting; coma; convulsions | Remove toxic material from skin and stomach; other therapy as for cyanide poisoning |
| Acetonitside | Solvent for preparation of acetamide | Nausea; vomiting; coma; convulsions; sweating; salivation; dyspnea; angina; diuresis; collapse | Remove toxic material from skin; other therapy as for cyanide poisoning |
| Acetrizoate (Urokon®) | Diagnostic agent | Nausea; vomiting | Gastric lavage |
| Acetylcysteine (Mucomyst®) | Mucolytic agent | Bronchospasm; fever; chills; nausea and vomiting; stomatitis; rhinorrhea | Discontinue use |
| Allopurinol (Zyloprim) | Hyperuricemia | Skin rashes of various types (maculopapular, exfoliative, urticarial or purpuric); eosinophilia; leukopenia; arthralgias; hepatitis; diarrhea. Reduce dosage of mercaptopurine (Purinethol) by 75 per cent with concomitant use of allopurinol | Reduce dosage or discontinue use |
| Amantadine HCL (Symmetrel) | Antiviral (A.[2] Asian influenza) | Nausea; vomiting; anorexia. CNS effects: hyperexcitability, tremors, ataxia, blurred vision, lethargy, depression, slurred speech, convulsions | Discontinue use; symptomatic therapy |
| Ambenonium Chloride (Mytelase®) | Anticholinesterase agent (myasthenia gravis) | Acute cholinergic crises (muscle weakness, inability to swallow, paralysis, etc.). Both muscarine and nicotinic effects | Discontinue use; give atropine for muscarine effects and pralidoxime chloride for nicotinic manifestations |
| Amidoazotoluene (toluazotoluidine) | Dye for epithelization and granulation | Hypersensitization; urticaria, erythema and papulovesicular eruptions | Discontinue use of dye |
| Aminocaproic Acid (Amicar®) | Antifibrinolytic agent (inhibits plasminogen activators which convert plasminogen into plasmin and digest the fibrinclot) | Hypotension; nausea, vomiting and diarrhea; skin rash; pruritus; diuresis; hyperkalemia; conjunctival and nasal suffusion; may potentiate a thrombotic disorder | Use only when hemorrhage results from overactivity of the fibrinolytic system; contraindicated when bleeding occurs in closed spaces (pericardium, ureter, kidney) since it may prevent lysis of clots |
| Aminoglutethimide (Elipten®)* | Anticonvulsant in epilepsy | Skin rash within first week of treatment; drowsiness; ataxia; nausea; gastroenteritis; leukopenia; ulcerative stomatitis | Reduce dosage or discontinue use if rash persists after five to eight days |
| *p*-Aminohippurate | Diagnostic agent | Nausea; vomiting; sudden warmth | Gastric lavage |
| Aminometradine (Mictine) | Cardiovascular drug | Nausea; vomiting; diarrhea; headache | Discontinue use |
| Aminopterin* | Antineoplastic agent | Lymphopenia; fetal death or abnormalities; stomatitis | Discontinue use |
| *p*-Aminosalicylic Acid (PAS) | Chemotherapy | Fever; pruritis; acidosis; laryngeal edema; hypopotassemia; leukocytosis | Discontinue use |
| Amiphenazole | Stimulant | Convulsions | Discontinue use |

TABLE 128—*Continued*
MISCELLANEOUS DRUG COMPOUNDS

| *Drug* | *Use* | *Toxic Effect* | *Treatment* |
|---|---|---|---|
| Amisometradine (Rolicton®) | Cardiovascular drug | Nausea; vomiting; diarrhea; headache | Discontinue use |
| Amitriptyline (Elavil) | Antidepressant | Drowsiness; vertigo; nausea; headache; excitement; hypotension; convulsions; visual hallucinations | Do not use in glaucoma, urinary retention or with amine oxidase inhibitor; force diuresis; use inhalation anesthetics for seizures; barbiturates can potentiate depression |
| Ammoniated Mercury | Antiseptic | Urticaria; anemia; mercury salt poisoning | Discontinue use; mercury therapy |
| Ammonium Chloride | Diuretic; expectorant | Nausea; vomiting; restlessness; stupor; acidosis | IV fluids for hydration or acidosis; discontinue use of drug |
| Amodiaquin Hydrochloride (Camoquin® hydrochloride) | Chemotherapy | Nausea; vomiting' diarrhea; salivation; ataxia; convulsions | Discontinue use |
| Amphenidone (Dornwal)* | Tranquilizer | Agranulocytosis | Discontinue use |
| Amylene Hydrate (tertiary amyl alcohol) | Narcotic | Headache, drowsiness and coma; dilated pupils; respiratory depression | *See* section on Amyl Alcohol |
| Amyl Nitrite | Vasodilator | Flushing; vertigo; yellow vision; lassitude; dyspnea; cyanosis | *See* section on Nitrates |
| Anthralin | Fungicide; psoriasis | Gastroenteritis; alopecia; renal irritation | Discontinue use |
| Apiol | Abortifacient | Vomiting; diarrhea; toxic hepatitis; nephritis | Discontinue use |
| Arecoline (Betel Nut) | Diaphoretic; vermifuge | Salivation; vomiting; diuresis; convulsions | Discontinue use |
| Arnica | Volatile oil | Local application causes severe skin irritation, while ingestion produces vomiting, diarrhea and respiratory distress | Wash skin thoroughly; mineral or castor oil by mouth followed by lavage |
| Arsthinol (Balarsen®) | Chemotherapy | Nausea; vomiting; severe diarrhea with mucus and later with blood; hemorrhagic nephritis and hepatitis may also occur | Discontinue use |
| Artane® | Parkinsonism | Mouth dryness; blurred vision; nausea; vomiting; vertigo and hallucinations | Discontinue use |
| Aspidium | Anthelmintic | Vomiting; diarrhea; vertigo; yellow vision; delirium; convulsions; hepatitis | Gastric lavage; demulcents; discontinue use |
| Auramine | Dye; antiseptic (veterinary medicine) | Local application causes severe skin irritation and destruction. Vomiting; fever; headache; yellow vision | Remove from environmental source and skin |
| Aurantia | Dye | Severe dermatitis due to sensitization | Discontinue use |
| Azapetine | Sympathetic blocking agent | Nasal congestion; miosis; tachycardia; vertigo; indigestion; weakness; vasomotor collapse | Discontinue use |
| Azathioprine (Imuran®) | Antimetabolite, immunosuppressive agent (prevention of rejection in renal homotransplantation) | Hematopoietic toxicity | Complete blood counts including platelets should be done frequently; discontinue use if blood changes indicate |
| Azulfidine (salicylazo | Chronic ulcerative colitis | Fever; dermatitis; hepatitis; acidosis; hematuria; peripheral neu- | Discontinue use or reduce dosage |

TABLE 128—*Continued*
MISCELLANEOUS DRUG COMPOUNDS

| *Drug* | *Use* | *Toxic Effect* | *Treatment* |
|---|---|---|---|
| sulfapyridine) | | ritis; agranulocytosis; hemolytic anemia | |
| Benzethonium, Chloride (benzalkonium chloride) | *See* Cationic Detergents | | |
| Benzoic Acid | Antiseptic | Ingestion of 50 gm causes gastric upset | Discontinue use |
| Benzyl Benzoate | Antiseptic | Ingestion of 1 gm/kg causes incoordination, excitement, convulsions | Discontinue use |
| Betahistine, hydrochloride (Serc®) | Vertigo; Ménière's syndrome | Histamine-like activity; exacerbates peptic ulcer | Discontinue use or reduce dosage |
| Betazole (Histalog®) | Antineoplastic agent | Flushing; headache; syncope; respiratory difficulty | Discontinue use |
| Bishydroxycoumarin (Dicumarol®) | Anticoagulant | Hemorrhage | Discontinue use; give water-soluble vitamin K immediately |
| Bonadoxin® (meclizine and pyridoxine HCL) | Antiemetic; antispasmodic | Drowsiness and other atropine-like effects | Discontinue use or reduce dosage |
| Bromoform (tribromomethane) | Sedative | Burning sensation in mouth; CNS and respiratory depression | *See* section on Barbiturates |
| Bunamiodyl, Sodium (Orabilex)* | Diagnostic agent in cholecystography and cholangiography | Oliguria; renal insufficiency and failure | Do not use in patients suspected of having renal disease |
| Butamben Picrate (Butesin® picrate) | Anesthetic and antiseptic ointment | Severe dermatitis due to sensitization | Discontinue use |
| Caffeine | Stimulant | Vomiting; ringing in ears; diplopia; constricted pupils; headache; palpitation; in severe cases, tremors, opisthotonus and convulsions | Emetic or gastric lavage; force fluids; sedation if necessary |
| Cantharidin (Cantharone™) | Counterirritant | Skin contact causes erythema, vesiculation and exfoliation. Ingestion produces dysphagia, salivation, diarrhea, dysuria, corrosion of mucous membranes of mouth, nephritis and collapse. Severe conjunctivitis follows eye contamination | Wash skin and irrigate eyes; gastric lavage; levarterenol; treat cardiovascular collapse with blood transfusion; IV fluids |
| Capreomycin Sulfate (Capastat® Sulfate) | Antituberculous | Nephrotoxic; ototoxic; hypokalemia; eosinophilia | Discontinue use |
| Capsicum | Irritant | Irritating to skin; ingestion of large amounts causes vomiting and diarrhea | Ingestion: gastric lavage; skin: thorough irrigation |
| Carbarsone | Treatment of amebiasis and trichomonas vaginalis | Pruritic eruptions of the skin, followed by scaling, arsenical dermatitis, keratoses of the palms and loss of hair | *See* section on Arsenic |
| Carbimazole | Hyperthyroidism | In several instances, especially in allergic patients, prolonged medication with this drug has caused purpuric eruptions, arthralgias, hemorrhages, fever, thrombocytopenia and agranulocytosis with aplasia of the bone marrow | Discontinue use |

TABLE 128—*Continued*
MISCELLANEOUS DRUG COMPOUNDS

| *Drug* | *Use* | *Toxic Effect* | *Treatment* |
|---|---|---|---|
| Carbolic Acid | Antiseptic; disinfectant; surface anesthesia | *See* section on Phenol | |
| Carbromal | Sedative; hypnotic | Purpuric eruptions, more or less marked depression of the CNS, ranging from excitement to somnolence and from stupor to coma | Gastric lavage and cathartics; in severe cases, same as outlined for barbiturate poisoning |
| Carisoprodol (Soma®) | Muscle relaxant; analgesic | Drowsiness; skin rashes | Discontinue use |
| Cashew Nut Oil | Irritant | Blisters skin; vomiting; diarrhea | Skin contamination: wash in running water for at least fifteen minutes |
| Chenopodium | Anthelmintic | Nausea; vomiting; headache; acute depression; low back and flank pain due to kidney damage; convulsions | Discontinue use; anticonvulsive therapy |
| Chloral Hydrate | Sedative | Constricted pupils; respiration weak and shallow; pulse barely perceptible; cold clammy skin; lowered temperature and blood pressure | Gastric lavage; discontinue use |
| Chlorambucil (Leukeran®) | Antineoplastic agent | Vomiting; convulsions; coma | Discontinue use |
| Chloramine-T | Drinking water disinfectant | Rapid onset of respiratory embarrassment and cyanosis; marked hypotension; subnormal temperature; abdominal pain; convulsions | Discontinue use; gastric lavage |
| Chloramphenicol (Chloromycetin®) | Antibiotic | Nausea; vomiting; distention; diarrhea; enanthema; exanthema; blood dyscrasias (thrombocytopenia, granulocytopenia, aplastic and hypoplastic anemia) | Discontinue use or reduce dosage one-half |
| Chloriodized Oil | Antineoplastic agent | Irritation or sensitivity reaction | Discontinue use |
| Chloroguanide Hydrochloride (Paludrine®) | Antimalarial agent | Irritation of the skin; itching and puffiness of the eyelids and face; erythema followed by desquamation and urticaria have been reported in rare cases; also dizziness; abdominal discomfort | Discontinue use |
| Chloroquine Phosphate (Aralen® phosphate) | Chemotherapy | Fever; headache; lassitude; nausea; leukocytosis; vomiting; skin rash | Discontinue use |
| Chlorosalicylic Acid Anilide | Tinea capitis | Adults have been known to develop pruritic, maculopapular, erythematous contact dermatitis of hands and forearms because of sensitization to this material | Discontinue use |
| Chlorothiazide (Diuril®) | Diuretic and hypertensive agent | Hypokalemia; hypochloremic alkalosis; azotemia; nausea; vomiting; diarrhea; pulmonary edema; glycosuria, diabetogenic; dizziness: paresthesias; skin rash; urticaria; photosensitivity; necrotizing vasculitis; blood dyscrasias | Discontinue use; should be used cautiously in advanced renal or hepatic disease |
| Chlorphenesin Carbamate (Maolate®) | Muscle relaxant | Drowsiness; dizziness; insomnia; headache; gastrointestinal disturbances | Discontinue use or reduce dosage |

TABLE 128—*Continued*
MISCELLANEOUS DRUG COMPOUNDS

| *Drug* | *Use* | *Toxic Effect* | *Treatment* |
|---|---|---|---|
| Chlorphentermine HCI (Pre-Sate®) | Anorexic | Sympathomimetic amine effects | Discontinue use or reduce dosage |
| Chlorpromazine (Thorazine) | Tranquilizer | Drowsiness; somnolence; apathy and muscular weakness; hepatic dysfunction and jaundice; skin sensitization | Discontinue use |
| Chlorpropamide (Diabinese®) | Oral hypoglycemic agent | Jaundice; hypoglycemia; anorexia; skin eruptions; erythema multiforme and exfoliative dermatitis; depression of bone marrow with leukopenia and thrombocytopenia; induced granulomas; hyponatremia and water intoxication | Discontinue use; corticosteroid therapy |
| Chlorquinaldol (Sterosan®) | Antiseptic | Skin sensitization | Discontinue use |
| Chlortetracycline Hydrochloride | Antibiotic | Vesicopapular eruptions; diarrhea; moniliasis | Discontinue use or reduce dosage |
| Cholestyramine (Cuemid®) | Antipruritic in biliary cirrhosis | Nausea; diarrhea; abdominal distention | Reduce dosage; fat-soluble vitamins A, D and K |
| Chrysarobin | Fungicide; psoriasis | Nausea; vomiting; gastric pain; diarrhea; renal irritation; eye contact produces severe conjunctivitis | Discontinue use; thorough washing of the eyes |
| Cinnamon Oil | Flavoring agent in foods | Cheilitis and dermatitis in sensitive persons | Discontinue use |
| Citric Acid | In beverages | Irritation of the gastrointestinal tract | Discontinue use; IV administration of calcium salts |
| Cocillana | Irritant | Vomiting; diarrhea; collapse; headache; rhinorrhea | Skin contamination: wash in running water for at least fifteen minutes |
| Colocynth | Hydragogue; cathartic; diuretic | Abdominal pain; diarrhea with watery and bloody stools; tenesmus; meteorism; vomiting; irritation of kidneys; irritation of liver and pancreas | Discontinue use |
| Coparaffinate | Antiseptic | Skin irritation | Discontinue use |
| Crotamiton (Eurax®) | Antiseptic | Skin irritation | Discontinue use |
| Croton Oil | Cathartic | Burning sensation in the mouth; severe stomach pain with nausea and vomiting; severe purging—diarrhea which may be bloody; collapse and coma | White of egg or flour mixed with water, by mouth; discontinue use |
| Cubeb | Urinary antiseptic | Nausea; vomiting; abdominal pain; diarrhea; severe muscle and joint pain; muscular fibrillation and twitching; miosis; delirium, followed by coma and death from respiratory failure | Activated charcoal; discontinue use |
| Curare | Muscle relaxant | Prolonged apnea; bradycardia and vascular collapse | Discontinue use |
| Cyclamate, Calcium (Sucaryl®) | Synthetic sweetening agent | Diarrhea; flatulence | Decrease dosage or discontinue use |
| Cyclandelate (Cyclospasmol®) | Antispasmodic | Flushing; tingling; dizziness; sweating; nausea; headache | Decrease dosage or discontinue use |
| Cycrimine Hydrochloride (Pagitane® | Antispasmodic in treatment of parkinsonism | Rapid pulse and respiration; flushed face; lowered body temperature; restlessness; impaired | Gastric lavage; administration of sedatives; discontinue use |

TABLE 128—*Continued*
MISCELLANEOUS DRUG COMPOUNDS

| *Drug* | *Use* | *Toxic Effect* | *Treatment* |
|---|---|---|---|
| Hydrochloride) | | speech and vision | |
| Cyproheptadine Hydrochloride (Periactin®) | Antipruritic; appetite stimulant | Drowsiness; dry mouth; dizziness; nausea; ataxia | Discontinue use or diminish dosage |
| Dantrolene, Sodium (Dantrium®) | Muscle relaxant for spasticity | Drowsiness; vertigo; general malaise; diarrhea; hepatitis | Discontinue use after four to five days if no great benefit; monitor liver enzymes |
| Decamethonium Iodide | Muscle relaxant | May cause alarming fall of blood pressure | Discontinue use. *See,* Tricyclics |
| Desipramine Hydrochloride (Pertofrane, Norpramin) | Antidepressant | A metabolite derivative of imipramine with less frequent and severe side-effects | |
| Dextrothyroxine, Sodium (Choloxin®) | Hypercholesterolemia | Insomnia; nervousness; tremors; palpitation (inc. metabolism); weight loss; lid lag; sweating; hyperthermia; diuresis; menstrual irregularities | Discontinue use or reduce dosage |
| Diamethazole* | Antiseptic | Intensive skin application may cause hallucinations, muscle tremors and convulsions | Discontinue use |
| Diatrizoate | Antineoplastic agent | Feeling of generalized warmth; nausea and vomiting; fall of blood pressure; generalized itching and weakness; edema of the glottis | Discontinue use |
| Diazepam (Valium®) | Psychomotor relaxant | Fatigue; drowsiness; diplopia; hypotension; slurred speech; alopecia; dizziness; ataxia; nausea; skin rash; paradoxical reactions such as excitement, depression, stimulation, sleep disturbance and hallucination; ego-alien suicidal ideation | Discontinue use or reduce dosage; simultaneous use of other drugs and alcohol should be avoided; contraindicated in those with glaucoma; levarterenol drip for hypotension; dialysis uneffective |
| Dibenamine® | Sympathetic blocking agent | Nausea; vomiting; cerebral stimulation | Discontinue use |
| Dibenzyline | Hypotensive agent | Severe fatigue; marked persistent tachycardia; postural hypotension; persistent stuffy nose | Discontinue use |
| Dichlorophene | Antiseptic in dentifrices; antiperspirants; deodorant creams, etc. | In exceptional cases its use in dentifrices has been followed by stomatitis, glossitis, cheilitis, perlèche and circumoral dermatitis | Discontinue use |
| Dicodid® | Sedative; analgesic | Toxic reactions similar to morphine | *See* section on Morphine |
| Diethylcarbamazine (Hetrazan®) | Vermifuge | Fever; headache; lassitude; leukocytosis; nausea; vomiting; skin rash | Discontinue use |
| Dihydrostreptomycin | Antibiotic | Dermatitis; exfoliative dermatitis; vertigo; nystagmus; deafness | Reduce dosage or discontinue use |
| Diiodohydroxyquin (Diodoquin®)* | Chemotherapy | Iodism, neurological deficits; optic atrophy | Discontinue use |
| Dimenhydrinate (Dramamine®) | Motion sickness | Nausea; drowsiness; paresthesias | Discontinue use |
| Diphenhydramine (Hydrochloride (Benadryl) | Antihistamine | Drowsiness; dizziness; restlessness; nervousness; disorientation; epigastric distress | Discontinue use; gastric lavage |
| Diphenidol (Vontrol®) | Antiemetic | Auditory and visual hallucinations; disorientation; confusion; drowsiness; dry mouth; dizziness | Discontinue use or reduce dosage |

TABLE 128—*Continued*
MISCELLANEOUS DRUG COMPOUNDS

| *Drug* | *Use* | *Toxic Effect* | *Treatment* |
|---|---|---|---|
| Diphenoxylate Hydrochloride with Atropine Sulfate (Lomotil) | Antidiarrheal agent (narcotic exempt) | Nausea; drowsiness; dizziness; vomiting; pruritus; skin rashes and insomnia; respiratory depression with other narcotic effects; atropine effects early | Discontinue use or reduce dosage; risk of addiction with prolonged use; narcotic antagonist (naloxone) and supportive measures |
| Diprotrizoate | Antineoplastic agent | Nausea; vomiting; urticaria; fall in blood pressure; edema of the glottis; bouts of coughing | Discontinue use |
| Dulcin (Sucrol®) | Sweetening agent | Vertigo; swaying and ataxic gait; nausea | Discontinue use |
| Dyazide® (triamterene plus hydrochlorothiazide) | Diuretic | Nausea and vomiting; rash; dry mouth; vertigo; headache; electrolyte imbalance | Discontinue use or reduce dosage |
| Echothiophate Iodide (Phospholine® iodide) | Glaucoma (eye drops) | Cilary spasm; cysts of iris; a potent inhibitor of cholinesterase; systemic absorption can produce nausea, vomiting, diarrhea and salivation. (Succinylcholine is hydrolized by pseudocholinesterase and should be avoided in patients who have received echothiophate iodide within six weeks prior to surgery) | Discontinue use or reduce dosage; atropine; pralidoxime chloride |
| Emetine | Emetic; expectorant | Nausea; vomiting; acute stomach pains; intestinal cramping; diarrhea; cardiac depression and collapse | Discontinue use; absolute rest |
| Erythrityl Tetranitrate | Hypertension | Methemoglobinemia; lowering of the blood pressure; perspiration; fainting spells | Discontinue use; methylene blue for methemoglobinemia |
| Estrogens | Endocrine drug | Headache, nausea; vomiting; excessive vaginal bleeding; breasts enlarged from inhalations during manufacture or application to skin as hormone cream | Discontinue use |
| Ethacrynic Acid (Edecrin) | Diuretic | Abdominal pain; anorexia; nausea; diarrhea; malaise; may precipitate gout; hypokalemia; hyponatremia and hypotension; ototoxic with transient (and permanent) deafness, tinnitus and vertigo | Discontinue use or reduce dosage |
| Ethamivan (Emivan®) | CNS stimulant; analeptic | Sneezing; coughing; laryngospasm; restlessness; muscular twitching; tremor and convulsions | Reduce rate of administration; discontinue use |
| Ethchlorvynol (Placidyl) | Hypnotic; sedative | GI symptoms: hypothermia; bradycardia; hypotension; drowsiness; coma with toxic doses; pungent aromatic breath | Reduce dosage; force diuresis; peritoneal or hemodialysis for coma; adequate pulmonary ventilation and care |
| Ethyl Chloride | Inhalation; freezing (local) anesthetic | Sudden circulatory and respiratory failure; burning of the eyes; twitchings and tremors | Discontinue use |
| Ethylmorphine Hydrochloride | Sedative; analgesic; antispasmodic | Itching of the skin; swelling of the face; somnolence | Discontinue use |
| Ethyl Nitrite | Vasodilator | Headache; rapid pulse rate; cyanosis; nausea; vomiting; diarrhea | Discontinue use; *see* Nitrates |
| Eucaine | Local anesthetic | Lacrimation; blepharospasm; mydriasis | Discontinue use |

TABLE 128—*Continued*
MISCELLANEOUS DRUG COMPOUNDS

| *Drug* | *Use* | *Toxic Effect* | *Treatment* |
|---|---|---|---|
| Eucalyptol | Household remedies | Nausea; vomiting; dizziness; mental confusion; miosis; dyspnea; cyanosis; stupor | Discontinue use |
| Fowler's Solution (potassium arsenite solution equivalent to 1% arsenic trioxide) | Hematinic | *See* section on Arsenic | |
| Furaltadone (Altafur)* | Antibacterial agent | Nausea; vomiting; diarrhea; urticaria; maculopapular lesions; diplopia; purpura | Give drug with meals; decrease dosage or discontinue use |
| Furosemide (Lasix) | Diuretic | Nausea; vomiting; diarrhea; rash; pruritus; postural hypotension; hypokalemia; visual blurring; dizziness; muscle weakness and cramps; hyperuricemia; hyperglycemia (in diabetics); leukopenia; rare thrombocytopenia | Discontinue use or reduce dosage. Concomitant use with chloral hydrate may produce adverse effects. |
| Gelsemine | Antineuralgic | Great weakness; vertigo; intense tremors; ataxic gait; dryness of the mouth | Discontinue use; gastric lavage |
| Gelsemium (yellow jessamine) | Antineuralgic; antispasmodic | Great weakness; unsteady gait; aphasia; paralysis of the tongue with inability to swallow | Discontinue use; gastric lavage |
| Gentian Violet (methylrosaniline chloride) | Local antiseptic (Gentian Violet is a cationic [basic] chemical mixture of at least three rosaniline dyes, mainly crystal violet. It is used in diverse products and as a drug in human and veterinary [fungicide, vermicide, bactericide] medicine) | Methemoglobinemia after large doses; cardiovascular collapse and death from respiratory failure from large doses orally; nausea; vomiting; kidney irritation; epistaxis in occupational apple packers (from use of salvaged newspapers); hyperemia; hemorrhage of tissue and mucous membranes | Discontinue use; aniline therapy |
| Glutamic Acid (glutamate, sodium and disodium) | Flavoring in food | Allergic reactions characterized by epigastric fullness; vomiting; eructation; distention and upper abdominal discomfort (? Chinese restaurant syndrome) | Discontinue use |
| Glycobiarsol (Milibis®) | Intestinal diseases; amebicide | Sensitivity reactions; hepatitis; rare exfoliative dermatitis; arsenical hemorrhagic encephalitis | Discontinue use; BAL therapy |
| Griseofulvin (Grifulvin®, Fulvicin®) | Oral antifungal antibiotic | GI symptoms; headache; urticaria; other allergic skin rashes; hyperpigmentation; gynecomastia; antagonizes anticoagulant action of warfarin (Coumadin) | Discontinue use |
| Guaiacol | Analgesic; expectorant | Burning in the mouth and throat, with a whitish discoloration of the tongue and mucous membrane of the throat; nausea; vomiting; severe abdominal pain; slow weak pulse; faintness; coma; collapse | Discontinue use; phenol therapy |
| Guanethidine Sulfate | Antihypertensive | Dizziness; fatigue; dyspnea; postural hypotension; diarrhea; | Discontinue use or reduce dosage |

TABLE 128—*Continued*
MISCELLANEOUS DRUG COMPOUNDS

| *Drug* | *Use* | *Toxic Effect* | *Treatment* |
|---|---|---|---|
| (Ismelin®) | | polyarteritis syndrome; inhibition of ejaculation | |
| Haloperidol (Haldol®) | Tranquilizer | Dystonia; akathisia or dyskinesia; transient jaundice; teratogenic in mice | Discontinue use or reduce dosage |
| Heparin | Anticoagulant | Purpura; ecchymosis; hematuria; itching; rhinitis; bronchial asthma; multiple fractures | Discontinue use; protamine sulfate therapy |
| Heroin | Narcotic | Same as for Morphine | *See* section on Morphine |
| Hexamethonium Salts | Cardiovascular drug | Prolonged fall of blood pressure; failure of renal function; cardiac infarction; abdominal distention; tremor; psychosis | Discontinue use |
| Hexylresorcinol | Local and urinary antiseptic | Numbness of the tongue; blanching of the mucous membranes; occasionally very slight corrosion; stomatitis; cheilitis | Discontinue use |
| Homatropine | Mydriatic | Slow pulse; dysphagia; vertigo; weakness; excitement; collapse; mydriasis | Discontinue use |
| Honey | Food; vehicular syrup | May cause poisoning if it is ingested from certain plants; vomiting; diarrhea; headache; weakness | Discontinue use if honey obtained from toxic sources |
| Hydralazine Hydrochloride (Apresoline) | Antihypertensive | Flushed face; headache; stuffy nose; edema; palpitation; tachycardia and occasionally anginal pain; pyridoxine deficiency neuropathy | Discontinue use |
| Hydrochlorothiazide (HydroDIURIL) | Antihypertensive | Twelve times more potent by weight than chlorothiazide | |
| Hydrogen Peroxide 3% | Antiseptic | Congestion and irritation of mucous membranes; distention of abdomen from release of gas. Hydrogen peroxide as a 1% colonic irrigation agent is hazardous because major oxygen embolization with temporary portal venous obstruction may occur | Discontinue use |
| Hydroxydione Succinate Sodium (Viadril®) | Antineoplastic agent | Thrombophlebitis after IV injection | Discontinue use |
| Hydroxyprogesterone Caproate (Delalutin®) | Endocrine drug | Edema; exacerbation of epilepsy; migraine; asthma | Discontinue use |
| Hydroxystilbamidine | Chemotherapy (blastomycosis, etc.) | Transitory fall of blood pressure; rapid pulse; dizziness; nausea; vomiting; renal irritation from old solutions; trigeminal neuropathy | Use only fresh solutions; store drug away from heat and light; discontinue use |
| Hydroxyzine Pamoate or Hydrochloride (Vistaril®) | Ataractic | Dryness of the mouth; drowsiness; involuntary motor activity | Discontinue use |
| Hyoscine | *See* Atropine | | |
| Hyoscyamus | *See* Atropine | | |
| Ibuprofen (Motrin®) | Anti-inflammatory (nonsteroidal), analgesic | G-I symptoms; skin rashes; vertigo; fluid retention and edema | Discontinue use |
| Ichthammol (Ichthyol®) | Antiseptic; fungicide | Nausea and diarrhea after ingestion | Discontinue use; remove by gastric lavage |

TABLE 128—*Continued*
MISCELLANEOUS DRUG COMPOUNDS

| *Drug* | *Use* | *Toxic Effect* | *Treatment* |
|---|---|---|---|
| Idoxuridine (IDU) | Keratitis | No systemic toxic effects from local use | Keep refrigerated and do not use after expiration date |
| Imipramine Hydrochloride (Tofrānil) | Antidepressant | Atropine-like effects; agitation; parkinsonian symptoms; speech interference; visual hallucinations; coma; convulsions; cardiac disturbance with arrhythmias, EKG change and hypotension; respiratory depression | Intermittent gastric lavage for two to four days and activated charcoal. Drug reexcreted in stomach for several days from the intestinal tract. (Forced diuresis by IV fluids saved two infants with lethal doses.) *See,* Tricyclics |
| Indomethacin (Indocin®) | Antirheumatic | Nausea; vomiting; diarrhea; epigastric distress (gastric ulcer); headache; vertigo; may mask signs and symptoms accompanying infectious disease and may increase susceptibility to infection; questionable toxic hepatitis | Discontinue drug or reduce dosage. Interacts with coumarin anticoagulants and probenecid |
| Insulin | Diabetes mellitus | Hypoglycemia; anaphylaxis | Give glucose; discontinue use temporarily |
| Iodipamide (Cholografin®) | Diagnostic agents; renograms, etc. | Nausea; vomiting; diarrhea; possible renal involvement (dose related); other reactions include a feeling of generalized warmth and flushing of face and neck; urticaria; fall of blood pressure; hyperpnea; generalized itching and weakness; lacrimation; salivation; edema of the glottis; bouts of coughing (symptoms usually disappear in fifteen to thirty minutes but may progress rapidly and result in fatalities from bronchial constriction or cardiovascular collapse) | Discontinue use; give epinephrine 1:1000 solution; shock therapy (Hippuran is superior to iodopyracet, 10 to 15 per cent of which is collected in the liver) |
| Iodoalphionic Acid (Priodax®) | Diagnostic agent | *See* Iodipamide above | |
| Iodoform | Antiseptic | Skin irritation; in chronic poisoning, the heart, kidney and liver are involved. | Discontinue use |
| Iodohippurate (Hippuran®) | Diagnostic agent | *See* Iodipamide above | |
| Iodomethamate (Neo-Iopax®) | Diagnostic agent | *See* Iodipamide above | |
| Iodopanoic Acid (iopanoic acid, Telepaque®) | Diagnostic agent | *See* Iodipamide above; thrombocytopenic purpura | |
| Iodopyracet (Diodrast®) | Diagnostic agent | *See* Iodipamide above | |
| Iodopyracet Compound | Diagnostic agent | *See* Iodipamide above | |
| Iodopyracet Concentrated | Diagnostic agent | *See* Iodipamide above | |
| Iophendylate | Diagnostic agent | Reactions after intraspinal injection include backache and transient fever; the bulk of the injected material should be removed if possible | Discontinue use |
| Iothiouracil (Itrumil®) | Antithyroid | Drug fever; skin rashes; granulocytopenia | Discontinue use |
| Isoniazid (Nydrazid®) | Chemotherapy (tuberculosis, etc.) | Dizziness; headache; fever; arthralgia; paresthesias; twitching; deafness; polyneuritis; toxic | Discontinue drug or reduce dosage below 5 mg/kg/day; anticonvulsives; peritoneal dialysis; pyri- |

TABLE 128—*Continued*
MISCELLANEOUS DRUG COMPOUNDS

| *Drug* | *Use* | *Toxic Effect* | *Treatment* |
|---|---|---|---|
| | | hepatitis; paralysis and convulsions; elevated SGOT | doxine (large doses) |
| Isuprel® Hydrochloride | Asthma | Tachycardia; irregularities of blood pressure; palpitation; precordial pain; nervousness; headache; sweating; tremors | Discontinue use |
| Ketobemidone | Narcotic agent | Euphoria with prolonged use; nervousness; inability to concentrate, disturbances of memory and impairment of the mental functions | Discontinue use |
| Khellin | Cardiovascular drug | Nausea; vomiting; diarrhea; dermatitis; dizziness and sleepiness or wakefulness | Discontinue use |
| Knockout Drops | *See* section on Chloral Hydrate | | |
| Kynex® (sulfamethoxypyridazine) | Chemotherapy | *See* section on Sulfonamides | |
| Lactic Acid | Acidifier for variable uses | Severe burning of the mouth, pharynx, esophagus and stomach; nausea and vomiting | *See,* Acids |
| Laudanum (tincture of opium) | *See* section on Morphine | (A 10% solution of opium in alcohol, equivalent to about 1% morphine. This is not paregoric) | |
| Levothyroxine | Endocrine drug | Tachycardia; headache; excessive sweating; thyrotoxicosis after massive ingestion | Discontinue use; Propranolol |
| Liquiprin | Antipyretic; analgesic | Acetaminophen | *See* Acetaminophen |
| Lobeline | Stimulant | Dryness in the throat; nausea; vomiting; abdominal pain; diarrhea | Discontinue use |
| Lucanthone Hydrochloride | Treatment of schistosomiasis | Giddiness; vertigo | Discontinue use |
| Lututrin | Endocrine drug for dysmenorrhea | Drowsiness | Discontinue use or reduce dosage |
| Lypressin (50 U.S.P. posterior pituitary units) | Diabetes insipidus | Water retention with possible water intoxication | Discontinue use; meralluride or mannitol |
| Mandelic Acid | Antiseptic | Gastric irritation; nausea; renal irritation; acidosis | Discontinue use |
| Mechlorethamine (nitrogen mustard, Mustargen®) | Antineoplastic agent | Lymphopenia; thrombosis at site of injection; necrosis following extravascular injections; precipitation of uric acid; renal irritation | Discontinue use |
| Menthol (Mentholated American cigarettes contain 1 to 2 mg of menthol. The maximum quantity inhaled per cigarette is 0.7 mg) | Volatile oil | Severe abdominal pain; nausea and vomiting; dizziness and staggering gait; slow respiration; flushed face; sluggishness and sleepiness; large amounts in children produce coma | Discontinue use |
| Meperidine Hydrochloride (Demerol®) | Analgesic; substitution for morphine | Dyspnea; abrupt and marked fall of blood pressure; soft and rapid pulse | Discontinue use |
| Mephenesin (Tolseram®) | Muscle relaxant | Leukopenia; fever; allergic reactions | Discontinue use |

TABLE 128—*Continued*
MISCELLANEOUS DRUG COMPOUNDS

| *Drug* | *Use* | *Toxic Effect* | *Treatment* |
|---|---|---|---|
| Meprobamate | Antianxiety agent | Hypersensitivity reactions; urticaria; erythematous maculopapular skin rashes; chills; fever; peripheral edema and nonthrombocytopenic purpura with petechiae and ecchymosis; convulsions on withdrawal | Discontinue use |
| Merbromin (Mercurochrome®) | Antiseptic | Occasional urticaria progressing to weeping dermatitis; rarely anemia | Discontinue use; *see* section on Mercury |
| Mercamylamine (Inversine® hydrochloride) | Ganglion-blocking agent | Constipation; muscular weakness; dryness of the mouth; blurred vision; impotence; postural hypotension | Discontinue use |
| Mercocresol | Antiseptic | Leukopenia and liver damage; ingestion may cause symptoms of mercury salt poisoning | *See* section on Mercury |
| Mercury Protoiodide | Antiseptic | Skin rash; repeated ingestion may cause symptoms of chronic mercury poisoning | As for mercury poisoning |
| Methacholine Chloride (Mecholyl®) | Parasympathomimetic agent | Nausea; vomiting; precipitation of asthmatic attacks in susceptible persons; momentary heart block | Discontinue use; atropine as antagonist |
| Methadone Hydrochloride (Dolophine®) | Narcotic | Withdrawal symptoms are characterized by weakness, restlessness, diarrhea and lack of energy | Discontinue use; as for morphine poisoning |
| Methamphetamine Hydrochloride | Central nervous system stimulant | Hypertension; tachycardia; euphoria | Discontinue use |
| Methantheline Bromide (Banthine® bromide) | Parasympatholytic agent | Pruritus; papular erythema; xerostomia; urinary retention; mydriasis | Discontinue use |
| Methaqualone (Quaalude®) | Hypnotic | Nausea; vomiting; dry mouth; drowsiness; transient paresthesia ("pins and needles"); serious effects from overdosage include the following: motor excitation followed by deep coma; rapid variations in pupillary width and reaction to light; increased muscle tone with overstretching of the extremities; hyperreflexia and muscle fasciculations. Less frequent are tonic-clonic convulsions, vomiting, salivation and lacrimation. Emergence from coma is usually accompanied by recurrence of motor excitation. Characteristic is the *nachschlaf,* sleep from which the patient can be roused and which persists for twenty-four or more hours after regression of all other signs of the toxic condition. The causes of death are acute cardiac failure and pneumonia with terminal shock | As for barbiturate<br>Purgation and colonic lavage advisable since there is protracted absorption of this compound from the GI tract. It has been recovered four days after ingestion, and methaqualone metabolites have been recovered as many as seven days after ingestion. Hemodialysis |
| Methenamine (Mandelamine®) | Antiseptic | Skin rash; kidney and bladder irritation; hematuria; nausea and vomiting | Discontinue use |

TABLE 128—*Continued*
MISCELLANEOUS DRUG COMPOUNDS

| *Drug* | *Use* | *Toxic Effect* | *Treatment* |
|---|---|---|---|
| Methetharimide (Megimide) | Stimulant | Delirium; hallucinations; convulsions; psychotic symptoms | Discontinue use |
| Methimazole | Antithyroid; hyperthyroidism | Urticaria; rash; fever; nausea; vomiting; stomatitis; pain in the joints | Discontinue use |
| Methixene Hydrochloride (Trest®) | Antispasmodic | Anticholinergic effects (dry mouth, blurred vision, urinary retention, etc.) | Discontinue use or reduce dosage |
| Methocarbamol | Muscle relaxant | Drowsiness; vertigo; blurred vision; fever and headache | Discontinue use |
| Methorphinan Hydrobromide (Dromoran®) | Narcotic | Subcutaneous injection of excessive overdoses produces lethargy and coma with slow respiration of the Biot type | Discontinue use |
| Methotrimeprazine (Levoprome®) | Analgesic | Orthostatic hypotension; sedation; dry mouth; nasal congestion; leukopenia; agranulocytosis | Discontinue use or reduce dosage |
| Methyldopa (Aldomet®) | Antihypertensive | Drowsiness; parkinsonism; nausea; abdominal distention; dryness of mouth; nasal stuffiness; fever; positive direct Coombs' test with or without hemolysis and interference with blood cross matching; mentation difficulties; hypersensitivity myocarditis (?) | Discontinue use |
| Methylparafynol (Dormison®) | Hypnotic | Overdosage has resulted in unconsciousness, rapid and shallow respiration, low blood pressure, slow pulse, coma and acute psychosis | Discontinue use |
| Methylphenidate† (Ritalin®) | Stimulant | Anorexia; dizziness; headache; nausea; insomnia; hallucinosis; increased pulse and blood pressure; tics | Discontinue use |
| Methylrosaniline Chloride | | *See* Gentian Violet | |
| Methyltestosterone | Endocrine drug | Jaundice from bile stasis; enlarged liver | Discontinue use |
| Methylthiouracil | Hyperthyroidism; thyrotoxicosis | Prolonged medication causes agranulocytosis | Discontinue use |
| Methyprylon (Noludar) | Hypnotic | Ingestion of 30 (200 mg) tablets has been followed by unconsciousness and coma, grayish-blue discoloration of the face and nail beds, areflexia; rapid pulse; hypotension and pyrexia | *See* section on Barbiturates; hemodialysis |
| Metronidazole (Flagyl) | Trichomoniasis; amebiasis | Nausea; vomiting; glossitis: dysuria; dark urine; leukopenia; jaundice; disulfiram (Antabuse) effects | Discontinue use |
| Mickey Finn Drops (¼ to ½ tsp. croton oil or tartar emetic mixed with drink) | In bars to get rid of offensive customers | Acute burning sensation in the mouth; nausea and violent vomiting associated with severe abdominal pain; diarrhea and tenesmus; cold and clammy skin; weak pulse; hypotension; collapse and | Supportive and symptomatic |

†Retinopathy due to talc and cornstarch emboli has been reported in drug addicts following repeated intravenous injections of crushed methylphenidate hydrochloride tablets taken for their stimulatory effects. IV doses have produced atrial fibrillation.

TABLE 128—*Continued*
MISCELLANEOUS DRUG COMPOUNDS

| *Drug* | *Use* | *Toxic Effect* | *Treatment* |
|---|---|---|---|
| | | sometimes death from respiratory and/or circulatory failure if an excessive amount has been administered | |
| Movellan | Tonic; criminal use for abortion | Cramping pain in the extremities; excitability; muscular twitchings; parathesias; convulsions | *See* section on Strychnine |
| Nalidixic Acid (NegGram®) | Urinary infections | Nausea; vomiting; drowsiness; weakness; skin manifestations; pruritus; eosinophilia; phototoxic; convulsions; false positive urine test for glucose, but true glycosuria has been reported; reversible increased intracranial pressure | Discontinue use or reduce dosage |
| Neomycin Sulfate | Antibiotic | Nephrotoxic and ototoxic | Discontinue use |
| Neostigmine Bromide | Myasthenia gravis | Nasal secretion; slight salivation; restlessness; giddiness; fainting and great anxiety; respiratory depression | Discontinue use and administer atropine |
| Neostigmine Methylsulfate | Parasympathetic stimulant | General convulsive seizures; salivation; marked depression of respiration; death | Discontinue use and administer atropine |
| Nicotinic Acid (Niacin®) | Hypercholesterolemia | Flushing; itching and temporary feeling of heat after intravenous administration; fall of blood pressure may be severe; anaphylactic reactions occasionally occur | Discontinue use and give epinephrine for anaphylactoid reactions |
| Nitrofurantoin (Furadantin) | Antiseptic | Maculopapular erythematous eruption; anemia; leukopenia; granulocytopenia; polyneuritis | Discontinue use |
| Nitrofurazone (Furacin®) | Antiseptic | Weeping dermatitis | Discontinue use |
| Nitromersol (Metaphen®) | Antiseptic | Occasional urticaria progressing to weeping dermatitis | Discontinue use; *see* section on Mercury |
| Norpramin® | *See* section on Tricyclics | | |
| Nortriptyline HCl (Aventyl) | Antidepressant | Dry mouth; drowsiness; blurred vision; constipation | Discontinue use or reduce dosage |
| Nux Vomica | *See* section on Strychnine | | |
| Nystatin (Mycostatin®) | Antibiotic | Nausea; vomiting; diarrhea | Reduce dosage |
| Octin® | Antispasmodic | Dizziness and headache; malaise; vertigo; palpitation; dryness in the mouth | Discontinue use |
| Oil of Bitter Almond | *See* section on Cyanides | | |
| Oil of Mustard‡ (allyl isothiocyanate) | Irritant; rubefacient | Blistering and corrosion of skin or gastrointestinal tract; a single drop in the eye has caused blindness. Used in some glue cements to deter "glue sniffers" | Ingestion: lavage; skin contamination: wash in running water for at least fifteen minutes |
| Oil of Wintergreen (methyl salicylate) | *See* section on Salicylate (also known as *Betula lenta,* gaultheria and sweetbirch oil) | | |

‡Occurs naturally in black mustard seed and in raw cabbage, where it is a weak goitrogen.

TABLE 128—*Continued*
MISCELLANEOUS DRUG COMPOUNDS

| *Drug* | *Use* | *Toxic Effect* | *Treatment* |
|---|---|---|---|
| Orphenadrine Citrate (Norflex®) | Muscle relaxant | Anticholinergic effects; dryness of mouth; tachycardia; blurred vision; dilation of pupils, etc. | As for atropine |
| Oxanamide (Quiactin®) | Tranquilizer | *See* section on Tranquilizers | |
| Oxazepam (Serax®) | Tranquilizer | Drowsiness; rash; syncope; ataxia; hypotension; hyperglycemia | Discontinue use or reduce dosage |
| Oxophenarsine Hydrochloride (Mapharsen®) | Anti-infective agent; syphilis | Severe fall of blood pressure | Discontinue use |
| Oxtriphylline (Choledyl®) | *See* section on Aminophyllin | | |
| Oxymorphone HCl (Numorphan®) | *See* section on Morphine | | |
| Oxyphencyclimine Hydrochloride (Daricon®) | Anticholinergic | Dryness of mouth; blurring of vision; dizziness; drowsiness; constipation | Discontinue use |
| Oxyphenonium Bromide (Antrenyl® bromide) | Anticholinergic agent | *See* section on Atropine | |
| Pamaquine Naphthoate | Chemotherapy | Hemolytic anemia; postural hypotension; weakness; methemoglobinemia; gastric distress | Discontinue use or reduce dosage |
| Pantopon® | Narcotic; analgesic | Respiratory disturbances of the Cheyne-Stokes type | Discontinue use |
| Paraldehyde | Sedative; antispasmodic | Flushing of the face; dryness in the mouth; nausea; vomiting | Morphine therapy |
| Paregoric (camphorated tincture of opium) | (A tincture of 0.4% opium or 0.04% morphine) | *See* section on Morphine | Morphine therapy |
| Pargyline Hydrochloride (Eutonyl®) | Antihypertensive | *See* Tranylcypromine (Parnate®) | |
| Paris Green | *See* section on Arsenic | | |
| Pelletierine Tannate | Chemotherapy | Dizziness; visual disturbances; headaches; weakness; vomiting and diarrhea; muscular cramps progressing to twitching, convulsions and paralysis | Discontinue use |
| Pennyroyal (hedeoma plant) | Infusions used as carminatives and stimulants | Retching; unconsciousness; collapse; rapid pulse | Discontinue use |
| Pentaquine Phosphate | Chemotherapy | Hemolytic anemia; postural hypotension; weakness; methemoglobinemia; gastric distress | Discontinue use |
| Pentazocine (Talwin®) | Analgesic | Nausea; vomiting; dizziness; euphoria; respiratory depression; rhinorrhea; hives; fever; secondary muscular atrophy from repeated injections; neonatal withdrawal symptoms | Methylphenidate (Ritalin®) as respiratory stimulant; naloxone is specific for respiratory depression |
| Peru Balsam | Indolent wounds and ulcers | Dermatitis and nephritis | Discontinue use |
| Phenaglycodol (Ultran®) | Muscle relaxant | Drowsiness | Reduce dosage |
| Phenarsone Sulfoxylate (Aldarsone®) | Chemotherapy | Severe fall of blood pressure; *see* section on Arsenic | Discontinue use |
| Phenazopyridine HCl (Pyridium®) | *See* Pyridium | | |

TABLE 128—*Continued*
MISCELLANEOUS DRUG COMPOUNDS

| *Drug* | *Use* | *Toxic Effect* | *Treatment* |
|---|---|---|---|
| Phenindione (Danilone®) | Anticoagulant | Red discoloration of the urine; dryness of the mouth; thirst; polyuria; tachycardia | Discontinue use |
| Phentolamine (Regitine®) | Sympathetic blocking agent | Nasal congestion; miosis; tachycardia; vertigo; indigestion; weakness; vasomotor collapse | Discontinue use |
| Phenylbutazone (Butazolidin®) | Arthritis; gout | Edema; vertigo; stomatitis; hypertension; agranulocytosis; thrombocytopenia; toxic hepatitis | Discontinue use; avoid in senile patients |
| Phenylhydrazine | Polycythemia vera | Fatigue and headache; edema of the upper extremities, occasionally of the eyelids; toxic hepatitis and anemia; acute gastritis with or without diarrhea | Discontinue use |
| Phenylmercuric Salts | Antiseptic | Occasional urticaria progressing to weeping dermatitis; rarely, anemia, leukopenia and liver damage; ingestion may cause symptoms of mercury salt poisoning | Discontinue use; *see* section on Mercury |
| pHisoHex®* (3% hexachlorophene) | Antiseptic | Accidental introduction of small amounts in the eye, unless removed promptly, may result in protracted keratitis with photophobia. Do not use as wet dressing for extensive burns | Discontinue use; symptomatic |
| Physostigmine | Parasympathetic stimulator | Bradycardia; intense salivation; miosis; twitching of skeletal muscles; coma; collapse | Discontinue use; give the physiologic antagonist Pro-Banthine®. |
| Picric Acid | Antiseptic ointment | Intense bitter taste; nausea; vomiting; abdominal and epigastric tenderness and pain; bright yellow color of the skin; bladder tenesmus; severe liver and kidney damage | *See* section on Picric Acid |
| Picrotoxin | Analeptic | Burning sensation in the mouth; pallor; cold sweat; nausea and vomiting; shallow respiration | Discontinue use |
| Pilocarpine | *See* Physostigmine | | |
| Pipamazine | *See* section on Tranquilizers | | |
| Piperazine | Vermifuge | Convulsions in doses above 1 gm/kg; vomiting; blurred vision; weakness | Discontinue use |
| Piperoxane | Sympathetic blocking agents | Nasal congestion; miosis; tachycardia; vertigo; indigestion; weakness; vasomotor collapse | Discontinue use |
| Pipradrol (Meratran®) | Stimulant | Anorexia; insomnia; increase in excitement and anxiety in disturbed patients | Discontinue use |
| Podophyllum | Laxative | Inflammatory reaction; toxic alopecia | Discontinue use |
| Polythiazide (Renese®) | Diuretic; antihypertensive | Weakness; nausea; vertigo; skin rash | Discontinue use |
| Potassium Chloride | Cardiac arrhythmias | Enteric-coated tablets may cause ulcerating and obstructing small bowel lesions | Discontinue use or substitute natural food sources of potassium; sodium lactate for arrhythmias |

*Regulatory action of the FDA has made this preparation a prescription item. In addition, hexachlorophene is excluded from cosmetics, except as part of a preservative system, in levels not to exceed 0.1%. There is a firm basis of concern, especially in infants, about indiscriminate and prolonged exposure of humans to hexachlorophene.

TABLE 128—*Continued*
MISCELLANEOUS DRUG COMPOUNDS

| *Drug* | *Use* | *Toxic Effect* | *Treatment* |
|---|---|---|---|
| Primaquine Phosphate | Antimalarial | Hemolytic anemia; postural hypotension, weakness; methemoglobinemia; agranulocytosis; gastric distress | Discontinue use |
| Primidone (Mysoline®) | Antiepileptic | Drowsiness; ataxia; psychotic episodes; irritability or lethargy; vertigo | Discontinue use |
| Privine® | Vasoconstrictor | Severe headache; excitement; acute anxiety; cold perspiration; cyanosis, especially of lips and fingertips; respiratory failure | Discontinue use |
| Probenecid (Benemid®) | Gout | Nausea; skin rash; rarely liver necrosis; anaphylactoid reaction; renal colic; hematuria; reducing substance in the urine | Discontinue use |
| Progesterone | Endocrine drug | Porphyria | Discontinue use |
| Promazine Hydrochloride (Sparine®) | *See* section on Tranquilizers | | |
| Promoxolane | Muscle relaxant | Gastrointestinal upset | Discontinue use |
| Prophenpyridamine Maleate (Trimeton®) | *See* section on Antihistaminics | | |
| Propanolol HCL (Inderal) | β-adrenergic blocking agent (for cardiac arrhythmias) | Nausea; vomiting; diarrhea; vertigo; insomnia; weakness and fatigue; hypotension; bradycardia; agranulocytosis | Discontinue use or reduce dosage; glucagon for bradycardia and hypotension |
| Propylthiouracil | Antithyroid | Drug fever; skin rashes; granulocytopenia; purpura; hypoprothrombinemia | Discontinue use |
| Protriptyline HCL (Vivactil®) | Antidepressant | Tachycardia and postural hypotension; dry mouth; dilated pupils and blurring of vision; dystonia; ataxia; tremor; fatigue; weakness; dizziness; vertigo; insomnia; tingling of extremities; allergic skin reaction; MAO drugs may potentiate effects | Discontinue use or reduce dosage |
| Pyrethyldione (Sedulon, Presidon) | Hypnotic, cough sedative | Flushing; headache; fatigue; dizziness; staggering; unconsciousness | Discontinue use |
| Pyridine | Solvent | Headache; insomnia and restlessness; vertigo; muscular incoordination; disturbances in hearing; severe peripheral neuritis | Discontinue use |
| Pyridium | Antiseptic | Methemoglobinemia; hepatitis; hemolytic anemia; vomitus and urine deeply red stained; urinary tract calculi | Discontinue use; force fluids |
| Pyrimethamine | Antimalarial | Anemia; leukopenia | Discontinue use |
| Quinacrine Hydrochloride | Antimalarial | Headache; hepatitis; aplastic anemia; psychosis; yellow skin | Discontinue use |
| Rauwolfia Alkaloids (Rauwiloid®) | Cardiovascular drug | Lassitude; diarrhea; nasal stuffiness; cardiac pain; extrasystoles; edema; congestive failure; thrombocytopenia; tremors and muscular spasm; depression | Discontinue use |
| Resorcinol | *See* section on Phenol | | |
| Rhubarb | *See* section on Oxalates | | |

TABLE 128—*Continued*
MISCELLANEOUS DRUG COMPOUNDS

| *Drug* | *Use* | *Toxic Effect* | *Treatment* |
|---|---|---|---|
| Rosemary Oil | Rubefacient | Rapid, weak pulse; nausea and vomiting; unconsciousness; hyperactive reflexes; marked albuminuria; pulmonary edema | Discontinue use |
| Saccharin (anhydro-o-sulfamine benzoic acid) | Sweetening agent | 5 gm has caused nausea, vomiting and diarrhea; large daily doses may produce gastric hyperacidity | Discontinue use or reduce dosage |
| Saffron | Coloring and flavoring agent | Severe gastric pain; vomiting sometimes bloodstained; diarrhea, with or without blood; rapid weak pulse; hematuria; convulsions; coma | Gastric lavage |
| Sage | Carminative | Marked dyspnea; weak rapid pulse; lowered blood pressure; symptoms of shock; generalized convulsions | Discontinue use; short-acting barbiturates for convulsions |
| Salicylamide | Analgesic; antipyretic | Toxicity compares with that of other salicylates; can be used safely in those allergic to aspirin | Gastric lavage or emesis |
| Saltpeter (potassium nitrate) | *See* section on Nitrates | | |
| Santonin | Anthelmintic | Amblyopia; amaurosis; restriction of visual field | Discontinue use |
| Scarlet Red (amino-azotoluene) | To promote epithelization of skin | Nausea and vomiting; fever and general malaise; hypotension; severe abdominal pain; sometimes diarrhea | Discontinue use; gastric lavage if ingested |
| Sedicin | Sedative | Widespread purpuric eruptions with pruritus | Discontinue use |
| Sedormid | Sedative; hypnotic | Polyneuritis; thrombocytopenia; coma; convulsions | Symptomatic and supportive |
| Selenium Sulfide (Selsun®) | Seborrhea (In industries for the manufacture of glass, photoelectric cells, etc.) | Diffuse hair loss; metallic taste; dermatitis; weight loss; weakness; depression | Discontinue use or exposures |
| Somnifene | Sedative; hypnotic | Vomiting and immediate deep sleep | Gastric lavage |
| Spirit of Niter | *See* section on Nitrites | | |
| Spironolactone (Aldactone-A®) | Diuretic | Electrolyte imbalance (hyponatremia and hyperkalemia); drowsiness; ataxia; skin rashes; gynecomastia | Discontinue use |
| Stanozolol (Winstrol®) | Anabolic steroid | Hirsutism; acne; voice change; edema; menstrual irregularities | Discontinue use |
| Stibamine Glucoside (Neostam®) | Chemotherapy | Vomiting; diarrhea; fall in blood pressure; respiratory depression; sensitivity reactions; liver damage, contraindicated in liver, kidney or pulmonary disease | Discontinue use |
| Stibophen (Fuadin®) | Chemotherapy | As above | Discontinue use |
| Stilbamidine Isethionate | Chemotherapy | Trigeminal nerve damage; liver or kidney damage from old solutions; do not use in the presence of liver or kidney disease | Discontinue use |
| Stramonium | *See* section on Atropine | | |
| Streptokinase- | Enzymes for remov- | Chills; restlessness; profuse per- | Discontinue use |

TABLE 128—*Continued*
MISCELLANEOUS DRUG COMPOUNDS

| *Drug* | *Use* | *Toxic Effect* | *Treatment* |
|---|---|---|---|
| streptodornase (Varidase®) | al of clotted blood or purulent material | spiration; pain in chest, shortness of breath; anaphylactic shock | |
| Strophanthin | Cardiovascular | Anxiety; labored respiration; contracted pupils; pulse either rapid or slow and thready | Discontinue use |
| Succinylcholine Chloride | Myoneural blocking agent;short-acting muscle relaxant | Muscular fasciculation; apnea; elevated blood pressure; cardiac irregularities such as auricular standstill, nodal rhythm or ventricular tachycardia may appear | Discontinue use |
| Sulfobromo-phthalein Sodium (BSP) | Liver function tests* | Anxiety; oppression in the chest; dyspnea; vomiting; circulatory collapse | Discontinue use |
| Para-sulfonedi-chloramidobenzoic Acid (Halazone®) | Sterilization of drinking water | Loss of consciousness; tremors; convulsions | Supportive and symptomatic for anoxia and convulsions |
| Sulfonmethane (Sulfonal) | Sedative | Deep sleep which may pass into stupor; vomiting with acetone odor; and later thirst, constipation and coproporphyrinuria | Discontinue use |
| Sulfur | Dermatology | Symptoms of hydrogen sulfide poisoning; headache; vertigo; excitement | Discontinue use |
| Tacobromine | Diuretic and myocardial stimulant | Violent headache; insomnia; excitement; bradycardia or tachycardia; oliguria; tremors; nausea; vomiting; diarrhea | Discontinue use |
| Tartar Emetic | Effervescent powders of antimony and potassium tartrate | Nausea and vomiting; severe abdominal cramping and pain; diarrhea; circulatory collapse | Discontinue use; antimony therapy |
| Tartaric Acid | *See* Tartar Emetic | | |
| Tempra | Antipyretic; analgesic | N-acetyl-*p*-aminophenol (major metabolic end product of acetanilid and phenacetin) | |
| Terpenes | Volatile oil | Some of the terpenes may cause severe injury to the skin | Discontinue use |
| Tetraethylammonium Bromide and Chloride | Hypertension | Severe and sudden lowering of the blood pressure associated with vascular collapse; signs of cerebral anoxia and respiratory arrest | Discontinue use |
| Tetraethylammonium Salts | *See* Tetraethylammonium | | |
| Tetrahydrozoline HCL (Tyzine®) | Nasal decongestant | Drowsiness; profuse sweating; marked hypotension; shock | Discontinue use |
| Thihexinol Methylbromide (Entoquel®)* | Parasympatholytic agent | Xerostomia; mydriasis; flushing of the skin; dysuria | Reduce dosage |
| Thimerosal (Merthiolate®) | Antiseptic | Occasional urticaria progressing to weeping dermatitis; rarely anemia; leukopenia and liver damage; ingestion may cause symptoms of mercury salt poisoning | Discontinue use; mercury therapy |
| Thiocyanates | Hypertension | Nausea and vomiting; diarrhea; acute gastric pain; edema of the glottis or larynx; acute depression and exhaustion; signs of hypothyroidism | Discontinue use |

*Drugs found to interfere with BSP tests are barbiturates, chlortetracycline, contraceptives (oral estrogens), heparin, iodine-containing radiologic contrast media, meperidine, methadone, phenazopyridine, phenolphthalein and probenecid.

TABLE 128—*Continued*
MISCELLANEOUS DRUG COMPOUNDS

| *Drug* | *Use* | *Toxic Effect* | *Treatment* |
|---|---|---|---|
| Thioglycerol | Promotion of wound healing | Marked sensitizing action, said to be greater than that of thioglycolic acid | Discontinue use |
| Thiopental Sodium | Sedative | Intravenous injection action of 0.3 to 1.0 gm has been followed by vomiting, respiratory depression, coughing and choking because of laryngeal spasm | Reduce dosage or discontinue use |
| Thiosemicarbazone | Chemotherapy | Liver damage; skin eruptions; anemia; leukopenia | Discontinue use |
| Thiosinamine | To promote the absorption of fibrous tissue such as scars | Gastric irritation; garlicky odor of breath; hemorrhages from the mucous membranes | Reduce dosage or discontinue use |
| Thiouracil | Hyperthyroidism; thyrotoxicosis | Nausea; dizziness; abdominal pain | Discontinue use |
| Thiourea | Thyrotoxicosis | Enlargement of the spleen; maculopapular eruptions with monocytosis and leukopenia | Discontinue use |
| Thorotrast (thorium dioxide) | Diagnostic agent; declared unsafe by FDA | Renal damage and local inflammatory reactions; progressive myelopathy; thorotrastoma | Discontinue use; surgical removal of thorotrastomas |
| Thymol | Antiseptic | Feeling of warmth in stomach; dizziness and ataxia; nausea and vomiting; excitement; severe epigastric pain; marked generalized weakness | Discontinue use |
| Thyroid§ | Endocrine drug | Ingestion of 0.3 gm/kg desiccated thyroid has caused fever, tachycardia, hypertension, hyperactivity and cardiovascular collapse. Recovery followed† | Gastric lavage |
| Tolazoline Hydrochloride (Priscoline® HCl) | Adrenolytic; sympatholytic; vasodilator | Flushing; paresthesia; tingling; chilliness; tachycardia; nausea; epigastric distress; postural hypotension; severe cardiac pain | Discontinue use |
| Tolbutamide (Orinase®) | Diabetes mellitus | Leukopenia; thrombocytopenia; nephrosis; impaired liver function; hypoglycemia; nausea and vomiting; weakness; intolerance to alcohol; skin eruptions | Discontinue use; concurrent antibacterial sulfonamides may provoke severe hypoglycemia |
| Tranylcypromine (Parnate)* | Antidepressant | Postural hypotension; dizziness; agitation; confusion and incoherence (psychotic episodes); paradoxical hypertensive reaction when used with Tofrānil, Elavil, MAO inhibitors or ingestion of cheese | Discontinue use; do not use in combination with Tofrānil, Elavil, or MAO inhibitors; omit cheese from diet; avoid alcohol |
| Treburon | Anticoagulant | Large doses have resulted in alopecia of the scalp, and to a lesser extent, of the eyebrows, suprapubic and axillary areas; diarrhea; nosebleed | Discontinue use |

§Fortunately, it requires a great deal of thyroid hormone to cause a devastating reaction. There is a report (Schottstaedt, E. S., and Smoller, M.: *Ann Intern Med, 64*:847, 1966) of a very serious illness resulting from the ingestion of 48 gm of desiccated thyroid. It produced a kind of thyroid storm. The reason for the rarity of self-inflicted thyroid storm is simply that it requires enormous amounts of hormone. In the natural disease hyperthyroidism, several hundred micrograms of thyroxine and triiodothyronine are manufactured each day for months or years. Since the half-life of thyroxine is relatively long (four to six days even when speeded by the hyperthyroid state), it tends to cumulate and this leads to progressively more severe symptoms. On the other hand, in accidental cases of thyroid ingestion, only a single dose is taken and no cumulation occurs.

TABLE 128—*Continued*
MISCELLANEOUS DRUG COMPOUNDS

| *Drug* | *Use* | *Toxic Effect* | *Treatment* |
|---|---|---|---|
| Triamterene (Dyrenium®) | Diuretic | Nausea and vomiting; diarrhea; weakness; dry mouth; headache; rash | Discontinue use or reduce dosage |
| Triethylene Melamine (T.E.M.) | Antineoplastic agent | Lymphopenia | Discontinue use |
| Triparanol (MER/29)* | Hypercholesterolemia | Loss of body hair; baldness; dry itchy skin; exfoliation; ichthyosis; impotency; leukopenia | Discontinue use |
| Tybamate (Solacen®, Tybatran®) | Tranquilizer | Drowsiness; dizziness; nausea; vomiting; dry mouth; blurred vision; glossitis; euphoria; paresthesia | Discontinue use or reduce dosage |
| Undecylenic Acid | Antiseptic | Exudative dermatitis; nausea; fever; headache after ingesting | Discontinue use |
| Urethane | Antineoplastic | Vomiting; coma; hemorrhages; kidney and liver damage | Discontinue use |
| Vasopressin (Pitressin®) | Diabetes insipidus; portal variceal bleeding | Myocardial injury; tremor; sweating; vertigo; circumoral pallor; nausea and vomiting | Discontinue use. This drug should never be given IV to patients with vascular disease, especially disease of the coronary arteries |
| Vitamin A (20 to 100 times daily requirement) | Vitamin | Painful nodular periosteal swelling; itching; skin eruptions; anorexia; and occasionally, liver enlargement | Discontinue use |
| Vitamin $B_1$ | Vitamin | Drug fever and anaphylaxis after intravenous administration | Discontinue use |
| Vitamin D (150,000 IU or more daily) | Vitamin | Weakness; nausea; vomiting; diarrhea; anemia; decrease in renal function with polyuria and moderate elevation of blood pressure. Serum calcium and BUN are raised. X-rays show metastatic calcification in the kidney, heart, blood vessels and skin | Discontinue use |
| Vitamin K | Vitamin | Hemolytic anemia, hyperbilirubinemia, icterus, enlargement of liver and death in newborn infants from excessive doses | Discontinue use or reduce dosage |
| Warfarin (Coumadin®) Panwarfin®) | Anticoagulant (vs other drugs, *see* Table 129) | Hemorrhages; urticaria; hypersensitive reactions; alopecia; experimentally in dogs, certain drugs such as glutethimide, amobarbital, secobarbital and meprobamate reduce the warfarin plasma half-life and increase the amount of warfarin required to maintain adequate anticoagulation. A syndrome of congenital anomalies has been attributed to maternal consumption of Coumadin during pregnancy. | Vitamin K and fresh whole blood for uncontrolled bleeding. Diazoxid; ethacrynic, mefenamic and nalidixic acids may potentiate anticoagulant effect. *See* Table 129. |
| Xylene | Organic solvent | Exposures to the vapors of xylene frequently result in fatigue, headache and conjunctivitis | Discontinue use or exposure |
| Zephiran® Chloride | Antiseptic | Somnolence; unconsciousness; circulatory disturbances; nystagmus; polyuria | Discontinue use |
| Zoxazolamine (Flexin)* | Muscle relaxant | Nausea; vomiting; anorexia; headache; skin rash; malaise; renal and hepatic injury | Discontinue use |

*Drugs indicated by an asterisk have been removed from the market or are obsolete.

TABLE 129
ORAL ANTICOAGULANTS VS. OTHER DRUGS

**Drugs that diminish anticoagulant response**

| *By enzyme induction* | *By stimulation of clotting factor synthesis* |
|---|---|
| phenobarbital | phytonadione |
| butabarbital | estrogens |
| heptabarbital | |
| amobarbital | |
| secobarbital | |
| glutethimide | |
| ethchlorvynol | |
| meprobamate | |
| griseofulvin | |

**Drugs that increase anticoagulant response**

| *By enzyme inhibition* | *By depression of clotting factor synthesis* |
|---|---|
| phenyramidol | salicylate |
| methylphenidate | acetaminophen |
| disulfiram | quinidine |
| chloramphenicol | mercaptopurine |
| | |
| *By displacement of anticoagulant from plasma albumin* | *By reducing availability of vitamin $K_1$* |
| phenylbutazone | broad-spectrum antibiotics |
| oxyphenbutazone | mineral oil |
| clofibrate | |
| chloral hydrate | |
| | |
| *By increasing receptor site affinity* | *Mechanism unknown* |
| dextrothyroxine | norethandrolone |
| | methandrostenolone |

**Drugs whose effects are increased by anticoagulants**

oral hypoglycemic agents: tolbutamide
chlorpropamide
diphenylhydantoin

Based on: Solomon, H. M., Barakat, M. J., Ashley, C. J.: "Mechanisms of drug interaction," *JAMA*, Vol. 216, No. 12.

# DRUG INFORMATION CENTERS

It is obviously impossible for any busy clinician to stay abreast of all advances being made every day in drug therapy. To help fill this information gap, drug information centers (DICs) throughout the United States maintain specialized libraries containing comprehensive data about United States, foreign and investigational drugs—including their identification, side-effects, adverse effects, interactions, indications, drugs of choice for given conditions (with alternatives), drug-induced alterations of laboratory test values, United States equivalents of foreign drugs, bioavailability data, etc. You can phone or write the DIC nearest you for the information you want (*see* Table 130).

Two valuable and useful drug and toxicological information publications are: (1) *Physicians' Desk Reference* (PDR) which most physicians have readily available on their desk, and (2) *Facts and Comparisons* published by Facts and Comparisons, Inc. of 111 West Port Plaza, St. Louis, MO 63141. This large loose leaf volume offers prescribing information in comprehensive drug monographs which may be presented (i.e. Thiazide Diuretics) as a group monograph while specific information relating to a particular drug is presented in an individual drug monograph under the generic drug name. Actions, indications, contra-indications, warnings and precautions, drug interactions, adverse reactions, overdosage and administration and dosage are all briefly summarized for each listed drug. Monthly revisions are issued to keep drug information up to date, and the index is completely revised and reissued every three months.

TABLE 130
DRUG INFORMATION CENTERS*

| *City* | *Name, Address and Phone* | *Hours* | *Services* |
|---|---|---|---|
| | **ALABAMA** | | |
| Birmingham | G. Edward Collins<br>Drug Information Center<br>University of Alabama Hospitals<br>Birmingham 35233<br>Phone: (205) 934-2162 | Mon.-Fri. 8 AM-5 PM | Provides newsletters, lectures, etc.<br>No fee charged. |
| | **CALIFORNIA** | | |
| Berkeley | Lawrence Fleckenstein<br>Alta Bates Hospital<br>Drug Information Service<br>Berkeley 94705<br>Phone: (415) 845-7110 Ext. 209 | Mon.-Sun. and Hol. 8:30 AM-5 PM | Provides drug abuse information and also newsletters, lectures, etc.<br>No fee charged. |
| Long Beach | Byron F. Schweigert<br>Drug Information Center<br>Memorial Hospital Medical Center of Long Beach<br>Long Beach 90801<br>Phone: (213) 595-2303 | Mon.-Sun. and Hol. 8 AM-5 PM (24 hr. emergency service) | Provides drug abuse information and also newsletters, lectures, etc.<br>Charges fee. |
| Los Angeles | G. Thompson<br>Drug Information Center<br>LAC-USC Medical Center | Mon.-Fri. and Hol. 8 AM-5 PM | Provides newsletters, lectures, etc.<br>Charges fee. |

*As this information is put to press, there are reports of four new centers opening in New Orleans (Louisiana College of Pharmacy of Xavier University); Annapolis, Maryland (Anne Arundel General Hospital); Omaha, Nebraska (University of Nebraska); and Royal Oaks, Michigan (William Beaumont Hospital).

TABLE 130—*Continued*
DRUG INFORMATION CENTERS

| *City* | *Name, Address and Phone* | *Hours* | *Services* |
|---|---|---|---|
| | 1200 N. State St.<br>Los Angeles 90033<br>Phone: (213) 226-7741 | | |
| San Francisco | Gary McCart<br>Drug Information Analysis Service<br>University of California<br>San Francisco 94131<br>Phone: (415) 666-4346 | Mon.-Fri. 8 AM-6 PM | Provides newsletters, lectures, etc.<br>No fee charged. |
| Ventura | William B. Mead<br>Community Memorial Hospital<br>2800 Loma Vista Rd.<br>Ventura 93003<br>Phone: (805) 648-8711 Ext. 226 | Mon.-Fri. 6 AM-10 PM<br>Sat., Sun. and Hol. 7 AM-4:30 PM | Provides drug abuse information and also newsletters, lectures, etc.<br>No fee charged. |
| | **CONNECTICUT** | | |
| Farmington | Alex A. Cardoni<br>Drug Information Service<br>University of Connecticut Health Center<br>Farmington 06032<br>Phone: (203) 674-2782 or (203) 674-2783 | Mon.-Fri. 8 AM-5 PM<br>(24 hr. emergency service) | Provides drug abuse information and also newsletters, lectures, etc.<br>No fee charged. |
| New Haven | Arthur G. Lipman<br>Yale-New Haven Hospital<br>789 Howard Avenue<br>New Haven 06504<br>Phone: (203) 436-4880 | Mon.-Sun. and Hol.<br>24 hr. service | Provides newsletters, lectures, etc.<br>No fee charged. |
| | **DISTRICT OF COLUMBIA** | | |
| Washington, D.C. | Jay Barbaccia<br>Drug Information Center<br>Washington Hospital Center<br>110 Irving St. NW<br>Washington 20010<br>Phone: (202) 541-6646 | Mon.-Fri. 8 AM-4 PM | Provides newsletters, lectures, etc.<br>No fee charged. |
| | **FLORIDA** | | |
| Gainesville | M. Peter Pevonka<br>Drug Information and Pharmacy Resource Center<br>MSB 779<br>J. Hillis Miller Health Center<br>University of Florida<br>Gainesville 32610<br>Phone: 1-800-342-1106 Toll free | Mon.-Fri. 9 AM-5 PM | Provides newsletters, lectures, etc.<br>No fee charged. |
| Miami | Harry Keusch<br>Victoria Hospital Drug Information Service<br>955 N.W. Third St.<br>Miami 33628<br>Phone: (305) 545-8050 | Mon.-Sun. and Hol.<br>7 AM-11 PM | Provides drug abuse information and also newsletters, lectures, etc.<br>No fee charged. |
| | **GEORGIA** | | |
| Augusta | Merle W. Riley<br>Drug Information Center<br>Medical College of Georgia<br>Augusta 30902<br>Phone: (404) 828-2887 | Mon.-Fri. 9 AM-5 PM | Provides newsletters, lectures, etc.<br>No fee charged. |

TABLE 130—*Continued*
DRUG INFORMATION CENTERS

| *City* | *Name, Address and Phone* | *Hours* | *Services* |
|---|---|---|---|
| | **ILLINOIS** | | |
| Chicago | Marilyn Leonian<br>Drug and Poison Information Center<br>South Chicago Community Hospital<br>2320 E. 93rd St.<br>Chicago 60617<br>Phone: (312) 978-2000 | Mon.-Fri. 8 AM-4:30 PM | Provides newsletters, lectures, etc.<br>No fee charged. |
| Chicago | Susan Mendelewski<br>University of Chicago Hospitals and Clinics<br>950 E. 59th St.<br>Chicago 60637<br>Phone: (312) 947-6046 | Mon.-Fri. 8:30 AM-5 PM | Provides newsletters, lectures, etc.<br>No fee charged. |
| Chicago | Ernest Gurwich<br>University of Illinois Hospital Drug Information Center<br>840 S. Wood St.<br>Chicago 60612<br>Phone: (312) 996-6885 | Mon.-Fri. 8:30 AM-5 PM | Provides newsletters, lectures, etc.<br>No fee charged. |
| Normal | Terry W. Trudeau<br>Drug Information and Poison Control Center<br>Brokaw Hospital<br>Virginia and Franklin Sts.<br>Normal 61761<br>Phone: (309) 829-7685 Ext. 223 | Mon.-Sun. and Hol.<br>6:45 AM-11:30 PM | Is also a major poison information center, provides drug abuse information, and newsletters, lectures, etc.<br>No fee charged. |
| Rockford | Donald Mickalski<br>Rockford Drug Information Center<br>Swedish American Hospital<br>1316 Charles St.<br>Rockford 61101<br>Phone: (815) 968-6898 Ext. 54 | Mon.-Sun. and Hol.<br>24 hr. service | Is also a major poison information center, provides drug abuse information, and newsletters, lectures, etc.<br>No fee charged. |
| | **KENTUCKY** | | |
| Lexington | Ann B. Amerson<br>Drug Information Center<br>Albert B. Chandler Medical Center and College of Pharmacy<br>University of Kentucky<br>Lexington 40506<br>Phone: (606) 233-5320 | Mon.-Fri. 8 AM-5 PM | Provides newsletters, lectures, etc.<br>No fee charged. |
| | **LOUISIANA** | | |
| Monroe | John J. Guerriero, Jr.<br>St. Francis Hospital Drug Information and Poison Control Center<br>309 Jackson St.<br>Monroe 71201<br>Phone: (318) 325-6454 | Mon.-Sun. and Hol.<br>7:30 AM-10 PM | A major poison information center, also provides newsletters, lectures, etc.<br>No fee charged. |
| | **MICHIGAN** | | |
| Ann Arbor | Stewart B. Siskin<br>Drug Information Center<br>University of Michigan Hospital Pharmacy | Mon.-Sun. and Hol.<br>24 hr. service | Provides newsletters, lectures, etc.<br>No fee charged. |

TABLE 130—*Continued*
DRUG INFORMATION CENTERS

| *City* | *Name, Address and Phone* | *Hours* | *Services* |
|---|---|---|---|
| | 1405 E. Ann St.<br>Ann Arbor 48104<br>Phone: (313) 763-0243 | | |
| Detroit | Gerald Zieg<br>The Grace Hospital Drug Information Center<br>The Grace Hospital<br>4160 John R. St.<br>Detroit 48201<br>Phone: (313) 494-6083 | Mon.-Sun. and Hol. 7 AM-11 PM | Provides newsletters, lectures, etc.<br>No fee charged. |
| Ionia | Richard L. Munschy<br>Pharmacy Clinic Riverside Center<br>Riverside Center<br>777 W. Riverside Dr.<br>Ionia 48846<br>Phone: (616) 527-0110 Ext. 255 | Mon.-Fri. 9 AM-5 PM | Is also a major poison information center, provides drug abuse information, and newsletters, lectures, etc.<br>No fee charged. |
| Kalamazoo | John H. Trestraid III<br>Bronson Methodist Hospital<br>Drugs and Poison Information Center<br>252 W. Lovell St.<br>Kalamazoo 49006<br>Phone: (616) 383-6409 | Mon.-Sun. and Hol. 6 AM-11:30 PM | Is also a major poison information center, provides drug abuse information, and newsletters, lectures, etc.<br>No fee charged. |
| Saginaw | Dale F. Schultz<br>Saginaw General Hospital<br>1447 N. Harrison St.<br>Saginaw 48602<br>Phone: (517) 753-3411 Ext. 253 | Mon.-Fri. 7 AM-8 PM<br>Sat., Sun. and Hol. 8 AM-6 PM | A major poison information center, also provides drug abuse information.<br>No fee charged. |
| Southfield | Robert C. Barger<br>Providence Hospital Drug Information Center<br>16001 W. Nine Mile Rd.<br>Southfield 48075<br>Phone: (313) 424-3125 | Mon.-Fri. 9 AM-5 PM<br>Sat. 9 AM-12 noon | Provides newsletters, lectures, etc.<br>No fee charged. |
| | **MINNESOTA** | | |
| Minneapolis | Roger D. Schroeder<br>Drug Information<br>University of Minnesota Hospitals<br>412 Union St. SE<br>Minneapolis 55455<br>Phone: (612) 373-8888 | Mon.-Fri. 8 AM-11 PM<br>Sat., Sun. and Hol. 10 AM-8 PM | Provides drug abuse information and also newsletters, lectures, etc.<br>No fee charged. |
| | **MISSOURI** | | |
| Kansas City | Thomas J. Garrison<br>Lakeside Hospital<br>8701 Troost<br>Kansas City 64131<br>Phone: (816) 363-6380 Ext. 267 | Mon.-Fri. and Sun. 7 AM-11 PM; Sat. 7 AM-8 PM; Hol. 7AM-6 PM | Provides newsletters, lectures, etc.<br>No fee charged. |
| | William G. Troutman<br>Western Missouri Area Health Education Center Drug Information Service<br>Rm. M3-102<br>WMKC School of Medicine | Mon.-Fri. 8 AM-5 PM | Provides drug abuse information.<br>No fee charged. |

TABLE 130—*Continued*
DRUG INFORMATION CENTERS

| City | Name, Address and Phone | Hours | Services |
|---|---|---|---|
| | 2411 Holmes St.<br>Kansas City 64108<br>Phone: (816) 471-1895 | | |
| | The following eight hospitals are associated with this drug information center. | | |
| | Freeman Hospital<br>Joplin 64801<br>Phone: (417) 623-2801 | Same as above | Same as above |
| | St. John's Medical Center<br>Joplin 64801<br>Phone: (417) 781-2727 | Same as above | Same as above |
| | Methodist Hospital and Medical Center<br>St. Joseph 64501<br>Phone: (816) 232-8461 | Same as above | Same as above |
| | St. Joseph Hospital<br>St. Joseph 64501<br>Phone: (816) 279-0821 | Same as above | Same as above |
| | John H. Bothwell Memorial Hospital<br>Sedalia 65301<br>Phone: (816) 826-8833 | Same as above | Same as above |
| | Lester E. Cox Medical Center<br>Springfield 65802<br>Phone: (417) 836-3000 | Same as above | Same as above |
| | St. John's Hospital<br>Springfield 65802<br>Phone: (417) 881-8811 | Same as above | Same as above |
| | Johnson County Memorial Hospital<br>Warrensburg 64093<br>Phone: (816) 747-3181 | Same as above | Same as above |
| St. Louis | Kenneth R. Keefner<br>St. Louis College of Pharmacy<br>Euclid Ave and Parkview Pl.<br>St. Louis 63110<br>Phone: (314) 367-8700 | Mon.-Fri. 9 AM-5 PM | Also a drug abuse information center, provides newsletters, lectures, etc.<br>No fee charged. |
| | **NEBRASKA** | | |
| Omaha | Paul D. Groth<br>Creighton University Drug Information Services<br>Creighton University<br>School of Pharmacy<br>2500 California<br>Omaha 68124<br>Phone: (402) 536-3000 | Mon.-Fri. 8 AM-5 PM | Provides newsletters, lectures, etc.<br>Charges fee. |
| | **NEW JERSEY** | | |
| Ridgewood | Jack M. Rosenberg<br>The New Jersey Regional Medical Program Pharmaceutic and Therapeutic Drug Information Center<br>The Valley Hospital<br>Ridgewood 07451<br>Phone: (201) 445-4900 Ext. 131 | Mon.-Fri. 9 AM-5 PM | Provides newsletters, lectures, etc.<br>No fee charged. |

TABLE 130—*Continued*
DRUG INFORMATION CENTERS

| *City* | *Name, Address and Phone* | *Hours* | *Services* |
|---|---|---|---|
| Ocean County | Millard B. Hall<br>Community Memorial Hospital<br>Rte. 37 West<br>Toms River 08753<br>Phone: (201) 349-8000 Ext. 209 | Mon.-Fri. 7:30 AM-4:30 PM | No fee charged. |
| | **NEW MEXICO** | | |
| Albuquerque | Diana F. Rodriguez-Calvert<br>New Mexico Poison and Drug Information Center<br>Bernalillo County Medical Center<br>2211 Lomas Blvd. NE<br>Albuquerque 87131<br>Phone: (505) 266-5503 | Mon.-Sun. and Hol. 24 hr. service | Has a formal training program for medical students, interns and residents. A major poison information center, also provides drug abuse information, newsletters, lectures, etc.<br>No fee charged. |
| | **NEW YORK** | | |
| Buffalo | Robert E. Pearson<br>Drug Information Service<br>Department of Pharmacy<br>State University of New York at Buffalo<br>60 High St.<br>Buffalo 14203<br>Phone: (800) 462-1076 or (716) 842-3819 | Mon.-Fri. 8 AM-5 PM (24 hr. emergency service) | Provides newsletters, lectures, etc.<br>No fee charged. |
| New York City | Jack M. Rosenberg<br>The Arnold and Marie Schwartz Inter-Regional Pharmaceutic and Therapeutic Drug Information Center of the Brooklyn College of Pharmacy<br>600 Lafayette Ave.<br>Brooklyn 11216<br>Phone: (212) 622-8989 or (212) 636-7535 | Mon.-Fri. 9 AM-4:30 PM | Provides newsletters, lectures, etc.<br>No fee charged. |
| | H.M. Silverman<br>Drug Information Service<br>Lenox Hill Hospital<br>100 E. 77th St.<br>New York 10021<br>Phone: (212) 794-4280 | Mon.-Fri. 9 AM-5 PM | No fee charged |
| | Eugene Weiss<br>Drug Information Service<br>Montefiore Hospital and Medical Center<br>111 E. 210th St.<br>Bronx 10467<br>Phone: (212) 920-4511 and (212) 920-4103 | Mon.-Fri. 8:30 AM-5 PM (24 hr. emergency service) | Has a formal training program for medical students, interns and residents. Provides newsletters, lectures, etc.<br>No fee charged. |
| Rockville Centre | William S. Tomasulo<br>Drug Information Center<br>Mercy Hospital<br>1000 N. Village Ave.<br>Rockville Centre 11570<br>Phone: (516) 255-2407 | Mon.-Fri. 8 AM-4 PM | Provides drug abuse information and also newsletters, lectures, etc.<br>No fee charged. |

TABLE 130—*Continued*
DRUG INFORMATION CENTERS

| *City* | *Name, Address and Phone* | *Hours* | *Services* |
|---|---|---|---|
| | **NORTH CAROLINA** | | |
| Chapel Hill | Benjamin O. Williams<br>Drug Information Program<br>University of North Carolina<br>School of Pharmacy<br>N.C. Memorial Hospital<br>Chapel Hill 27514<br>Phone: (919) 966-2371 | Mon.-Fri. 9 AM-6 PM | Provides newsletters, lectures, etc.<br>No fee charged. |
| Charlotte | Jerry S. Curry<br>Drug Information Center<br>Charlotte Memorial Hospital<br>1000 Blythe Blvd.<br>Charlotte 28201<br>Phone: 1-704-373-2434 Toll free | Mon.-Fri. 8 AM-4:30 PM | Provides drug abuse information and also newsletters, lectures, etc.<br>No fee charged. |
| | **OHIO** | | |
| Cincinnati | Leonard Sigell<br>Cincinnati Drug and Poison Information Center<br>Rm. E7-8<br>234 Goodman St.<br>Cincinnati 45267<br>Phone: (513) 872-5111 | Mon.-Sun. and Hol. 24 hr. service | A major poison information center, also provides drug abuse information, and newsletters, lectures, etc.<br>No fee charged. |
| Columbus | James A. Visconti<br>The Ohio State University Drug Information Center<br>Ohio State University Hospital<br>410 W. 10th Ave<br>Columbus 43210<br>Phone: (614) 422-8733 | Mon.-Fri. 7 AM-6 PM | Provides drug abuse information and also newsletters, lectures, etc.<br>No fee charged. |
| Zanesville | Steve Deedrick<br>Bethesda Hospital<br>Drug Information Center<br>Maple Ave.<br>Zanesville 43701<br>Phone: (614) 454-4203 | Mon.-Sun. and Hol. 8 AM-10 PM | A major poison information center, also provides drug abuse information, and newsletters, lectures, etc.<br>No fee charged. |
| | **OREGON** | | |
| Corvallis | Freya Hermann<br>Drug Information Service<br>Oregan State University<br>School of Pharmacy<br>Corvallis 97331<br>Phone: (503) 754-3535 | Mon.-Fri. 8 AM-5 PM | Provides newsletters, lectures, etc.<br>No fee charged. |
| | **PENNSYLVANIA** | | |
| Erie | William N. Kelly<br>Pharmacy and Drug Information Service<br>Hamot Medical Center<br>4 E. Second St.<br>Erie 16512<br>Phone: (814) 455-6711 Ext. 529 | Mon.-Sun. and Hol. 7 AM-11PM | Provides drug abuse information and also newsletters, lectures, etc.<br>No fee charged. |

TABLE 130—*Continued*
DRUG INFORMATION CENTERS

| *City* | *Name, Address and Phone* | *Hours* | *Services* |
|---|---|---|---|
| Philadelphia | Joseph A. Linkewich<br>Pharmacy Service<br>Hospital of University of Pennsylvania<br>Philadelphia 19104<br>Phone: (215) 662-2903 | Mon.-Fri. 8 AM-5 PM; Sat. 8 AM-4 PM (24 hr. emergency service) | Provides newsletters, lectures, etc.<br>No fee charged. |
| | Thomas T. Culkin<br>Thomas Jefferson University Hospital Drug Information Center<br>11th and Walnut Sts.<br>Philadelphia 19107<br>Phone: (215) 829-6736 | Mon.-Fri. 8 AM-5 PM | Provides drug abuse information and also newsletters, lectures, etc.<br>No fee charged. |
| | Frank F. Williams<br>Pharmacy Department<br>Drug Information Service<br>Temple University Hospital<br>3401 N. Broad St.<br>Philadelphia 19140<br>Phone: (215) 221-3462 | Mon.-Fri. 9 AM-4:30 PM | Provides newsletters, lectures, etc.<br>No fee charged. |
| Pittsburgh | John G. Lech<br>Drug Information Center<br>Mercy Hospital<br>Pride and Locust Sts.<br>Pittsburgh 15219<br>Phone: (412) 232-7903 | Mon.-Sun. and Hol. 24 hr. service | Provides newsletters, lectures, etc.<br>No fee charged. |
| | **RHODE ISLAND** | | |
| Providence | Philip Johnson<br>Drug Information Center<br>Rhode Island Hospital<br>593 Eddy St.<br>Providence 02902<br>Phone: (401) 277-4000 | Mon.-Fri. 8:30 AM-5 PM | A major poison information center, also provides drug abuse information, and newsletters, lectures, etc.<br>No fee charged. |
| | **SOUTH CAROLINA** | | |
| Charleston | J.L. Brueggeman<br>Medical University Poison and Drug Information Service<br>80 Barre St.<br>Charleston 29401<br>Phone: Drug Info: (803) 792-3896<br>Poison Info: (803) 792-4201 | Mon.-Fri. 8 AM-5 PM | A major poison information center, also provides drug abuse information, and newsletters, lectures, etc.<br>No fee charged. |
| Columbia | Brooks C Metts, Jr.<br>Drug and Poison Information Center<br>College of Pharmacy<br>University of South Carolina<br>Columbia 29208<br>Phone: (803) 777-4151 | Mon.-Fri. 8:30 AM-5 PM (24 hr. emergency service) | A major poison information center, also provides drug abuse information, and newsletters, lectures, etc.<br>No fee charged. |
| | **TENNESSEE** | | |
| Memphis | Domingo Martinez<br>Drug and Toxicology Information Center | Mon.-Fri. 8 AM-5 PM (24 hr. emergency service) | Provides newsletters, lectures, etc.<br>No fee charged. |

TABLE 130—*Continued*
DRUG INFORMATION CENTERS

| *City* | *Name, Address and Phone* | *Hours* | *Services* |
|---|---|---|---|
| | 800 Madison Ave.<br>Memphis 38163<br>Phone: (901) 528-5555 | | |
| | **TEXAS** | | |
| San Antonio | Ronald P. Evens<br>University of Texas Drug Information Service<br>7703 Floyd Curl Dr.<br>San Antonio 78284<br>Phone: (512) 696-6410 | Mon.-Fri. 7 AM-11 PM; Sat. 8 AM-8 PM; Sun. and Hol. 12 noon-8 PM | Provides drug abuse information and also newsletters, lectures, etc.<br>Did not reply about fees. |
| | **VIRGINIA** | | |
| Hampton | N.D. Kennedy,<br>Hampton General Hospital<br>Drug Information Center<br>3120 Victoria Blvd.<br>Hampton 23669<br>Phone: (804) 722-7921 Ext. 396 | 24 hr. service | Provides drug abuse information and also newsletters, lectures, etc.<br>No fee charged. |
| Richmond | Fred Salter<br>Virginia Drug Information and Consultative Service<br>MCV Hospitals<br>Box 42<br>Richmond 23298<br>Phone: (804) 770-4656 | 24 hr. service | Provides newsletters, lectures, etc.<br>No fee charged. |
| | Thomas A. Fox<br>Drug Information Service<br>St. Mary's Hospital<br>5801 Bremo Rd.<br>Richmond 23226<br>Phone: (804) 285-2011 Ext. 213 | 24 hr. service | Provides newsletters, lectures, etc.<br>No fee charged. |
| | **WASHINGTON** | | |
| Pullman | Philip D. Hansten<br>Drug Information Center<br>Washington State University College of Pharmacy<br>Pullman 99163<br>Phone: (509) 335-1402 | Mon.-Fri. 8 AM-5 PM | Provides newsletters, lectures, etc.<br>No fee charged. |
| Seattle | Gary H. Smith<br>Drug Information Center<br>University of Washington School of Pharmacy<br>Seattle 98195<br>Phone: (206) 543-9487 | Mon.-Fri. 8 AM-5 PM | Provides newsletters, lectures, etc.<br>No fee charged. |
| | **WEST VIRGINIA** | | |
| Morgantown | Art Jacknowitz<br>West Virginia University Drug Information Center<br>School of Pharmacy<br>West Virginia University Medical Center<br>Morgantown 26506<br>Phone: (800) 352-2501 | Mon.-Fri. 8 AM-9 PM; Sat. 8 AM-1 PM | Provides newsletters, lectures, etc.<br>No fee charged. |

TABLE 130—*Continued*
DRUG INFORMATION CENTERS

| *City* | *Name, Address and Phone* | *Hours* | *Services* |
|---|---|---|---|
| | **WISCONSIN** | | |
| Madison | Monte S. Cohon<br>Drug Information and Poison Control Center<br>University Hospitals<br>University of Wisconsin<br>1300 University Ave.<br>Madison 53706<br>Phone: Drug Info: (608) 262-1315<br>Poison Info: (608) 262-3702 | 24 hr. service | A major poison information center, also provides drug abuse information, and newsletters, lectures, etc.<br>No fee charged. |

TABLE 131
BLOOD LEVELS

| *Compound* | *Therapeutic or Normal* | *Toxic* | *Lethal* |
|---|---|---|---|
| Acetaminophen (Tylenol) | 1-2 mg% | 40 mg% | 150 mg% |
| Acetazolamide (Diamox) | 1-1.5 mg% | — | — |
| Acetohexamide (Dymelor) | 2.1-5.6 mg% | — | — |
| Acetone | — | 20-30 mg% | 55mg% |
| Aluminum | 0.013 mg% | — | — |
| Ammonia | 50-170 μg% | — | — |
| Aminophylline (Theophylline) | 1-2 mg% | — | — |
| Amitriptyline (Elavil) | 5-20 μg% | 40 μg% | 1.0-2.0 mg% |
| Amphetamine | 2-3 μg% | — | 0.2 mg% |
| Arsenic | 0.0-0.002 mg% | 0.1 mg% | 1.6 mg% |
| Barbiturates | | | |
| Short-acting | 0.1 mg% | 0.7 mg% | 1 mg% |
| Intermediate-acting | 0.1-0.8 mg% | 1-8 mg% | 3 mg% and> |
| Phenobarbital | 1.0 mg% | 4-6 mg% | 8-15 mg% and> |
| Barbital | 1.0 mg% | 6-8 mg% | 10 mg% and> |
| Benzene | — | any measurable | 0.094 mg% |
| Beryllium | Tissue levels generally used (lung & lymph) | — | — |
| Boron (Boric acid) | 0.08 mg% | 4 mg% | 5 mg% |
| Bromide | 5.0 mg% | 50-150 mg% (17 mEq/liter) | 200 mg% |
| Brompheniramine (Dimetane) | 0.8-1.5 μg% | — | — |
| Cadmium | 0.01-0.02 μg% | 0.005 mg% | — |
| Caffeine | — | — | 10 mg% and> |
| Carbamazepine (Tegretol) | 0.2 mg% | 0.8-1.0 mg% | — |
| Carbon monoxide | 1% | 15%-35% | 50% |
| Carbon tetrachloride | — | 2-5 mg% | — |
| Carisoprodol (Rela, Soma) | 1.0-4.0 mg% | — | — |
| Chloral hydrate (Noctec) | 1.0 mg% | 10 mg% | 25 mg% |

TABLE 131—*Continued*
BLOOD LEVELS

| *Compound* | *Therapeutic or Normal* | *Toxic* | *Lethal* |
|---|---|---|---|
| Chloroform | — | 7-25 mg% | 39 mg% |
| Chlordiazepoxide (Librium) | 0.1-0.3 mg% | 0.55 mg% | 2 mg% |
| Chlorpheniramine | — | 2-3 mg% | — |
| Chlorpromazine (Thorazine) | 0.05 mg% | 0.1-0.2 mg% | 0.3-1.2 mg% |
| Chlorpropamide (Diabinese) | 3.0-14.0 mg% | — | — |
| Chlorprothixine (Taractan) | 0.004-0.03 mg% | — | — |
| Codeine | 2.5 μg% | — | 20-60 μg% |
| Copper | 100-150 μg% | 540 μg% | — |
| Cyanide | 0.015 mg% | — | 0.5 mg% and > |
| DDT | 1.3 μg% | — | — |
| Desipramine (Norpramin) | 0.059-0.14 mg% | — | 1-2 mg% |
| Dextropropoxyphene (Darvon) | 5-20 μg% | 0.5-1 mg% | 5.7 mg% |
| Diazepam (Valium) | 0.05-0.25 mg% | 0.5-2.0 mg% | 2.0 mg% and> |
| Dieldrin | 0.15 μg% | — | — |
| Digitoxin | 2-3.5 μg% | — | 32 μg% |
| Digoxin | 0.06-0.13 μg% | 0.20-0.90 μg% | — |
| Dinitro-o-Cresol | — | 3-4 mg% | 7.5 mg% |
| Diphenhydramine (Benadryl) | 0.5 mg% | 1 mg% | — |
| Diphenylhydantoin (Dilantin) | 0.5-2.2 mg% | 5 mg% | 10 mg% and > |
| Divinyl oxide | — | — | 70 mg% |
| Doxepin (Sinequan) | — | — | 1.0 mg% and > |
| Ethanol | — | 150 mg% | 350 mg% and |
| Etchlorvynol (Placidyl) | ~0.5 mg% | 2 mg% | 15 mg% |
| Ethinamate (Valmid) | 0.5-1.0 mg% | — | — |
| Ethosuximide (Zarontin) | 2.5-7.5 mg% | — | — |
| Ethyl chloride | — | — | 40 mg% |
| Ethyl ether | 90-100 mg% | — | 140-189 mg% |
| Ethylene glycol | — | 150 mg% | 200-400 mg% |
| Fluoride | 0-0.05 mg% | — | 0.2 mg% |
| Glutethimide (Doriden) | 0.02 mg% | 1-8 mg% | 3-10 mg% |
| Gold (Sodium aurothionalate) | 300-600 μg% | — | — |
| Halothane (Fluothane) | 0.18 mg% | — | 20 mg% |
| Hydrogen sulfide | — | — | 0.092 mg% |
| Hydromorphone (Dilaudid) | — | — | 0.01-0.03 mg% |
| Imipramine (Tofranil) | 0.005-0.016 mg% | >0.07 mg% | 0.2 mg% |
| Isopropanol | — | 340 mg% | — |
| Iron | 50 mg% (RBC) | 0.6 mg% (serum) | — |
| Lead | 0.005-0.07 mg% | 0.13 mg% | — |
| Lidocaine | 0.2 mg% | 0.6 mg% | — |
| LSD (lysergic acid diethylamide) | — | 0.1-0.4 μg% | — |
| Lithium | 0.42-0.83 mg% (0.6-1.2 mEq/liter) | 1.39 mg% (2.0 mEq/liter) | 1.39-3.47 mg% (2.0-5.0 mEq/liter) |

TABLE 131—*Continued*
BLOOD LEVELS

| *Compound* | *Therapeutic or Normal* | *Toxic* | *Lethal* |
|---|---|---|---|
| Magnesium | 1.5-2.5 mg% | —— | 5 mg% |
| Manganese | 0.015 mg% | 0.46 mg% | —— |
| Meperidine (Demerol) | 60-65 µg% | 0.5 mg% | ~3 mg% |
| Meprobamate | 1 mg% | 10 mg% | 20 mg% |
| Mercury | 0.006-0.012 mg% | —— | —— |
| Methadone | 48-86 µg% | 0.2 mg% | 0.4 mg% and > |
| Methamphetamine | —— | 0.5 mg% | 4 mg% |
| Methanol | —— | 20 mg% | 89 mg% and > |
| Methapyrilene | 0.2-0.4 mg% | 3-5 mg% | 5 mg% and > |
| Methaqualone (Quaalude) | 0.5 mg% | 1-3 mg% | 3 mg% and > |
| Methsuximide (Celontin) | 0.25-0.75 mg% | —— | —— |
| Methylene chloride | —— | —— | 28 mg% |
| Methylenedioxyamphetamine (MDA) | —— | —— | 0.4-1.0 mg% |
| Methyprylon (Noludar) | 1.0 mg% | 3-6 mg% | 10 mg% |
| Morphine | 0.01 mg% | —— | 0.005-0.4 mg% (free morphine from heroin) |
| Nickel | 0.041 mg% | —— | —— |
| Nicotine | —— | 1 mg% | 0.5-5.2 mg% |
| Nitrofurantoin (Furadantin) | 0.18 mg% | —— | —— |
| Nortriptyline (Aventyl) | 12-16 µg% | 0.5 mg% | 1.3 mg% |
| Orphenadrine | —— | 0.2 mg% | 0.4-0.8 mg% |
| Oxalate | 0.2 mg% | —— | 1.0 mg% |
| Papaverine | 0.1 mg% | —— | —— |
| Paramethoxyamphetamine (PMA) | —— | —— | 0.2-0.4 mg% |
| Paraldehyde | ~5.0 mg% | 20-40 mg% | 50 mg% |
| Pentazocine (Talwin) | 0.014-0.016 mg% | 0.2-0.5 mg% | 1-2 mg% |
| Perphenazine (Trilafon) | —— | 0.1 mg% | —— |
| Phencyclidine | —— | —— | 0.1 mg% |
| Phenmetrazine | —— | —— | 0.4 mg% |
| Phensuximide (Milontin) | 1-1.9 mg% | —— | —— |
| Phenylbutazone (Butazolidin) | ~10 mg% | —— | —— |
| Phosphorus | Tissue levels usually used | | |
| Primidone (Mysoline) | 1.0 mg% | 5-8 mg% | ~10 mg% |
| Probenecid (Benemid) | 10-20 mg% | —— | —— |
| Procainamide | 0.6 mg% | 1 mg% | —— |
| Prochlorperazine (Compazine) | —— | 0.1 mg% | —— |
| Promazine (Sparine) | —— | 0.1 mg% | —— |
| Propoxyphene | 5-20 µg% | 0.5-2 mg% | 5.7 mg% |
| Propranolol (Inderal) | 0.0025-0.02 mg% | —— | 0.8-1.2 mg% |
| Propylhexedrine (Benzedrex) | —— | —— | 0.2-0.3 mg% |
| Quinidine | 0.03-0.6 mg% | ~1.0 mg% | 3-5 mg% |
| Quinine | —— | —— | 1.2 mg% |

TABLE 131—*Continued*
BLOOD LEVELS

| *Compound* | *Therapeutic or Normal* | *Toxic* | *Lethal* |
|---|---|---|---|
| Salicylate (Acetylsalicylic acid) | 2-10 mg% | 15-30 mg% | 50 mg% |
| Sulfadiazine | 8-15 mg% | — | — |
| Sulfadimethoxine (Madribon) | 8-10 mg% | — | — |
| Sulfaguanidine | 3-5 mg% | — | — |
| Sulfanilamide | 10-15 mg% | — | — |
| Sulfisoxazole (Gantrisin) | 9-10 mg% | — | — |
| Strychnine | — | 0.2 mg% | 0.9-1.2 mg% |
| Theophylline | 1-2 mg% | — | — |
| Thioridazine (Mellaril) | 0.10-0.15 mg% | 1.0 mg% | 2-8 mg% |
| Tin | 0.012 mg% | — | — |
| Tolbutamide (Orinase) | 5.3-9.6 mg% | — | — |
| Toluene | — | — | 1.0 mg% |
| Tribromoethanol | — | — | 9 mg% |
| Trichloroethane | — | — | 10-100 mg% |
| Trimethobenzamide (Tigan) | 0.1-0.2 mg% | — | — |
| Uric acid | 3-7 mg% | — | — |
| Warfarin | 0.1-1.0 mg% | — | — |
| Zinc | 68-136 μg% | — | — |
| Zoxazolamine (Flexin) | 0.3-1.3 mg% | — | — |

From Charles L. Winek, Injury by Chemical Agents. In C. G. Tedeschi, L. G. Tedeschi and W. G. Eckert (Eds.), *Forensic Medicine,* © 1977 by W. B. Saunders Company, Philadelphia, Pennsylvania.

# Chapter 7

# SOAP, DETERGENT, POLISHING AND SANITIZING AGENTS

This group of compounds includes the various types of kitchen and bathroom soaps, detergents, bleaches, fabric cleaners, polishes, waxes, grease solvents, etc. The number of different products involved in this category runs into many thousands (*also see* Table 37).

The large variety of silver-polishing and cleaning substances available today varies from the relatively innocuous liquids and creams with mild inert abrasives, through the electrolytic types of cleaners, to the very potent dip-type cleaners which contain thiourea, sulfuric or phosphoric acid, plus a detergent and water. Ingestion of this strongly corrosive solution necessitates dilution with water or milk and gastric lavage. The former use of cyanide salts as a silver-polishing agent has been practically discontinued. The furniture polishes, metal cleaners and abrasives usually contain petroleum distillates, mineral seal oil, cedar oils, industrial alcohols, silica, alkali, etc.

A number of potentially toxic products are on the market for removing grease from ovens, grills and stoves. Some of these contain sodium hydroxide in concentrations up to 10%. If ingested, these agents can cause severe damage to mucous membranes of the mouth, pharynx, upper respiratory tract, esophagus and stomach. Small infants have developed severe burns with scarring about the mouth by playing with brushes used for grease removal. *Treatment* is similar to that for caustic alkali.

Steam iron cleaners are also often ingested by children. These agents contain organic acid salts adjusted to a pH of 3.0; at the present time all evidence indicates that they have a low toxicity. They may produce gastric irritation such as that produced by the intake of a large amount of concentrated citrus fruit juice. *Treatment* should consist of administering milk as a diluent and demulcent, and then using supportive measures as indicated. In the event that a large quantity is ingested, emptying of the stomach should be considered.

## DETERGENTS

Because they are such necessary and familiar household items, cleaners are not usually regarded as hazardous substances. However, in 1976, 5323 incidents involving ingestion of detergents, as well as soaps and cleaners, in children under five years of age were reported to the National Clearinghouse for Poison Control Centers. This represented 5.9 per cent of all the reported accidental ingestions in this age-group. Although severe toxic effects occur infrequently and fatalities are rare, these are still rather significant statistics for a potential cause of injury that is largely preventable by handling and storing these products properly to keep them out of reach of children.

Unfortunately, the terms "soap" and "detergent" are synonymous to many laymen;

there was an incident, for example, in which significant injury occurred from the misuse of a detergent instead of a soapsuds enema. To prevent this type of erroneous substitution, the physician should give very careful and specific instructions if he orders a soapsuds enema.

An additional problem, the widespread pollution of surface and ground water by synthetic detergents, has been of grave concern to public health and sanitary officials in the United States and other countries. Detergents themselves in concentrations found in water supplies are not harmful. The health problem associated with detergents is caused by the sewage which accompanies them in waste waters and which reaches water supplies under certain conditions. The high percentage of phosphates in detergents causes a continuous buildup of nutrients, resulting in algae and water plant growth, a complex process called eutrophication, which is undesirable in many waters since it can produce slimes, sludges and marshes. Detergents, however, are not the only source of phosphates. The most common organic surface-active agent in these products is an alkyl benzene sulfonate (ABS) derived from tetrapropylene. This molecule is relatively resistant to biological degradation in conventional

TABLE 132
CHEMICAL CLASSIFICATION OF DETERGENTS

| *Type* | *Contents* | *Added agents* | *Effects* | *Lethal dose* | *Treatment* |
|---|---|---|---|---|---|
| Anionic | Na, K, and $NH_4$ salts of fatty acids<br>Sulfonated hydrocarbons | Water softener (sodium phosphate)<br>Bleach | Irritates skin by removing oils causing papular dermatitis. Ingestion causes vomiting, diarrhea, & intestinal distention | Over 2 gm/kg according to animal experiments | Remove exposure to skin. No Rx necessary for ingested soap except demulcents and Rx of diarrhea as needed |
| | Phosphorylated hydrocarbons<br>Hydrophilic part of molecule is neg. and releases Na+ or K+ in $H_2O$ | | | Not known. 20 gm—no signs or symptoms | No Rx |
| Non-Ionic | Alkyl aryl polyether<br>Sulfates<br>Alcohols or sulfonates<br>Alkyl phenol polyglycol<br>Polyethylene glycol alkyl<br>Aryl ethers | | Slightly irritating | Up to 20 gm tolerated | No Rx necessary except dilute with demulcents |
| Cationic | Hydrophilic part of molecule is pos. rather than neg. Detergents release an anion ($Cl^-$ or $Br^-$) | | Readily absorbed. Interferes with many cellular functions. Vomiting, collapse, coma, early death | 1–3 gm | Inactivated by tissues or ordinary soaps. Remove unabsorbed detergent by lavage. Ordinary soap inactivates unabsorbed residual. Maintain respiration and treat convulsions |

From Lawrence, R.A. and Haggerty, R.J., Household Agents and Their Potential Toxicity. *Modern Treatment:* Vol. 8, No. 3, August, 1971.

waste treatment plants and in streams. Substitution of more readily biodegradable detergents, which are now in development, may help to solve some of the water pollution hazards that exist today. LAS-based detergents (linear alkylate sulfonate), which are also known as soft or biodegradable detergents, are more rapidly decomposed by organisms in the soil and sewage treatment processes. LAS is directionally less toxic than ABS, but the difference is not considered statistically significant. Therefore, present information on detergent toxicity still hold. It is understood that when the change occurs, the concentration of LAS in formulations will be approximately the same as that of the ABS it replaces.

Luminol™ (5-amino-2,3-dihydro-1,4-phthalazinedione) phosphoresces for detergents at an acidity of pH 5 to 6 and can be used as a chemical test for its identification.

In general, the term "detergent" refers to synthetic products (liquid or granules) that are "non-soap" cleaners; they promote detergency, wetting and emulsification by lowering surface tension. There are three types of these surface-active agents (surfactants): cationic, anionic and nonionic.

### *Cationic Detergents*

The cationic detergents or quaternary ammonium compounds such as benzethonium chloride (Phemerol® Chloride), benzalkonium chloride (Zephiran® Chloride), methylbenzethonium chloride (Diaparene® Chloride) and cetylpyridinium chloride (Ceepryn® Chloride) are synthetic derivatives of ammonium chloride.

Their toxicity has not been definitely established, but the human fatal dose by ingestion has been estimated to be between 1 and 3 gm. These compounds are rapidly inactivated by tissues and ordinary soaps. The principal manifestations of poisoning from ingestion of these agents are vomiting, collapse and coma.

*Treatment* consists first of giving milk, egg whites or a mild soap solution by mouth, then an emetic or gastric lavage with weak soap solution. Respiration should be supported. If convulsions occur, short-acting barbiturates should be given parenterally; central nervous system stimulants are likely to aggravate the convulsive state.

### *Anionic and Nonionic Detergents*

There are numerous anionic surface-active agents (sodium alkyl aryl sulfates, sodium alkyl sulfates and alkyl sodium isothionates). All are only moderately toxic; the $LD_{50}$ values in animal vary from 1 to 5 gm/kg. The maximum safe amount for children has been estimated at 0.1 to 1.0 gm/kg. They may cause skin and eye irritation.

The nonionic surfactants (alkylphenyl polyethoxyethanol, polyalkaline glycol, fatty acid alkanolamine amide) are less toxic and are no more hazardous than the anionic agents (*see* Table 132).

### *Household Detergent Products*

PACKAGED DETERGENT GRANULES. Manufacturers classify these products as (1) light-duty for dishes and baby clothes, (2) all-purpose sudsing products for laundry and general use, and (3) washday low-sudsing detergents made especially for automatic washers. However, with respect to their toxicity and the treatment of patients who have ingested them, all of these products may be considered as a single group. Building ingredients in modern detergent formulations are designed to chelate or otherwise remove the elements responsible for water hardness (mostly calcium and magnesium) and in this way prevent the inactivation of substances that serve as surface-active agents (surfactants). Granular household detergent products are composed largely of builders. These builders are of two general types: those which hold calcium in solution as soluble chelates and those which precipitate it. In the first category are found polyphosphates (especially sodium tripoly-phosphates) and nitrilotriacetate (NTA). The second category includes sodium carbonate, sodium bicarbonate, sodium sesquicarbonate, sodium silicate and sodium metasilicate.

Each product formulation usually includes some but not all of the following substances: anionic surfactants, fatty acid amides, nonionic surfactants, sodium tripolyphosphate, tetrasodium pyrophosphate, sodium orthophosphate, sodium metaphosphate, sodium silicate, sodium sulfate and sodium carbonate. Small quantities of other substances such as protective colloids, corrosion inhibitors, coloring agents and perfumes may be included, but these should affect toxicity only slightly, if at all.

Although the systemic toxicity of carbonates and silicates is low, their solutions can be very alkaline and may produce corrosive burning of the mucous membranes. The alkalinity of household detergent granules is adjusted to a pH which is not irritating to the skin; however, like soaps, they may be irritating to mucous membranes. Various alkaline phosphate salts also may cause irritation of mucous membranes.

The ingestion of sodium tripolyphosphate and hexametaphosphate has caused severe gastroenteritis with vomiting and diarrhea, and at least one child has developed an esophageal stricture. Rarely, hypocalcemia may occur after the ingestion of appreciable amounts of polymeric polyphosphates, possibly because of the binding of ionized serum calcium by the polyphosphate anions. The intravenous administration of calcium may be necessary for hypocalcemic effects. The emphasis on the impact of polyphosphate laundry detergent formulations on the environment has resulted in the marketing of a number of phosphate-free compounds. A sodium carbonate complex is the most frequent substitute in the newer products. In some cases, the carbonates represent as much as 60 to 70 per cent of the formulation. If weak acids are used to neutralize the product, there is a potential for release of large quantities of carbon dioxide gas, which possibly could lead to gastric distention, dilation and rupture. Therefore, the use of milk or water is recommended as a diluent when these products are ingested.

The acute oral toxicities of various detergent granule formulations in animals vary considerably. A child weighing 10 kg who has ingested 1 oz., by weight, of packaged detergent granules could become quite ill. By weight, 1 oz. of many of these products occupies approximately the same volume as 3 oz. of fluid.

*Treatment* consists of the immediate administration of milk or water to dilute the material. Demulcents such as milk or vegetable oil should be given liberally. Lavage is unnecessary unless appreciable amounts are ingested; in many cases, vomiting is apt to occur spontaneously. When vomiting or diarrhea is excessive, appropriate measures must be taken to maintain the fluid and electrolyte balance. Further treatment depends upon what other manifestations are encountered. The possibility that esophageal stricture may develop, although remote, should be kept in mind.

ELECTRIC DISHWASHER DETERGENT GRANULES. These products, although similar in composition to other household detergents, are capable of damaging mucous membranes because of their greater alkalinity. In cases of ingestion, *treatment* should include immediate dilution with copious quantities of water or milk and administration of demulcents such as olive oil. The decision to empty the stomach must be based both on the amount ingested and the presence or absence of damage to the oropharyngeal mucous membranes. The induction of vomiting is contraindicated. Gastric lavage may be done after cautious passage of a small-bore well-oiled tube.

Further treatment depends upon the extent of tissue damage and the development of local or systemic manifestations. The physician must be alert for evidence indicating possible involvement of the esophagus, stomach and the respiratory tract.

LIQUID DETERGENTS. The formulations of the liquid household detergent preparations are similar to those of the detergent granules.

TABLE 133
TOXICITY OF SOAPS AND DETERGENTS

| *Agent* | *Contents* | *Toxicity* | *Symptoms* | *Treatment* |
|---|---|---|---|---|
| Toilet soap bars | Soap<br>Salts of fatty acids<br>Synthetic surface-active agents | Low | GI irritation, vomiting & diarrhea | Demulcents: milk, etc.; emptying stomach unnecessary |
| Packaged detergent granules | Light-duty for dishwashing by hand —anionic detergent 25%<br>All-purpose for laundry (low sudsing)<br>Anionic surfactants<br>Carbonates<br>Silicates | Moderate (1–5gm/kg) | GI irritation, vomiting & diarrhea | Dilute with milk or water; lavage only for large amounts |
| | Na tripolyphosphate | Low systemic toxicity | Mucous membrane damage | Follow for stricture (esophageal) |
| Electric dishwasher detergent granules | Inorganic salts<br>Very high pH & small amount of surfactant<br>Na carbonate<br>Na tripolyphosphate | Moderate | Severe mucous membrane damage. Can cause hypocalcemia with shock, cyanosis | Immediate dilution, vinegar, citrus, demulcents; emesis contraindicated; 5 ml of 10% Ca gluconate for tetany |
| Liquid household detergents | Aqueous or hydroalcoholic solutions of anionic detergents | Lower than of powders | GI irritation | Dilute with milk or water |
| Liquid general purpose cleaners | May contain pine oil or petroleum distillates as kerosene | Moderate | Hydrocarbon pneumonitis. Irritates GI and/or GU tract | Same as for petroleum distillates |
| Detergents with bleach or bactericidal agents | Chlorine compounds<br>Antiseptics | | Although additives are mod. toxic, their conc. is low. No influence on overall toxicity | As for specific detergent |

From Lawrence, R.A. and Haggerty, R.J., Household Agents and Their Potential Toxicity. *Modern Treatment:* Vol. 8, No. 3, August, 1971.

The main difference is that they are in aqueous or hydroalcoholic solution; only low concentrations of alcohol are used in the hydroalcoholic solutions. The toxicity of these liquid detergents, in general, is lower than that of the powders. Manifestations associated with the swallowing of appreciable quantities are no different than those expected from the ingestion of detergent granules, and similar *treatment* should be instituted.

However, several highly advertised general purpose liquid cleaning agents contain petroleum distillates or pine oil (a mixture of terpene alcohols, hydrocarbons and ethers) made soluble by the addition of synthetic surfactants. When such a preparation has been ingested, care should be taken to determine whether it was merely "pine scented" or whether it contained pine oil as an active ingredient. Unlike the latter type, the pine-scented preparations usually contain pine oil only in small quantities.

Aspiration of petroleum distillates, which may occur at the time of ingestion or later in association with vomiting, may produce pneumonitis; involvement of the lungs has not been reported in cases in which the ingested product did not contain substantial amounts of this substance. Pine oil causes irritation of the eyes, mucous membranes and gastrointestinal and genitourinary tracts and depression of the central nervous system with hypothermia and respiratory failure. When large quantities of these cleaning agents are swallowed, the stomach should be emptied by means of careful gastric lavage rather than by

TABLE 134
COMPOSITION OF SOAP AND DETERGENT PRODUCTS

BAR SOAP

*Major Ingredients*
Sodium (or potassium) soaps from tallow, coconut oil, etc.

*Occasional Ingredients*
Hexachlorophene
Trichlorocarbanilide
Tribromosalicylanilide
Glycerin
Lanolin
Sodium Silicate

BEAUTY BAR (Detergent)

*Major Ingredients which may be present*
Sodium alkyl sulfate
Fatty acid isothionates
Free fatty acids
Sulfated fatty acid monoglyceride
Sodium linear alkylate sulfonate (LAS)
Sodium soaps

*Minor Ingredients*
Glyceryl esters
Sodium sulfate
Sodium chloride

*Occasional Ingredients*
Sodium tripolyphosphate

SOAP POWDER (Heavy Duty)

*Major Ingredients which may be present*
Sodium tallow soap
Tetrasodium pyrophosphate
Trisodium orthophosphate

*Minor Ingredients*
Sodium silicate
Sodium carbonate

SOAP FLAKES (Light Duty)

*Major Ingredients*
Sodium soaps from tallow, coconut oil, etc.

*Minor Ingredients*
Sodium chloride
Sodium tripolyphosphate

ALL-PURPOSE DETERGENT
(Granular) Heavy-duty, High-sudsing

*Major Ingredients which may be present*
Sodium linear alkylate sulfonate (LAS)
Sodium alkyl sulfate
Fatty alkanolamide
Sodium tripolyphosphate
Tetrasodium pyrophosphate
Trisodium orthophosphate
Sodium sulfate
Sodium sesquicarbonate

*Minor Ingredients*
Sodium silicate

*Occasional Ingredients*
Sodium tetraborate
Sodium perborate
Sodium carbonate

ALL-PURPOSE DETERGENT (Granular)
Heavy-duty, Low-sudsing

*Major Ingredients which may be present*
Sodium linear alkylate sulfonate (LAS)
Alkylphenol ethylene oxide condensate (nonylphenol polyethoxyethanol)
Alkanol ethylene oxide condensate (lauric and myristic polyethoxyethanol)
Fatty alkanolamide
Sodium tripolyphosphate
Tetrasodium pyrophosphate
Sodium sulfate
Sodium carbonate

*Minor Ingredients*
Sodium toluenesulfonate
Sodium soap
Trisodium orthophosphate
Sodium silicate

*Note:* Most products also contain water and small amounts of perfumes, colors and other minor ingredients that do not contribute significantly to the toxicological properties of the products.

TABLE 134—*Continued*
COMPOSITION OF SOAP AND DETERGENT PRODUCTS

*Occasional Ingredients*
Sodium tetraborate
Sodium perborate

FINE-FABRIC DETERGENT
(Granular) Light-duty, Hand-dishwashing, etc.

*Major Ingredients which may be present*
Sodium linear alkylate sulfonate (LAS)
Fatty alkanolamide
Sodium sulfate

*Minor Ingredients*
Sodium tripolyphosphate
Trisodium orthophosphate
Tetrasodium pyrophosphate
Sodium silicate

GENERAL HOUSEHOLD CLEANER
(Crystalline)
Walls and Hard-surface cleaning

*Major Ingredients which may be present*
Sodium tripolyphosphate
Sodium carbonate
Sodium bicarbonate
Trisodium orthophosphate
Sodium sesquicarbonate

*Minor Ingredients*
Sodium linear alkylate sulfonate (LAS)
Nonylphenol polyethoxyethanol
Ammonium chloride

ALL-PURPOSE DETERGENT
(Liquid)
Heavy-duty; recommended for regular laundry

*Major Ingredients which may be present*
Sodium linear alkylate sulfonate (LAS)
Alkylphenol ethylene oxide condensate
Fatty alkanolamide
Sodium potassium toluene (xylene) sulfonate
Polyoxyethylene fatty acid amide
Tetrapotassium pyrophosphate
Potassium tripolyphosphate
Tripotassium orthophosphate

*Minor Ingredients*
Sodium silicate
Alcohol
Sodium sulfate

GENERAL HOUSEHOLD CLEANER
(Liquid)
Walls, Hard-surface cleaning

*Major Ingredients which may be present*
Sodium linear alkylate sulfonate (LAS)
Fatty alkanolamide
Sodium (potassium) toluene (xylene) sulfonate
Sodium lauryl sulfate
Tetrapotassium pyrophosphate
Sodium tripolyphosphate
Soda or potassium soap
Alkanol ethylene oxide condensate
Stoddard solvent

*Minor Ingredients*
Sodium sulfate

*Occasional Ingredients*
Pine oil
Ammonium hydroxide
Glycol ethers

HAND DISHWASHING DETERGENT
(Liquid)
Light-duty, Dishes and delicate fabrics

*Major Ingredients which may be present*
Sodium linear alkylate sulfonate (LAS)
Fatty alcohol ethylene oxide sulfate
Sodium lauryl sulfate
Fatty alkanolamide
Sodium (potassium) toluene (xylene) sulfonate
Alcohol
Sodium (potassium) soaps
Alkylphenol ethylene oxide sulfate

*Minor Ingredients*
Sodium sulfate

FABRIC SOFTENER (Liquid)

*Major Ingredients which may be present*
Distearyldimethylammonium chloride
Ditallow-dimethylammonium methyl sulfate
Fatty quaternary ammonium compounds
Fatty acid ethylene oxide condensates
Ethylene oxide condensates of di-coco amine

BORAX (Crystalline)

*Major Ingredient*
Sodium tetraborate

BLEACH (Granular)

*Major Ingredients which may be present*
Sodium perborate
Calcium hypochlorite
Sodium tripolyphosphate
Potassium or sodium dichloroisocyanurate (dichloro-s-triazinetrione)
Potassium monopersulfate
Sodium sulfate

TABLE 134—*Continued*
COMPOSITION OF SOAP AND DETERGENT PRODUCTS

Sodium chloride
Trisodium orthophosphate

*Minor Ingredients*
Sodium linear alkylate sulfate (LAS)

BLEACH (Liquid)

*Major Ingredients*
Sodium hypochlorite
Sodium chloride

HAND CLEANER (Waterless)

*Major Ingredients which may be present*
Mild abrasive
Sodium, ammonium, or triethanolamine soaps
High flash naphtha

AUTOMATIC DISHWASHER DETERGENT

*Major Ingredients which may be present*
Sodium tripolyphosphate
Tetrasodium pyrophosphate
Glassy phosphate
Sodium metasilicate or other sodium silicates
Trisodium orthophosphate
Chlorinated trisodium phosphate
Sodium carbonate

*Minor Ingredients*
Alkylphenol ethylene oxide condensate
Alkanol ethylene oxide condensate
Potassium or sodium dichloroisocyanurate (dichloro-s-triazinetrione)
Sodium hypochlorite

*Occasional Ingredients*
Dichloramine–T

WINDOW AND GLASS CLEANERS
(Liquid)

*Major Ingredients which may be present*
Alcohol (ethyl or isopropyl)
Glycol ethers
Sodium linear alkylate sulfonate (LAS)
Ammonium hydroxide

SHAMPOO (Soap Type) LIQUID

*Major Ingredients*
Potassium coconut oil soap
Alcohol

SHAMPOO (Detergent Type) LIQUID

*Major Ingredients which may be present*
Alkanolamine lauryl sulfate
Alkanolamine alkylate sulfonate, linear, (LAS)
Triethanolammonium ether sulfate
Fatty acid alkanolamide
Alcohol

*Minor Ingredients*
Lanolin
Zinc

CREAM HAIR RINSE

*Major Ingredients*
Stearyldimethylbenzylammonium chloride

SCOURING POWDER

*Major Ingredients which may be present*
Ground silica
Pumice
Feldspar

*Minor Ingredients*
Sodium linear alkylate sulfonate (LAS)
Sodium tripolyphosphate
Trisodium orthophosphate
Sodium sulfate

Sodium (potassium) dichloroisocyanurate (sodium dichloro-s-triazinetrione)

*Occasional Ingredients*
Sodium perborate

DRAIN CLEANERS
(Crystalline)
(Hazardous Compounds)

*Major Ingredients*
Sodium bisulfate
Sodium bioxalate
Sodium hydroxide
Aluminum powder

DRAIN CLEANERS
(Liquid)
(Hazardous Compounds)

*Major Ingredients*
Trichloroethane

TOILET BOWL CLEANERS
(Crystalline)
(Hazardous Compounds)

*Major Ingredients*
Sodium acid sulfate

TOILET BOWL CLEANERS
(Liquid)
(Hazardous Compounds)

Sulfuric Acid

the induction of vomiting. Further treatment is based on the patient's individual responses.

DETERGENTS WITH BLEACHING AND BACTERICIDAL PROPERTIES. Bleaching agents (chlorine-releasing agents) or bactericidal agents (mild concentrations of quaternary ammonium compounds) have been included in the formulation of a number of these products. Recent reports reveal that these additives are only moderately toxic. Furthermore, since the concentrations are low, these agents should not influence the toxicity of the product significantly.

Deleterious effects have been reported from the simultaneous use by housewives of acid-type toilet bowl cleaners and sodium hypochlorite bleaches. Such a mixture produces chlorine gas, which causes respiratory irritation with coughing and labored breathing and inflammation of the eyes and mucous membranes.

DETERGENTS WITH ENZYMES. The large number of laundry products containing detergents and enzymes in combination, once released and later taken off the market, exceeded 10 per cent of the total detergent market and amounted to almost 5 billion pounds annually. These products included presoak preparations such as Amaze®, Axion®, Biz®, and Sure®, and regular laundry detergents with enzymes added such as Ajax®, Bold®, Drive®, Gain®, Punch® and Tide XK®. The enzymes used in these products are obtained from spore-forming bacteria *Bacillus subtillis* and are mainly proteolytic, although some concentrates used in laundry products contain amylase as well. Enzymes are relatively ineffective for general laundering when used alone. However, when used in combination with compatible surfactants and builders as in presoaks and other enzyme-detergent combinations, they were found to aid greatly in soil removal, especially in material of protein composition such as found in stains from blood, milk, chocolate, excrement, etc. Liquid formulations have been found to be unstable. Concentrated formulations of the enzymes can be irritating to the skin, but in the amounts used with detergent products, they did not appear to cause any greater skin irritation than would be expected from the detergent formulations alone. Home laundry products, as has already been indicated, are frequently reported in childhood ingestions with very little evidence of producing substantial injury. As with other detergent formulations, the enzyme detergent combinations could be expected to cause vomiting when ingested. The addition of enzymes and brighteners in the concentrations used did not add to the toxicity of these agents. If ingested, it may be detrimental to make these patients vomit with syrup of ipecac because the detergent may froth, and the frothing could block the airway.

## *Abrasive Cleaners*

Abrasive cleaners are largely composed of an abrasive such as pumice or silica and have a low order of toxicity. Gastrointestinal irritation is possible from ingestion and should be treated by administering milk or water and giving symptomatic care.

## *Toilet Soap Bars*

These include all bars ordinarily found on the washstand and used in shower or tub. Some are made entirely from soap (salts of fatty acids), while others contain synthetic surface-active agents alone or in combination with soap. Some deodorant soaps contain photosensitizing compounds. In general, toilet bars have a low toxicity. When ingested in sufficient quantity, soap may cause gastrointestinal irritation, and vomiting and diarrhea may ensue. *Treatment* includes administration of demulcents and symptomatic measures for diarrhea, should it occur. Because of the low toxicity, emptying the stomach is unnecessary.

## *Toilet Bowl Cleaners*

Toilet bowl agents are sold as either solids or liquids. Both forms, because of their potential toxicity, must be kept in places where they cannot be reached by small children.

By far the largest number of the solid cleaners are essentially sodium acid sulfate, with sodium hydroxide a poor second. Sodium acid sulfate in aqueous solution is strongly acidic. The liquid preparations usually contain either hydrochloric or phosphoric acid. All of these are corrosive to body tissue with superficial destruction of skin and mucous membranes. The estimated lethal human dose of sodium acid sulfate is 1 ounce (30 gm).

Mixing household cleaners of various types is a common practice among American housewives. They are usually unaware of the dangers from inhalation, especially in poorly vented spaces, of the fumes of their own bathroom or kitchen cocktails.

The use of acid-type toilet bowl cleaners with vinegar, lye, ammonia, sodium hypochlorite bleaches and other alkaline compounds, coincidentally or concomitantly, produces chlorine (MAC 1 ppm) or ammonia gas (MAC 100 ppm). Either mixture when inhaled causes respiratory tract irritation with coughing and labored breathing and pulmonary edema, along with inflammation of the eyes and other mucous membranes. Headache, vertigo, cyanosis and hypotension may also occur. (No deleterious effects, however, occur from the simultaneous use or mixing of a liquid or powdered hypochlorite bleach with lye, laundry detergents or soaps.)

The cake deodorants for toilet bowls, on the other hand, are not cleaners; they usually contain paradichlorobenzene, which is a much less dangerous chemical than naphthalene.

TABLE 135
CLEANING, POLISHING AND SANITIZING AGENTS

| *Trade Name** | *Contents* | *Page Reference* |
|---|---|---|
| Acco Emulsifer #5 | Polyethylene glycol ester of fatty acids | |
| Acidol 25-A | Salt of a fatty acid tertiary amine | |
| Acidolate | Sulfonated oils, etc. | |
| Acidose | Alkyl aryl sulfonate | |
| ACTO 450 | Alkyl aryl sulfonate | |
| 500 | Mol. wt. 465—480 | |
| 600 | | |
| 630 | | |
| 700 | | |
| AD | Anionic | |
| Advawet 10 | Alkyl aryl polyether alcohol | |
| Advawet 25 | Sodium salt of a sulfonated mineral oil | |
| Advawet 33 | Polyglycol ester | |
| Aerosol AY | Diamyl ester of sulfosuccinic acid | |
| Aerosol C-61 | An ethanolated alkyl guanidine amine complex | |
| Aerosol MA | Dihexyl ester of sodium sulfosuccinic acid | *See Index* |
| Aerosol OS | Isopropyl naphthalene sodium sulfonate | |
| Aerosol OT | Dioctyl ester of sodium sulfosuccinic acid | |
| Aerosol SE | Stearamidopropyldimethyl B-hydroxyethyl-ammonium chloride | |
| Aerosol 18 | N-octa decyl tetrasodium (1, 2-dicarboxyl ethyl sulfosuccinamate) | |
| Agrimul 70-A | Alkyl aryl polyether alcohol | |
| Agrimul C | Aromatic sulfonate-oxide condensate blend | |
| Agrimul GM | Aromatic sulfonate-oxide condensate blend | |
| Agrimul T | Aromatic sulfonate-oxide condensate blend | |
| Ahcovel E | Fatty carbamide derivatives | |
| Ahcowet ANS | Alkyl aryl sodium sulfonate | |

*All products listed below are registered trademarks. Since trade names and formulations are frequently and unexpectedly changed, consult labels for definite contents.

TABLE 135—*Continued*
CLEANING, POLISHING AND SANITIZING AGENTS

| *Trade Name* | *Contents* | *Page Reference* |
|---|---|---|
| Ahcowet N | Ethylene oxide condensate | |
| Ahcowet RS | Sulfated fatty acid ester | |
| Ajax | Silica, alkyl aryl sulfonate, phosophate, chlorinated bleach | |
| Albasol BF | A potassium soap, solubilized with glycol | |
| Albatex POK Paste | Benzimidazole compounds | |
| Albino Bleach Solution "A" | Caustic alkali | |
| Albino Bleach Solution "B" | Mineral acid | |
| Alexyl Disinfectant | Phenols | |
| All Detergent | Ethylene glycol, sodium and other phosphate salts, fatty acid esters | |
| Arnofos Detergent | Sodium polyphosphate | |
| Axurwhite Bleach | Sodium perborate, alkali | |
| Bacilicide Disinfectant | Hypochlorites | |
| Beacon Paste Wax | Waxes, terpene, and paraffin solvents | |
| Beacon "Quick Gloss" Wax | Water, wax emulsion | |
| Bell's Cleaning Fluid | Carbon tetrachloride | |
| Bionol Disinfectant | Cetyl dimethyl ammonium chloride | |
| B-K Liquid Bleach | Sodium chlorate | |
| B-K Powder Disinfectant | Calcium hypochlorite | |
| Black Flag Disinfectant | Potassium chlorphenyl phenate, pine oil soap, et al. | |
| Bleachette Laundry Blue | Ultramarine blue | |
| Blind-X Cleaner | Trisodium phosphate, quadrafos | |
| Bowlclene | Mineral acid | |
| Bowlene | Sodium bisulfite | |
| Breath-O-Pine Disinfectant | Distilled pine oil, soap, water | See Index |
| Breeze | Sodium alkyl aryl sulfonate plus binders | |
| Bright Sail Air Deodorant and Purifier | Petroleum distillates | |
| Bright Sail Bleach | Sodium hypochlorite | |
| Bright Spot Bleach | Sodium hypochlorite | |
| Bromat Disinfectant | Cetyl trimethyl ammonium bromide | |
| Bruce Cleaning Wax | Petroleum solvent, waxes | |
| Bruce Floor Cleaner | Petroleum solvent, zinc stearate, waxes | |
| Bruce Self Polishing Wax | Waxes, resins, emulsifiers | |
| Bruce Tuf Lustre Wax | Petroleum solvent, waxes | |
| Burton Cesspool Cleaner | Sodium bisulfite | |
| Butcher's Boston Polish | Sovasol (petroleum solvent), turpentine, waxes, hydrocarbons | |
| Buti-Glow Silicone Polish | Petroleum solvent, silicone oil | |
| Calgon | Sodium phosphate, sodium carbonate, sodium bicarbonate | |
| Calgonite | Calgon and alkaline sodium silicate | |
| Camp Instant Drain Pipe Cleaner | Potassium hydroxide, potassium carbonate, sodium hydroxide | |
| Carbona Cleaning Fluid | Trichloroethylene, petroleum hydrocarbons | |
| Carbon Met Metal Cleaner | Methylated hydrocarbon | |
| Carogol | Sodium hexametaphosphate | |
| Cee-Dee Disinfectant | Quaternary ammonium compound | |
| Cetol Disinfectant | Dimethyl benzyl ammonium chloride | |
| Cetylon Disinfectant | Cetyl dimethyl benzyl ammonium chloride | |
| Cheer | Alkyl aryl sodium sulfonate | |
| Chiffon Liquid | A formulated product | |
| Chlor-Clean | Chlorine | |
| Chlorfectant | Hypochlorite | |
| Chrome Kleen | Phosphates, abrasives, soaps | |
| Cleanesco | Sodium metasilicate | |

TABLE 135—*Continued*
CLEANING, POLISHING AND SANITIZING AGENTS

| *Trade Name* | *Contents* | *Page Reference* |
|---|---|---|
| Cleanser 400 | Sodium metasilicate, trisodium phosphate, soda ash | *See Index* |
| Clearpine Disinfectant | Pine oil | |
| Clor-O-Tol Bleach | Hypochlorite | |
| Cloroben | O-dichlorobenzene | |
| Clorox Bleach | Sodium hypochlorite | |
| C-N Disinfectant | Coal tar neutral oil, coal tar, phenols, soaps | |
| Copper Brite | Hydrochloric acids, phosphoris acid, silica | |
| Copper Coin Cleaner ("CCC") | Phosphoric acid | |
| Creol Disinfectant | Coal tar neutral oil, cresylic acid, soap | |
| Creoletta | Coal tar phenols | |
| Creotex | Creosote concentrate | |
| Creozone | Coal tar phenols | |
| Cresanol | Coal tar phenols | |
| Cresolene | Coal tar phenols | |
| Cresophan | Tertiary butyl cresol | |
| Cristy Cooling System Cleaner | Oxalic acid | |
| Crosley Special Furniture Polish | Silicones | |
| Crystamet | Sodium metasilicate, pentahydrate | |
| Dactin Bleach & Germicide | Dichloro dimethyl hydantoin | |
| Dan-Dee Floor Polish | Industrial alcohols, mineral spirits | |
| Dash | Anionic | |
| Dazzle Bleach & Disinfectant | Sodium hypochlorite | |
| Des-Tex Dry Cleaner | Carbon tetrachloride | |
| Dexodine Metal Cleaner | Phosphoric acid | |
| Dial Soap | Hexachlorophene 0.75%, 0.75% triclocarbon (TCC) | |
| Dichloran Disinfectant | Quaternary ammonium compound | |
| Dip-It-Stain Remover | Sodium phosphate, sodium metasilicate, sodium perborate, magnesium sulfate | |
| Dippo Silver Cleaner | Potassium chlorate, sodium bicarbonate, alkyl aryl sulfonate | |
| Dirilyte Polish | Naphtha, ammonia | |
| Dowclene Dry Cleaner | Trichloroethane | |
| Drano Disinfectant | Sodium hydroxide | |
| Dryloene Dry Clean | Petroleum solvent | |
| Ducozone Bleach | Sodium peroxide | |
| Du Pont Dry Clean | Trichloroethylene | |
| Easy Aid Silver Cleaner | Phosphoric acid, thiourea | |
| Easy Bleach | Sodium hypochlorite | |
| Easy Off Oven Cleaner | Sodium hydroxide, aluminum stearate | |
| Electro-Silicon Polishing Cream | Diatomaceous earth, jelling soap | |
| Electro-Sol Dishwashing Compound | Sodium tripolyphosphate, sodium carbonate, sodium metasilicate | |
| Elkay-s Klens-All | Carbon tetrachloride | |
| Emulphogene Detergent | Ethylene oxide condensate | |
| Energine Cleaning Fluid | Trichloroethane | |
| Fab | Alkyl aryl sulfonate plus binders | |
| Fixit Scratch Cover Furniture Polish | Petroleum distillate | |
| Fluid-Cress Disinfectant | Cresol | |
| Formcolor Disinfectant | Hypochlorite | |
| Furniture Doctor | Petroleum distillate | |
| Fyne-Tex Disinfectant | Pine oil, soap | |
| Gardsite Rust Remover | Oxalic acid | |
| Germ-I-Tol Deodorizer | Quaternary ammonium compound | |
| Germa-Pine Disinfectant | Pine oil | |
| Glamorene Rug Cleaner | Trichloroethylene, ethylene dichloride, heavy naphtha | |
| Glass Wax | Isopropyl alcohol, mineral spirits | |
| Go-Fecto Disinfectant | Pine oil | |

TABLE 135—*Continued*
CLEANING, POLISHING AND SANITIZING AGENTS

| *Trade Name* | *Contents* | *Page Reference* |
|---|---|---|
| Gold Seal Snowy Bleach | Alkali | |
| Gorham Silver Polish | Diatomaceous earth | |
| Guardsman Cleansing Polish | Liquid petroleum | |
| Holly Pine Cleaner | Sodium hydroxide | |
| H-T-H Bleach | Calcium hypochlorite | |
| I.C. Degreaser | Sodium tetra pyro phosphate | |
| Insecticidal Freewax for Floors | Gamma BHC, petroleum distillates | |
| Instant Dip Silver Cleaner | Thiourea, dilute sulfuric acid | |
| Johnson's Carnu Gloss | Petroleum distillate | |
| Johnson's Carplate Auto Wax | Petroleum naphtha, silicone fluid | |
| Johnson's Cream Wax | Petroleum distillate | |
| Johnson's Glo-Coat | Petroleum waxes | |
| Johnson's Jubilee | Petroleum naphtha | |
| Johnson's Liquid Wax | Petroleum naphtha | |
| Johnson's Paste Wax | Petroleum distillate | |
| Johnson's Pride | Petroleum naphtha, silicone fluid | |
| Karith Cleaning Fluid | Carbon tetrachloride | |
| Kemtex Cleaner | Alkali | |
| Klean Spot Kit | Carbon tetrachloride | |
| Kleenal | Sodium metasilicate, sodium hexametaphosphate | |
| Kleenize Disinfectant | Hypochlorite | |
| Kot-O-Fom Cleaner | Soaps | |
| Lemcke's Dip-N-Rinse | Potassium cyanide | |
| Linco | Sodium hypochlorite | |
| Lycons Cleaner | Sodium hydroxide, sodium carbonate | |
| Lysol Disinfectant† | Phenylphenol, benzyl-*p*-chloro-phenol, alcohol, soap | |
| Maid Easy Stain Remover | Alkali, phosphates | |
| M-E Cleaner | Alkali | |
| Merphenyl Disinfectant | Phenyl mercuric compound | |
| Microlin Disinfectant | Hypochlorite | |
| Mufti Spot Remover | Naphtha, chlorothene | *See Index* |
| Myro Range & Porcelain Cleaner | Alkali | |
| Mystic Foam Cleaner for Fabrics | Soaps | |
| N.S.C. Detergent | Sodium hydroxide, sodium phosphate | |
| Naccolene Dry Clean Detergent | Alkyl aryl sodium phosphate | |
| Natco Fabric Cleaner | Carbon tetrachloride | |
| Nice Room Deodorant | Triethylene and propylene glycol | |
| Nopocide K Disinfectant | Quaternary ammonium compound | |
| Norway Penetrating Oil | Petroleum distillate | |
| No Worry Household Bleach | Sodium hypochlorite | |
| Noxon Metal Polish | Dilute ammonium oxalate | |
| Nuplate Silver Cleaner | Potassium cyanide | |
| O-Cedar All Purpose Polish | Mineral seal oil | |
| O-Cedar Dri-Glo | Petroleum naphtha | |
| O-Cedar Glass Polish | Monoethyl ether or ethylene glycol | |
| O-Cedar Paste Wax | Mineral seal oil | |
| O-Cedar Self Polishing Wax | Solid wax | |
| O-Cedar Touch Up Furniture Polish | Petroleum naphtha | |
| O-Cedar Upholstery & Rug Cleaner | Alkyl aryl sulfonate | |
| Old English Red Oil Polish | Mineral seal oil, petroleum distillates | |
| Old English Scratch Cover Polish | Mineral seal oil, petroleum distillates | |
| Onyx Disinfectant & Deodorant | Alkyl dimethyl, benzyl ammonium chloride | |
| Orpine Disinfectant | Pine oil | |
| Orthosil Detergent | Sodium subsilicate | |
| Oxydol | Anionic | |
| Oxygenate Bleach | Hypochlorite | |
| Oxylapine Disinfectant | Pine oil | |
| Pearl Range, Refrigerator and Metal Polish | Petroleum solvent, ammonia triethanolamine | |

† Methemoglobinemia, Heinz bodies and massive intravascular hemolysis can occur in serious poisoning.

TABLE 135—*Continued*
CLEANING, POLISHING AND SANITIZING AGENTS

| *Trade Name* | *Contents* | *Page Reference* |
|---|---|---|
| pHisoHex | Hexachlorophene, 3% | |
| Pine Sol | Pine oil | |
| Pinuseptol | Pine oil | |
| Plumite Drain Opener | Sodium hydroxide | |
| Preen | Stoddard solvent | |
| Preenet | Petroleum waxes | |
| Prelim | Tall oil (petroleum distillate) | |
| Pronton Detergent | Sodium hydroxide | |
| Purex Dry Bleach | Calcium hypochlorite | |
| Purex Pipe and Drain Cleaner | Sodium hydroxide | |
| Purex Toilet Bowl Detergent | Sodium bisulfite | |
| Quick-N-Brite | Sodium hydroxide | |
| Rad Cleaner | Trisodium phosphate | |
| Radiant Lemon Oil Polish | Petroleum distillates | |
| Rawleigh's Car Cleaner | Petroleum hydrocarbons, silicone | |
| Rawleigh's Car Polish | Silicone, petroleum hydrocarbons | |
| Rawleigh's Cleanser | Trisodium phosphate | |
| Re-Clean for Fabrics | Petroleum distillates | |
| Red Cap Refresh-R Germicide & Deodorant | Ethyl alcohol | |
| Renofab | Chlorothene | |
| Renuzit All Purpose Dry Clean | Petroleum distillates | |
| Renuzit Spot & Stain Remover | Petroleum distillates | |
| Reviva Spot Remover | Ethylene glycol | |
| Rid-O-Spot | Carbon tetrachloride | |
| Roccal Detergent | Quaternary ammonium compound | |
| Rodalon Disinfectant | Quaternary ammonium compound | |
| Rose X-Bleach | Sodium hypochlorite | |
| Safeguard Soap | Tribromsalan, triclocarban, cloflucarban | |
| Sage Dry Bleach | Dichloro-dimethyl hydantoin | |
| Sage-O Pine Disinfectant | Pine oil | |
| Sani-Chlor | Sodium hypochlorite | *See Index* |
| Sani-Flush | Sodium bisulfite | |
| Sani-Stod Dry Clean | Petroleum distillate | |
| Savol Purified Bleach | Sodium hypochlorite | |
| Shasta | Anionic | |
| Shop-Rite Bleach | Sodium hypochlorite | |
| Silver Dust | Anionic | |
| Simoniz Hi-Lite Furniture Polish | Petroleum distillate | |
| Sno-Bol Liquid Bowl Cleaner | Hydrochloric acid | |
| Sodisil Detergent | Sodium silicate | |
| Solozone Bleach | Sodium peroxide | |
| Solvoterge Metal Cleaner | Stoddard solvent | |
| Spandy Disinfectant | Dodecylamine lactate, salicylate, alcohol | |
| Speed Up Bleach | Sodium hypochlorite | |
| Speed Up Cleaner, Disinfectant | Pine oil | |
| Sta-Kleen Toiletabs | Trisodium phosphate | |
| Stanson Laundry Detergent | Trisodium phosophate | |
| Staphene | Isopropyl alcohol | |
| Star Water Deodorant | Sodium hypochlorite | |
| Stop Spot | Petroleum hydrocarbon | |
| Sudia Deodorant | Pine oil | |
| Super Alkali Detergent | Sodium hydroxide | |
| Superoxol Bleach | Sodium peroxide | |
| Suprep Metal Cleaner | Phosphoric acid | |
| Swift Metal Cleaner | Petroleum solvent | |
| Sylpho-Nathol | Coal tar neutral oil | |
| Take-Off | Carbon tetrachloride | |
| Tavern Spot Remover | Carbon tetrachloride | |
| Tenn-Creo Disinfectant | Creosotes | |
| Texatone Bleach | Sodium chlorate | |

TABLE 135—*Continued*
CLEANING, POLISHING AND SANITIZING AGENTS

| *Trade Name* | *Contents* | *Page Reference* |
|---|---|---|
| Texize Foaming Action Bleach | Sodium hypochlorite | |
| Texize Laundry Starch | Corn starch, borax, o-phenyl phenol sodium salt (Dow A) | |
| Texize Rug Cleaner | Sodium alkyl aryl sulfonate, ethylene oxide alkyl | |
| Textolit Bleach | Sodium chlorate | |
| Tide | Anionic | |
| Titan Oil Disinfectant | Pine oil | |
| Tri-Clene Dry Clean | Trichloroethylene | |
| Triad Metal Cleaner | Trichloroethylene | |
| Triad Metal Polish | Trichloroethylene | |
| Vanish Detergent | Sodium acid sulfate | *See Index* |
| Vel | Anionic | |
| Vernax Beauty Cream for Furniture | Turpentine, waxes, soaps | |
| West Pine Deodorant | Pine oil | |
| Whitepine Disinfectant | Pine oil | |
| Wilbert's Fresh Pine Deodorant | Pine oil | |
| Wilson Cleaner | Carbon tetrachloride | |
| Windex | Isopropyl alcohol | |
| Woodbrite Furniture Polish | Petroleum distillates | |
| Wright's Silver Cream | Diatomaceous earth, soda ash | |
| X-O Deodorant | Quaternary ammonium compound | |
| Zest Soap | Tribromsalan, triclocarban | |

*Chapter 8*

# COSMETICS AND TOILET ARTICLES

Beauty may be only skin deep but that does not stop Americans from spending over $5 billion a year on the quest for beauty. According to *Drug Topics,* the money was spent like this in 1976: shaving products, $498 million; face and body powder, $262 million; lipstick, $458 million; cleansing creams, eye makeup and face lotions, $374 million; oral hygiene, $1 billion; hair products, $1.7 billion; hand products, $300 million; and other toiletries such as perfumes, bath salts, soaps and deodorants, $1.8 billion. Current unavailable figures must be considerably higher. In addition, anyone can market a new cosmetic at any time without submitting it to any authority for testing and evaluation. In Arlington, Virginia, some questions about the safety of these cosmetics were asked at a conference sponsored by the American Medical Association and the Society of Toxicology. One of the big problems today, noted Doctor Paul Lazar, Assistant Professor of Dermatology, Northwestern University Medical School, is photosensitivity. Some toiletries, particularly certain soaps, have made many women sensitive to sunlight. In fact, some of these consumers have remained "persistent light reactors" even after they have stopped using the product. Nail hardeners and hair dyes have also brought injury to some users.

These cosmetic and toilet articles include various types of preparations intended for application to the skin, hair and nails, More than 15,000 reports of poisonings due to accidental ingestion of chemicals were received by the Committee on Toxicology of the American Medical Association over a two-year period from various sources. A review of these data revealed that cosmetics were involved in 3 per cent of the cases. While most products are quite safe when used as directed, some contain chemicals that can be dangerous if ingested in large quantity or otherwise misused. Moreover, through an allergic or photodynamic process, many of these compounds frequently cause an inflammatory reaction in living tissue on contact in susceptible individuals and become strong sensitizers. For beauticians who handle these chemicals as well as other defatting and irritating agents such as detergents, hydrogen peroxide, etc., rubber gloves are mandatory to prevent dermatitis. Fortunately, the chemicals are regulated under federal and many state laws, and their potential hazards and toxicity are well controlled.

The acute oral $LD_{50}$ test performed on white rats does not result in data directly translatable to humans. Yet this test does establish a range in toxicity that is useful in determining the probable hazard to man. The effect of the test substance on the animal varies widely with the product under test, although there are similarities within any class of cosmetic products. Cosmetics in general show acute oral $LD_{50}$s in rats in excess of 10 gm/kg, which for a 10 kg child extrapolates to 100 gm or more before life is endangered.

## SHAMPOOS

The liquid shampoos usually consist of various oils such as castor oil, cottonseed, almond, soy bean, olive oil, etc., saponified with an alkali (sodium, potassium or ammonium salts). The vast majority of shampoos at the present time are composed of synthetic detergents with or without soap. It is practically impossible to find an all-soap shampoo. Soapless shampoos are synthetic detergent products. Unless large amounts of liquid shampoo are ingested, danger of ill effects or toxicity is practically nil. Many, however, are irritating to the eyes and may need to be discontinued because of the chemical conjunctivitis produced. Dry shampoos, on the other hand, can be quite dangerous. These usually amount to dry-cleaning agents for the hair and may contain carbon tetrachloride, alcohol, salts of sulfonate oils or salts of sulfonated fatty alcohols. Those with carbon tetrachloride or isopropyl or methyl alcohol, of course, can be extremely toxic and dangerous, while the shampoos with the sulfonated oils or alcohol (ethyl) are fairly innocuous unless substantial amounts are ingested.

## HAIR-WAVING PREPARATIONS

Both the electrically heated permanent or machine wave and the "cold" home permanent wave solutions utilize chemicals strong enough to react chemically with the keratin in the hair. This action is produced by employing fairly strong alkaline solutions. Ammonium hydroxide, sodium and potassium carbonate and bicarbonate, sodium borate, triethanolamine and monoethanolamine are among those used for commerical curling solutions. The "cold" wave products, on the other hand, are usually made from the various alkaline salts of thioglycolic acid, which are strong irritants. These keratolytic agents, since they are used at room temperature, must be more potent compounds, and to achieve this, sufficient ammonium or sodium hydroxide is added to develop a pH of 9.0 to 9.5. This facilitates the softening and dissolving of the keratin in the hair shaft. Antagonizing or neutralizing solutions are therefore used to arrest the intense action of the thioglycolate before too much damage is done to the hair. These neutralizing solutions are generally weak oxidizing agents in a weak acidic medium and include peroxides, perborates, bromates and citric or acetic acid. Most manufacturers have voluntarily removed bromate from their products because of its potential toxicity. Home permanent wave users should exercise the following precautions. Contact between the skin and the thioglycolate solution should be kept at a minimum. The solution should also be kept away from the eyes and the ears or else severe inflammation may occur.

## HAIR-STRAIGHTENING SOLUTIONS

Thioglycolates are also used in hair straighteners. In fact, the process is very similar to hair curling except that the hair is held in a straight position instead of being wound on curlers. This method is much safer than those formerly used where basically caustic agents such as sodium carbonate, sodium or barium hydroxide and other strong alkaline solutions were employed. In this process, however, a supplementary procedure is added once the hair has been straightened. The addition of a fixing agent such as a 10% solution of formaldehyde or a 1:1000 solution of potassium permanganate is necessary to hold the hair in the straight position as long as possible.

## HAIR TINTS AND DYES

Hair-coloring agents are of five major types: (1) the rather safe organic vegetable tints such as indigo, henna and various wood extracts (redwood, logwood, etc.); (2) the more toxic metallic preparations such as cobalt, copper, cadmium, iron, lead, nickel, silver, bismuth and tin; (3) a combination of groups 1 and 2; (4) oxidation dyes, the synthetic organic types of the aniline, amine or sulfonated azo dyes which have largely supplanted the other groups. One of the more widely used of these is para-phenylenediamine, which usually requires an oxidizing agent (hydrogen peroxide, sodium persulfate or perborate) in order to become a dye. Unfortunately, this preparation has become a notorious strong sensitizing agent. The synthetic para dyes, because of their carcinogenic effect in animals, are now under close federal supervision and control. All coloring agents containing para-phenylenediamine or one of its homologues must include a caution statement on the package relative to the sensitizing properties of para-phenylenediamine and its ability to cause blindness if it contacts the eyes. The law also requires that patch tests be conducted twenty-four hours before such a dye is applied. Modern oxidation dyes are high sophisticated products containing as many as twenty ingredients, which include in the liquid or cream carrier or base, dye-forming intermediates, color stabilizers and modifiers, antioxidants, keratin-swelling agents and other additives. (5) Semipermanent color with synthetic dyes which do not reduce oxidation (high-intensity rinses, etc.).*

No discussion of hair coloring would be complete without at least a single reference to the most familiar bleach, hydrogen peroxide, which is the safest and least expensive bleaching agent on the market. However, concentrated solutions of 20% to 30% can be strong irritants to the skin or mucous membranes, and repeated use of hydrogen peroxide leaves the hair brittle, difficult to manage and perhaps even impossible to permanent wave. Solutions of hydrogen peroxide 5% to 6% which liberate 17 to 20 volumes of oxygen are most satisfactory for hair bleaching. Ammonia is often added to hasten and intensify the bleaching action. Pure ammonia water (28% solution) purchased in the drugstore, not household ammonia water, should be used. The average used is 20 to 30 drops/oz. of peroxide. Stronger concentrations often leave the hair with an undesirable red tinge.

Recent reports of various *in vitro* tests have raised questions regarding the safety of hair dyes. In particular, the potential carcinogenicity of such products has been questioned. A major cause of these doubts has been the highly publicized findings of Doctor Bruce Ames, a University of California biochemist, who announced that genetic damage was caused by many aromatic compounds when mixed with a special strain of Salmonella bacteria (the Ames test).

A number of other studies also have been run, including dominant lethal studies, teratology studies, reproduction studies and chronic toxicities in rats and micronucleus assays on twelve hair dye ingredients at Huntington Research Labs in England. None of these studies have shown positive correlation to results shown by the Ames bacterial mutagenicity test.

Carmine, which is used primarily to color foods, drugs and cosmetics, is derived from an insect. This dye occasionally contains *Salmonella cubana* and incidents of salmonellosis have been reported.

Phenylenediamines are aromatic diamines related to aniline. The ortho- isomer (Diolen®) is less toxic than the para-isomer (Orsin®, Ursol D®). These compounds are used for dyeing hair and fur, giving a long-lasting natural color ranging from light yellow to jet black. They are potent skin sensitizers, producing urticaria, severe dermatitis, exfoliation and deep staining. Chemosis, lacrimation, exphthalmos, ophthalmia and even permanent blindness may occur as eye complications. Systemic effects include asthma (particularly from inhalation of particulates), vertigo, hypertension, gastritis (regardless of portal of entry), transudation into serous cavities, methemoglobinemia, tremors, convulsions and coma. Phenylenediamines are prime suspects as a cause of bladder tumors in aniline workers.

---

*The ingestion of 2 oz. of Roux Fancifull Rinse® (quaternary ammonium compound) has been reported to have caused the death of a two-year-old child.

*Treatment* consists of discontinuing the exposure immediately and removing the dye from the skin with copious quantities of water. Antihistamines and corticosteroids are helpful in controlling the allergic manifestations, while symptomatic and supportive therapy may be required for pulmonary edema. Methemoglobinemia can be treated with 1% methylene blue.

## HAIRSPRAYS

Present hair spray products contain synthetic and natural resins. Polyvinylpyrrolidone (PVP) is a relatively high molecular weight, synthetic, water-soluble polymer prepared by reacting acetylene, ammonia and formaldehyde under high pressure. It is essentially inert, exceptionally soluble, nontoxic and compatible with a great number of other substances, including body fluids. Because of these characteristics, PVP has found wide acceptance in such diverse fields as medicine, cosmetics and toiletries, textiles, dyestuffs, paper, paints, lithography, inks, protective coatings, agricultural chemicals and beverage clarification.

Hairsprays, when inhaled, have been reported to produce hilar lymphadenopathy and diffuse pulmonary infiltration or storage disease (thesaurosis). Animal experimentation so far does not fully support this danger of hairsprays. Ocular irritation followed by keratitis has also been documented.

Female cosmetologists exposed to aerosol hairsprays are at increased risk of developing pulmonary dysfunctions, according to the National Institute for Occupational Safety and Health. A controlled study of 262 student cosmetologists and 213 graduate cosmetologists in Utah revealed that practicing cosmetologists have a greater chance of developing chronic respiratory disease and atypical sputum cytology which may progress toward more severe changes. The thesaurosis-sarcoidosis syndrome was demonstrated in 22.5 per cent of the graduate cosmetologists, 12 per cent of students and 14 per cent of controls.

Length of time in the industry was an important variable in the development of respiratory disease, graduate cosmetologists showing more dysfunction than students. Symptoms correlating with aerosol use, including wheezing, sputum, cough and phlegm production, were reported by 84 per cent of practicing cosmetologists, 13 per cent of students and only 3 per cent of controls.

Since the evidence linking hairsprays and breathing difficulty is suggestive but still equivocal, healthy young men and women were exposed to timed exposures of three brands of hairspray and their respiratory function measured. Three preparations caused significant decreases in maximum expiratory flow rates at low lung volumes. Peak expiratory flow rates were reduced slightly after use of one brand only. The findings suggest that hairsprays cause acute reversible narrowing of small airways. Although the chemical nature of the responsible ingredients is not known, it is suggested that the mechanism involves histamine release from lung tissue or a direct effect on airway smooth muscle or both (Zuskin, E., and Bouhuys, A.: Acute Airway Response to Hair-spray Preparations. *N Engl J Med, 290*:660, 1974).

Though strict precautionary measures are probably unwarranted for casual use, it would not be amiss to spray such products with eyes closed at a distance of twelve inches from the hair and inhale as little of the mist as possible.

## DEPILATORIES

Chemical depilatories usually have the soluble sulfides (barium sulfide and sodium sulfide) or calcium thioglycolate as the active ingredients. Concentration and pH of thioglycolate are regulated so that the hair is destroyed. In view of the similarity between the chemical composition of the hair and skin, a preparation that is effective in destroying hair may be irritating to the skin. However, many persons use these preparations quite satisfactorily. There is no reason to suspect that this chemical is absorbed through the skin or that its use alters the character or rate of future hair growth. If ingested, the alkalinity of the sulfides may cause irritation of the GI tract with salivation, vomiting and the odor of "rotten eggs" on the breath. Systemic absorption could conceivably cause convulsions and respiratory failure. *Treatment* consists of gastric lavage or emesis and demulcents.

## DEODORANTS

There are basically two types of deodorants: simple deodorants and antiperspirants. A simple deodorant consists of an antibacterial agent in a cream base; an antiperspirant contains aluminum salts, which reduce the flow of perspiration. These agents are in use in one of four forms: cream, liquid (spray), powder or stick. They have the following ingredients: aluminum salts, titanium dioxide, oxyquinoline sulfate, zirconium salt, formaldehyde, antibacterial agents, etc. The amounts present in these products are usually small, and unless a large quantity were ingested, no ill effect should ensue. However, sensitization occurs frequently, which may require discontinuing their use. The stick type of deodorant with zirconium salt, producing chronic granulomatous lesions in the axilla which bear a superficial resemblance to the lesions of tuberculosis, is no longer used in cosmetic deodorants; however, insoluble zirconium oxide in proprietary dermatitis ointments is still a source of disfiguring granulomas. Zirconium-containing aerosol antiperspirants, which have become popular products, have the potential of producing granulomatous lung disease if inhaled over long periods of time; the FDA is considering banning their use.

## ROYAL JELLY

This substance created in beehives by worker bees for the queen bee contains primarily B-complex vitamins, although small amounts of vitamins A and C are also sometimes present. A highly touted miracle cosmetic, it is great for the queen bee and advertising claims to that effect are entirely accurate, but the alleged value of royal jelly for humans has never been confirmed by any reputable scientific studies.

## SUNTAN PREPARATIONS

These articles contain alcohol, sodium, methyl- or ethyl-*p*-aminobenzoate, titanium dioxide, iron oxide pigments, etc. In vogue at present is the use of lotions which when applied to the skin give a suntanned appearance. Chemical constituents of these products are ethyl alcohol, brucine sulfate and other organic solvents. Ingestion of such preparations may be followed by manifestations of acute ethyl alcohol intoxication—exhilaration, nausea, vomiting and central nervous system depression. *Treatment* of established poisoning depends upon the severity of the presenting symptoms (*see* ethyl alcohol).

## "SUNTAN PILLS" (PSORALENS)

Early publicity labeling the psoralens "suntan pills" has led many physicians and patients to regard these compounds as an equivalent to proprietary suntan lotions. Psoralens are furocoumarin compounds present in various plants (bishop's weed, etc.) that have long been know to possess photosensitizing properties. They accelerate pigmentation of the skin when exposed to the sun, ultraviolet or fluorescent light and other sources of radiant energy by increasing production and retention of melanin. Casual prescribing, inadequate instructions, passing around the medications and experimentation by patients have all led to instances of severe blistering dermatitis. In addition, nausea, vomiting, vertigo and mental excitation have been produced. There has been considerable concern over changes in liver function tests during psoralen therapy, and for the present, it should not be used in patients with obvious or incipient liver disease. Despite the drawbacks, it is probably the best treatment for vitiligo at the present time.

*Treatment.* If overdosage occurs, the drug should be removed by gastric lavage or emetics, and the patient kept in a darkened room for twelve hours.

## MISCELLANEOUS COSMETIC PRODUCTS

A glance at Table 37 will give the contents of other miscellaneous cosmetic items of interest that are frequently misused or accidentally ingested by children. Special emphasis, however, should be directed to the common household product hydrogen peroxide, since solutions of 20-30 percent concentration can be strong irritants to the skin and mucous membranes, and corrisive esophagitis may occur with ingestion of such strengths. Experimental studies have demonstrated that Polident® and Efferdent® tablets and Ansodent® powder can produce focal and diffuse caustic burns of the esophagus due to the concentration of hydrogen peroxide liberated by these compounds.

# Chapter 9

# POISONOUS PLANTS, REPTILES, ARTHROPODS, INSECTS AND FISH*

## POISONOUS PLANTS

Much folklore surrounds the subject of plant intoxication, yet the vast majority of the many thousands of known kinds of plants are not only harmless if swallowed, but represent, directly or indirectly, the food source of all living animals. A small number of these plants, however, may be mildly toxic, and a very few can be extremely so and even fatal if ingested in any great quantity. Some plants are harmful only when eaten at certain stages of their growth, while others may be toxic in all stages of development. Thus, both the species of the plant and its stages of growth or the season of the year may be important factors in determining the potential hazard. The noxious chemicals present in plants are alkaloids, glucosides, resins, phenols, alcohols, oxalates and phytotoxins.

It is hearsay that one should beware of all plants with milky sap. This fear is groundless, for the material is not always an indication of toxicity. It is present in abundance in many edible plants as well as in poisonous species. Contrary to popular belief, what a bird eats is not necessarily safe for human consumption, for they often feed on toxic berries and seeds without deleterious effects. In the tropics or jungles, the feeding habits of monkeys or apes would be a safe guide for humans.

Every year more than a million people in the United States experience painful aftereffects from contact with poisonous weeds—in almost all cases, poison ivy, poison oak and poison sumac. The skin irritant of all three is the resin urushiol, containing the allergen pentadecylcatechol. It is present in the sap, which is found in the leaves, roots, stems, pollen and flowers. The painful skin condition results from contact with the exudate that is released by a bruised portion of the plant. The danger of poisoning is greatest in spring and summer when the sap is abundantly produced and accessible.

Aside from direct skin contact with the plants, the irritant may be spread by dogs or other animals; by contaminated clothing, tools or sports equipment such as golf clubs; by smoke from the burning plants; or by accidental ingestion of the fruit buds. After contact, the first symptoms of itching and burning may appear in a matter of a few hours or may take five days, depending on the individual. Severe dermatitis, with vesiculation and local edema, usually develops under the skin and may remain for several days.

*It is not within the scope of this book nor within my competency to describe in detail the enormous number of plant and animal hazards to which humans are subjected. Nevertheless, a brief discussion with tables including the more common species may be helpful to those who are in great need for a ready reference on an emergency basis.

Persistent symptoms are generally due to new contacts with plants or previously contaminated clothing or to spread of the irritant from scratched affected skin areas. Secondary infections may occur when the vesicles are broken. Proper identification and knowledge of the plants with a healthy respect for their potential morbidity are essential in prevention, but eradication of their growth by means of digging or through chemical herbicides is, of course, the most effective method of preventing weed poisoning.

Poison ivy *(Rhus radicans)* is sometimes called three-leaved ivy,† poison creeper, climbing sumac, markweed, picry or mercury. The leaf shapes may vary, but one identifying feature remains constant: there are always three leaflets, two of which are directly opposed; only one leaflet leads off the node of each stem. White waxy flowers and fruit cluster among the smaller branches even after the leaves have fallen. Poison ivy commonly takes the form of a sturdy vine climbing into trees and hedges, over stone walls and up the sides of brick and stone houses. Often, however, it may appear as a shrub, particularly along fence rows or in open fields.

Poison oak *(Rhus toxicodendron),* otherwise referred to as oakleaf ivy or eastern oakleaf poison ivy, usually does not appear as a vine but as a low-growing shrub. The slender upright branches bear leaflets that resemble oak leaves and grow in threes in the same manner as poison ivy. As with poison ivy, there is a wide variation in the shape and size of the leaves. Usually the underside of the leaves is distinctively lighter in color because of the presence of fine hairs on the surface. The fruit resembles that of the poison ivy plant.

Western poison oak, often called yeara, appears along the coastal areas of California, Washington and Oregon. Actually, it is related to poison ivy rather than to poison oak, and the physical resemblance is marked. In open fields, western poison oak usually grows in spreading clumps up to several feet tall. The plant may grow as a vine in wooded areas.

Poison sumac *(Rhus vernix)* is identified as a coarse woody shrub or a small tree. It never assumes the vinelike form of its poison ivy relatives. It is also known as swamp sumac, poison elder, poison ash, poison dogwood and thunderwood. Most frequently growing alongside wet, swampy ground, it ranges in height from five or six feet to twenty-five feet. The leaves of poison sumac are divided into seven to thirteen leaflets that grow in pairs and have a single leaflet at the end of the stem. At first appearance in the spring, the leaves are bright orange and velvet-like. Later they become dark green and glossy on the upper surface and pale green on the lower. Early in the fall they take on a red-orange or russet color. Little yellow-green flowers may be found in clusters among the smaller branches.

Although usually the reaction is not as intense, other plants are capable of producing similar reactions in sensitive individuals. This is more likely a seasonal dermatitis affecting the exposed surface (face, hands, legs and often the genitals). Indirect exposure may occur through the media of animals, insects, clothing and smoke. The following list includes some of the other weeds which produce contact dermatitis.

| | |
|---|---|
| Bittersweet | Marsh elder |
| Broom weed | Pasture sage |
| Burweed | Ragweed, short, giant and western |
| Buttercup | |
| Cocklebur | Sneezeweed |
| Gaillardia (Blanket flower) | Timothy |

The farmer is usually familiar with plants having poisonous seed, which can contaminate grain or flour made from grain. These include corn cockle, mustards, flax, lupines and jimson weed. Cattle grazing in or out of pasture may ingest wild onions, garlic, yarrow, buttercup, dock, tansy, ragweed, mustards and chickory, which give a pungent, unpleasant flavor to milk. The white snakeroot *(Eupatorium rugosum* or *Eupatorium urticaefolium)* and rayless goldenrod *(Aplopappus het-*

† Leaves of three
Quickly flee
Berries white
Poisonous sight

*erophyllus)* produce trematol, an alcohol which causes trembles and muscular weakness in cattle and in human beings who unfortunately drink milk thus contaminated.

Illness in animals, chiefly cattle, is called trembles and results usually from their eating the plant in the fresh state during dry summers and falls when natural food becomes scarce. Occasionally, illness comes from the eating of an affected animal. As animals become sick, they lose their appetite, become weak, frequently fall, tremble noticeably, especially when made to exercise, and become stiff; gaseous abdominal distention develops and they lose consciousness. Death can occur within a few days; on the other hand, the disease may become chronic with periods of remission and exacerbation. The weakness is thought to be due chiefly to hypoglycemia and death to ketosis and acidosis, marked fatty degeneration of liver, kidney and sometimes muscle being noted at post mortem.

In man, the sequence of development of symptoms is anorexia, listlessness, weakness, vague pains, stiffness of muscles, vomiting, abdominal discomfort, constipation often to the degree suggesting obstruction, ketosis, acidosis, occasionally hypoglycemia and lipemia and finally coma. As in animals, death can come quickly, or the disease can become chronic and latent, with exacerbations brought on by fatigue, starvation or intercurrent infection. In man, the disease is almost always the result of drinking raw milk or eating butter made from such milk secreted by trematol-poisoned cows.

Heating only somewhat reduces the toxicity of poisoned milk. Oxidation readily destroys the toxic properties of trematol. Since only a small number of cows are likely to be secreting toxic milk at one time, human illness is seen chiefly when milk from a single animal or small herd is consumed. The dilution which occurs in the usual dairy acquisition and distribution of milk from a large milk shed, rather than pasteurization, is thought to be the reason for failure of the disease to develop in urban areas.

Many ornamental garden plants contain known toxins. Common foxglove *(Digitalis purpurea)*, oleander *(Nerium oleander)*, and lily of the valley *(Convallaria majalis)* all have cardiac glycosides in their leaves.

Although it has been known since ancient times that the leaves, flowers, bark, wood and roots of the common ornamental bush *N. oleander* of the *Apocynaceae* or dogbane family are toxic and that ingestion results in severe and fatal poisonings, the general population unfortunately has not been aware of this fact. Symptoms of oleandrin toxicity include severe abdominal pain, nausea, vomiting, bloody diarrhea, hypotension, hypothermia, cyanosis, cardiac irregularities, convulsions, respiratory paralysis, coma and death. Dipotassium rather than calcium EDTA is the antidote of choice, since it effectively chelates calcium in the body and thus reduces the synergistic action of calcium and oleandrin on the heart.

A common garden flower, the opium poppy *(Papaver somniferum)*, contains the alkaloid opium in its capsule juice. Thebaine obtained from the poppy *Papaver bracteatum* can be readily converted to codeine, and this could be an independent source of codeine to meet United States medical needs if it were allowed to be cultivated in specific quantities. The fragrant yellow jessamine *(Gelsemium sempervirens)* has a toxic alkaloid in all parts that is capable of causing muscular weakness, profuse sweating, convulsions and respiratory failure. Narcissus bulbs, daphne berries, privet berries, larkspur seed, castor bean, jequirity bean, fava bean and Jerusalem cherry are all toxic or potentially toxic depending on the amount taken. Flour made of the bulb of the camas lily *(Zygadenus* and *Camassia)* produced violent intestinal symptoms in the expedition forces of Lewis and Clark. Two alkaloids in the death camas are zygadenine and veratrine. The latter chemical is also found in the false hellebore *(Veratrum viride)*, another member of the lily family which is a strikingly pretty but poisonous green-petaled flower found alongside buttercups and skunk cabbage in swamp and meadow. (A recently improved drug, germine diacetate, has been derived from the dried roots of hellebore and is being used effectively against myasthenia gravis without hypotensive reactions.) The stinging acrid taste of this herb seems to protect all but the hungriest of animals and the most curious of children. The roots of monkshood *(Aconitum)* have been mistaken for horseradish and the shoots of mountain laurel for wintergreen, and when ingested, have produced severe gastrointestinal symptoms. Honey made from laurel or other members of the heath family can also be poisonous.

Jequirity bean *(Abrus precatorius)* has a variety of other names, such as the rosary pea, prayer bead, Buddhist rosary bead, crab's eye, mienie-mienie, Indian bead, Seminole bead, love bean, weather plant and lucky bean. It is a small beautiful bean, measuring 6 mm (¼ in.) long, scarlet or bright orange in color, with a

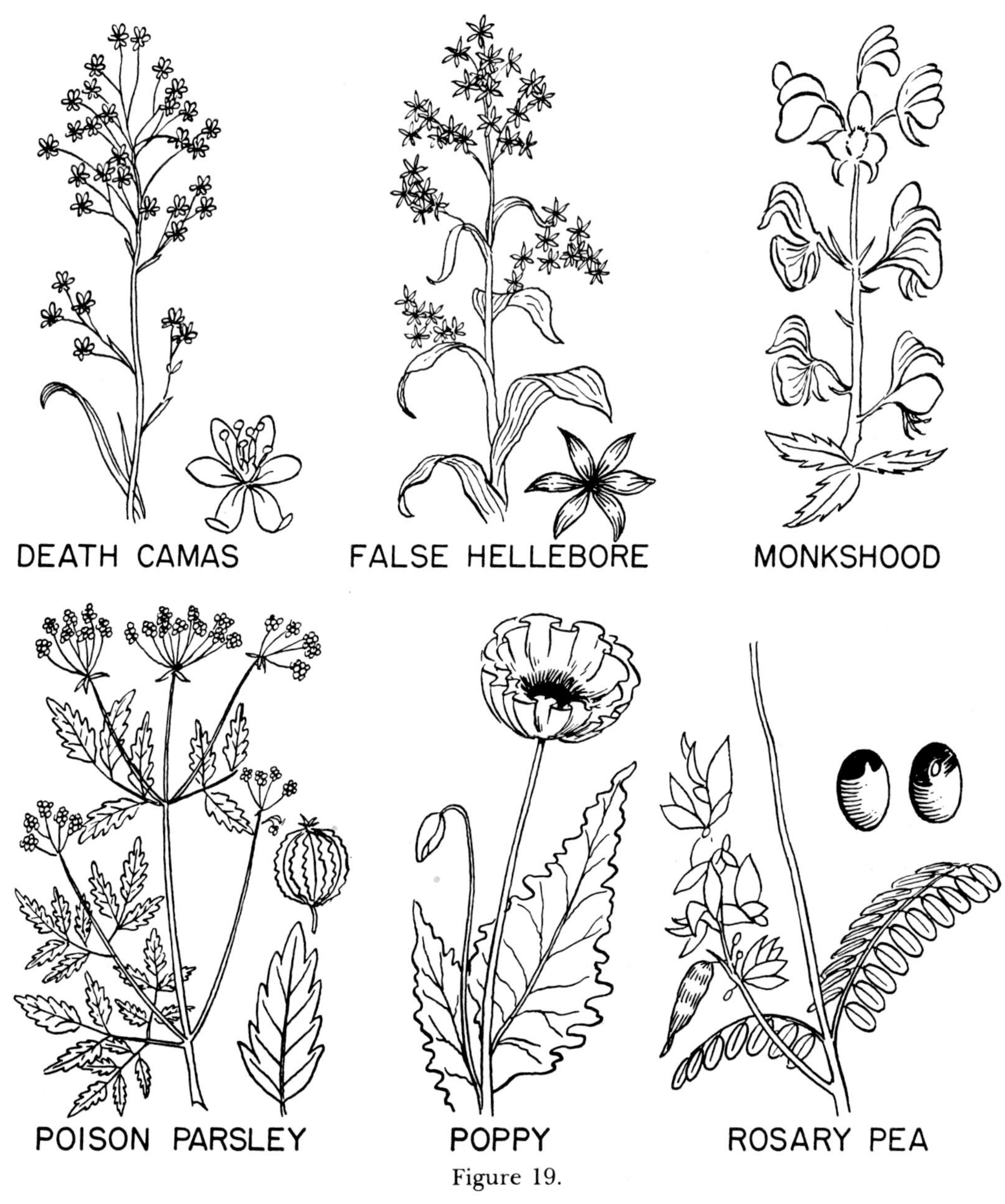

Figure 19.

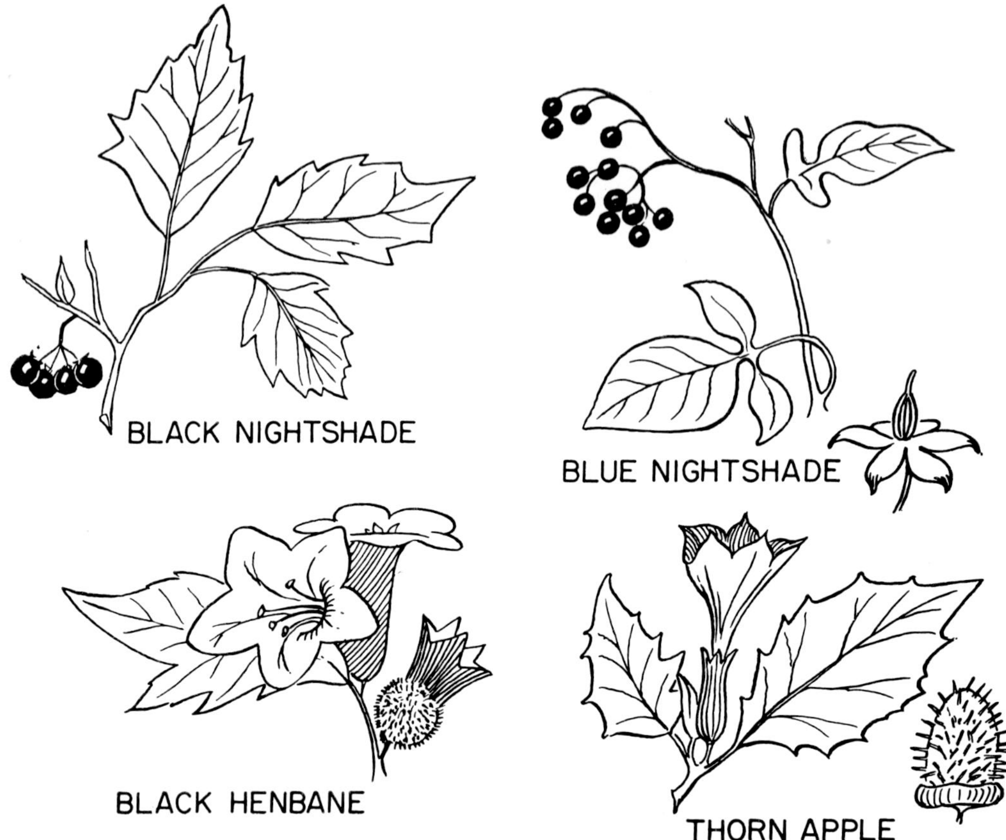


Figure 20.

black "eye" at the hilus, indigenous to tropical and subtropical areas throughout the world. Because of its intense colors and beauty, it is used extensively in inexpensive beadwork and jewelry (necklaces, belts, bead bags, rosaries, brooches, earrings, etc.) for the tourist trade. Unaware of the potential toxicity of these beans, tourists have introduced them, via these products, to many areas in which exposure could not otherwise occur.

The jequirity bean contains a toxic albumin abrin, which has a long history as a poison in both animals and humans. Apparently there is great variability of species toxicity, the dog being considerably less susceptible than the horse and about a hundred times less so than the cat. There are no well-documented toxicity levels in man, and the seriousness of this type of poisoning may very well be overrated in the literature. The toxic effects of abrin are similar to those of ricin, a related toxic albumin obtained from the castor bean, seed of the castor oil plant *(Ricinus communis).* Effects consist of red cell agglutination (hemolysis, thrombus and embolus formation); a direct toxic action on parenchymal cells, the nature of which is poorly understood; severe gastroenteritis; focal necrosis in the liver and kidneys; and occasionally retinal hemorrhages.

Symptoms of jequirity bean poisoning consist of gastroenteritis with nausea, vomiting and diarrhea leading to dehydration, convulsions, circulatory collapse and perhaps death. Symptoms are often delayed one to three days after the ingestion. If the beans are swallowed whole, poisoning is unlikely, since the hard outer coat is unaffected by digestive secretions. However, chewing, grinding or drilling holes in the bean allows contact to occur between the intestinal secretions and the core of the bean, permitting disintegration, absorption and possible poisoning. The immature bean, whose coat is soft and easily broken, is always a potential hazard, especially for children who are attracted by the brilliant colors.

*Treatment* is supportive and symptomatic with parenteral fluids, electrolytes and blood transfusions if needed. Gastric lavage or emetics should be used with caution owing to the necrotizing action of abrin. Saline cathartics for removal may be advisable if used early, but one must keep in mind the subsequent gastrointestinal effects of this toxin. Alkalinization of the urine with sodium bicarbonate may prevent precipitation of hemoglobin and its products in the kidney tubules. Obviously, prevention is better than therapy, and this can only be accomplished by educating the public to the potential dangers of this colorful bean.

Castor beans are also attractive to children. The seeds are about three-eighths to three-quarters of an inch in length, mottled brown or gray or black and glossy. They have toxic potential similar to the jequirity bean, but again, like the jequirity bean, they must be chewed.

*Dieffenbachia* is a small genus of tropical plants belonging to the Araceae, a family which also includes such common ornamental plants as the jack-in-a-pulpit, *Philodendron, Pothos, Anthurium,* calla lily and *Monstera.* Many of these plants are shade loving and have thick, waxy, resistant leaves and are therefore popular as houseplants. *Dieffenbachia* plants are tall, reaching a height of four to eight feet. The fleshy stems are as much as an inch thick, with conspicuous joints. They may be green or somewhat striped with white. The alternate leaves are stalked and have dark green ovate blades, up to twelve to eighteen inches long, sometimes splashed with white markings. Kelade (yarn) belonging to this genus is used for food in Malaya, as a dart poison by the Chinese and as a counterirritant by the aborigines. The common name of the genus, dumbcane, arises from the fact that ingestion of portions of the stem causes extreme irritation of the mouth and throat, with paralysis of the vocal cords. The inflammation and irritation may be prolonged. Greenhouse workers have been known to feed bits of stem to their fellows as a "practical joke," and with the great popularity of the plants for household decoration, cases of poisoning among the general public are now occurring. The action of *Dieffenbachia* has generally been attributed to the microscopic, needle-like calcium oxalate raphides which are common in the tissues of many Araceae. Experimental work with *D. picta* and *D. seguine,* however, showed that accidental contact of the juice of the stem of these species caused intense irritation of the skin on the backs of the hands of the experimenters. Rabbits and guinea pigs treated by placing 1 or 2 ml of fresh *Dieffenbachia* juice in the mouth showed edematous swelling of the lips and tongue. This was followed by dyspnea and suffocation due to constriction of the glottis. These effects were attributed to the portion of the juice which was insoluble in water. The filtrate or centrifuge of the juice contained raphides and a toxic protein. Portions of the filtrate treated with trypsin to digest the protein were still able to provoke the usual initial effects of *Dieffenbachia,* i.e. swelling and irritation of the mouth and tongue. Respiratory embarrassment, however, did not follow. It was concluded from these studies that the respiratory effects of *Dieffenbachia* were therefore due to the protein fraction of the juice, the free amino acid and asparagin, rather than to crystals of calcium oxalate. The possibility of a proteolytic enzyme or protease is also likely. Dyspnea could be prevented or relieved in experimental animals by subcutaneous injection of diphenhydramine hydrochloride or epinephrine. In severe cases, tracheotomy was necessary.

The bird-of-paradise *(Strelitzia)* is another showy plant used for decorative purposes. It is a shrub with a few large leaves and many small leaflets, scarcely one-half inch long, obtuse and glabrous. The flowers are light yellow, with brilliant red stamens protruding four to five inches in terminal racemes. The seed pods bear a close resemblance to the green pea pod and usually appear during the month of June. Ingestion of the seeds or pods can cause severe gastrointestinal symptoms characterized by nausea, vomiting and profuse diarrhea due to an irritant which as yet has not been identified. *Treatment* is symptomatic and supportive.

The *Pyracantha coccinea,* because of its bright red berry-like fruit, is an attractive shrub for children. During the fruit-bearing season (November to March) of this plant, many inquiries are received as to its potential toxicity. From animal experimental studies, it appears that *Pyracantha* berries are not harmful, especially in the relatively small amounts which might be consumed by children. However, the hazards of garden sprays used to combat red spiders on these shrubs must not be overlooked. Lindane, malathion and DDT were common constituents of these sprays.

Several familiar trees are capable of producing toxic symptoms from their bark, leaves, nuts or fruit. The nut of the buckeye or horse chestnut tree, the bean of the Kentucky coffee tree, the leaves of fox bushes, the inner bark of black locusts and all parts of the yew tree are poisonous. Cultivation of tung nut trees in the Gulf states has caused an increase of poisoning from the ingestion of the Brazil-nut-like fruit. The patients have great pain, prostration, intestinal gripings, delirium and weak, rapid pulse. The major GI symptoms such as nausea, vomiting, thirst and diarrhea appear to be caused by toxic albumin. *Treatment* includes oral magnesium sulfate, parenteral fluid and electrolyte replacement, central nervous system stimulants when necessary and oxygen. The tung nut oil, however, is nontoxic other than its potential irritating effect on the skin.

Ackee poisoning or the "vomiting sickness" of Jamaica is caused by eating the unripe or spoiled fruits (ackees) of the *Blighia sapida,* Koenig tree, which is a native of West Africa but also grows in the West Indies and the Canal Zone. The immature seeds contain peptides which have hypoglycemic properties and, in addition, unidentified ninhydrin-positive compounds. The unripe fruits contain a toxic water-soluble substance (hypoglycine) which is not found in water extracts after the fruit reaches maturity. Manifestations of poisoning are violent vomiting followed by drowsiness, stupor, coma and convulsions. Marked hypoglycemia occurs, and in addition to symptomatic and supportive measures in the *treatment,* the intravenous administration of glucose is an important part of therapy.

*Metopium toxiferum,* the poisonwood tree, is abundant in many areas along the borders of hammocks and pine woods. This, as well as the manchineel, are the two most poisonous trees in Florida. The milky sap produces severe dermatitis similar to that of poison ivy.

The nightshade family of plants includes such familiar members as the Irish potato, wild tomato, tobacco, belladonna (deadly nightshade) and the ornamental potted plant, Jerusalem cherry. Uncultivated members of this species are the "angel's trumpet" *(Datura suaveolens),* a pretty flowering shrub of the Southeastern United States and the jimsonweed *(Datura stramonium),* which is also occasionally referred to as the thornapple, stinkweed and Jamestown weed, found particularly around livestock pens and lots or wherever rich soil is available. The early settlers of Jamestown, Virginia, used *Datura stramonium* as a "pot herb" with fatal results, thus establishing one of its common names.

In 1676, a rather hungry contingent of British redcoats arrived in Jamestown, Virginia, to quell an uprising known as Bacon's Rebellion. While bivouacked there, the soldiers gathered some young plants and cooked themselves a tasty pot herb. The consequences of this historic meal are to be found in Robert Beverly's book, *History and Present State of Virginia.*

> The James-Town Weed (which resembles the Thorny Apple of Peru, and I take to be the Plant so call'd) is supposed to be one of the greatest Coolers in the World. This being an early Plant, was gather'd very young for a boil'd salad, by some of the Soldiers sent thither, to pacifie the Troubles of *Bacon;* and some of them eat plentifully of it, the

Effect of which was a very pleasant Comedy; for they turn'd natural Fools upon it for several Days; One would blow up a Feather in the Air: another would dart Straws at it with much Fury; and another stark naked was sitting up in a Corner, like a Monkey, grinning and making Mows at them; a Fourth would fondly kiss and paw his Companions, and snear in their Faces, with a Countenance more antick than any in a *Dutch* Droll. In this frantick Condition they were confined, lest they should in their Folly destroy themselves; though it was observed, that all their Actions were full of Innocence and good Nature. Indeed, they were not very cleanly; for they would have wallow'd in their own Excrements, if they had not been prevented. A Thousand such simple Tricks they play'd, and after Eleven Days, return'd themselves again, not remembering any thing had pass'd.

Thus the hallucinogenic properties of *Datura stramonium* (and *Datura suaveolens*) just now being discovered and used by the drug-cultists (sometimes with fatal results) was historically documented as early as the mid-seventeenth century.

The total belladonna alkaloid of the leaves is 0.35% and that of the seeds 0.40%; the main constituents are atropine and hyoscyamine, the latter being in excess. During the summer months and early fall, the green thorn-covered apples ripen and open, exposing the numerous black seeds. Although the leaves are also poisonous, it is the seeds which are most frequently ingested by children, resulting usually in some manifestation of intoxication and at times a fatal reaction.

The grafting of tomato plants on jimsonweed roots in order to produce large tomatoes that would be resistant to cold has resulted in severe intoxication in several members of a family in Hawkins County, Tennessee, after ingestion of the raw tomatoes. Transient dilation of the pupil has been reported in cornpickers from jimsonweed dust after using a machine in fields where the plant was growing.

*Datura* is a genus under the Solanaceae, and the species *D. stramonium* is a widespread wild plant; but it is one of many species, selections and hybrids of this genus or the very closely related genus *Brugmansia* found as herbs or (in the Deep South and in tropical climates) even as shrubs and small trees. Many forms are cultivated, but wild or cultivated, they are all toxic without exception. Each contains some, if not most, of the following alkaloids, varying somewhat in amount by location in the plant: hyoscyamine, hyoscine, ditiglyteloidine, cuscohygrine, meteloidine, nor-hyoscyamine and unknown alkaloids. The seeds of stramonium may be tan colored.

Other members of the family which are poisonous have the toxic alkaloid solanine in the fruit. The black nightshade *(Solanum nigrum)* is one to two feet high. It has small, white, star-shaped blossoms and black or purple berries. The blue nightshade *(Solanum dulcamara)* has blue or purple wheel-shaped flowers with red berries. The wild tomato *(Solanum carolinense)* is an herb with spiny stem and leaves, lavender or white blossoms and yellow berries.

The parsley family is known by the botanical name of *Umbelliferae*. It is so designated because its many tiny flowers are clustered together in an umbrella-like clump at the top of a stem or branch. Parsley, of course, is not poisonous. The two deadly members of this genus are water hemlock *(Cicuta maculata)* and poison hemlock *(Conium maculatum)*. These plants are three to six feet high, much taller than regular parsley, and have smooth greenish stems speckled with purple spots. They are often mistaken for parsnips, artichokes and other roots. The water hemlock roots contain the toxic resin cicutoxin, which produces convulsions, among other symptoms. The alkaloid coniine, on the other hand, which is present in all parts of the poison hemlock, can cause respiratory depression with paralysis.

A tea popular with Chicanos and some native American Indian tribes called "gordolobos," known also by the common names of tansy ragwort, fat wolf herb, groundsel and mullen, has been recently reported to have caused several deaths in children and adults. The plants* grow throughout Mexico, as well as in the southwestern and western United States, and the teas are commercially distributed to Latino groceries and pharmacies.

---

**Gnaphalium* (gordolobo) and *Senecio longilobus*

TABLE 136
HERBAL PREPARATIONS WITH PSYCHOACTIVE EFFECTS

| *Ingredient* | *Botanical Source* | *Pharmacologic Principle* | *Use* | *Effects* |
|---|---|---|---|---|
| African Yohimbe Bark; Yohimbe | *Corynanthe yohimbe* | Yohimbe | Smoke or tea as stimulant | Mild hallucinogen |
| Broom; Scotch Broom | *Cytisus* spp. | Cytisine | Smoke for relaxation | Strong sedative-hypnotic |
| California Poppy | *Eschscholtzia californica* | Alkaloids and glucosides | Smoke as marihuana substitute | Mild euphoriant |
| Catnip | *Nepeta cataria* | Nepetalactone | Smoke or tea as marihuana substitute | Mild hallucinogen |
| Cinnamon | *Cinnamomum camphora* | ? | Smoke with marihuana | Mild stimulant |
| Damiana | *Turnera diffusa* | ? | Smoke as marihuana substitute | Mild stimulant |
| Hops | *Humulus Lupulus* | Lupuline | Smoke or tea as sedative and marihuana substitute | None |
| Hydrangea | *Hydrangea paniculata* | Hydrangin, saponin, cyanogenes | Smoke as marihuana substitute | Stimulant |
| Juniper | *Juniper macropoda* | ? | Smoke as hallucinogen | Strong hallucinogen |
| Kavakava | *Piper methysticum* | Yangonin, pyrones | Smoke or tea as marihuana substitute | Mild hallucinogen |
| Kola Nut | *Cola* spp. | Caffeine, theobromine, kolanin | Smoke, tea, or capsules as stimulant | Stimulant |
| Lobelia | *Lobelia inflata* | Lobeline | Smoke or tea as marihuana substitute | Mild euphoriant |
| Mandrake | *Mandragora officinarum* | Scopolamine, hyoscyamine | Tea as hallucinogen | Hallucinogen |
| Mate | *Ilex paraguayensis* | Caffeine | Tea as stimulant | Stimulant |
| Mormon Tea | *Ephedra nevadensis* | Ephedrine | Tea as stimulant | Stimulant |
| Nutmeg | *Myristica fragrans* | Myristicin | Tea as hallucinogen | Hallucinogen |
| Passion Flower | *Passiflora incarnata* | Harmine alkaloids | Smoke, tea, or capsules as marihuana substitute | Mild stimulant |
| Periwinkle | *Catharanthus roseus* | Indole alkaloids | Smoke or tea as euphoriant | Hallucinogen |
| Prickly Poppy | *Argemone mexicana* | Protopine, bergerine, isoquinilines | Smoke as euphoriant | Narcotic-analgesic |
| Snakeroot | *Rauwolfia serpentina* | Reserpine | Smoke or tea as tobacco substitute | Tranquilizer |
| Thorn Apple | *Datura stramonium* | Atropine, scopolamine | Smoke or tea as tobacco substitute or hallucinogen | Strong hallucinogen |
| Tobacco | *Nicotiana* spp. | Nicotine | Smoke as tobacco | Strong stimulant |
| Valerian | *Valeriana officinalis* | Chatinine, velerine alkaloids | Tea or capsules as tranquilizer | Tranquilizer |
| Wild Lettuce | *Lactuca sativa* | Lactucarine | Smoke as opium substitute | Mild narcotic-analgesic |
| Wormwood | *Artemisia absinthium* | Absinthine | Smoke or tea as relaxant | Narcotic-analgesic |

From Ronald K. Siegel, *JAMA, 236 (5)*:474, 1976. Copyright 1976, American Medical Association.

Pyrrolizidine alkaloids present in the tea have been responsible for acute and chronic liver disease that occurs. Veterinarians have known for years that such poisoning is a common problem with cattle grazing in the semiarid southwestern states. The ethnic practice of drinking gordolobos tea in Arizona may account for the 20 to 25 per cent higher liver cirrhosis death rate in that state.

Chemical structures of naturally occurring plant alkaloids vary considerably, but the essential feature of hepatotoxicity appears to be a double bond in the pyrrolizidine moiety and the primary allylic hydroxyl esterified with a branched-chain acid. Despite differences in chemical structure, the various hepatotoxins appear to affect an essential cell constituent, probably a mitotic hormone of steroidal nature. Each substance may interfere with a particular stage in biosynthesis of the mitotic factors. The hepatotoxic alkaloids have produced liver injury in all species tested, including rats, mice, hamsters, rabbits, chickens and monkeys. In rats, large doses produce acute liver necrosis and death. Small quantities, even in single doses, cause chronic forms of liver damage and occasional hepatomas which do not become apparent for up to two and one-half years. Traditional usage of local plants should be investigated as possible hepatotoxic factors, particularly in isolated primitive communities where endemic liver disease appears to be related to viral or genetic causes.

Artificial plants consisting of delicate lacy leaves made of plastic are capable of giving off nitrogen dioxide, which can be dangerous if they are kept in a confined area or a person's breathing zone. In addition, they ignite with ease and present a potential fire hazard. Of all plastic flowers and plants, 90 per cent will ignite if a lighted match is held close to them for a few seconds. The plastics usually burn like paraffin and produce dripping balls of fire or puddles of burning liquid.

In photosensitization produced by plants, the photodynamic substance may come directly and unchanged from the plant (primary), or it may be a normal breakdown product in digestion, eliminated by the liver (hepatogenic). Some photosensitization is associated with types of vegetation (algae, fungi, etc.) rather than with individual species of plants.

Rhubarb leaves have a much greater content of oxalic acid than rhubarb stalks. The report of a fatality in a five-year-old girl who ate a large number of the raw leaves would indicate that a potential hazard exists albeit an unusual and uncommon one.

Symptoms are those of oxalic acid intoxication and include burning sensation in the mouth, nausea, vomiting, diarrhea, abdominal pain, muscular tremors, convulsions and collapse. Acute renal failure can occur from the blocking of renal tubules by calcium oxalate crystals. Microscopic examination of the urine shows proteinuria as well as envelope-shaped calcium oxalate crystals and red blood cells. *Treatment* is similar to that for oxalic acid.

### *Mushroom*

There are old mushroom hunters,
And bold mushroom hunters,
But there are no
Old, bold mushroom hunters.

This is an age of a return to natural things, including natural foods. Well, nothing can be any more natural, more available, than mushrooms—or any more dangerous, for that matter. Over the past few years about 500 people annually have been poisoned by mushrooms, some fatally. "Ten persons have died and hundreds have been hospitalized in Italy's worst epidemic of mushroom poisoning in a decade. . . . A number . . . have picked a common, highly toxic mushroom, amanita phalloides, that is easily mistaken for safe varieties," according to Associated Press, September 25, 1975.

In this country almost all cases of mushroom poisoning (mycetismus) are caused by fungi of the *Amanita* genus, particularly *Amanita muscaria* and *Amanita phalloides,* commonly referred to as toadstools. Other less

TABLE 138
PLANTS PRODUCING PHOTOSENSITIZATION

| | | | | | |
|---|---|---|---|---|---|
| | *Hypericum perforatum* | | | St. Johnswort; klamath weed | |
| | *Fagopyrum sagittatum* | | | buckwheat | |
| **Fungi** | | **Algae** | | **Hepatogenic** | |
| *Medicago sativa* | alfalfa | *Avena sativa* | oats | *Agave lecheguilla* | lechugilla |
| *Polygonum* spp. | smartweeds | *Euphorbia maculata* | milk purslane | *Brassica napus* | cultivated rape |
| *Kochia scoparia* | summer cypress | | | *Lantana* spp. | lantana |
| *Sorghum vulgare sudanense* | Sudan grass | | | *Nolina texana* | sacahuiste |
| | | | | *Panicum* spp. | panic grasses |
| *Trifolium* spp. | clovers | | | *Tetradymia* spp. | horsebrush |
| *Vicia* spp. | vetches | | | *Tribulus terrestris* | puncture vine |

TABLE 139
POISONOUS PLANTS

| *Name* | *Part of Plant and Active Principle* | *Symptoms* | *Treatment* |
|---|---|---|---|
| Ackee *(Blighia sapida)* | Unripe fruit (hypoglycin) | Severe vomiting, drowsiness, stupor, coma and convulsions, marked hypoglycemia | Intravenous glucose and supportive |
| Arnica *(Arnica montana, sororia, cordifolia)* | Flowers, roots | Severe GI symptoms; drowsiness and coma | Gastric lavage or emesis; symptomatic |
| Arum family: calla lily, dumbcane, elephant's ear *(Dieffenbachia, Caladium, Alocasia, Colocasia, Philodendron, Dracunculus, Amorphophallis)* | All parts (calcium oxalate, unidentified principles) | Severe burning of mucous membranes with swelling of tongue and throat; nausea; vomiting; diarrhea; salivation; rare direct systemic effects | Gastric lavage or emesis; symptomatic; give demulcents; cold packs to lips and mouth |
| Baneberry, snakeberry *(Actaea spicata, rubra, alba)* | Berries, roots, stock, sap | Severe gastroenteritis; dizziness; circulatory failure | Symptomatic |
| Beechnut *(Fagus sylvatica)* | Seeds | Severe GI symptoms; weakness | Gastric lavage or emesis; symptomatic |
| Betel nut *(Areca catechu)* | Seed (arecoline) | GI symptoms; miosis; dyspnea; convulsions | Gastric lavage or emesis; give atropine, 2 mg SC; repeat p.r.n. |
| Bird of paradise *(Strelitzia)* | Seeds, pods | GI symptoms; vertigo; drowsiness | Gastric lavage or emesis; symptomatic |
| Bittersweet *(Solanum dulcamara)* | Leaves, fruit (solanine) | Abdominal pain; vomiting; diarrhea; shock and depression | |
| Black henbane *(Hyoscyamus niger)* | All parts (alkaloid hyoscyamine) | *See* section on Atropine | *See* section on Atropine |
| Black locust *(Robinia pseudoacacia)* | Bark, foliage, seeds (phytotoxin) | Nausea; vomiting; weakness; and depression | Symptomatic |
| Black nightshade *(Solanum nigrum)* | Leaves, green fruit (solanine) | Abdominal pain; vomiting; circulatory and respiratory depression; diarrhea | Gastric lavage or emesis; symptomatic |
| Bleeding heart, Dutchman's breeches *(Dicentra pusilla, cucullaria)* | Foliage; roots (isoquinoline-type alkaloids such as apomorphine, protoberberine, protopine) | Trembling; ataxia; respiratory distress; convulsions | Symptomatic |

| | | | |
|---|---|---|---|
| Blood root *(Sanguinaria canadensis)* | All parts and especially rhizome (sanguinarine) | GI symptoms; fainting; shock and coma | Gastric lavage or emesis; symptomatic |
| Box *(Buxus sempervirens)* | Leaves, twigs (alkaloid buxine) | GI symptoms; convulsions may occur | Gastric lavage or emesis; symptomatic |
| Buckeye *(Aesculus)* | Flowers, seeds, nuts (glucosides) | GI symptoms; inflammation of mucous membranes; depression; weakness and paralysis | Gastric lavage or emesis; symptomatic |
| Burning bush, wahoo *(Euonymus atropurpureus)* | Fruit, leaves | GI symptoms; weakness; chills; coma or convulsions | Gastric lavage or emesis |
| Calabar bean *(Physostigma venenosum)* | Bean (physostigmine) | Dizziness; faintness; vomiting; diarrhea; pinpoint pupils | Gastric lavage or emesis; give atropine 2 mg IM repeat q.2 to 4hr. p.r.n. |
| Cashew nut *(Anacardium occidentale)* | Oil (mono and polyhydric phenols) | Contact dermatitis with edema and vesiculation | Apply wet dressing; symptomatic |
| Cassava *(Manihot utilissima)** | Root (amygdalin) | A soluble cyanogenetic glycoside in the juice causes cyanide poisoning unless removed | Treat as for cyanide poisoning |
| Castor bean *(Ricinus communis)* | Seed (ricin), if chewed; if swallowed whole, hard seed coat prevents absorption and poisoning | Severe GI symptoms; convulsions; uremia | Immediate gastric lavage or emesis; supportive; alkalinize urine with 5 to 15 gm of sodium bicarbonate daily |
| Celandine *(Chelidonium majus)* | All parts and especially root (chelidonine) | GI symptoms; fainting and coma | Gastric lavage or emesis; supportive |
| Cherry, black (*Prunus serotina, demissa, melanocarpa,* etc.) | Bark, leaves but especially the seed (amygdalin which breaks down into hydrocyanic acid) | Stupor; vocal cord paralysis; twitching; convulsions and coma from chewing seeds | Treat as for cyanide poisoning |
| China berry *(Melia azedarach)* | All parts | Narcotic effects; GI symptoms | Gastric lavage or emesis; symptomatic |
| Chrysanthemum | All parts (a resin) | Contact dermatitis from sensitivity, with erythema and vesiculation | Wash skin thoroughly |
| Cockles, corn *(Agrostemma githago)* | Seeds (githagin) | GI symptoms; dizziness; weakness; slow respiration | Gastric lavage or emesis; supportive |
| Colchicum: meadow saffron, autumn crocus, naked ladies *(Colchicum autumnale)* | Seeds, leaves, flowers (colchicine) | Burning pain in mouth and stomach; GI symptoms; prostration; hematuria; anuria | *See* Colchicum |
| Croton *(Croton tiglium)* | Seed (croton oil) | Burning pain in mouth and stomach; tachycardia; bloody diarrhea; coma and death | Gastric lavage, milk for demulcent; symptomatic |
| Crowfoot family: crowfoot or buttercup *(Ranunculaceae)* | All parts (anemenol) | Paresthesia; burning sensation of the mouth and skin; nausea; vomiting; hypotension; weak pulse; convulsions | Atropine, 2 mg IM and repeat p.r.n.; maintain blood pressure; artificial respiration |
| Christmas rose *(Hellebous niger)* | All parts (alkaloids, veratrin, etc.) | As above | As above |
| Golden seal *(Hydrastis canadensis)* | All parts (berberine, canadine, hydrastine) | As above | As above |
| Larkspur (*Delphinium* sp.) | All parts (delphinine, etc.) | As above | As above |

*The toxicity of cassava has long been recognized. However, it remains an important food plant in certain parts of South America because the people using it have learned means of preparation that serve to remove or hydrolyze the linamarin and lotaustralin and to destroy the β-glucosidase that is present.

TABLE 139—*Continued*
POISONOUS PLANTS

| *Name* | *Part of Plant and Active Principle* | *Symptoms* | *Treatment* |
|---|---|---|---|
| Marsh marigold *(Caltha palustris)* | All parts (volatile oil, protoanemonin) | As above | As above |
| Monkshood *(Aconitum napellus)* | All parts, but especially roots and seed (aconitine and related alkaloids) | As above | As above |
| Daffodil, jonquil *(Narcissus pseudonarcissus, jonquilla)* | Bulb | GI symptoms | Gastric lavage or emesis |
| Daphne *(Daphne mezereum)* | All parts (daphnin) | Abdominal pain; vomiting; convulsions; nephritis | Gastric lavage or emesis; symptomatic |
| Darnel *(Lolium temulentum)* | Seed (temuline) | Vertigo; ataxia; vomiting; visual disturbances; tremors; dysphagia; prostration | Gastric lavage or emesis; supportive |
| Deadly nightshade *(Atropa belladonna)* | Berries, leaves, roots (atropine and related alkaloids) | *See* section on Atropine | *See* section on Atropine |
| Death camas *(Zygadenus)* | Bulb or root (zygadenine, veratrine, others) | Salivation; GI symptoms; muscular weakness; hypotension; bradycardia | *See* section on Veratrum |
| Elderberry, black and scarlet elder *(Sambucus canadensis, pubens)* | Leaves, shoots, bark (sambunigrin, a cyanogenetic glycoside) | *See* section on Cyanide | *See* section on Cyanide |
| False hellebore *(Veratrum viride)* | All parts (veradridene, veratrine, others) | Craniofacial (teratogenic) malformation in animals (lambs); *see* section on Veratrum | *See* section on Veratrum |
| Fava bean, broad bean, horse bean, Windsor bean *(Vicia faba, Canavalia gladiata)* | Pollen, bean | Onset 2 to 3 hr. after inhalation of pollen or 2 to 3 days after ingestion; headache; GI symptoms and severe hemolytic anemia may occur. (Seen in families of Italian and Mediterranean origin with G-6-PD deficiency.) | Gastric lavage or emesis; blood transfusions, if necessary; keep urine alkaline |
| Finger cherry *(Rhodomyrtus macrocarpa)* | Fruit | Blindness within 24 hours which can at times be complete and permanent | Gastric lavage or emesis; symptomatic |
| Fish berries *(Cocculus indicus)* | Dried fruit (picrotoxin) | GI symptoms; restlessness; fever; convulsions and coma | Gastric lavage or emesis; cold pack for hyperthermia; treat convulsion |
| Four o'clock *(Mirabilis jalapa)* | Root, seed (alkaloid trigonelline) | Laxative effect; irritant to skin and mucosa | Symptomatic |
| Foxglove *(Digitalis purpurea, D. lanata)* | Leaves (digitalis, glycosides) | *See* section on Digitalis | *See* section on Digitalis |
| Gloriosa or climbing lily *(Gloriosa superba)* | All parts, particularly tuber (colchicine and mixture of alkaloids) | *See* section on Colchicine | *See* section on Colchicine |
| Henbane, black *(Hyoscyamus niger)* | All parts (atropine and related alkaloids) | *See* section on Atropine | *See* section on Atropine |
| Holly, black alder *(Ilex aquifolium, opaca, verticillata)* | Berries (ilicin) | GI symptoms; narcosis | Gastric lavage or emesis; symptomatic |
| Hyacinth† *(Hyacinthus orientalis)* | Bulb | Severe GI symptoms | Gastric lavage or emesis; symptomatic |

| | | | |
|---|---|---|---|
| Hydrangea, wild hydrangea | Under normal conditions this plant is nontoxic. However, formation of hydrocyanic acid is possible and may cause symptoms | *See* section on Cyanide | *See* section on Cyanide |
| Indian tobacco *(Lobelia inflata)* | All parts (α-lobeline) | Progressive vomiting; weakness; stupor; tremors; miosis and coma | Gastric lavage or emesis; artificial respiration; give atropine, 2 mg IM and p.r.n. |
| Iris *(Iridaceae)* | Root | Nausea; severe diarrhea; abdominal burning and pain | Gastric lavage or emesis; symptomatic |
| Jack-in-the-pulpit *(Arisaema triphyllum)* | All parts, especially the rhizome (calcium oxalate) | Severe GI symptoms; irritation and burning of the mouth | Symptomatic; aluminum hydroxide for neutralizing and demulcent effects |
| Jequirity bean, love bean, rosary bead, lucky bean, prayer bead *(Abrus precatorius)* | Bean (abrin) must be thoroughly chewed; if swallowed whole, poisoning is unlikely since hard seed coat prevents rapid absorption; causes agglutination and hemolysis of red cells in extreme weak dilution | After 1 to 3 days severe GI symptoms; drowsiness; coma; circulatory collapse; hemolytic anemia; oliguria and fatal uremia | Gastric lavage or emesis; maintain circulation and correct hemolytic anemia with blood transfusions; keep urine alkaline |
| Jerusalem cherry *(Solanum pseudocapsicum)* | Fruit (solanine) | GI symptoms; convulsions; respiratory and central nervous system depression | Support respiration; symptomatic |
| Jessamine or yellow jessamine *(Gelsemium sempervirens)* | All parts (gelsemine, gelseminine) | Profuse sweating; muscular weakness; convulsions; respiratory depression | Gastric lavage or emesis; atropine 2 mg IM and p.r.n.; artificial respiration |
| Jet berry bush *(Rhodotypos)* (an ornamental bush with black berries) | Berries (amygdaline, other cyanogenetic glycosides) | Vomiting; abdominal rigidity and pain; fever; convulsions and coma; *see* section on Cyanide | Gastric lavage or emesis; lower temperature by cold applications; treat as for cyanide poisoning |
| Jimson weed, thornapple, stinkweed, etc. *(Datura stramonium)* | All parts (atropine and related alkaloids) | *See* section on Atropine | *See* section on Atropine |
| Jute *(Corchorus olitorius, C. capsularis)* | Fibrous stem | Allergic reaction from sensitivity (asthma, hayfever, contact dermatitis) | Avoid further exposure; symptomatic |
| Kentucky coffee tree *(Gymnocladus dioica)* | Seed (cytisine) | GI symptoms | Symptomatic |
| Laburnum, golden chain *(Cytisus laburnum)* | Leaves, seeds (cytisine) | Dysphagia; nausea; severe vomiting; diarrhea; prostration; irregular pulse and respiration; delirium; twitching and coma (similar to nicotine effects); renal damage may occur | Gastric lavage or emesis; *see* section on Nicotine |
| Lady's slipper *(Cypripedium hirsutum)* | Hairs of stems, leaves (fatty acids) | Contact dermatitis | Symptomatic |
| Lantana, red sage, wild sage *(Lantana camara)* | All parts (lantanin), especially the green berries | Photosensitization, with increase in severity from sunlight; acute symptoms resemble belladonna alkaloid (atropine) poisoning | Gastric lavage or emesis; *see* section on Atropine |
| Laurel: Mountain, Black, Sheep, American, etc. *(Kalmia)* | All parts (andromedotoxin) | Salivation; lacrimation; rhinorrhea; vomiting; convulsions; slowing of pulse; hypotension; paralysis; *see* Veratrum | *See* section on Veratrum. Atropine |
| Lecythis: monkey pod, coco de mono | Nuts (almonds) | Nausea; malaise; chills; loss of hair | Symptomatic |

†The hyacinth bean, *Dolichos lablab* (papapa bean, Hawaii), is used by the Filipinos for food, after having boiled them and decanted the *cyanide* in the discard water.

TABLE 139—*Continued*
POISONOUS PLANTS

| *Name* | *Part of Plant and Active Principle* | *Symptoms* | *Treatment* |
|---|---|---|---|
| Lily of the valley *(Convallaria majalis)* | Leaves, flowers (convallatoxin and other glycosides) | *See* section on Digitalis | *See* section on Digitalis |
| Lima bean *(Phaseolus limensis, P. lunatus)* | Beans | Colored varieties of the lima bean contain cyanogenetic glycosides. Many instances of cyanide poisoning have occurred in New Guinea from eating raw lima beans (cooking is preventive) | *See* section on Cyanide |
| Lupin *(Lupinus* sp.) | All parts but specifically the berries (lupinine and related alkaloids) | Paralysis; weak pulse; respiratory depression; convulsions | Gastric lavage or emesis; artificial respiration; treat convulsions |
| Manchineel *(Hippomane mancinella)* | Sap, fruit | Contact dermatitis with severe irritation; blistering; peeling of skin from contact with sap; GI symptoms | Gastric lavage or emesis; wash skin with soap and water |
| Mango *(Mangifera indica)* | Skin of fruit, sap of tree | Dermatitis; GI symptoms | Avoid eating the peel |
| Marihuana, Indian hemp *(Cannabis sativa)* | Leaves, flowers, sap (cannabinol‡, and related compounds) | Exhilaration; hallucinations; delusions; blurred vision; ataxia; stupor; coma | Gastric lavage or emesis |
| Mayapple *(Podophyllum peltatum)* | Green fruit, foliage, roots (resin podophyllin) | Laxative effect with severe purging; local contact produces dermatitis | Symptomatic |
| Mescal, peyote *(Lophophora williamsii)* | Button (mescaline) | Nausea; headache; hallucinations and illusions; early vomiting usually prevents serious poisoning | Gastric lavage or emesis, if vomiting does not occur |
| Mexican poppy *(Argemone mexicana)* | Seed, expressed oil (protopine and berberine alkaloids) | Myocardiopathy; edema; GI symptoms; visual disturbances | Symptomatic |
| Mistletoe *(Phoradendron flavescens)* | All parts, but especially the berries (beta-phenylethylamine and tyramine) | GI symptoms and bradycardia similar to digitalis. Leaves have been used for tea, as coffee substitute with apparently no ill effect. | *See* section on Digitalis |
| Moonseed *(Menispermum canadense)* | Roots, fruit (bitter alkaloid) | GI symptoms; the rough, sharp ridges of the fruitpits may cause mechanical injury to the intestines | Symptomatic |
| Morning glory, heavenly blue, pearly gates, etc. *(Ipomoea violacea)* | Seeds (alkaloids, ergine, isoergine, elymoclavine, etc. all related to LSD) | From 50 to 200 powdered seeds have produced LSD effects | *See* section on LSD |
| Mulberry, red *(Morus rubra)* | Green berries and sap from stems and leaves | Contact dermatitis; CNS stimulation and hallucination reported from eating green berries | Gastric lavage or emesis; wash with soap and water |
| Mushrooms *(Amanita, Muscaria* and *Phalloides)* | *See* section on Mushrooms | *See* section on Mushrooms | *See* section on Mushrooms |
| Nutmeg *(Myristica fragrans)* | Seeds (myristicin) | *See* section on Nutmeg | *See* section on Nutmeg |
| Oleander *(Nerium oleander)* | Leaves (oleandrin, nerioside) | Same as for Digitalis | *See* section on Digitalis |

| | | | |
|---|---|---|---|
| Peas, sweet pea *(Lathyrus odoratus)* | All parts, but especially seeds (beta-aminopropionitrile, alpha-gamma-aminobutyric acid) | Paralysis; slow and weak pulse; respiratory depression; convulsions | Gastric lavage or emesis; symptomatic |
| Physic nut *(Jatropha* sp.) | Seed | Nausea; vomiting; bloody diarrhea; coma | Gastric lavage or emesis; symptomatic |
| Poinsettia *(Euphorbia pulcherrima)* | Leaves, stem, milky sap | Contact dermatitis; GI symptoms | Gastric lavage or emesis |
| Poison hemlock, deadly hemlock, poison parsley *(Conium maculatum)* | All parts (alkaloid coniine) allergen α-pentadecylcatechol | GI symptoms; necrosis; muscular weakness; respiratory paralysis; convulsions | Gastric lavage or emesis; saline cathartic; keep airway clear; oxygen and artificial respiration; anticonvulsive therapy |
| Poison ivy, poison oak, poison creeper, picry, "mercury" *(Rhus toxicodendron)* | All parts (resin urushiol) | Skin lesions due to sensitivity; no systemic symptoms | Symptomatic |
| Poison sumac, poison dogwood, poison elder, poison ash, swamp sumac, thunderwood *(Rhus vernix)* | All parts (resin urushiol) | Skin lesions due to sensitivity; no systemic symptoms | Symptomatic |
| Poison tree, coral sumac, doctor gum *(Metopium toxiferum)* | Sap | Severe dermatitis leaving black stains | Wash skin with soap and water |
| Pokeweed, pokeberry, scoke, inkberry *(Phytolacca americana)* | All parts, but especially root (saponins and glycoprotein); gylcoproteins in species of pokeweed in Africa produce lymphocytes that strongly resemble (by electronmicroscope) those found in Burkitt's lymphoma | Burning and bitter taste in the mouth; persistent vomiting; amblyopia; slowed respiration; dyspnea; weakness; tremors and convulsions; peripheral blood plasmacytosis (potential immunosuppressive properties); not as innocuous as sometimes indicated in the literature | Gastric lavage or emesis; symptomatic |
| Poppy *(Papaver somniferum)* | Unripe seed capsule (opium alkaloids) | *See* section on Morphine | *See* section on Morphine |
| Potato *(Solanum tuberosum)* | Green tubers, new sprouts (solanine) | Severe GI symptoms; headache; cold and clammy skin; circulatory and respiratory depression | Gastric lavage or emesis; symptomatic |
| Primrose *(Primula* sp.) | Stems, leaves (primin) | Contact dermatitis | Symptomatic; wash skin thoroughly with soap and water |
| Privet, common *(Ligustrum vulgare)* | Berries, leaves (andromedotoxin) | Gastrointestinal irritation; hypotension and renal damage; *see* section on Veratrum | Gastric lavage or emesis; treat as for veratrum |
| Pyracantha, firethorn *(Pyracantha coccinea)* | Shrub bearing clusters of small bright red and orange berry-like fruit | The ingestion of large numbers of berries by animals and children has not produced any serious symptoms | None |
| Rayless goldenrod *(Aplopappus heterophyllus)* | All parts (trematol) | Drinking milk from animals which have been fed on white snakeroot or rayless goldenrod causes nausea, severe vomiting, anorexia, constipation, weakness, tremors, jaundice, and convulsions; there may be oliguria or anuria from kidney damage | Symptomatic; treat liver damage and anuria |
| Rhododendron (*Rhododendron albiflorum, macrophyllum,* etc.) | All parts (andromedotoxin) | Salivation; lacrimation; nasal discharge; vomiting; convulsions; bradycardia; lowering of blood pressure; paralysis | As for veratrum. Atropine |

‡The active chemical synthesized principle tetrahydrocannabinol was made available for research purposes in 1966.

TABLE 139—*Continued*
POISONOUS PLANTS

| *Name* | *Part of Plant and Active Principle* | *Symptoms* | *Treatment* |
|---|---|---|---|
| Rhubarb *(Rheum rhaponticum)* | Leaves only (oxalic acid) | Nausea; vomiting; abdominal pain; anuria; hemorrhages; *see* Oxalic acid | Treat as for oxalic acid |
| Skunk cabbage *(Symplocarpus foetidus)* | Leaves, rhizomes (calcium oxalate) | *See* jack-in-the-pulpit above | |
| Snakeroot, white *(Eupatorium urticae folium)* | All parts (trematol) | *See* rayless goldenrod above | Treat as for rayless goldenrod above |
| Spanish broom, Scotch broom *(Sparteus junceum, Sarothamnus scoparius)* | Seeds or leaves (sparteine) | Weak pulse; intestinal paralysis; weakness; fall of blood pressure | Treat as for quinidine |
| Spindle-tree *(Euonymus europaeus)* | Fruits, leaves | GI symptoms; weakness; chills; coma or convulsions | Gastric lavage or emesis; symptomatic |
| Staggerbush *(Lyonia mariana)* | All parts (andromedotoxin) | Salivation; increased tear formation; nasal discharge; vomiting; convulsions; bradycardia; hypotension; paralysis | Treat as for veratrum |
| Star anise, Japanese *(Illicium anisatum)* | All parts | GI symptoms; coma; convulsions | Gastric lavage or emesis; symptomatic |
| Star of Bethlehem *(Ornithogalum umbellatum)* | All parts, bulbs, leaves, fresh or dried (alkaloids) | GI symptoms | Symptomatic |
| Tung nut *(Aleurites fordii)* | Seed (sapotoxin) | Nausea; vomiting; abdominal pain; weakness; hypotension; shallow respiration | Symptomatic |
| Water hemlock, cowbane, beaver poison *(Cicuta maculata, virosa)* | Roots (resin cicutoxin) | GI symptoms; convulsions; respiratory depression | Gastric lavage or emesis; symptomatic; control convulsions with parenteral short-acting barbiturates |
| Wild grape *(Rhiocissus cuneifolia)* | Root | GI symptoms; respiratory depression | Gastric lavage or emesis; artificial respiration |
| Wild monkshood *(Aconitum uncinatum)* | All parts (alkaloid aconitine) | Dysphagia and numbness in the mouth and throat; colicky abdominal pain; vomiting; bloody diarrhea; ataxia; convulsions; coma; respiratory failure | Gastric lavage or emesis; artificial respiration |
| Wild tobacco *(Nicotiana glauca)* | All parts of plant (nicotine) | *See* section on Nicotine | *See* section on Nicotine |
| Wild tomato, horse nettle, bull nettle, sand briar *(Solanum carolinense)* | Green fruit (solanine) | GI symptoms; abdominal pain; circulatory and respiratory depression | Gastric lavage or emesis; symptomatic |
| Wisteria *(Wisteria sinensis)* | Pods (resin and glucoside, wisterin) | Severe GI symptoms; collapse | Gastric lavage or emesis; symptomatic |
| Yellow nightshade *(Urechites suberecta)* | Fruit | Burning of the mouth and throat; drowsiness; paralysis; convulsions; respiratory failure | Gastric lavage or emesis; symptomatic |
| Yew *(Taxus baccata)* | All parts (alkaloid taxine) | GI symptoms; mydriasis; muscular weakness; coma; convulsions; cardiac and respiratory depression | Gastric lavage or emesis; control pain with meperidine (Demerol); otherwise symptomatic |

well known mushrooms, such as the *Galerina venenata, Halvella esculenta, Lactarius vellereus* and *Lepiota morgani,* contain muscarine and phalloidine which can also produce symptoms. Poisoning occurs only rarely from the false morel *(Gyromitra esculenta)* and other species. It must be recognized that diverse opinions exist as to the specificity and toxicity of the various types; undoubtedly the content of toxin in any species of mushrooms may vary with the seasons, individual susceptibilities, environmental factors and geographic location.

Mushrooms are unpredictable. Some species are consistently poisonous, although they cause symptoms of varying severity; other species are occasionally poisonous. Some are poisonous only when eaten raw, others when eaten during certain seasons or stages of maturity. The variations within the same species seem to be due to genetic differences as well as differences in the soil and climate.

Then, too, man is unpredictable. One person may be poisoned severely by a mushroom species that another eats with no ill effect. For some people, drinking alcohol before, during or after eating mushrooms causes a reaction similar to that of disulfiram (Antabuse) and alcohol. Also, use of certain drugs, hydroxychloroquine for example, may make an ordinarily harmless mushroom toxic for certain people.

Rapid intoxication (a few minutes to two hours) is caused by the ingestion of muscarine contained in *A. muscaria.* Depending on the amount of muscarine present, which is variable and may even be insignificant, the symptoms are lacrimation, miosis, salivation, sweating, dyspnea, abdominal cramps, diarrhea, vomiting and circulatory failure. Mental disturbances, coma and convulsions are also characteristic.

A delayed intoxication (usually six to twenty-four hours) and more deadly type of poisoning is caused by phalloidine or other toxins in *A. phalloides.* This long asymptomatic latent period is often puzzling to the physician, and unless he is aware of this possibility, an erroneous diagnosis may be made. Gastrointestinal symptoms are similar to those due to muscarine. In addition, liver damage and oliguria or even anuria may result, secondary to renal tubular damage. Circulatory failure and coma usually follow within a week.

The highly lethal mushroom toxins phalloidine and phalloin have been isolated and identified by ultraviolet absorption spectral characteristics and by chromatographic separation of liver extracts. A thin-layer chromatographic assay of vomitus, intestinal aspirate, stool and uneaten specimens can rapidly and reliably detect the presence of amanitin and phalloidine. Toxicologic analysis of tissue in fatal cases of suspected mushroom poisoning is promising and actually may be the only method for making the correct diagnosis in a puzzling situation. Muscarine, myceto-atropina (levohyoscyamine), bufotenin, amanita toxins (five in number), helvellic acid, psilocybin, disulfiram and gastrointestinal irritants have been identified so far in mushrooms.

It should be noted that cooking does not destroy all the toxins in poisonous mushrooms and thus does not protect against the lethal effects of failure of proper identification. Nor is there any truth in the statements that a silver spoon or coin added to the pan in which mushrooms are cooked will darken if poisonous species are present nor that if the skin can be peeled from the cap of a mushroom, and/or that if they fail to turn color when broken, they are nonpoisonous.

*Treatment* consists of gastric lavage with tannic acid 1:200 or potassium permanganate 1:5000 solution, followed by a saline purgative. Atropine sulfate given subcutaneously or intravenously in a dose of 0.1 to 0.5 mg (1/640 to 1/120 gr) specifically antagonizes the overstimulation of the parasympathetic nervous system caused by muscarine. Larger doses are tolerated and repeated as necessary. Toxins similar to atropine, producing atropine-like symptoms, would obviate the use of atropine in therapy. A high-protein diet and protein hydrolysate should be administered intravenously to help prevent severe liver damage caused by phalloidine. Corticosteroids may prove useful as therapeutic agents

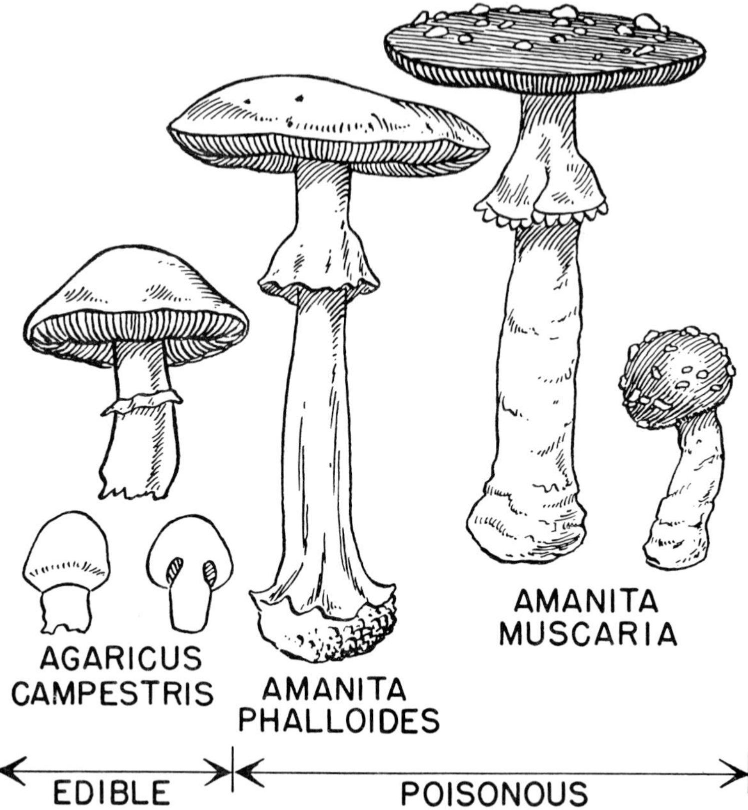


Figure 21. Edible Four are: the puffball or Calvatia family (sphere without gills that look like seamless softballs and sometimes grow as large as 15 inches in diameter and weigh several pounds; the chicken mushroom (yellow, grows on trees in wrinkled, flat, layered clumps and tastes like chicken); the morel (brown, hollow inside, unmistakable because of its spongy, pitted exterior, grows only in the spring near old trees); and the shaggy-mane Coprinus comatus (elongated cap with yellowish, hairy scales, hollow stem with delicate white cord suspended in the cavity, found in rich earth near roads, in pastures and at dumps).

and should be given a trial. Both peritoneal dialysis and hemodialysis have been successful in preventing kidney failure in patients who had developed renal tubular necrosis, and there should be no hesitation in using these measures. Activated charcoal by mouth should be used for *A. phalloides* ingestion. Antiphalloidine serum was ineffective and is no longer available. A clinical impression persists that the sooner and the more vigorous the purging, whether spontaneous or induced by treatment, the less severe is the late injury to vital organs. Supportive therapy should be given as required.

During the past ten years, the use of thioctic acid (alpha-lipoic acid) in the successful treatment of *Amanita phalloides* mushroom poisoning has been enthusiastically reported in the European literature. In the United States, the first reported case of thioctic acid therapy for mushroom poisoning was described in 1968 by Finestone. Since then, eleven other cases of *Amanita* or *Galerina* poisoning in the United States are known to have received thioctic acid. Nearly all of these patients had chemical and clinical evidence of hepatocellular damage. Ten have survived and recovered without major sequelae. The only observed side-effect of thioctic acid to date has been hypoglycemia. Whether the hypoglycemia was a consequence of the drug or from the severe hepatic abnormalities

## WHICH OF THESE LOOK-ALIKES IS POISONOUS?

One of each pair is poisonous; the other, edible. As you can see, they are indistinguishable, so never try to identify them yourself.

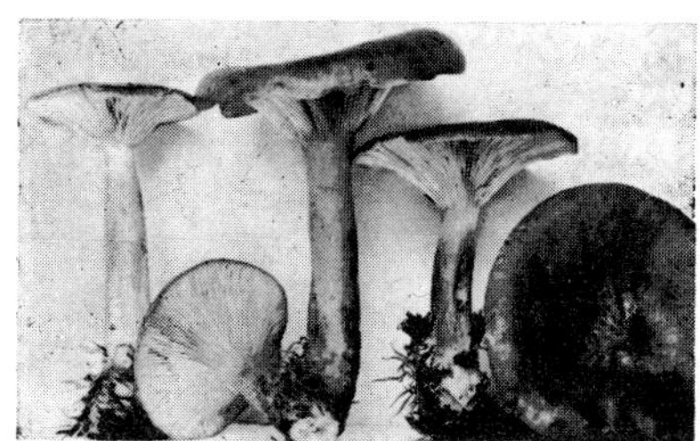
1A—Lactarius helvus

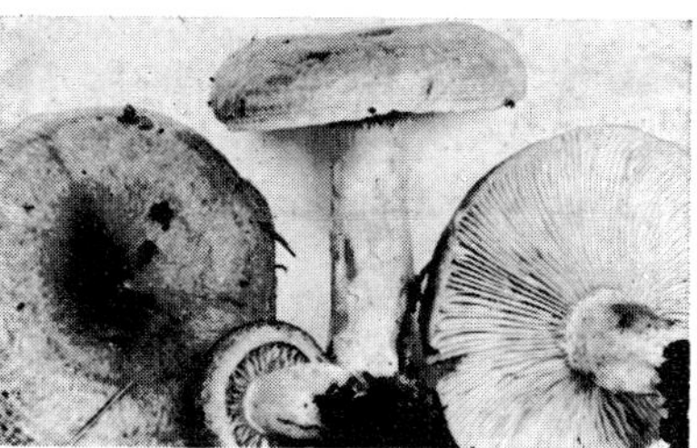
1B—Lactarius deliciosus

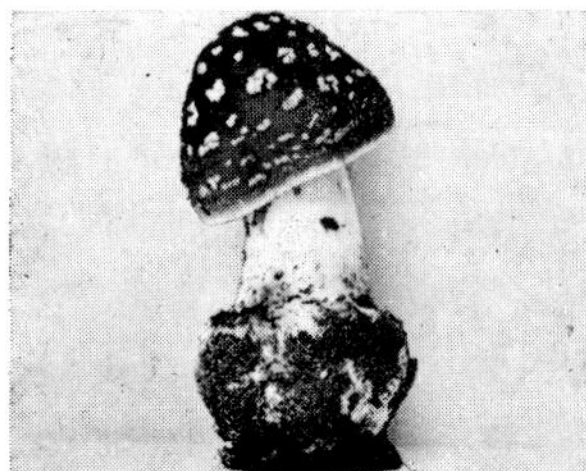
2A—Amanita brunnescens

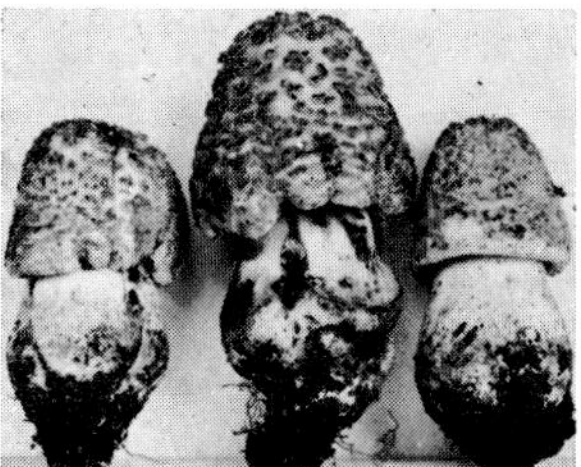
2B—Amanita rubescens

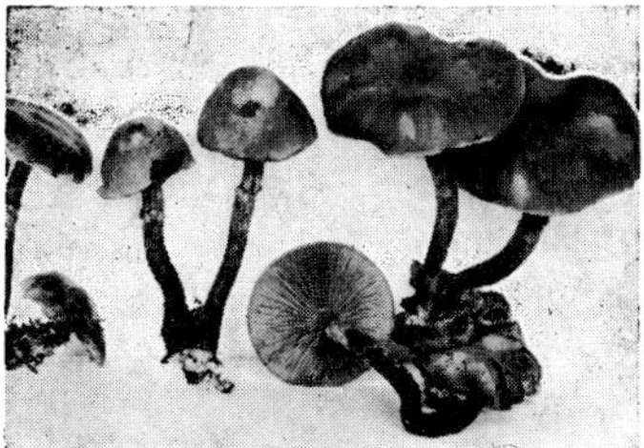
3A—Pholiota curvipes

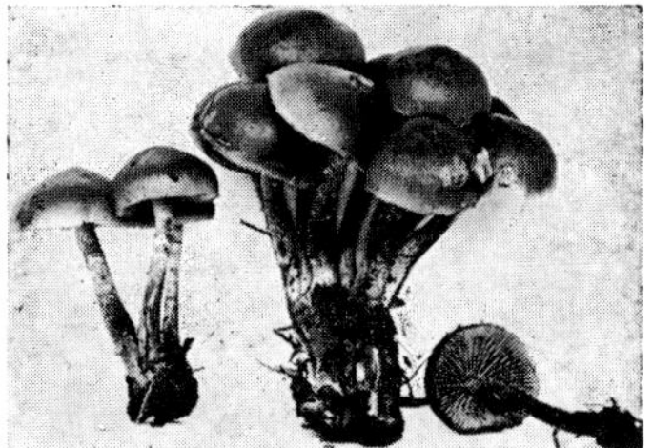
3B—Galerina autumnalis

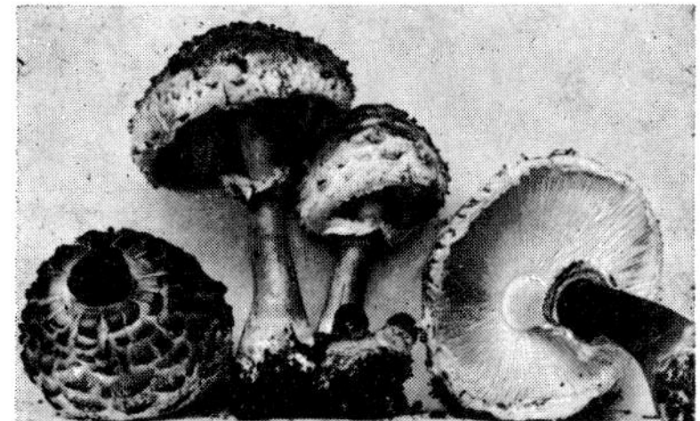
4A—Lepiota rhachodes

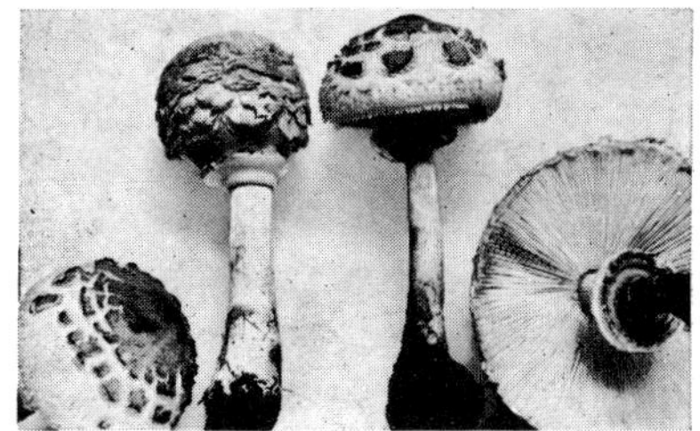
4B—Lepiota molybdites

(Numbers 1A, 2A, 3A, and 4B are poisonous)

---



Figure 22.

secondary to the mushroom poisoning remains unclear. The mechanism of the action of thioctic acid in amanitin poisoning is still unresolved. It is thought that since lipoic acid is a component of coenzymes necessary to oxidize keto-acids such as pyruvate, the thioctic acid protective effect may be produced at the level of the Krebs cycle. Thioctic acid is also known to be a cofactor for the decarboxylation of alpha-ketoacids; therefore, it has been postulated that it exerts a protective effect upon liver enzymes against the action of toxic cyclopeptides. It has also been speculated that the disulfide group of thioctic acid forms a complex with the cyclopeptides to modify their toxicity. Thioctic acid in a small series of animals (dogs) made toxic with amanitin failed to provide any significant protection. It appears that the early administration of thioctic acid in cases of amanitin poisoning may be important for it to produce its protective or regenerative effect. Patients who have not responded favorably to thioctic acid invariably received it late during the clinical course.

The investigational drug protocol developed by the Food and Drug Administration for the experimental administration of thioctic acid states that this drug should be used in patients only who are known or strongly suspected of having ingested *Amanita phalloides, Amanita verosa* or *Amanita verna* mushrooms. Initially, 25 mg of thioctic acid given four times a day may be infused in a solution of glucose and water or saline. The dose may be increased to 75 mg four times a day on the second day of treatment and infused as rapidly as necessary depending upon the patient's clinical status. SGOT, SGPT, LDH, creatinine, BUN and glucose levels and urinalysis should be measured at least once daily and more frequently if clinical presentation warrants their evaluation. Because thioctic acid is light and heat sensitive, protective coverings of the bottles and infusion lines that contain the solution are necessary. Any physician with a patient poisoned by *Amanita phalloides* may call the National Institute of Health (NIH) Clinical Center twenty-four hours a day, 201-656-4000, for use of experimental thioctic acid as well as advice concerning its use.

Natural hepatotoxic substances in plants and fungi may be significant factors in the etiology of chronic liver diseases and hepatomas. Several hepatotoxins are commonly used as medicines or are accidentally ingested, especially among primitive communities in tropical and subtropical countries. Tropical climates favor growth of fungi on food, which then acquires hepatotoxic properties. Toxicity of yellow rice has been traced to contamination with *Penicillium islandicum* and that of ground nut meal to contamination with *Aspergillus flavus.* The toxins may be excreted in milk of cows fed contaminated food. Plant hepatotoxins commonly used as food in primitive countries include nuts from *Cycas circinalis,* which contains the toxin methylazoxymethanol, the aglycone of cycasin. Pyrrolizidine alkaloids are particularly prevalent in numerous unrelated botanical families and genera widely distributed throughout the world. Several of these plants which contain toxic alkaloids are recommended for medical purposes in various nations, particularly as emmenogogues and abortifacients.

## POISONOUS SNAKES (OPHIDISM)*

The World Health Organization estimates that 40,000 persons are killed by snakebites every year, with perhaps 70 per cent of such deaths occurring in Asia. Approximately 6600 victims of venomous snakes are treated annually in the United States, and 138 deaths were reported from the years 1950 through 1959 (an average of 15 per year). Of the 2500 different varieties of snakes known to exist,

* It is unjust that when we have done
All that a serpent should,
You gather our poisons, one by one,
And break them down to your good.
—Kipling

TABLE 137
MUSHROOM POISONING*

| | *Genus and Species* | *Toxins* | *Comments* |
|---|---|---|---|
| Cellular Toxins | *Amanita* (spp. *A. phalloides, A. verna, A. virosa*) | Amanitin<br>Phalloidine | These species of *Amanita* account for nearly 90 per cent of all cases of lethal mushroom poisoning. Found mostly in wooded areas, more frequently during late summer and fall seasons. Neither taste nor smell obnoxious. As little as one-third of a single cap has been fatal to a child. Symptoms of gastrointestinal disturbance occur after a delay of six to twenty-four hours following ingestion. A transient period of improvement is followed by metabolic disturbances and renal and hepatic impairment. Most fatalities occur within several days. The mortality rate varies from 40 to 90 per cent. |
| | *Galerina* (spp. *G. autumnalis, G. marginata, G. venenata*) | | *Galerina* is an inhabitant of the western United States. Can be found on lawns, meadows, etc. Produces symptoms similar to those of *Amanita.* |
| | *Gyromita*<br>*Helvella* (spp. *H. esculenta, H. underwoodii*) | Helvellic acid | These mushrooms produce symptoms similar to intoxication by amanitin but less severe. Appearing six to twelve hours or more after ingestion, symptoms are primarily gastrointestinal. Hemolysis and central nervous system effects have been associated with ingestion of this genus of mushrooms. Exact identity of chemical nature of helvellic acid not known. Certain individuals are resistant to its effect. Fatalities have been reported. Estimated mortality is 2 to 4 per cent. |
| CNS Toxins | *Inocybe*<br>*Clitocybe* (some).<br>*Boletus* and others | Muscarine | "Muscarinic" effects, e.g. salivation, lacrimation, nausea, abdominal pain, vomiting, diarrhea and miosis, occur within fifteen to thirty minutes following ingestion. Death is rare, and treatment is primarily supportive and to provide symptomatic relief. There appears to be specie differences, since only some *(Inocybe)* have caused death. |

TABLE 137—*Continued*
MUSHROOM POISONING

| | *Genus and Species* | *Toxins* | *Comments* |
|---|---|---|---|
| | *Amanita* (spp. *A. Muscaria, A. pantherina*) | Plizatropine | These mushrooms produce symptoms resembling those central nervous system effects of atropine. The principle toxin is still not identified, and its presence cannot be chemically detected. Symptoms occur within one to two hours after ingestion and frequently resemble alcohol intoxication. These symptoms sometimes are accompanied by "muscarinic" effects. Common inhabitant of western United States appearing in spring and fall, these mushrooms can be found in wooded areas, especially conifer forests. Said to taste bitter, these mushrooms have unusual and unexplained attraction for flies, thus are also known as "fly mushrooms" or "fly agarics." These are also the "magic mushrooms" in *Alice in Wonderland.* |
| | *Psilocybe*<br>*Panaeolus*<br>*Conocybe*<br>*Psathyrella* | Psilocybin | Psychotropic "LSD-like" manifestations begin about thirty to sixty minutes and may continue for several hours. Recovery is spontaneous and usually within a day. Treatment is symptomatic. |
| GI Irritants | *Agaricus*<br>*Boletus*<br>*Clitocybe*<br>*Lepiota* and others | ? | Mild to severe nausea, vomiting, diarrhea and other gastrointestinal symptoms occur one-half to two hours after ingestion and may persist for several hours. No fatalities have been reported. Treatment is supportive. |
| Disulfiram-like Effects | *Coprinus*<br>*Atramentarius* | ? | Flushing, palpitation, hyperventilation and tachycardia occur after one-half to two hours and last for a short time when these mushrooms are consumed along with alcohol. These symptoms may occur even when alcohol is consumed several hours following ingestion of the mushrooms. Gastrointestinal symptoms are infrequent. Treatment is supportive and avoidance of alcohol. |

*From material in *Toxic and Hallucinogenic Mushroom Poisoning:* Lincoff, G. and Mitchell, D. H.: Van Nostrand Reinhold Co., New York, 1977.

fewer than 200 are considered dangerous to humans. In the United States there are approximately 115 species of snakes, of which only 19 are venomous.

Snakebite is most common and more severe in early spring when the reptiles, having hibernated for several months, emerge from their winter retreats with poison glands (one on either side of the head) containing large amounts of venom. The fangs of a poisonous snake produce two distinct punctures. A row of minute wounds from the small teeth of the lower jaw may or may not be present. The teeth of nonpoisonous species produce marks similar to scratches, which can occur in two uniform rows. Herpetologists place much emphasis on detecting definitive odors about the habitat of snakes. The key to diagnosis, however, lies first in identification of the reptile, which should be killed, if possible, and examined.

Only four varieties of poisonous snakes occur in this country: the rattlesnake, the copperhead, the water moccasin (all three are pit vipers, which are responsible for 99.6% of poisonous snakebites) and the coral snake.

### *Crotalus (True Rattlesnakes)*

Only five of the more than twenty species and varieties included in this genus are an important menace to human beings.

*The Florida diamondback (C. adamanteus),* the largest and one of the most dangerous, ranks among the world's deadliest snakes. Large adults may measure from six to eight feet long, with a circumference of twelve inches. This species attains the greatest weight of any North American viperine snake; six-foot specimens may weigh twelve to fifteen pounds. The fangs may be three-fourths of an inch long or more. *C. adamanteus* occurs in the low coastal areas of southeastern United States, from North Carolina south to and including all of Florida and westward almost to the Mississippi. The Florida diamondback prefers regions of scrub palmetto and low brush, frequently close to water, and it can swim. The body is a dark olive or olive-brown marked with a chain of symmetrical, pale-edged, blackish rhombs with light centers ("diamonds"). When coiled amidst vegetation it is well camouflaged, for the vivid blotches blend with the lights and shadows of the tangled stems and debris of the ground. It advances rather than retreats, and it strikes with remarkable accuracy.

*The Texas diamondback (C. atrox),* common to the arid and semiarid regions of southwestern United States from central Arkansas and Texas to California, reaches a length of five to seven feet and weighs up to fifteen pounds. Bold and aggressive, it often crawls in the open and commonly is seen in cultivated areas or even in or near farm buildings. Its bite causes as many deaths as those of all other species combined. When disturbed it quickly coils, almost always gives warning, and strikes, often simultaneously with the sound of the rattle. The general coloration is paler than in *C. adamanteus,* and the tail is chalky white with clear black rings.

*The timber rattlesnake (C. horridus),* ranging from New England to northern Florida and westward to eastern Minnesota, eastern Kansas and Texas, is partial to hilly regions in the north and east, but in the south it lives on the flat coastal plain. The average length of an adult is three feet, six inches; the largest specimen reported is six feet, two inches. It may stray into farm lands, especially during the haying or harvesting season. The typical specimen is yellow or tan with chevron-shaped crossbands of black or dark brown. In the north some of these may be entirely black; females are seldom black, but males frequently are. Ordinarily this snake retreats if disturbed, but if unable to escape it usually gives warning before it strikes. The male is usually less irritable than the female.

*The prairie rattlesnake (C. viridis)* is generally about two and one-half to three and one-half feet long and has a wide distribution on the Great Plains of the United States, extending westward to the Rockies and ranging from

Canada to Mexico. The coloring is usually greenish gray, olive green or greenish brown, with a symmetrical row of darker, rounded and well-separated blotches on the back.

*The Pacific rattlesnake (C. oreganus)* is the most important rattler found on the Pacific coast, extending from British Columbia southward to lower California and eastward into Idaho. There is also an isolated colony in Arizona. It averages three to four feet and may reach five feet in length. The body background varies from brown to grayish or greenish; some are nearly black. Markings are dorsal blotches edged with a paler hue and a wide dark bar through the eye.

### *Sistrurus (Ground Rattlers)*

*The pigmy rattler (S. miliarius),* smallest crotaline snake in the United States (rarely more than eighteen or twenty inches long), is common from the Carolinas to and including Florida, and westward to southeastern Missouri, Oklahoma and Texas. It thrives in dry areas with low vegetation. The body is usually slate colored with rounded, widely separated black blotches along the midline of the back, with similar smaller markings on the sides, and a reddish band between the dorsal blotches. Its tiny rattle produces a faint, insect-like buzzing which may be heard at a distance of six to eight feet. The buzz of insects ceases as the intruder draws closer, whereas that of *S. miliarius* grows more persistent.

*The massasauga (S. catenatus),* a larger species, ranges from southern Ontario and central New York throughout the central and prairie states to Texas and Arizona. It prefers prairie areas, either wet or dry, but usually shuns the water. It also has been reported in woodpiles, in cellars of houses and under steps, in hay fields and on mossy ground under bushes and evergreen trees. The massasauga is gray-brown, with a dark belly heavily blotched with black. There is a series of squarish, dark brown or black blotches, usually with a narrow white border, along the midline of the back; two alternating rows of similar but smaller markings are along each side. The maximum length is three feet, six inches; the average is about two feet. When excited, it strikes repeatedly.

### *Agkistrodon (Moccasins, Copperheads)*

Members of this genus are especially dangerous, for they lack the telltale rattle and may be easily confused with some harmless snakes.

*The venomous copperhead or highland moccasin (A. mokeson),* within its range, is one of the most common of American poisonous snakes. Rarely more than three feet long, it occurs from Massachusetts to northern Florida, westward to extreme southeastern Nebraska, Oklahoma and western Texas. In the north it prefers wooded mountains, hills and wild damp meadows and sometimes is seen along old stone walls or in sawdust or slab piles about abandoned sawmills. In the south it frequents both lowland swamps and uplands. The body is usually pale pinkish and reddish brown, marked with large crossbands of chestnut brown resembling dumbbells or hourglasses. The coppery tinge of the head, without conspicuous markings, has prompted the popular name. Those found in Texas have wider bands than those that occur farther east.

The more pugnacious *water moccasin or cottonmouth (A. piscivorus)* is usually about four feet long. It is semiaquatic and infests swamps, lakes, lagoons and sluggish waterways of southeastern United States, from the Dismal Swamp in southeastern Virginia southward to and including Florida, and westward throughout the Gulf states into eastern Oklahoma and Central Texas. It extends up the Mississippi Valley to southern Illinois and central Missouri. The body is usually dingy brown or olive, crossed with darker blotches boldly defined on the sides but barely showing on the back. Large specimens may be nearly black, with little trace of markings. The snake has a heavy body and a broad, flat head. With the jaws open to strike, the white mouth parts are revealed, hence the popular name, "cottonmouth." Characteristically, the moccasin rests, crawls and swims with the head raised at an angle of 45°.

### *Micrurus fulvius (Coral or Harlequin Snakes)*

This is a common reptile of the southeastern part of the United States. They measure about three feet in length and three-fourths of an inch in diameter at the thickest part of the body. The snout is black. The head is blunt and flattened, with minute beady eyes. A yellow band crosses it followed by a black ring. The head has the same width as the neck. The scales are highly polished and opalescent; the pattern consists of regularly disposed broad scarlet and black rings, separated by narrow rings of yellow. Ranging into Mexico, the coral snake undergoes a considerable variation in pattern with an increase in the size of the red rings, a constriction of the black ones and almost total obliteration of the yellow. The coral snake lives among decaying leaves and moist humus and usually feeds on small snakes and lizards. They are usually quiet and do not attack man unless they are provoked, but then they attack suddenly; because the wound is slight, it is often neglected and may prove fatal due to absorption of the neurotoxic venom. False coral snakes, which are nonpoisonous, have pink or yellow snouts.

In general, the poisonous snakes, with the exception of the coral snake, have the following characteristic identifying marks: (1) a triangular-shaped head; (2) a pit between the eye and the nostril from which pit viper derives its name; (3) elliptical pupils (also present in some nonpoisonous varieties); (4) single caudal plates; (5) well-developed fangs

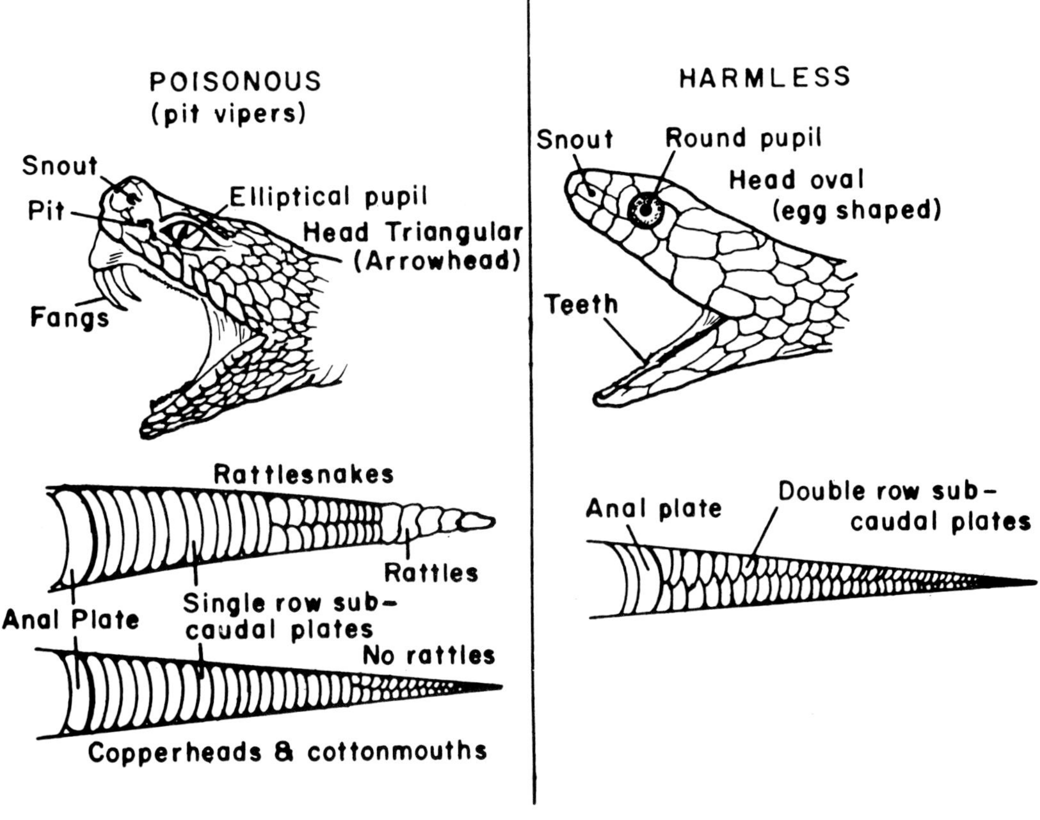


Figure 23. Some identifying features of poisonous (pit vipers) and harmless snakes.

which protrude from the maxillae when the snake's mouth is opened; and (6) only rattlesnakes have rattles attached to their tails. The notion that the number of rattles on the tail indicates the number of years the snake has lived is false. A rattle is added each time the snake sheds its skin, which occurs three or four times a year in the young predator. The life span of the rattlesnake is approximately ten years, although some have been reported to have lived up to twenty years. The coral snake and the nonpoisonous type, on the other hand, show characteristic features such as these: (1) an oval or blunt-shaped head; (2) absence of pit between the eye and the nostril; (3) round pupils; and (4) double caudal plates with no rattles. A snake without fangs may reliably be regarded as harmless. However, fangs often fold back into the roof of the mouth and may be difficult to detect. Patterns vary somewhat depending upon the locality in which they are found. Nevertheless, color may be helpful in differentiation, especially between the coral and the king snakes. Both have red, yellow and black stripes, but in a different order. A mnemonic saying frequently used is as follows:

> Red against yellow, kill the fellow;
> Red against black, venom lack.

Several harmless snakes resemble coral snakes, but their snouts are usually gray or red. It is important to remember that *the coral snake's snout is always black!*

Rather closely allied to the king snakes, the scarlet snake, *Cemophora coccinea,* is a secretive, gentle and very colorful species. The pattern is composed of black-edged red blotches separated by yellow or grayish interspaces and

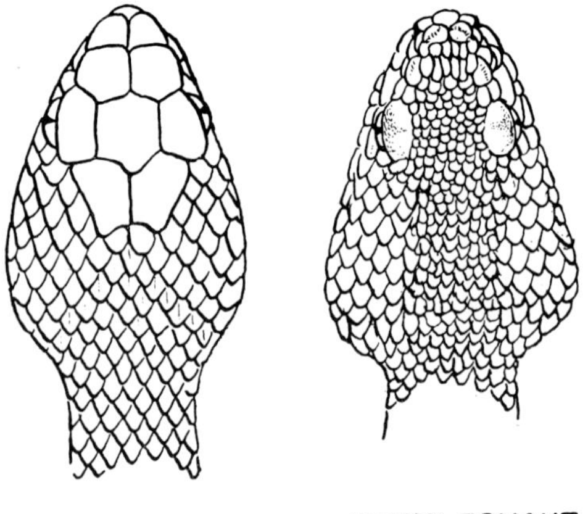


Figure 24. Pigmy or ground *(Sistrurus)*: Top of head covered well back of the eyes with large plates usually nine in number. True rattlesnake *(Crotalus)*: Top of head covered with smaller scales of varying size. If large scales present, they do not extend back of the eyes. Water moccasin or cottonmouth *(Agkistrodon)*: Has broad flat head with larger scales than those seen in the rattler. Copperhead derives its name from the coppery tinge of the head, without conspicuous markings. Members of this genus have blunt tails without rattles.

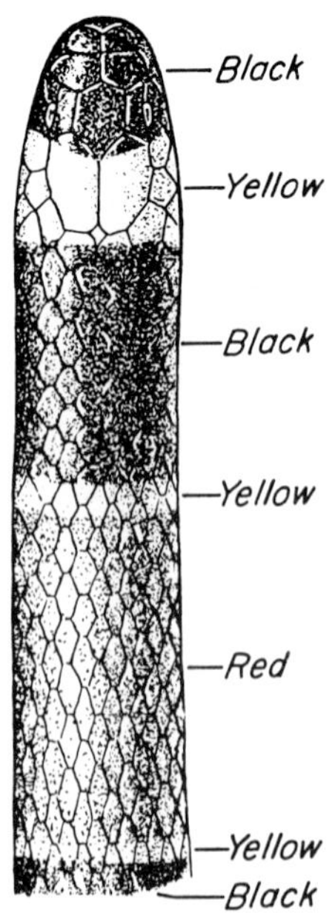


Figure 25. Coral or harlequin *(Micrurus fulvius)*: Head has the same width and is blunt and flattened with minute beady eyes. Snout is always black. A yellow band crosses it followed by a black ring. The scales are highly polished and opalescent.

is brightest in younger specimens. The snout is red and the underside of the body is unmarked. The nose is pointed and well adapted for burrowing in sandy and loamy soils. The scarlet snake and scarlet kingsnake are sometimes confused with the venomous coral snake. To further complicate matters, the three species may often be found in the same general habitat.

However, in both harmless forms *the snout is red, and the red and black areas of the body touch. The snout of the poisonous coral snake is black, and the red and yellow rings are in contact.* In addition, the underside of the scarlet snake is white and unmarked, since the pattern is composed of blotches and not rings. Scarlet snakes average about fifteen inches in length, but a few specimens slightly exceeding thirty inches have been recorded.

## *Poisonous Snakebite Symptoms*

If the bite is poisonous, unmistakable symptoms rapidly appear. There is burning pain, often excruciating, occurring at the site of the injury in three to five minutes, and within ten minutes a distinct swelling develops which increases and advances up the limb. In a serious bite on the hand, the entire arm becomes extremely swollen in the first hour. The skin of the bitten area becomes dark and purplish, and bloody fluid oozes from the wound. The patient becomes weak, dizzy and faint, perspires profusely, is nauseated and often vomits bloodstained material. Subcutaneous and internal hemorrhages may occur, with bleeding from the nose, bladder and intestine. The pulse is weak, pupils are dilated (or constricted) and respiration is difficult. Later there may be loss of vision, paralysis, unconsciousness, coma and complete collapse.

Systemic anaphylaxis to venom *per se* and not from its toxic effects can produce severe manifestations and even sudden death in individuals who are snake handlers or who have had a previous history of snakebite.

The venoms of snakes are complex mixtures, chiefly proteins, many of which have enzymatic activities. During recent years, it has been shown that the lethal and perhaps more deleterious fractions of snake venoms are certain peptides and proteins of relatively low molecular weight. They range in molecular weight from less than 6000 to approximately 30,000; some of them are five to twenty times more lethal than the crude venom. The peptides appear to have very specific receptor sites, both chemically and physiologically. Some of the more important enzymes are proteinases; L-arginine-ester hydrolases; transaminase; hyaluronidase; L-amino acid oxidase; cholinesterase; phospholipase A, B, C and D; ribonuclease; deoxyribonuclease; phosphomonoesterase; phosphodiesterase; 5′-nucleotidase; adenosine triphosphatase; alkaline phosphatase; acid phosphatase; nicotinamide-adenine dinucleotidase; and endonucleases.

Two main effects occur in snakebite depending on which of the two types of toxin is predominantly present.

NEUROTOXIC (AS PRODUCED BY *Micrurus fulvius*). Venoms consisting of a neurotoxin produce weakness, paralysis of the muscles of the mouth and throat and then paralysis of the muscles of respiration. The clinical neurotoxic effects are drowsiness, difficulty in breathing and swallowing, slow weak pulse, drooping of eyelids, muscular pain and weakness, trismus, nausea, vomiting, coma and eventual respiratory and cardiac failure. Convulsions may occur.

Cobra venom, in addition to the paralysis, also may cause severe convulsions. Often little or no immediate tissue reaction occurs at the site of injury, and pain results only from the fang punctures. Initial symptoms may be delayed for an hour or more, giving a false sense of security. Contrary to popular opinion, however, and comforting to know, the majority of bites from the dreaded cobra are not particularly harmful. A significant percentage have severe local reactions with necrosis, but very few develop systemic neurotoxic effects, and only about one in twenty dies.

HEMOTOXIC (AS PRODUCED BY *Crotalus*). If the

snake venom has hemotoxins (cytolysins), enzymatic destruction of cell walls and tissues and hemolysis will result, producing hemorrhage into vital organs. The hemorrhagic consequences of snakebite are due to one of three types of hypofibrinogenemia: with neither thrombocytopenia nor fibrinolysis, without thrombocytopenia but with fibrinolysis, and with thrombocytopenia, which may be caused by disseminated intravascular coagulation (DIC) or a DIC-like syndrome. Hemotoxins (cytolysins) cause marked local swelling and pain, necrosis, discoloration and hemorrhages at the site of the bite. The area of necrosis and hemorrhage spreads rapidly from the bite, and collections of lymph or serum appear under the skin. Bleeding from the mucous membranes of the mouth, nose, eyes and gastrointestinal tract is also common. Hematuria generally occurs. Nausea, vomiting and collapse follow as poisoning progresses. Circulatory failure is the usual cause of death. Blood coagulation studies must be done daily for four or five days even in cases of seemingly minor envenomation. The plasma fibrinogen level may fall to undetectable levels, and the platelet count may fall below 50,000/cu. mm. These levels usually return to normal within four or five days postbite. Fibrinogen– or platelet-rich plasma or both correct these low levels when bleeding problems are present. (Usually no bleeding problems occur with these low levels of fibrinogen and platelets.)

So far, the following components of venom have been recognized.

1. *Blood coagulants, anticoagulants and agglutinins.* These affect the red cells and coagulation of the blood.
2. *Cytolysins, proteolysins and antibactericidin.* These affect cellular blood components as well as the endothelium of the vessels. The latter contributes to uncontrolled suppuration, paralyzing the phagocytic activity of the white blood cells.
3. *Neurotoxins.* Type A affects the nervous system, particularly the cardiorespiratory higher centers, while type B usually affects the myoneural junction.
4. *Cholinesterase and anticholinesterase.* These components also affect the myoneural junction.
5. *Cardiotoxin.* This substance stimulates the heart.
6. *Hyaluronidase.* This facilitates the spread of the venom through the tissue.

All the above fractions are contained in the venom of poisonous snakes, but in varying proportions. The venom of pit vipers is high in the hemopathic components, causing damage to blood, tissues and vessels, while the venom from coral snakes is rich in neurotoxins, primarily producing neurologic symptoms.

### *Treatment of Snakebite*

Treatment consists of using all local and specific measures that are available. Have the patient lie down as soon as possible, and carry him to the hospital. *Do not let him walk.* If available, use an ice pack (cryotherapy, however, is a controversial measure, and no valuable time should be lost in applying its use) on the part bitten, and apply a wide tourniquet (preferably not a string or ligature) immediately and continuously two to four inches proximal to the bite. The tourniquet should be tight enough to occlude the lymphatics, but not the arterial supply or venous return. As long as the tourniquet does not occlude the arterial circulation, loosening the tourniquet at intervals is not necessary. As the swelling about the bite spreads, the tourniquet should be moved proximally. After an interval of six to twelve hours, the tourniquet can be loosened for gradually longer intervals if generalized symptoms have not occurred.

If the area of the bite becomes swollen with considerable reaction about it, incision and suctioning (by mouth suction or breast pumps, syringes, etc.) should be carried out at the first opportunity and always before antivenin is given. The incisions should be one-half inch long and not more than one-eighth inch deep. They should be placed one or two inches apart at the edge of the swollen area and suction applied. A thirty-minute period of suction extracts about 90 per cent of the available venom even though delayed as long as two hours after the bite. If the swelling continues to progress, new lines of incisions are recommended by some, approximately every three or four inches, followed by suction. However, in the balance of severe local effect, incision and suctioning are not helpful and, in fact, may even be contraindicated if the venom is predominantly neurotoxic, since incision can increase the rapidity of absorption. Many authorities prefer a single straight incision through the fang marks instead of the multiple incision method, or immediate debridement and fasciotomy if indicated (if muscle is edematous, hemorrhagic or necrotic) to prevent the local destructive effects (bleeding and necrosis) of the venom. Also recommended is the cutting of a silver dollar sized plug of skin and surface tissue around the bite, which is said to remove 90 to 95 per cent of the venom, provided that it is done within two hours and that a tourniquet has been applied. If the bite is on the trunk, incision, ice packs and rest must be relied upon to slow absorption of the venom.

It has been recently reported that the chelating agent EDTA (edetate), when infiltrated about the bite, has a braking effect on local tissue destruction. If this agent, after further testing, proves effective in dampening or eliminating deleterious enzyme activity without causing any tissue damage itself, it should be an additional therapeutic measure of considerable value.

Immobilization without incision and suctioning is recommended and indeed preferred by some experts in this field. In a recent study, envenomation of experimental animals showed that the best results were obtained by the swiftest possible administration of antivenin without the use of incision-suction or local cooling. Therefore, it is imperative in the treatment of bites by crotalids that first aid measures should in no way substitute for, nor delay in any manner, the giving of the three A's: "antivenin," "antibiotic," and "antitoxin" or toxoid (tetanus).

Specific therapy consists of the immediate administering of polyvalent serum to neutralize the absorbed venom and prevent or minimize its effects. Antivenin (from Wyeth, Merck Sharp & Dohme and others) is the only known specific agent for the treatment of bites by the crotaline snakes of North America, and the prompt and sufficient injection of this antiserum prevents death in most patients, relieves pain, aborts the serious effects and shortens convalescence. Crotaline antivenin, polyvalent, is administered subcutaneously, intramuscularly or intravenously in doses of 10 to 50 ml of reconstituted serum, depending on severity of symptoms, lapse of time after bite, size of snake and size of patient (the smaller the body of the victim in relation to the size of the snake, the larger the dose required). The freeze-dried serum should be reconstituted immediately prior to use. Preliminary intradermal and conjunctival tests for sensitivity to horse serum should be carried out before administration of the antivenin with or without a history of allergy.

Since there is only a two– to fifteen-minute "incubation" or latent period between the time the snake injects its venom and the appearance of clinical symptoms, intravenous antivenin therapy is probably the most efficient way of neutralizing the venom before it is absorbed and is considered by most experts as the route of choice. When given subcutaneously or intramuscularly, it is impossible to titrate the amount needed. With the intravenous route, the physician can control dosage more accurately, while observing progression or regression of symptoms. To prevent severe reactions (anaphylaxis), antivenin for intravenous administration should be mixed with saline in a 1:50, 1:100 or even greater dilution. Mephentermine sulfate (Wyamine®) 60 mg in 1 liter of saline and adrenalin should be available for immediate use. A few drops of the dilute antivenin solution are allowed to drop into the vein. If no reaction occurs in five minutes, about 2 ml of antivenin solution is given. After another wait of five to ten minutes, the dose of antivenin solution is infused rapidly.

An alternate though less effective method

of therapy can be used. If desensitization is not required, the estimated dose is administered IM by separate injections, not to exceed 10 ml at any one site. If the victim is treated within two hours, a small quantity of the serum may be injected around the wound (except for bites on the digits); otherwise, the entire dose should be administered higher on the bitten limb. The initial dose is the most important one, since viper venoms rapidly break down blood vessels and thus impede systemic absorption of the serum; therefore, the initial dose should be large enough to saturate the system and overwhelm the toxin. If symptoms such as swelling or pain persist or recur, additional doses may be injected every thirty minutes to two hours, as necessary. Although the serum frequently may be administered by laymen as an emergency procedure, it should not be given intravenously except by a physician. All patients should be hospitalized if possible, and blood typing for transfusions should be performed as soon as possible, because alteration of the blood pattern by the venom soon may make accurate cross-matching impossible.

If an *immediate* untoward reaction develops, apply a tourniquet above the injected site. Administer an appropriate dose of epinephrine proximal to the tourniquet or into another extremity. Wait at least thirty minutes. Then administer the next dose of serum in the same amount as the last dose which did not produce a reaction.

ACTH and cortisone may be used as a supplement to specific treatment to control urticaria and similar *delayed* manifestations of allergy to horse serum, antibiotics and the venom itself. Such agents, however, do not of themselves influence the outcome of snake poisoning. Doses of 25 mg cortisone have been administered by mouth, beginning with the first injection of serum and continuing every six hours until all symptoms of envenomation were under control, and no further doses of serum were required. Such treatment has aided in reducing morbidity and has prevented evidences of serum sensitivity, even in known serum-sensitive patients. In severe cases, cortisone may be administered intramuscularly or by vein if necessary. IV heparin should be used for disseminated intravascular coagulation or a DIC-like syndrome. General measures include the use of 1% procaine containing 1 minim of epinephrine solution 1:1000 to each 6 ml, injected about the bite to relieve pain and nervousness. Opiates and barbiturates should be used with caution, although analgesics and mild sedatives can be given as needed. Antibiotics (preferably a broad-spectrum one) and tetanus antitoxin or toxoid are indicated as for any other puncture wound. Antihistamines appear to enhance the toxicity of crotaline venoms and are contraindicated for treatment of crotaline envenomation. Supportive therapy for shock and respiratory depression should be instituted immediately. *Alcohol should never be given, as this only increases the absorption of the venom.*

The crotaline polyvalent serum is of no value for the neutralization of venom following bites inflicted by noncrotaline snakes, such as the American coral snake, the true vipers, including the puff adder, the cobra and the mamba, or any of the venomous spiders or scorpions. Coral snake antivenin, however, can be obtained from Wyeth Laboratories, Center for Disease Control, Atlanta, Georgia, 30333 (phone 404-633-3311; off-duty hours 404-633-2176) and C. Amaral and Cia L.T.D.A., Gloria 34, P.O. Box 2123, São Paulo, Brazil. An Antivenin Index Center has recently been established in Oklahoma City. It provides a current catalog of antivenins available for treatment of snakebites (from both native and exotic species) that are stocked in North American zoos, laboratories, and related institutions. A 24-hour retrieval service gives emergency information. The index is limited to sera currently stocked by participating institutions; full data are provided so the inquirer can obtain the nearest supply of antivenin as quickly as possible. To use this service, the inquirer should obtain both the scientific name (genus and species) and the common name of the snake involved and call the center at (405) 271-5454. The center was established by a cooperative effort of the

Oklahoma Poison Information Center and the Oklahoma City Zoo and is a program of the Oklahoma State Department of Health.

The panic that results when a snakebite occurs, with the patient in a state of partial shock from fright, often makes it most difficult for the physician to evaluate his true condition. Table 140 can be a useful guide in this regard.

TABLE 140
OPHIDISM: A GUIDE TO THERAPY

| | *Grades of Poisoning* | *First Aid* | *Hospital Management* |
|---|---|---|---|
| O | *None*<br>Fang marks; minimal pain, wheal 1″ or less in first 12 hours. | Observe 12 hours to rule out delayed venom reaction. | Antibiotic plus antitetanus therapy. |
| I | *Minimal*<br>Moderate pain; edema extending 1–6″ along limb within 12 hours; erythema. | Apply tourniquet (tight enough to impede the superficial venous and lymphatic return but not so tight as to obstruct the arterial supply or produce ischemia. The tourniquet should admit a finger beneath it easily and may remain in place for an hour); make linear incision at fang marks and use suction for 30 minutes; observe 12 hours. | Type, cross-match blood; test for horse serum sensitivity. Administer antibiotic plus antitetanus therapy. Observe 12 hours. |
| II | *Moderate*<br>Severe pain, tenderness; edema extending 10–15″ within 12 hours; erythema→petechiae→ecchymosis; weakness, nausea, vomiting; bloody ooze at fang marks. | Same as for Grade I. | Same as Grade I, plus intravenous administration antivenin in 5% glucose until advance of edema is halted; observe; if edema recurs give more antivenin; antihistamines may be useful but steroids are questionable at this time (use after 3rd day in event of serum sickness). |
| III | *Severe*<br>Widespread pain, tenderness; edema extending 10–20″ within 12 hours; petechiae→ecchymosis. Grade I and II signs appear rapidly and proceed to systemic signs, including vertigo. | Same as for Grade I. If hospital treatment unavailable for hours, administer antivenin* intramuscularly, or use tight tourniquet with prospect of possible amputation.<br>*Not in bite area. | Same as Grade II, plus attention to maintenance of serum electrolyte and fluid balance. (Important: give antivenin before loosening tourniquet.) |
| IV | *Very severe*<br>Rapid swelling, sometimes affecting trunk; ecchymosis→bleb formation; weakness; vertigo; vomiting, perhaps hematemesis; tingling about face, head; fasciculation; muscle cramping; possibly paralysis; yellow vision, blindness, shock, convulsions. | Same as Grade I. Death may occur within 40 minutes. Antivenin *must* be given if available, preferably IV which will permit rapid absorption. Otherwise, occlusive tourniquet may prevent death, although it will most certainly predispose to amputation if kept in place too long. | Same as Grade III, plus attention to possible kidney involvement within 24 hours. Start physiotherapy as soon as feasible to prevent contractures. Heparin should be used for disseminated intravascular coagulation (DIC) |

GRADED SYSTEM for diagnosing degree of severity of pit viper poisoning, originated by Drs. J. T. Wood, W. W. Hoback and T. W. Green, adapted for *Image* by Dr. Newton McCollough, Orlando, Fla., and Dr. J. F. Gennaro, venom chemist, at Gainesville, Fla. Courtesy of *Image* (Roche Medical).

### *Gila Monster*

The Gila monster (*Heloderma suspectum*) has a stout body (eighteen inches long), broad blunt head and stumpy tail and lives in the desert areas of southwestern United States and northern Mexico. This poisonous lizard has grooves in the front teeth instead of fangs, which carry the venom and inflict a wound with multiple lacerations. Poisoning is due to the enzymatic tissue destruction and curare-like muscular weakness, or paralysis, that occurs from its neurotoxic venom.

The principal manifestations of toxicity include nausea, vomiting, edema and inflammation about the bite, cyanosis, respiratory depression, weakness and paralysis. *Treatment* is similar to that recommended for snakebites as to general measures and the use of cryotherapy, tourniquet and suctioning. No specific antivenin is available. The mortality rate is greater in children (5%) than in adults (1%), but fatalities fortunately are rare since the lizard is infrequently encountered and is not likely to bite unless handled.

## ARTHROPODS AND INSECTS

### *Black Widow Spider*

An epidemiologic study of deaths from bites and stings of venomous animals and insects in the United States indicated that spider bites were responsible for thirty-nine fatalities in the period of 1950 to 1954. The black widow spider (genus *Latrodectus,* species *mactans* and *curacaviensis*) presumably caused most or all of these deaths.

The black widow spider is found in nearly all of the United States, although it is most common in the Middle and South Atlantic States, the Gulf States, and in the area west of the Rocky Mountains. It is also prevalent in Mexico, Central America, the Antilles and the western part of South America.

The adult female black widow spider has a coal-black, almost spherical body about one-half inch long and a leg span of about two inches. It has a red or orange hourglass-shaped marking on the ventral surface of the body. The immature female has, in addition, three spots of similar color on the dorsal surface of the body. The adult male spider is less than half as large as the adult female.

The web is a disorderly tangle of coarse, irregular strands put together without definite pattern. Webs are built in outbuildings or in protected spots out of doors, often between masses of stone or across openings such as the seats of outdoor toilets, waste cans, stopcock vents and manholes. The spider may be seen hanging in the web, but in the daytime it usually remains out of sight in a protected corner or under a rock. Appearance in cities has been reported.

The bite of a black widow spider usually produces a sharp pain similar to that caused by puncture with a needle; however, some patients do not realize they have been bitten. This initial pain may continue for several hours but ordinarily disappears rapidly. The patient may feel no serious discomfort until local muscular cramps begin from fifteen minutes to several hours after the bite. The exact sequence of symptoms depends somewhat on the location of the bite. The venom is neurotoxic and acts on the myoneural junctions or on the nerve endings, causing an ascending motor paralysis or destruction of the peripheral nerve endings. The groups of muscles most frequently affected at first are those of the thigh, shoulder and back. After a varying length of time, the pain spreads to the abdomen and becomes more severe, and weakness, tremor and exquisite pain usually develop. The abdominal muscles assume a boardlike rigidity, but tenderness is slight. Respiration is thoracic. The patient is restless and anxious. Feeble pulse, cold clammy skin, labored breathing and speech, light stupor and delirium may follow. Convulsions may also occur, particularly in small children. The temperature may be slightly elevated or normal. Urinary retention, shock, cyanosis, nausea and vomiting, insomnia and cold sweats have also been reported. The syndrome following the bite of the black widow spider may be easily confused with any medical or surgical condition with acute abdominal symptoms.

The symptoms of black widow spider bite increase in severity for several hours, perhaps a day, and then very slowly become less severe, gradually passing off in the course of two or three days, except in fatal cases. Residual symptoms such as general weakness, tingling, nervousness and transient muscle spasm may persist for weeks or months after recovery from the acute stage.

As soon as a diagnosis of arachnidism due to the black widow spider is made, the patient should receive IM the contents of one restored "Vacule" vial (2.5 ml) of Lyovac® antivenin *(Latrodectus mactans),* which is prepared from blood serum of horses and can be obtained from any branch location of Merck Sharp & Dohme. Symptoms usually subside in one to three hours. Although one dose of serum is usually adequate, it has been found necessary in some cases to administer two doses of the antivenin over a period of time.

It is important that tests for serum sensitivity be made, because serious reactions and even death can result from the administration of horse serum. The intradermal skin test and the eye test are the procedures most commonly employed. The following outline of these procedures may be used.

Intradermal Skin Test. Inject into (not under) the skin not more than 0.02 ml of the test material (1:10 dilution in physiologic saline of normal horse serum). Evaluate result in ten minutes. A positive reaction consists of an urticarial wheal surrounded by a zone of erythema.

Eye Test. Evert the lower lid of one eye and place a few drops of the test material on the conjunctiva. Release lid of eye. During the following ten minutes occasionally evert both lids and compare tested with untested eye. A positive reaction consists of congestion of conjunctival vessels, lacrimation and itching. Apply a few drops of epinephrine solution 1:1000 immediately to the test eye showing a positive reaction.

Desensitization should be attempted only when the administration of antivenin is considered necessary to save life. Epinephrine must be available in case of untoward reaction.

Associated Treatment. The patient should be hospitalized if possible to insure adequate nursing care. In addition to the use of the specific antivenin, the measures giving greatest relief from the symptoms appear to be prolonged warm baths and intravenous injection of 10 ml of 10% solution of calcium gluconate; this may be repeated as necessary to control muscle pain. Morphine may also be required for this purpose. Barbiturates may be used for extreme restlessness. However, as the venom is a neurotoxin, it can cause respiratory paralysis. This must be borne in mind when the administration of morphine or a barbiturate is considered. Adrenocorticosteroids have been used with varying degrees of success. Muscle relaxants such as methocarbamol have been reported to give striking relief of pain and muscle spasm when calcium therapy failed to do so. Supportive therapy should be given as indicated by the condition of the patient. Local treatment of the site of the bite is of no value. Nothing is gained by applying a tourniquet or by attempting to remove venom from the site of the bite by incision and suction as in bites by poisonous snakes.

### *Brown Recluse Spider (Loxosceles reclusa)*

The brown spider *(Loxosceles reclusa),* whose venom is chiefly cytotoxic and hemotoxic, can produce a local necrotic lesion and severe systemic symptoms including disseminated intravascular coagulation (DIC). It can be readily distinguished from other spider genera first by its color, which ranges from fawn to dark brown, and next by its cephalothorax, which tends to be depressed and is decorated on top by a frying pan or violin-shaped spot in contrasting dark color. The legs are long and capable of high speed. Body length of the female measures 9 mm on the average, and the male is a little shorter. On close examination, a set of six white eyes (instead of eight, as expected in spiders) can be seen just anterior to the violin marking and just above the deadly chelicerae. The eyes are arranged in a semicircle, which is also distinctive. All species of *Loxosceles* spin coarse, scanty, irregular webs, most often found in dark dry cellars, closets, garages, attics or sheds. The spiders like to hide in the folds of clothes or bedding. They are reclusive and not aggressive but bite in self-defense when disturbed or when the clothes are donned or the bed is occupied. Three enzymes have been recently identified as the major components of the venom: a protease, an esterase and a hyaluronidase. Volume-for-volume, this venom is more toxic than that of the poisonous snakes (15 μg kills a rabbit). The brown recluse, native to the south central part of the United States, has been found in northern sections of Illinois in recent years. Since the spider does not tolerate temperatures below 40° F, it has adapted itself to an indoor environment. A specific test for loxoscelism with radioactive thymidine can facilitate diagnosis.

The initial pain of a brown spider bite is less intense than that caused by wasps or bees but becomes progressively more severe and may be agonizing in eight hours or so. By this time, a bleb has formed and is surrounded by an erythematous area. As the bleb sloughs off, it reveals a zone of intense ischemia, with ecchymosis and radiating edema.

In the course of the next day or two, the erythema often becomes violaceous and the central zone darkens, usually forming a tough, black eschar by the end of the first week. The eschar then separates within two to five weeks, leaving an ulcer with irregular walls and a necrotic base. This may be slow to heal and there may be residual scarring and keloid formation, sometimes requiring plastic surgery.

In severe cases (many are mild), there may be a generalized pruritic morbilliform eruption with arthralgia, vomiting and fever as high as 39.4° to 40° C (103° to 104° F), occurring within thirty-six hours and lasting as long as a week. These patients may be relatively incapacitated and prone to syncope for a short time. Hemoglobinuria is prominent in the most serious cases, and some degree of hemolysis can be detected by examination of the serum in virtually all cases. Hemoglobinuria may be accompanied by jaundice (in 30%) and extensive organic damage, and the patient may go into shock. However, fatalities are rare in the United States. The most dangerous of South American brown spiders, *L. laeta,* for which an antivenom has been developed, has more potent venom than *L. reclusa,* and most of the deaths have been reported from that region.

*Treatment.* There is no specific antivenin available for use against the species *(Loxosceles*

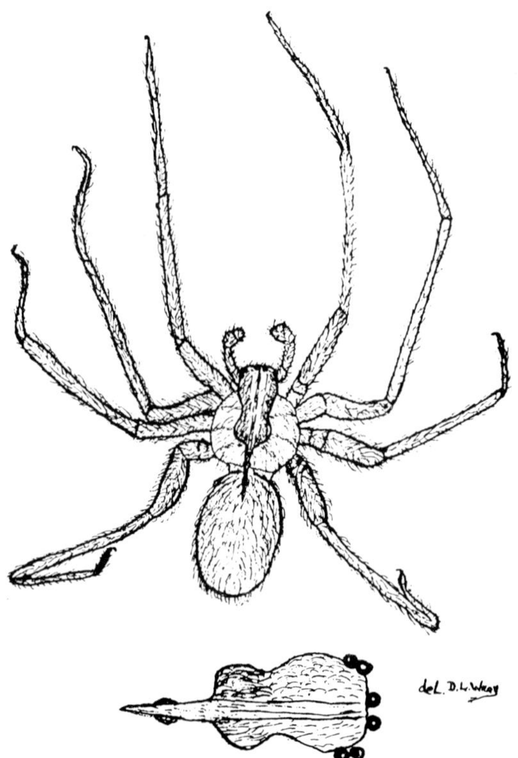


Figure 26. Brown recluse spider. (Courtesy of David L. Wray.)

*reclusa)* responsible for practically all the brown spider bites in this country. Presumably, antisera made for other species (as in South America) of *Latrodectus* would give protection. It would be unlikely that any South American preparations, even if considered, could be readily obtained for any emergency therapy. Since the venom contains levarterenol, local infiltration of phentolamine (Regitine), provided it can be administered early, may limit the edema and necrosis. Antihistamines may be of particular value for loxoscelism. Oral hydroxyzine pamoate (Vistaril®) has been reported to be effective for its muscle relaxant, antihistaminic and tranquilizing properties. Corticosteriods are considered specific for combatting hemolysis, severe sensitization and other systemic complications; they are the drugs of choice in treatment when given early and in adequate doses.

Immediate total excision of all apparently

TABLE 141
NORTH AMERICAN SPIDERS AND INSECTS POTENTIALLY HARMFUL TO MAN

| | *Identification* | *Type of Emergency** | *Treatment* |
|---|---|---|---|
| **Spiders** | | | |
| Black widow *Latrodectus mactans* | shiny, black body; red hourglass on abdomen *bite:* proximal muscle spasm; intense abdominal cramps | systemic envenomation: neurotoxicity, muscle spasm, shock, delirium | IV calcium ±corticosteroids: antivenin if severe |
| Brown recluse *Loxosceles reclusa* | small brown; violin-shaped coloring on cephalothorax *bite:* late necrosis | local necrosis; systemic symptoms with hemolysis, weakness, possible kidney failure | corticosteroids early; supportive for hemolysis |
| Running spiders *Chiracanthium* species | tiny; greenish-white or pale yellow *bite:* proximal muscle pain | local pain; neurotoxic; systemic symptoms usually mild | supportive; consider local steroid injection |
| Black and yellow garden spiders *Argiope aurantia* | black, yellow, and silver markings *Bite:* little pain except at site | similar to above | same as above |
| **Insects** | | | |
| Scorpions *Centruroides (or Vejovis)* species | crablike; long, segmented tail ending in bulbous sac and stinger | local effects or systemic neurotoxin | immobilization; antivenin if available; IV calcium |
| Blister becties *Meloidae* | blisters at sites of contact | bullae due to vesicant | cleansing, local steroids |
| Puss-moth caterpillar *Megalopyge opercularis* | teardrop shape; furry pointed tail *lesion;* gridlike track; papules and vesicles; desquamation in hours or days | local irritation: vesicles, intense pain from "hair" contact | symptomatic local treatment |
| Bees, wasps, hornets *Hymenoptera* | biwinged, three body segments; antenna; black and yellow | painful sting; allergic; toxicity resembling black widow envenomation with many bites | epinephrine; then antihistamine for allergy; calcium IV for toxicity |
| Fire ants | large, bright red *bite:* intense burning, multiple bites in clusters | local pustule; systemic effect usually allergic or like black widow | same as above |

*Allergic reactions possible with all; mentioned here only if sole or principal threat. From Alan K. Done, *Emergency Medicine, 5*:251, 1973. Courtesy of publishers.

involved tissue, with primary closure, appears to be the only effective means of preventing the eventual massive cutaneous necrosis produced by the bite of the brown recluse spider. Once established, the entire necrotic area—always confined to the skin and immediately adjacent subcutaneous tissue—must be excised at the fascial level. Split-thickness skin grafts provide excellent coverage for the excised area, and use of pedicled tissue is seldom necessary. Other supportive measures are similar to those as outlined for the black widow spider.

### *Tarantulas*

The widespread fear of the tarantulas of the southwestern United States seems unfounded. They belong to various genera of the family Aniculariidae, and their bites usually produce moderate to severe local reaction with erythema, edema and ecchymosis, without systemic symptoms. The giant crab-spiders belonging to the species heteropodidae, often found in bunches of bananas, however, can inflict painful stings with marked local swelling.

### *Scorpions*

In the United States the species of poisonous scorpions are the *Centrurorides gertschii* and *sculpturatus.* Adult specimens range from 2 to 20 cm in length. They have powerful claws for seizing spiders and insects upon which they prey. Glands in the terminal segment produce venom which is injected into the victim by a stinger located on the tip of the tail. Scorpions often enter dwellings. During the day they retreat into crevices, commonly in the attic or beneath the floor. Emerging at night, they frequently get into shoes and clothing not being worn, and even into bedding. They do not deliberately attack man, but accidental contact results in a sting.

Their habitat is mainly the arid Southwest, being fairly well limited to Arizona and portions of neighboring states. Fatalities from stings are rare, and most always small children and old people are the victims. Scorpion venom is much more toxic than that of the snake since it contains neurotoxins, cardiotoxins and agglutinins. Fortunately only minute amounts are injected with the sting, and if absorption can be delayed, serious systemic symptoms are not usually encountered.

The venom causes muscular stimulation and hemorrhages. Symptoms are a stinging or burning at the site of the sting, often with very little edema or inflammation about the area. There is a progressive muscular spasm and fibrillation, a choking sensation in the throat, hyperesthesia, thick tongue, abdominal pain and cramps, irritability, convulsions and respiratory depression. Within forty-eight hours the symptoms usually subside.

*Treatment* consists of applying a tourniquet proximal to the sting to limit absorption. This should be loosened for one minute out of every ten; if no symptoms occur, the time interval should be increased. At the same time, ice packs should be placed over the bite. A 2% procaine-epinephrine solution infiltrated locally relieves the pain. In infested areas, specific antiserum should be available for immediate use. Intravenous calcium gluconate (10 ml of 10% solution) helps relieve the muscular spasm. Muscle relaxants also are useful for this purpose. Specific measures for respiratory depression and convulsions must be used as needed. Morphine should be used cautiously in adults and not at all in children.

### *Centipedes*

These insects have a pair of hollow jaws which serve as fangs to inject into the skin toxic substances elaborated in their heads. The venom is relatively weak and at most produces an inflammatory reaction at the puncture site with mild lymphangitis. *Treatment* with compresses is all that is needed for relief. *Scolopendra morsitans,* whose habitat is in the southern United States, is the only centipede dangerous to man in North America. The toxin is a cytolysin. The bite causes local inflammation, erythema, edema and occasionally purpura and systemic symptoms which usually disappear in four to five hours without sequelae. *Treatment* is symptomatic with a cool saline wet dressing and analgesics or sedatives as required.

### *Bee Sting (Wasp, Yellow Jacket)*

Stings from bees and wasps can be as deadly as snakebites. In fact, these insects kill more Americans than snakes. In a five-year period, bees, wasps, hornets and yellow jackets killed eighty-six persons, snakes seventy-one, and poisonous spiders, thirty-nine. Victims of fatal bee stings are usually adults who have gradually developed a serious allergy to the venom of the insects. These reactions are only forewarnings of more violent ones—perhaps even death—to come.

The stinger of the honeybee *(Apis mellifera)* is located in the posterior abdominal wall and is connected with a sac in which the venom is produced by specialized glands. When the stinger is driven into the skin of a victim, the barbs anchor it firmly. As the bee hurries to escape, the stinger apparatus is torn free and continues pumping venom into the wound. The bee dies later from the injury. Queen bees have a large stinger without barbs, while the drones (males) are stingless. Unlike the honeybee, which can only sting once, the wasps and hornets can sting more than once and are therefore potentially more dangerous.

Bee venom resembles snake venom, having hemolytic and neurotoxic properties. In addition, it has a strong histamine-like action upon living tissue. There is some evidence that an antigenic substance is present also in the body of the bee.

Normal individuals, that is, those who are not hypersensitive, react to a single bee or wasp sting with pain followed by a wheal and erythema. There is annoying pruritus. If the sting is on loose tissue like that of the eyelid or genitalia, considerable local edema may develop. This edema is dangerous only in exceptional cases when a bee is swallowed or inhaled so that the sting occurs in the hypopharynx or glottis, causing respiratory obstruction. Ordinarily, the reaction subsides spontaneously in a few hours, or at most in a day or two, and requires only palliative treatment. The stinger itself is usually brushed away by the patient on rubbing the itchy area.

In hypersensitive patients, a bee sting causes no more than the usual local reaction. Within a few minutes, however, there is tingling of the skin and generalized urticaria with extreme pruritus developing. Nausea, vomiting and abdominal cramps may occur; uterine cramping and bleeding have also been recorded. Sometimes there is cough and asthmatic breathing. Angioneurotic edema follows quickly, involving the face, especially the lips and eyelids, sometimes the hands and genitalia and the glottis. Dyspnea and cyanosis appear; respiratory obstruction increases rapidly. Encephalopathy and papilledema can occur. Shock supervenes with cold, clammy extremities, unconsciousness, rapid or imperceptible pulse and precipitously falling blood pressure. Death may occur. Multiple hornet bites can produce muscle necrosis and myoglobinuria with resulting fatal renal failure unless prompt dialysis is used.

*Treatment.* Epinephrine may be lifesaving in the anaphylactic type of reaction. In mild cases, subcutaneous administration of 0.3 to 0.5 ml of a 1:1000 solution may suffice, the dose being repeated at intervals of twenty minutes to an hour or more as symptoms recur. In severe cases, the initial dose should be 0.5 ml injected IM or 0.3 ml given IV. Corticosteroid therapy (100 ml hydrocortisone sodium succinate IV) results in dramatic improvement and should be used early in the treatment. Oxygen is indicated until the respiration is normal, since hypoxia may itself contribute to vascular collapse and cerebral edema. When the acute symptoms have subsided, ephedrine should be given orally in doses of 25 mg three times daily for two or three days, or antihistaminic drugs might be used to prevent recurrence of symptoms. Recovery is usually complete in forty-eight

## HABITS AND EFFECTS OF VARIOUS ARTHROPODS

| INSECT | AVERAGE LENGTH IN MM (10 mm = 3/8 in.) | USUAL LOCATION | METHOD OF ATTACK | | TIME OF ACTIVITY | | | | LOCAL REACTION | | | | | DISTRIBUTION OF LESIONS | | | RESIDUA |
|---|---|---|---|---|---|---|---|---|---|---|---|---|---|---|---|---|---|
| | | | | | | | | | ONSET | | DURATION | | | | | | |
| | | | BITE | STING | DAY | NIGHT | DUSK | DAWN | IMMEDIATE | DELAYED | HOURS | DAYS | WEEKS | SINGLE | SCATTERED | GROUPED | |
| BUMBLEBEE | 20–25 | FLOWERS | | X | X | | | | X | X | X | X | | X | | | NONE |
| HONEYBEE | 10–15 | FLOWERS | | X | X | | | | X | X | X | X | | X | | | NONE |
| MUD-DAUBER WASP | 20–25 | ORCHARDS GARBAGE PAILS | | X | X | | | | X | | | X | | X | | | NONE |
| YELLOW JACKETS | 10–15 | ORCHARDS GARBAGE PAILS | | X | X | | | | X | | X | | | X | | | NONE |
| HORNET | 20–30 | WOODS FLOWERS | | X | X | | | | X | | X | | | X | | | NONE |
| HARVESTER ANT | 7– 9 | VEGETATION KITCHEN | | X | X | | | | | | | X | | X | | | NONE |
| FIRE ANT | 6– 7 | FIELDS | | X | X | | | | X | | | X | | | | X | PIGMENTED MACULES OCCASIONALLY NODULES |
| STABLE FLY | 6– 7 | BARNS | X | | X | | | | X | | X | | | X | | | NONE |
| HORSE FLY | 10–20 | BARNS | X | | X | | | | X | | X | | | X | | | NONE |
| DEER FLY | 7– 9 | CATTLE | X | | X | | | | X | | X | | | X | X | | NONE |
| BLACK FLY | 1– 5 | WOODLANDS RUNNING WATER | X | | X | | | X | | X | | | X | | X | | NODULES SCARS |
| SAND FLY | 1– 4 | WOODLANDS | X | | | X | | | X | | | X | | | X | | BLUISH SPOTS |
| BITING MIDGES | 0.6– 5 | MARSHLANDS | X | | | | X | | X | | X | | | | X | | NONE |
| CHIGGER MITE | 0.2– 1 | VEGETATION | X | | X | | | | | X | | X | | | | X | HYPERPIGMENTATION |
| TICKS | 5–15 | VEGETATION | X | | | | | | | | X | X | | X | X | | GRANULOMAS |
| BROWN RECLUSE SPIDER | 10–15 | CLOSETS ATTICS | X | | | | | | X | | X | X | | X | | | SCAR |
| BLACK WIDOW SPIDER | 10 | BASEMENTS OUTHOUSES | X | | | | | | X | | X | X | | X | | | NONE |
| TARANTULAS | 15–20 | VEGETATION | X | | | | | | | | | | | X | | | NONE |
| SCORPIONS | 15–200 | STONES AND SAND | | X | | X | | | X | | X | | | X | | | NONE |
| WHEEL BUG | 20+ | VEGETATION | X | | X | | | | X | | X | | | X | | | NONE |
| KISSING BUG | 20+ | BEDROOM | X | | | X | | | | X | | X | | | | X | NONE |

Figure 27.

hours. Desensitization has been accomplished by repeated injections of single and polyvalent extracts. It has been established that all members of the Hymenoptera group (honeybee, wasp, hornet, yellow jacket) have common antigens and that cross-sensitivity to the various members of the group is a distinct possibility. If desensitization is not practical, contact with bees should be avoided. A fully equipped emergency treatment kit with specific instructions as to use should be available at all times.

The following questions about immunization as answered by Doctor Mary Hewitt Loveless, an authority on the subject, clarify some of the variable and inconsistent reports in the literature.

1. Which insect ranks as the chief offender?

Among patients we have treated, the yellow jacket has been by far the most common cause of severe sting allergy. Next in order are the Polistes wasp, the bald-faced hornet, the bumblebee and finally the honeybee.

Where beekeeping is more prevalent, the honeybee ranks much higher. But both types of bees are generally friendly, not given to stinging unless provoked. By contrast, yellow jackets and bald-faced hornets are very aggressive. The abundant Polistes wasp is not aggressive but retaliates if disturbed.

People commonly fail to distinguish between the bee and the yellow jacket, which lives in the ground or in sides of buildings rather than in paper nests of their own construction. Most "bee stings" reported to us have really been yellow jacket stings.

2. What methods of immunization can be used?

Patients showing extreme allergy to stings can, with rare exceptions, tolerate a therapeutic dose of specific venom (the amount obtained from six venom sacs), given during one office visit. Whole-body extracts should not be used since they are immunologically ineffective antigens (*see* page 742 for further discussion). Venom-specific IgE titers are not significantly affected by treatment with stinging-insect whole-body extracts, and titer decreases appear to be a function of time, with no stimulation of total antibodies reacting with bee venom or bee venom phospholipase $A_2$ (PLA).

Venom in fluid form can be injected intracutaneously in five to seven divided doses over a period of one and one-quarter to four hours or more. A second method is to prepare the venom in emulsion form and place this repository under the skin in a single subcutaneous injection. This repository dose provides complete cross-immunity for a year.

3. Does immunization with one venom protect against stings by other insects?

Venom from the Polistes wasp protects the patient who is allergic to stings from the yellow jacket, which is closely related to the Polistes. As yet, no other such cross-protective action among venoms has been scientifically studied in man.

4. What precautions should be used in determining sensitivity?

All insect preparations should be used with great caution since they can incite allergy even

TABLE 142
REACTIONS TO HYMENOPTERA STINGS

| *Types of Reaction* | *Signs and Symptoms* |
|---|---|
| Local | Tenderness, itching, swelling, redness |
| Generalized | Generalized urticaria, itching, malaise and anxiety, sometimes accompanied by generalized edema, chest constriction, wheezing, abdominal pain, nausea and vomiting, dizziness |
| Severe generalized | Any of those listed above plus two or more of the following: dyspnea, dysphagia, hoarseness or thickened speech, confusion, feeling of impending disaster |
| Shock (systemic) | Any of those listed above plus two or more of the following: cyanosis, fall in blood pressure, collapse, incontinence, unconsciousness |
| Delayed | Erythema, vesicles, local skin necrosis, papular urticaria, anaphylactoid reaction |

in the normal person. Insect sting allergy is comparable to serum disease and to penicillin anaphylaxis.

Routine testing should be avoided. We question the patient about the circumstances of the previous stinging and his reactions. If he has an extreme allergy and if the decision is made to begin immunization therapy, then we test carefully to determine the lowest concentration of the offending venom that produces a reaction when instilled into the eye or injected superficially into the skin.

However, because bee venom is inherently irritating, conjunctival testing with it should not be done.

5. How soon does immunization become effective? How long does protection last?

Injections of fluid venom become effective within seven to ten days; injections of emulsified venom, in about two months.

Either form of injection provides immunity against one to three stings for at least four to six months. If year-round immunity is necessary, therapy can be repeated every six months. Conversely, the duration of protection can be extended indefinitely by planned stinging under the physician's supervision.

Emergency kits for treatment of allergic reaction to insect stings should include the following equipment (Doctor Joseph H. Shaffer).

1. Tourniquet: Apply to arm or leg above site of sting.
2. Tweezers: Remove stinger promptly, using care not to squeeze venom sac.
3. Disposable syringe and needle with epinephrine solution: Inject contents into cleaned skin area above tourniquet in upper arm or thigh. Or use aerosol inhaler with epinephrine or isoproterenol solution: Inhale three or four whiffs; repeat at three– to four-minute intervals as necessary.
4. Isoproterenol tablets: Place under tongue and let dissolve; repeat in five to ten minutes if necessary.
5. Antihistamine: Take orally.
6. Cold packs: Apply to sting area.

Several types of commercial emergency kits with detailed instructions for their use are available to combat severe allergic reactions caused by insect stings.* Persons with a history of severe reactions should have these materials with them at all times for emergency treatment. Such kits have also been recommended for persons over forty years old who are engaged in outdoor occupations, especially if they have any cardiac disease.

If you are allergic to insect stings, take these precautions whenever you must be in stinging insect territory.

1. Wear white, tan or green clothes.
2. Avoid flowery prints and flower colors.
3. Wear light, smooth fabrics rather than dark, rough ones.
4. Use insect repellent on clothing and exposed parts of the body and always keep it handy, especially during picnics and outings.
5. Avoid picking flowers.
6. Walk cautiously near bushes, hedges, tall grass, garbage areas, eaves, attics, boathouses and abandoned buildings.
7. Avoid touching insect nests. Warn your children not to touch them either.
8. Don't walk barefoot or in sandals.
9. Don't use scented substances such as hair dressings, deodorants, powders, soaps, perfumes or lotions.
10. Avoid wearing jewelry.
11. Avoid perspiring, if possible, as that tends to lure insects.

*Blister beetles* produce a painful blister with erythema when their juices are brought in contact with the skin. These beetles of the Meloidae family *(Epicanta fabricii)* are common in the Midwest and eastern United States. They contain significant amounts of cantharidin and are capable of producing symptoms from accidental ingestion or from skin absorption.

---

*Ana-Kit® is a compact and well-designed kit containing a preloaded epinephrine syringe with a package life of eighteen months or more and available only by prescription. Hollister-Stier Laboratories, Spokane, Washington, 99220. A similar kit is available from Center Laboratories, Incorporated, Port Washington, New York, 11050, and from other sources.

The *moth* and *hairy caterpillars* elaborate venom at the base of some of their hairs which, when in contact with the skin, often causes large areas of erythema, wheals and pruritus. *Megalopyge opercularis,* a stinging caterpillar, (commonly called "asp," "puss caterpillar" or "wooly worm") has been a public health problem throughout the southern states and Mexico.

The caterpillar is 20 to 30 mm long, 10 to 20 mm in height and width and looks like a blob of neatly combed brownish fur, similar in shape to a Brazil nut. It appears in elm, plum, sycamore and oak trees. Venom is polypeptide in nature and is elaborated in specialized unicellular glands that empty into corresponding spiney, hollow setae on the dorsal surface of the worm. Survey of an "epidemic" in southern Texas showed a high percentage of severe symptoms, including constitutional reactions that required hospitalization in three cases. In fact, severity of reactions observed in some patients suggest the possibility that death could result from these stings, although no deaths were reported in the survey made. The symptoms most frequently observed were marked local pain, local swelling, lymphadenopathy and headache; shock-like symptoms and convulsions were also noted. Hypersensitivity phenomena appeared to be uncommon.

In the *treatment,* it has been found that immediate light application of adhesive or Scotch® tape over the sting may be effective in removing broken-off spines. Early application of ice packs has been of some help in relieving pain. The use of an atropine-containing ophthalmic ointment has been found to be specific in aborting the local skin effects, while parenteral atropine has produced prompt relief of the systemic symptoms. Antihistamines and corticosteroids appear to be of only questionable value so far. Intravenous calcium gluconate may be of distinct benefit in patients with severe generalized reactions. Epinephrine hydrochloride has helped to control symptoms in severe cases. Mild analgesics such as aspirin generally fail to control pain and/or associated headache, and meperidine, morphine sulfate or codeine is usually required for control of intense pain.

Other irritative species are range and saddleback caterpillars and io, tussock, brown-tail, white and buck moths.

Many insects such as mosquitoes, stable and other flies, fleas, bedbugs, ants, lice and assassin bugs introduce saliva which contains an anticoagulant and sensitizing agent into the skin before taking a blood meal. This foreign protein causes hypersensitization and allergic manifestations in many individuals, producing various skin disorders as well as typical systemic symptoms of serum sickness.

The large desert ant, *Pogonomyrmex barbatus,* is distributed widely over the entire desert Southwest with numerous subspecies being found in California, Arizona, New Mexico and Texas. The ant, about one centimeter long and weighing 12 to 18 mg, is colored black when located at altitudes of about three thousand feet and is colored brown thereabove. Its stinger is located in the extreme posterior tip of the abdomen.

When one is stung, the usual site for the sting is on an extremity. Severe pain is immediately felt, which radiates quickly up and down the limb. Deep aching pain is experienced within minutes even into the trunk. The actual site of the sting develops wheal and flare within three to five minutes. Intensive inflammation, sweating and piloerection over the flare area occur, and this continues for up to forty-eight hours. The flare continues for up to four days with mild itching, inflammation and sensitivity to touch. When multiple stings are experienced, systemic toxicity ensues, with a few cases of death in children on record. *Treatment* is symptomatic and supportive. A paste of Adolph's® Meat Tenderizer applied to the area of an insect bite often reduces the swelling and itching by its enzymatic action. Unprocessed pineapple juice which contains the proteolytic enzyme bromelain (used successfully for phytobezoar), if available, could be used for this purpose.

The venom of *P. barbatus* is cholinergic, and its protein component has yielded sixteen amino acids, of which those with the highest concentrations were aspartic acid, glutamic acid, leucine and lysine.

### *Ticks and Mites (Acarina, Trombicula)*

Five tick-borne diseases of man are known to be in existence in the United States: Rocky Mountain spotted fever, tularemia, relapsing fever, tick paralysis and Q fever.

Some species of ticks and several species of mites cause serious local irritation and itching at the sites of the skin where they bite. The most notorious mites are the chigger ("red bug") and the rat mite. Dusting of DDT into socks and pants or applying a repellent such as dimethylphthalate on the ankles and legs may help prevent infestation with these mites.

Certain ticks, such as the Rocky Mountain wood tick *(Dermacentor andersoni)* and others, introduce saliva which may produce flaccid ascending motor paralysis which begins in the lower extremities. Recovery is usually rapid and complete if the tick is removed quickly, but if it is allowed to remain, death may result from respiratory paralysis. The most common sites of attachment are the pubic region, axilla and especially the back of the neck or scalp. Contrary to "old wives tales," the pajaroello tick *(Ornithodoros coriaceus),* whose habitat is on the west coast from California to southern Mexico, does not produce severe systemic symptoms. They are nuisances usually causing local effects only.

Tick Protection.

1. The best individual protection from ticks is wearing adequate clothing and inspecting the body thoroughly once or twice daily when in tick-infested areas.
2. When venturing into tick-infested areas, wear high shoes, boots or leggings, tucking trousers tightly into boots.
3. Inspect naked body carefully on returning from a field trip and remove ticks. Pay particular attention to the armpits, neck nape, crotch and groin areas. In heavily infested tick areas, children should be inspected twice daily. If ticks do attach, they usually feed several hours before infecting man.
4. Hang up field clothing in the open after returning home. Ticks still on your clothes will walk off eventually.
5. Remove attached ticks with forceps, eyebrow tweezers or a piece of paper or cotton held between the fingers. Do not use bare hands. A drop of alcohol, ether, gasoline, etc., may be used to force ticks to release their hold. Coating the tick with vaseline or applying fingernail polish (acetone) produces asphyxia and easy withdrawal of the tick. Do not leave the tick head or mouth parts embedded in the skin. Ticks mashed between fingernails or onto the fingers can infect man.
6. Be sure to paint the tick bite with an available antiseptic after removing the tick. Man can be infected through tick feces as well as the bites, so disinfection of bite and surrounding area is advisable.
7. Clothing (trousers, socks) can be dipped or sprayed with several repellents which are quite effective in warding off ticks. There are several chemicals on the market which may be readily purchased such as indalone or dibutyl adipate.
8. If your work necessitates frequent travel into tick-infested areas, obtain the spotted fever vaccine several weeks before tick season starts. To be effective, the vaccine must be given before spotted fever infection is acquired. Vaccination protects for one year only and must be repeated annually and there is now some question of its overall effectiveness.
9. If you become ill with fever, headache and rash, be sure you inform your doctor of any tick bite you may have received. This will help him to diagnose your case and prescribe specific treatment early.

Protection from acarids, insects and annelids is achieved mainly by treatment of the clothing with repellents. When properly used, they provide a high degree of protection in the presence of large numbers of blood-sucking arthropods. None of the present repellents are completely satisfactory, but the better repellents for ticks are DEET (N,N-diethyl-m-toluamide), butopyronoxyl (butyl-3,4-dihydro-2,2-dimethyl-4-oxo-2H-pyran-6-carboxylate), dimethyl carbamate and benzyl benzoate; for fleas, DEET and benzyl benzoate; for chiggers (larvae of Trombiculid mites), dimethylphthalate, ethyl hexanediol or any of the tick repellents; for leeches, DEET and benzyl benzoate. The only chigger repellent remaining effective after rinsing and washing in water is benzyl benzoate.

Vendex® (hexakis distannoxane) is a selective organotin miticide with high activity against foliage-feeding mites. It is only slightly toxic to animals and birds by ingestion, but highly toxic to fish. Human poisoning from Vendex ingestion is unlikely, but it can cause severe irritation of the eyes (particularly) and skin. The eyes should be thoroughly flushed or irrigated for fifteen minutes, while skin contamination should be washed with soap and water, after removing contaminated clothing.

## POISONOUS FISH

Illness produced by eating decomposed fish, whether in the natural state or canned, belongs to the general problem of food poisoning. However, true fish poisoning (ichthyosarcotoxism) is in no way related to putrefactive processes. Some fish produce a variety of profound neurotoxic or physiologic effects similar to compounds like aconite, muscarine and curare. Four general types of fish poisoning are recognized: ichthyosarcotoxins, of which there are at least nine kinds; ichthyotoxism; ichthyohemotoxism; and ichthyoacanthotoxism. The pharmacology and chemistry of fish poisons have not been characterized or well documented as yet.

Paralytic shellfish poisoning occurs worldwide and results from ingestion of shellfish that have ingested toxic species of dinoflagellates. The potent neurotoxin elaborated by the dinoflagellate is concentrated in the digestive glands of the shellfish. This toxin has been referred to as a saxitoxin, having been extracted from the Alaskan butterclam *Saxidomus giganteus.*

Dinoflagellates and other phytoplankton are important producers of the primary food supply of the sea. At certain times of the year in certain weather conditions, the dinoflagellates "bloom" in excessive numbers, coloring the water from light green to deep amber. Often there is a distinctive reddish tinge to the water, hence the name "red tide." Red tides occur in coastal waters (since offshore waters are less favorable to the growth of dinoflagellates) and may be fatal to massive numbers of fish when the dinoflagellates exhaust the oxygen supply of the water. Other animal life in the affected areas may die after consuming the shellfish.

Perhaps the first reference is recorded in Exodus 7:20-21: "And all the waters that were in the river were turned to blood. And the fish that was in the river died; and the river stank, and the Egyptians could not drink of the water of the rivers." Ancient Greek authors applied the name "red sea" to the coasts of Arabia presumably because of red water blooms in this region.

Centuries before Europeans reached the shores of the Pacific, the Indians watched the sea at night for luminescence, a phenomenon caused by the dinoflagellate *Noctiluca.* Indian guards were posted to warn the unwary not to eat shellfish during this period of luminescence; this might have been the earliest effort to maintain a public health quarantine. The first large epidemic recorded in the United States was in San Francisco in 1927, in which 102 persons were ill and 6 died. Today, illness associated with the red tide is uncommon.

The meat of approximately three hundred species of fish causes poisoning when ingested. The most common form of fish poisoning that occurs in the Caribbean area is called *ciguatera.* (It also occurs in other areas.) This syndrome is usually, but not always, caused by the meat of the moray eel or *Sphyraena* barracuda and is due to a toxin produced by benthic blue-green algae which is ingested by the small herbivores of the reef, which in turn are eaten by carnivorous fish. The grouper, snapper and members of the wrasse family are other fishes frequently involved. The incidence of *ciguatera* cannot be accurately determined since in many cases the symptoms are too mild to be considered important. A fat-soluble, heat-stable toxin has been isolated from the flesh of barracudas. Symptoms, which appear thirty minutes after ingestion, consist of nausea, vomiting, diarrhea, abdominal cramps, circumoral tingling, sweating, muscle weakness and incoordination. *Treatment* is mainly symptomatic and supportive; however, recent animal experimentation has demonstrated that cholinesterase activity is definitely inhibited by the toxin and that the administration of pralidoxime chloride, a cholinesterase reactivator, is an effective antidote. There should be no hesitation in the use of this preparation in humans, for it has already been tried successfully.

Scombroid poisoning is caused by a histamine-like substance called saurine, which produces in its human victims the symptoms of a severe allergy. Many reported cases of "fish sensitivity" are more correctly instances of scombroid poisoning following the ingestion of spoiled mackerel-like fishes, and even commercially canned tuna has occasionally been responsible.

Normally, fish tissue contains the histamine-precursor histidine. When histidine is acted upon by bacteria, as may occur when these fish are exposed to the sun or left to stand at room temperature for an extended period of time, saurine is produced. For some unknown reason, possibly because the scombroid fish contain greater amounts of histidine in their musculature, they seem to be especially susceptible to this kind of putrefication. The symptoms are similar to those of histamine poisoning. Within a few minutes after eating the toxic fish, which reportedly has a "peppery" or sharp taste, victims develop nausea and vomiting, flushing of the face, intense headache, epigastric pain, burning of the throat with difficulty in swallowing, thirst and swelling of the lips. Soon they also develop massive red welts and intense itching. The symptoms usually subside within twelve hours. *Treatment* should encompass evacuation of the stomach contents and catharsis. Administration of one of the common antihistamines (diphenhydramine HCL) often relieves the victim's distress. Scromboid poisoning can be readily prevented by adequately refrigerating fresh fish.

The consumption of mussels (shellfish) has sporadically given rise to epidemics of poisoning in this country and abroad. In some instances, the toxic effects are apparently caused by an allergic idiosyncrasy; in others, infection with *Salmonella* organisms; and in many, poisoning due to toxic compounds (saxitoxin), probably quaternary or tertiary amines, which are especially concentrated in mollusks during the spawning season. The ingestion of the latter acts as an autonomic ganglion blocking agent and results in nausea, vomiting and diarrhea, numbness of the lips, tongue and mouth, tingling sensation in the fingers and toes, followed by incoordination, ataxia, and in severe cases, paralysis and respiratory failure. Related species of Buccinidae found in the North Pacific, including *Buccinum leucostoma, Neptunea arthritica, Neptunea intersculpta,* and *Neptunea antiqua* (red whelk), all secrete tetramines. In the process of cooking, it is claimed that the addition of one tablespoon of sodium bicarbonate per quart of water inactivates the toxic compounds which accumulate in the broth. *Treatment* consists of gastric lavage with sodium bicarbonate and administration of saline cathartics. Artificial respiration and oxygen may be necessary for the pulmonary involvement.

There is a group of fish which poison by their sting or bite. Fish of the genus *Muraeva* have well-developed teeth which are adjacent to a sac, the venom of which is injected into the wound following a bite. In the stingrays (Dasyatidae), the tail is armed on the upper side with a barbed spine that is connected with the poison sac. Some of the stingrays, because of their deep penetrating wounds, are capable of introducing tetanus bacilli and producing tetanus.

Salt-water and skin divers and swimmers have a special group of undersea enemies which they should be prepared to recognize and avoid. These are the animals which can cause serious illness or death by biting or stinging. Halstead, in an intriguing and comprehensive study of the subject, states that probably the marine animals most generally feared by swimmers and skin divers are sharks. There are approximately 350 known kinds of sharks, but only 20 or less are thought to attack human beings. Those believed to be of most concern are, in the order of their danger, the mackerel or man-eaters, the requiem sharks, the sand sharks and the hammerheads. The physical appearance of all types of sharks is so characteristic that recognition should be no problem, and most authorities agree that any shark should be considered dangerous regardless of its family name and reputation. Their multiple rows of sharp teeth and their tremendously strong jaws inflict severe bites; death is caused by massive hemorrhage and shock. The skin of the shark, like that of the manta ray and some other orders of marine life, is so rough that it can cause major abrasions. *Treatment* of shark bites must be prompt, directed first at control of hemorrhage and shock, followed by measures applicable to management of any other large wound or traumatic amputation, including tetanus prophylaxis and antibiotics.

According to Halstead, making loud noises, blowing bubbles, splashing and creating commotion is of doubtful value in keeping a shark away if he really means business. Some noises attract the beasts. It has occasionally been observed that sharks investigate an unwounded person who remains motionless and then leave. You get nowhere with attempts to wound an attacker, but striking him on the snout, gills or eyes or shoving him away with a large club called a "shark billy" may be effective. Bright-colored garments and swimsuits however, which contrast sharply with light skin are likely to attract sharks, as do wounded fish and jettisoned garbage.

"Shark Chaser," the repellent developed by the United States Naval Research Laboratory as part of the survival equipment issued to airmen who traversed shark-infested waters, was composed 20 percent of copper acetate, which has some chemical properties resembling decayed shark flesh, and 80 percent of a highly soluble ammonium derivative of nigrosine dye that simulates the ink that the octopus or squid sends out to protect itself. This repellent performed well in initial tests; but later airmen and skin divers came up with conflicting reports, and its true value is therefore questionable.

Other biting underwater creatures are the barracudas and the moray eels, whose bites are treated in the same way as shark wounds. The giant grouper or sea bass can be dangerous, but not to the extent of the shark; male sea lions during the mating season may snap at a swimmer but are not usually ferocious. Killer whales, widely distributed in oceans and seas, are vicious and swift to attack; divers should get out of the water at once if killer whales are spotted. Another ocean animal to be shunned is the giant clam, or tridacna. While it does not truly bite, it can attain a weight of several hundred pounds and traps an unwary diver by closing its valves upon a foot or hand. This rarely happens, but if it does, the victim can be released by severing both adductor muscles of the clam with a knife.

### *Stinging Marine Animals (Invertebrates)*

Marine animals that sting are of many kinds, sizes, shapes and colors, and there are many ways in which they injure swimmers and divers. They fall into two general classes: the invertebrates and the vertebrates. The former include four major categories: coelenterates, mollusks, annelid worms and echinoderms.

There are three classes of coelenterates. The hydroids grow on rocks, weeds, pilings and sunken vessels, and among them are the fire coral of tropical waters and Portuguese man-of-war *(Physalia palagica)* which floats at the surface, trailing stinging tentacles several feet long. The tentacles, dangling beneath the surface, are covered with thousands of stinging cells capable of emitting microscopic organelles, the nematocytes, each of which consists of a small sphere containing a coiled hollow thread. When activated by touch the thread is uncoiled with such force that it can penetrate skin and even rubber gloves. On contact, venom in the cyst is injected into the victim through the thread. The toxic reaction depends upon the number of stings and the degree of the victim's sensitivity. In most cases, the sting is extremely painful, somewhat akin to the sting of hornets. Severe pain is often associated with signs of clinical shock. Cardiac arrhythmias occur and can be demonstrated by EKG.

Scyphozoa, or jellyfish, include the dangerous sea wasp, the sea nettle and sea blubber. Anthozoa are the elk horn coral and members of the sea anemone group.

The coelenterates sting by releasing venom from cells on the tentacles through minute stinging thread-like tubules when a diver brushes against them. Results of contact vary from mild to severe, local to general, and sometimes are fatal. As is the case in most stinging marine animals, there is no known specific antidote; Halstead suggests morphine to relieve pain, calcium gluconate for muscle spasm, antihistamines, topical creams and lotions, and for severe systemic reactions, cardiac and respiratory stimulants, artificial respiration and other supportive measures as needed.

Corals that sting produce symptoms similar to those produced by jellyfish, but only to the mildest degree. Coral cuts, however, are another problem altogether. Their initial mildness is totally deceptive, and it's this deceptiveness that often brings them to the attention of American physicians. Except around the Florida Keys, coral is not a major hazard in the United States. The large majority of cuts requiring attention here are acquired in the Caribbean. But because they seem benign at first, many tourists ignore them; it is only when they get back to the States that they learn the ill wisdom of their unconcern. All coral abrasions contain pieces of calcareous material and animal protein. If untreated, a mere scratch can turn into a painfully festering ulcer that recurs periodically for years.

The initial reaction to the coral cut, sometimes called coral poisoning, is the appearance of red welts and itching or burning around the wound—the danger signals that should call for further treatment. Prompt application of antiseptic agents, such as 2% tincture of iodine, or preferably Zephiran, go a long way toward preventing later difficulty.

Another but unconventional approach has been found quite effective: cleanse the wound with a brush or coarse cloth, water, and pHisoHex® or soap. Then dry the wound and clean it with alcohol; dry again and rinse with hydrogen peroxide. These measures should remove foreign material and bacteria. While the wound is still wet, empty the contents of a tetracycline capsule onto the area, and pat it into a paste with a tongue blade. Allow this to dry and use no further covering. The paste forms a false eschar that retards the growth of organisms underneath. This protective barrier sloughs as the wound heals from the edges.

In severe cases, the patient may have to be put on complete bedrest with the affected limb elevated. Kaolin poultices should be used, dressings should be saturated with magnesium sulfate in glycerin solution and antibiotics should be administered. Antihistamines, given orally or applied locally, help relieve the pain.

The mollusks are of two types: the gastropods (univalve mollusks), of which only the genus *Conus* need concern the diver, and the cephalopods, such as the octopus, squid, nautilus and cuttlefish. The shells of most cones have interesting and often beautiful color patterns and are prized by seashell collectors. Their venom is introduced by radular teeth. It causes numbness, cyanosis or a sharp burning sensation at the site of the wound, followed by spreading of these symptoms to the entire body. In severe cases paralysis may occur. Of the cephalopods, only the octopus is considered to be of medical importance, and many are surprised to learn that these animals carry venom which is introduced by biting. The symptoms of octopus envenomation are seldom severe, usually localized to one extremity, and recovery is smooth. There is, however, one reported death from the bite of a small octopus when the diver who captured it allowed it to crawl over his arms and shoulders. He was bitten on the neck and in a few minutes began to vomit, lost muscular control, developed difficulty in breathing and died two hours later in a hospital.

The third main class of invertebrate stingers, the annelid worms, are usually segmented and carry bristles which in some species cause an inflammatory reaction. Whether this is the result of a toxin is unknown. Other types of the annelids do their damage by biting with chitinous jaws.

The fourth group consists of the sea urchins, starfish and sea cucumbers. These echinoderms are characterized by having radial symmetry, with the body usually of five radii around an oral-suboral axis, comprised of calcareous plates which form a more or less rigid skeleton, or with plates and spicules embedded in the body wall. Very painful wounds can be made by the long-spined tropical sea urchins. Symptoms and treatment are the same as for any other stinging invertebrate.

### *Stinging Vertebrates*

Marine vertebrates consist of two groups: the fishes and the sea snakes. There are many kinds of venomous fishes, but only a few species of sea snakes. Some of the fishes capable of stinging or wounding man are the spiny dogfish, elephantfish or ratfish; catfish; weaverfish; scorpionfish, which include zebrafish, waspfish and stonefish; toadfish; sturgeonfish; dragonfish; stargazers; and the many types of rays. Most of these introduce their venom through spines located on various parts of the body. In others, venom apparatus has not been found, although sharply pointed or razor-edged spines and fins can produce serious wounds.

Stingrays are an important menace, and about 1500 attacks are reported annually in the United States. Such injuries usually occur when a person steps on a ray buried in a sandy or muddy bottom. The pressure on the back of the fish provokes him to whip his tail up and forward, driving the stinger, located on the caudal appendage, into the foot or leg of the victim. Hand and arm injuries are more common among commercial fishermen who are stung while emptying nets and seines. Stings on the trunk usually occur when a diver swims against a ray half covered in sand. The stinging weapon is a caudal spine covered by an integumentary sheath which holds the venom. The sheath is frequently left in the wound, and sometimes the entire stinger remains. The wounds are either laceration or puncture type, and pulling out the stinger may cause extensive damage to surrounding tissues. There is no known antidote and treatment is outlined below.

### *Treatment of Fish Stings*

Efforts in treating venomous fish stings should be directed toward (1) alleviating pain, (2) combating effects of the venom and (3) preventing secondary infection. The severe lacerations of ray and catfish stings are the result of the recurved spines or barbs of the stinger. These wounds should be irrigated immediately with sterile saline solution or hot salt water if available. Puncture-type wounds are usually small, making it difficult to remove venom; incision and suction may be required, and possibly irrigation. Prompt suction is recommended, but it is not likely to be very satisfactory.

TABLE 143
POISONOUS FISH

| Name | Region | Diagnosis | Treatment |
|---|---|---|---|
| Great barracuda (*Sphyraena barracuda*) | Florida, West Indies, Brazil, Indo-Pacific region | Straight razor-like lacerations without tissue removal; most attacks occur on beaches, near dusk, in murky water, on a cloudy day; they are usually related to poor visibility and the victims having been mistaken for food fish | Tourniquet (greatest danger is blood loss); prompt suture of wounds, tendons, nerves and large arteries; tetanus prophylaxis and antibiotics |
| Sharks<br>Mackerel, mako, white (Isuridae family) | Fast-swimming open water sharks | Tissue removal with loss of entire area of bite in a crescent or disc-shaped area; most deaths are due to hemorrhage | Prompt tourniquet and control of shock; tetanus prophylaxis and antibiotics<br>PREVENTION<br>A. *Swimmers*—Do not swim alone, in dirty water, with a wound, or areas in which sharks have been sighted.<br>B. *Divers*—Do not provoke sharks, even the small ones. Remove bleeding fish from water as soon as they have been speared. Leave the water quickly and quietly when sharks are sighted. Remember that sharks have been discouraged by beating the head, gills and snout.<br>C. *Sea Disasters*—Do not abandon your clothing as this protects against the rough skin of a shark. Place the bleeding wounded in a raft. Keep your arms and legs in the raft. Do not throw out garbage, blood, or bait for fish if sharks are sighted. Remain quiet and use rhythmic strokes if you must remain in the water. |
| Requiem sharks: tiger, lemon, bull, white-tipped, blue, Lake Nicaragua (Carcharinidae family) | In shore and open water | | |
| Sand, gray nurse, ganges (Carcharinidae family) | Shore-feeding sharks | | |
| Hammerhead (Sphyrnidae family) | In all the warm waters in the world and believed to locate their prey by keen senses of smell and hearing | | |
| Killer whales (*Orcinus orca*) | In all seas.<br>(*Warning:* Never frequent any area in which they have been reported. They have accounted for several deaths off the California coast.) | Ferocious and large (30 ft.) killer whales attack in packs and have been known to slaughter entire herds of seals | Symptomatic and supportive |
| Moray eel (*Gymnathorax mordax*) | In tropical seas and about reefs | Severe lacerations with spiny teeth. Generally, provoked when a diver's hand enters the hole in which it lives. Danger of infection. The powerful eel can hold a diver down long enough to suffocate him. | Irrigation, hemostasis, and suture of the wound; tetanus prophylaxis and antibiotics |

| | | | |
|---|---|---|---|
| Electric fishes | | | |
| Eels (*Electrophorus*) | Freshwater inhabitants of the tropics | The shock may temporarily disable the swimmer; it is believed to range about 200 volts | No treatment is necessary other than possible aid in reaching shore |
| Rays (*Torpedo, Hypnos, Narcine*) | Temperate and tropic ocean dwellers | | |
| Stingray (*Urobatis halleri* and others) | Inhabit most of the world; representative species include diamond, butterfly, European, eagle, California and South American freshwater stingray; all large freshwater varieties are dangerous | Penetration of the skin by the barb in the tail of the stingray causes intense local pain, swelling, nausea, vomiting, abdominal pain, dizziness, weakness, generalized cramps, sweating, fall of BP; recovery occurs in 24 to 48 hours; fatalities have occurred when the barb has penetrated the chest or abdomen | Cleanse wound by irrigation and remove foreign material; soak wound in hot water (as hot as tolerable) for 30 to 60 minutes; surgical debridement and closure of wound; tetanus prophylaxis and antibiotics |
| Scorpion fish (*Scorpaena guttata*) | Temperate and tropic zones of all seas | Spines of the gill-covers may penetrate skin and cause severe local pain and swelling, with extension of pain and swelling to involve the entire extremity | Treat as for stingray; infiltrate wound with 2% procaine if pain is severe |
| Jellyfish or Portuguese man-of-war (*Physalia palagica*) | Atlantic coast and Indo-Pacific region | Contact with these jellyfish causes urticarial wheals, numbness and pain of the extremities, severe chest and abdominal rigidity, and dysphagia | Inject 10 ml of 10% calcium gluconate IV to relieve muscular cramps or give muscle relaxants (methocarbamol, etc.) |
| Sea urchins (The black long-spined urchin, *Diadema setosum* is the most venomous variety; The red sea urchins such as *Toxpneustes elegans* and *Asthenosoma jimoni* produce milder symptoms.) | In warm waters around pilings, rocks, wrecks, etc. | The spines penetrate soft tissues and produce redness, swelling, and intense burning; the venomous spine or pedicellariae have poisonous tips and tooth-like 3 pronged biting teeth which cling long after detachment | Remove spines immediately with forceps; pedicellariae must be searched out and also promptly removed; brittle tips may break off and if not absorbed within 48 hours must be surgically excised; purple discoloration at the point of injury is a pigment of the spine and is not dangerous although often worrisome to the patient; shoes and gloves offer little protection from the spines; the diver or swimmer should avoid contact with these urchins |
| Annelid Worms | | | |
| *Glycera*, biting jaws (resembles centipede) | North Carolina to Canadian coast | Glycera produces an oval bite which becomes erythematous, inflamed, and later numb and itching; bristle worm stings produce swelling, inflammation, and numbness | Bites should be thoroughly cleansed; bristles are best removed with adhesive tape |
| *Eurythoë, Hermodice,* stinging hairs | Gulf of Mexico and Pacific | | |
| **Sea snakes** | See section on Sea snakes | | |

TABLE 143—*Continued*
POISONOUS FISH

| Name | Region | Diagnosis | Treatment |
|---|---|---|---|
| Stinging shells | Indo-Pacific | The cone shells of the Indo-Pacific are prized by collectors and several human deaths have been noted from stings on the hand; the gastropod uses its sting to kill other gastropods and secretes a toxin which competes for acetylcholine at the motor end plate; symptoms consist of weakness, ataxia, depressed respiration, coma, and finally death | *See* Stingray |
| Octopus | | Bites from the beak-like mouth of the octopus and infiltration in the area of a poison from the salivary glands which is used to paralyze the small crustacea on which it feeds have caused at least one known human death; symptoms usually are burning, swelling, redness, heat and free bleeding from the wound | Generalized supportive care; treat the bite as for fish stings |
| Lionfish (*P volitans*) | Shoals of the beaches in Barbados | Site of bite is inflamed, edematous and very painful; systemic symptoms may consist of tachycardia, dyspnea, profuse perspiration, vomiting, diarrhea, and intense colicky abdominal pain | Supportive and symptomatic; local anesthetic (2% solution of procaine, etc.) can be used to infiltrate the wounded area for relief of pain |

If ligation is used, and there is difference of opinion among physicians as to its value, the ligature should be applied at once proximal to but as close as possible to the sting, and it should be loosened every few minutes. Soaking the injured extremity in the hottest water that can be tolerated for one-half to one hour is recommended therapy (the venom is heat labile). Hot, wet compresses should be applied to face or body wounds. Adding epsom salts or magnesium sulfate to the water is thought to be useful, and infiltration of the area with 0.5% to 2% procaine has brought good results. Intramuscular or intravenous meperidine usually relieves pain. After soaking the wound, it may be desirable to employ debridement and additional cleansing. Lacerations should be closed with dermal sutures. Antibiotic therapy is usually not required if treatment is begun early, but tetanus toxoid or antitoxin is necessary. Treatment of shock resulting from stingray venom acting on the cardiovascular system should be prompt and vigorous and aimed at maintenance of cardiovascular tone and prevention of other complications. Respiratory distress may require the use of suitable stimulants. The familiar ligature-cryotherapy method of treatment has also been effective in some stings by rays. The Commonwealth Serum Laboratories in Melbourne, Australia, has developed a specific antivenom for stonefish stings.

### *Sea Snakes*

The venom of all species of sea snakes is extremely toxic; in some, the venom is said to be fifty times more powerful than that of the king cobra. The mortality rate is estimated at about 25 per cent. However, the venom apparatus is not well developed in most species, and they are a fairly docile group. They are true snakes, with lidless immovable eyes and a typical forked tongue. Most species are three to four feet in length, but some grow to a length of nine feet or more. They are found chiefly in the tropical Pacific and Indian oceans. Although considered to be generally peaceful, they should not be handled or approached carelessly.

Sea snake venom is primarily myotoxic, and myoglobinuria becomes evident early. The onset of symptoms after a bite is usually within one hour and they are generalized. They consist initially of thickening of the tongue and overall stiffness of muscles, which develop gradually. There may be pain upon movement, and an ascending general paralysis soon follows. Trismus is an outstanding symptom, as is drooping eyelids. The pulse weakens and becomes irregular; the pupils are dilated; talking and swallowing are difficult; and sometimes there is thirst or dryness of the throat, nausea and vomiting. Spastic movements have been observed. In severe cases the symptoms grow gradually more marked, the skin is cold and clammy, cyanosis appears, convulsions begin and respiratory difficulty becomes more and more intense. The victim finally becomes unconscious.

*Treatment* is little different from that employed after the bites of land snakes. Any exertion is to be discouraged. A tourniquet is applied to the thigh in leg bites and to the upper arm in bites on the hand or wrist. It must be loosened every half hour. The patient should be carried to a hospital immediately. The snake should be captured if possible and identified because it may turn out to be a harmless water snake. At the hospital or first aid station, the patient should receive immediate administration of antivenin, using a polyvalent antiserum containing a krait fraction. After doing sensitivity tests, inject 20 ml slowly by vein. Cortisone has been given to prevent possible severe anaphylaxis. If cortisone fails to control the serum therapy reaction, epinephrine may be required. Tetanus toxoid or antitoxin should be given as for any puncture wound. Bedrest is a requisite until all signs of poisoning subside. Adequate maintenance of fluid and electrolyte balance is imperative. Antibiotics should be used in case of infection. For sedation, if needed, intramuscular paraldehyde or barbiturates are recommended. Morphine is contraindicated, as are any of its derivatives. If respiratory paralysis occurs, the patient may require intubation, tracheotomy and a respirator. Hemodialysis has been used successfully for renal failure from tubular necrosis. Delayed effects from sea snake venom are unknown, and if recovery occurs, it is rapid and complete.

In the electric rays (Torpedinidae), the dorsal surface is electrically positive and the ventral one negative. To receive a shock one must contact the torpedo species at two distinct points. Some of these electric rays can temporarily paralyze the arm of a man. Two of the best known poisonous fishes are *Trachnius draco* and *Scorpaena scropha. T. draco* has the appearance of a trout with blue and brown stripes. Passing through each of its gill covers is a grooved spine which contains the poison gland. Another poison gland also connects the dorsal fin. *S. scropha* is an ugly red fish with a large head and prominent fins. The poison apparatus is connected with the first three rays of the dorsal fin. Bathers or swimmers who strike against these fins experience stabbing, burning pains in the affected part. The area about the bite is swollen and ecchymotic and later may become necrotic and slough. Systemic symptoms are dyspnea and delirium, and at times circulatory collapse and respiratory depression may occur, resulting in death. Vigorous *treatment* not unlike that for snakebite is necessary. The flesh of these fishes is wholesome as food and may be eaten with impunity.

The species *Pterois volitans* (the lionfish) is frequently found in the shoals of the beaches in Barbados, where it hides in weed-covered crevasses of the coral; bathers may be struck by its sharp spines or by stepping on them. This often produces very severe symptoms such as profuse perspiration, tachycardia, dyspnea, vomiting, diarrhea and intense abdominal, colicky pain. The site of the bite is inflamed, edematous and very painful. The pain often extends the entire length of the extremity. The *treatment* is mainly supportive and symptomatic. If available, a local anesthetic (2% solution of procaine, etc.) can be used to infiltrate the area around the wound to relieve the pain.

The sting of the jellyfish or Portuguese man-of-war can produce urticarial wheals, numbness, pain, severe chest and abdominal pain, abdominal rigidity and dysphagia. In addition to supportive therapy already mentioned, the administration of 10 ml of a 10% solution of calcium gluconate or a muscle relaxant often relieves the muscular cramps. Alcohol and compresses of aromatic spirits of ammonia or 1:20 Clorox bleach (Dakin's solution) and Adolph's Meat Tenderizer are reported to be effective in relieving discomfort and irritation. Lathering and shaving affords relief by removing organelles and tentacular material.

Severe stings and dermatitis may be received from the so-called sea lice, which are small crustaceans known scientifically as cymothoids because they are members of the suborder Cymothoid of the order Isopoda. They live in tropical and temperate ocean waters close to the shore where they eat or live on higher marine organisms. They often burrow into the sand just below water level. Their biting parts are well developed, and the crustaceans readily attach themselves to the bodies of fish or to the extremities of mammals that approach them. Although they are only one-quarter inch long, they cause the death of cod and other large fish and inflict painful wounds with ulceration on humans.

### *Kokoi Frog*

The venom from the skin of the kokoi frogs has been used as a deadly arrow poison for centuries by the Cholo Indians of Colombia. It causes an irreversible block of transmission of nerve impulses to the musculoskeletal system, producing death within minutes. It is ten times as deadly as tetrodotoxin, the venom of the Japanese puffer fish, up to now the most active venom known. Investigations have found that the molecular structure of the kokoi toxin is chemically related to the steroid hormones secreted by the adrenal gland.

*Bufus marinus,* a giant (one to one and one-half pounds) tropical night-feeding toad, produces a neurotoxic venom which can be lethal to pets and small animals, with multiple effects on humans such as nausea, vomiting, increased blood pressure and pulse, severe headache and paralysis.

## ZOONOSES

Over 600,000 humans are bitten and treated for animal bites each year, and probably two or three times that number are never reported.

Poison Control Centers are often asked for advice not only concerning the proper handling of animal bites, but also about diseases transmitted to man by pets and other animals. There are at least 150 different diseases which we now know can be transmitted naturally from animals to humans; these are known as "zoonoses."

The animal population of the world is exploding, just as is the human population. It is estimated that there are more than 3 billion domestic animals and over 4 billion domestic fowl in the world in addition to the unknown billions of wild animals and birds. In the United States, the calculated annual animal production is enormous: about 110 million swine, 100 million cattle, 30 million sheep, 4 million horses, 3 million fowl and 1 million goats. The number of pets, which has doubled since 1945, is an equally astounding figure, with an estimated 25 million dogs (two-dog families may soon become as common as two-car families), 25 million cats and 12 million birds in American homes.

The zoonoses have certain characteristics in common. The human incidence of the diseases is higher in those people having closer contact with animals. If the portal of entry of the causative agent is the same, the resulting disease will be similar in both man and animals. On the other hand, the disease is rarely transmitted from man to man. The etiologic agents responsible may be parasites, fungi, bacteria or viruses, and the mode of transfer is through direct or indirect contact with animals, their excretions or secretions.

The organism *Pasteurella multocida* is frequently found in the mouths of domestic and wild animals, and therefore the threat of infection from bites can be a problem.

Among the serious effects that can be caused by this organism, especially from a cat bite, is a progressive osteomyelitis. The disorder is associated with cats because this pet has very sharp teeth and tends to bite about the hands where bone and tendon are very close to the surface. An acute, inflammatory cellulitis, however, is a more common manifestation of *P. multocida* infection in humans, which responds to penicillin although it is a gram-negative organism.

Ecthyma contagiosum, or orf, is a comparatively uncommon zoonosis, but when it occurs in man, it may present considerable diagnostic difficulty. This viral disease causes epithelial hyperplasia, and the lesions may be easily mistaken for precancerous ones. The name "orf" derives from the Anglo-Saxon word for cattle, but the disease is endemic among sheep and is also found in goats. Usually it is contracted from diseased animals, but as the virus is quite hardy, it may also be transmitted by objects such as fences and barn doors that have been in contact with affected sheep.

The risk of man's acquiring zoonoses is actually not great, yet the possibility is ever present, and particularly in children, it is important to consider these diseases when the diagnosis is not clear or esoteric. Persons engaged in commercial processing of animals for food (abattoir) and other products undergo significant risks of infections which also should not be overlooked. Cat-scratch disease is often a perplexing diagnostic problem, particularly in children. After a two-day incubation period, the first sign may be fever and malaise, followed in a few days by a papule or ulcer at the scratched area and enlargement of the regional lymph nodes for two weeks to six months. Of the involved nodes, 50 per cent eventually become fluctuant and 30 per cent suppurate. A pink macular rash may follow. Epidemics have been reported. Thrombocytopenic purpura, coma, convulsions, encephalitis and osteolytic lesions rarely occur. Skin (cat-scratch antigen) and complement fixation tests with a virus from the cat's claws are positive. A puppy bite can cause similar signs and symptoms. Parinaud's oculoglandular conjunctivitis, which is due to tuberculosis, *Leptothrix,* virus or sarcoidosis, also is spread by cats.

Dogs suffer from and harbor a number of diseases that may be transmitted to man as a result of contamination by dog feces. These diseases include amebiasis, ancylostomiasis (dog hookworm), balantidiasis, echinococcosis (hydatid cyst), visceral larva migrans (toxocariasis), cutaneous larva migrans and salmonellosis. *Toxocara canis* is a roundworm whose eggs, when swallowed by man, hatch in the intestine with migration of the larvae through the bloodstream to other organs, creating the disease visceral larva migrans. The cutaneous form of larva migrans on the other hand, results from skin invasion of larvae of the dog (and cat) hookworm. Echinococcosis and toxocariasis, in particular, are diseases transmitted to man when mature eggs have been ingested as a result of contamination by dog excrement. Airborne infection from dried fecal dust is unlikely.

There are some dog diseases that are transmissible to man by urine; the principal disease in this category is leptospirosis, which occasionally produces disease in persons whose food has been contaminated with dog urine.

Most of the diseases that can be communicated from dog to man occur under unusually unhygienic conditions. Young children, however, are frequently in much closer contact with animal excrement than are adults and are consequently exposed to a greater risk of communicable diseases from this source. Fortunately, dog distemper is not transmitted to humans.

Not a single human case of rabies was reported in the United States in 1967 (one death of a thirteen-year-old boy in 1968 and 8 human cases from 1969 to 1973), yet over 30,000 persons received rabies vaccine prophylactically in varied amounts. Over 3500 rabid dogs, cats, foxes, raccoons, skunks and bats are recorded annually, and this figure probably represents only a small percentage of the actual number. Rabbits and rodents (squirrels, chipmunks, mice, rats) seldom, if ever, transmit rabies, and prophylactic therapy is usually unnecessary. As long as this large reservoir of rabies exists in nature, concern over rabies after every mammalian bite will continue, in spite of the rarity of human rabies. The disease is apparently transmitted rarely, if at all, from one person to another. Most fatal cases occur in young men, nearly one-fourth in children, and in boys three times more often than in girls. Dog bites account for 51 per cent of fatal cases, although since 1960 skunks as rabid animals are being frequently reported as a common source of human rabies in the United States. No history of animal exposure is available in a surprisingly large number of cases, however.

Upper extremities, face and lower extremities are bitten, in decreasing order of frequency. Distance of bite from brain does not correlate with duration of incubation period, which ranges from twenty to one hundred fifty days, with a mean of fifty-seven days. After onset of symptoms, death occurs within hours or as many as thirty-eight days; the average is a week. Likelihood of fatal disease depends on severity of bite and amount of tissue destruction.

Without history of exposure, diagnosis may be missed and psychoneurosis, frank psychosis, malingering or upper respiratory infection suspected. Neuritic pain, often referred to the bite site, is the initial complaint in nearly half of the patients. Nonspecific symptoms including chills, fever, nausea, anxiety, malaise, dyspnea, headache, paresthesia, paresis and vertigo are the first clinical signs in others. As the disease progresses, fever, psychiatric manifestations and dysphagia become prominent. Hydrophobia occurs in 43 per cent of patients. Mode of death is a generalized seizure in only 28 per cent.

The usual surgical principles should be followed in *treatment* of a bite: suturing, if necessary, and administering tetanus toxoid

TABLE 144
GUIDE FOR SPECIFIC ANTIRABIES PROPHYLAXIS*

| | *Status of Biting Animal (Whether Vaccinated or Not)* | | *Recommended Treatment* | |
|---|---|---|---|---|
| *Nature of Exposure* | *At Exposure* | *During 10 Days Observation* | *Rabies Prevalent* | *Rabies Not Prevalent* |
| No lesions; indirect contact | Healthy or rabid | Healthy or rabid | None | None |
| Licks: | | | | |
| 1. Unabraded skin | Rabid | — | None | None |
| 2. Abraded skin, scratches and unabraded or abraded mucosa | a. Healthy | Clinical signs of rabies or proven rabid (laboratory) | Start vaccine (twice daily 1st week; once daily 2nd week) at first signs of rabies in the *bitting animal* | Start vaccine at first signs of rabies in the biting animal |
| | b. Signs suggestive of rabies | Healthy | Start vaccine immediately; stop at 5 days | None† |
| | c. Rabid, escaped, killed or unknown | Rabid | Start vaccine immediately | Start vaccine immediately |
| Bites: 1. Mild exposure | a. Healthy | Clinical signs of rabies or proven rabid (laboratory) | Serum immediately; start vaccine when diagnosis *positive* | Start vaccine when diagnosis positive |
| | b. Signs suggestive of rabies | Healthy | Serum and vaccine immediately; stop at 5 days | Serum and vaccine immediately; stop at 5 days |
| | c. Rabid, escaped, killed or unknown | — | Start vaccine immediately | Vaccine immediately |
| | d. Wild wolf, jackal, fox, bat or skunk | — | Serum and vaccine immediately | Serum and vaccine immediately |
| 2. Severe exposure (multiple, or face, hand, finger or neck) | a. Healthy | Clinical signs of rabies or proven rabid (laboratory) | Serum immediately; start vaccine at first sign of rabies in the biting animal | Vaccine immediately |
| | b. Signs suggestive of rabies‡ | Healthy | Serum and vaccine immediately; stop at 5 days | Serum and vaccine immediately; stop at 5 days |
| | c. Rabid, escaped, killed or unknown | Rabid | Serum and vaccine immediately | Serum and vaccine immediately |
| | d. Wild wolf, jackal, fox, bat or skunk | — | Serum and vaccine immediately | Serum and vaccine immediately |

Three booster vaccine doses should be given at 7, 14 and 21 days after the 21st dose (2 weeks).

*The avianized (duck) embryo vaccine (DEV) is used instead of the Semple vaccine (nervous tissue origin, no longer available in United States) because there are fewer neurologic complications. The dose of equine antirabies serum is 1000 U./55 lb. of body weight given IM within twenty-four hours after the bite. If more than twenty-four to seventy-two hours have elapsed, two to three times this amount should be administered. If available, rabies immune globulin (RIG), human, should be used (20 I.U./kg) instead of the equine serum. Up to half the dose should be thoroughly infiltrated around the wound, and the rest given IM in the buttocks.

†In areas where rabies is not prevalent, the physician may recommend no treatment. Rabies should be considered prevalent in an area if one or more cases in animals have been reported within one year prior to the accident. This recommendation must be interpreted in the light of circumstances. A bite by a pet dog in an area of low prevalence would not require treatment, whereas a bite by a wild animal such as a fox, skunk or bat (unless proven negative by laboratory examination) would be an indication for treatment. Rats, squirrels and mice do not usually transmit rabies. The extent and location of the bite should also be considered.

American and Iranian researchers have developed a new rabies vaccine (HDCV, human diploid cell vaccine) which offers protection with fewer injections. The new vaccine, which is highly immunogenic and causes virtually no side-effects, protects with six injections compared with fourteen to twenty-one shots of vaccine produced from other animal tissue. The HDCV vaccine does not confer immunity until about the seventh to tenth day after the initial dose, so antirabies serum is recommended to provide passive immunity during the critical postexposure period. When available, this vaccine will supplant the avianized (duck) embryo vaccine; however, at present, it can be obtained only from the Center for Disease Control for use in patients with demonstrated allergy to the duck embryo vaccine or for those who have not achieved antibody levels considered protective from DEV.

‡Suggested in judgment of a veterinarian.

TABLE 145
EPIDEMIOLOGICAL ASPECTS OF SOME ZOONOSES
(Zoonoses are infections and infestations shared by lower vertebrate animals and man.)

| *Disease* | *Causative Organism* | *Principal Animals Affected* | *Geographical Distribution* | *Probable Vector or Means of Spread* |
|---|---|---|---|---|
| | | 1. BACTERIAL DISEASES | | |
| Anthrax | *Bacillus anthracis* | Cattle, sheep, goats, swine | Worldwide | Occupational exposure; ingestion of contaminated meat; occasionally airborne or biting insects |
| Bacterial food infections and intoxications | Various bacteria and their toxins, including Arizona organisms, *Salmonellae*, *Staphylococci*, *Clostridium perfringens*, *Clostridium botulinum* (toxin types A, B, D, E, & F), *Bacillus cereus* | Cattle, swine, fowl | Worldwide | Ingestion |
| Brucellosis | *Brucella abortus*, *Brucella suis*, *Brucella melitensis* | Cattle, sheep, goats, horses, reindeer, swine | Worldwide | Occupational exposure and by ingestion of contaminated milk products and other foods; occasionally airborne |
| Colibacillosis | *Escherichia* spp. | Cattle, swine, domestic fowl | Worldwide | Ingestion |
| Erysipeloid | *Erysipelothrix insidiosa* | Swine, fowl, fish | Worldwide | Occupational contact |
| Gas gangrene | *Cl. perfringens* and other Clostridia | Cattle, sheep | Worldwide | Soil |
| Glanders | *Actinobacillus mallei* | Horses, mules, asses | Asia, Africa and South America | Occupational contact |
| Leptospirosis | *Leptospira serotypes* | Rodents, dogs, swine, cattle, and a variety of wildlife | Worldwide | Occupational contact, immersion, exposure and contaminated food |
| Listeriosis | *Listeria monocytogenes* | Sheep, cattle, chinchilla, swine, goats, fowl | Worldwide | Unknown |
| Lung abscess | *Bordetella bronchiseptica* | Rodents | Worldwide | Contact |
| Malignant edema | *Cl. septicum* | Cattle | Worldwide | Wound infection |
| Melioidosis | *Pseudomonas pseudomallei* | Rodents, rabbits | Asia, Australia, Guam and Philippine Islands | Exposure and ingestion |
| Pasteurellosis | *Pasteurella multocida* | Mammals and birds | Worldwide | Exposure and ingestion |
| Plague | *Pasteurella pestis* | Rodents | Worldwide | Infected fleas and airborne |
| Pneumococcal mastitis | *Diplococcus pneumonia* | Cattle | Northern and Central Europe | Contact |
| Pneumonia | *Diplococcus pneumonia* | Calves (transmitted from man) | Europe and North America | Airborne |
| Pseudotuberculosis | *Pasteurella pseudotuberculosis* | Guinea pigs and other rodents, pigeons, turkeys and canaries | Worldwide | Occupational exposure |
| Ratbite fever | *Spirillum minus*, *Streptobacillus moniliformis* | Rodents and wild animals | Worldwide | Rodent bites |

| | | | | |
|---|---|---|---|---|
| Relapsing fever, endemic | *Borrelia* spp. | Rodents and wild animals | Worldwide | Infected ticks and body lice |
| Salmonellosis[*] | *Salmonella serotypes* | Cattle, swine, fowl | Worldwide | Ingestion, airborne, and contact |
| Staphylococcic disease[**] | *Staphylococcus* spp. | Cattle, swine, fowl | Worldwide | Ingestion and contact |
| Streptococcosis[***] | *Streptococcus* spp. | Cattle and fowl | Worldwide | Ingestion and contact |
| Tetanus | *Cl. tetani* | Principally herbivorous, but all animals may harbor the agent | Worldwide | Wounds |
| Tuberculosis | *Mycobacterium tuberculosis* | | Worldwide | Ingestion, inhalation, and occupational exposure |
| | var. *bovis* | Cattle | | |
| | var. *hominis* | Monkeys | | |
| | var. *avium* | Fowl | | |
| Tularemia | *Francisella tularensis* | Rabbits, sheep and wild rodents | North America, Europe, and Asia | Occupational exposure, handling, ingestion, and bite of infected insects and ticks |
| Vibriosis | *Vibrio fetus* | Cattle and sheep | Europe, North and South America | Unknown |
| | | **2. FUNGUS DISEASES** | | |
| Actinomycosis | *Actinomyces bovis*[****] | Cattle, swine, horses, dogs | Worldwide | Endogenous |
| Aspergillosis | *Aspergillus* spp. | Birds, fowl and many mammals | Worldwide | Contact with organisms in nature |
| Candidiasis (moniliasis) | *Candida* spp. | Birds, fowl, calves, pigs, rodents, dogs, cats, foals and other mammals | Worldwide | Endogenous |
| Coccidioidomycosis | *Coccidioides immitis* | Cattle, dogs, wild rodents, sheep, horses | Southwestern United States, areas of Mexico, Central and South America | Contact with organisms in nature |
| Cryptococcosis | *Cryptococcus neoformans* | Cattle, horses, cats, dogs, pigs and other mammals | Worldwide | Contact with organisms in nature |
| Dermatophilosis | *Dermatophilus congolensis* | Cattle, horses, sheep, deer and other mammals | Worldwide | Not fully understood |
| Geotrichosis | *Geotrichum candidum* | Cattle | Worldwide | Endogenous or exogenous |
| Histoplasmosis | *Histoplasma capsulatum* | Dogs, cats, cattle, horses, rodents and other mammals | Probably worldwide | Contact with organisms in nature |
| Maduromycosis | Several species and genera of fungi | Horses and dogs | Worldwide, chiefly tropical areas | Contact with organisms in nature |
| Nocardiosis | *Nocardia* spp. | Cattle, dogs and other mammals | Worldwide | Contact with organisms in nature |
| North American Blastomycosis | *Blastomyces dermatitidis* | Dogs, horses and sea lions | North America (occasional human infections in Africa and South America) | Probably contact with organisms in nature |

[*] Arizona organisms cause similar infections.

[**] Some strains occur commonly in man and some are common to animals, while others appear in both man and animals.

[***] Group A streptococci have been found in man only.
Group B streptococci: common cause of bovine mastitis; other strains cause infection in man; no evidence of interchange.
Group C streptococci: strains isolated from both human and animal infections.
Group D streptococci found only in animal infections.

[****] *Actinomyces bovis* is the cause of actinomycosis in lower animals. It does not cause this disease in man. The agent of actinomyces in man is *Actinomyces israeli,* a different species.

TABLE 145-*Continued*
EPIDEMIOLOGICAL ASPECTS OF SOME ZOONOSES

| *Disease* | *Causative Organism* | *Principal Animals Affected* | *Geographical Distribution* | *Probable Vector or Means of Spread* |
|---|---|---|---|---|
| Phycomycosis | Several species and genera of phycomycosis | Cattle, pigs, dogs and other mammals | Probably worldwide | Contact with organisms in nature |
| Piedra | *Piedraia hortai* | Lower primates and other mammals | South and Central America, Java, Asia, and Africa | Contact with organisms in nature |
| | *Trichosporon cutaneum* | Lower primates and horses | Rare, reported from England and Latin America | Contact with organisms in nature |
| Rhinosporidiosis | *Rhinosporidium seeberi* | Horses, cattle, mules | Endemic in India, Ceylon, and areas of western hemisphere Sporadic in rest of world | Unknown |
| Ringworm | *Microsporum* and *Trichophyton* spp. | All mammals and birds | Worldwide | Direct contact and fomites; contact with organisms in nature |
| Sporotrichosis | *Sporotrichium schenckii* | Horses, mules, dogs, cats, rats, mice and swine | Worldwide | Contact with organisms in nature |
| | | 3. PARASITIC DISEASES<br>a. Protozoan Diseases | | |
| Amoebiasis | *Entamoeba histolytica* | Dogs, primates | Worldwide | Ingestion |
| Babesiasis* | *Babesia* sp. | Wild and domestic animals | Worldwide | Bite of infected ticks |
| Balantidiasis | *Balantidium coli* | Swine | Worldwide | Ingestion |
| Coccidiosis | *Isospora* spp. | Dogs | Worldwide | Ingestion of oocysts |
| Endemic pneumocystis | *Pneumocystis carinii* | Rabbits, guinea pigs, rats, dogs, cats, mice, sheep, monkeys | Europe, United States | Unknown |
| Leishmaniasis | | | | |
| American | *Leishmania braziliensis* | Dogs, cats, and spiny rat | Central and South America | Bite of infected sand flies (*Phlebotomus*) |
| Oriental sore (cutaneous) | *Leishmania tropica* | Dogs, cats, and gerbils | Asia, Africa, and Europe | Bite of infected sand flies (*Phlebotomus*) |
| Visceral | *Leishmania donovani* | Dogs, cats, and rodents | South America, Africa, Europe, Asia | Bite of infected sand flies (*Phlebotomus*) |
| Pneumocystis infection | *Pneumocystis carinii* | Dogs | Worldwide | Unknown |
| Simian malaria | *Plasmodium knowlesi* | Monkeys | Borneo | *Anopheles* spp. |
| | *Plasmodium malariae* | Chimpanzees | Africa | |
| | *Plasmodium cynomolgi* | Macaques | Malaya | |
| | *Plasmodium simium* | Howler monkeys | South America | |
| | *Plasmodium inui* | Macaques | Southeast Asia | |
| | *Plasmodium brazilianum* | New world monkeys | South America | |
| Toxoplasmosis | *Toxoplasma gondi* | Birds and mammals | Worldwide | Probably contact and ingestion although exact route is not known |

* Symptoms resemble malaria. Can be differentiated by the appearance of the parasite and the absence of circulating gametocytes and malarial pigments. Like malaria, responds to therapy with chloroquine.

| | | | | |
|---|---|---|---|---|
| Trypanosomiasis African Sleeping Sickness | *Trypanosoma rhodesiense* | Wild and domestic ruminants | Africa | Bite of infected tsetse fly (*Glossina* spp.) |
| Chagas' disease | *Trypanosoma cruzi* | Dogs, cats, swine, foxes, bats, rodents, and monkeys | North, Central, and South America | Fecal material of triatomid bug |
| | *Trypanosoma rangeli* | Dogs and opossums | Northern part of South America | Fecal material of triatomid bug |

b. Trematode Diseases

| | | | | |
|---|---|---|---|---|
| Amphistomiasis | *Gastrodiscoides hominis* | Swine | Asia | Unknown Snails (?) |
| Clonorchiasis | *Clonorchis sinensis* | Dogs, cats, swine, wild animals | Asia | Ingestion of raw or partially cooked infected fresh water fish |
| Fascioliasis | *Fasciola hepatica* | Cattle and sheep | Worldwide | Ingestion of contaminated greens |
| | *Fasciola gigantica* | Cattle and sheep | Worldwide | |
| Fasciolopsiasis | *Fasciolopsis buski* | Swine and dogs | Asia | Ingestion of raw aquatic plants |
| Heterophyiasis | *Heterophyes heterophyes* (and other heterophids) | Cats, dogs, foxes, fish | Nile Delta, Turkey, and the Far East | Eating uncooked fish |
| Metagonimiasis | *Metagonimus yokogawai* | Cats, dogs, other fish-eating mammals and fish | Asia, Europe, and Siberia | Eating uncooked fish |
| Opisthorchiasis | *Opisthorchis felineus* | Cats and dogs | Eastern Europe, Asia, Siberia | Raw or uncooked fish ingested containing metacercariae |
| | *Opisthorchis viverrini* | Dogs, cats and fish-eating mammals | Thailand and Laos | Eating uncooked fish containing metacercariae |
| Paragonimiasis | *Paragonimus westermani* | Dogs, cats, wild animals | Asia and Africa | Ingestion of raw or partially cooked infected crayfish |
| Schistosomiasis | *Schistosoma japonicum* | Cattle, swine, dogs, rodents | Asia | Penetration of unbroken skin by cercariae in water |
| Swimmer's itch | *Schistosoma mansoni* | Baboons and rodents | Africa | |
| | *Schistosoma* spp. | Birds and rodents | Worldwide | Penetration of unbroken skin by cercariae in fresh and salt water |

c. Cestode Diseases

| | | | | |
|---|---|---|---|---|
| Beef tapeworm | *Taenia saginata* | Cattle | Worldwide | Ingestion of measly beef |
| Dog tapeworm | *Dipylidium caninum* | Dogs and cats | Worldwide | Ingestion of dog or cat flea |
| Fish tapeworm | *Diphyllobothrium latum* | Dogs and fish-eating animals | Worldwide | Ingestion of raw or partially cooked infected fish |
| Hydatidosis | *Echinococcus granulosus* | Dogs, sheep, cattle, swine, rodents | Worldwide | Ingestion of tapeworm eggs |
| | *Echinococcus multilocularis* | Foxes, microtine rodents, dogs | North America, Russia, Europe | Ingestion of tapeworm eggs |
| Pork tapeworm and cysticercosis | *Taenia solium* *Cysticercus cellulosae* | Swine | Worldwide | Ingestion of measly pork and autoinfection |
| Dwarf tapeworm | *Hymenolepis nana* | Rodents | Worldwide | Ingestion of tapeworm eggs in food, fleas, mealworms |
| Mouse or rat tapeworm | *Hymenolepis diminuta* | Rats, mice | Worldwide | Ingestion of tapeworm eggs in food, fleas, mealworms |

TABLE 145-*Continued*
EPIDEMIOLOGICAL ASPECTS OF SOME ZOONOSES

| *Disease* | *Causative Organism* | *Principal Animals Affected* | *Geographical Distribution* | *Probable Vector or Means of Spread* |
|---|---|---|---|---|
| Sparganosis | *Diphyllobothrium* spp. *Spirometra* spp. (pseudophyllidean tapeworms) | Monkeys, cats, pigs, weasels, rats, chickens, snakes, frogs, mice | Mostly Far East | Ingestion of *cyclops* or poultices from infected animals |
| | | d. Nematode Diseases | | |
| Capillariasis | *Capillaria hepatica* | Rodents | Worldwide | Unknown |
| Dracunculiasis | *Dracunculus medinensia* | Dogs, racoons | Worldwide | Bites of infected cyclops |
| Filariasis | | | | |
| Dirofilariasis | *Dirofilaria* spp. | Dogs | Worldwide | Bites of infected mosquitoes |
| Malayan filariasis | Brugia Malayi | Dogs and cats | Asia | Mosquito |
| Tropical eosinophilia | Brugia spp.; *Dirofilaria* spp. | Lower primates and mammals | Worldwide, Tropical | Bites of infected mosquitoes |
| Giant kidney worm | *Dioctophyme renale* | Dogs and other carnivores | Europe, North America | Ingestion of infected fish |
| Gnathostomiasis | *Gnathostoma spinigererum* | Dogs, cats, wild carnivores | Far East, India | Ingestion of infected fish or amphibian |
| Larva migrans | | | | |
| Ancylostomiasis (cutaneous larva migrans or "creeping eruption") | *Ancylostoma braziliense* | Dogs and cats | Worldwide | Contact with infective larvae which penetrate the skin |
| Anisakiasis | Anisakis spp. | Herring, other marine fish | Europe | Ingestion of raw or partially cooked herring |
| Parasitic meningo-encephalitis | *Angiostrongylus cantonensis* | Rats | Pacific and Orient | Raw prawns and prawn juice, latter used on vegetables; slugs that contaminate raw vegetables and are accidentally ingested |
| Visceral larva migrans (Toxocariosis) | *Toxocara canis* | Dogs | Worldwide | Ingestion of dog and cat roundworm eggs |
| Strongyloidiasis | *Strongyloides stercoralis* | Dogs | Worldwide | Contact with infective larvae which penetrate the skin |
| Thelaziasis | *Thelazia* spp. | Dogs, cats, sheep | California, and Far East | Infected insects |
| Trichinosis | *Trichinella spiralis* | Swine, rodents, wild carnivores | Worldwide | Ingestion of pork and other flesh containing viable cysts |
| Trichostrongylosis | *Trichostrongylus colubriformis* and occasionally other species | Domestic and wild herbivorous animals | Worldwide | Ingestion of contaminated vegetation |
| | | e. Annelid Diseases | | |
| Hurudiniasis | *Limnatis nilotica* and related spp. | Cattle, buffaloes, horses, sheep, dogs, and pigs | Africa, Asia, Europe. and Chile | Direct contact with leech |

| | | | | |
|---|---|---|---|---|
| | | **4. ARTHROPOD DISEASES** | | |
| Acariasis (Mange) | *Sarcoptes* spp. | Domestic Animals | Worldwide | Contact with infected individuals or animals and contaminated clothing |
| Myiasis | *Cochliomyia Cordylobia, Dermatobia, Gastrophilus, Hypoderma, Oestrus,* and other genera | Mammals | Worldwide | Invasion of living tissues by fly larvae |
| Pentastomid infections | *Linguatula* spp. *Armillifer* spp. *Porocephalus* spp. (Tongue worms) | Dogs, snakes, and other vertebrates | Worldwide | Ingestion of infected animal tissues |
| Tunga infections | *Tunga penetrans* | Man, dog, pig and other mammals | Western Hemisphere and Africa | Contact with contaminated soil |
| | | **5. RICKETTSIAL DISEASES** | | |
| Boutonneuse fever | *Rickettsia conori* | Dogs and rodents | Europe and Africa | Bite of infected ticks |
| Murine typhus | *Rickettsia mooseri* | Rats | North America | Infected rodent fleas |
| Q fever | *Coxiella burnetii* | Sheep, cattle, goats, fowl and other mammals | Worldwide | Mainly airborne, although milk may be a vehicle and occasionally ticks |
| Queensland tick typhus | *Rickettsia australis* | Bandicoots, rodents | Australia | Bite of infected tick |
| Rickettsial pox | *Rickettsia akari* | Mice | Eastern USA and USSR | Bite of infected rodent mites |
| Scrub typhus | *Rickettsia tsutsugamushi* | Rodents | Asia, Australia and East Indies | Bite of infected larval mites |
| Spotted fever | *Rickettsia rickettsii* | Rabbits, field mice and dogs | North and South America | Bite of infected ticks or their crushing on the skin |
| | | **6. VIRUS DISEASES** | | |
| | | a. Arthropod-borne | | |
| Chikungunya | Group A virus | | East and South Africa | Mosquito (*Culex* and *Aedes* spp.) |
| Eastern encephalitis | Group A virus | Wild birds, domestic fowl, horses, mules, donkeys | Eastern Canada, USA, Mexico, Panama, Trinidad, Colombia, Brazil, and Philippines | Mosquito (*Culiseta melanura* and *Aedes* sp.) |
| Mayaro | Group A virus | | Trinidad, Colombia, and Brazil | Unknown |
| Middelburg | Group A virus | Sheep | South Africa | Mosquito (*Aedes* spp.) |
| Mucambo | Group A virus | Rodents, wild birds, monkeys | Brazil | Mosquito |
| O'nyong-nyong | Group A virus | | Uganda | Mosquito |
| Sindbis | Group A virus | Birds | Africa and India | Culicine mosquitoes |
| Venezuelan encephalitis | Group A virus | Rodents, wild birds, domestic fowl, horses, mules, donkeys | Venezuela, Colombia, Brazil, and Trinidad | Mosquito (*Mansonia titillans*) |
| Western encephalitis | Group A virus | Wild birds, domestic fowl, horses, mules, donkeys | Canada, USA, Mexico, Trinidad, British Guiana, and Argentina | Mosquito (*Culex tarsalis, Culiseta melanura*) |
| Bat salivary gland | Group B virus | Bats | Western United States | Unknown; laboratory infections in man |

TABLE 145-*Continued*
EPIDEMIOLOGICAL ASPECTS OF SOME ZOONOSES

| *Disease* | *Causative Organism* | *Principal Animals Affected* | *Geographical Distribution* | *Probable Vector or Means of Spread* |
|---|---|---|---|---|
| Central European encephalitis | Group B virus | Cattle, goats (serological evidence only) and wild birds | Central and Eastern Europe from the Baltic to the Balkans | Tick (milk) |
| Dengue, type 1 | Group B virus | | South and Southeast Asia, Oceania, and Pacific | Mosquito |
| Dengue, type 2 | Group B virus | Monkeys and bats (serological evidence only) | Circumglobal in the Tropics | Mosquito (*Aedes aegypti* and *Aedes* spp.) |
| Dengue, type 3 | Group B virus | | Philippines and Thailand | Mosquito (*Aedes aegypti* and *Aedes* spp.) |
| Dengue, type 4 | Group B virus | | Philippines | Mosquito (*Aedes aegypti* and *Aedes* spp.) |
| Diphasic meningo-encephalitis | Group B virus | Cattle and sheep | USSR | Tick (milk) |
| Ilheus | Group B virus | Wild birds | Northern South America, Trinidad, and Central America | Mosquito |
| Japanese B encephalitis | Group B virus | Wild birds, swine, horses, cattle | Japan, China, Taiwan, Thailand, Malaya, Burma, India, Guam, Philippines Australia and New Guinea | Mosquito (*Culex tritaenorhynchus* and *Culex gelidus*) |
| Kunjin | Group B virus | Unknown | Australia | Mosquito |
| Kyasanur Forest disease | Group B virus | Monkeys, small mammals | Mysore, India | Tick (*Haemaphysalis spinigera*) |
| Louping III | Group B virus | Sheep, goats and grouse | Great Britain | Tick (*Ixodes ricinus*) |
| Murray Valley encephalitis | Group B virus | Wild birds | Australia and New Guinea | Mosquito (*Culex annulirostris*) |
| Negishi | Group B virus | Rodents | Japan | Ticks suspected |
| Omsk hemorrhagic fever | Group B virus | Rodents, muskrats, goats | Omsk, Siberia, USSR | Tick (*Dermacentor pictur*, *Dermacentor marginatus*), goat milk borne |
| Powassan | Group B virus | Squirrels | Ontario, Canada | Tick |
| Russian spring-summer encephalitis | Group B virus | Birds, small mammals and sheep | USSR | Tick |
| St. Louis encephalitis | Group B virus | Wild birds and domestic fowl | USA, Caribbean Islands, and Northern South America | Mosquito (*Culex tarsalis* and *Culex pipiens, quinquefasciatus* complex, *Culex nigri palpus*) |
| Spondweni | Group B virus | Serological evidence in domestic and wild animals | Southern Africa | Mosquito |
| Wesselsbron | Group B virus | Sheep | East and South Africa | Mosquito (*Aedes* spp.) |
| West Nile | Group B virus | Wild birds and horses | Africa, Near East, and South Asia | Mosquito (*Culex univittatus;* Egypt, *Culex pipiens*) |

| | | | | |
|---|---|---|---|---|
| Yellow fever | Group B virus | Monkeys and marmosets | Tropical, Central and South America and Africa | Mosquito [*Aedes aegypti*, *Haemagogus* sp., *Aedes leucocelanenus* (S.A.); *Aedes africanus* (Africa), *Aedes simpsoni* (Africa)] |
| Zika | Group B virus | Monkeys | Nigeria and Uganda | *Aedes africanus* |
| Apeu, Caraparu, Itaqui, Marituba, Murutucu, Oriboca | Group C virus | Rodents, possibly monkeys | Brazil | Mosquito |
| Madrid, Ossa | Group C virus | Rodents | Panama | Mosquitoes suspected |
| Restan | Group C virus | Rodents | Trinidad, Surinam | Mosquitoes, *Culex* (Melanoconion) |
| Bunyamwera | Group Bunyamwera virus | | East and South Africa | Mosquito |
| Germiston | Group Bunyamwera virus | | South Africa | Mosquito |
| Guaroa | Group Bunyamwera virus | | Colombia and Brazil | Mosquito |
| Ilesha | Group Bunyamwera virus | | Nigeria | Mosquito |
| Wyeomyia complex | Group Bunyamwera virus | | Colombia, Brazil, Trinidad, Panama | Mosquito |
| Bwamba | Bwamba virus | Monkeys | East, Central and West Africa | Mosquito (*Aedes* spp.) |
| California encephalitis virus | Group California virus | Hares and squirrels | Western and Central United States | Mosquito (*Aedes* spp.) |
| La Crosse virus | Group California virus | Rabbits | Midwestern and Southern United States | Mosquito (*Aedes* spp.) |
| Tahyna | Group California virus | Domestic animals, hares | Southern United States, Czechoslovakia, Yugoslavia | Mosquito (*Aedes* spp.) |
| Catu | Group Guama virus | Rodents, monkeys | Brazil | Mosquito |
| Guama | Group Guama virus | Rodents | Brazil | Mosquito |
| Oropouche | Group Simbu virus | Monkeys | Trinidad and Brazil | Mosquito |
| Argentinian hemorrhagic fever | Tacaribe group (Junin virus) | Rodents | Argentina | Rodent mite |
| Bolivian hemorrhagic fever | Tacaribe group (Machupo virus) | Rodents | Bolivia | Rodent urine |
| Hemorrhagic uremic syndrome | Tacaribe group virus | | Argentina | Unknown |
| Colorado tick fever | Ungrouped virus | Squirrels, porcupines, small rodents | Western United States | Tick (*Dermacentor andersoni*) |
| Crimean hemorrhagic fever | Ungrouped virus | Hares | Southern USSR | Tick (*Hyaloma marginatum*) |
| Kemerovo | Ungrouped virus | Cattle, horses, rodents | Siberia | Tick (*Ixodes persulcatus*) |
| Nairobi sheep disease | Ungrouped virus | Sheep | East Africa | Tick |
| Piry | Ungrouped virus | Rodents, opossum | Brazil | Laboratory infections have occurred |
| Quaranfil | Ungrouped virus | Wild birds, pigeons | Nile Delta of Egypt | Ticks *Argas* (persicargas) *arboreus* |
| Rift Valley fever | Ungrouped virus | Sheep, goats, cattle | Africa | Mosquito (*Aedes caballua*, *Aedes* spp.); contact on autopsy or handling fresh meat |
| Vesicular stomatitis | Ungrouped virus | Swine, cattle, horses | North and South America | Contact exposure and insect bites |

TABLE 145-*Continued*
EPIDEMIOLOGICAL ASPECTS OF SOME ZOONOSES

| *Disease* | *Causative Organism* | *Principal Animals Affected* | *Geographical Distribution* | *Probable Vector or Means of Spread* |
|---|---|---|---|---|
| | | **b. Not Arthropod-borne** | | |
| African Green Monkey disease | Virus | African Green Monkey (*Cercopithecus aethiops*) | Unknown | Contact with infected tissues |
| Contagious ecthyma | Virus | Sheep and goats | Worldwide | Occupational exposure |
| Cowpox | Virus | Cattle | Worldwide especially where smallpox exists | Contact exposure |
| Encephalomyocarditis | Virus | Rats, mice, squirrels, swine, monkeys, baboons | Worldwide | Environmental contamination |
| Foot-and-mouth disease | Virus | Cattle, swine and related species | Europe, Asia, Africa, and South America | Contact exposure; man is quite resistant |
| Herpes virus, Simian virus (both B virus and T virus) | Virus | Monkeys | Worldwide | Bites of monkeys, occupational exposure |
| Infectious hepatitis (human) | Virus | Subhuman primates | Worldwide | Contact exposure |
| Influenza and parainfluenza including Type A (swine and equine) and Sendai (Type D) | Virus | Swine and rodents | Asia and Europe, North America | Contact exposure |
| Lymphocytic choriomeningitis | Virus | Rodents, swine, dogs | Worldwide | Virus contaminates food and environment |
| Newcastle disease | Virus | Fowl; psittacine birds | Worldwide | Occupational exposure |
| Pseudo cowpox | Virus | Cattle | Worldwide | Occupational exposure |
| Psittacosis, ornithosis (Bedsonia infections) | Virus | Birds, related virus found in cattle, cats and sheep | Worldwide | Contact and occupational exposure |
| Rabies | Virus | Dogs and biting vertebrate animals | Worldwide except Australia, New Zealand, Great Britain, Scandinavia and Japan; a number of smaller islands are also free | Bites of diseased animals |
| Yaba | Virus | Monkeys | Unknown | Contact |
| Cat-scratch fever | Unknown (virus suspected) | Cats and dogs | Worldwide | Wounds and scratches |

*Note:* Many proved zoonoses, particularly helminth infections of relatively rare occurrence have been omitted, as well as those diseases caused by fish and reptile toxins.
*Prepared by Veterinary Public Health Section, National Communicable Disease Center, U.S. Public Health Service, Atlanta, Georgia.*
Revised June 1968 by James H. Steele, D.V.M.

or antitoxin (human), whichever is indicated. The recommendations of the World Health Organization Expert Committee on Rabies, as modified and outlined in Table 144, should be the standard guide for rabies prevention and treatment. However, prudence and good judgment may alter these suggestions after considering whether rabies is present in the community, or if the animal has been adequately immunized and is available for observation, or whether the patient has previously been immunized against rabies.

Microscopic detection of characteristic lesions and isolation of the virus by animal passage are reliable in postmortem diagnosis. Lesions include cerebral congestion, perivascular cuffing, inflammatory exudates primarily in the gray substance of the brainstem and Negri bodies. With Seller's methylene blue/basic fuchsin stain, a Negri body by definition has inner basophilic granules, heterogenous matrix, magenta tinge and less refractility than other viral inclusions. When Negri bodies are not found, histology is that of any viral encephalitis, with important predisposition to infect gray matter. Predilection for gray matter is the most important point in differentiating rabies encephalitis from allergic encephalomyelitis secondary to rabies vaccine.

PREEXPOSURE RABIES PROPHYLAXIS. The relatively low frequency of severe reactions to DEV has made it practical to offer preexposure immunization to persons in high-risk groups: veterinarians, animal handlers, certain laboratory workers and persons—especially children—living in places where rabies is a constant threat. Others whose vocational or avocational pursuits bring them into contact with potentially rabid dogs, cats, foxes, skunks or bats should also be considered for preexposure prophylaxis.

Two 1 ml injections of DEV given subcutaneously in the deltoid area one month apart are followed by a dose six to seven months after the second dose. This series of three injections can be expected to produce neutralizing antibody in 80 to 90 per cent of persons so vaccinated.

For more rapid immunization, three injections of DEV, 1 ml each, should be given at weekly intervals and a fourth dose three months later. This schedule elicits an antibody response in about 80 per cent of those immunized.

All who receive the preexposure vaccination should *have serum collected for rabies antibody testing three to four weeks after the last injection.* Testing for rabies antibody can be arranged by state health department laboratories. If no antibody is detected, booster doses should be given until a response is demonstrated. Persons with continuing exposure should receive boosters every two years.

When an immunized person with previously demonstrated rabies antibody is bitten by a rabid animal, he or she should receive five daily doses of vaccine plus a booster dose twenty days after the fifth dose. Passive immunization should not be given in this case; it might inhibit a rapid anamnestic response. For nonbite exposures, an immunized person with antibody needs only one 1 ml dose of vaccine.

When the immune status of a previously vaccinated person is not known, postexposure antirabies treatment may be necessary. In such cases, if antibody can be demonstrated in a serum sample collected before vaccine is given, treatment can be adjusted accordingly.

*Pasteurella multocida* is a common cause of infection following bites or scratches caused by dogs and cats. It is rarely reported and apparently often overlooked as a pathogen. It causes the typical clinical manifestations of a rapidly developing cellulitis at the site of injury. The infection is potentially dangerous and can cause a chronic local infection of deep tissues and septicemia. However, it responds well to several antimicrobials, with penicillin being the drug of choice (*see* Cat-scratch disease).

# VETERINARY TOXICOLOGY

Approximately 5 per cent of the calls received each year at the Duke Poison Control Center concern the poisoning of animals of all kinds, domesticated and nondomesticated. Information regarding symptoms and treatment are often urgently requested by both laymen and veterinarians. The following discussion and Table 146 may be helpful when such an emergency arises. However, though sources, symptoms and even treatment of poisoning are often not unlike those in humans, the diagnosis and handling of an ill animal is always best left in the competent hands of the veterinarian, and information from the center, when available, should be given only on a consultative basis.

On the other side of the coin, the veterinarian has a responsibility of his own in preventing human poisoning by not dispensing drugs for ill animals in plain envelopes or containers without some identification and explanation of the drugs' potential toxicity, so that these compounds may be kept out of sight and reach of small children. We have experienced a severe and almost fatal digitalis poisoning in a two-year-old child who took all the digitalis tablets from a small envelope which the veterinarian had given the parents for an ailing dog, without discussing with the parents the nature or toxicity of the compound. Because the parents were unaware of the facts, the drug was left in an area easily accessible to this small child. The wide range of pet care products now available makes it vital for physicians and veterinarians to warn parents not to confuse animal medications with human medications and to take the same precautions with them as they would with their own drugs.

The great majority of poisonings in animals results from their taking the toxic material in food or water. Aflatoxin in peanut meal, for example, is a toxic and carcinogenic metabolite of the *Aspergillus flavus* mold, which has been implicated in deaths of rats, trout and turkey and duck poults. Human toxicity, however, has not been demonstrated. Yet circumstantial evidence is impressive. Human liver cancer appears to be concentrated in areas of the world where climate and food storage methods favor the mold *Aspergillus flavus.* One such area is in Africa, where the liver cancer rate of Bantu men in Mozambique is 500 times that of United States males, black and white. Occasionally intoxication may result from absorption, through a wound or even the unbroken skin (sheep dipping, etc.). Malicious poisoning is most frequently carried out against dogs and cats, although horses and ruminants are also sometimes involved. The use of various chemicals to control rabbits, foxes, rats, mice, etc. is of course common practice, and domesticated animals can be poisoned easily by this bait or by eating the sick or dead vermin that result from its ingestion.

Similarities and differences in toxicologic diagnoses are apparent when various regions are compared. Rodenticide poisoning, particularly strychnine and warfarin, is frequently diagnosed throughout the United States. The frequency of use and ease of acquisition make these two poisons hazardous from both home and industrial exposure. In the Midwest, strychnine is often implicated in malicious poisoning.

Pesticides are a great problem in the agriculturally oriented Midwest and Southwest. Agricultural use of chlorinated hydrocarbon insecticides is a significant factor in the Midwest. Arsenical dips, insect sprays and crabgrass killers are common sources of arsenic across the nation. The greatest number of pesticide accidents, however, are due to organophosphates, often when used for oral or dermal ectoparasite control. In the southwestern and western United States, a large amount of metaldehyde is used as snail or slug bait, and this compound is a commonly reported poison in those regions. Lead poisoning is most often recognized in the northeastern and midwestern states, particularly in large cities with older housing. Snake and toad poisoning is greatest in the Southwest and Southeast.

TABLE 146
COMMON ANIMAL POISONS

| *Poison* | *Source* | *Symptoms and Treatment* |
|---|---|---|
| Arsenic | Dips, dusts, or sprays | *See* section on Arsenic poisoning |
| Lead | Lead arsenate sprays, lead paint, discarded storage batteries, contaminated vegetation in vicinity of lead smelters or residue from evaporation of leaded gasoline | *See* section on Lead poisoning |
| Strychnine | Poisoned bait or ingestion of poisoned animals | *See* section on Strychnine poisoning |
| Fluoride | Drinking water, phosphatic limestones; contamination of forage from gases and dusts from chemical factories | *See* section on Fluoride |
| Cyanides | Fumigants, soil sterilants, fertilizers, rodenticides | *See* section on Cyanides |
| Mercury | Mercurial antiseptics and fungicides | *See* section on Mercury |
| Molybdenum | Molybdenum control of forage below 5 ppm | Poor performance, diarrhea, weight loss and anemia; the use of 1% of copper sulfate in salt on forage usually provides satisfactory control |
| Selenium<br>Alkali type<br>Blind staggers type | Highly seleniferous (accumulator) plants | Alkali or chronic: emaciation, loss of hair and cracking of the hoofs<br>Blind staggers: wandering, staggering, paralysis and death from respiratory failure<br>Treatment: selenium free or low forages and grain; symptomatic |
| Salt | Consuming excessive quantities and unavailability of fresh drinking water | |
| Nitrate and nitrite | Nitrate fertilizers, forages, food, well water of high content, antirust tablets | *See* section on Nitrites |
| Pitch (clay pigeon or coal tar poisoning) | Ingestion of expended clay pigeons | Weakness, ataxia, icterus with enlarged liver and death from hepatic failure<br>Treatment: symptomatic |
| Trichloroethylene | Ingestion of soy bean, oil meal defatted with trichloroethylene | Hemorrhage, aplastic anemia; *see* section on Trichloroethylene |
| Chlorinated naphthalene | Ingestion of or exposure to contaminated food or the chemical additive | *See* section on Naphthalene |
| Herbicides | *See* section on Herbicides | |
| Rodenticides | *See* section on Rodenticides | |
| Insecticides<br>Chlorinated hydrocarbons<br>Organic phosphates<br>Botanical | *See* section on Chlorinated hydrocarbons<br>*See* section on Phosphates<br>*See* section on Botanical insecticides | |

TABLE 146-*Continued*
COMMON ANIMAL POISONS

| *Poison* | *Source* | *Symptoms and Treatment* |
|---|---|---|
| Sulfur (lime, sulfur) | Contaminated food | Rarely toxic. Lethal dose 5 gm/kg; may produce irritation and blistering of skin<br>Treatment: symptomatic |
| Fescue | Ingestion of tall fescue grass | Resembles ergot poisoning in that it produces lameness in hind feet which may progress to necrosis of the parts; *see* Ergot |
| Bracken fern (Pteridium aquilinum, Pteris aquilina) | Ingestion of the plant (leaves and rhizomes) containing thiaminase, an enzyme which inactivates thiamine | Symptoms are delayed 1–3 months and are those associated with thiamine deficiency<br>Treatment: large doses of parenteral thiamine |
| Sweet clover | Ingestion of large quantities of spoiled sweet clover, hay or silage | Hemorrhages with hypoprothrombinemia<br>Treatment: parenteral synthetic vitamin K and blood transfusions |
| Plant poisoning | *See* Table 139 | |
| Fungal toxicoses | | |
| Stachybotrys | Stachybotrysatra | Hemorrhages |
| Aspergillus | *Aspergillus* (varied strains) | Hemorrhages |
| Moldy corn | *Aspergillus flavus*<br>*Penicillium rubrum* | Hemorrhages |
| Paspalum staggers | *Claviceps paspali* | Fasciculation of muscles |
| Ergotism | *Claviceps purpurea* | *See* section on Ergot |
| Snakebite | *See* section on Snakebites | |

Garbage intoxication or food poisoning is reported frequently from all sections and states. The incidence of access to spoiled food closely parallels the freedom which pets are allowed in a given community. This is true of many rodenticide poisonings also, since a source of both rodenticides and garbage is commercial establishments such as grain elevators, lumber yards, junkyards, packing houses and restaurants.

Problems related to toxic plants such as mushrooms are greatest in the spring. Occasionally ingestion of philodendron causes poisoning, especially in cats (*see* Table 146 for Seleniferous Plants).

The effects of the first frost on certain plants can result in prussic acid poisoning in grazing cattle, creating a personal problem for cattlemen.

The cattle get the prussic (hydrocyanic) acid from a number of plants. However, under practical conditions, only a few plants are actually dangerous. Those that commonly cause the poisoning are black cherry, Johnsongrass, arrow grass, Queen's root, sorghum, Sudan grass and Sudan-sorghum hybrids. Free hydrocyanic acid as such is not found in any appreciable quantities in healthy growing plants. The acid develops only when the normal growth of plants has been retarded or stopped. The factors that can affect the quantity of hydrocyanic acid in plants are drought, bruising, trampling, wilting, mowing and frost. The best way to prevent this type of animal poisoning is to stop grazing during periods when poison is suspected. Prevent cattle access to sorghum and Sudan grass plants after the first killing frost. If one animal shows symptoms of poisoning, all animals should be removed immediately from the pasture.

Hydrocyanic acid acts rapidly, frequently killing the animal within a few minutes. However, the animal may live for several hours after the symptoms develop. First there is a period of stimulation, followed by depression and paralysis. Signs of colic often appear. Stupor, difficult breathing and convulsions result from the action of the poison on the central nervous system (*see* Cyanide for treatment).

## Chapter 10

# MISCELLANEOUS COMPOUNDS

There is a vast miscellaneous and heterogenous group of compounds, substances and agents that are capable of producing toxic symptoms. The following chapter is devoted to the more important ones, and some of the disorders they produce, that fall under this classification.

## ACRODYNIA (MERCURY, COPPER)

Acrodynia is a complex, multisystem disorder of infancy and early childhood with varied symptoms which mimic many other pediatric diseases. Unfortunately, many pediatricians feel that acrodynia is extinct and rarely think of this possibility when suddenly faced with some of its bizarre manifestations. The recent report of a five-year-old boy with severe acrodynia from the use of a paint containing mercury and the fact that many instances remain undiagnosed indicate that acrodynia is not extinct. Chronic copper poisoning has also produced clinical acrodynia. Warkany, Hubbard and others have assembled convincing data that most, if not all, cases of acrodynia are the result of an unusual sensitivity or idiosyncrasy to mercury. The source of mercury in this age-group occurs usually from the use of calomel (mercurous chloride) as a teething powder or lotion, mercurial ointments, mercurial diaper rinses, or from the inhalation of mercury present in some paints. Phenyl mercuric propionate is incorporated into many of the outdoor water-based paints as an antimildew additive (to prevent mold growth). It is a source of potential danger of mercury intoxication either from ingestion or inhalation of its toxic vapors.

To inactivate the mercury already absorbed, therapy with BAL, which has a greater affinity for the mercuric ion than do the sulfhydryl groups, has been until recently the *treatment* of choice. One of the penicillamine derivatives (Cuprimine), a new group of chelating agents, is now available for the treatment of mercury and other heavy metal poisoning. The clinical and experimental results compare favorably with BAL, and the use of an oral antidote sounds intriguing. However, since vomiting occurs early and frequently in acrodynia, this preparation may find little use in children. The side-effects to BAL are well known. Those reported from the penicillamine derivatives are fever, nausea and vomiting, myalgia, stupor, leukopenia, thrombocytopenia and nephrosis and optic axial neuritis which are both reversible *(see* Mercury and Copper).

## AEROSOLS

Aerosol is a trademark name for a series of commercial surfactants. These are a group of anionic surface-active agents, with dioctyl sodium sulfosuccinate being the most prominent one. In concentrations of 1%, they are irritating to the eyes but not to the skin. Zinc, copper and lead are some of the substances contained in aerosol spray paints in one degree or another and are among the most toxic poisons whether inhaled or eaten. Furthermore, these heavy metals have a cumulative effect and are only minimally excreted from the body tissues once there. But there are a number of other dangerous substances in addition to the propellants (Freon™, etc.) contained in spray paints and other aerosols, such as toluene, acetone, propane, trichloroethane, isobutane, xylene and benzene, as well as aliphatic, aromatic and halogenated hydrocarbons. When inhaled or ingested in sufficient quantities, these can cause many serious physiological side-effects, some irreversible and fatal (*see* Aerosol Sprays and Freon).

## ALPHAZURINE 2 G

This compound is a triphenylmethane dye which stains only viable tissues, thus enabling immediate differentiation of second– and third-degree burns. An immediate fatal anaphylactic reaction has been reported in one patient, so it should be used with caution until its toxicity and antigenicity are established.

## AQUA FORTIS

A weak nitric acid solution once employed as a cauterizing agent for the immediate sterilization of dangerously infected wounds and animal bites (*see* Acids), it is now obsolete.

## AQUARIUM PRODUCTS*

With the growing popularity of tropical fish in home aquariums and the resultant increase in products used to maintain them has come an increase in the number of calls requesting information concerning accidental ingestion of these products. The following material is an overview and not all-inclusive.

Aquarium products may be divided into four major categories:

1. Antimicrobials
   a. Algaecides
   b. Fungicides
   c. Antibacterials
   d. Antiparasitics
2. Antichlorine compounds
3. pH indicators and adjustors
4. Miscellaneous

Although some of the individual ingredients used in these products are potentially toxic to humans, they are also toxic to marine animals. With few exceptions, the concentration of these ingredients is low, and therefore, overall product toxicity is low.

Antimicrobials include tetracycline, penicillin, streptomycin, malachite green, mafenide, 9-aminoacridine, methylene blue (tetramethylthionine), sulfathiazole, acriflavine, merbromin, paratoluene sulfonchloramide, benzethonium chloride, monuron, atrazine and simazine. (This list is probably not all-inclusive). Antimicrobials are used to treat conditions such as ich, shimmy, fungus, tail and fin rot, algae, velvet and gill diseases. Most of these products are supplied in dropper bottles for home use. Generally the active ingredient is in trace amounts and the container is small. Notable exceptions are penicillin tablets and tetracycline capsules which contain a therapeutic dosage for humans. However, neither penicillin nor tetracycline exhibit true acute toxicity and would not be expected to present

---

*This material is courtesy of the National Clearinghouse for Poison Control Centers.

medical problems unless an idiosyncratic hypersensitivity reaction occurs. With tetracycline, the age of the product is important as a Fanconi-type syndrome is possible. A few algaecides are available in tablet form and might possibly cause symptoms if a large amount were ingested. Treatment for ingestion of antimicrobials consists of giving milk and observing for the possible hypersensitivity reaction.

Antichlorine compounds usually contain sodium thiosulfate, but some contain potassium permanganate or silver salts, such as silver oxide (also used as an antimicrobial). The ingredients are usually in small dropper bottles and in low concentrations, making the product of low toxicity.

Bromothymol blue is the most commonly used pH indicator. Once again, due to low concentration and small container size, the products in this category are considered to be of low toxicity. Some pH test kits contain sodium hydroxide, which is potentially hazardous due to its causticity.

The miscellaneous category includes vitamins, tonics, aquarium salts, quinine and copper sulfate. Vitamins and tonics are of low toxicity in the quantities available. Aquarium salts are potentially hazardous due to the major ingredient, sodium chloride. Quinine in small amounts has caused extreme allergic-type reactions. Copper sulfate is very toxic, if retained. Both quinine and copper sulfate are available as capsules.

When a call is received concerning the ingestion of an aquarium product, the caller should be directed to read the product's label to determine if ingredients are listed. Should the product contain any potentially toxic ingredients, the appropriate treatment should be given. If the product is of low toxicity, milk should be given to deter the gastrointestinal irritation that may occur.

As a rule of thumb, liquid products are of low potential hazard due to small container size and/or low concentration of ingredients (sodium hydroxide is an exception). Liquids are available in both dropper and nondropper containers. The dropper bottles are usually more concentrated (dispensed by the drop) and have less volume than the nondropper type (dispensed by teaspoonful or tablespoonful).

## AROMATICS

This term is used to refer to substances with a fragrant, spicy or pungent odor. They are usually complex mixtures of plant origin, the so-called volatile oils. Since they are present in commercial products only in small quantities, they rarely produce toxic signs or symptoms other than those due to sensitization. This group should not be confused with the aromatic hydrocarbons or the aromatic solvents, which are all potentially dangerous compounds.

## BALSAM OF PERU (PERUVIAN, INDIAN BALSAM)

This is an oleoresin consisting chiefly of esters of cinnamic and benzoic acids. In humans, cinnamic acids are excreted in the urine as benzoic and hippuric acids. This is an innocuous, mildly antiseptic compound which has been ingested without ill effects. However, prolonged use on the skin has produced dermatitis.

## BATTERIES

Batteries are of two types: the dry cell conventional (flashlight) and the mercury cell battery (hearing aids, penlights, small transistor radios).

Battery Contents

| | |
|---|---|
| *Dry Cell* | |
| Carbon | 3.00 gm |
| Manganese dioxide | 26.00 gm |
| Ammonium chloride | 13.00 gm |
| Zinc chloride | 5.00 gm |
| Mercuric chloride | 0.02 gm |
| Cornstarch | 0.75 gm |
| Zinc (container) | 20.00 gm |
| Water | |
| *Mercury Cell* | |
| Mercuric oxide | 5.0 gm |
| Mercury (metallic) | 0.5 gm |
| Zinc | 2.0 gm |
| Potassium hydroxide | 1.5 gm |
| Zinc oxide | 0.5 gm |

Since the dry cell battery contains only 0.02 gm of mercuric chloride (1/5 of a toxic dose), it would be unusual for any degree of toxicity to result from the swallowing (very unlikely) or ingestion of a single whole battery. On the other hand, if the nickel case of the mercury cell battery should be ruptured or dissolved on ingestion, the 5 gm of mercuric oxide could very easily produce serious toxic symptoms, since this amount is potentially dangerous.

Mercury dry cell batteries can explode forcefully, especially after they are spent, and these precautions should be taken.

1. Never throw a spent battery in a fire or waste container the contents of which might be burned.
2. When a battery becomes too weak to do an adequate job, remove it from the equipment and discard it immediately.
3. Store batteries in a well-ventilated place and discard any which are older than the "place in use before" date stamped on them.
4. After removing batteries from equipment, place tape across the end terminal to prevent accidental short circuit, or replace the battery in its original cardboard container.
5. To discard, submerge the battery in water and pierce the steel jacket of each cell to prevent accumulation pressure.
6. Deposit the harmless battery in a garbage container where it can be carried away. Don't burn it at home because it contains mercury which could spread toxic vapors.

## BENZENE (BENZOL)

A coal tar distillate, benzene is a mixture of short-chain aliphatic hydrocarbons that was often used in hospitals for removing adhesive tape and for miscellaneous cleansing jobs; this should not be confused with "benzine" or "benzin," a petroleum ether discussed under petroleum distillates.

## BENZOIC ACID U.S.P.

This compound has been widely used as a food preservative. It is relatively nontoxic and almost tasteless and therefore is ideal for this purpose. In an acid medium, concentrations of 0.1% prevent bacterial growth. Benzoate salts are formed with an alkaline pH and therefore are far less effective for bacteriostasis. A daily intake of 4 to 6 gm produces no toxic symptoms aside from a slight gastric irritation. Larger doses have systemic effects not unlike those of the salicylates. After ingestion, the benzoic acid is combined with glycine and excreted in the urine as hippuric acid.

## BLUE VELVET

This is a mixture of concentrated paregoric and blue-colored tripelennamine (Pyribenzamine®) tablets that has been gaining popularity for its euphoric effects among addicts, since these preparations are inexpensive and readily available. Unfortunately the intravenous use of this concoction has been responsible for fatalities. Severe pulmonary hypertension occurs due to arteritis and thrombosis of small pulmonary arteries, arterioles and capillaries from the mechanical trauma to the vascular endothelium by sharp, irregular crystals of talc in the Pyribenzamine tablets. Physicians should be alerted to the manifestations of "Blue Velvet" effects and its likely disastrous results.

## BORAX (SODIUM TETRABORATE)

Solutions of borax are alkaline, but the toxicity is essentially the same as that of boric acid. This compound is used as an antiseptic and cleaning agent.

## BORDEAUX MIXTURE

A foliage fungicide consisting usually of equal parts of copper sulfate and unslaked lime, freshly prepared, this compound is less astringent and less toxic than copper sulfate *per se.*

## BOROGLYCERIN

Boroglycerin consists of two parts of boric acid and three parts of glycerin. (Boroglycerin glycerite NF is approximately 50% boroglycerin.)

## BROWN MIXTURE

A compound mixture of opium and glycyrrhiza NF, this is an antiquated cough and sedative preparation that contains 0.6 ml paregoric, 1.2 mg tartar emetic and 0.15 ml ethyl nitrite spirit per teaspoonful dose. Symptoms of toxicity due to overdosage produce systemic antimony poisoning or severe vomiting from the tartar emetic.

## BUROW'S SOLUTION

Aluminum acetate solution U.S.P. is an aqueous solution of aluminum acetate (5% to 6%) that is used as a wet dressing because of its astringent and antiseptic properties for pyodermias and eczema. If ingested in appreciable amounts, the astringent action may produce considerable irritation to the mucous membranes of the mouth and oropharynx.

## CALAMINE U.S.P.

Calamine is a pink powder of zinc oxide, not less than 98%, and 0.5% ferric oxide. A common official preparation is calamine lotion U.S.P. Ingestion of large quantities of this compound has caused gastritis with vomiting. In the *treatment,* gastric lavage would not be necessary if vomiting has occurred. Milk or other demulcents may be soothing and allay pain.

## CATARIA (CATNEP, CATNIP, CATMINT)

Cataria is a perennial herb of the dried flowering tops of *Nepeta cataria,* which is common near dwellings in the United States but is indigenous to Europe. It has been cultivated on a large scale in New Hampshire. It is called catnep on account of the fondness which cats show for it, either in the fresh or dried state. It is employed as a "tea" in domestic practice, as an emmenagogue, carminative and antispasmodic. In the southern United States, certain segments of the population use it as a popular home remedy for infant colic.

This plant contains tannin and volatile oils of alpha– and beta-citral, limonene, dipentene, geraniol, citronellal, nerol, a levorotatory sesquiterpene, acetic acid, butyric acid and valeric acid.

A dose of 5 to 15 ml of the infusion (1 oz. of the dried leaves to 1 pt. of warm water) or 5 ml of the NF fluid extract is usually used.

Reports of toxic manifestations from this preparation are difficult to find in the literature. However, the author knows of a two-week-old infant who had severe convulsions following an overdose, which could not be explained on any other basis. Cataria has been reported recently to have been used for psychedelic effects by smoking its leaves or by spraying its extract on tobacco.

## CELLOSOLVES (METHYL, ETHYL, BUTYL, DIETHYL)

These are monoalkyl ethers of ethylene glycol. Butyl cellosolve is the most toxic of the group, the oral $LD_{50}$ being 1.5 ml/kg in rats. They are readily absorbed through the skin and therefore can produce poisoning by absorption as well as by inhalation. Signs and symptoms of toxicity are irritation of mucous membranes, central nervous system depression, dyspnea, anemia, renal damage, hemoglobinuria and hematuria. Hemolysis of red blood cells has also been reported.

*Treatment* consists of removing the individual from the exposure and washing the skin thoroughly with soap and water for cutaneous exposure. In anuric patients, fluids and electrolytes must be restricted to cover daily requirements and those being lost. Support respiration and give other symptomatic treatment as necessary.

## CHALK

A calcium carbonate compound occurring naturally as limestone, coral, marble, etc., chalk is used as an antacid and antidote for acids, particularly oxalic acid.

## CHEMISTRY SETS*

Elmer was a chemist.
But Elmer is no more,
For what Elmer thought
Was $H_2O$, was $H_2SO_4$.

Chemistry sets have been designed so that the young hobbyist can perform experiments based on chemical reactions. Proper procedures are presumed to be written into the instruction books accompanying these sets, and common sense dictates that the sets should be given only to those children who can read the directions and will follow them. An obvious hazard exists, however, in the possible ingestion of the chemicals by younger, less discriminating siblings.

*This material is courtesy of the National Clearinghouse for Poison Control Centers.

TABLE 147
CHEMISTRY SETS
A. VERY LOW TOXICITY

| | | | |
|---|---|---|---|
| 1. Bean seed | | 9. Nichrome wire | |
| 2. Calcium carbonate | Chalk; not harmful | 10. Nickel steel wire | |
| 3. Cochineal | Dried, ground insects | 11. Phenolphthalein solution | Catharsis; children have tolerated single oral doses as large as 8 gm without distress |
| 4. Copper wire | | 12. Powdered chloride | |
| 5. Diatomaceous earth | Not harmful unless inhaled | 13. Starch | |
| 6. Gum arabic | Little danger of distress except allergic reaction, diarrhea, flatulence, or rarely, fecal impaction | 14. Strontium chloride | Strontium less toxic than calcium |
| 7. Iron metal (powdered) | Iron dust can cause conjunctivitis, choroiditis, and retinitis | 15. Zinc metal | Nontoxic; fumes produced by heating may be toxic and produce "metal fume fever" |
| 8. Log wood | Wood containing hematoxylin dye; mild astringent devoid of irritating properties | | |

CHEMISTRY SETS
B. LOW TOXICITY

| | | | |
|---|---|---|---|
| 1. Acetic acid | Dependent on concentration | 9. Sodium bicarbonate | Large doses may cause alkalosis |
| 2. Ammonium chloride | Diuresis, possible acidosis | 10. Sodium bisulfite | Moderate toxicity; may cause irritation of stomach by liberating sulfurous acid |
| 3. Calcium chloride | Acute oral LD in rats 4 gm/kg; possible gastrointestinal irritation | 11. Sodium chloride | Ingestion of large amounts of sodium chloride can cause irritation of the stomach and vomiting |
| 4. Calcium monophosphate | Toxicity expected to be that of calcium, hence, low | 12. Sodium ferrocyanide, ferricyanide (salts—sodium, potassium) | Probable acute, human lethal dose orally, 0.5–5.0 gm/kg; comparatively benign; these salts are not decomposed to cyanide; they are rapidly excreted in the urine without metabolic alterations |
| 5. Chrome alum (chromium potassium sulfate | Probable acute, human lethal dose orally, 0.5–5.0 gm/kg; 1.5 gm has been lethal to a 14-year-old boy * | 13. Sodium iodide | Acute toxicity low; oral MLD of iodide about 50 gm for a 150-lb. man |
| 6. Gypsum (calcium sulfate, hydrous) | Probable acute, human lethal dose orally, 0.5–5.0 gm/kg; may cause obstruction | 14. Sodium thiosulfate | Probable acute, human lethal dose orally, 0.5–5.0 gm/kg; osmotic cathartic |
| 7. Magnesium sulfate | Probable acute, human lethal dose orally, 0.5–5.0 gm/kg; slowly absorbed; may cause purging | 15. Three minerals | |
| 8. Manganese sulfate | Probable acute, human lethal dose orally, 0.5–5.0 gm/kg; poorly absorbed; no acute systemic toxicity | | |

* Severe gastroenteritis, toxic hepatitis, bleeding diathesis, and renal failure followed by death was observed. Early use of BAL and dialysis is recommended.

TABLE 147-*Continued*
CHEMISTRY SETS
C. POTENTIALLY TOXIC

|  |  |
|---|---|
| 1. Aluminum sulfate | Toxicity probably similar to aluminum ammonium sulfate, 30 gm of which was the lethal dose in two adult ingestions, probably due to corrosive action; evidence of nephritis from concentrated solutions |
| 2. Ammonium hydroxide | Vapor irritating to skin, eyes, and mucous membranes; corrosive to gastrointestinal tract, depending on concentration |
| 3. Azurite (basic copper sulfate) | Acute, oral $LD_{50}$ in rat about 159 mg/kg |
| 4. Benedict's solution (alkaline copper sulfate) | Copper sulfate: oral MLD about 15 gm for a 150-lb. man |
| 5. Borates, etc. | Estimated acute, human lethal dose orally is 0.5–5.0 gm/kg for borax and borate salts and 50–500 mg/kg for boric acid |
| 6. Calcium hypochlorite | Corrosive: MLD is approximately 15 ml for a child |
| 7. Calcium nitrate | Estimated acute lethal dose of nitrate in the human is 0.5–5.0 gm/kg orally; nitrate salts, as such, are no more toxic than neutral salts, but may be reduced to nitrites (lethal dose 50–500 mg/kg) in the bowel |
| 8. Calcium oxide | Produces thermal and caustic burns: estimated fatal dose is 36 gm |
| 9. Cobalt chloride | Estimated acute, human, lethal dose orally is 50–500 mg/kg; gastrointestinal irritation, pain, vomiting, vasodilation of face, hypotension, rash, tinnitis, nerve deafness |
| 10. Diglycolstearate | Estimated human lethal dose is 2 gm/kg; central nervous system depression, liver and kidney damage, gastrointestinal irritation |
| 11. Ferric ammonium sulfate | Toxicity due to iron salts, 2 to 5 gm of which have been fatal to a 2-year-old child |
| 12. Ferrous ammonium sulfate | See Ferric ammonium sulfate |
| 13. Nickel ammonium sulfate | Lethal dose is probably 50–500 mg/kg; nickel salts have a stringent, irritant action and are emetic; systemic poisoning rare |
| 14. Ninhydrin | Irritating to skin and mucous membranes |
| 15. Potassium chloride | Acute potassium intoxication from oral administration is highly improbable because of pylorospasm and vomiting from the large doses required, but cardiac arrhythmia may occur; lethal dose is 0.5–5.0 gm/kg |
| 16. Sodium bisulfate | Aqueous solutions are strongly acidic and corrosive to body tissue; estimated fatal human dose, 30 gm; superficial destruction of skin and mucous membranes |
| 17. Sodium carbonate | Estimated fatal human dose is 30 gm; strong irritant, causing erythema, blistering; corrosion of gastrointestinal tract; local necrosis of skin and eyes |
| 18. Sodium salicylate | Toxic dose, 100–259 mg/kg |
| 19. Sodium silicate solution | Alkaline, producing irritation of mucous membranes and skin |
| 20. Strontium nitrate | Nitrate lethal dose is 0.5–5.0 gm/kg; nitrite salts as such are no more toxic than neutral salts but may be reduced to nitrites (lethal dose 50–500 mg/kg) |
| 21. Sulfur | Lethal dose is 0.5–5.0 gm/kg; may cause hydrogen sulfide |

TABLE 147-*Continued*
CHEMISTRY SETS
C. POTENTIALLY TOXIC

| | | | |
|---|---|---|---|
| | production due to bacterial action in the colon | 24. Trisodium phosphate | Aqueous solutions are alkaline and may produce caustic burns |
| 22. Tannic acid | Estimated acute lethal dose orally in humans is 0.5–5.0 gm/kg; astringent of moderately low toxicity, but large doses may produce gastritis, vomiting, pain, diarrhea, or constipation | 25. Zinc sulfate | Estimated acute lethal dose orally in humans is 50–500 mg/kg; irritation and corrosion of alimentary tract, pain, emesis |
| 23. Tartaric acid | 30 gm can cause gastrointestinal symptoms, circulatory disturbances, and possible death | | |

In Table 147 are listed fifty-five ingredients which may be found in one or more of three popular chemistry sets. The substances have been grouped into three categories: those from which no toxicity is expected, those of moderate toxicity and those which could produce more severe toxic effects when taken in the available quantities. In general, a container in a chemistry set holds about 15 gm of an ingredient, but this is not constant and cannot be counted on in any individual case of ingestion.

Some ingredients are considered essentially nontoxic. Many of the items are not easily absorbed and may be considered simply as foreign bodies. Others have very little systemic activity but might cause gastrointestinal symptoms.

Other compounds are of low toxicity, and ingestion of large amounts would be required before symptoms would appear. The acetic acid would be corrosive if in a concentrated form.

Although the chemicals in the last list are considered more toxic than those in the previous two, each ingestion must be evaluated according to the actual amount and concentration involved. With the acids, for example, the concentration is more critical than the volume, and the local effect is usually more grave than the systemic. *Treatment* of this last group of chemicals, therefore, must be individualized. In every case more comprehensive toxicity data should be sought. However, the general principles of treatment apply. Skin and eyes should be washed thoroughly after contact with an irritating, caustic or corrosive substance. Ingested acids or alkalis should be diluted with water or milk, and demulcents are recommended to protect the mucous membranes. Emesis is contraindicated following ingestion of caustics, acids, alkalis or in comatose or convulsing patients; gastric lavage should be used only when there is little danger of perforating damaged tissue. Other than these precautions, emptying the stomach should be performed only when necessary after the ingestion of these chemicals. Iron salts, salicylates, nitrites and others all have their individual toxicologic traits and should be treated specifically.

Usually arts and crafts material and home chemistry sets have such small quantities of chemicals with low concentrations that they do not pose a serious threat.

## CHLORACETOPHENONE

Chloracetophenone (U.S. Army designation CN) is a severe irritant to the entire respiratory system, in addition to the eyes, and is capable of producing a fatal acute pulmonary edema. First– and second-degree burns of the skin can occur from exposure to high concentrations. The estimated human fatal MAC for a 10 min. exposure is a concentration of 0.85 oz./1000 cu. ft. Other extensively used tear gases are chloroacetylenone, bromoacetone, ethylbromoacetate, bromomethylethylketone, bromobenzylcyanide and orthochlorobenzylidene malononitrile (U.S. Army designation CS).

*Treatment* is symptomatic and supportive for the pulmonary edema. Corticosteroids should be given a trial, if the respiratory distress is severe. Artificial respiration and oxygen may be necessary. Thoroughly irrigate the eyes and apply soothing ophthalmic ointment. The exposed skin should be completely washed and contaminated clothes removed (*see* Mace and Tear Gas).

## CHLOROTHEN (CHLOROMETHAPYRILENE)

This antihistaminic, more effective and less toxic than Pyribenzamine, produces slightly more sedation. Side-effects occur in about 25 per cent of those who use it.

## CITRONELLA OIL (LEMON GRASS OIL)

Citronella oil is a fragrant volatile oil consisting of geraniol, citronella, methyl heptenone and terpenes. It is used as a perfume and as a repellent against insects. Little is known of its toxicity, but it is presumed to be low. Lemon grass is from different species of Indian grasses.

## CLOVE OIL U.S.P.

A volatile oil with approximately 80 per cent eugenol (a phenol), clove oil is used for its antiseptic and local anesthetic properties. It is popularly used by the public for relief of toothaches. Its systemic effects are much lower than phenol, because of its insolubility in water; however, severe gastroenteritis can follow ingestion of appreciable amounts. (For *treatment, see* Phenol.)

## COCILLANA

Cocillana is an irritant produced from the bark of a Bolivian tree, *Guarea rusbyi,* and widely used as an expectorant and nauseant. Symptoms of intoxication are severe vomiting, diarrhea, collapse, headache and rhinorrhea. *Treatment* requires gastric lavage or emesis and symptomatic and supportive therapy as needed.

## COLLODION U.S.P.

A solvent compound of 70 per cent ether, 24 per cent absolute ethyl alcohol and 4 per cent pyroxylin (dinitrocellulose). (For symptoms of poisoning and *treatment, see* Ether and Ethyl Alcohol.)

## CRAYONS (ART MATERIAL)

Children's crayons are usually made from mixtures of stearic acid and paraffin, colored with harmless pigments. The only harmful colors are those containing para reds, which are used by some manufacturers in the red and orange crayons. Cyanosis and methemoglobinemia caused by the formation of paranitroaniline have been reported in a few instances from the ingestion of these particular colored crayons. Industrial crayons such as lumber or textile marking crayons, on the other hand, are loaded with permanent pigments containing lead chromate, which could be toxic if any appreciable amount were ingested.

Crayons, chalk, clay, paste and water colors which bear seals with the letters AP or CP, or are marked CS 130-46, are nontoxic. Products so identified do not contain more than 0.05 per cent of lead, arsenic or other toxic materials, in accordance with Bureau of Standards recommendations.

There are, however, some nontoxic crayons, chalk, clay, paste and water colors which do not bear these seals or markings. These also meet the specifications of the Bureau of Standards.

Therefore, when art materials identified with AP or CP seals or marked CS 130-46 are ingested, there is no need for alarm or therapy; these substances are nontoxic. However, if the package of the ingested material does not bear the seals, the marking or a toxicity statement, composition of the product should be determined. The unmarked product may or may not be toxic.

## CREOSOTE (CREOSOTE OIL)

Creosote is a mixture of phenols, creosols, guaiacol, etc. obtained from coal or wood tar. The bactericidal potency of creosote varies, but in general it is about two or three times that of phenol. Creosote NF and creosote carbonate are used infrequently as antiseptics but are employed mainly as expectorants. Creosote is also used for preserving wood. Its inhalation in strong concentrations has been reported to produce severe reversible neurological disturbances, although its MAC threshold has not been established (*see* Phenol).

## DICHLOROISOCYANURATES, SODIUM OR POTASSIUM

These are chlorine-releasing agents used for bleaching. Toxicity studies in rats show the oral $LD_{50}$ to be 1.67 gm for sodium and 1.2 gm/kg for the potassium salt, with corrosive action on the gastrointestinal mucosa rather than systemic effects.

Symptoms of intoxication are weakness, lethargy, tremors, salivation, lacrimation, dyspnea and coma. The pathological findings consist of gastrointestinal irritation and inflammation, tissue edema and liver and kidney congestion.

*Treatment* should include cautious gastric lavage if ingested, followed by milk or other demulcents. Avoid carbonates and bicarbonates because of gas formation. For skin or eye contact, copious washing with water is necessary, otherwise the treatment is symptomatic and supportive.

## DIMETHYL SULFOXIDE (DMSO)

Dimethyl sulfoxide, synthesized in 1867, is a clear, colorless, hygroscopic liquid (acetone related) with a distinctive garlic– or oyster-like odor. It acts as a powerful solvent, dissolving most aromatic and unsaturated hydrocarbons, organic nitrogen compounds and many other substances. Today it is available in crude form as a by-product of the paper pulp industry and has found extensive use as an industrial solvent. Its value in protecting biologic specimens against freezing damage is well recognized.

Sensational publicity in the lay press as to its miraculous pain-relieving and anti-inflammatory properties when rubbed on the skin has led those afflicted with musculoskeletal disorders to expect imminently a nontoxic, wonder drug which will take away their pain and improve their activity by a simple topical application. This compound so far has been found to be relatively nontoxic to animals and humans. The following summary should be kept in mind.

1. The physiological and pathological effects of dimethyl sulfoxide (DMSO) on the skin and health of adult men have been extensively studied.
2. Concentrated solutions of dimethyl sulfoxide, 70% and above, markedly increase the penetration of various dyes, steroids and antiperspirants. The enhancement of penetration is not dependent on irreversible damage to the horny layer. Skin anesthesia was not achieved by 2% solutions of procaine hydrochloride and lidocaine hydrochloride in 90% dimethyl sulfoxide.
3. Dimethyl sulfoxide possesses potent histamine-liberating properties at the site of application. The circulating basophils are decreased after extensive topical use but remain within normal limits.
4. Dimethyl sulfoxide is mildly antifungal and antibacterial. Concentrated solutions reduce the resident microflora by 95 per cent. Dimethyl sulfoxide is a promising vehicle for antifungal agents in the treatment of ringworm infections.
5. When injected, dimethyl sulfoxide produces hemolysis of RBC and reduces the clearance of soluble substances from the skin, chiefly by reducing diffusion through the dermis. The resorption of saline wheals is promoted by 90% dimethyl sulfoxide.
6. Dimethyl sulfoxide (90%) neither hindered nor helped experimental thermal burns, contact dermatitis and ultraviolet burns.
7. Dimethyl sulfoxide (90%) was not systemically injurious when applied once daily to the trunks of healthy subjects for six months. Twice daily applications of 90% dimethyl sulfoxide caused a mild scaling dermatitis in certain subjects. The skin rapidly becomes tolerant to the irritant effects of dimethyl sulfoxide, even upon continuous exposure. Occlusive exposure causes death of the outer epidermis, followed by rapid regeneration despite continued application.
8. Because of its distinctive odor, double-blind studies have been difficult to conduct.
9. Contact with clothing may destroy the fabric.

## DIOCTYL SODIUM SULFOSUCCINATE

This is probably the most potent wetting compound now available and therefore the most popular anionic surfactant on the market. Other than gastroenteritis, no toxic symptoms have been reported in humans or animals. However, eye irritation resulting in chemical conjunctivitis can be produced when used locally in concentrations above 0.1%. This agent can increase the absorption, and therefore the possibility of toxicity, of other compounds such as danthron and oxyphenisatin, which are often used as combinations.

## DONOVAN'S SOLUTION

*Liquor arseni et hydrargyri iodidi* contains 1 per cent each of arsenious iodide and mercuric iodide. Once used for syphilitic skin lesions, lymphadenitis and chronic joint diseases, this preparation is rarely used in present day therapeutics. If ingested, toxic symptoms from both arsenic and mercury would be expected, since the solution has equal parts of each. The mercuric ion has a greater emetic effect and may produce enough vomiting to empty the stomach thoroughly and thereby reduce the danger of toxicity (*see* section on Mercury and Arsenic Poisoning).

## ELECTRIC SHOCK

Electrocution accounts for approximately 1000 deaths/year in the United States. Although morbidity figures are not available, it is estimated about 7000 to 9000 nonfatal accidents occur in the same period of time. Nonfatal injury frequently is associated with severe tissue destruction, especially extensive body burns. Current markings—painless, grayish-white tracks of skin changes—are common and may be of specific diagnostic value. Intense tetanic muscular contraction sometimes causes muscle rupture or bone fracture.

The current actually flowing through the body, rather than the voltage, determines the effects of electric shock. The critical level of current at which permanent nerve damage occurs is 300 ma/3 mm of nerve diameter for five seconds. Pathologically, the myelin sheath balloons and the axon fragments. The current seems always to choose the shortest path from contact to contact without deflection by anatomic landmarks. Alternating current is three times as dangerous as direct current of the same voltage. In hand-to-hand contact, fatalities are high due to cervical spinal injury. Hand-to-foot contacts are less often fatal. Actual effects depend upon the amount of current passing between the contacts, which varies inversely with the body resistance.

Immediate result of high-voltage injuries is coma or sudden death. Cause of death is unknown and may be secondary to ventricular fibrillation or respiratory paralysis. Patients should be *treated* for respiratory paralysis; prolonged artificial respiration has been the most satisfactory form of immediate therapy. Unconsciousness may vary from moments to days. Immediately after injury, the patient may have temporary quadriparesis or slight monoparesis. Dysesthesia, hyperesthesia and hypesthesia are usually transient. Tremors, myoclonic twitches and respiratory irregularity sometimes occur. Secondary effects are those which persist for five days after the injury and include muscular pain in the trunk and extremities, temporary paralysis, autonomic disturbances and headache.

Late effects on the central nervous system are often due to arterial disease and may develop days or weeks after injury. Pathologically, blood vessel damage is common, especially involving the basal vessels, often with rupture. Unexplained fissuring of the cortex is seen, with occasional splitting apart of cortical layers. Petechial and subarachnoid hemorrhage is frequently seen. In the spinal cord, hemorrhage in the gray matter is common. A wide separation of pia and arachnoid occurs. Myelin degeneration, glial proliferation and chromatolysis may be evident. Many patients have postinjury psychoneurotic reactions.

## EPOXY RESIN GLUES*

Cold-setting epoxy resin adhesives contain ingredients which cause serious skin, eye and respiratory irritations and allergic sensitization. Toxic hepatitis can also occur. The resin base in home kits consists of oligomers, short to intermediate chains of the monomer molecules. The epoxy oligomer, with or without a diluent, comes in one compartment and a curing agent in another. Measured

*The federal Consumer Product Safety Commission temporarily banned thirteen spray adhesive products for fear of birth defects linked to chromosome breaks. These findings, however, were not confirmed by precise investigation or data, and the ban was lifted.

portions are mixed and allowed to harden at room temperature for two to twenty-four hours.

Oral toxicity of oligomeric resins is relatively slight, but ingestion of curing agents causes symptoms of alkaline poisoning. Most commonly used hardeners for cold-setting adhesives for household use are primary and tertiary amines which possess volatile and caustic alkaline properties. Spillage may induce contact dermatitis and allergic skin reactions; vapors may cause respiratory and eye damage. Similar skin, eye and lung irritations are caused by exposure to the viscous portion containing resin and diluent. Reaction after mixture of resin and curing agent is usually exothermic, producing fumes of unreacted amines and phenols which can induce severe pruritus of the face, periorbital edema and conjunctivitis. Vapors may cause coughing and provoke asthmatic attacks. The mixture may stick in skin crevices, and transfer from hands to sensitized skin, eye and mucous membranes may result in serious irritation. After hardening, the adhesive is inert and harmless but capable of inducing allergic reactions in susceptible persons.

*Treatment.* Soap and water and organic solvents such as acetone should be used to clean skin crevices, nail beds and mucous membranes. Burow's solution and acid mantle cream neutralize residual free amines. Deep necrotizing injuries are treated like caustic burns. Eye injuries are washed with copious amounts of water. Acute respiratory inhalation is treated like ammonia exposure. In oral intoxication, alkaline material in the gastrointestinal tract must be well diluted with water or milk.

Control of exposure demands essentially good housekeeping, personal cleanliness and adequate ventilation. Disposable overlay papers should be used where bench and floor contamination is likely. Disposable paper towels should be used for cleanup. Workers should wear protective clothing and gloves. The best gloves are those which can be discarded when contaminated. Spills of resin, curing agents and diluent should be removed immediately with mild soap and water. Adequate ventilation should be supplied to the work area. In some operations, exhaust ventilation may be necessary to remove excessive concentrations of the vapors of the curing agent or diluent.

## FERBAM (FERMATE)

Ferric dimethyl dithiocarbamate is used both agriculturally and medicinally as a fungicide.

Alcohol should be avoided, as it greatly increases the toxicity of the thiocarbamates.

## FERTILIZERS AND PLANT FOODS

Fertilizers (plant foods) contain one or more of the three chemical elements (nitrogen, phosphorus, potassium) necessary for plant growth. They are often formulated from ingredients such as nitric acid, phosphoric acid, anhydrous ammonia and caustic potash. These basic ingredients react to form complex salts which do not have the same toxic properties as the basic ingredients. Nitrogen-containing components include ammonium nitrate, sodium nitrate, ammonium sulfate, ammonium phosphate, urea, cottonseed meal, linseed meal and soybean meal. Calcium cyanamide is also employed as a source of nitrogen to a limited extent in agricultural fertilizers. Phosphorus is usually present in the form of superphosphate (monobasic calcium phosphate and calcium sulfate), or sometimes as tribasic calcium phosphate (phosphate rock, animal bone meal) or potassium phosphate. Potassium may be present as the carbonate (cotton hull ashes), chloride (muriate), phosphate, sulfate or potassium-magnesium sulfate. Tankage (dried meat and

TABLE 148
TOXICITY OF EPOXY RESIN ELEMENTS

| *Elements* | *Chemicals* | *Toxicity* | *Skin Irritation* | *Comments* |
|---|---|---|---|---|
| 1. Oligomeric Resin | Diglycidyl ether of bisphenol A | Moderate | Mild | *Medium Molecular Weight (Liquids):* CNS depression from large doses. High skin irritancy. Sensitization. Precipitation of asthmatic attacks. |
| | Resorcinol diglycidyl | Moderate | Moderate to Severe | *High Molecular Weight (Solids):* Practically non-toxic. Skin irritancy mild or absent. Sensitization relatively rare. |
| 2. Curing agents | Amines (probably 90% of products) | Moderate | Severe | More active, physiologically, than epoxy resins themselves. |
| | Polyamides (most of remaining 10%) | Low | Mild | Produce respiratory tract and eye irritation. |
| | Organic acids (uncommon) | Moderate | Moderate | |
| 3. Partially Polymerized Resins | Uncured mixtures of 1 and 2. Low molecular weight. Slight excess of curing agent. Fewer free active groups. | Moderate | Mild to Moderate | With a decrease in volatility goes a partial loss of biological activity (see 1 and 2). |
| 4. Fully Cured Resins | High molecular weight, unreactive | Low | None | Sensitivity reactions relatively rare. No bone marrow depression or carcinogenic effects in experimental animals. |
| 5. Active Diluents (Contained in Oligomer) | Styrene oxide N-butyl glycidyl (monofunctional epoxy groups) | Moderate | Moderate to Severe | Solubilizer in oligomer system. Sensitization common; respiratory tract irritants. |
| 6. Accelerators (Contained in hardeners) | Phenol<br>Resorcinol | High | Mild to Moderate | Usually only a small percentage of the curing agent. Toxic hepatitis from methylenedianiline has been reported. |

bone from slaughterhouses or fish) contains both nitrogen and phosphorus.

The majority of fertilizers on the market are premixed combinations of several of these materials containing the three necessary elements. Some, in addition, contain small amounts of other elements such as magnesium, boron, cobalt, copper, iron, manganese, molybdenum or zinc. Liquid fertilizers usually employ water as the main vehicle. A few fertilizers are composed solely of dried cow or sheep manure. Some also contain herbicides or insecticides.

The label of a premixed fertilizer customarily bears a series of three numbers. For example, "X Brand Fertilizer, 8-6-4," indicates that the product contains nitrogen compounds equivalent to 8 per cent elemental nitrogen, phosphorus compounds equivalent to 6 per cent phosphoric acid anhydride ($P_2O_5$) and potassium compounds equivalent to 4 per cent potash ($K_2O$).

Acute oral toxicity studies on a few liquid and granular fertilizer products have indicated a low degree of toxicity in the products tested. The acute oral $LD_{50}$ value, as a rule, was more than 5 gm/kg in rats. However, nitrates which are present in most products may cause methemoglobinemia. The few products containing calcium cyanamide, borates, herbicides, insecticides or other additives may exhibit toxicity due to these ingredients. Calcium cyanamide, which does not produce free cyanide, is an irritant and has an estimated fatal adult human dose of 40 to 50 gm. Borates have an estimated fatal dose of 30 gm in adults.

Ingestion usually causes no symptoms other than nausea, with possible vomiting and diarrhea. However, methemoglobinemia (manifested by cyanosis) may occur, particularly in children under one year of age, due to conversion of nitrates to nitrites by bacterial action in the intestine. Some commercial baby foods, especially beets and spinach, have been found to contain as much as 0.8 per cent nitrate nitrogen. An infant fed a standard 2 oz. jar gets about 40 mg of nitrate, which is over three times his recommended daily intake. Nitrates in open jars of baby food could presumably be converted to nitrites by bacteria whose gross effect would fall short of obvious spoilage. Symptoms applicable to specific ingredients present in a few fertilizer products include those by calcium cyanamide, a powerful irritant which may cause ulceration of the skin from contact, pulmonary edema from inhalation of the dust, headache, vertigo, congestive hyperemia, tachypnea, hypotension and shock. Borates can cause gastroenteritis, CNS depression and congestion of all organs.

For *treatment,* give milk and demulcents. If spontaneous vomiting has not occurred, induce emesis or perform gastric lavage. Give fluids. The salts present in these products should produce laxative action, therefore administration of a saline cathartic is probably unnecessary. Observe for methemoglobinemia, particularly in infants, and if needed give methylene blue as a 1% solution intravenously, 1 to 2 mg/kg; if severe, consider exchange transfusion. Further treatment, if required, is symptomatic and supportive. In the case of products containing additional ingredients, such as those enumerated above, treat accordingly.

## FIBERGLASS AND RESIN PLASTICS

The use of polymerized resins and fiberglass coatings has developed rapidly during the last few years. The appearance on the market of many brand name products composed of these plastics has made them available to the public, and they are bought for a wide variety of uses. The ability of most of these plastics to take on a smooth polish and hold paint without primers or fillers makes them especially useful to the do-it-yourselfer. In the family garage, the products are accessible to children; particularly hazardous is when the hardener is packaged in small plastic bottles closely resembling the nursing bottles found in toy baby kits.

The resins and the fiberglass are considered nontoxic, but the hardeners used in polymerization are toxic in varying degrees. Four substances are in general use as hardeners; three are peroxides and the fourth is dimethylaniline. The peroxides are, in order of decreasing toxicity, methyl ethyl ketone peroxide, cyclohexanone and benzoyl peroxide.

1. *Methyl ethyl ketone peroxide* has by far the greatest toxicity. The principal manifestations are the chemical burns and their effects, which parallel the course following ingestion of a corrosive such as lye.
2. *Cyclohexanone* is considerably less toxic.
3. *Benzoyl peroxide* is reasonably benign. It is often used topically for burns and dermatitis as a dusting powder, in 10% ointment or 2% olive oil solution, and for poison ivy as a paste.
4. *Dimethylaniline* has a toxicity similar to aniline.

Chemically, the peroxides' action is similar to hydrogen peroxide, giving off oxygen under certain conditions. Care must be taken to prevent inhalation. Contact with the skin and especially the eyes should be avoided, as these peroxides are corrosive. They are also flammable and should be handled with caution.

After the oxygen, with its corrosive action, has been given off, the residuals, namely methyl ethyl ketone, cyclohexanol and benzoic acid, have toxicities of their own. If the hardeners are in solution, the solvent is usually a phthalate ester, which, in turn, is a toxic compound.

Immediate *treatment* should be directed against development of esophageal scarring, as well as toward correction of the ketosis and acidosis which can develop following absorption of the toxic substances from the gastrointestinal tract, producing the effects of acetone-like poisoning. It is believed that it would be almost impossible to swallow any great quantity of methyl ethyl ketone peroxide accidentally because of its burning taste. However, if one purposely swallows it for suicidal intent, then absorption of large amounts via the gastrointestinal tract could result in decreased respiration, pulse and temperature, dyspnea, stupor and in extreme cases, death from ketosis. *Treatment* here requires immediate gastric lavage or an emetic and supportive measures as indicated.

Special Precautions. Since activated resins can produce severe dermatitis and their activators are strong bases, which can cause chemical burns in contact with the skin, proper handling methods should be strictly adhered to.

1. The materials should be used with adequate ventilation.
2. Rubber gloves should be worn at all times and cleaned soon after use.
3. Skin areas that have been contaminated should be thoroughly cleansed immediately. Methyl ethyl ketone removes resin and uncured activated resin. Soap and water removes activator. Soap and water cleansing should follow solvent cleansing.
4. If the material is splashed in the eyes, flush with water for fifteen minutes.
5. Work areas contaminated during normal use should be cleaned as soon as possible.
6. Vaseline™ petroleum jelly or silicone preparations are good protective skin ointments.

## FREON (DICHLORODIFLUOROMETHANE)

Freon is a nonflammable gas used as a refrigerant and propellant for sprays and aerosol cans. Inhalation of a 20% concentration can cause drowsiness, mental confusion and pulmonary irritation. Sniffing of Freon propellants (fluorocarbons) for their intoxicating effects from products such as dry hair shampoos or Freon refrigerants, as in cocktail glass chillers, has produced over one hundred documented deaths (perhaps others not reported). Death is usually sudden and may occur in individuals who experienced inhalation of fluorocarbons (Freon) only once or who have repeated these inhalations on different occasions. The cause of death has not been defined. There is speculation of laryngeal edema, freezing damage to the respiratory epithelium and oxygen displacement, sensitization of the myocardium to circulating epinephrine causing ventricular fibrillation (since the propellant is a halogenated hydrocarbon) and other cardiac arrhythmias or a marked increase in carbon dioxide producing a reflex effect and a sudden cessation of respiration and heart rate. However, animal (dogs) experimentation indicates that sinus node suppression develops within seconds after aerosol inhalation. This chain of events most frequently included sinus bradycardia, A-V dissociation with progressive lower escape rhythms and ultimate electric asystole or ventricular fibrillation. Whatever the mechanism, the result is immediate and tragic. It appears that the victim is lulled into a false sense of security by having had, or knowing others who had, previous "harmless" experiences. Sniffing of a cocktail glass chilling Freon product (fluorocarbon 12) for its toxic and lethal effects needs more publicity. When exposed to heat, Freons may decompose into many irritant and toxic gases such as chlorine, fluorine, hydrogen fluoride and chloride and even phosgene. Freon use as a propellant in aerosol has now been phased out by the FDA.

*Treatment* consists of resuscitative efforts with cardiac massage, defibrillation and pacing. Epinephrine or isoproterenol is contraindicated.

## GAS (NATURAL, MANUFACTURED, PROPANE)

Natural gas consists chiefly of volatile hydrocarbons (85% methane), ethane and hydrogen, inert and of low toxicity. Natural gas contains no carbon monoxide unless contaminated. It can be formed, however, whenever carbonaceous material is burned with insufficient oxygen. Exhaust or flue gases often have corrosive oxides of nitrogen and sulfur present. Manufactured or artificial gas is a combustible gas produced from coal, coke or oil, or by reforming natural or liquid petroleum gases, and may have up to 10 per cent carbon monoxide, although now most have none.

Propane gas is the principal ingredient of bottled gas in northern states, whereas butane with its considerably higher boiling and freezing points is more widely used in warmer southern states.

Propane gas, in low concentrations, is physiologically inert. However, high concentrations may cause narcosis. Brief exposure to 10,000 ppm (1% of vol) causes no symptoms in man. A concentration of 100,000 ppm (10%) causes slight dizziness in a few minutes. This concentration of propane is not noticeably irritating to the eyes, nose and throat. Displacement of air by this gas may lead to shortness of breath, unconsciousness and death by hypoxemia. The greatest potential hazard of propane is its flammability. The flammable limits are from 22,000 to 95,000 ppm (2.2% to 9.5%). If gas were leaking into a house trailer and a source of ignition were present, an explosion would result when the concentration reached 2.2%. Propane cylinders for homes and trailers are equipped with fusible plugs. If fire is present, the plug melts at a designated temperature, releasing a small volume of gas which burns slowly, thus preventing an explosion. Most bottled gases also contain ethyl mercaptan, the odor of which serves as a warning for leaks. Spray-type oven-cleaning products containing propane gas may cause explosions when used on hot surfaces or near a pilot light. The principal toxic effects from gases are from carbon monoxide.

## GIBBERELLIC ACID

This substance is highly diluted when sold as a plant nutrient, and it is quite unlikely that enough nutrient could be ingested to be harmful. Ingestion of 25 gm/kg orally failed to cause death or produce more than minor toxic symptoms in mice.

## GLYCERIN (GLYCEROL)

Glycerin is a trihydric alcohol which is a clear, colorless, sweet, syrupy liquid miscible with water and alcohol but insoluble in chloroform, ether and fixed or volatile oils. It is extensively used as a vehicle for many drugs applied to the skin. Concentrated solutions are irritating to mucous membranes, while the ingestion of large amounts is capable of inducing hemolysis, convulsions and paralysis. Various congeners of glycerin are much more toxic than the parent compound (*see* Glycol, etc.).

## GLYCYRRHIZIN (LICORICE)

This agent is a demulcent, mild laxative and expectorant and often is used to disguise the taste of other medications. It exerts an action similar to that of deoxycorticosterone, increasing extracellular fluid, excreting potassium and retaining sodium. Overindulgence in eating licorice candy has produced hypertension, muscle weakness, myoglobinuria, hypokalemia and sodium retention with waterlogging and increased weight in humans. The hypertensive state is reversible and is related to the steroid-like compound, glycyrrhetinic acid. The similarity of the effects of excess licorice ingestion to primary hyperaldosteronism can be striking.

## GOLF BALLS

Old golf balls are occasionally splintered and dissected by children. Their centers, which may contain castor oil, honey, glycerin, clay, calcium, calcium carbonate, potassium or sodium hydroxide (rarely used now, if at all), barium sulfate and zinc sulfide occasionally are splashed in the eyes or are swallowed. None of the contents, however, are in sufficient strength to produce ill effects, except for the hydroxides, which can result in chemical conjunctivitis and esophagitis. The danger in these accidents appears to be from the mechanical trauma to the eye rather than from the contents of the golf ball.

## GRAPHITE (PLUMBAGO)

Artificial graphite made from coke is 99 per cent carbon and contains no free silica. Pneumoconiosis from exposure to this form of graphite has not been reported and probably rarely occurs. On the other hand, pneumoconiosis (silicographitosis) has been documented following excessive exposure to natural graphite (plumbago), which is a crystalline form of carbon containing free silica. (Lead pencils are made with graphite and their ingestion would not ordinarily produce lead poisoning, since pencils manufactured in this country adhere to stringent Pencil Makers Association regulations. *See* section on Pencils.)

## HEXACHLOROPHENE

Hexachlorophene, a chlorinated phenolic hydrocarbon, is albumin bound and fat stored, with an estimated blood half-life of ten hours, with excretion in the stool and urine. It is an odorless white powder, insoluble in water but freely soluble in alcohol. It is incorporated into soaps, detergents, creams, oils and other vehicles for topical application to reduce the number of, and to inhibit the metabolism of, microorganisms that occur naturally and pathologically as the skin bacterial flora. It is particularly effective against gram-positive organisms.

Irritant and toxic effects of hexachlorophene on the skin surface, even after long continued daily use, have been reported infrequently, but its application for detergent purposes on extensive burns has produced severe convulsions and death.

When preparations containing hexachlorophene are left in contact with denuded skin (such as extensive wounds, lacerations or severe burns), sufficient hexachlorophene may be absorbed to cause toxic symptoms manifested by signs of stimulation (irritation) of the central nervous system, sometimes with convulsions. In the few reported cases, the latter were attributable to cerebral edema and subsided with no neurologic or other sequelae on discontinuation of the prolonged contact method of application of the hexachlorophene preparation.

After each washing of a lacerated or burned area with pHisoHex, thoroughly rinse off the cleansed site with copious amounts of sterile saline solution or water to prevent the absorption of a toxic quantity of hexachlorophene from the broken skin. Pat dry with sterile gauze. Do not leave pHisoHex diluted or undiluted on broken or denuded skin nor apply pHisoHex as a wet or impregnated dressing. Do not immerse a burned patient, particularly a child, for prolonged periods in baths containing substantial quantities of hexachlorophene.

Systemic effects following the accidental ingestion of proprietary compounds of hexachlorophene classed as antiseptic detergents have also been reported. These symptoms, sometimes severe, were nausea, vomiting, diarrhea, abdominal cramps, convulsions, neuromuscular responses (encephalopathy), dehydration and shock. The fatal adult dose has been estimated to be between 2 and 5 gm (300 mg/kg). A single dose of 250 mg/kg hexachlorophene is fatal in children. Vacuolization of the white matter of the brain is a characteristic pathological finding.

*Treatment* should consist of immediate gastric lavage or measures to produce emesis. Subsequently the problem is that of adequate fluid and electrolyte replacement and the prevention of shock. Sedation, anticonvulsants and vasoconstrictors may be needed. Since most of the poisoning has occurred in hospitals where a milky preparation of a hexachlorophene-containing product had been placed in cups or glasses and mistakenly taken for milk of magnesia, hospital personnel should be made aware of the potential hazard of this procedure.

The use of these agents in the home for the bathing of infants and children has gained wide popularity. This presents an additional danger of accidental ingestion unless parents are forewarned to keep these attractive preparations out of the reach of children. A six-year-old child died nine hours after taking 4 to 5 oz. of one of these preparations, in spite of thorough gastric lavage within fifteen minutes after ingestion (*Med J Aust, 1*:737, 1963). The inadvertent use of 6% hexachlorophene, instead of 3%, in infant talcum powder produced over twenty tragic deaths in France recently.

## HEXACHLOROPHENE AND SKIN CARE OF NEWBORN INFANTS

The question of safety has been raised by the recent evidence that levels of hexachlorophene in the blood of newborn infants receiving daily baths with a 3% solution are close to levels which are neurotoxic for adult rats. Hexachlorophene was widely used in newborn nurseries, but techniques varied considerably; they ranged from meticulous, double, early bathing followed by daily baths to alternate-day washing with a diluted solution followed by rinsing off.

With chronic oral administration, blood

levels associated with leg weakness progressing to paralysis in the adult rat have ranged from 0.985 to 1.48 ppm. The chemical is readily absorbed from the skin, resulting in blood levels of 0.009 to 0.646 ppm. The compound is excreted as a monoglucuronide in the bile and feces. Convulsions have been reported in an infant four days after repeated application of the 3% emulsion to the skin without subsequent rinsing; and, toxic manifestations have been observed in burn patients, but at relatively high serum levels (29 μg/ml), after denuded areas have been washed with hexachlorophene.

Although the symptoms observed in adult man and adult rats are similar, the actual blood levels at which symptoms are produced in man appear to be much higher. Symptomatology in the rat with chronic oral administration was accompanied by brain lesions, cerebral edema and cystic spaces in the white matter of the brain; these lesions were reversible over a period of six weeks when hexachlorophene was discontinued. Similar lesions have been produced in experimental intoxication of monkeys following both subcutaneous administration and application of hexachlorophene to the skin. The animals did not demonstrate abnormal neurological signs even with plasma levels of 3.1 μg/ml, although papilledema was found at autopsy in some instances. It is not presently known whether the lesions are reversible when hexachlorophene is discontinued. Australian investigators (*Med J Aust, 1*:897–903, 1972) report no toxic reactions or CNS changes (as seen in experimental animals) in 24,322 infants from 1960 to 1971.

For a number of reasons, it appears that, at this time, there is little justification on microbiological grounds for routine, daily hexachlorophene baths for the newborn infant. With the "meticulous" techniques, the rate of colonization with coagulase-positive staphylococci and the incidence of skin lesions is reduced. However, there is no documented experience where this technique has arrested a serious nursery epidemic. It is also well established that the use of hexachlorophene increases colonization with gram-negative organisms as well as the incidence of gram-negative disease. Finally, for reasons that have not been defined, the problem of serious staphylococcal disease in the nursery has not been of major importance during the last five years, as it was ten to fifteen years ago, whether or not hexachlorophene has been used for skin care of newborn infants.

The Committee on Fetus and Newborn of the American Academy of Pediatrics has recommended (sec. 1974) that skin care of newborns should consist of the following points.

1. Cleansing of the newly born infant should be delayed until the infant's temperature has stabilized after the cold stress of delivery.
2. Cotton sponges (not gauze) soaked with sterile water are used to remove blood from the face and head and meconium from the perianal area. As an alternative, a mild nonmedicated soap can be used with careful water rinsing. Potential bacterial contamination of bar or liquid soaps should be remembered.
3. The remainder of the skin should be untouched unless grossly soiled. There is evidence to indicate that vernix caseosa may serve a protective function, some evidence to indicate it has no effect and no evidence to indicate it is harmful.
4. For the remainder of the infant's stay in the hospital nursery, the buttocks and perianal regions should be cleansed with sterile water and cotton. As an alternative, a mild soap with water rinsing may be used as required at diaper changes and more often if indicated.
5. There is no single method of cord care which has been proven to limit colonization and disease. Several methods currently in use include local application of alcohol, triple dye* and antimicrobial agents.

---

*Triple dye is composed of 2.29 gm of brilliant green, 1.14 gm of proflavine hemisulfate, 2.29 gm of crystal violet and enough water to make 1000 ml.

During nursery outbreaks of infection, a total program of infection control is indicated. This should include institution of a program of surveillance and epidemiologic investigation, possible tracking changes and institution of cohorts. Since hand transmission is the primary means of acquisition of most organisms by newly born infants, emphasis must be placed on hand-washing techniques as recommended in AAP *Standards of Recommendations of Hospital Care of Newborn Infants.*

In the case of staphylococcal outbreaks, several measures may be undertaken. These might include treatment of the cord or the cord and nose with an antibiotic ointment, treatment of the cord with triple dye or even brief institution of a program of total body bathing with a solution of not more than 3% hexachlorophene. (This application must be limited to full-term infants, must be thoroughly washed off after the application and applied no more than two times to each infant.) In serious outbreaks, the technique of bacterial interference or the administration of systemic antibiotics to all infants may be required.

## JAVELLE WATER

A weakened solution of potassium hypochlorite containing approximately 2.5 per cent active chlorine in fresh preparation which is one-half strength of the official NF solution (*see* Hypochlorite).

## LABARRAQUE'S SOLUTION

A solution of about 2 per cent sodium hypochlorite and sodium chloride with 0.1 to 0.5 per cent sodium hydroxide or carbonate. Because of the addition of the latter, the potential corrosive action of this solution is increased (*see* Hypochlorite).

## LANOLIN

Lanolin is wool fat mixed with 25 to 30 per cent water to give it more cohesive and adherent properties. This is an innocuous product if ingested, since it contains cholesterol esters of higher fatty acids and alcohols (cetyl) and is not readily absorbed from the gastrointestinal tract.

## LIME

Quicklime (unslaked lime, calcium oxide) liberates heat on contact with water. It is a very powerful caustic and may cause serious damage if ingested, extensively inhaled or allowed to come in contact with any portion of the eyes.

By mouth, the signs, symptoms and treatment are approximately the same as for any strongly caustic alkali.

In the eye it may cause (1) hyperemia, edema and corneal ulcers and/or opacities; (2) extensive erosion, sometimes with complete loss of vision.

For *treatment* (*see* Chemical Burn), immediately wash with large amounts of water and refer at once to an ophthalmologist.

Slaked lime (calcium hydroxide) is a simple alkali, and because of its low solubility in aqueous solutions, it is not greatly corrosive. *Treatment* therefore is usually unnecessary.

Lime sulfur (calcium polysulfide) used in agriculture as an insecticide and fungicide is irritating on contact with skin, eyes and mucous membranes. On ingestion, hydrogen sulfide is formed.

*Treatment* consists of thorough irrigation of eyes and skin with copious quantities of water (after the dry lime has been brushed away, so that the calcium oxide does not unite with water to form calcium hydroxide, a reaction that produces considerable heat). If taken internally, treat as for hydrogen sulfide intoxication.

## LINSEED OIL (FLAXSEED OIL)

Linseed oil is a vegetable oil consisting of glycerides of linoleic, oleic, stearic, palmitic and myristic acids. It is used as a drying oil in paints. Though digestible and nutritious, ingestion of large amounts is laxative. *Boiled linseed oil,* however, is usually toxic since lead and other chemical agents have been added to enhance its hardening properties.

## LITHIUM SALTS

Lithium closely resembles sodium, chemically and pharmacologically. It had no great therapeutic application in this country for many years, while in Europe, lithium carbonate was successfully being employed in the treatment of manic psychoses by a number of psychiatrists. It was employed in the past as a salt substitute, until reports of fatalities from its use led to its abandonment. Signs and symptoms of toxicity include anorexia, nausea, diarrhea, weight gain, alopecia, dysarthria, pretibial edema (sodium retention), metallic taste, dryness of the mouth, skin anesthesia, glycosuria, leukocytosis, tremor, ataxia, muscle spasm, seizures, apathy, blurring of vision, confusion, coma and death.

The mechanism whereby lithium produces its toxic and lethal effects is not clear, although the principal toxic action appears to be on the kidney. This toxicity is markedly increased in the presence of low sodium intake and when doses are close to therapeutic levels. Toxic reactions are seldom encountered at serum lithium levels below 1.5 mEq/liter. Mild to moderate toxic reactions can occur at levels from 1.5 to 2.5 mEq/liter; and moderate to severe reactions may be seen at levels from 2.0 to 2.5 mEq/liter. The normal half-life of lithium is twenty-four hours.

Lithium should *not* be administered to patients who have renal or cardiac disease, or during early or late pregnancy. Experiments have shown the teratogenic effects of lithium in many animal species. Neurologically depressed states have been reported in infants born to mothers under therapy with lithium. It is excreted in concentration from 30 to 100% of mother's serum in breast milk, and if the infant is nursing, he should be monitored closely for signs of toxicity.

Among other changes, lithium causes flattened or inverted T wave and prolonged QRS complex; ECG monitoring, as well as determining the serum sodium, potassium and lithium levels, should be an important part of management. A diet with normal or high sodium levels is necessary to accelerate renal elimination of lithium and prevent intoxication.

Lithium hydride only recently has been found to be useful in industrial and nuclear technology. Explosion of lithium hydride produces lithium hydroxide, which is reported to have produced severe burns of the mucous membrane that caused scarring of the corneas; stricture of the larynx, trachea and bronchi; and marked stricture of the esophagus.

*Treatment* includes emesis or gastric lavage for ingestion of toxic doses and the administration of sodium chloride.

Replace water and electrolytes as needed (sodium, potassium, calcium, magnesium). Total daily fluid should be at least 5 to 6 liters.

TABLE 149
SIDE-EFFECTS ASSOCIATED
WITH LITHIUM THERAPY

| |
|---|
| A. Innocuous<br>(low serum $Li^+$)<br>**Early onset**<br>Thirst, nausea<br>Dizziness<br>Fine tremor<br>Jerky movements<br>Loose stools<br>Increased urine volume<br>**Later onset**<br>Hand tremor<br>Polyuria<br>Polydipsia<br>Weight gain<br>Edema<br>Hypothyroidism and goiter |
| B. Imminent toxicity<br>(high serum $Li^+$)<br>Vomiting and diarrhea<br>Coarse tremor of hand<br>Sluggishness<br>Sleepiness<br>Vertigo<br>Dysarthria |
| C. Lithium toxicity<br>(very high serum $Li^+$)<br>Impairment of consciousness<br>Muscle fasciculation<br>Hyperreflexia, nystagmus<br>Epileptic seizures<br>Coma<br>Oliguria, anuria |

do not oversalinize,* and avoid abrupt changes in electrolyte intake. Monitor if changes are made.

*In patients who develop a lithium-induced nephrogenic diabetes insipidus like condition, inability to concentrate urine in the presence of a continuing salt load may lead to hypernatremia and hyperosmolality. Plasma sodium concentration and osmolality should be carefully monitored.

Promote lithium excretion by means of urea, 20 gm IV, two to five times daily (urea contraindicated if severe renal impairment antedates toxicity), or mannitol 50 to 100 gm IV total daily dose.

Increase lithium clearance with aminophylline (which also suppresses tubular reabsorption and increases blood flow). Dosage is 0.5 gm by slow IV administration (may cause a sharp but transitory hypotension).

Alkalinization of urine with IV sodium lactate has been recommended as an adjunctive measure.

If toxicity is severe, the patient should be dialyzed (peritoneal dialysis or artificial kidney), especially if the patient has seizures or is comatose, or has a serum level of 3 mEq/liter or greater.

The use of lithium carbonate for the treatment or prophylaxis of manic-depressive illness in pregnant women is associated with two kinds of danger: (1) the possible induction of morphogenetic abnormalities in the developing fetus as a result of intrapartum exposure to lithium; and (2) the induction of maternal or neonatal lithium toxicity (or both) as a result of excessive maternal lithium concentrations. When it is necessary to give lithium throughout a pregnancy, the dose should be the smallest amount possible to achieve the desired therapeutic effect.

## MACE

This compound, used mainly by law enforcement officers, is a chemical disabling agent that when sprayed on the face and in the eyes, produces numbness and excessive tearing with temporary blindness. It consists of a solution of (0.9%) chloroacetophenone (tear gas) in a mixed solvent of 1,1,2-trichloro-1,2,-2-trifluoroethane (approximately 70% to 80%), 1,1,1-trichloroethane (approximately 5%) and a mixture of hydrocarbons resembling kerosene (approximately 4%).

Although effects are transient, there is some concern as to permanent eye injury from heavy exposure.

## MATÉ

Maté is a tea-like beverage consumed in parts of South America, and is produced by boiling the dried leaves of the shrub *Ilex paraguayensis.* The infusions from these leaves contain about 24 mg of caffeine and about 4 mg of theobromine per 100 ml, plus varying amounts of choline, folic acid, vitamin C, fluorine, purines and a mixture of tannins. It has not been documented in the literature that these products are harmful or that they are advantageous. The product is prepared in a manner similar to that of tea and is apparently used in the same general manner.

## MESCAL (PEYOTE)

Mescaline and other alkaloids are found in the dumpling cactus, a small, carrot-shaped, spineless cactus which grows in the Rio Grande Valley. The ingestion of this plant by members of the youth-drug subculture or the drinking of its wine by Mexicans and Indians at religious rituals has produced bizarre symptoms. These are manifested by vivid hallucinations which are usually visual and consist of brightly colored lights and geometric designs of animals and occasionally people. Anxiety and muscular tremors and twitchings often occur. The sensorium, however, is usually clear. A recent survey of Huichol Indians indicated that multigenerational ingestion of peyote was not associated with abnormalities in lymphocyte chromosomes, and there was no increase in the incidence of congenital malformations in the offspring of users.

*Treatment* is mainly supportive and symptomatic since complete recovery without permanent ill effects occurs in six to eight hours.

## METHYLBENZETHONIUM CHLORIDE (DIAPARENE)

This is a derivative of benzethonium chloride in which a methyl radical is substituted on the benzene ring of the phenoxy group. It is widely used as a germicide and disinfectant, especially in solutions and ointments for diaper rash (*see* Quaternary Compounds).

## METHYLPARABEN U.S.P. (METHYL-P-HYDROXYBENZOATE, METHYL PARASEPT)

This substance is not toxic in the small amounts found in most commerical products (0.05% to 0.2%) where it serves as a preservative and antiseptic. It is less toxic than salicylic acid and its derivatives.

## MIRBANE, ESSENCE OR OIL (NITROBENZENE)

Mirbane is a solution obtained from mixing benzol and nitric acid. It is used as a substitute for oil of bitter almonds and in the manufacturing of aniline dyes. This preparation is toxic by all routes including skin absorption (*see* Aniline and Nitrobenzene).

## MONSEL'S SOLUTION

This is an externally used styptic solution of basic ferric sulfate or subsulfate containing approximately 20 per cent iron used in the control of external hemorrhage, especially for fighters (boxers).

## MURIATIC (HYDROCHLORIC) ACID

Muriatic acid is an aqueous solution of hydrogen chloride gas dispensed in concentrations of 10%, 32% and 38%. It is often supplied to and used by plumbers.

## NEATSFOOT OIL

This is the oil extracted from ox feet which contains glycerides of oleic and palmitic acid. It is used as a lubricant to soften and waterproof leather. The ingestion of this preparation should produce no ill effects.

## OIL OF SASSAFRAS

This is a volatile oil containing safrene and safrole used chiefly as a flavoring agent at present, although at one time it was used in the treatment of syphilis and skin diseases. Safrole is a hepatocarcinogen in rats, and its use in food has been prohibited. Ingestion can cause severe vomiting and diarrhea as well as circulatory collapse. *Treatment* is symptomatic and supportive.

## PARIS GREEN (SCHWEINFURTH GREEN)

This is a copper acetoarsenite compound of complex composition, having an arsenic trioxide content equivalent to about 60 per cent. It is used as a paint pigment, insecticide and wood preservative (*see* Arsenic).

## PENCILS

The "lead" in lead pencils is not elemental lead. The material is graphite, which is crystalline carbon chemically and biologically inert, and as such is not harmful. Indelible pencils contain methyl or crystal violet and, other than staining skin and clothing, are innocuous. However, tattooing the skin may leave permanent markings. Colored pencils for art and office use, particularly the yellows and greens, may contain lead chromate; however, the other colors usually are made of harmless dyes.

The Pencil Makers Association standards ("PMA Mark") require that the entire pencil cannot contain more than 1.2 mg of lead (Pb) and no component (lacquer, core, ferrule, etc.) can contain more than 0.06 per cent lead by weight. Although the maximum allowable quantity of lead per pencil is 1.2 mg, very few could have more than 0.3 mg and still qualify under other sections of requirements. A pencil or any of its components may not contain compounds of antimony, arsenic, cadmium, mercury or selenium, of which the metal content individually or in total (calculated as Sb, As, Cd, Hg, Se respectively) exceeds 0.06 per cent by weight. Likewise, a pencil, or any of its components, may not contain barium compounds of which the water-soluble barium (calculated as Ba) exceeds 1 per cent total barium by weight.

## PERMANGANATE, POTASSIUM

This drug is a strong oxidizing compound, highly caustic and capable of causing great tissue destruction. In dilute concentrations of 1:5000 or 1:10,000 it is frequently used as an oxidizing agent in the treatment of strychnine, nicotine, physostigmine, quinine and many other poisons. Its value and importance for this purpose are greatly exaggerated, and ordinary tap water may be equally as effective and certainly far safer. Far too often, particularly in children, stronger concentrations than necessary are used.

Oral potassium permanganate poisonings chiefly result from either accidental ingestions or suicidal attempts. The clinical manifestations vary with the dose ingested and the concentration. In low or moderate concentrations, 1% solutions, the usual symptoms are burning in the throat, nausea, vomiting, moderate gastroenteritis and some difficulty in swallowing, with no systemic manifestations. In higher concentrations, i.e. 2% to 3% solutions, in addition to the above symptoms, the patient also appears anemic, the pharynx becomes edematous and the patient may experience difficulty in swallowing and speaking. There is a dryness of the mucous membranes of the mouth due to the tanning by potassium permanganate; the patient also has difficulty in salivation. In severe cases when 4% to 5% solutions are taken, there may be kidney involvement associated with albuminuria. Salivation may be either excessive or become entirely suppressed; the salivary glands become edematous due to the reduction of saliva. In addition to the gastroenteritis, in the serious cases the stools may become bloody, and the patient may also present a picture of circulatory collapse with low blood pressure and rapid and shallow pulse. At times, these symptoms may be accompanied by paresthesia and disorientation. If death occurs, it is usually due to circulatory failure or pulmonary complications.

The misuse of this drug as a local abortifacient, instead of producing the desired effects, causes severe trauma, serious injury to the vaginal walls with ulceration, massive vaginal hemorrhage, and quite often, a secondary infection.

The *treatment* of potassium permanganate poisoning includes gastric lavage with 3% hydrogen peroxide (10 ml in 100 ml of water), copious amounts of fluid, careful observation and supportive therapy. Milk and dilute alcohol solutions are suggested to provide oxidizable organic material.

## PHENYL SALICYLATE (SALOL)

This is an insoluble compound used for enteric coating of pills, and at one time, as an intestinal antiseptic. It probably is hydrolyzed by the alkaline intestinal juices and enzymes to phenol and salicylic acid. The toxic effects are chiefly those of phenol but much less severe; therefore corrosive damage is rare (*see* Phenol).

## PHOTOGRAPHIC (POLAROID™) MATERIAL

### Pod Jelly

*Description*

This is a viscous highly alkaline solution contained in sealed foil envelopes called pods, which are part of each positive roll or pack of Polaroid film. There is one pod picture, each containing about 1 ml of solution. During processing the pod is ruptured, spreading the contents between the positive and the negative portion, which is subsequently discarded.

The solution in the pod and the excess that remains on and around the picture area of the negative discard continues to be highly alkaline for an hour or two following processing; contact with it should be avoided.

The SX-70™ product, on the other hand, does not normally expose the user to processing jelly. Should the picture structure be taken apart, however, it is possible to come in contact with the alkaline processing jelly.

*Ingredients*

The pods contain a highly caustic jelly consisting of up to 9 per cent alkali metal hydroxides; the pH of this jelly is 13 to 14.

*Toxicity*

Toxicity results primarily from the high alkalinity of the solution. The jelly may cause an alkali burn if left on the skin for a few minutes. It is an extreme eye irritant and causes severe burns to the eye or mouth if not rinsed immediately.

*Treatment*

Treatment should be the same as for contact with lye.

CONTACT WITH SKIN. Wash immediately with lots of water. Treat as any alkali burn.

CONTACT WITH EYES. Flood the eye immediately with lots of water. The patient should consult an ophthalmologist as quickly as possible.

CONTACT ORALLY. Rinse mouth thoroughly with water. Drink water or milk if available to dilute any alkali that may have been swallowed. Some burning of the mucous membranes and possible stricture of the esophagus could occur. Stomach tube and induced vomiting are not recommended.

## Print Coater™ Solution

*Description*

This is a solution used to treat the surface of black and white pictures which is applied from a cotton swab packaged in a plastic vial. Each swab contains about 8 ml of solution. Print coaters are included with many types of Polaroid black and white Land™ film.

*Ingredients*

The print coater is a nontoxic solution of water, alcohol, acetic acid, inert plastic and traces of other inert materials. The concentration of acetic acid is similar to that in vinegar (5%).

*Toxicity*

The solution is strongly irritating to the eyes but is otherwise nontoxic. If taken orally it may cause mouth irritation, as could vinegar. It is not normally a skin irritant.

*Treatment*

Wash eyes with copious amounts of water. If taken orally, rinse mouth with water.

## Dippit™ Solution

*Description*

This is a solution contained in a plastic dispenser that is used to treat Polaroid black and white transparent pictures. The dispenser is sold as a separate item with sufficient solution to treat six rolls of film. This film is used primarily for industrial and educational purposes.

*Ingredients*

The treatment solution is a 50/50 solution of isopropanol and water with a small amount of stannic chloride. This solution is very acidic with a pH of one.

*Toxicity*

It is an extreme eye irritant and a mild skin irritant. Toxicity results primarily from the acid nature of the solution.

*Treatment*

If the material gets into the eyes, flood the eyes immediately wth lots of water. The patient should consult an ophthalmologist as quickly as possible. If swallowed, prompt dilution with water and demulcents followed by lavage with a stomach tube is recommended.

## Polaroid Prints

Occasionally a Polaroid print may be eaten by a child. The extremely small amount of chemicals present poses no toxicity problem in either black and white or color, but if too many pictures are consumed, there may be difficulties because of intestinal blockage, as would be the case if an excess of any cellulosic product were ingested.

SX-70 pictures are also nontoxic. However, if the image structure is taken apart before it has thoroughly dried, contact with the residual alkaline pod jelly is possible.

## PINE OIL

Pine oil is a volatile oil consisting of terpene alcohols, ethers and hydrocarbons, capable of producing serious toxic effects if ingested or aspirated. Symptoms are due to the severe gastritis and central nervous system and respiratory depression that occur. In addition, it is markedly irritating to the eyes and mucous membranes. The chemical pneumonitis produced by aspiration can end in a fatality, and corticosteroid therapy may be beneficial. (For detailed *treatment,* see Volatile Oils.)

## PLASTER OF PARIS (GYPSUM)

Plaster of paris is anhydrous calcium sulfate or dihydrate with approximately 5 per cent water. The ingestion of this material may result in obstruction of the patient's upper intestinal tract, especially at the pylorus, since this compound hardens quickly after absorption of moisture. *Treatment* consists of giving glycerin or gelatin solutions or large volumes of water to delay the setting process. Surgical removal of the material may be necessary.

## PLASTIC CEMENT

Sniffing of plastic model cement for its euphoric effect has been reported as a fad among teen-agers. The accidental inhalation of the fumes while using these agents in a closed room can also produce deleterious effects (*also see* Xylene and Toluene).

The solvents contained in these cements are generally volatile hydrocarbons, aromatic or aliphatic, and include acetone, toluene, xylene, benzene, amyl acetate, butyl alcohol and isopropyl alcohol. In addition, plastic cements may contain carbon tetrachloride, chloroform or ethylene dichloride. The last three of these may have extensive toxicities involving the central nervous system, heart, gastrointestinal tract, liver and kidneys. All of these solvents are central nervous system depressants; many can cause central nervous stimulation also; and most can sensitize the myocardium sufficiently to produce ventricular fibrillation. Probable lethal doses by ingestion of benzene, toluene, xylene and carbon tetrachloride are 50 to 500 mg/kg, and other solvents fall into the .05 to 0.5 gm/kg range. Industrial tolerances for the vapors of these solvents vary from 25 ppm (benzene) to 1000 ppm (acetone).

It appears that the contents of these cements are theoretically capable of causing severe poisoning and, in fact, there have been some reports of their producing a reversible syndrome resembling acute alcoholic intoxication. These cases, however, have not as yet been well documented and, to date, no serious or permanent residual effects from contact with them have been reported.

## POMEGRANATE

The root bark and the bark of the tree contain the alkaloid pelletierine, which has been used as an anthelmintic. It is officially listed in the U.S.P. as "granatum."

## POLYMER FUME FEVER

Polymer fume fever is a short-lived influenza-like syndrome due to the inhalation of products of pyrolysis of polytetrafluoroethylene (Teflon®) during heating or machining the polymer or to contamination of cigarettes and pipes. It is characterized by a tight, gripping sensation in the chest associated with shivering, sore throat, fever and weakness.

Since this material has widespread use as a coating for cooking utensils, some concern has been aroused in regard to its safety. Thermal degradation of polytetrafluoroethylene occurs only at temperatures above 300° to 350°C. It has been demonstrated that the maximum temperatures reached in cooking a variety of foods in such pans are between 130° to 195°C. The scorching temperature or smoke point of cooking oils is approximately 200°C. This is obviously well below the decomposition range of Teflon. Should such a pan be neglected on the burner of a stove, it is comforting to know that the average pan is coated with only 2 gm of this plastic. The pyrolysis residue that would be released from this amount of resin into an average-sized kitchen would not reach harmful concentrations.

Unlike metal fume fever, this condition is usually benign with similar but milder symptoms and requires only symptomatic treatment after removal from the exposure (*see* Teflon).

## PROPANE, LIQUID

There are apparently no ill effects from remaining for several hours in an atmosphere containing this gas in concentrations as high as 3% to 5% or from repeated exposures, but the combustion of this hydrocarbon with an inadequate supply of air leads to the formation of carbon monoxide and risk of asphyxia. When used for heating purposes, combustion of the gas to carbon dioxide and water is usually complete. If, however, the supply of gas is turned down until one or more of the burners may go out or be easily blown out while some of the other burners continue to burn, the gas from the unlit burners may undergo a flameless and incomplete combustion and produce dangerous amounts of aldehydes and carbon monoxide.

## PRUSSIC ACID

This is a 2% aqueous solution of hydrocyanic acid, and 2 or 3 ml may be lethal. (*See* Cyanide for treatment, which should be carried out immediately.)

## PUMICE

This compound is made up of complex silicates and used as a polishing material. The silicates are insoluble and chemically inert and would hardly be toxic in any amounts. However, mechanical obstruction or perforation may conceivably occur in the gastrointestinal tract.

## QUINCE SEED

This is the seed of a rosaceous tree or shrub *(Cydonia oblonga)*. Quince seed gives off a mucilage-containing amygdalin which is used as a demulcent. Enzymes hydrolyze amygdalin into benzaldehyde, cyanide and glucose. The available cyanide produced, however, is so small that signs of toxicity rarely appear.

## RADIATION SYNDROME

The acute radiation syndrome after whole-body exposure to external ionizing radiation can be diagnosed with fair accuracy from the postirradiation sequence of events. When nausea and vomiting, usually the first symptoms, are severe, prolonged and accompanied by erythema and a depressed absolute lymphocyte count, the patient probably was exposed to a high and fatal dose of radiation; when nausea and vomiting are moderate and brief, succeeded by a period of well-being, the dose may have been lethal; and when initial symptoms are minor or missing, the dose probably was sublethal. The most important aid to diagnosis is the total white cell count, which should be correlated with the differential white cell count and absolute granulocyte and lymphocyte values. When the absolute lymphocyte count is 500 per cu. mm or less in the first two days, the prognosis is grave; when the count remains above 1000, some optimism is warranted; and when the value shows an upward trend after the first week, the prognosis is good.

*Treatment* is not necessary if the dose was less than 100 roentgens and probably is useless if the dose was more than 700 R. Slight sedation is indicated for doses of 100 to 200 R; hospitalization is advisable if the dose was more than 150 R. Therapy, which is symptomatic, is of greatest value in the 200 to 700 R range. Bone marrow replacement may be beneficial if the dose was more than 600 R. Fresh blood or platelet-enriched plasma should not be given unless clearly indicated, since sublethally irradiated patients often have spontaneous hematologic recovery. Since death invariably is associated with sepsis, infection should be watched for and treated promptly.

From 1300 to 6000 cancer deaths annually are caused by exposure of the American public to present levels of diagnostic x-rays. In addition, ill health results from genetic damage caused by the exposure. These conclusions were reached by the National Academy of Sciences/National Research Council through its study on *The Effects on Populations of Exposure to Low Levels of Ionizing Radiation.*

Shielding of any part of the body may modify significantly the response to ionizing radiation and change the course, prognosis and therapy. The protection afforded by shielding of critical organs may be sufficient to permit survival at high dose levels.

Clinical demands for diagnostic x-ray services has increased at a rapid rate. X-ray film consumption nearly doubled between 1947 and 1963. There is every indication that the total volume of medical radiology in the United States will continue to grow at a rate that exceeds the rate of population growth. The effect of this increase should be beneficial since doctors depend on radiological examinations. At the same time, the radiation exposure of the public will presumably increase unless improved techniques and equipment can offset the greater volume.

No cause for alarm is seen at the present level of genetically significant dose from medical diagnostic procedures; it is only half as large as the dose from natural background sources. Still, there is evidence that the dose could be further reduced without interfering with the very substantial benefits the public now derives from medical x-rays; for example, according to a PHS study, more than half of the genetically significant dose is now being delivered by radiation which is outside the film area. By careful attention to the available safety factors, the medical profession can prevent the radiation dose to the population from rising to a level that would cause concern, while still reaping the benefits of the expanding capabilities of diagnostic radiology.

The critical analyses of radiation exposure published in recent years demonstrate very well that fluoroscopy provides a relatively high dose rate to the patient as compared with diagnostic films. Both are of great value, but the making of films is more laborious and always has been chiefly the field of radiologists. On the other hand, large numbers of fluoroscopes are operated throughout the United States by nonradiologists, whose chief interest is other than diagnostic radiology.

The careful operation of a fluoroscope is a difficult task in the light of today's knowledge; and the occasional user must, therefore, shoulder the same responsibility as the specialist in using this tool of such potential danger. Every operator of a fluoroscope must feel obligated to apply to the method the same degree of caution and care as the physician who sterilizes his syringes or the surgeon who counts his sponges.

A Philadelphia study revealed that 50 per cent of fluoroscopes exceed the minimum recommended dose delivery of 10 R/min.; that the dose rate throughout the surveyed geographical area is from 2 to 64 R/min.; and that, although some radiologists, regrettably, are in the high ranges, the average dose rate used by radiologists is half that used by other practitioners. Therefore, the following cautions may be considered timely and practical.

### *Specific Precautions*

A. Have the fluoroscope dealer renovate and modernize your machine according to state requirements.

B. Have a radiation physicist calibrate your machine and inspect it for overall safety.

C. In the meantime, use strict principles of operation of the machine.

1. Be dark adapted (ten to fifteen minutes) before starting fluoroscopy, since perception is better and faster in this manner.
2. Use high kilovoltage (80 to 90 for adults, 60 to 70 for children).
3. Use low milliamperage current (1 to 3 for adults, 1/2 to 1 for children). Have your milliamperes locked at 3 maximum.
4. Use small fluoroscope screen aperature (4 x 4 in.) and do not allow shutters to open anywhere near full screen dimension, since the image will be much sharper, perception better and protection much greater.
5. Use short time of fluoroscopy. Keep foot off the pedal switch when you are not actively inspecting a tissue. A stomach or colon study on a baby can be done by an experienced worker in one minute of actual fluoroscopy, using only 1 R of total fluoroscopic dose. For an adult, a good fluoroscopy of the chest can be done usually on ten to thirty seconds of actual exposure, producing 0.6 to 2 R total at the skin surface.

D. Choose your patients carefully and protect them.

1. Fluoroscope only those in whom fluoroscopy is really essential and will yield the best and most valuable data. Do not use this for survey or multiple follow-up work. Have the other patients examined by other means which are safer (film study).
2. Avoid fluoroscopy for infants, children and pregnant women. Since most diagnostic radiation does not approach 10 rads, most authorities agree that therapeutic abortion is not indicated when diagnostic radiation has occurred during any stage of pregnancy from two weeks until term. During the first two weeks of gestation, however, 10 rads increases the risk of fetal abnormalities and embryonic death. Use it sparingly on all under forty-five.
3. Cover the pelvis with a lead apron if your examination approaches the abdomen.
4. Have a time clock wired to your machine and allow yourself only one minute/patient of actual fluoroscopy. If absolutely necessary, reset for another minute, and so on.

E. Protect yourself.

1. Wear a generous cover-all lead apron from neck to knees; preferably with sleeves attached.
2. Wear full-weight radiologist's lead gloves.
3. Be well adapted to dark with red goggles (ten to fifteen minutes).

4. Obey your time clock.
5. Use a fluoroscopic screen that is equipped with lead glass and lead protection around the borders.
6. Wear a film-monitoring badge for all radiation work and have it measured by a reputable physicist or monitoring institution.

F. Protect your office force.
1. Cover all walls separating the fluoroscopic room from all persons with 1/32 inch lead sheeting, or occupy an equivalent concrete or masonry room.
2. Exclude from the fluoroscopic room any assistant or observer not gowned in generous lead apron or protected behind lead screen.

TABLE 150
RADIATION EFFECTS AT VARIOUS DOSES*

| *Organ or System Irradiated* | *Amount* | *Radiation Dose Area* | *Time* | *Type of Reaction or Damage* |
|---|---|---|---|---|
| Total body or trunk | 50 rads | — | short | Possible radiation sickness; malaise; nausea and vomiting; diarrhea |
| | 200 rads | — | short | Severe radiation sickness plus possible skin and mucous membrane hemorrhages; hematopoietic depression; possible death |
| | 200 rads | — | 20 years at 10 rads a year | No apparent effect on anyone |
| Skin | 100 rads | small | short | No visible effect |
| | 200–700 rads | small | 1 week or less | Sunburn type of reaction with tanning later; possible hair loss and regrowth |
| | 2,000–3,000 rads | limited | 1 month or less | Permanent tanning; permanent hair loss; destruction of sweat glands |
| | 3,000 or more rads | hands or other small area | several years small daily doses (1–5 rads) | No early or intermediate changes<br>Late changes manifested by dry cracked skin; nails curled and cracked; intractable ulcers; possibly cancerous ulcers |
| Blood forming organs | 25 rads | whole body | short | Possible transitory leukopenia |
| | 50 rads | whole body | short | Temporary leukopenia |
| | 100 rads | whole body | short | Possible prolonged leukopenia |
| | 200–500 rads | spinal bone marrow | short | Possible development of leukemia<br>Increased incidence with increased dose |
| Eyes | several hundred rads | lens | short | Cataract formation; over a long period the dose must be considerably higher before lens changes occur |
| Gonads | 200–300 rads | — | short | Temporary sterility |
| | 500 rads | — | short | Permanent sterility |
| | 2–5 rads weekly | — | years | Reduced fertility |
| Fetus | 40 rads at 18–48 days of pregnancy | pelvis of mother | short | Possible congenital abnormalities |
| | 1,000 rads in first 8 weeks | pelvis of mother | short | Possible miscarriage or still birth; the later the pregnancy, the less likely are congenital defects |

* Radioisotopes in Medicine, pamphlet, Abbott Laboratories

*Safety of Color Television Receivers*

To insure that the television contribution to the population gonad dose will only be a small fraction of that due to natural background radiation, the National Council on Radiation Protection and Measurement (NCRP) recommends that the exposure dose rate at any readily accessible point 5 cm from the surface of any home television receiver shall not exceed 0.5 milliroentgen (mr)/hr. under normal operating conditions.

The recommended operating voltage for most color receivers is 25 kv. At this voltage level, the x-ray output from the picture tube is usually well below the 0.5 mr/hr. level. If the operating voltage is set higher, say to 30 kv, the x-ray production is increased tenfold to twentyfold and could exceed the recommended maximum value. It is important, therefore, that a color set is operating at its recommended voltage. This level can be accurately checked and adjusted by authorized servicemen.

To eliminate the x-ray leakage from voltage-regulating devices, the television industry is presently engineering solid-state devices to control voltage and is developing better shielding of the high-voltage sections. Quality control in manufacture and assembly of color sets is monitored by the industry and the Underwriters Laboratory. Prototype and

TABLE 151
REPRESENTATIVE RADIOISOTOPE DIAGNOSTIC PROCEDURES

| *Isotope Employed* | *Organ and Process Investigated* |
|---|---|
| Radioiodine* | Thyroid function |
| Radioiodine-labeled compounds | |
| Radio-L-thyroxine | Thyroid-binding protein |
| Radioiodinated serum albumin | Circulation time |
| | Plasma volume |
| | Cardiac output |
| | Edema |
| Radioiodinated rose bengal | Liver function |
| | Cardiac output |
| Radio-iodopyracet | Kidney function |
| Radioiodinated insulin | Insulin requirements |
| Radioiodinated fat | Pancreatic function |
| | Gastrointestinal malabsorption |
| | Steatorrhea |
| Radio-L-triiodothyronine | Thyroid function (*in vitro*) |
| Radiochromium | Red cell mass |
| | Red cell survival |
| | Red cell sequestration (spleen) |
| Radioiron | Iron metabolism |
| | Absorption |
| | Utilization |
| | Hemoglobin formation |
| Radio-cyanocobalamin (vitamin $B_{12}$) | Pernicious anemia |
| | Malabsorption disorders |
| | Anemia following gastrectomy |
| | Chronic myelogenous leukemia |
| Radiosodium and radiopotassium | Water and electrolyte metabolism |
| Radiosulfate sodium | Extracellular fluid volume |
| Radio-iodohippurate sodium | Renal function |

*Incidence of hypothyroidism after $I^{131}$ therapy is greater than generally recognized. Rate of increase is practically a linear function from the third to at least the fifteenth year.

production models are tested for x-ray leakage at all stages of production. Some manufacturers unpack sets ready for shipment and completely retest them in order to ensure that their quality control methods are effective.

New standards effective on October 16, 1969, limited x-ray emissions to a maximum of 0.5 mr/hr. 5 cm from any external surface of a set operating at a maximum of 130 line volts under three operating conditions, each of which has a high x-ray generation potential. Receivers now have to be manufactured to meet the maximum under even more rigid operating conditions.

## RADIOACTIVE ISOTOPE POISONING

For the person who has inadvertently ingested radioactive substances, a purgative is the best single agent available to speed elimination of the material from the body. Plutonium ($^{239}Pu$) poisoning can be treated with diethylene triamine penta-acetic acid (DTPA), a chelating agent. The radiotoxicity of plutonium is such that one should work toward as near zero retention and absorption of plutonium in the body as possible. The most common known absorption source is from contaminated wounds, which should be treated by early excision of the entire wound. When surgical removal is not possible or ineffective, it would be highly desirable to increase chemically the absorption and translocation of plutonium from the injection site by use of intravenous DTPA. Inhaled plutonium is difficult to detect because the isotope emits no radiation that can be monitored from outside the body. However, plutonium's carcinogenicity (lung) has been reported to be seriously underestimated from inhalation.

The important forms of plutonium undergo decay by the emission of α particles. That α particles produce bronchogenic cancer in man is now an established medical fact, from the tragic experiences of the United States uranium miners. Since the α particles from plutonium are approximately of the same energy as those from the radon daughter products that provoked lung cancer in the miners, it follows that plutonium α particles must necessarily be capable of provoking lung cancer. Corresponding gonadal α radiation raises the possibility of severe genetic defects in future generations. Clearly plutonium is the most potentially toxic substance handled in quantity by man. However, the magnitude of the public health hazard of plutonium should be qualified by the following considerations.

DETECTABILITY. Plutonium is detectable both in the environment and *in vivo.* Unlike other carcinogens, therefore, persons potentially exposed to plutonium can be routinely monitored and removed from exposure when indicated.

DISTRIBUTION OF PRODUCTION SITES. If production is limited to few easily monitored sites, control is facilitated and risk is minimized. The handling of plutonium will be limited to a relatively few facilities for reprocessing and fuel synthesis. Shipments between facilities, should plutonium recycling begin, will increase the hazard of accident and accidental release; health consequences of road accidents will be small, however, since little dispersion, if any, would occur.

BIOCONCENTRATION. There is far less contamination of plant and animal tissues with plutonium than with many fission products. This is the corollary of poor gastrointestinal absorption.

INTRINSIC VALUE. The high commercial value of plutonium creates an economic incentive for careful management that is missing for other toxic materials of no intrinsic value.

Release of plutonium into the environment in the respirable form seems possible only in the very unlikely event of a reactor core melt, where sufficient heat is available to drive large quantities of plutonium into the air. Yet, because most of the plutonium would plate out on metal surfaces of the reactor, only a small part of the health impact of a reactor

TABLE 152
IMPORTANT RADIOISOTOPES USED IN MEDICINE AND BIOLOGY

| *Isotope (Symbol and Mass Number)* | *Half-Life* | *Type of Radiation* | *Uses* |
|---|---|---|---|
| $^{3}H$ | 12.46 yr | Beta | Total body water |
| $^{14}C$ | 5600 yr. | Beta | Protein metabolism |
| $^{24}Na$ | 15.06 hr. | Beta and gamma | Fluid balance |
| $^{32}P$ | 14.30 days | Beta | Rx polycythemia, tumor localization, immunologic expts. |
| $^{35}S$ | 87.1 days | Beta | Extracell. fluid, protein metabolism |
| $^{36}Cl$ | 4.4 x $10^{5}$ yr. | Beta (neg.) Beta (pos.) | Fluid partition |
| $^{38}Cl$ | 37.29 m. | Beta and gamma | Fluid partition |
| $^{42}K$ | 12.44 hr. | Beta and gamma | Fluid partition, renal function |
| $^{45}Ca$ | 152 days | Beta | Bone metabolism |
| $^{51}Cr$ | 27.8 days | Gamma | RBC survival and mass, splenic function in anemia |
| $^{52}Mn$ | 6.0 days | Beta and gamma | Localize brain tumors |
| $^{15}N$ | Stable isotope | Not radioactive | Protein and uric acid metabolism |
| $^{59}Fe$ | 45.1 days | Beta (and gamma) | Iron turnover |
| $^{60}Co$ | 5.27 yr. | Beta (and gamma) | $B_{12}$ absorption, teletherapy |
| $^{64}Cu$ | 12.8 hr. | Beta (neg.) Beta (pos.) Gamma | Tumor localization |
| $^{72}Ga$ | 14.3 hr. | Beta and gamma | Localize bone tumors |
| $^{74}As$ | 17.5 days | Beta (neg.) Beta (pos.) Gamma | Localize brain tumors |
| $^{85}Sr$ | 65 days | Gamma | Bone metabolism |
| $^{90}Sr$ | 19.9 yr. | Beta | Bone metabolism |
| $^{90}Y$ | 61 hr. | Beta | Bone metabolism |
| $^{137}Cs$ | 33 yr. | Beta and gamma | Teletherapy |
| $^{198}Au$ | 2.69 days | Beta (and gamma) | Tumor Rx, esp. effusions |
| $^{232}Th$ | 1.4 x $10^{10}$ yr. | Alpha (beta and gamma) | R-E blockade expts., localization of metastases (dangerous), radioautography |
| $^{226}Ra$ | 1620 yr. | Alpha, beta, and gamma | Tumor therapy |
| $^{131}I$ | 8.141 days | Beta and gamma | Thyroid function, localization of antibodies, insulin metab., blood vol., GI absorp., cardiac output, and Rx of thyrotox. and cancer |

meltdown would be anticipated from release of the plutonium inventory of the core. The population at greatest risk, therefore, will probably be those occupational groups handling large quantities of plutonium. The excellent record of the past thirty years provides assurance that this can be done safely.

Many other isotopes can be identified by analysis of the wave height on a counter, measuring radiation from the isotope excreted in the urine. *Caution!* One should always remember that radiation emitted by radioactive isotopes, even when administered in tracer doses, can damage living tissue in the same manner as do x-rays. Likewise, constant vigilance is required when radioactive substances are handled. Firm knowledge of the effects of radiation on man is still so meager that prudence dictates one should always avoid unnecessary radiation. A close parallel can be drawn with the many precautions required when handling highly infectious material. The hazards, in both instances, are directly influenced by the user: carelessness and untidy technic increase them; awareness and cleanliness greatly reduce them. Properly selected, applied and safeguarded, radioactive isotopes have become valuable aids in the diagnosis of many diseases and in some instances are now regarded as essential. It has been recently documented that aluminum phosphate gel, the antacid, inhibits the absorption of radioactive strontium in man.

## ROCKET FUELS (BORON HYDRIDE)

Exposure to fumes from high-energy rocket fuels in the processing and handling of these agents for the space program may produce pulmonary irritation with pneumonitis, central nervous system depression and hepatic and renal injury. The chemicals usually involved are diborane, pentaborane and decaborane. Diborane ($B_2H_6$), the most noxious of these compounds, is a highly reactive gas that hydrolyzes the boric acid and hydrogen within seconds of contact with water. The odor is described as nauseating.

Considerable heat released during the process may produce an exothermic reaction in the lungs. Tightness, heaviness and burning in the chest, nonproductive cough, dyspnea and precordial pain are noted. Chest films show transient infiltration. Prolonged exposure to low concentrations can produce headache, dizziness, chills and fever. Fatigue and transient muscle weakness and fasciculations may occur.

TABLE 153
RADIOISOTOPES AND ORGANS CURRENTLY SUBJECT TO SCANNING

| *Organ* | *Radioisotope and Symbol* | *Pharmaceutical* | *Physical Half-Life* | *Dose μc* | *Scan Performed* |
|---|---|---|---|---|---|
| Bone | $^{47}Ca$ | Calcium chloride | 4.8 days | 50 | 48 hr. |
| | $^{85}Sr$ | Strontium chloride | 65 days | 50–100 | 24–48 hr. |
| | $^{87m}Sr$ | Strontium chloride | 2.8 hours | 100–1000 | 40 min. |
| Bowel | $^{197}Hg$ | Chlormerodrin | 2.7 days | 1000 | 24 hr. |
| Brain | $^{74}As$ | Sodium arsenate | 17.5 days | 1000–1500 | 20 min. |
| | $^{99m}Tc$ | Technitate | 6 hr. | 10,000 | 10 min. |
| | $^{131}I$ | Human serum albumin | 8.1 days | 300–600 | 18–24 hr. |
| | $^{197}Hg$ | Chlormerodrin | 2.7 days | 700–1000 | 1–2 hr. |
| | $^{203}Hg$ | Chlormerodrin | 45.7 days | 700 | 2–4 hr. |
| Kidney | $^{99m}Tc$ | Technitate | 6 hr. | 1000 | Immediately |
| | $^{131}I$ | Hippuran | 8.1 days | 100–800 | Immediately |
| | $^{197}Hg$ | Chlormerodrin | 2.7 days | 100–150 | 1 hr. |
| | $^{203}Hg$ | Chlormerodrin | 47.9 days | 70–100 | 1–2 hr. |
| Liver | $^{198}Au$ | Colloidal gold | 2.7 days | 150 | 1–6 hr. |
| | $^{131}I$ | Cholografin rose bengal | 8.1 days | 50–150 | ½–1 hr. |
| Lung | $^{131}I$ | Colloidal human serum albumin | 8.1 days | 200 | Immediately |
| Mediastinum | $^{131}I$ | Cholografin or albumin | 8.1 days | 250 | 10 min. |
| Pancreas | $^{75}Se$ | Selenium methionine | 120 days | 200 | 30 min. |
| Parathyroid | $^{75}Se$ | Selenium methionine | 120 days | 200 | 2–8 hr. |
| Placenta | $^{131}I$ | Human serum albumin | 8.1 days | 3–5 | 10 min. |
| Spleen | $^{51}Cr$ | Sodium chromate | 27.8 days | 200 | 24 hr. |
| | $^{197}Hg$ | Bromomercuri-2-hydroxypropane | 65 hr. | 150 | 2 hr. |
| Thyroid | $^{131}I$ | Sodium iodide | 8.1 days | 50–100 | 24 hr. |

Pentaborane ($B_5H_9$) is a powerful reducing volatile liquid compound with a sweet odor. Hydrolysis to boric acid and hydrogen requires several hours. MAC is 0.05 ppm. Pulmonary symptoms are rare in poisoned persons. Neurologic signs may ensue rapidly after exposure or may not appear for forty-eight hours. Headache, dizziness, hiccups, drowsiness and post-prandial nausea are the usual initial symptoms. Nervousness and progressive incoordination are common. More severe symptoms include muscular pain and cramps, abdominal muscle spasm, fine tremor and convulsions. Slight hypertension may be noted.

Decaborane ($B_{10}H_{14}$) is a solid compound that hydrolyzes in about thirty days. Unlike the smells of diborane and pentaborane, the bitter chocolate-like odor of decaborane is detectable in subtoxic concentrations. Toxic reaction to the chemical is relatively slight, with headache and nausea the most frequent symptoms.

Liver function values may be abnormal in persons with boron hydride poisoning, and blood urea nitrogen levels are frequently elevated. The phenolsulfonphthalein excretion, urine, blood count, sedimentation rate, hematocrit value and prothrombin time are usually normal.

*Treatment* is symptomatic and supportive. Oxygen for the pulmonary symptoms is practically always necessary. In the more severe involvement with pneumonitis, corticosteroids and antibiotics may be beneficial. For the intense muscle pain and spasm, a skeletal muscle relaxant such as methocarbamol often gives prompt relief. Since these agents are potent reducing compounds, the use of methylene blue for its oxidizing capacity should be given a trial. Animal experiments have been promising.

## ROSIN (ABIETIC ANHYDRIDE, YELLOW RESIN, COLOPHONY)

This is the resinous substance that remains after the distillation of oil of turpentine from the fresh pitch of pine wood. It is now being used mainly as an adhesive (sticky fly papers, etc.), although at one time it was used therapeutically in ointments for the skin. Rosin oils are frequently used in lubricants, varnishes, paints and inks. The potential toxicity of these compounds is very low. A bezoar following ingestion is a possible complication.

## SAFFRON

Saffron is used almost exclusively for its yellow coloring and for flavoring of foods (*see* Volatile Oils). This agent (*Crocus Sativus*) has no toxic effects.

## SALT (SODIUM CHLORIDE)

The occurrence of mass accidental salt poisoning of infants in a hospital population where salt was inadvertently substituted for cane sugar (sucrose) has produced new concepts in the pathogenesis, neuropathology, symptoms and treatment of this physiological disturbance. Severe salt poisoning increases both the plasma sodium concentration and total sodium in the body, whereas hypertonic dehydration from other sources such as diarrhea increases the plasma sodium concentration but decreases total body sodium.

Early symptoms are referable to the gastrointestinal tract, with nausa, vomiting and refusal of feeding. Later there is evidence of central nervous system involvement either by frank convulsions or by muscular twitchings. Temperature elevation is common, and severe respiratory distress with tachypnea and dyspnea may be the predominating finding and deserves more emphasis as a pathognomonic sign. Renal damage is well documented and occurs often in hypernatremia. Actual damage resulting from temporary redistribution of water in infants is predominantly in the brain, and those who have died from salt poisoning have all shown extensive hemorrhagic phenomena in the central nervous system, as well as in the kidney tubules. A level teaspoonful of table salt contains more sodium and chloride ions (about 350 mEq) than does a 5 kg baby. This amount for a newborn is equivalent to about a pound for an adult. A more subtle way of intoxication with salt in a neonate is the continuous use of skim milk, which contains considerable natural sodium and chloride. When allowed to take skim milk ad lib, the sodium load/calorie is very high. An ill infant is least able to cope with this because he usually has increased water losses and a temporary impairment of renal concentrating ability.

Peritoneal dialysis may be a lifesaving procedure and is the *treatment* of choice for salt-poisoned infants.

1. It is a remarkably safe and simple technique.
2. It produces a striking reduction in the level of salt serum accompanied by a marked clinical improvement in the patient's condition.
3. The solutions used for dialysis should closely approximate the concentration of the serum in order to forestall excessive absorption of fluid from the peritoneal cavity, which can put undue strain on the cardiovascular and renal system. Glucose water, 7% or 8% without the addition of potassium appears to be the ideal solution. Other measures should be symptomatic and supportive for the respiratory distress, temperature elevation, etc.

The present practice of recommending the use of table salt as an emetic in first aid charts and on labels should be discontinued. There have been several reported deaths from hyponatremia in both adults and children from this use, when the desired effect (vomiting) did not occur. If retained, 1 tbsp. of salt can raise the serum sodium level approximately 25 mEq/liter in a three-year-old child with 10 liters of body water.

## SELENIUM DERIVATIVES

Selenium is a metallic element found widely in the soil and vegetation west of the Mississippi and produces more animal than human poisoning. The sulfide salt is commonly used for the treatment of seborrhea of the scalp. These are general protoplasmic poisons like arsenic, presumably involving sulfhydryl enzymes, producing degenerative lesions in the liver, kidneys, heart, spleen, stomach, intestine and lungs. The following is the approximate order of decreasing toxicity: soluble selenites, selenates, insoluble inorganic salts (selenium sulfide) and various organic derivatives, of which some are volatile. Metallic selenium is insoluble and not toxic unless finely divided as a fume. Selenium sulfide, since it is a water-insoluble compound, is not decomposed, and only traces are absorbed through the skin. Though selenium is far less toxic than the soluble salts, if ingested, the stomach should be thoroughly lavaged, followed by a saline cathartic. Oils and alcohol should be avoided since they increase absorption. The soluble selenium salts, on the other hand, give signs and symptoms similar to arsenic poisoning. The *treatment* is identical except that BAL should not be given as an antidote since there is some evidence that symptoms are aggravated instead of improved by its use. Bromobenzene 1 gm by mouth increases the urinary excretion of selenium and should be added to the treatment.

## SESAME OIL

This is a volatile oil extracted from the seeds of *Sesamum indicum L.* It is used as a vehicle for intramuscular medications as well as a synergist for pyrethrins. Ingested in large amounts, it has a laxative action; otherwise, it has very little toxic effect.

## SHELLAC

A variety of lac from India, produced on various plants by the insect *Coccus lactis,* shellac is processed for marketing by the paint industry. A small amount of rosin and arsenic trisulfide is added for coloring. White shellac, however, is free of arsenic. Methyl alcohol is the usual solvent; this as well as arsenic can produce symptoms of intoxication if appreciable amounts are ingested.

## SILICA (SILICONE DIOXIDE)

Silica is a chemically and biologically inert compound that is innocuous unless chronically inhaled, thereby occasionally producing a progressive pneumoconiosis (silicosis) (*see* Pneumoconioses).

## SILICONES (METHYL POLYSILOXANE)

These are polymeric substances in which the basic structure is a chain of silicon and oxygen atoms, to each of which is generally attached an organic radical. They are extremely inert materials, owing their usefulness to their physical properties, and are being used for their defoaming and deflatulent action in the gastrointestinal tract. The possibility of intoxication from such agents is highly improbable.

Silicone's inert properties, which by design make it ideal for local tissue prosthetic augmentation, can have long-term side-effects, such as migration, hypopigmentation, hepatic disease manifested as granulomatous hepatitis and even death.

## SMOKE POISONING

It has been suggested that patients overcome with smoke experience gastrointestinal rather than respiratory toxicity and that calcium carbonate and glycine should be used in treatment.

During exposure to irritating fumes, one may well swallow smoke containing toxic materials, but the stomach can only accommodate a limited gas volume. Furthermore, the gastric contents are normally highly acidic. Thus, it is unlikely that the suspended particles in the air that are swallowed can materially alter gastric pH.

Significant quantitative differences between wood and kerosene smokes are seen in the CO and aldehydes. There is ten times more CO and fifteen times more aldehydes in wood smoke than in kerosene smoke. Since CO is nonirritating, aldehydes are considered the likely etiologic gases in the production of exudative pulmonary edema.

The relatively high concentration of aldehyde gases in wood smoke, as well as in smoke from burning cotton clothing and household furniture, is one of the major causes of acute pulmonary injury in the smoke poisoning syndrome.

Smoke from burning synthetic (nylon,

TABLE 154
PRINCIPAL TOXIC COMBUSTION PRODUCTS OF COMMON SUBSTANCES*

| *Substance* | *Pulmonary Irritants* | *Other Toxic Gases* |
|---|---|---|
| Wood, cotton, newspaper | Acetaldehyde, formaldehyde | Acetic acid, methane, formic acid |
| Petroleum products | Acrolein | Similar to wood |
| Wool, silk | Ammonia | Hydrogen sulfide, hydrogen cyanide |
| Nitrocellulose film | Oxides of nitrogen | Similar to wood |
| Cellulose acetate film | None | Similar to wood |
| Polyester resins | Hydrogen chloride | |
| Polyurethane foam | Isocyanates | Hydrogen cyanide |
| Polyvinylchloride (PVC)** | Hydrogen chloride, phosgene, chlorine | |
| Polyfluorocarbons (e.g., Teflon) | Octafluoroisobutylene | |
| Phenolic resins | Ammonia, formaldehyde | Hydrogen cyanide |
| Melamine resins | Ammonia | Hydrogen cyanide |
| Rubber latex foam, neoprene foam | Unknown, but exposed rats die from pulmonary edema | |

*Carbon monoxide and carbon dioxide are produced in all cases.
Thomas, D.M., and Conner, E.H.: *J. Ky. M.A., 66*:1051–1056, 1968.
**PVC containers (beer and soda-pop) throw off hydrochloric acid when incinerated, becoming an irritant to the respiratory tract and skin, and creating a potential (and often unrecognized) hazard in apartment and city incinerators.

acrylic) carpets is particularly dangerous and highly toxic. Inhalation of burning fats can produce lipoid pneumonia and can be an occupational hazard.

The inhalation of highly irritating vapors such as certain war gases and oxides of nitrogen is known to cause severe respiratory distress. The clinical picture resembles acute pulmonary edema. Histologic examination of the lung at this stage demonstrates edema and bronchiolitis. The value of oxygen inhalation for pulmonary edema is well established. Its use is definitely indicated in pulmonary edema secondary to toxic fume inhalation.

Since severe degrees of pulmonary damage following moderate fume inhalation are rare, there is probably little need for oxygen in the management of the average smoke inhalation case. Nevertheless, oxygen should be readily available for treatment whenever required. The use of calcium carbonate and glycine, however, does not appear to have any merit. In extreme and serious smoke inhalation, it is particularly important to recognize the six– to forty-eight-hour latent period which may ensue before complications of acute bronchial obstruction, pneumonia, pulmonary edema and eventual cardiopulmonary failure develop. Standard roentgenography often fails to show smoke damage to fire victims' lungs which can be detected by perfusion scans. Management may require tracheostomy, prolonged intermittent positive-pressure breathing with appropriate concentrations of oxygen and high humidity and, when indicated, administration of systemic antibiotics and steroids. Frequent arterial blood gas measurements are essential for proper evaluation in these cases, both to delineate the status of the patients and to guide and determine the effectiveness of therapy. If victims of smoke inhalation can be managed through the acute phases of their illness, they often make a complete recovery. Thermal injury to the upper respiratory tract from the smoke or fire's heat aggravates all symptoms and produces a more serious condition.

## SMOKING DETERRENTS

Lobeline sulfate is by far the most frequently used active ingredient in smoking deterrents. Lobeline is the principal alkaloid of the plant *Lobelia inflata* (Indian tobacco). Pharmacologically it closely resembles nicotine although less toxic, and there is a strong cross-tolerance between the two. In theory, lobeline should produce a satiety effect which would decrease the desire for tobacco. It has the same kinds of effects on the central nervous system as does nicotine: first stimulation, then depression. It also stimulates certain medullary centers, especially the emetic center and the respiratory center, and in sufficient quantity, has a curare-like paralyzing action on the nerves to the voluntary muscles. Lobeline had been used as an emetic, respiratory stimulant and expectorant in the past but has now been largely discarded except for its use as a nicotine deterrent.

Even with the smaller doses used today, side-effects may sometimes be encountered. The most common are nausea, epigastric discomfort, dizziness and headache. These symptoms are especially noted after a cigarette is smoked and may add to lobeline's effectiveness as a deterrent. These symptoms tend to disappear even with continued use of the drug. The toxic symptoms of massive overdoses of lobeline mimic those of toxic doses of nicotine, e.g. nausea, vomiting, giddiness, abdominal pain and diarrhea, tremors, respiratory failure, convulsions and death.

Other smoking deterrent agents are benzocaine, silver acetate and numerous flavoring compounds. Benzocaine is a local anesthetic of low toxicity, but it has considerable allergenic potential. Silver acetate is usually incorporated in lozenges in very small doses to make smoking unpleasant because of the bad taste it produces. The hazard of acute poisoning from these is unlikely because of the dosage involved, but there is always the risk of argyria from the prolonged use of silver. A definite time limit should be placed on the use of silver salt as a deterrent.

*Treatment* of the accidental or deliberate ingestion of a large number of these products is gastric lavage or emesis. Otherwise therapy is symptomatic and supportive.

## SODIUM ALGINATE (ALGIN)

This is an agent widely used as an emulsifier and stabilizer in commercial ice cream. It is prepared from various seaweeds (kelp). Apparently it is not greatly absorbed or decomposed when ingested, and therefore it is a compound of minor toxic potential.

## SOLOX™

Solox is the trade name for a shellac solvent made according to the following formula: ethyl alcohol, 100 gal.; denatured grade wood alcohol, 5 gal.; gasoline, 1 gal.; ethyl acetate, undenatured, 1 gal.; methyl isobutyl ketone, 1 gal.

Ingestion of Solox in appreciable amounts produces coma, a foul chemical odor of the breath (similar to wood alcohol with a superimposed, sweetish, acetone-like quality), acidosis, and of particular importance, hypoglycemia. There is a peculiar extensor rigidity of the extremities, apparently correlated with the hypoglycemia.

*Treatment* consists of thorough gastric lavage or emesis with specific therapy for the acidosis or hypoglycemia that may occur.

## SPERMACETI

This is an emollient consisting chiefly of cetyl palmitate and used primarily for ointment bases. No toxicity has been reported from the ingestion of this compound.

## STARCH

Laundry starch eating is often the undiagnosed cause of iron deficiency anemia in blacks (*also see* Chap. 1). Southern blacks have eaten native red clay for years. The move to the cities deprived them of this source (unless obliging relatives shipped some north), so many blacks switched to eating Argo Gloss® Laundry Starch, a crude chunky form of cornstarch.

The craving for laundry starch or clay can begin at any age but typically affects only children and women. Why adult males do not develop the desire is a question. Mostly it is acquired by women during pregnancy. In areas like Mississippi, Texas and North and South Carolina, up to 30 per cent of the obstetric population eats starch.

The effects of daily ingestion of laundry starch are still unknown because virtually no studies have been done. About the only thing known is that it causes iron deficiency anemia and depletes the iron stores in bone marrow. Possibly it leads to hypertrophy of the parotid glands as they work overtime to counteract the dryness of the starch. Cholesterol levels in these people are low, perhaps because the starch absorbs bile acids in the intestinal tract. But there have been no studies on the effect of starch consumption on the fetus or whether it results in premature, malnourished or low-birth-weight babies.

## STEARIC ACID (OCTADECANOIC ACID)

This acid is a basic ingredient in cosmetic preparations of all kinds. It has a very low potential for toxicity and is a constituent of many neutral fats.

## STODDARD SOLVENT (VARSOL)

This is a solvent distillate (petroleum naphtha fraction) used in dry cleaning establishments. Mineral spirits and varsol are common synonyms. See *page* 225 for a detailed discussion.

## SULFOSALICYLIC ACID

This colormetric reagent (qualitative proteinuria testing) is usually dispensed as a 20% solution and often used in a more dilute form (3% to 5%). Ingestion of this product can cause intense vomiting, hyperpnea, rapid pulse, confusion, acidosis, coma, convulsions and shock. Allergic reactions can occur from any amount, and there may be some irritation to the skin and mucous membranes subsequent to chronic local exposure.

*Treatment* consists of emesis or gastric lavage unless previous severe vomiting precludes this. There is no specific antidote, and the remaining therapy should be supportive and symptomatic with correction of electrolyte disturbances when they occur.

## SULFUR

This compound and its varied preparations have been used by the medical profession for a variety of purposes. Probably the only valid use of sulfur is as a fungicide and for the treatment of various skin disorders.

Sulfur has few systemic actions. When taken by mouth it may be partially converted to sulfide, thereby producing a laxative action and rarely sulfhemoglobinemia. On the other hand, the parenteral administration of colloidal sulfur may cause fever, malaise, fatigue, headache, myalgia and drowsiness.

*Treatment* of intoxication from this drug consists of discontinuing its use and administering symptomatic and supportive measures as the need arises.

## SWEETENING AGENTS

*Saccharin* (anhydro-o-sulfamine benzoic acid) is a white crystalline substance which is about four hundred times as sweet as sugar without having any food value. American consumers eat or drink more than 5 million pounds of saccharin a year.

Ordinarily this is a harmless product, but in hypersensitive persons even small doses may cause gastrointestinal symptoms such as vomiting and diarrhea and allergic skin manifestations. The ingestion of large amounts can produce toxic symptoms with more pronounced vomiting, diarrhea, abdominal pain, frothing at the mouth, muscle spasm, convulsions and stupor. High levels of saccharin used for over twenty-five years did not increase the risk of cancer among diabetics in a study reported from Oxford University in England. Nevertheless, the Food and Drug Administration announced a ban on saccharin (March 9, 1977), the only artificial sweetener approved in the United States, because it causes cancer in laboratory animals.

*Treatment* necessitates gastric lavage or an emetic for large doses, followed by a saline cathartic; otherwise, supportive and symptomatic measures should be used as indicated.

Sucaryl is sodium or calcium cyclamate with a sweetening effect of 125 mg approximately equivalent to one teaspoonful of sugar (sucrose). A bitter taste becomes noticeable when the quantity in foods approaches 0.5 per cent. This is overcome by combining the agent with a suitable proportion of saccharin.

There is no evidence that the cyclamates are toxic when taken at levels up to 5 gm/day for seven and one-half months, but at this level the stools may become mushy. At 7 gm/day, a slight increase in frequency of bowel movements may occur. The level at which some softening of the stools occurs varies, and in some subjects 0.1 gm/day may produce some effect. There is no indication that this formation of mushy stools is related to any functional change in the gastrointestinal tract. The softening is probably due to an increase in fecal bulk arising from osmotic effects of unabsorbed cyclamate. Photosensitization, probably on a photoallergic rather than on a phototoxic effect, has been reported.

Cyclamates were removed from a list of substances recognized as safe in food and drink by the Secretary of Health, Education and Welfare on October 18, 1969, because of their carcinogenic effects on animals. It is impossible to assess the carcinogenic hazard to humans from the information currently available from studies in animals. The research which prompted the action to greatly restrict the availability of cyclamates was a two-year toxicologic study with rats fed three levels of a 10:1 cyclamate-saccharin mixture. Rats fed 2500 mg/kg of body weight developed malignant bladder tumors. No tumors were found in animals fed 500 or 1200 mg/kg of body weight. The Secretary of Health, Education and Welfare, when made aware of this information, had no choice under the provisions of the so-called Delaney clause (prohibits the use of any substance in any amount whatever, which, when fed to man or animals, induces cancer) of the Food, Drug and Cosmetic Act other than to remove cyclamates from the list of food chemicals generally regarded as being safe.

*Treatment,* if unusually large amounts are ingested, consists of gastric lavage or emesis.

## SWIMMING POOL DISINFECTANTS (PURIFIERS)

The recent rapid rise in popularity and increased construction of backyard swimming pools have brought forth many inquiries concerning the misuse and/or accidental ingestion of agents used as water purifiers or disinfectants. Practically all of these compounds, in tablet or powder form, such as Pittchlor, Pittabs, HTH, etc., have over 70 per cent calcium hypochlorite (70% available chlorine) in their formulation, and 15% liquid sodium hypochlorite is a common substitute for this purpose.

Calcium hypochlorite is a strong oxidant and should be stored in a cool, dry place, as exposure to high temperatures or contact with organic matter or acids may cause active decomposition with the release of heat, free chlorine and oxygen, creating a fire hazard.

The list of agents which can turn an innocent-looking drum of pool cleaning powder, granules or tablets into an inferno includes such household materials as cleansing and general disinfecting agents, mineral oils, kerosene, turpentine, lubricants and greases, beverages, tobacco, paper, rags and other similar products.

And it is not necessary to intentionally mix these items with calcium hypochlorite to produce fire. A pool owner who dipped a measuring cup that had previously been used to dispense an insecticide into a pool sanitizer created a reaction that immediately started a fire. In a similar incident, particles of grass seed left in a measuring cup dipped into a pool cleaning material started a fire. Scoops should be clean and dry and made of enamel, glass or porcelain. Moisture is also a threat. When the chemical is sprinkled over pool water or dropped into a pool in tablet form, there is no danger with proper stirring. But if water is spilled on the chemical in its container, it can burst into flames.

Certain types of metals are also a danger when dealing with calcium hypochlorite. Iron or manganese oxides, when put in contact with it, result in a reaction which produces oxygen. Pressure builds up within the container and eventually an explosion occurs. The most suitable containers are lined with rubber, ceramic or glass.

Never expose pool sanitizers to heat. Their containers should never be rolled, dropped or skidded while being moved. The resulting friction and heat buildup could ignite the contents.

If a fire should break out, it should be fought only with large quantities of water capable of drenching the area. The fire department should always be called even after immediate attempts to extinguish the blaze have begun. Never use a vaporizing liquid type fire extinguisher.

Ingestion of these compounds causes severe gastritis. Skin contact can produce drying and localized dermatitis due to the removal of skin oils and moisture. The fumes from decomposition are intensely irritating to the eyes and respiratory tract; leaks in chlorinators occasionally affect a group of people in the immediate area (*see* Chlorine, p. 245, for symptoms and treatment.)

*Treatment.* In case of ingestion, the stomach should be emptied by either gastric lavage or an emetic, followed by milk or another available demulcent. Where the skin or eyes are involved, it is essential that prolonged and thorough irrigation with tap water be carried out immediately. Methyl cellulose drops are effective for swimming pool conjunctivitis. Swimmers exposed to fresh water, whether chlorinated or not, do develop a conjunctivitis after prolonged exposure. This results from both the hypotonic effects of water and the direct action of chlorine on the sensitive eye.

Some swimmers are unusually sensitive to chlorine and are not able to participate in a swimming program in a chlorinated pool. A high concentration of chlorine contributes to maintaining the pool water in a bactericidal state but also predisposes to eye irritation. Chlorine undergoes gradual degradation, and the concentration is tested daily to maintain the desired level. Testing requirements vary from state to state, according to health regulations. The desirable pH of the water ranges from 7.4 to 7.8.

Preliminary investigations show that bromine is an adequate disinfectant for swimming water when present in excess of 2.0 ppm. Its antimicrobial effect is independent of free chlorine residuals. Bromination of pool water using bromochlorodimethyl-hydantoin in which residuals of free and combined bromine were maintained above 4.0 ppm achieved inactivation of coliform bacteria and enterococci. Only when the levels fell below 2.0 ppm were these organisms detected again. Relatively high bromine concentrations up to 9.0 ppm caused no discomfort to the bathers, nor was there any appreciable odor in the vicinity of the pool.

Armazide, basically a detergent compound, is a pool algicide and sanitizer which consists of 12% W/V each of dodecylamine hydrochloride, trimethyl alkyl ammonium chloride and methyl alkyl dipolyoxypropylene ammonium methyl sulfate. This preparation is only moderately irritating to the skin in its undiluted form and is nonirritating when diluted according to directions.

## TALC (TALCUM) U.S.P.

Talc is a finely powdered, native hydrous magnesium silicate with many obvious uses. Although no toxicity is recognized, the danger of pneumoconiosis after chronic inhalation should not be minimized (*see* Talcosis). Aspiration and inhalation by infants can produce serious pulmonary involvement and even death (fatality in a twenty-two-month-old child). The use of a talcum powder container as a favorite plaything for small children should be vehemently discouraged and parents must be informed and warned of this potential danger.

## TANNIC ACID NF

This is an astringent acid of moderately low toxicity. The ingestion of large doses can produce severe gastroenteritis with abdominal pain, while the injection of tannic acid has caused collapse, convulsions and death. It is a potent toxic compound to the liver.

The addition of 0.25% to 3.0% tannic acid to barium sulfate suspensions employed in the roentgenographic examination of the colon has been recommended by a number of roentgenologists and is widely used. The rationale is based on the following considerations: tannic acid as an astringent stimulates contracture of the colon, inhibits the secretion of mucin and causes precipitation of the protein of the superficial layers of the mucosa. It also facilitates the adherence of barium sulfate to the bowel wall and probably inhibits absorption of substances from the colon.

The fact that tannic acid is a potent hepatotoxin has been well established, both clinically and experimentally. Five deaths in children and three in adults have been reported from hepatic necrosis due to use of tannic acid in barium enema examinations, and this procedure should not be used in children or adults with hepatic disease. It probably should be discarded completely or replaced with ammonium alum, which has been demonstrated to be a far safer additive.

*Treatment* is symptomatic and supportive. Give milk or water to dilute, and perform gastric lavage for ingested tannic acid. Gelatin or beaten egg whites should then be administered to form insoluble tannates, which later should be removed by gastric lavage.

## TEAR GASES

The most commonly used preparations are chloroacetophenone (CN), ethylbromoacetate, bromoacetone, bromomethylethylketone and orthochlorobenzylidene malononitril (CS) (*see* page 250.)

Alpha-chloroacetophenone, even though called a "gas," is actually a fine powder. In commercial blast-dispersion cartridges, it is mixed half and half with silica anhydride, and a standard shotgun primer is used as a propellant. The mixture is an effective lacrimator in concentrations as low as 2 ppm of air. It can cause extreme irritation and edema of the mucous membranes of the nose and eyes if discharged into the face, and temporary blindness may result. The eyes should be irrigated for fifteen minutes with normal saline or water, if this occurs. Removing clothing and showering for decontamination of the skin is advisable. Defective tear gas pistols which have exploded in the hands have produced severe muscle and nerve injury.

## TEFLON, KEL-F

Teflon (polytetrafluoroethylene) and Kel-F are macromolecule resins which are pharmacologically inert. The many desirable qualities of Teflon have led to its wide use in industrial, domestic and medical application. These compounds are nontoxic when ingested, nonirritating to the skin and nonsensitizers. However, while stability (resistance to chemicals and heat) is one of its outstanding qualities, at very high temperatures (over 506° C) toxic fumes are produced. Symptoms consist of dyspnea, cyanosis of variable degree, chest pain and pulmonary edema ("polymer fume fever") similar to the syndrome of "metal fume fever."

Teflon-coated frying pans present no greater health hazard than the ordinary cooking oils used in metal cooking utensils (*see* Polymer Fume Fever).

## THIOCYANATES

Sodium and potassium thiocyanate are obsolete hypertensive drugs that have been largely replaced by safer and more effective compounds. These salts have a low therapeutic index, the fatal serum level being 20 mg/100 ml. Thiocyanate is reabsorbed by the renal tubules, and renal excretion is the only method for eliminating these ions from the body. Even when diuresis is forced, renal excretion is quite slow, and days or weeks may be required for elimination.

The principal manifestations of thiocyanate poisoning are caused by stimulation of the central nervous system. Symptoms include mental confusion, hallucinations, delirium, psychotic behavior, hypotension, muscular spasms and convulsions.

Chronic poisoning due to prolonged use of the drug may produce urticaria, dermatitis, abnormal bleeding and thyroid enlargement.

Current methods of *treatment* are supportive in nature. If kidney function is normal, urinary output is kept at high levels so as to hasten excretion. If psychotic behavior is seen or if the serum level is 14 mg% or higher, thiocyanates should be removed by peritoneal dialysis or by hemodialysis. Thiocyanate has a molecular weight of 58. Furthermore, its ions are almost totally distributed throughout the extracellular fluid, with about one-third reversibly bound to protein and lipid. These properties enable the thiocyanate ions to be easily dialyzed. It has been clearly demonstrated that hemodialysis is about eighty times more effective than urinary excretion in removing thiocyanate and can be a lifesaving procedure.

## THIOGLYCOLATE SALTS

The toxic dose of thioglycolate salts is estimated to be in excess of 30 gm. The quantities usually present in hair-waving lotions are generally too small to cause serious effect. When ingested in toxic amounts, however, the alkalinity (pH 9) is capable of producing a severe caustic burn. Hypoglycemia, central nervous system depression, convulsions and dyspnea have been reported in experimentally poisoned animals.

*Treatment* is similar to that used for caustic alkalis, albeit less vigorous.

## THUJA (YELLOW CEDAR, ARBOR VITAE)

This is an evergreen tree of eastern North America largely cultivated for ornamental purposes and as a hedge. A fluid extract from this plant has been used in the past as an expectorant, emmenagogue, anthelmintic and abortifacient. Symptoms of poisoning consist of severe abdominal pain with diarrhea, dyspnea, frothing at the mouth, pulmonary depression and tonic and clonic convulsions. If seen early, gastric lavage should be carried out immediately. Short-acting barbiturates should be given to prevent or terminate convulsive seizures. *Treatment* otherwise is symptomatic and supportive.

## TOBACCO

Deaths have been reported from the ingestion and rectal administration of a few grams of tobacco. Many infants, however, have chewed and swallowed tobacco and cigarettes with impunity. Nevertheless, it is estimated that the nicotine content in the tobacco of some American cigarettes varies from about 15 to 20 mg. Within any one brand, however, the nicotine content remains quite constant but low tar cigarettes are now the vogue. There is considerable individual variation in minimally toxic doses, but oral ingestion of as little as 2 to 5 mg may cause nausea. The oral lethal dose, ingested at one time, has been estimated to be between 40 and 60 mg.

It would not take much imagination to foresee in a small child the possible toxic effects from the ingestion of three or four cigarettes. Fortunately, the gastrointestinal absorption of nicotine, as it is present in tobacco, is so slow that spontaneous vomiting removes much unabsorbed alkaloid. The remaining nicotine is poorly absorbed because of the acidity of the stomach contents (*see* Nicotine).

## TRICALCIUM PHOSPHATE

Besides its presence in dentifrices as an abrasive, tricalcium phosphate also is added as an anti-caking, flow-promoting agent to a variety of food powders, salt and products for industrial application. Dicalcium phosphate, an abrasive in many toothpastes, is of different crystalline structure, harder and almost as insoluble as the tricalcium salt.

Often repeated, inadvertent inhalation or unusual ingestion of these agents has been reported, in at least one case, to have produced systemic and pulmonic granulomatous lesions, which were puzzling and a diagnostic perplexity.

## TRICHLOROACETIC ACID

This is a corrosive organic acid which is used for penetrating and fixing tissues. The toxic effects are due to the gastrointestinal injury and acidosis rather than to the trichloroacetate ion, which apparently has a low inherent toxicity.

## TRIS-BP

Tris-BP (tris [2,3-dibromopropyl] phosphate) is widely used as a flame retardant in children's clothing and other materials as a consequence of federal regulations designed to reduce injuries and deaths that result from children's clothing catching fire. Two reports suggest that this agent is mutagenic in bacterial test systems used to screen chemicals for carcinogens and may also be carcinogenic. Although the data implicating Tris-BP as a carcinogen are inconclusive, the possible consequences of the widespread use of Tris-BP are serious, since it comes off fabric, can be absorbed topically, is a strong mutagen and may contain a potent carcinogen. Ingestion of the agent could result when infants and young children suck their clothing. Washing Tris-treated clothing three times appears to remove 95 per cent of the chemical without significantly reducing the overall flame-retardant properties. The use of Tris-BP as a flame retardant in children's clothing has now been banned by the United States Consumer Product Safety Commission.

## TURKEY RED OIL

This is an anionic surfactant prepared by sulfating castor oil and consisting mainly of the ammonium salt of ricinoleic sulfuric acid ester. It is used in agriculture and the textile industry and has a low toxic potential.

## UVA URSI

This is a volatile oil containing a glucoside, arbutin, tannin and gallic and malic acids. Arbutin is broken down into hydroquinone, which appears in the urine after large doses. Now obsolete, it once was used as an antiseptic and diuretic.

## VITRIOLIC ACID

This is a commercial sulfuric acid agent containing 95 per cent hydrogen sulfate and 5 per cent water. The estimated lethal dose of this mineral acid is 1 oz.

## WATER GLASS

This is a slightly alkaline compound of variable composition, containing mainly sodium silicate, which has a low inherent toxicity. Skin contact causes irritation.

## WELDING HAZARDS

Toxic gases or fumes may be produced during gas-shielded arc welding and can be the most insidious, because unseen, hazards of the industry. They are toxic oxides of nitrogen, ozone by action of ultraviolet rays on oxygen in the air, irritant and toxic breakdown products by action of ultraviolet rays or chlorinated hydrocarbon vapors in the area, and toxic fumes from the melting of toxic metals or metal alloys. Toxic fume constituents are produced by all electrodes, ferrous and nonferrous, consumable and nonconsumable, coated and noncoated. Used in submerged arc, inert gas, metal arc, Heliarc, and Aircomatic processes filler materials (mild steel, stainless steel, silicone, bronze, copper, aluminum, nickel, monel and aluminum bronze); used in atomic hydrogen welding with thoriated tungsten electrodes; and used in carbon arc welding with copper-filled metal, the toxic fume constituents may produce the following symptoms.

Copper causes fume fever, chills, sweating and dry throat.

Chromium causes severe nasal irritation and nasal ulcers.

Fluorides cause nasal and throat irritation, severe reactions.

Iron oxide in a large quantity in the lungs may cause impaired breathing. Reddish-brown fumes may impair visibility.

Ozone causes irritation in eyes and respiratory tract and headache. Ozone is generated when ultraviolet radiation of sufficient intensity and wavelength from the arc activates oxygen molecules in the surrounding air. Substantial concentrations of this gas can form several feet from the arc, the amount depending on the metals involved in the weld, the type of gas used as the shield—argon produces a greater amount of ozone than helium—and the temperature of the arc.

Ozone levels of 2 to 9 ppm have been reported to cause pulmonary congestion in shielded arc welders, whereas at 0.2 ppm this effect was not apparent. Substantial changes in lung function have occurred in other humans during prolonged exposure (three hours/day and six days/week for twelve weeks) at 0.5 ppm. The American Conference of Governmental Industrial Hygienists has accordingly recommended that the time-weighted average exposure for an eight-hour working day be limited to 0.1 ppm so as to prevent any discernible injury. It is highly advisable, therefore, that adequate ventilation be provided. Preferably, some type of local exhaust should be in close proximity to the weld areas at all times.

Thoriated tungsten causes impaired breathing.

Atmospheric studies at the breathing zone of the worker must be made to determine whether the gases or fumes are produced in sufficient quantities to cause symptoms.

Argon used as a shield gas in welding presents no hazard. The gas is a simple asphyxiant and is physiologically inert. It is only hazardous at the point of production or in a closed storage room containing cylinders of the gas.

Excessive concentrations of gases or fumes can be controlled by properly designed local exhaust ventilation. If such ventilation is impractical for the job situation, the worker should wear personal protective respiratory equipment.

During gas-shielded arc welding there may be hazards from intense ultraviolet, visible and infrared radiation. The ultraviolet light generated can cause keratoconjunctivitis. The action of infrared rays is thermal, and although such action gives warning in the skin, in the eye there is no warning. Proper standard lenses worn under the helmet protect against stray flashes, reflected ultraviolet light and radiant energy.

## WITCH HAZEL (HAMAMELIS, WINTER BLOOM, SNAPPING HAZEL, STRIPED OR SPOTTED ALDER, TOBACCO WOOD)

The term "witch hazel" is commonly employed to mean witch hazel extract.

WITCH HAZEL. The dried leaves of *Hamamelis virginiana* contain tannin (2% to 9%), gallic acid, volatile oil and bitter principle. It has been used in suppositories in therapeutic doses of 2 gm as an astringent.

WITCH HAZEL EXTRACT (WITCH HAZEL WATER). A saturated aqueous distillate from the twigs and leaves of *Hamamelis virginiana* to which about 15 per cent alcohol has been added. In addition to the constituents listed above, this preparation contains small amounts of terpenes (sesquiterpenes). It is used externally as an astringent.

WITCH HAZEL FLUIDEXTRACT, NF IX. An extract of *Hamamelis* leaf contains 70 to 78 per cent ethyl alcohol. It has been used in therapeutic doses of 2 to 4 ml.

The toxic symptoms from ingestion of any of the above products are due to their tannin (tannic acid) and ethyl alcohol content. Witch hazel (dried leaves) has an estimated lethal dose of 5 to 15 gm/kg for man. The leaves contain less than 10 per cent tannin. Tannin is an irritant and has an estimated adult lethal dose of 500 to 5000 mg/kg, while ethyl alcohol has an estimated lethal dose of 250 to 500 ml. Ingestion produces mucous membrane and gastrointestinal irritation due to the tannin, and large amounts may produce exhilaration or central nervous system depression due to the ethyl alcohol. In cases reported to the National Clearinghouse for Poison Control Centers, young children and adults ingesting witch hazel extract in amounts up to 240 ml exhibited no symptoms other than irritation or burning of the upper gastrointestinal tract and in one young child, dizziness.

For *treatment,* give milk or demulcents. Observe for possible symptoms of ethyl alcohol intoxication if the fluid extract or great amounts of the extract have been ingested. Emptying of the stomach is probably not necessary unless the quantity taken is unusually large.

## XYLENE (BENZENE, TOLUENE, CUMENE, MESITYLENE)

These are aromatic hydrocarbon solvents widely used in industry and around the home in paint removers, lacquers, degreasing cleaners, insecticides and pesticides. They are toxic by all portals of entry, but percutaneous absorption is generally too slow to produce acute systemic poisoning. Essentially the same train of symptoms follows the ingestion of liquid and the inhalation of vapor, but in respiratory exposures bronchial and laryngeal irritation are usually more prominent. All of these aromatic hydrocarbons produce basically similar toxic reactions, namely local irritation, central nervous system excitation and depression and bone marrow inhibition. The lethal dose of xylene is not known but is probably about 15 ml by mouth. Symptoms consist of burning sensation in the mouth, nausea, vomiting, salivation, substernal pain, cough and hoarseness. In vapor exposures transient euphoria is sometimes observed. Headache, giddiness, vertigo, ataxia and tinnitus occur often with confusion, stupefaction and coma. Associated with coma are tremors, motor restlessness, hypertonus and hyperactive reflexes. Frank convulsions rarely occur except with terminal asphyxia. Death is from respiratory failure or from sudden ventricular fibrillation. Contact with liquid may cause erythema and blisters of the skin and hemorrhagic inflammatory lesions of mucous membranes.

### *Glue Sniffing*

Deliberate inhalation by children and adolescents of model cement (glue) vapors has recently become a major problem. This practice results in an initial sense of exhilaration and euphoria which progresses to disorientation and coma if continued. In many ways the symptoms are similar to those produced by ethyl alcohol. Toxic hallucinations, bizarre and inappropriate behavior and antisocial acts frequently result from glue sniffing. Thus, it has become a prominent contributing factor in delinquency, which is causing increasing concern to juvenile authorities. The favorite glue implicated to date is Testor's® Polystyrene Plastic Cement, which contains 100 per cent toluene.

Glue sniffing is done in the following manner. About one half of a tube of model glue is squeezed into a cloth, rag, sock or plastic bag; the vapors are inhaled either through the mouth or nostril until the desired results are obtained.

So far no residual toxic effects have been found in the individuals involved, but in addictive chronic sniffers toxic polyneuritis may occur. The MAC of toluene is 200 ppm. Toluene is initially oxidized to benzoic acid, which in turn is conjugated with glycine and is excreted in the urine as hippuric acid. Glue sniffers may have a rise in the blood toluene concentration and a corresponding increase in urinary hippuric acid excretion. The variable effects of toluene on the hematopoietic system (bone marrow depression and hepatic enlargement) have been well documented in the literature. Two decades ago toluene often contained as much as 20 per cent benzene; however, a recent survey of commercial toluene reveals less than a 0.5 per cent contamination of benzene. Although the physical consequences from glue sniffing may not appear serious, the chronic effects have not as yet been determined. The major stimulus, however, is toward increasing delinquency and creating a juvenile problem of increasing magnitude. A coordinated approach to this problem should include the following measures: efforts aimed at correcting the underlying emotional disorder when one exists; a community program to educate parents and children to the potential risk of such sniffing; making these preparations less available on the open "serve yourself" shelves of stores, substituting less toxic organic solvents wherever possible; and adding special odor retardants to these compounds. The Testor Corporation, a leading manufacturer of quick-drying plastic glue for hobbyists, has now added mustard oil (allylisothiocyanate) to its product to make it obnoxious to sniffers. The oil affects the nasal area with the impact of a mouthful of mustard or horseradish and hopefully will be so disagreeable to sniffers that one experience will suffice.

The toxicity of toluene di-isocyanate (TDI) is well known to persons who handle this chemical, which is widely used in industry as a polymerizing agent in the production of foam plastics and other polyurethane materials. Symptoms caused by TDI vapor can be misdiagnosed as influenza, bronchitis, asthma or bronchopneumonia. Physicians responsible for preemployment and placement examinations of workers should constantly be aware of any possible exposure to this toxic vapor and should pay particular attention to the pulmonary status of workers to be engaged in operations where TDI is used. Exposure to TDI vapors can lead to protracted respiratory disease. Successful treatment depends upon removal of the patient from exposure to the agent.

### *Treatment of Toluene Toxicity*

1. Cautious gastric lavage with warm water. Mineral oil, 1 or 2 oz., may be instilled and left in the stomach at the completion of lavage.
2. Sodium or magnesium sulfate (15 to 30 gm dissolved in water) as a saline cathartic.
3. Ascorbic acid (50 to 100 mg IV) has been reported as beneficial in the treatment of benzene poisoning.
4. General supportive measures, including oxygen administration, artificial respiration and parenteral fluids, as indicated.
5. Avoid epinephrine because of its possible adverse effect on the sensitized myocardium. Abstain from all digestible fats and oils and alcohol, which might promote intestinal absorption.
6. If eyes or skin are affected, wash thoroughly and apply a bland analgesic ointment. An ophthalmic ointment with added corticosteroid is far more effective if the eyes are severely involved.
7. *Also see* Benzene (Toluene).

*Chapter 11*

# PUBLIC SAFETY EDUCATION

In recent years there has been repeated publicity relating to deaths due to suffocation in plastic bags among infants and children, to fatalities and morbidity from lead poisoning due to the ingestion of paint flakes which have fallen from rooms in old and dilapidated homes and to inadequate ventilation for widely used space heaters, leading to carbon monoxide poisoning, particularly in house trailers. The recognition of unused refrigerators as asphyxiating hazards to children dates back only a few years and is a continuing potential hazard.

The substitution of detergents for soap has enhanced the efficiency of many cleansing operations, but it has also increased irritative and allergic reactions and introduced a new hazard of poisoning. Useful but caustic chemicals have helped to keep drains and soil pipes cleaner but continue to be a source of possible poisoning or caustic injury to delicate tissues such as conjunctivae or mucous membranes. Garden chemicals for weed and pest control present an ever increasing problem in accidental poisoning, especially when these are carelessly stored in milk or soft drink bottles.

The hazard of carbon monoxide poisoning is not limited to trailers and shack homes. Even the modern heating system, if improperly vented, may feed back carbon monoxide into the home, as may gasoline motors left running unattended in closed attached garages.

The dangers created by the increased use of potent drugs, particularly self-medication with barbiturates and tranquilizers, are increasing rather than diminishing despite warnings by medical and public health authorities.

Food and fruits potentially contaminated by chemicals and insecticides focus more attention on the possible hazards resulting from weed and pest control sprays and from food additives.

The multiplicity of labor-saving devices now fills the home with heavier electric currents and more rapidly moving machinery. Do-it-yourself equipment, particularly power tools, creates additional dangers, especially in the hands of the unskilled. The homemade extension and frayed electric cord continue to threaten electrocution of the unwary.

A look at safety in the home and environment is certainly indicated, in a spirit of inquiry, evaluation and prevention rather than panic. The responsibility is particularly great on the manufacturers and distributors of potentially dangerous substances and devices, on the public officials charged with the responsibility for their control and on the medical profession for devising and publicizing means of prevention as well as for developing effective treatment.

Physicians therefore should take a more active role in safety education through existing local organizations, civic clubs and churches. Office visits and particularly house calls, rare though they may be, provide excellent opportunities for directing parents in this regard, since the obvious hazards in and about the home can be readily pointed out. The following items of information and preventive measures are presented solely as a basis for civilian and lay group instruction and patient education.

## POISON CONTROL CENTERS

In 1976, approximately 5000 persons died from accidental poisoning (including gases and vapors) in the United States, with an incidence of well over 2 million. However, since poisoning is not a reportable condition, these figures may be just the "tip of the iceberg." If the facts were known, there are adults and many children who die from poisoning who are never correctly diagnosed and therefore not tabulated statistically. In addition, many other children and adults are either crippled, made seriously ill or require some treatment for accidental nonfatal poisoning. With the large number of new, potentially toxic household products being developed, the problem of accidental poisoning becomes increasingly complex.

To treat an accidental poisoning properly, the nature of the offending substance must be known. What few specific antidotes are available can thus be utilized. Although most cases of poisoning are managed according to a few principles—termination of exposure, evacuation, dilution, support and symptomatic management—it is helpful if the identity of the poison or chemicals in the ingested agent is known. Pesticides, caustics, drugs and cosmetics containing coal tar derivatives are required by law to bear labels listing ingredients.

However, until 1960 many household products were not so labeled. The busy practitioner of medicine could not be expected to be familiar with ingredients or formula changes of trade name products and the 250,000 household agents, many with potentially toxic chemicals. Thus, since 1953 poison control centers have been helping physicians in dealing with poisoning, and now there are approximately 600 poison control centers in the United States.

Poison control centers perform a number of functions. Chemical and toxicity information on almost any toxic or potentially toxic product is available to physicians in cases of poisoning. The centers keep abreast of current methods of therapy for poisoning and can advise inquiring physicians accordingly. Such information is available to physicians twenty-four hours a day and is ordinarily dispensed by a physician at the center (usually a resident physician if the center is located in a hospital). In some centers, pharmacists, nurses or sanitarians working under a physician's supervision give this information.

If a lay person calls a nontreatment center for help (such as the distraught mother whose child just swallowed some sleeping pills), only immediate first aid instructions are given, and the person is advised to call his physician at once.

Besides giving information, many of the centers are set up to give treatment for poisoning or are affiliated with a cooperating hospital or hospitals where treatment can be obtained. However, poison control centers are not the only foci for poison treatment activity. Any well-equipped emergency room can properly administer emergency treatment.

Other poison control activities include research into the problem of accidental poisoning. Many of the centers keep records on all poisoning cases coming to their attention. Follow-up on poisoning cases is often achieved in cooperation with local health departments.

The poison control center can and does serve in many communities as a stimulus to prevention activities. Here lies the crux of the problem of accidental poisoning, of all accidents—prevention.

Poison control centers are usually sponsored by or affiliated with local or state health departments, medical schools, local medical societies and state chapters of the American Academy of Pediatrics. Almost all of these centers are located in hospitals.

It is not easy to develop and operate a poison control program. Providing a twenty-four-hour telephone information service on the toxicity of almost any product or substance which an infant is likely to ingest is no small operation. The information must be at hand or almost immediately available to center personnel. Regardless of whether they are physicians, nurses, sanitarians or pharmacists, these individuals must be trained to utilize the informational sources available to them in an intelligent and effective manner.

In 1957, the National Clearinghouse for Poison Control Centers (Bureau of Medicine, Department of Health, Education and Welfare, Washington, D.C., 20204) was established with the United States Public Health Service as a service unit for the centers. The National Clearinghouse performs those functions which aid in the successful operation of the local center, such as furnishing toxicity and treatment information on household products to the various centers. It also codes, tabulates and analyzes the poisoning reports from those centers requesting the service.

The effectiveness of the local poison control center depends on the number of physicians in the area who use the services. To learn the location of your local, or the nearest, poison control center, *see* Table 155, United States Directory of Poison Control Centers.

TABLE 155
UNITED STATES DIRECTORY OF POISON CONTROL CENTERS, 1977*

| *City* | *Name and Address* | *City* | *Name and Address* |
|---|---|---|---|
| | **ALABAMA** | | |
| STATE COORDINATOR | Department of Public Health<br>Montgomery 36104<br>(205) 832-3194 | | |
| Anniston | N. E. Alabama Regional Medical Center<br>400 E. 10th St. 36201<br>(205) 237-5421 Ext. 307 | Gadsden | Baptist Memorial Hospital<br>1007 Goodyear Avenue 35903<br>(205) 492-1240 Ext. 205 |
| Auburn | Auburn University School of Pharmacy 36830<br>(205) 826-4037<br>(Night) 887-6778, 887-3235 | Huntsville | Huntsville Hospital<br>101 Sivley Rd. 35801<br>(205) 539-9411 |
| Birmingham | Children's Hospital<br>1601 6th Ave., S. 35233<br>(205) 933-4050 | Mobile | Mobile General Hospital<br>2451 Fillingim St. 36617<br>(205) 473-3325 |
| Dothan | Southeast Alabama General Hospital 36301<br>(205) 794-3131 Ext. 521 | Opelika | Lee County Hospital<br>2000 Pepperill Parkway 36801<br>(205) 745-4611 |
| Florence | Eliza Coffee Memorial Hospital<br>600 W. Alabama St. 35630<br>(205) 764-8321 Ext. 206, 207 | Tuskegee | John A. Andrew Hospital<br>Tuskegee Institute 36088<br>(205) 727-8485 |
| | **ALASKA** | | |
| STATE COORDINATOR for Administration | Department of Health and Social Services<br>Juneau 99811<br>(907) 465-3100 | | |
| STATE COORDINATOR for Epidemiology and Reporting | Alaska Native Health Service<br>Anchorage 99510<br>(907) 279-6661 Ext. 308, & 380 | | |

*U.S. Department of Health, Education and Welfare, Public Health Service, Food and Drug Administration, John J. Crotty, M.D., Director, 5401 Westbard Avenue, Bethesda, Maryland, 20016.

This Directory of Poison Control Centers has been compiled from information received from the centers and state departments of health. It is revised periodically in an attempt to keep it up-to-date. Since changes occur frequently, it is impossible for the directory to be completely current; indeed, some of the material (1977) may already be incorrect.

TABLE 155—*Continued*
UNITED STATES DIRECTORY OF POISON CONTROL CENTERS, 1977*

| *City* | *Name and Address* | *City* | *Name and Address* |
|---|---|---|---|
| | **ALASKA** *(Continued)* | | |
| Anchorage | Providence Hospital<br>3200 Providence Dr. 99504<br>(907) 274-6535 | Ketchikan | Ketchikan General Hospital<br>3100 Tongass Ave. 99901<br>(907) 225-5171 Ext. 31 |
| Fairbanks | Fairbanks Memorial Hospital<br>1650 Cowles 99701<br>(907) 456-6655 Ext. 15 | Sitka<br>Mt. Edgecumbe | PHS Alaska Native Hospital<br>Box 577 99835<br>(907) 966-2411 |
| Juneau | Bartlett Memorial Hospital<br>Box 3-3000 99802<br>(907) 586-2611 | | |
| | **ARIZONA** | | |
| STATE<br>COORDINATOR | College of Pharmacy<br>University of Arizona<br>Tucson 85721<br>(602) 882-6300 | | |
| Douglas | Cochise County Hospital<br>Rural Route #1 85607<br>(602) 364-7931 | Prescott | Yavapai Community Hospital<br>1003 Willow Creek Rd. 86301<br>(602) 445-2700 Ext. 25, 6 |
| Flagstaff | Flagstaff Hospital<br>1215 N. Beaver St. 86001<br>(602) 744-5233 Ext. 255, 4,232 | Tucson | Kino Community Hospital<br>(Pima County General)<br>2800 E. Ajo Way 85713<br>(602) 294-4471 Ext. 170, 1, 2, 3 |
| Ganado | Navajo Health Foundation<br>Sage Memorial Hospital<br>P. O. Box 457 86505<br>(602) 755-3411 | | St. Mary's Hospital<br>1601 W. St. Mary's Rd. 85703<br>(602) 622-5833 Ext. 625, 6, 623 |
| Kingman | Mohave General Hospital<br>3269 Stockton Hill Rd. 86401<br>(602) 757-2101 Ext. 117, 8, 9 | | Tucson General Hospital<br>3838 N. Campbell Ave. 85719<br>(602) 327-5431 Ext. 111 |
| Nogales | St. Joseph's Hospital<br>Target Range Road<br>P. O. Box 1809 85621<br>(602) 287-2771 Ext. 94 | | Tucson Medical Center<br>East Grant Rd. and<br>Beverly Bvd. 85716<br>(602) 327-5461 Ext. 482 |
| Phoenix | Good Samaritan Hospital<br>1033 E. McDowell Rd. 85006<br>(602) 257-4545 | | University of Arizona<br>College of Pharmacy 85721<br>(602) 882-6300 |
| | Maricopa County General Hospital<br>2601 E. Roosevelt 85008<br>(602) 267-5011 Ext. 5411 | Winslow | Winslow Memorial Hospital<br>1500 Williamson Ave. 86047<br>(602) 289-4691 |
| | Memorial Hospital<br>1201 S. 7th Ave. 85007<br>(602) 252-5911 Ext. 391 | Yuma | Yuma Regional Medical Center<br>Avenue A and 24th St. 85364<br>(602) 344-2000 Ext. 321 |
| | St. Joseph's Hospital<br>350 W. Thomas Rd. 85013<br>(602) 277-6611 Ext. 3581 | | |
| | St. Luke's Hospital<br>Medical Center<br>525 N. 18th St. 85006<br>(602) 253-3334 | | |

TABLE 155—*Continued*
UNITED STATES DIRECTORY OF POISON CONTROL CENTERS, 1977*

| *City* | *Name and Address* | *City* | *Name and Address* |
|---|---|---|---|
| | **ARKANSAS** | | |
| STATE COORDINATOR | Department of Health<br>Little Rock 72201<br>(501) 661-2397 | | |
| El Dorado | Warner Brown Hospital<br>460 West Oak St. 71730<br>(501) 863-2266 Ext. 221 | Helena | Helena Hospital<br>Hospital Drive 72342<br>(501) 338-6411 Ext. 271 |
| Fort Smith | St. Edward's Mercy Hospital<br>7301 Rogers Ave. 72903<br>(501) 452-5100 | Little Rock | University of Arkansas Medical Center<br>4301 W. Markham St. 72201<br>(501) 661-6161 |
| | Sparks Regional Medical Center<br>1311 S. Eye St. 72901<br>(501) 441-4381 | Osceola | Osceola Memorial Hospital<br>611 Lee Ave. West 72370<br>(501) 563-2611 Ext. 53 |
| Harrison | Boone County Hospital<br>620 N. Willow St. 72601<br>(501) 365-6141 Ext. 120 | Pine Bluff | Jefferson Hospital<br>1515 W. 42nd Ave. 71601<br>(501) 535-6800 Ext. 4706 |
| | **CALIFORNIA** | | |
| STATE COORDINATOR | Department of Health<br>Sacramento 95814<br>(916) 322-2300 | | |
| Fresno | Fresno Community Hospital<br>Fresno and R Sts.<br>P.O. Box 1232 93715<br>(209) 233-0911 Ext. 2431 | Sacramento | Emergency Medical Services<br>Sacramento Medical Center<br>University of California, Davis<br>2315 Stockton Blvd. 95817<br>(916) 453-3692, 453-3797 |
| Los Angeles | Thos. J. Fleming Memorial Center<br>Children's Hospital of Los Angeles<br>P.O. Box 54700<br>4650 Sunset Blvd. 90054<br>(213) 664-2121 | San Diego | University Hospital<br>225 W. Dickinson St. 92103<br>(714) 294-6000 |
| Oakland | Alameda-Contra Costa Medical Association<br>6230 Claremont Ave. 94618<br>(415) 652-8171 | San Francisco | Central Emergency Medical Service<br>San Francisco County Health Department<br>135 Polk St. 94102<br>(415) 553-1574, 558-3881 |
| | Children's Hospital of the East Bay<br>51st and Grove Sts. 94608<br>(415) 654-5600 | San Jose | Santa Clara Valley Medical Center<br>751 S. Bascom Ave. 95128<br>(408) 393-0262 Ext. 318, 9 |
| Orange | University of California<br>Irvine Medical Center<br>101 City Drive South 92668<br>(714) 634-5988 | | |
| | **CANAL ZONE** | | |
| Balboa Heights | Gorgas Hospital<br>Box 0<br>2-2600 | | |

TABLE 155—*Continued*
UNITED STATES DIRECTORY OF POISON CONTROL CENTERS, 1977*

| *City* | *Name and Address* | *City* | *Name and Address* |
|---|---|---|---|
| **COLORADO** | | | |
| STATE COORDINATOR | Department of Health<br>Denver 80220<br>(303) 388-6111 | | |
| Denver | Rocky Mountain Poison Center<br>Denver General Hospital<br>W. 8th Ave. and Cherokee St. 80204<br>(303) 629-1123 | | |
| **CONNECTICUT** | | | |
| STATE COORDINATOR | University of Connecticut Health Center<br>Farmington 06032<br>(203) 674-3456 | | |
| Bridgeport | Bridgeport Hospital<br>267 Grant St. 06602<br>(203) 334-3566 | New Britain | New Britain General Hospital<br>100 Grand St. 06050<br>(203) 224-5672 |
| | St. Vincent's Hospital<br>2820 Main St. 06606<br>(203) 334-1081 | New Haven | The Hospital of St. Raphael<br>1450 Chapel St. 06511<br>(203) 772-3900 |
| Danbury | Danbury Hospital<br>95 Locust Ave. 06810<br>(203) 774-2300 | | Yale-New Haven Hospital<br>789 Howard Ave. 06504<br>(203) 436-1960 |
| Farmington | University of Connecticut Health Center 06032<br>(203) 674-3456 | Norwalk | Norwalk Hospital<br>24 Stevens St. 06852<br>(203) 838-3611 |
| Middletown | Middlesex Memorial Hospital<br>28 Crescent St. 06457<br>(203) 347-9471 | Waterbury | St. Mary's Hospital<br>56 Franklin St. 06702<br>(203) 756-8351 |
| **DELAWARE** | | | |
| Wilmington | Poison Information Service<br>501 W. 14th St. 19899<br>(302) 655-3389 | | |
| **DISTRICT OF COLUMBIA** | | | |
| STATE COORDINATOR | Department of Human Resources<br>Washington, D.C. 20009<br>(202) 629-3052 | | |
| Washington, D.C. | Children's Hospital<br>111 Michigan Ave., N.W. 20010<br>(202) 745-2000 | | |
| **FLORIDA** | | | |
| STATE COORDINATOR | Department of Health and Rehabilitative Services<br>Jacksonville 32201<br>(904) 354-3961 | | |

TABLE 155-*Continued*
UNITED STATES DIRECTORY OF POISON CONTROL CENTERS, 1977*

| City | Name and Address | City | Name and Address |
|---|---|---|---|
| | **FLORIDA** *(Continued)* | | |
| Apalachicola | George E. Weems Memorial Hospital<br>P.O. Box 610<br>Franklin Square 32320<br>(904)653-3311 | Melbourne | Brevard Hospital<br>945 Hickory Street 32901<br>(305) 727-7000 Ext. 704 |
| Bartow | Polk General Hospital<br>2010 E. Georgia St.<br>P.O. Box 81 33830<br>(813) 533-1111 Ext. 237 | Miami | Jackson Memorial Hospital<br>Att: Pharmacy<br>1611 N.W. 12th Ave. 33136<br>(305) 325-6799 |
| Bradenton | Manatee Memorial Hospital<br>206 2nd St. E. 33505<br>(813) 746-5111 Ext. 466 | Naples | Naples Community Hospital<br>350 7th St. N. 33940<br>(813) 649-3131 Ext. 221 |
| Daytona Beach | Halifax District Hospital<br>Clyde Morris Blvd.<br>P.O. Box 1990 32015<br>(904) 255-0161 Ext. 256 | Ocala | Munroe Memorial Hospital<br>1410 S.E. Orange St. 32670<br>(904) 732-1111 Ext. 15 |
| Ft. Lauderdale | Broward General Hospital<br>1600 S. Andrews Ave. 33316<br>(305) 525-5411 Ext. 513 | Orlando | Orange Memorial Hospital<br>1416 S. Orange Ave. 32806<br>(305) 841-8411 Ext. 656 |
| Fort Myers | Lee Memorial Hospital<br>2776 Cleveland Ave.<br>P.O. Drawer 2218 33902<br>(813) 334-5286 | Panama City | Memorial Hospital of Bay County<br>600 N. MacArthur Ave. 32401<br>(904) 769-1511 |
| Ft. Walton Beach | General Hospital of Ft. Walton Beach<br>1000 Mar-Walt Drive 32548<br>(904) 242-1111 Ext. 106 | Pensacola | Baptist Hospital<br>1000 W. Moreno St. 32501<br>(904) 434-4011 Ext. 4811 |
| Gainesville | Alachua General Hospital<br>912 S.W. 4th Ave. 32601<br>(904) 372-4321<br><br>J. Hillis Miller Health Center<br>University of Florida 32601<br>(904) 392-3261 | Plant City | South Florida Baptist Hospital<br>Drawer H 33566<br>(813) 752-1188 |
| Jacksonville | St. Vincent's Hospital<br>Barrs St. and St. Johns Ave.<br>(904) 389-7751 Ext. 315 | Pompano | N. Broward Hospital<br>201 Sample Rd. 33064<br>(305) 941-8300 Ext. 710 |
| Key West | Florida Keys Memorial Hospital<br>Stock Island 33040<br>(305) 294-5531 | Punta Gorda | Medical Center<br>809 E. Marion Ave.<br>P.O. Box 1507 33950<br>(813) 639-3131 Ext. 129 |
| Lakeland | Lakeland General Hospital<br>Lakeland Hills Blvd.<br>P.O. Box 480 33801<br>(813) 683-0411 | Rockledge | Wuesthoff Memorial Hospital<br>110 Longwood Ave. 32955<br>(305) 636-2211 Ext. 506 |
| Leesburg | Leesburg General Hospital<br>600 E. Dixie 32748<br>(904) 787-7222 Ext. 221 | St. Petersburg | Bayfront Medical Center, Inc.<br>701 6th St., S.<br>P.O. Box 1438 33701<br>(813) 821-5858 Ext. 242 |
| | | Sarasota | Memorial Hospital<br>1901 Arlington Ave. 33579<br>(813) 955-1111 Ext. 1241 |
| | | Tallahassee | Tallahassee Memorial Hospital<br>Magnolia Drive and<br>Miccosukee Rd. 32303<br>(904) 599-5100 |

TABLE 155—*Continued*
UNITED STATES DIRECTORY OF POISON CONTROL CENTERS, 1977*

| City | Name and Address | City | Name and Address |
|---|---|---|---|
| **FLORIDA** *(Continued)* | | | |
| Tampa | Tampa General Hospital<br>Davis Islands 33606<br>(813) 253-0711 | West Palm Beach | Good Samaritan Hospital<br>1300 N. Dixie Hwy. 33402<br>(305) 655-5511 Ext. 341 |
| Titusville | Jess Parrish Memorial Hospital<br>951 N. Washington Ave. 32780<br>(305) 269-1100 Ext. 474 | Winter Haven | Winter Haven Hospital, Inc.<br>200 Avenue F., N.E. 33880<br>(813) 293-1121 Ext. 222 |
| **GEORGIA** | | | |
| STATE COORDINATOR | Department of Human Resources<br>Atlanta 30308<br>(404) 894-5068 | | |
| Albany | Phoebe Putney Memorial Hospital<br>P.O. Box 115 31701<br>(912) 883-1800 Ext. 158 | Rome | Floyd Hospital<br>P.O. Box 233 30161<br>(404) 232-1541 Ext. 223 |
| Athens | Athens General Hospital<br>797 Cobb St. 30601<br>(404) 549-9977 Ext. 357 | Savannah | Memorial Medical Center<br>P.O. Box 6688, Sta. C. 31405<br>(912) 355-3200 Ext. 455 |
| Atlanta | Grady Memorial Hospital<br>80 Butler St., S.E. 30303<br>(404) 659-1212 Ext. 4893 | Thomasville | John D. Archbold Memorial Hospital<br>900 Gordon Ave. 31792<br>(912) 226-4121 Ext. 169 |
| Augusta | University Hospital<br>1350 Walton Way 30902<br>(404) 724-7171 Ext. 2176 | Valdosta | S. Georgia Medical Center<br>Pendleton Park 31601<br>(912) 242-3450 Ext. 717 |
| Columbus | The Medical Center<br>19th St. and 18th Ave. 31902<br>(404) 324-4711 Ext. 431 | Waycross | Memorial Hospital<br>410 Darling Ave. 31501<br>(912) 283-3030 Ext. 240 |
| Macon | Medical Center of Central Georgia<br>777 Hemlock St. 31201<br>(912) 742-1122 Ext. 3144 | | |
| **GUAM** | | | |
| STATE COORDINATOR | Bureau of Environmental Health and Consumer Protection<br>Agana 96910<br>742-4158 | | |
| Agana | Pharmacy Service, Box 7696<br>U.S. Naval Regional Medical Center (GUAM)<br>FPO San Francisco, CA 96630<br>746-9171 | | |
| **HAWAII** | | | |
| STATE COORDINATOR | Department of Health<br>Honolulu 96801<br>(808) 531-7776 | | |
| Honolulu | Kauikeolani Children's Hospital<br>226 Kuakini St. 96817<br>(808) 537-1831 | | |

TABLE 155—*Continued*
UNITED STATES DIRECTORY OF POISON CONTROL CENTERS, 1977*

| *City* | *Name and Address* | *City* | *Name and Address* |
|---|---|---|---|
| | **IDAHO** | | |
| STATE COORDINATOR | Department of Health and Welfare<br>Boise 83701<br>(208) 384-2125 | | |
| Boise | St. Alphonsus Hospital<br>1055 N. Curtis Rd. 83704<br>(208) 376-1211 Ext. 707 | Pocatello | St. Anthony Hospital<br>650 North 7th St. 83201<br>(208) 232-2733 Ext. 244 |
| Idaho Falls | Idaho Falls Hospital<br>Emergency Department<br>900 Memorial Dr. 83401<br>(208) 522-3620 | | |
| | **ILLINOIS** | | |
| STATE COORDINATOR | Department of Public Health<br>Springfield 62761<br>(217) 785-2087 | | |
| Alton | Alton Memorial Hospital<br>Memorial Drive 62202<br>(618) 463-7475 | Carthage | Memorial Hospital<br>South Adams St. 62321<br>(217) 357-3131 Ext. 84, 85 |
| Aurora | Copley Memorial Hospital<br>Lincoln and Weston Aves. 60507<br>(312) 897-6021 Ext. 725<br>(312) 896-3911 Direct Line | Centralia | St. Mary's Hospital<br>400 N. Pleasant Ave. 62801<br>(618) 532-6731 Ext. 716 |
| Belleville | Memorial Hospital<br>4501 N. Park Dr. 62223<br>(618) 233-7750 Ext. 250 | Champaign | Burnham City Hospital<br>407 S. 4th St. 61820<br>(217) 337-2533 |
| Belvidere | Highland Hospital<br>1625 State St. 61008<br>(815) 547-5441 Ext. 367 | Chanute AFB | USAF Hospital<br>Chanute Air Force Base 61868<br>(217) 495-3133<br>(Limited for treatment of military personnel and families, except for indicated civilian emergencies) |
| Berwyn | MacNeal Memorial Hospital<br>3249 Oak Park Ave. 60402<br>(312) 797-3159 | | |
| Bloomington | Mennonite Hospital<br>807 N. Main St. 61701<br>(309) 828-5241 Ext. 395 | Chester | Memorial Hospital<br>1900 State St. 62233<br>(618) 826-4581 |
| | St. Joseph's Hospital<br>2200 E. Washington 61701<br>(309) 662-3311 Ext. 356 | Chicago | Rush-Presbyterian St. Luke's Medical Center<br>1753 W. Congress Pkwy. 60612<br>(312) 942-5969 |
| Cairo | Padco Community Hospital<br>2020 Cedar St. 62914<br>(618) 734-2400 Ext. 42 | | Children's Memorial Hospital<br>2300 Children's Plaza 60614<br>(312) 649-4161 |
| Canton | Graham Hospital Association<br>210 W. Walnut St. 61520<br>(304) 647-5240 Ext. 240 | | Cook County Children's Hospital<br>700 South Wood St. 60612<br>(312) 633-6542, 633-6543, 633-6544 |
| Carbondale | Doctors Memorial Hospital<br>404 W. Main St. 62901<br>(618) 549-0721 Ext. 341 | | |

TABLE 155—*Continued*
UNITED STATES DIRECTORY OF POISON CONTROL CENTERS, 1977*

| City | Name and Address |
|---|---|
| | **ILLINOIS** *(Continued)* |
| | Mercy Hospital and Medical Center<br>Stevenson Expressway at<br>King Drive 60616<br>(312) 567-2017 |
| | Michael Reese Medical Center<br>29th and Ellis Ave. 60616<br>(312) 791-2810 |
| | Mt. Sinai Hospital<br>California at 15th St. 60608<br>(312) 542-2030 |
| | Resurrection Hospital<br>7435 W. Talcott Ave. 60631<br>(312) 774-8000 Ext. 401 |
| | St. Mary of Nazareth<br>Hospital Center<br>2233 W. Division 60622<br>(312) 770-2419 |
| | South Chicago Community<br>Hospital<br>2320 E. 93rd St. 60617<br>(312) 978-2000 |
| | University of Illinois<br>Hospitals<br>840 S. Wood St. 60612<br>(312) 996-6885, 996-6886 |
| | Wyler Children's Hospital<br>950 E. 59th St. 60637<br>(312) 947-6231 |
| Danville | Lake View Memorial Hospital<br>812 N. Logan Ave. 61832<br>(217) 443-5221 |
| | St. Elizabeth's Hospital<br>600 Sager Ave. 61832<br>(217) 442-6300 Ext. 647,<br>674, 736 |
| Decatur | Decatur Memorial Hospital<br>2300 N. Edward St. 62526<br>(217) 877-8121 Ext. 676 |
| | St. Mary's Hospital<br>1800 E. Lakeshore Dr. 62521<br>(217) 429-2966 Ext. 731,<br>732, 733, 742 |
| De Kalb | Kishwaukee Community Hospital<br>Route 23 and Bethany Rd.<br>P.O. Box 707 60115<br>(815) 756-1521 Ext. 491 |
| Des Plaines | Holy Family Hospital<br>100 N. River Rd. 60016<br>(312) 297-1800 Ext. 1000 |
| East St. Louis | Christian Welfare Hospital<br>1509 Martin Luther King<br>Drive 62201<br>(618) 874-7076 Ext. 216, 232 |
| | St. Mary's Hospital<br>129 N. 8th St. 62201<br>(618) 274-1900 Ext. 204, 268 |
| Effingham | St. Anthony's Memorial<br>Hospital<br>503 N. Maple 62401<br>(217) 342-2121 Ext. 211, 212 |
| Elgin | St. Joseph's Hospital<br>77 Airlite St. 60120<br>(312) 695-3200 Ext. 348 |
| | Sherman Hospital<br>934 Center St. 60120<br>(312) 742-9800 Ext. 681 |
| Elmhurst | Memorial Hospital of<br>Du Page County<br>209 Avon Rd. 60126<br>(312) 833-1400 Ext. 550 |
| Evanston | Evanston Hospital<br>2650 Ridge Ave. 60201<br>(312) 492-6460 |
| | St. Francis Hospital<br>355 Ridge Ave. 60202<br>(312) 492-2440 |
| Evergreen Park | Little Company of<br>Mary Hospital<br>2800 W. 95th St. 60642<br>(312) 445-6000 Ext. 221 |
| Fairbury | Fairbury Hospital<br>519 S. 5th St. 61739<br>(815) 692-2346 Ext. 248 |
| Freeport | Freeport Memorial Hospital<br>420 S. Harlem Ave. 61032<br>(815) 235-4131 Ext. 228 |
| Galesburg | Galesburg Cottage Hospital<br>695 N. Kellogg St. 61401<br>(309) 343-8131 Ext. 336,<br>356, 386 |
| | St Mary's Hospital<br>333 North Seminary 61401<br>(309) 343-3161 Ext. 255, 256 |

TABLE 155—*Continued*
UNITED STATES DIRECTORY OF POISON CONTROL CENTERS, 1977*

| *City* | *Name and Address* | *City* | *Name and Address* |
|---|---|---|---|
| | **ILLINOIS** *(Continued)* | | |
| Granite City | St. Elizabeth Hospital<br>2100 Madison Ave. 62040<br>(618) 876-2020 Ext. 421 | Lincoln | Abraham Lincoln Memorial Hospital<br>315 Eighth St. 62656<br>(217) 732-2161 Ext. 346 |
| Harvey | Ingalls Memorial Hospital<br>One Ingalls Dr. 60426<br>(312) 333-2300 Ext. 5295 | Macomb | McDonough District Hospital<br>525 E. Grant St. 61455<br>(309) 833-4101 Ext. 433 |
| Highland | St. Joseph's Hospital<br>1515 Main St. 62249<br>(618) 654-2171 Ext. 297, 8 | Mattoon | Memorial Hospital<br>District of Coles County<br>2101 Champaign Ave. 61938<br>(217) 234-8881 Ext. 29 |
| Highland Park | Highland Park Hospital<br>718 Glenview Ave. 60035<br>(312) 432-8000 | Maywood | Loyola University Hospital<br>2160 1st Ave. 60153<br>(312) 531-3000 |
| Hinsdale | Hinsdale Sanitarium and Hospital<br>120 N. Oak St. 60521<br>(312) 887-2600 | McHenry | McHenry Hospital<br>3516 W. Waukegan Rd. 60050<br>(815) 385-2200 Ext. 602 |
| Hoopeston | Hoopeston Community Memorial Hospital<br>701 E. Orange St. 60942<br>(217) 283-5531 | Melrose Park | Westlake Community Hospital<br>1225 Superior St. 60160<br>(312) 681-3000 Ext. 226, 239 |
| Jacksonville | Passavant Memorial Area Hospital<br>1600 W. Walnut St. 62650<br>(217) 245-9541 | Mendota | Mendota Community Hospital<br>Rt. 51 and Memorial Dr. 61342<br>(815) 539-7461 Ext. 225 |
| Joliet | St. Joseph's Hospital<br>333 N. Madison St. 60435<br>(815) 725-7133 Ext. 679, 80<br><br>Silver Cross Hospital<br>1200 Maple Rd. 60432<br>(815) 729-7563, 729-7565 | Moline | Moline Public Hospital<br>635 10th Ave. 61265<br>(309) 762-3651 Ext. 233 |
| | | Monmouth | Community Memorial Hospital<br>1000 W. Harlem Ave. 61462<br>(309) 734-3141 Ext. 224 |
| Kankakee | Riverside Hospital<br>350 N. Wall St. 60901<br>(815) 933-1671 Ext. 606<br><br>St. Mary's Hospital<br>500 West Court 60901<br>(815) 936-4111 Ext. 735 | Mt. Carmel | Wabash General Hospital<br>1418 College Dr. 62863<br>(618) 263-3112 Ext. 211 |
| | | Mt. Vernon | Good Samaritan Hospital<br>605 N. 12th St. 62864<br>(618) 242-4600 Ext. 521 |
| Kewanee | Kewanee Public Hospital<br>719 Elliott St. 61443<br>(309) 853-3361 Ext. 219 | Naperville | Edward Hospital<br>S. Washington St. 60540<br>(312) 355-0450 Ext. 326 |
| Lake Forest | Lake Forest Hospital<br>660 N. Westmoreland Rd. 60045<br>(312) 234-5600 Ext. 684, 685, 683 | Normal | Brokaw Hospital<br>Franklin and Virginia Aves. 61761<br>(309) 829–7685 Ext. 274 |
| | | Oak Lawn | Christ Community Hospital<br>4440 W. 95th St. 60453<br>(312) 425-8000 Ext. 382 |
| La Salle | Illinois Valley Community Hospital<br>La Salle Division<br>1015 O'Conor Ave. 61301<br>(815) 223-0607 Ext. 14 | Oak Park | West Suburban Hospital<br>518 N. Austin Blvd. 60302<br>(312) 383-6200 |

TABLE 155—*Continued*
UNITED STATES DIRECTORY OF POISON CONTROL CENTERS, 1977*

| *City* | *Name and Address* | *City* | *Name and Address* |
|---|---|---|---|
| | **ILLINOIS** *(Continued)* | | |
| Olney | Richland Memorial Hospital<br>800 Locust St. 62450<br>(618) 395-2131 Ext. 226, 8 | | Swedish-American Hospital<br>1316 Charles St. 61108<br>(815) 968-6898 Ext. 534 |
| Ottawa | Community Hospital of Ottawa<br>1100 E. Norris Dr. 61350<br>(815) 433-3100 Ext. 227 | Rock Island | Rock Island Franciscan Hospital<br>2701 17th St. 61201<br>(309) 793-1000 Ext. 2106 |
| Park Ridge | Lutheran General Hospital<br>1775 Dempster St. 60068<br>(312) 696-5151 | St. Charles | Delnor Hospital<br>975 N. 5th Ave. 60174<br>(312) 584-3300 Ext. 229 |
| Pekin | Pekin Memorial Hospital<br>14th and Court Sts. 61554<br>(309) 347-1151 Ext. 241 | Scott Air Force Base | USAF Medical Center 62225<br>(618) 256-7595 |
| Peoria | Methodist Hospital of Central Illinois<br>221 N.E. Glen Oak Ave. 61603<br>(309) 672-5500, 672-4950 | Springfield | Memorial Medical Center<br>1st and Miller Sts. 62701<br>(217) 528-2041 Ext. 460 |
| | Proctor Community Hospital<br>5409 N. Knoxville 61614<br>(309) 691-4702 Ext. 791 | | St. John's Hospital<br>800 East Carpenter 62701<br>(217) 544-6464 Ext. 210 |
| | St. Francis Hospital Medical Center<br>530 N.E. Glen Oak Ave. 61603<br>(309) 672-2109, 672-2110, 672-2111 | Spring Valley | St. Margaret's Hospital<br>600 East 1st St. 61362<br>(815) 663-2611 Ext. 464, 466 |
| | | Streator | St. Mary's Hospital<br>111 E. Spring St. 61364<br>(815) 673-2311 Ext. 221 |
| Peru | Illinois Valley Community Hospital<br>Peru Division<br>925 West St. 61354<br>(815) 223-3300 Ext. 253 | Urbana | Carle Foundation Hospital<br>611 W. Park Ave. 61801<br>(217) 337-3311 |
| | | | Mercy Hospital<br>1400 W. Park Ave. 61801<br>(217) 337-2131 |
| Pittsfield | Illini Community Hospital<br>640 W. Washington St. 62363<br>(217) 285-2113 Ext. 238 | Waukegan | St. Therese Hospital<br>2615 W. Washington St. 60085<br>(312) 688-4181 |
| Princeton | Perry Memorial Hospital<br>530 Park Ave. E. 61356<br>(815) 875-2811 Ext. 311 | | Victory Memorial Hospital<br>1324 N. Sheridan Rd. 60085<br>(312) 688-6181 |
| Quincy | Blessing Hospital<br>1005 Broadway 62301<br>(217) 223-5811 Ext. 255 | Winfield | Central DuPage Hospital<br>O North, 025 Winfield Rd. 60190<br>(312) 653-6900 Ext. 556 |
| | St. Mary's Hospital<br>1415 Vermont St. 62301<br>(217) 223-1200 Ext. 260 | Woodstock | Memorial Hospital of McHenry County<br>527 W. South St. 60098<br>(815) 338-2500 Ext. 215, 232 |
| Rockford | Rockford Memorial Hospital<br>2400 N. Rockton Ave. 61103<br>(815) 968-6861 Ext. 441 | Zion | Zion-Benton Hospital<br>Shiloh Blvd. 60099<br>(312) 872-4561 Ext. 239, 40 |
| | St. Anthony's Hospital<br>5666 E. State St. 61108<br>(815) 226-2041 | | |

TABLE 155—*Continued*
UNITED STATES DIRECTORY OF POISON CONTROL CENTERS, 1977*

| *City* | *Name and Address* | *City* | *Name and Address* |
|---|---|---|---|
| | **INDIANA** | | |
| STATE COORDINATOR | State Board of Health<br>Indianapolis 46206<br>(317) 633-4830 | | |
| Anderson | Community Hospital<br>1515 N. Madison Ave. 46012<br>(317) 646-5198 | Frankfort | Clinton County Hospital<br>1300 S. Jackson St. 46041<br>(317) 654-4451 |
| | St. John's Hickey Memorial Hospital<br>2015 Jackson St. 46014<br>(317) 649-2511 Ext. 251 | Gary | Methodist Hospital of Gary, Inc.<br>600 Grant St. 46402<br>(219) 886-4710 |
| Angola | Cameron Memorial Hospital, Inc.<br>416 East Maumee St. 46703<br>(219) 665-2141 Ext 42, 665-2166 | Goshen | Goshen General Hospital<br>200 High Park Ave. 46526<br>(219) 533-2141 Ext. 462 |
| | | Hammond | St. Margaret Hospital<br>25 Douglas St. 46320<br>(219) 932-2300 |
| Columbus | Bartholomew County Hospital<br>2400 East 17th St. 47201<br>(812) 376-5277 | Huntington | Huntington Memorial Hospital<br>1215 Etna Ave. 46750<br>(219) 356-3000 |
| Crown Point | St. Anthony Medical Center<br>Main at Franciscan Rd. 46307<br>(219) 738-2100 | Indianapolis | Methodist Hospital of Indiana, Inc.<br>1604 N. Capitol Ave. 46202<br>(317) 924-8355 |
| East Chicago | St. Catherine Hospital<br>4321 Fir Street 46312<br>(219) 392-1700, 392-7203 | | Wishard Memorial Hospital<br>1001 West 10th St. 46202<br>(317) 639-6671 |
| Elkhart | Elkhart General Hospital<br>600 East Blvd. 46514<br>(219) 294-2621 | Kendallville | McCray Memorial Hospital<br>Hospital Drive 46755<br>(219) 347-1100 |
| Evansville | Deaconess Hospital<br>600 Mary St. 47710<br>(812) 426-3405<br>St. Mary's Hospital<br>3700 Washington Ave. 47715<br>(812) 477-6261 | Kokomo | Howard Community Hospital<br>3500 S. LaFountain St. 46901<br>(217) 453-0702 Ext. 444 |
| | Welborn Memorial Baptist Hospital<br>401 S.E. 6th St. 47713<br>(812) 426-8000 | Lafayette | St. Elizabeth Hospital<br>1501 Hartfort St. 47904<br>(317) 742-0221 Ext. 428, 421 |
| Fort Wayne | Lutheran Hospital<br>Emergency Dept.<br>3024 Fairfield Ave. 46807<br>(219) 458-2211 | LaGrange | LaGrange County Hospital<br>Route #1 46761<br>(219) 463-2144 |
| | Parkview Memorial Hospital<br>220 Randalia Dr. 46805<br>(219) 484-6636 Ext. 7800 | LaPorte | LaPorte Hospital, Inc.<br>1007 Lincolnway 46350<br>(219) 362-7541 Ext. 212 |
| | St. Joseph's Hospital<br>700 Broadway 46802<br>(219) 423-2614 | Lebanon | Witham Memorial Hospital<br>1124 N. Lebanon St. 46052<br>(317) 482-2700 Ext. 44 |

TABLE 155—*Continued*
UNITED STATES DIRECTORY OF POISON CONTROL CENTERS, 1977*

| *City* | *Name and Address* | *City* | *Name and Address* |
|---|---|---|---|
| | **INDIANA** *(Continued)* | | |
| Madison | King's Daughter's Hospital<br>112 Presbyterian Ave.<br>P.O. Box 447 47250<br>(812) 265-5211 Ext. 14 | Shelbyville | Wm. S. Major Hospital<br>150 W. Washington St. 46176<br>(317) 392-3211 Ext. 52 |
| Marion | Marion General Hospital<br>Wabash and Euclid Ave. 46952<br>(317) 662-4692 | South Bend | St. Joseph's Hospital<br>811 E. Madison St. 46622<br>(219) 234-2151 Ext. 253, 264 |
| Mishawaka | St. Joseph's Hospital<br>215 W. 4th St. 46544<br>(219) 259-2431 | Terre Haute | Union Hospital, Inc.<br>1606 N. 7th St. 47804<br>(812) 232-0361 Ext. 397, 398 |
| Muncie | Ball Memorial Hospital<br>2401 University Ave. 47303<br>(317) 747-3241 | Valparaiso | Porter Memorial Hospital<br>814 LaPorte Ave. 46383<br>(219) 464-8611 Ext. 232, 312, 334 |
| Portland | Jay County Hospital<br>505 W. Arch St. 47371<br>(317) 726-7131 Ext. 159 | Vincennes | The Good Samaritan Hospital<br>520 S. 7th St. 47591<br>(812) 885-3348 |
| Richmond | Reid Memorial Hospital<br>1401 Chester Blvd. 47374<br>(317) 692-7010 Ext. 622 | | |
| | **IOWA** | | |
| STATE COORDINATOR | Department of Health<br>Des Moines 50319<br>(515) 281-3826 | | |
| Des Moines | Iowa Methodist Hospital<br>1200 Pleasant St. 50308<br>(515) 283-6212 | Fort Dodge | Trinity Regional Hospital<br>Department of Pharmacy<br>Kenyon Rd. 50501<br>(515) 573–3101 |
| Dubuque | Mercy Medical Center<br>Mercy Drive 52001<br>(319) 588-8210 | Iowa City | University of Iowa Hospital and Clinics<br>Pharmacy Department 52240<br>(319) 356-1616 |
| | **KANSAS** | | |
| STATE COORDINATOR | Department of Health and Environment<br>Topeka 66620<br>(913) 296-3708 | | |
| Atchison | Atchison Hospital<br>1301 N. 2nd St. 66002<br>(913) 367-2131 | Fort Riley | Irwin Army Hospital<br>66442<br>(913) 239-2323 |
| Dodge City | Trinity Hospital<br>1107 6th St. 67801<br>(316) 227-8133 | Fort Scott | Mercy Hospital<br>821 Burke St. 66701<br>(316) 223-2200<br>Night: 0476 |
| Emporia | Newman Memorial Hospital<br>12th and Chestnut Sts. 66801<br>(316) 342-7120 Ext. 330 | | |

TABLE 155—*Continued*
UNITED STATES DIRECTORY OF POISON CONTROL CENTERS, 1977*

| *City* | *Name and Address* | *City* | *Name and Address* |
|---|---|---|---|
| | **KANSAS** *(Continued)* | | |
| Great Bend | Central Kansas<br>Medical Center<br>3515 Broadway 67530<br>(316) 793-3523<br>Night: 792-2511 | Lawrence | Lawrence Memorial Hospital<br>325 Maine St. 66044<br>(913) 843-3680 |
| Hays | Hadley Regional<br>Medical Center<br>201 E. 7th St. 67601<br>(913) 628-8251 | Parsons | Labette County<br>Medical Center<br>S. 21st St. 67357<br>(316) 421-4880 |
| Kansas City | University of Kansas<br>Medical Center<br>39th and Rainbow Blvd. 66103<br>(913) 831-6633 | Salina | St. John's Hospital<br>139 N. Penn St. 67401<br>(913) 827-5591 Ext. 112 |
| | Bethany Medical Center<br>51 N. 12th St. 66102<br>(913) 287-8881 | Topeka | Stormont-Vail Hospital<br>10th and Washburn Sts. 66606<br>(913) 234-9961 Ext. 150 |
| | | Wichita | Wesley Medical Center<br>550 N. Hillside Ave. 67214<br>(316) 685-2151 Ext. 7515 |
| | **KENTUCKY** | | |
| STATE COORDINATOR | Department For Human Resources<br>Frankfort 40601<br>(502) 564-4935 | | |
| Ashland | King's Daughters Hospital<br>2201 Lexington Ave. 41101<br>(606) 324-2222 | Louisville | Norton-Children's Hospital<br>Pharmacy Department<br>200 E. Chestnut St. 40202<br>(502) 589-8222 |
| Berea | Porter Moore Drug, Inc.<br>124 Main St. 40403<br>(606) 986-3061 | Murray | Murray-Calloway<br>County Hospital<br>803 Popular 42071<br>(502) 753-7588 |
| Fort Thomas | St. Lukes Hospital<br>85 N. Grand Ave. 41075<br>(606) 292-3215 | Owensboro | Owensboro-Daviess<br>County Hospital<br>811 Hospital Court 42301<br>(502) 683-3511 Ext. 275<br>Night: Ext. 232 |
| Lexington | Central Baptist Hospital<br>1740 S. Limestone St. 40503<br>(606) 278-3411 Ext. 152 | Paducah | Western Baptist Hospital<br>2501 Kentucky Ave. 42001<br>(502) 444-6361 Ext. 284<br>Night: Ext. 541 |
| | University of Kentucky<br>Medical Center<br>40506<br>(606) 233-5320 | Whitesburg | Quillen Rexall Drug<br>Store<br>41858<br>(606) 633-2160 |
| | **LOUISIANA** | | |
| STATE COORDINATOR | Office of Health Services and<br>Environmental Quality (DHHR)<br>New Orleans 70160<br>(504) 568-5413 | | |

TABLE 155—*Continued*
UNITED STATES DIRECTORY OF POISON CONTROL CENTERS, 1977*

| City | Name and Address | City | Name and Address |
|---|---|---|---|
| **LOUISIANA** *(Continued)* | | | |
| Alexandria | Rapides General Hospital<br>211 Fourth St.<br>P.O. Box 7146 71306<br>(318) 487-8111 Ext. 231 | Monroe | St. Francis Hospital<br>309 Jackson St. 71201<br>(318) 325-6454<br>Night: 325-2611 |
| Bogalusa | Washington-St. Tammany Charity Hospital<br>400 Memphis St. 70427<br>(504) 735-1322 | New Orleans | Charity Hospital<br>Pharmacy Department<br>1532 Tulane Ave. 71040<br>(504) 524-3617, 524-3618, 524-3619 |
| Lake Charles | Lake Charles Memorial Hospital<br>P.O. Drawer M 70601<br>(318) 478-1310 Ext. 210 | Shreveport | Schumpert Medical Center<br>915 Margaret Place 71101<br>(318) 222-0709 |
| **MAINE** | | | |
| STATE COORDINATOR | Department of Health and Welfare<br>Augusta 04330<br>(207) 623-4511 | | |
| Portland | Maine Medical Center<br>Emergency Division<br>22 Bramhall St. 04102<br>(207) 871-2381 | | |
| **MARYLAND** | | | |
| STATE COORDINATOR | Department of Health and Mental Hygiene<br>Baltimore 21201<br>(301) 383-2668 | | |
| Baltimore | Johns Hopkins Hospital<br>601 N. Broadway 21205<br>(301) 955-5000 | Cumberland | Sacred Heart Hospital<br>900 Seton Drive 21502<br>(301) 722-6677 |
| | University of Maryland<br>School of Pharmacy<br>636 W. Lombard St. 21201<br>(301) 528-7701<br>(800) 494-2414 | Easton | Memorial Hospital<br>S. Washington St. 21601<br>(301) 822-5555 |
| Bethesda | Suburban Hospital<br>Emergency Room<br>8600 Old Georgetown Rd. 20014<br>(301) 530-3880 | Hagerstown | Washington County Hospital<br>King and Antietam Sts. 21740<br>(301) 797-2400 |
| **MASSACHUSETTS** | | | |
| STATE COORDINATOR | Department of Public Health<br>Boston 02111<br>(617) 727-2670 | | |
| Boston | Boston Poison Information Center<br>300 Longwood Ave. 02115<br>(617) 232-2120 | Fall River | Union Truesdale Hospital<br>Highland Ave. at New Boston Rd. 02720<br>(617) 674-5789 |

TABLE 155—*Continued*
UNITED STATES DIRECTORY OF POISON CONTROL CENTERS, 1977*

| *City* | *Name and Address* |
|---|---|
| **MASSACHUSETTS** *(Continued)* | |
| New Bedford | St. Luke's Hospital<br>101 Page St. 02740<br>(617) 997-1515 |
| Springfield | Bay State Medical<br>Springfield Unit<br>759 Chestnut St. 01107<br>(413) 787-3233 |
| | Mercy Hospital<br>233 Carew St. 01104<br>(413) 781-9100 |
| | Wesson Memorial Hospital<br>150 High St. 01105<br>(413) 787-2562 |
| Webster | Hubbard Regional Hospital<br>of Webster<br>Thompson Rd. 01570<br>(617) 943-2600 |
| Worcester | Worcester City Hospital<br>26 Queen St. 01609<br>(617) 756-1551 |
| **MICHIGAN** | |
| STATE COORDINATOR | Department of Public Health<br>Lansing 48909<br>(517) 373-1448 |
| Adrian | Emma L. Bixby Hospital<br>818 Riverside Ave. 49221<br>(517) 263-2412 |
| Ann Arbor | University Hospital<br>1405 E. Ann St. 48104<br>(313) 764-5102 |
| Battle Creek | Community Hospital<br>183 West St. 49016<br>(616) 963-5521 |
| Bay City | Bay Medical Center<br>100 15th St. 48706<br>(517) 892-6589 |
| Berrien Center | Berrien General Hospital<br>Dean's Hill Rd. 49102<br>(616) 471-7761 |
| Coldwater | Community Health Center<br>of Branch County<br>274 E. Chicago St. 49036<br>(517) 278-7361 |
| Detroit | Children's Hospital<br>of Michigan<br>3901 Beaubien 48201<br>(313) 494-5711 |
| | Mount Carmel Mercy<br>Hospital<br>6071 W. Outer Dr. 48235<br>(313) 864-5400 Ext. 416 |
| Eloise | Wayne County General<br>Hospital<br>30712 Michigan Ave. 48132<br>(313) 722-3748<br>Night: 274-3000 Ext. 6231 |
| Flint | Hurley Hospital<br>6th Ave. and Begole 48502<br>(313) 766-0111 |
| Grand Rapids | St. Mary's Hospital<br>201 Lafayette, S.E. 49503<br>(616) 774-6794 |
| | Western Michigan<br>Poison Center<br>1840 Wealthy, S.E. 49502<br>(800) 442-4571, 632-2727 |
| Hancock | Portage View Hospital<br>200-210 Michigan Ave. 49930<br>(906) 482-1122 Ext. 209 |
| Holland | Holland Community Hospital<br>602 Michigan Ave. 49423<br>(616) 396-4661 |
| Jackson | W.A. Foote Memorial<br>Hospital<br>205 N. East St. 49201<br>(517) 788-4816 |
| Kalamazoo | Borgess Hospital<br>Ambulatory Care Service<br>1521 Gull Rd. 49001<br>(616) 383-4815 |
| | Bronson Methodist Hospital<br>252 E. Lovell St. 49006<br>(616) 383-6409 |
| Lansing | St. Lawrence Hospital<br>1210 W. Saginaw St. 48914<br>(517) 372-5112, 372-5113 |

TABLE 155—*Continued*
UNITED STATES DIRECTORY OF POISON CONTROL CENTERS, 1977*

| *City* | *Name and Address* |
|---|---|
| **MICHIGAN** *(Continued)* | |
| Marquette | Marquette General Hospital<br>425 W. Fisher St. 49855<br>(800) 562-9723 |
| Midland | Midland Hospital<br>4005 Orchard Dr. 48640<br>(517) 631-7700 Ext. 304 |
| Petoskey | Little Traverse Hospital<br>416 Connable 49770<br>(616) 347-7373 |
| Pontiac | St. Joseph Mercy Hospital<br>900 Woodward Ave. 48053<br>(313) 858-3000 |
| Port Huron | Port Huron Hospital<br>1001 Kearney St. 48060<br>(313) 987-5555, 987-5000 |
| Saginaw | Saginaw General Hospital<br>1447 N. Harrison 48602<br>(517) 755-1111 |
| Traverse City | Munson Medical Center<br>Sixth St. 49684<br>(616) 947-6140 |
| **MINNESOTA** | |
| STATE COORDINATOR | State Department of Health<br>Minneapolis 55440<br>(612) 296-5276 |
| Bemidji | Bemidji Hospital<br>56601<br>(218) 751-5430 |
| Brainerd | St. Joseph's Hospital<br>56401<br>(218) 829-2861 Ext. 211 |
| Crookston | Riverview Hospital<br>320 S. Hubbard 56716<br>(218) 281-4682 Ext. 202 |
| Duluth | St. Luke's Hospital<br>Emergency Department<br>915 E. First St. 55805<br>(218) 727-6636 |
| | St. Mary's Hospital<br>407 E. 3rd St. 55805<br>(218) 727-4551 Ext. 359 |
| Edina | Fairview-Southdale Hospital<br>6401 France Ave., S. 55435<br>(612) 920-4400 |
| Fergus Falls | Lake Region Hospital<br>56537<br>(218) 736-5475 |
| Fridley | Unity Hospital<br>550 Osborne Rd. 55432<br>(612) 786-2200 |
| Mankato | Immanuel-St. Joseph's Hospital<br>325 Garden Blvd. 56001<br>(507) 387-4031 |
| Marshall | Louis Weiner Memorial Hospital 56258<br>(507) 532-9661 |
| Minneapolis | Fairview Hospital<br>Outpatient Department<br>2312 S. 6th St. 55406<br>(612) 332-0282 |
| | Hennepin County Medical Center<br>701 Park Ave. 55415<br>(612) 347-3141 |
| | Minnesota Department of Health<br>717 Delaware St., S.E. 55440<br>(612) 296-5276 |
| | North Memorial Hospital<br>3220 Lowry North 55422<br>(612) 588-0616 |
| | Northwestern Hospital<br>810 E. 27th St. 55407<br>(612) 874-4233 |
| Morris | Stevens County Memorial Hospital 56267<br>(612) 589-1313 |
| Rochester | St. Mary's Hospital<br>1216 Second St., S.W. 55901<br>(507) 285-5123 |
| St. Cloud | St. Cloud Hospital<br>1406 6th Avenue, N. 56301<br>(612) 251-2700 Ext. 221 |
| St. Paul | Bethesda Lutheran Hospital<br>559 Capitol Blvd. 55103<br>(612) 224-9121 |

TABLE 155—*Continued*
UNITED STATES DIRECTORY OF POISON CONTROL CENTERS, 1977*

| *City* | *Name and Address* |
|---|---|
| **MINNESOTA** *(Continued)* | |
| | The Children's Hospital Inc.<br>311 Pleasant Ave. 55102<br>(612) 227-6521 |
| | St. John's Hospital<br>403 Maria Ave. 55106<br>(612) 228-3132 |
| | St. Joseph's Hospital<br>69 W. Exchange 55102<br>(612) 291-3348, 291-3139 |
| | United Hospitals, Inc.<br>St. Luke's Division<br>300 Pleasant Ave. 55102<br>(612) 298-8201 |
| | St. Paul-Ramsey Hospital<br>640 Jackson St. 55101<br>(612) 222-4260 |
| Virginia | Virginia Municipal Hospital<br>55792<br>(218) 741-3340 |
| Willmar | Rice Memorial Hospital<br>402 W. 3rd St. 56201<br>(612) 235-4543 |
| Worthington | Worthington Regional Hospital<br>1016 6th Ave. 56187<br>(507) 372-2941 |
| **MISSISSIPPI** | |
| STATE COORDINATOR | State Board of Health<br>Jackson 39205<br>(601) 354-6650 |
| Biloxi | Gulf Coast Community Hospital<br>4642 West Beach Blvd. 39531<br>(601) 388-6711 Ext. 233, 234, 235 |
| | USAF Hospital Keesler<br>Keesler Air Force Base 39534<br>(601) 377-2516, 377-6555, 377-6556 |
| Brandon | Rankin General Hospital<br>350 Crossgates Blvd. 39042<br>(601) 825-2811 Ext. 287, 288 |
| Columbia | Marion County General Hospital<br>39429<br>(601) 736-6303 Ext. 217 |
| Greenwood | Greenwood-LeFlore Hospital<br>River Road 38930<br>(601) 453-9751 Ext. 633 |
| Hattiesburg | Forrest County General Hospital<br>400 S. 28th Ave. 39401<br>(601) 544-7000 Ext. 565 |
| Jackson | Mississippi Baptist Medical Center<br>1225 N. State St. 39201<br>(601) 968-1704 |
| | St. Dominic-Jackson Memorial Hospital<br>969 Lakeland Dr. 39216<br>(601) 982-0121 Ext. 345 |
| | State Board of Health<br>Bureau of Disease Control 39205<br>(601) 354-6650 |
| | University Medical Center<br>2500 N. State Street 39216<br>(601) 354-7660 |
| Laurel | Jones County Community Hospital<br>Jefferson St. at 13th Ave. 39440<br>(601) 649-4000 Ext. 207, 218, 220, 248 |
| Meridian | St. Joseph's Hospital<br>Highway 39, North 39301<br>(601) 483-6211 Ext. 54, 71 |
| Pascagoula | Singing River Hospital<br>Highway 90 East 39567<br>(601) 762-6121 Ext. 654 |
| University | School of Pharmacy<br>University of Mississippi 38677<br>(601) 234-1522 |
| Vicksburg | Mercy Regional Medical Center<br>100 McAuley Dr. 39181<br>(601) 636-2131 Ext. 250, 276 |

TABLE 155—*Continued*
UNITED STATES DIRECTORY OF POISON CONTROL CENTERS, 1977*

| *City* | *Name and Address* |
|---|---|
| **MISSOURI** | |
| STATE COORDINATOR | Missouri Division of Health<br>Jefferson City 65101<br>(314) 751-2713 Ext. 221, 216 |
| Cape Girardeau | St. Francis Hospital<br>825 Good Hope St. 63701<br>(314) 335-1251 Ext. 217 |
| Columbia | University of Missouri Medical Center<br>807 Stadium Blvd. 65201<br>(314) 882-8091 |
| Hannibal | St. Elizabeth Hospital<br>109 Virginia St. 63401<br>(314) 221-0414 Ext. 101, 183 |
| Joplin | St. John's Hospital<br>2727 McClelland Blvd. 64801<br>(417) 781-2727 Ext. 393 |
| Kansas City | Children's Mercy Hospital<br>24th and Gillham Rd. 64108<br>(816) 471-0626 Ext. 383 |
| | Truman Medical Center W.<br>2301 Holmes St. 64108<br>(816) 556-3000 Ext. 3100 |
| Kirksville | Kirksville Osteopathic Hospital<br>800 W. Jefferson St. 63501<br>(816) 626-2266 |
| Poplar Bluff | Lucy Lee Hospital<br>330 N. 2nd St. 63901<br>(314) 785-7721 Ext. 166 |
| Rolla | Phelps County Memorial Hospital<br>1000 W. 10th St 65401<br>(314) 364-3100 Ext. 126 |
| St. Joseph | Methodist Hospital and Medical Center<br>8th and Faraon Sts. 64501<br>(816) 232-8461 Ext. 277 |
| St. Louis | Cardinal Glennon Memorial Hospital for Children<br>1465 S. Grand Blvd. 63104<br>(314) 772-5200 |
| | St. Louis Children's Hospital<br>500 S. Kingshighway 63110<br>(314) 367-6880 Ext. 220 |
| Springfield | Lester E. Cox Medical Center<br>1423 N. Jefferson St. 65802<br>(417) 836-3193 |
| | St. John's Hospital<br>1235 E. Cherokee 65802<br>(417) 881-8811 Ext. 248, 241 |
| West Plains | West Plains Memorial Hospital<br>1103 Alaska Ave. 65775<br>(417) 256-9111 Ext. 36, 22 |
| **MONTANA** | |
| STATE COORDINATOR | Department of Health and Environmental Sciences<br>Helena 59601<br>(406) 449-3895 |
| Bozeman | Bozeman Deaconess Hospital<br>15 West Lamme 59715<br>(406) 586-5431 |
| Great Falls | Montana Deaconess Hospital<br>1101 26th St. S. 59401<br>(406) 761-1200 |
| Helena | St. Peter's Hospital<br>59601<br>(406) 442-2480 Ext. 137 |
| **NEBRASKA** | |
| STATE COORDINATOR | Department of Health<br>Lincoln 68502<br>(402) 471-2122 |

TABLE 155—*Continued*
UNITED STATES DIRECTORY OF POISON CONTROL CENTERS, 1977*

| *City* | *Name and Address* | *City* | *Name and Address* |
|---|---|---|---|
| | **NEBRASKA** *(Continued)* | | |
| Lincoln | Bryan Memorial Hospital<br>4848 Sumner St. 68506<br>(402) 483-3244 | Omaha | Children's Memorial Hospital<br>44th and Dewey Sts. 68105<br>(402) 553-5400 |
| | **NEVADA** | | |
| STATE COORDINATOR | Department of Human Resources<br>Carson City 89710<br>(702) 885-4750 | | |
| Las Vegas | Southern Nevada Memorial Hospital<br>1800 W. Charleston Blvd. 89102<br>(702) 385-1277 | Reno | Washoe Medical Center<br>77 Pringle Way 89502<br>(702) 785-4129<br>Night: 785-4140 |
| | **NEW HAMPSHIRE** | | |
| Hanover | Mary Hitchcock Hospital<br>2 Maynard St. 03755<br>(603) 643-4000 | | |
| | **NEW JERSEY** | | |
| STATE COORDINATOR | Department of Health<br>Trenton 08625<br>(609) 292-5666 | | |
| Atlantic City | Atlantic City Medical Center<br>1925 Pacific Ave. 08401<br>(609) 344-4081 | East Orange | East Orange General Hospital<br>300 Central Ave. 07019<br>(201) 672-8400 |
| Belleville | Clara Maass Memorial Hospital<br>1A Franklin Ave. 07109<br>(201) 751-1000 Ext. 781, 782, 783 | Elizabeth | St. Elizabeth Hospital<br>225 Williamson St. 07207<br>(201) 527-5059 |
| Boonton | Riverside Hospital<br>Powerville Rd. 07005<br>(201) 334-5000 | Englewood | Englewood Hospital<br>350 Engle St. 07631<br>(201) 568-3400 |
| Bridgeton | Bridgeton Hospital<br>Irving Ave. 08302<br>(609) 451-6600 | Flemington | Hunterdon Medical Center<br>Route #31 08822<br>(201) 782-2121 |
| Camden | West Jersey Hospital<br>Evesham Ave. and Voorhees Turnpike 08104<br>(609) 795-5554 | Livingston | St. Barnabas Medical Center<br>Old Short Hills Rd. 07039<br>(201) 992-5161 |
| Denville | St. Clare's Hospital<br>Pocono Rd. 07834<br>(201) 627-3000 | Long Branch | Monmouth Medical Center<br>Dunbar and 2nd Ave. 07740<br>(201) 222-2210 |
| | | Montclair | Mountainside Hospital<br>Bay and Highland Aves. 07042<br>(201) 746-6000 |

TABLE 155—*Continued*
UNITED STATES DIRECTORY OF POISON CONTROL CENTERS, 1977*

| City | Name and Address |
|---|---|
| **NEW JERSEY** *(Continued)* | |
| Morristown | Community Medical Center<br>Emergency Department<br>95 Mount Kemble Ave. 07960<br>(201) 538-0900 Ext. 221 |
| Mount Holly | Burlington County<br>Memorial Hospital<br>175 Madison Ave. 08060<br>(609) 267-7877 |
| Neptune | Jersey Shore Medical<br>Center-Fitkin Hospital<br>1945 Corlies Ave. 07753<br>(201) 988-1818<br>(800) 822-9761 |
| Newark | Newark Beth Israel<br>Medical Center<br>201 Lyons Ave. 07112<br>(201) 926-7240, 41, 42, 43 |
| New Brunswick | Middlesex General Hospital<br>180 Somerset St. 08901<br>(201) 828-3000 |
| | St. Peter's Medical Center<br>254 Easton Ave. 08903<br>(201) 545-8000 Ext. 495 |
| Newton | Newton Memorial Hospital<br>175 High St. 07860<br>(201) 383-2121 Ext. 270,<br>71, 72, 73, 74 |
| Orange | Hospital Center at<br>Orange<br>188 S. Essex Ave. 07051<br>(201) 678-1100 |
| Passaic | St. Mary's Hospital<br>211 Pennington Ave. 07055<br>(201) 473-1000 |
| Perth Amboy | Perth Amboy General Hospital<br>530 New Brunswick Ave. 08861<br>(201) 442-3700 |
| Phillipsburg | Warren Hospital<br>185 Roseberry St. 08865<br>(201) 859-1500 |
| Point Pleasant | Point Pleasant Hospital<br>Osborn Ave. and River Front 08743<br>(201) 892-1100 |
| Princeton | Medical Center at<br>Princeton<br>253 Witherspoon St. 08540<br>(609) 921-7700 |
| Saddle Brook | Saddle Brook General<br>Hospital<br>300 Market St. 07662<br>(201) 843-6700 |
| Somers Point | Shore Memorial Hospital<br>Shore and Sunny Aves. 08244<br>(609) 653-3515 |
| Somerville | Somerset Hospital<br>Rehill Ave. 08876<br>(201) 725-4000 |
| Summit | Overlook Hospital<br>193 Morris Ave. 07901<br>(201) 522-2232 |
| Teaneck | Holy Name Hospital<br>718 Teaneck Rd. 07666<br>(201) 837-3070 |
| Trenton | Helene Fuld Medical Center<br>750 Brunswick Ave. 08638<br>(609) 396-1077 |
| Union | Memorial General Hospital<br>1000 Galloping Hill Rd. 07083<br>(201) 687-1900 |
| Wayne | Greater Paterson General<br>Hospital<br>224 Hamburg Tnpk. 07470<br>(201) 684-6900 Ext. 224,<br>225, 226 |
| **NEW MEXICO** | |
| STATE COORDINATOR | New Mexico Poison, Drug Information, and Medical Crisis Center<br>University of New Mexico<br>Albuquerque 87131<br>(505) 843-2551<br>1-800-432-6866 within New Mexico |

TABLE 155—*Continued*
UNITED STATES DIRECTORY OF POISON CONTROL CENTERS, 1977*

| City | Name and Address | City | Name and Address |
|---|---|---|---|
| | **NEW MEXICO** *(Continued)* | | |
| Alamogordo | Gerald Champion Memorial Hospital<br>1209 9th St. 88310<br>(505) 437-3770 | Clovis | Clovis Memorial Hospital<br>1210 Thornton St. 88110<br>(505) 763-4493 |
| Albuquerque | New Mexico Poison, Drug Information, and Medical Crisis Center<br>University of New Mexico 87131<br>(505) 843-2551 | Las Cruces | Memorial General Hospital<br>Alameda and Lohman 88001<br>(505) 522-8641 |
| Carlsbad | Carlsbad Regional Medical Center<br>Northgate Center<br>P.O. Box 1479 88220<br>(505) 887-3521 | Roswell | Eastern New Mexico Medical Center<br>405 Country Club Rd. 88201<br>(505) 622-8170 |
| | **NEW YORK** | | |
| STATE COORDINATOR | Department of Health<br>Albany 12210<br>(518) 474-3664 | | |
| Albany | Albany Medical Center<br>Hospital Emergency Room<br>New Scotland Ave. 12208<br>(518) 445-3131 | Glens Falls | Glens Falls Hospital<br>100 Park St. 12801<br>(518) 792-3151 |
| Binghamton | Binghamton General Hospital<br>Mitchell and Park Sts. 13903<br>(607) 772-1100 Ext. 431 | Ithaca | Tompkins County Hospital<br>1285 Trumansburg Rd. 14850<br>(607) 274-4011, 4383, 4411 |
| | Our Lady of Lourdes Memorial Hospital<br>169 Riverside Drive 13905<br>(607) 729-6521 | Jamestown | W.C.A. Hospital<br>207 Foote Ave. 14707<br>(716) 487-0141 |
| Buffalo | Children's Hospital<br>219 Bryant St. 14222<br>(716) 878-7000 | Johnson City | Wilson Memorial Hospital<br>33-57 Harrison St. 13790<br>(607) 773-6611 |
| Dunkirk | Brooks Memorial Hospital<br>10 West 6th St. 14048<br>(716) 366-1111 Ext. 414, 415 | Kingston | Kingston Hospital<br>396 Broadway 12401<br>(914) 331-3131 Ext. 250 |
| East Meadow | Nassau County Medical Center<br>2201 Hempstead Tnpk. 11554<br>(516) 542-2323, 24, 25 | New York | N.Y. City, Dept. of Health<br>Bureau of Laboratories<br>455 First Ave. 10016<br>(212) 340-4495 |
| Elmira | Arnot Ogden Memorial Hospital<br>Roe Ave. and Grove 14901<br>(607) 737-4194 | Niagara Falls | Niagara Falls Memorial Medical Center<br>621 Tenth St. 14302<br>(716) 278-4511 |
| | St. Joseph's Hospital<br>555 E. Market St. 14902<br>(607) 734-2662 | Nyack | Nyack Hospital<br>North Midland Ave. 10960<br>(914) 358-6200 Ext. 451 452 |
| Endicott | Ideal Hospital<br>600 High Ave. 13760<br>(607) 754-7171 Ext. 66 | Oswego | Oswego Hospital<br>110 West 6th St. 13126<br>(315) 343-1920 |

TABLE 155—*Continued*
UNITED STATES DIRECTORY OF POISON CONTROL CENTERS, 1977*

| *City* | *Name and Address* | *City* | *Name and Address* |
|---|---|---|---|
| | **NEW YORK** *(Continued)* | | |
| Rochester | Strong Memorial Hospital<br>260 Crittenden Blvd. 14620<br>(716) 275-5151 | Watertown | House of the Good Samaritan Hospital<br>Corner Washington and Pratt Sts. 13602<br>(315) 788-8700 |
| Syracuse | Upstate Medical Center<br>750 E. Adams St. 13210<br>(315) 476-3166, 473-5831 | | |
| | **NORTH CAROLINA** | | |
| STATE COORDINATOR | Duke University Medical Center<br>Durham 22710<br>(919) 684-8111 | | |
| Asheville | Memorial Mission Hospital<br>509 Biltmore Ave. 28801<br>(704) 255-4660 | Hendersonville | Margaret R. Pardee Hospital<br>Fleming St. 28739<br>(704) 693-6522 |
| Charlotte | Mercy Hospital<br>2001 Vail Ave. 28207<br>(704) 372-5100 | Hickory | Catawba Memorial Hospital<br>Fairgrove-Church Rd. 28601<br>(704) 328-2191 |
| Durham | Duke University Medical Center<br>Box 3007 27710<br>(919) 684-8111 | Jacksonville | Onslow Memorial Hospital<br>Western Blvd. 28540<br>(919) 353-1234 Ext. 211 |
| Greensboro | Moses Cone Hospital<br>1200 N. Elm St. 27401<br>(919) 379-4109 | Wilmington | New Hanover Memorial Hospital<br>2431 S. 17th St. 28401<br>(919) 763-9021 Ext. 311 |
| | **NORTH DAKOTA** | | |
| STATE COORDINATOR | Department of Health<br>Bismarck 58505<br>(701) 224-2388 | | |
| Bismarck | Bismarck Hospital<br>300 N. 7th St. 58501<br>(701) 223-4700 | Jamestown | Jamestown Hospital<br>419 5th St., N.E. 58401<br>(701) 252-1050 |
| Dickinson | St. Joseph's Hospital<br>Seventh Street, W. 58601<br>(701) 225-6771 Ext. 329, 259 | Minot | St. Joseph's Hospital<br>304 4th St. 58701<br>(701) 838-0341 Ext. 253 |
| Fargo | North Dakota State University<br>College of Pharmacy 58201<br>(701) 237-8115 | Williston | Mercy Hospital<br>1301 15th Ave. 58801<br>(701) 572-7661 |
| Grand Forks | Deaconess Unit United Hospitals<br>212 S. 4th St. 58201<br>(701) 775-4241 | | |

TABLE 155—*Continued*
UNITED STATES DIRECTORY OF POISON CONTROL CENTERS, 1977*

| City | Name and Address | City | Name and Address |
|---|---|---|---|
| | **OHIO** | | |
| STATE COORDINATOR | Department of Health<br>Columbus 43216<br>(614) 466-2544 | | |
| Akron | Children's Hospital<br>Buchtel at Bowery 44308<br>(216) 379-8562 | Dayton | U.S.A.F. Medical Center<br>Wright Patterson AFB 45431<br>(513) 878-6623 |
| Canton | Aultman Hospital<br>Emergency Room<br>6th and Clarenden Ave. S.W. 44701<br>(216) 452-9911 | Lorain | Lorain Community Hospital<br>3700 Kolbe Rd. 44052<br>(216) 282-2220 |
| Cincinnati | University of Cincinnati<br>Cincinnati General Hospital<br>234 Goodman St. 45267<br>(513) 872-5111 | Mansfield | Mansfield General Hospital<br>335 Glessner Ave. 44903<br>(419) 522-3411 Ext. 545 |
| Cleveland | Cleveland Academy of Medicine<br>10525 Carnegie Ave. 44106<br>(216) 231-4455 | Springfield | Community Hospital<br>2615 E. High St. 45501<br>(513) 325-0531 Ext. 371 |
| Columbus | Children's Hospital<br>17th at Livingston 43205<br>(614) 228-1323 | Toledo | Medical College Hospital<br>P.O. Box 6190 43614<br>(419) 382-7971 |
| Dayton | Children's Medical Center<br>P.O. Box 1000<br>1735 Chapel St. 45404<br>(513) 461-4790 | Youngstown | St. Elizabeth Hospital<br>1044 Belmont Ave. 44505<br>(216) 746-2222 |
| | | Zanesville | Bethesda Hospital<br>2951 Maple Ave. 43701<br>(614) 454-4000 |
| | **OKLAHOMA** | | |
| STATE COORDINATOR | Department of Health<br>Oklahoma City 73105<br>(405) 271-5454 | | |
| Ada | Valley View Hospital<br>1300 E. 6th St. 74820<br>(405) 332-2323 Ext. 200 | Oklahoma City | St. Anthony's Hospital<br>Emergency Room<br>1000 N. Lee 73102<br>(405) 271-5454 |
| Ardmore | Memorial Hospital of Southern Oklahoma<br>1011 14th Ave., NW 73401<br>(405) 223-5400 | | State Dept. of Health<br>N.E. 10th St. and Stonewall 73105<br>(405) 271-5454 |
| Lawton | Comanche County Memorial Hospital<br>3401 Gore Blvd. 73501<br>(405) 355-8620 | Ponca City | St. Joseph Medical Center<br>14th and Hartford 74601<br>(405) 765-3321 Ext. 372 |
| McAlester | McAlester General Hospital, Inc. West<br>P.O. Box 669 74501<br>(918) 426-1800 Ext. 240 | Tulsa | Hillcrest Medical Center<br>1120 South Utica 74104<br>(918) 584-1351 Ext. 598 |

TABLE 155—*Continued*
UNITED STATES DIRECTORY OF POISON CONTROL CENTERS, 1977*

| *City* | *Name and Address* |
|---|---|
| **OREGON** | |
| Portland | Pediatrics Department<br>University of Oregon<br>Medical School<br>3181 S.W. Sam Jackson<br>Park Rd. 97201<br>(503) 225-8500 |
| **PENNSYLVANIA** | |
| STATE COORDINATOR | Department of Health<br>Harrisburg 17120<br>(717) 787-2307 |
| Allentown | Leheigh Valley Poison<br>Control<br>Sacred Heart Hospital<br>17th and Chew St. 18102<br>(215) 433-2311 |
| Altoona | Altoona Region Poison<br>Center<br>Mercy Hospital of Altoona<br>2601 Eighth Ave. 16603<br>(814) 946-3711 |
| Bethlehem | St. Luke's Hospital<br>800 Ostrum St. 18015<br>(215) 691-4141 |
| Bloomsburg | The Bloomsburg Hospital<br>549 E. Fair St. 17815<br>(717) 784-7121 |
| Bradford | Bradford Hospital<br>Interstate Pkwy. 16701<br>(814) 368-4143 |
| Bryn Mawr | The Bryn Mawr Hospital<br>19010<br>(215) 527-0600 |
| Carlisle | Carlisle Hospital<br>246 Parker St. 17013<br>(717) 249-1212 |
| Chambersburg | The Chambersburg Hospital<br>7th and King St. 17201<br>(717) 264-5171 Ext. 431 |
| Chester | Sacred Heart General<br>Hospital<br>9th and Wilson St. 19013<br>(215) 494-0721 Ext. 232 |
| Clearfield | Clearfield Hospital<br>809 Turnpike Ave. 16830<br>(814) 765-5341 |
| Coaldale | Coaldale State General<br>Hospital 18218<br>(717) 645-2131 |
| Coudersport | Charles Cole Memorial<br>Hospital<br>RD #3, Route 6 16915<br>(814) 274-9300 |
| Danville | Susquehanna Poison<br>Center<br>Geisinger Medical Center<br>North Academy Ave. 17821<br>(717) 275-6116 |
| Doylestown | Doylestown Hospital<br>595 W. State St. 18901<br>(215) 345-2281 |
| Drexel Hill | Delaware County Memorial<br>Hospital<br>Lansdowne and Keystone Ave. 19026<br>(215) 259-3800 |
| East Stroudsburg | Pocono Hospital<br>206 E. Brown St. 18301<br>(717) 421-4000 |
| Easton | Easton Hospital<br>21st and Lehigh St. 18042<br>(215) 258-6221 |
| Erie | Doctors Osteopathic<br>252 W. 11th St. 16501<br>(814) 455-3961 |
| | Erie Osteopathic Hospital<br>5515 Peach St. 16509<br>(814) 864-4031 |
| | Hamot Medical Center<br>4 E. Second St. 16512<br>(814) 455-6711 Ext. 521 |
| | Northwest Poison<br>Center<br>St. Vincent Health Center<br>P.O. Box 740 16512<br>(814) 452-3232 |

TABLE 155—*Continued*
UNITED STATES DIRECTORY OF POISON CONTROL CENTERS, 1977*

| *City* | *Name and Address* | *City* | *Name and Address* |
|---|---|---|---|
| | **PENNSYLVANIA** *(Continued)* | | |
| Gettysburg | Annie M. Warner Hospital<br>S. Washington St. 17325<br>(717) 334-2121 | Lebanon | Good Samaritan Hospital<br>4th and Walnut Sts. 17042<br>(717) 272-7611 |
| Greensburg | Westmoreland Hospital Association<br>532 W. Pittsburgh St. 15601<br>(412) 837-0100 | Lehighton | Gnaden-Huetten Memorial Hospital<br>11th and Hamilton St. 18235<br>(215) 377-1300 |
| Hanover | Hanover General Hospital<br>300 Highland Ave. 17331<br>(717) 637-3711 | Lewistown | Lewistown Hospital<br>Highland Ave. 17044<br>(717) 248-5411 |
| Harrisburg | Harrisburg Hospital<br>S. Front and Mulberry St. 17101<br>(717) 782-3639 | Muncy | Muncy Valley Hospital<br>P.O. Box 340 17756<br>(717) 546-8282 |
| | Polyclinic Hospital<br>3rd and Polyclinic Ave. 17105<br>(717) 782-4141 Ext. 4132 | Nanticoke | Nanticoke State Hospital<br>W. Washington St. 18634<br>(717) 735-5000 |
| Hershey | Milton S. Hershey Medical Center<br>University Dr. 17033<br>(717) 534-6111 | Paoli | Paoli Memorial Hospital<br>19301<br>(215) 647-2200 |
| Jeannete | Jeannete District Memorial Hospital<br>600 Jefferson Ave. 15644<br>(412) 527-3551 | Philadelphia | Phildelphia Poison Information<br>321 University Ave. 19104<br>(215) 823-8460 |
| Jersey Shore | Jersey Shore Hospital<br>Thompson St. 17740<br>(717) 398-0100 | Philipsburg | Philipsburg State General Hospital 16866<br>(814) 342-3320 |
| Johnstown | Conemaugh Valley Memorial Hospital<br>1086 Franklin St. 15905<br>(814) 536-6671 | Pittsburgh | Children's Hospital<br>125 Desoto St. 15213<br>(412) 681-6669 |
| | Lee Hospital<br>320 Main St. 15901<br>(814) 535-7541 | Pittston | Pittston Hospital<br>Oregon Heights 18640<br>(717) 654-3341 |
| | Mercy Hospital<br>1020 Franklin St. 15905<br>(814) 536-5353 | Pottstown | Pottstown Memorial Medical Center<br>High St. and Firestone Blvd. 19464<br>(215) 327-1000 |
| Lancaster | Lancaster General Hospital<br>555 North Duke St. 17604<br>(717) 299-5511 | Pottsville | Good Samaritan Hospital<br>E. Norwegian and Tremont St. 17901<br>(717) 622-3400 |
| | St. Joseph's Hospital<br>250 College Ave. 17604<br>(717) 299-4546 | Reading | Community General Hospital<br>145 N. 6th St. 19601<br>(215) 376-4881 |
| Lansdale | North Penn Hospital<br>7th and Broad St. 19446<br>(215) 368-2100 | | |

TABLE 155—*Continued*
UNITED STATES DIRECTORY OF POISON CONTROL CENTERS, 1977*

| *City* | *Name and Address* | *City* | *Name and Address* |
|---|---|---|---|
| | **PENNSYLVANIA** *(Continued)* | | |
| | Reading Hospital and Medical Center 19603 (215) 378-6218 | State College | Centre Community Hospital 16801 (814) 238-4351 |
| Sayre | The Robert Packer Hospital Guthrie Square 18840 (717) 888-6666 | Titusville | Titusville Hospital 406 W. Oak St. 16354 (814) 827-1851 |
| Scranton | Moses Taylor Hospital 700 Quincy Ave. 18510 (717) 346-3801 | Tunkhannock | Tyler Memorial Hospital RD #1 18657 (717) 836-2161 |
| | Scranton State General Hospital 205 Mulberry St. 18501 (717) 961-4205 | Wellsboro | Soldiers and Sailors Memorial Hospital Central Ave. 16901 (717) 724-1631 |
| | Community Medical Center 316 Colfax Ave. 18510 (717) 343-5566 | Wilkes-Barre | Wilkes-Barre General Hospital N. River and Auburn St. 18702 (717) 823-1121 Ext. 222 |
| Sellersville | Grandview Hospital 18960 (215) 257-3611 | Williamsport | Williamsport Hospital 777 Rural Ave. 17701 (717) 322-7861 |
| Somerset | Somerset Community Hospital 225 South Center Ave. 15501 (814) 443-2626 | York | Memorial Osteopathic Hospital 325 S. Belmont St. 17403 (717) 843-8623 |
| | **PUERTO RICO** | | |
| STATE COORDINATOR | University of Puerto Rico Rio Piedras (809) 765-4880, 0615 | Mayaguez | Mayaguez Medical Center Department of Health P.O. Box 1868 00709 (809) 832-8686 |
| Arecibo | District Hospital of Arecibo 00613 (809) 878-3535 | Ponce | District Hospital of Ponce 00731 (809) 842-8354, 2080 |
| Fajardo | District Hospital of Fajardo 00649 (809) 863-0505 | Rio Piedras | Medical Center of Puerto Rico (809) 764-3515 |
| | **RHODE ISLAND** | | |
| STATE COORDINATOR | Department of Health Providence 02908 (401) 277-2401 | | |
| Kingston | College of Pharmacy University of Rhode Island (401) 792-2775, 2762 | Pawtucket | Memorial Hospital Prospect St. 02860 (401) 724-1230 |

TABLE 155—*Continued*
UNITED STATES DIRECTORY OF POISON CONTROL CENTERS, 1977*

| *City* | *Name and Address* | *City* | *Name and Address* |
|---|---|---|---|
| | **RHODE ISLAND** *(Continued)* | | |
| Providence | Rhode Island Hospital<br>593 Eddy St. 02902<br>(401) 277-4000 | | Roger Williams General Hospital<br>825 Chalkstone Ave. 02907<br>(401) 521-5055 |
| | **SOUTH CAROLINA** | | |
| STATE COORDINATOR | Department of Health and Environmental Control<br>Columbia 29201<br>(803) 758-5506 | | |
| Charleston | Medical University of South Carolina<br>80 Barre St. 29401<br>(803) 792-4201 | Columbia | Richland Memorial Hospital<br>3301 Harden St. 29202<br>(803) 765-7359 |
| | **SOUTH DAKOTA** | | |
| STATE COORDINATOR | Department of Health<br>Pierre 57501<br>(605) 224-3361 | | |
| Aberdeen | St. Luke's Hospital<br>305 S. State St. 57401<br>(605) 225-5110 | Sioux Falls | McKennan Hospital<br>800 East 21st St. 57101<br>(605) 336-3894 |
| | **TENNESSEE** | | |
| STATE COORDINATOR | Department of Public Health<br>Nashville 37216<br>(615) 741-7247 | | |
| Chattanooga | T.C. Thompson Children's Hospital<br>910 Blackford St. 37403<br>(615) 755-6100 | Johnson City | Memorial Hospital<br>Boone and Fairview Ave. 37601<br>(615) 926-1131 |
| Columbia | Maury County Hospital<br>1224 Trotwood Avenue 38401<br>(615) 381-4500 Ext. 458 | Knoxville | Memorial Research Center and Hospital<br>1924 Alcoa Highway 37920<br>(615) 971-3261 |
| Cookeville | Cookeville General Hospital<br>142 W. 5th St. 38501<br>(615) 528-2541 | Memphis | LeBonheur Children's Hospital<br>848 Adams Ave. 38103<br>(901) 522-3000 |
| Jackson | Madison General Hospital<br>708 W. Forest 38301<br>(901) 424-0424 | Nashville | Vanderbilt University Hospital<br>21st and Garland 37232<br>(615) 322-3391 |
| | **TEXAS** | | |
| STATE COORDINATOR | Department of Health<br>Austin 78756<br>(512) 458-7254 | | |

TABLE 155—*Continued*
UNITED STATES DIRECTORY OF POISON CONTROL CENTERS, 1977*

| City | Name and Address |
|---|---|
| **TEXAS** *(Continued)* | |
| Abilene | Hendrick Hospital<br>19th and Hickory Sts. 79601<br>(915) 677-3551 Ext. 266, 7 |
| Amarillo | Amarillo Hospital District<br>Amarillo Emergency Receiving Center Education<br>P.O. Box 1110<br>2203 W. 6th St. 79175<br>(806) 376-4431 Ext. 501, 2, 3, 4 |
| Austin | Brackenridge Hospital<br>14th and Sabine Sts. 78701<br>(512) 478-4490 |
| Beaumont | Baptist Hospital of Southeast Texas<br>P.O. Box 1591<br>College and 11th St. 77701<br>(713) 833-7409 |
| Corpus Christi | Memorial Medical Center<br>P.O. Box 5280<br>2606 Hospital Blvd. 78405<br>(512) 884-4511 Ext. 556, 7 |
| El Paso | R.E. Thomason General Hospital<br>P.O. Box 20009<br>4815 Alameda Ave. 79905<br>(915) 533-1244 |
| Fort Worth | W.I. Cook Children's Hospital<br>1212 Lancaster 76102<br>(817) 336-5521 Ext. 17<br>336-6611 |
| Galveston | Southeast Texas Poison Control Center<br>8th and Mechanic Sts. 77550<br>(713) 765-1420 |
| Grand Prairie | Grand Prairie Community Hospital<br>2733 Sherman Rd. 75050<br>(214) 641-1313 |
| Harlingen | Valley Baptist Hospital<br>P.O. Box 2588<br>2101 S. Commerce St. 78550<br>(512) 423-1224 Ext. 23 |
| Laredo | Mercy Hospital<br>1515 Logan St. 78040<br>(512) 724-8011 Ext. 29 |
| Lubbock | Methodist Hospital Pharmacy<br>3615 19th St. 79410<br>(806) 792-1011 Ext. 3315 |
| Midland | Midland Memorial Hospital<br>1908 W. Wall 79701<br>(915) 684-8257 |
| Odessa | Medical Center Hospital<br>P.O. Box 633 79760<br>(915) 337-7311 Ext. 250, 252 |
| Plainview | Plainview Hospital<br>2404 Yonkers St. 79072<br>(806) 296-9601 |
| San Angelo | Shannon West Texas Memorial Hospital<br>P.O. Box 1879<br>9 S. Magdalen St. 76901<br>(915) 653-6741 |
| San Antonio | Bexar County Hospital District<br>c/o Department of Pediatrics<br>University of Texas Medical School at San Antonio<br>7703 Floyd Dr. 78229<br>(512) 223-1481 |
| Tyler | Medical Center Hospital<br>1000 S. Beckham St. 75701<br>(214) 597-0351 Ext. 255 |
| Waco | Hillcrest Hospital<br>3000 Herring Ave. 76708<br>(817) 753-1412, 756-8611 |
| Wharton | Caney Valley Memorial Hospital<br>3007 N. Richmond Rd. 77488<br>(713) 532-2440<br>Night: 532-1440 |
| Wichita Falls | Wichita General Hospital<br>Emergency Room<br>1600 8th St. 76301<br>(817) 322-6771 |
| **UTAH** | |
| STATE COORDINATOR | Division of Health<br>Salt Lake City 84113<br>(801) 533-6191, 6131 |
| Salt Lake City | Intermountain Regional Poison Control Center<br>50 N. Medical Drive 84132<br>(801) 581-2151 |

TABLE 155—*Continued*
UNITED STATES DIRECTORY OF POISON CONTROL CENTERS, 1977*

| *City* | *Name and Address* | *City* | *Name and Address* |
|---|---|---|---|
| | **VIRGIN ISLANDS** | | |
| STATE COORDINATOR | Department of Health<br>St. Thomas 00801<br>(809) 774-1321 Ext. 275 | | |
| St. Croix | Charles Harwood Memorial Hospital<br>Christiansted 00820<br>(809) 773-1212, 1311 Ext. 221 | St. John | Morris F. DeCastro Clinic<br>Cruz Bay 00830<br>(809) 776-1469 |
| | Ingeborg Nesbitt Clinic<br>Frederiksted 00840<br>(809) 772-0260, 0212 | St. Thomas | Knud-Hansen Memorial Hospital 00801<br>(809) 774-1321 Ext. 266 |
| | **VIRGINIA** | | |
| STATE COORDINATOR | Department of Health<br>Richmond 23219<br>(804) 786-4265 | | |
| Alexandria | Alexandria Hospital<br>4320 Seminary Rd. 22314<br>(703) 370-9000 Ext. 555 | Lynchburg | Lynchburg Gen. Marshall Lodge Hospital, Inc.<br>Tate Springs Rd. 24504<br>(804) 528-2066 |
| Arlington | Arlington Hospital<br>5129 N. 16th St. 22205<br>(703) 558-6161 | Nassawadox | Northampton-Accomack Memorial Hospital<br>23413<br>(804) 442-8000 |
| Blacksburg | Montgomery County Community Hospital<br>Rt. 460, S. 24060<br>(804) 951-1111 | Norfolk | DePaul Hospital<br>Granby St. at Kingsley Lane 23505<br>(804) 489-5111 |
| Charlottesville | University of Virginia Hospital<br>Pediatric Clinic 22903<br>(804) 924-0211 | Petersburg | Petersburg General Hospital<br>Mt. Erin and Adams Sts. 23803<br>(804) 732-7220 Ext. 327, 328 |
| Danville | Danville Memorial Hospital<br>142 S. Main St. 22201<br>(804) 799-2100 Ext. 3869 | Portsmouth | U.S. Naval Hospital<br>23708<br>(804) 397-6541 Ext. 418 |
| Falls Church | Fairfax Hospital<br>3300 Gallows Rd. 22046<br>(703) 698-3600, 3111 | Richmond | Medical College of Virginia Hospital<br>Pediatric OPD, Box 874<br>MCV Station 23298<br>(804) 770-5123 |
| Hampton | Hampton General Hospital<br>3120 Victoria Blvd. 23661<br>(804) 722-1131 | Roanoke | Roanoke Memorial Hospital<br>Belleview at Jefferson St.<br>P.O. Box 13367 24033<br>(703) 981-7336 |
| Harrisonburg | Rockingham Memorial Hospital<br>738 S. Mason St. 22801<br>(804) 424-4421 Ext. 225 | Staunton | King's Daughters' Hospital<br>P.O. Box 2007 24401<br>(703) 885-0361 Ext. 209, 247 |
| Lexington | Stonewall Jackson Hospital<br>22043<br>(804) 463-9141 | | |

TABLE 155—*Continued*
UNITED STATES DIRECTORY OF POISON CONTROL CENTERS, 1977*

| City | Name and Address | City | Name and Address |
|---|---|---|---|
| | **VIRGINIA** *(Continued)* | | |
| Waynesboro | Waynesboro Community Hospital<br>501 Oak Ave. 22980<br>(703) 942-8355 Ext. 440, 500 | Williamsburg | Williamsburg Community Hospital<br>Mt. Vernon Ave.<br>Drawer H 23185<br>(804) 229-1120 Ext. 65 |
| | **WASHINGTON** | | |
| STATE COORDINATOR | Department of Social and Health Services<br>Olympia 98504<br>(206) 753-3468 | | |
| Aberdeen | St. Joseph's Hospital<br>1006 North H St. 98520<br>(206) 533-0450 Ext. 277 | Seattle | Children's Orthopedic Hospital and Medical Center<br>4800 Sandpoint Way, N.E. 98105<br>(206) 634-5252 |
| Bellingham | St. Luke's General Hospital<br>809 E. Chestnut St. 98225<br>(206) 676-8400 | Spokane | Deaconess Hospital<br>W. 800 5th Ave. 99210<br>(509) 747-1077 |
| Longview | St. John's Hospital<br>1614 E. Kessler 98632<br>(206) 636-5252 | Tacoma | Mary Bridge Children's Hospital<br>311 S. L St. 98405<br>(206) 272-1281 Ext. 59 |
| Madigan | Madigan Army Medical Center Emergency Room<br>(206) 967-6972 | Vancouver | St. Joseph Community Hospital<br>600 N.E. 92nd St. 98664<br>(206) 256-2064 |
| Olympia | St. Peter's Hospital<br>413 N. Lilly Rd. 98506<br>(206) 491-0222 | Yakima | Yakima Valley Memorial Hospital<br>2811 Tieton Dr. 98902<br>(509) 248-4400 |
| Richland | Kadlec Hospital<br>888 Swift Blvd. 99352<br>(509) 943-1283 | | |
| | **WEST VIRGINIA** | | |
| STATE COORDINATOR | Department of Health<br>Charleston 25305<br>(304) 348-2971 | | |
| Beckley | Beckley Hospital<br>1007 S. Oakwood Ave. 25801<br>(304) 252-6431 Ext. 213 | Huntington | Cabell-Huntington Hospital<br>1340 16th St. 25701<br>(304) 696-6160 |
| Belle | E.I. DuPont de Nemours and Company 25015<br>(304) 949-4314 Ext. 261 | | St. Mary's Hospital<br>2900 1st Ave. 25701<br>(304) 696-2224, 2573 |
| Charleston | Charleston Area Medical Center Memorial Division<br>3200 Noyes Ave. 25304<br>(304) 348-4211 | Martinsburg | City Hospital<br>Dry Run Rd. 25401<br>(304) 263-8971 |
| Clarksburg | United Hospital Center Inc.<br>Downtown Division<br>Washington and Chestnut Sts. 26301<br>(304) 623-3177 Ext. 251 | Morgantown | West Virginia University Hospital 26505<br>(304) 293-5341 |

TABLE 155—*Continued*
UNITED STATES DIRECTORY OF POISON CONTROL CENTERS, 1977*

| *City* | *Name and Address* | *City* | *Name and Address* |
|---|---|---|---|
| | **WEST VIRGINIA** *(Continued)* | | |
| Parkersburg | Camden-Clark Hospital<br>717 Ann St. 26101<br>(304) 424-2212 | Weirton | Weirton General Hospital<br>St. John's Rd. 26062<br>(304) 748-3232 Ext. 208 |
| | St. Joseph's Hospital<br>19th St. and Murdoch Ave. 26101<br>(304) 424-4251 Ext. 251 | Welch | Stevens Clinic Hospital<br>U.S. 52 East 24801<br>(304) 436-3161 Ext. 264 |
| Pt. Pleasant | Pleasant Valley Hospital<br>Valley Drive 25550<br>(304) 675-4340 Ext. 252 | Weston | Stonewall Jackson Hospital<br>507 Main Ave. 26452<br>(304) 269-3000 Ext. 201, 228 |
| Ronceverte | Greenbrier Valley Hospital<br>608 Greenbrier Ave. 24970<br>(304) 647-4411, 12, 13 | Wheeling | Wheeling Hospital<br>109 Main St. 26003<br>(304) 243-2381 |
| | **WISCONSIN** | | |
| STATE COORDINATOR | Department of Health and Social Services<br>Madison 53701<br>(608) 266-2661 | | |
| Eau Claire | Luther Hospital<br>310 Chestnut St. 54701<br>(715) 835-1511 | Madison | University Hospital<br>1300 University Ave. 53706<br>(608) 262-3702 |
| Green Bay | St. Vincent Hospital<br>835 S. Van Buren St. 54301<br>(414) 432-8621 | Milwaukee | Milwaukee Children's Hospital<br>1700 W. Wisconsin 53233<br>(414) 344-7100 |
| Kenosha | Kenosha Hospital<br>6308 8th Ave. 53140<br>(414) 656-2201 | | |
| | **WYOMING** | | |
| STATE COORDINATOR | Department of Public Health<br>Cheyenne 82001<br>(307) 777-7511 | | |
| Casper | Memorial Hospital of Natrona County<br>1233 E. 2nd St. 82601<br>(307) 577-7201 | Cheyenne | Laramie County Memorial Hospital<br>23rd and House Sts. 82001<br>(307) 634-3341 Ext. 220 |

## MANUFACTURERS AND OTHER SOURCES (HOT LINES)

**A. H. Robins**
*See* Robins

**Abbott Labs**
(317) 688-6100

**Alexandra de Markoff Products**
*See* Gillette

**American Cyanamid Agricultural Products**
(201) 835-3100

**Ames**
(219) 264-8901 (bus. hrs.)
(219) 264-8371 (other hrs.)

**Ansar Herbicides**
*See* Ansul

**Ansul Co.**
(715) 735-7411

**Avon**
(914) 357-2012

**Ayerst Labs**
(212) 986-1000

**Bain de Soleil Products**
*See* Gillette

**Best Food Products (Rit and Shinola)**
*See* CPC International

**Bon Ami Products**
(816) 421-7075 (bus. hrs.)
(816) 373-6321 (other hrs.)

**Borden Chemical Co.**
(607) 967-2111
ext. 216, B. Gorton
ext. 272, B. Volkert

**Boyle-Midway Products**
Cranford Research Lab.
(201) 276-3900, 732-8360 (bus. hrs.)
(201) 276-0170 (other hrs.)

**Bristol Labs**
(315) 432-2838, 432-2713 (bus. hrs.)
(315) 432-2121 (other hrs.)

**Burroughs Wellcome and Co.**
(919) 549-8371
ext. 437, Mr. Singleton

**Center for Disease Control**
(404) 633-3311 (bus. hrs.)
(404) 633-2176 (other hrs.)

**Charles of the Ritz Products**
*See* Gillette

**Chemtrec**
(800) 424-9300
(800) 483-7616 (from D.C.)
(202) 483-7616 (from outside continental U.S.)

**Chemagro Agricultural Products**
(816) 242-2000

**Chesebrough Pond's Products**
(203) 377-7100

**Chevron Chemical Co.**
(415) 233-3737 (collect)

**Churchill Chemical Co.**
(404) 872-0721 (bus. hrs.)
(404) 255-8167 (other hrs.)

**Ciba Pharmaceutical Co.**
(201) 277-5000

**Ciba-Geigy Agricultural Products**
(914) 478-3131

**Cincinnati Milacron**
(513) 841-8100

**Clairol Products**
(203) 357-5900

**Clinique Labs**
*See* Estee Lauder

**Colgate-Palmolive Co.**
(212) 751-1200 (bus. hrs.)
(201) 434-1300 (other hrs.)

**Conklin Co.**
(612) 445-6010 (bus. hrs.)
other hrs.
(612) 824-4465, James O'Hara
(612) 448-3760, James Leonard

**Cooper Labs**
(201) 540-8700 (bus. hrs.)
other hrs.
(201) 821-8846, J. F. Grattan
(201) 746-9543, F. C. Goble

**CPC International**
(317) 632-5321 (bus. hrs.), chief chemist
other hrs.
(317) 881-6691, L. M. Clark
(317) 786-4782, J. E. Miller
(317) 244-1636, R. G. Lanwelen
(317) 253-1819, D. B. Wilson
(317) 888-1311, P. T. Blackwell

**Dorsey Labs**
(402) 464-6311 (bus hrs.), medical director
(402) 488-0060 (other hrs.)

**Dow Chemical Co.**
(317) 873-7000

**Drackett Co.**
(513) 632-1500

**DuBois Chemicals**
(513) 769-4200 (bus. hrs.)
other hrs.
(513) 321-5358, W. J. Corbett
(513) 874-9271, R. R. Keast
(513) 984-8872, E. R. Loder

**DuPont Products**
(302) 774-1000

**Eastman Kodak Products**
(716) 458-1000
ext. 85566 (bus. hrs.)
ext. 74755 (other hrs.)

**Eaton Labs**
(607) 335-2111 (bus. hrs.)
(607) 335-2243 (other hrs.)

**E. I. DuPont DeNemours**
*See* DuPont

**Eli Lilly**
*See* Lilly

**Elanco Products** (agrichemical subsidiary of Eli Lilly Co.)
bus. hrs.
(317) 261-2586, Dr. F. M. Chernish
(317) 261-2918, Dr. J. Bader
(317) 261-2568, Dr. I. F. Bennett
other hrs.
(317) 636-2211

**Endo**
(516) 832-2210

**Estee Lauder, Inc.**
bus. hrs.
(516) 420-7040, Vincent Basmajian
(516) 420-7356, Joseph Gubernick
other hrs.
(212) 544-9132, Joseph Gubernick
(212) 357-3233, 454-9616, Vincent Basmajian

**Exxon Oil Products**
bus. hrs.
(713) 668-7024, J. W. Hammond
other hrs.
(713) 668-7024, J. W. Hammond
(713) 528-3346, J. G. Lione

MANUFACTURERS AND OTHER SOURCES
(HOT LINES) *Continued*

**Faberge Products**
bus. hrs.
(201) 945-5800
ext. 329, 331, Richard J. Witkowski
ext. 328, Joy Frank
ext. 316, 320, Maurice Siegel
other hrs.
(201) 288-6204, Richard J. Witkowski
(201) 939-7579, Joy Frank
(201) 666-3398, Maurice Siegel

**Fabmagic Inc.**
*See* Purex

**Faultless Starch Products**
(816) 421-7075 (bus. hrs.)
(816) 373-6321 (other hrs.)

**Food Poisoning**
(commercially processed)
(301) 443-4667 (bus. hrs.), R. Swanson, D. Brand
other hrs.
(703) 591-6409, R. Swanson
(301) 253-9510, D. Brand
Consumer complaints on food
(301) 443-1240, Doris Sandborn

**Ford Motor Co. Products**
(313) 323-0045, 322-1133

**Foretell, Inc.**
*See* Puritan Chemical

**Frances Denney Products**
(215) 729-8200 (bus. hrs.)
(609) 654-4146 (other hrs.)
Mr. Gallant

**Fuller Brush Co. Products**
(316) 792-1711 (bus. hrs.)
other hrs.
(316) 792-5493, Phyllis I. Franke
(316) 793-5816, Louis Gray
(316) 792-3265, John Mansfield
(316) 793-5174, Michael Zemanick

**G. D. Searle**
*See* Searle

**Geigy Pharmaceuticals**
(201) 277-5000

**General Motors Products**
(313) 635-5244 (bus. hrs.)
(313) 635-5281 (other hrs.)

**Gillette Co.**
**(617) 421-7000**
*includes:*
Papermate
Toiletries and Safety Razor Division
Hyponex Co.
Jafra Cosmetics
Cambridge Shaver Imports
Swiss Farms
Toni (617) 268-3200

**Glamorene Products**
bus. hrs.
(201) 778-2400, Howard Eisen
(914) 895-2933, Dr. C. J. Umberger
other hrs.
(914) 452-0400
(201) 797-5428, Howard Eisen

**Glidden-Durkee Products**
bus. hrs.
(216) 771-5121
ext. 2258, S. T. Bowell
(216) 771-5121
ext. 2291, J. G. Kingston
other hrs.
(216) 777-4061, S. T. Bowell
(216) 235-5364, J. G. Kingston

**Goddard Products**
(414) 554-2111 (collect)

**Gulf Products**
(713) 750-2811 (bus. hrs.)
Dr. F. M. Love
Dr. L. L. Pickett
Dr. D. T. Cline
Dr. W. H. Yates
(713) 226-1011, 750-2000 (other hrs.)
Dr. F. M. Love
Dr. L. L. Pickett
Dr. D. T. Cline
Dr. W. H. Yates
(412) 362-1600
ext. 2101, Dr. L. B. Barnes
ext. 2487, Dr. M. L. Gilberti
ext. 2673, Dr. H. N. MacFarland
other hrs.
(412) 487-4069, Dr. L. B. Barnes
(412) 781-5837, Dr. M. L. Gilberti
(412) 963-8598, Dr. H. N. MacFarland

**Hoffman LaRoche**
*See* Roche Labs

**Holmdel**
(201) 264-9000

**Hyponex Co. Products**
*See* Gillette

**ICI United States Products**
(302) 575-3305 (bus. hrs.)
(302) 575-3000 (other hrs.)

**Imperial Products**
*See* Gillette

**International Society of Aquatic Medicine**
(213) 481-0896, Dr. Rosco

**Ives Labs**
(212) 986-1000 (bus. hrs.)
(914) 769-9060 (other hrs.)

**Jafra Cosmetics**
*See* Gillette

**Jean Nate Products**
*See* Gillette

**Jewel Products**
(312) 381-2600
ext. 322 (bus. hrs.), Oliver E. Libman
(312) 824-2760 (other hrs.)

**Johnson and Johnson Products**
(201) 524-0400

**Johnson and Sons Co.**
American products (414) 554-2111 (collect)
Canadian products (519) 756-7900 (collect)

**Johnson's Wax Products**
*See* Johnson and Son Co.

**Kodak Products**
*See* Eastman Kodak

**Lanvin Products**
*See* Gillette

**Lederle Labs**
(914) 735-5000

**Lilly and Co.**
(317) 261-3714

**Luzier Cosmetic Products**
bus. hrs.
(913) 384-1000, ext. 290, director of technology
other hrs.
(913) 888-1928, Merlyn G. Flom
(913) 342-1165, Ted Tracz

**Mallinckrodt**
(314) 895-0123 (bus. hrs.)

**Max Factor**
bus. hrs.
(213) 462-6131, Dr. David Anderson
(213) 888-7258, Peter Kaufman

MANUFACTURERS AND OTHER SOURCES
(HOT LINES) *Continued*

**McNeil Labs**
(215) 836-4500

**Mead Johnson Labs**
(812) 426-6000

**Merck, Sharp and Dohme**
(215) 699-5311

**Merrell-National Labs**
(513) 948-9111, ext. 529

**Mushroom poisoning**
*See* Thioctic acid

**National Antivenin Index**
(405) 271-5454

**Nor-Am Agricultural Products**
(815) 338-1800 (bus. hrs.)
other hrs.
(815) 459-5391, Dr. Katsaros
(815) 459-3475, Dr. Lambert
(815) 459-4749, Dr. Martin
(312) 668-5428, Dr. Seven

**Norwich**
*See* Eaton Labs

**Ortho Insecticide and Chemical Products**
*See* Chevron Chemical

**Ortho Pharmaceutical Corp.**
(201) 524-2162 (bus. hrs.)
(201) 524-1566 (other hrs.)

**Papermate**
*See* Gillette

**Parke, Davis and Co.**
(313) 567-5300
(617) 864-6000, ext. 3338, Dr. Green

**Pesticide Poisoning Consultants**
(EPA contracted)
*Western States*
(319) 353-5558, 5559 (bus. hrs.), D. P. Morgan
(319) 338-8474 (other hrs.)
*Eastern States*
(803) 792-2281 (bus. hrs.), S. H. Sandifer
(803) 722-7760 (other hrs.)
(803) 792-2111, ext. 3305 (bus. hrs.), J. R. Reigart
(803) 556-5321 (other hrs.)
(803) 723-5352 (bus. hrs.), C. M. Cupp
(803) 792-2285 (other hrs.)

**Pesticide Safety Team Network**
*See* CHEMTREC

**Pfizer Labs**
(212) 573-2422

**Pitman Moore Products**
*See* Dow

**Polaroid Corp. Products**
bus. hrs.
(617) 354-9426, Dr. Briefer
(617) 864-6000, ext. 3338, Dr. Green
(617) 332-6515 (other hrs.)

**Proctor and Gamble Co.**
(513) 562-1100 (bus. hrs.)
other hrs.
(513) 521-3518, J. H. Benedict
(513) 825-8234, J. E. Weaver
(513) 761-5468, W. R. Michael
(513) 729-4314, C. A. Ivy

**Purex Corp.**
(213) 634-3300

**Puritan Chemical Co.**
(404) 872-0721 (bus. hrs.)
(404) 394-3227 (other hrs.), Robert Lynn

**Raid Products**
*See* Johnson and Sons

**Redken Labs**
(213) 992-2700 (bus. hrs.)

**Revlon**
(212) 824-9000 (bus. hrs. until 1:00 a.m.)
(212) 340-4494 (NYC PCC) (other hrs.)

**Rit**
*See* CPC International

**Robins Co.**
(804) 257-2000 (bus. hrs.)
(804) 643-7373 (other hrs.)

**Roche Labs**
(201) 235-2355

**Roerig**
*See* Pfizer

**Ross Labs**
*See* Abbott

**Sandoz Pharmaceuticals**
(201) 386-1000

**Searle Labs**
(312) 982-7000

**Sears, Roebuck and Co.**
(303) 623-5872

**Schering Corp.**
(201) 931-2000

**Shaklee Products**
(415) 786-1500

**Shell Chemical Co.**
(for decontamination)
(618) 254-7331

**Shell Oil Co. Agricultural, Chemical, and Consumer Products**
(513) 961-3337

**Sherwin Williams Products**
(216) 566-2917

**Shinola**
*See* CPC International

**Smith, Kline and French**
(215) 854-4900

**Snake antivenin**
*See* National Antivenin Index

**Stanley Home Products**
(413) 527-1000

**Sterling-Winthrop**
*See* Winthrop

**Stuart Pharmaceuticals**
*See* ICI United States Products

**Swiss Farms**
*See* Gillette

**Syntex Labs**
(415) 855-3881 (bus. hrs.)
other hrs.
(415) 855-3881
(415) 666-4346 San Francisco Health Dept.

**Texaco Products**
*New York*
(914) 253-4000 (bus. hrs.)
R. T. Richards
J. P. Licata
E. R. Stanton
other hrs.
(203) 744-3006, R. T. Richards
(201) 487-4130, J. P. Licata
(203) 531-4916, E. R. Stanton
*Texas*
(713) 666-8000 (bus. hrs.) Mr. Hobson, H. E. Hyder
other hrs.
(713) 467-9486, H. E. Hyder

**Texize Chemicals**
(803) 963-4261

MANUFACTURERS AND OTHER SOURCES (HOT LINES) *Continued*

**Thioctic acid** (mushroom poisoning) *(Amanita phalloides* only)
(301) 496-6268 (bus. hrs.), Dr. Bartter
(301) 656-4000, (202) 244-5562 other hrs.

**Toni**
*See* Gillette

**Union Carbide Products**
bus. hrs.
(212) 551-4785, Dr. Demehl
(304) 747-5975, Dr. Hall
(212) 551-4787, Dr. Lane
other hrs.
(304) 744-3487

**Upjohn Co.**
(616) 323-4000

**USV Labs**
(914) 779-6300

**Wallace Labs**
(609) 655-1100 (bus. hrs.)
(609) 799-1167 (other hrs.)

**Warner Chilcott**
(201) 540-2025

**Winthrop Labs**
(212) 972-4141

**Wyeth Labs**
(215) 688-4400

**Yves St. Laurent Products**
*See* Gillette

## *Guide to the Organization of a Poison Control Center*

A. General Objectives
Minimizing the damage from potentially toxic substances by improving efforts at prevention and treatment of poisoning.

B. Specific Objectives
1. *Treatment*
 a. Making initial treatment (primarily first aid) more prompt and effective.
 b. Improvement of overall treatment
 (1) Increasing knowledge of potentially toxic substances.
 (2) Increasing the knowledge of the type of general and specific treatment measures required in the hospital, the office and the patient's home.
 (3) Making resources for treatment readily and continuously available.
 (4) Stimulating research for specific antagonists or antidotes for more frequent and dangerous chemicals.
2. *Prevention*
 a. Developing a better knowledge of the distribution, type, and toxicity of the various poisons.
 b. Developing a more thorough knowledge of the circumstances in which the poison is likely to be taken.
 c. Interrupting the chain of circumstances that leads to poisoning.
 d. Using all available pertinent professional personnel such as physicians, nurses, pharmacists, veterinarians, botanists, agricultural and exterminator specialists, manufacturing chemists, etc. in increasing the efforts of prevention and proper treatment.
 e. Using all available community agencies and communication media for spreading information about poisoning, e.g. safety councils, service clubs, parent-teacher associations, junior chambers of commerce, the Red Cross, radio, television, newspapers, periodicals, etc.

C. Activities of Participants in Poison Control Centers
1. *Hospitals**
 a. Treatment

*Implementation of the hospitals' role in a poison control center will be greatly aided by the appointment of a poison control officer (and an alternate or associate officer) for each participating hospital to coordinate and direct the hospitals' efforts in this area. Part D gives suggested duties of such a poison control officer. Large hospitals that are major medical centers with more personnel, funds and facilities than smaller ones will have more extensive roles to play in the areas of professional education and research and will usually have more complete reference and information and treatment services. A pattern of "master centers" and less elaborate "daughter centers" may be desirable in some communities.

(1) Development of a twenty-four-hour-a-day poison *information* service to physicians on treatment of poisoning (information to parents limited to first aid instructions).
(2) Development of a twenty-four-hour-a-day emergency treatment facility.
(3) Research on most effective treatment methods.

b. Prevention
(1) Compilation of reports on the type of poisons encountered and of the response of patients to treatment.
(2) Periodic summaries and conferences to develop information for distribution to the general medical staff, to pharmacists, veterinarians, nurses, etc.

2. *Local Health Department*
a. To gather, tabulate and summarize the poisoning reports from the various participating hospitals.
b. To follow up poisoning cases wherever indicated for the purpose of preventing future poisoning in the same and other households.
c. To cooperate with the state health department in pooling information and resources.
d. To encourage and participate in community health education measures in the prevention and treatment of poisoning.
e. To facilitate toxicological laboratory analyses and telephone contacts with manufacturers.
f. To recheck death certificates where fatalities are due to poisoning to make sure their full educational and preventive possibilities have been obtained.
g. To consider investigating deaths associated with encephalitis, uremia, severe gastroenteritis and similar nonspecific conditions for possible poisons in cooperation with the medical examiner or coroner.

3. *State Health Departments*
a. The coordination, exchange and dissemination of information obtained from each of the local health departments and from the hospitals directly in areas where there are no local health departments; this could include the tabulation and summary of reports and the distribution of releases or other pertinent information on new poisoning hazards or on new or changed methods of treatment.
b. Providing report forms and reference material.
c. Assistance in both lay and professional health education regarding poisoning on a statewide basis.
d. Assistance and supplementation of activities of local health departments as indicated.
(1) Epidemiologic investigation of sudden increases in prevalence or toxicity of chemical products (such as cyanide, silver polish or 1080 rodenticide).
(2) Computer tabulation of reports for small health departments.
(3) Toxicologic analysis for lead, arsenic, morphine, thallium, etc., if specially indicated.
(4) Payment for emergency long-distance telephone calls to manufacturers if information not otherwise available.

e. Rechecking death certificates to make sure that actual and potential poisoning fatalities have been explored to obtain optimum educational and preventive values.
f. Considering proposing legislation for remedial or preventive purposes, if indicated.

4. *Local Branches of the Academy of Pediatrics and of the Medical Societies*

a. Review and support (and approval) of program, including assistance in planning and professional publicity to the program.
b. Periodic conferences or meetings to aid in the dissemination of the information obtained by participating hospitals, physicians and others.
c. Where facilities permit and where practical, to provide or supplement a central information service and card file for physicians and hospitals.

5. *Medical Colleges (similar functions by colleges of pharmacy and veterinary medicine)*
Participation by the departments of pediatrics, psychiatry, pharmacology and toxicology, internal medicine, etc. in the poisoning control program both by participating in hospital subcenters and by representation of selected personnel on the planning committee and the consultant staff of the overall poisoning control program; incorporating lessons learned in the respective teaching programs.
6. *Medical Examiner of the Coroner's Office*
Provide laboratory facilities for the examination and confirmation of suspected poisons in fatalities resulting from homicidal, suicidal or accidental ingestion of poison.
7. *Nursing, Veterinary, Medical and Pharmacy Associations* may have roles similar to that performed by other medical associations.
8. *Industrial Laboratory Facilities* may be a valuable supplement to the community's toxicological laboratories, and often the physicians and chemists associated with these industries are valuable as outstanding consultants in the field.
9. *Local Safety Councils, PTA, Service Clubs, Welfare Councils, etc.*
These agencies usually have special experience and already established channels for developing and implementing safety activities for the lay public, and they can frequently help with this aspect of the preventive activities.
10. *Individual Physicians*
a. Reporting cases treated outside hospital subcenters on a simple postage prepaid postcard.
(1) Those on which information from center is requested.
(2) Those on which no information is requested.
b. Treating patients for poisoning
11. *Individual Pharmacists*
a. Reporting cases that come to their attention.
(1) That receive later care by physicians.
(2) That do not get later care by physicians.
b. First aid information to parents
c. Information to physicians as requested
12. *Citywide Sponsoring and Planning Committee*
a. Membership
There is a possible disadvantage in having too large a membership; this disadvantage can be overcome by having a small steering or executive committee with specific responsibility for well-defined tasks assigned, or by starting with a relatively small committee and then enlarging later; the advantage of a large and representative committee is that there is much more widespread knowledge and cooperation. Membership should include
(1) State and local health department
(2) General and pediatric medical society—also pharmacy and veterinary society at beginning or later
(3) Medical colleges (pediatric,

pharmacology, psychiatry, internal medicine, etc. departments)

(4) Hospital association

(5) State pesticide law enforcement official

(6) Medical examiner or coroner's office

(7) Safety council

(8) Health division of welfare council

(9) Agricultural college (pesticides)

(10) Botanical specialist (plant poisons)

b. Planning and developing overall program and coordinating the constituent agencies.

c. Periodic evaluation of results and costs of program with revisions if indicated.

d. Notifying or alerting responsible federal or state agencies of unusual or unique or especially hazardous cases which occur.

D. Suggested Duties for Poison Control Officer of a Hospital

1. To familiarize himself with the poison control facilities in the community including both individuals and agencies.
2. To see that regular operating procedure for twenty-four-hour-a-day treatment of poisoning is developed; this includes determining initially, and by periodic checks, the easy availability of the necessary drugs, appliances, equipment and references.
3. To enlist the cooperation of the house and attending staff in treating and reporting cases of poisoning, including special orientation of emergency room personnel.
4. To be on call for consultation as needed. (For this duty particularly an alternate is desirable.)
5. To arrange periodic hospital conferences and to serve as a liaison person between the participating hospital and other participants in the community.

### *Standards for Poison Control Centers**

It is recognized that the establishment of poison control centers nationally will encompass both the large and the small hospitals. Information centers may be in any other facility. Accordingly, the following definitions and standards of poison treatment centers and information centers are intended to be used in their broadest sense, allowing for local adaptation. There are two major types, one which gives information only and one which gives information and treatment.

A. Definitions

1. *Information Center*

   This particular part of the overall Prevention of Accidental Poisoning Program shall mean—the accumulation of reference materials in one specified area of a hospital, or other facility, which will enable the center to offer twenty-four-hour-a-day poison information service. The center shall also act as a stimulus for an educational program to prevent accidental poisoning in the community.

2. *Poison Treatment Center*

   This particular part of the overall Prevention of Accidental Poisoning Program shall mean—the accumulation of reference materials in one specified area of a hospital, or other facility, which will enable the center to offer twenty-four-hour-a-day poison information service, and having readily available drugs, antidotes, appliances, and equipment necessary for the treatment of poisoning cases. The poison treatment center shall also act as a stimulus for an educational program to prevent accidental poisoning in the community.

---

*Approved by the American Association of Poison Control Centers (AAPCC).

B. Administration

1. *Information Center*
   a. The establishment of a twenty-four-hour-a-day poison information service.
   b. Sources and availability of antidotes shall be listed among the reference materials.
   c. Adequate record keeping of the number of calls received for information. The record shall contain the name, age and address of suspected case, type of toxic substance ingested, amount ingested, name of caller and information given.
   d. The center shall act as a stimulus for an educational program to prevent accidental poisoning in the community.
2. *Poison Treatment Center*

   One person shall be appointed to be in charge of the center, preferably a physician. This person need not necessarily be on duty, but available for consultation, with an alternate appointment to serve in his absence.

   The physician shall be responsible for
   a. Adequate orientation of emergency personnel in the treatment of poisoning cases.
   b. Establishing regular operating procedure for twenty-four-hour-a-day treatment of poisoning cases.

   A person shall be responsible for
   a. Maintaining and keeping up to date a supplemental card index file on poisonous substances, which will enable the center to offer twenty-four-hour-a-day poison information service.
   b. Adequate orientation of emergency personnel in reporting of all poisoning cases on forms provided for this purpose.
   c. The stimulation of an educational program to prevent accidental poisoning in the community.

C. Treatment in Poison Treatment Centers

1. The drugs, antidotes, appliances, and equipment shall be kept readily and continuously available.
2. There shall be established regular operating procedures twenty-four hours a day for treatment of poisoning cases.

D. Case Reporting by Poison Treatment Centers

Cases shall be reported on forms provided for this purpose. The reports shall give details as completely as possible and shall be sent to the designated agency.

*Recommendations*

Realizing that standards must be as specific as possible, the AAPCC feels that certain recommendations should be made which fall outside the strict definition of "standards" but nevertheless are important in the overall Poison Control Program. Accordingly, the following recommendations are offered.

1. The Information Center, if possible, should include on their records the outcome of the case on which information was given, particularly from the standpoint of whether or not the case was hospitalized, or if the patient died.
2. A plan should be developed for periodic conferences (such as monthly or quarterly conferences) in which individuals involved in the Poison Control Program participate.
3. Procedures should be developed for transmittal of information based on the operation of poison treatment centers and information centers, suitable for warning, advice and education to the general public.
4. Poison treatment centers and information centers should
   a. Cooperate with other official and non-official agencies in the community interested in the overall accident prevention program.
   b. Cooperate in medical and lay education in the prevention of accidental poisoning.
   c. Report to local or state health depart-

ments, as indicated, or directly to the National Clearinghouse for Poison Control Centers, all unusual cases of special hazards, in order that this information may be transmitted to other poison treatment centers, information centers and public health departments.

## STATUS OF HOUSEHOLD ARTICLES UNDER FEDERAL LAWS AS TO IDENTITY OF CONTENTS AND PRECAUTIONS IN LABELING

*Regulated*

1. Drugs
2. Disinfectants
3. Economic poisons (pesticides)
4. Caustic and corrosive acids and alkalis

*Regulated (since 1960 and 1967)*

1. Cosmetics
2. Heating, power and lighting fuels
3. Household care and repair articles, including water repellents, leather dressings, preservatives, etc.
4. Household cleaners (other than acids and alkalis mentioned), including soaps and other detergents, solvent cleaning fluids, polishes and waxes, deodorizers, etc.
5. Paint and accessories, including thinners, removers, etc.
6. Miscellaneous items, such as toys, inks and dyes, hobby supplies, novelties, etc.

Drugs and disinfectants intended for use on man or other animals are subject to the Federal Food, Drug and Cosmetic Act of 1938, enforced by the Food and Drug Administration. This agency is part of the United States Department of Health, Education and Welfare and is charged with the enforcement of the Federal Food, Drug and Cosmetic Act, the Caustic Poison Act and several other statutes. The Food and Drug Administration is directed by the Commissioner of Foods and Drugs and maintains district offices and laboratories in Boston, Buffalo, New York, Philadelphia, Baltimore, Atlanta, Cincinnati, St. Louis, Chicago, New Orleans, Kansas City, Minneapolis, Denver, Los Angeles, San Francisco and Seattle. The administrative offices and special laboratories are located in Washington.

The Federal Food, Drug and Cosmetic Act regulates the labeling of drug products, but its authority does not extend to advertising. Seizure of offending goods or criminal prosecution of responsible firms or persons in federal courts are among the methods used to enforce the provisions of the Act. In addition, repeated violations may be enjoined by the courts.

Violations may consist of either adulteration or misbranding or both. Adulteration refers to illegal deviations in the composition of an article which accompany the article either physically or as a result of coming to rest with the article in the hands of the consumer.

The Food, Drug and Cosmetic Act prohibits certain things from appearing in the labeling, i.e. any statement that is false or misleading. It also requires certain things to appear in the labeling, such as a statement of the quantity of contents; the name and address of the manufacturer, packer or distributor; the name and quantity of certain specific narcotic or habit-forming drugs together with a statement, *"Warning: May be habit-forming";* the common or usual name of each active ingredient and the quantities of certain specified ingredients; adequate directions for use; and adequate warnings against possible misuse. The Act further prohibits the distribution of drugs that may be dangerous to health under the conditions of use prescribed or recommended in the labeling or of drugs which are deceptively packaged. New drugs may not be introduced into interstate commerce unless an application has been permitted to become effective. Such an application must show by adequate scientific evidence that the new drug is safe for use under the conditions proposed for its use. To obtain an effective application, the petitioner must show that the new drug is safe, but he is not required to prove efficacy. A new drug distributed for study before an application for it has become effective must be labeled, *"Caution: New Drug—Limited by Federal law to investigational use."*

Certain drugs containing insulin, penicillin, streptomycin, bacitracin, tetracycline, chloramphenicol and chlortetracycline are subject to special control. Samples of each batch of these drugs are examined by the Food and Drug Administration for compliance with standards set forth in regulations issued by the Administration. Each batch must be certified as complying with these standards before the batch may be distributed. Such batches of these drugs are referred to as "certified drugs."

An amendment to the Food, Drug and Cosmetic Act requires that drugs that are not suitable for use in self-medication be restricted to prescription sale. These must be labeled, *"Caution: Federal law prohibits dispensing without prescription."* Prescriptions for these drugs cannot be refilled except as authorized by the physician, either by notation on the original prescription or by subsequent written or oral communication to the pharmacist.

Disinfectants for inanimate objects and pesticides are subject to the Insecticide, Fungicide and Rodenticide Act of 1947, enforced by the U.S. Department of Agriculture. Recently the Food and Drug Administration procedure for setting safe tolerances for pesticides on crops was revised and simplified. The twelve caustic and corrosive acids and alkalis in certain concentrations designated in the Federal Caustic Poison Act of 1927 are also controlled by the Food and Drug Administration. Although many new chemicals have been introduced since the enactment of the law, it has never been amended to provide for these developments.

All the federal laws cited have the common requirements that the active ingredients be declared on their labels by their common names, together with directions for use and warnings against injury under specified conditions of the use. In addition, the twelve caustics and corrosives and those pesticides (economic poisons) deemed highly toxic to man must carry the poison legend (skull and crossbones) and directions for emergency treatment.

## FEDERAL HAZARDOUS SUBSTANCES LABELING ACT

The above Act, the first to regulate the interstate distribution and sale of packages of a wide range of hazardous substances intended or suitable for household use, was enacted into law on July 11, 1960. This Act was effective immediately, although enforcement of penalties did not occur until suitable standards were achieved.

The law covers any substance that is toxic, corrosive, irritating, strongly sensitizing, flammable or which generates pressure through heat, combustion or other means, if it is capable of causing injury or illness to man. Substances covered by certain preexisting laws are excluded.

This law pertains specifically to the labeling of hazardous substances. It requires manufacturers of such materials as may be defined under the Act as hazardous to label the immediate containers of these materials with the following information: manufacturer's (or distributor's, etc.) name and address; all ingredients (by common, chemical or generic name) which contribute to the hazard; proper warning words in heavy type; affirmation of the principal hazard, e.g. "flammable," "causes burns," etc.; precautionary measures; handling and storage instructions; first aid instructions for injury or illness due to the product; the word "poison" for all "highly toxic" substances (defined explicitly in terms of ingestion, inhalation and skin contact on the basis of tests in laboratory animals, with the provision that data from human experience take precedence over the results of animal experiments in determining toxicity), and "danger," "warning" or "caution" labels in descending order for chemicals of lesser toxicity; and a warning to keep out of the reach of children. This information is to be printed prominently and clearly, as defined. All products not so labeled are considered misbranded.

The Secretary of Health, Education and Welfare is given latitude to decide what substances are considered hazardous and what labeling is required in any given instance.

Interstate traffic of misbranded substances is strictly prohibited by the Act, and the Secretary of HEW is invested with full authority to investigate, examine and inspect factories, warehouses, packages, etc., pursuant to the enforcement of this Act. He also is empowered to seize products that are labeled in violation of this law.

Full penalties are delineated to be awarded by the federal judiciary. The law is administered under provisions of the Federal Food, Drug and Cosmetic Act and is administered by the Food and Drug Administration.

It should be emphasized that the law recognizes precedence of human experience in the field of toxicity over the laboratory animal data. This underscores the importance of the experiences of Poison Control Centers and their system of reporting cases to the National Clearinghouse.

The Hazardous Substance Act was amended in 1967 to include "banned hazardous substances" such as (1) any toy or other article intended for use by children that is a hazardous substance or bears or contains a hazardous substance, or (2) substances, other than those exempted, which are intended for or packaged in a form suitable for household use and which the FDA commissioner finds and classifies by regulation as being so hazardous in nature that they cannot be made suitable for safe use in or around the household by any form of cautionary labeling. The Consumer Protection Act of 1972 establishes an independent agency which has authority to set and enforce safety standards applicable to various consumer products. This agency, however, is not responsible for duties assigned to the Food and Drug Administration.

Since the first reported successful use of safety closures (Arena, J.M.: *JAMA, 169*:1188, 1959), the history of safety packaging is one of persistent efforts by many groups culminating in the passage of the Poison Prevention Packaging Act of 1970 administered by the Consumer Product Safety Commission. This act provided that all potentially harmful household substances including prescription medication be marketed in safety packaging. One of the salient ideas incorporated into the legislation is that "the package is the message" and serves as a constant reminder of safety education in the marketplace as well as in the home. Although twenty years of educational programs succeeded in alerting the public to the problem of accidental poisoning and reduced mortality, the morbidity actually increased. The introduction of safety packaging marked an abrupt decline in accidental poisoning. For example, at the Omaha Children's Memorial Hospital Master Poison Control Center, analgesic ingestion decreased rapidly from a 1966 peak of 49 to 30 per cent in the four years after the aspirin limitation but declined to 12 per cent in the four years after the introduction of safety packaging. Previous studies of safety prescription packaging establish its efficacy: Three out of four poisonings will not occur when prescription safety packaging is used properly (i.e. resealing the package after use, etc.).

## FOOD ADDITIVES

While many chemical additives are essential to efficient agricultural production, others are vital to the manufacture of food products. There is no reason to believe that the present use of chemicals in foods is endangering the health of people. Responsible manufacturers

TABLE 156
STATE DRUG LAWS
(ENFORCEMENT AGENCIES AND PRINCIPAL PROVISIONS)*

| *States* | *Type of Law Enforced* | *Enforcing Agency* | *Modern New Drug Provisions* | *Device Law* | *Cosmetic Law* |
|---|---|---|---|---|---|
| Alabama | Food and Drug Act 1970 | Agriculture | | | Agriculture |
| Alaska | Uniform FD and C Act | Health | Health | Health | Health |
| Arizona | Uniform FD and C Act | Public Safety | Safety | Safety | |
| Arkansas | Uniform FD and C Act | Health | | Health | Health |
| California | Uniform FD and C Act | Health | Health | Health | Health |
| Colorado | Uniform FD and C Act | Health | | Health | Health |
| Connecticut | Uniform FD and C Act | Consumer Protection | Consumer Protection | Consumer Protection | Consumer Protection |
| Delaware | Food and Drug Act 1907 | | | | |
| Florida | Uniform FD and C Act | Health | | Health | Health |
| Georgia | Drug and Cosmetic Act | Pharmacy | | Pharmacy | Pharmacy |
| Hawaii | Uniform FD and C Act | Health | Health | Health | Health |
| Idaho | Uniform FD and C Act | Health | | Health | Health |
| Illinois | Uniform FD and C Act | Agriculture | Health | Health | Health |
| Indiana | Uniform FD and C Act | Health | Health | Health | Health |
| Iowa | Drug and Cosmetic Act | Pharmacy | | Pharmacy | Pharmacy |
| Kansas | Uniform FD and C Act | Health | Health | Health | Health |
| Kentucky | Uniform FD and C Act | Health | | Health | Health |

*Prepared by Program Development Branch, Division of Federal-State Relations, Office of the Executive Director of Regional Operations, July 1972, Revised March 1974.

Because of recurrent federal and state changes, some of the functions of these enforcement agencies may be altered.

TABLE 156—*(Continued)*
STATE DRUG LAWS

| *States* | *Type of Law Enforced* | *Enforcing Agency* | *Modern New Drug Provisions* | *Device Law* | *Cosmetic Law* |
|---|---|---|---|---|---|
| Louisiana | Uniform FD and C Act | Health | | Health | Health |
| Maine | Food and Drug Act 1907<br>Cosmetic Act 1938 | Agriculture | | | Health |
| Maryland | Uniform FD and C Act | Health | Health | | Health |
| Massachusetts | Uniform FD and C Act | Health | | Health | Health |
| Michigan | Pure Drugs Act 1909 | Pharmacy | | Pharmacy | |
| Minnesota | Drug Act 1907 | Pharmacy | | | |
| Mississippi | Food and Drug Act 1907 | State Chemist | | | |
| Missouri | Uniform FD and C Act | Health | | Health | Health |
| Montana | Uniform FD and C Act | Health | Health | Health | Health |
| Nebraska | Drug Law | Health | | | |
| Nevada | Uniform FD and C Act | Health | | Health | Health |
| New Hampshire | Uniform FD and C Act | Health | | Health | Health |
| New Jersey | Uniform FD and C Act | Health | | Health | Health |
| New Mexico | Uniform FD and C Act | Pharmacy | | Pharmacy | Pharmacy |
| New York | Uniform FD and C Act | Pharmacy | Pharmacy | Pharmacy | Pharmacy |
| North Carolina | Uniform FD and C Act | Agriculture | | Agriculture | Agriculture |
| North Dakota | Uniform FD and C Act | State Lab | State Lab | State Lab | State Lab |
| Ohio | Uniform FD and C Act | Agriculture-Pharmacy | | Agriculture-Pharmacy | Agriculture-Pharmacy |

TABLE 156—*(Continued)*
STATE DRUG LAWS

| *States* | *Type of Law Enforced* | *Enforcing Agency* | *Modern New Drug Provisions* | *Device Law* | *Cosmetic Law* |
|---|---|---|---|---|---|
| Oklahoma | Uniform Drug, Device and Cosmetic Act | Health | | Health | Health |
| Oregon | Drug Act 1907 | Pharmacy | | | |
| Pennsylvania | Uniform Drug, Device and Cosmetic Act | Health | | Health | Health |
| Rhode Island | Uniform FD and C Act | Health | | Health | Health |
| South Carolina | Uniform FD and C Act | Agriculture-Health | Health | | Agriculture |
| South Dakota | Drug Act 1907 | Agriculture | | | |
| Tennessee | Uniform FD and C Act | Agriculture | | Agriculture | Agriculture |
| Texas | Uniform FD and C Act | Health | Health | Health | Health |
| Utah | Uniform FD and C Act | Agriculture-Pharmacy | Agriculture-Pharmacy | Agriculture | Agriculture |
| Vermont | Uniform FD and C Act | Health | | Health | Health |
| Virginia | Uniform FD and C Act | Pharmacy | Pharmacy | Pharmacy | Pharmacy |
| Washington | Uniform FD and C Act | Agriculture-Pharmacy | | Agriculture-Pharmacy | Agriculture-Pharmacy |
| West Virginia | Food and Drug Act 1907 | Health-Pharmacy | | | Health-Pharmacy |
| Wisconsin | Food and Drug Act 1907 | Agriculture-Pharmacy | | | |
| Wyoming | Food and Drug Act 1907 | Agriculture | | | Agriculture |
| District of Columbia | Act Supplementing Federal Act | Health | | | Health |
| Puerto Rico | Uniform FD and C Act | Health | | | Health |

have made careful safety tests before the introduction of new chemicals, and the Food and Drug Administration is diligently and effectively protecting consumers from the presence of hazardous chemicals under existing federal laws.

Since the enactment of the revised Food, Drug and Cosmetic Act in 1938, three important amendments have broadened the scope of our food laws. Section 408 of the Food, Drug and Cosmetic Act (the Miller Bill of 1954) has provided for the establishment of tolerances in the safe use of pesticides on raw agricultural products. The New Food Additives Amendment of 1958 (Section 409) requires that new food additives be tested for safety prior to use, and that government approval must be obtained for their use. The Color Additive Amendment of 1960 regulates the listing and certification of colors which are to be used in foods, drugs and cosmetics, and in addition, provides for testing both existing colors and new colors for safety.

The Food Additives Amendment gives special consideration to additives used in food prior to January 1, 1958. Continued use of these additives is now permitted without toxicity tests if qualified experts generally recognize them as having been shown safe through either toxicologic tests or experience based on common use in food. Some chemicals used in foods had been evaluated prior to the enactment of the Food Additives Amendment and found to be safe. These are allowed at the present time by virtue of this prior sanction. However, experience based on common use in food does not prove the absence of chronic harmful effects. Both animal tests and experience with use are needed for evaluating safety. The food industry should be allowed adequate time to demonstrate the safety of new chemicals used in foods, and decisions to continue the use of additives should be based on demonstrations of their safety through scientific methods. All food additives are now getting a close scrutiny by the FDA as witnessed by the ban on cyclamates and investigation of monosodium glutamate (MSG).

### *Sodium Nicotinate*

This chemical additive is legal in thirty-seven states for use as a fresh meat color preservative, and it is estimated that over 400 million pounds of meat are treated with this agent each year. However, the amount added to meat without regard to patent privileges is not known and may be substantial. This additive has been responsible for several outbreaks of food poisoning in the United States, producing the following symptoms: cutaneous vasodilatation; a diffuse feeling of heat with redness and flushing of the face and extremities; dryness of the mouth; and swelling of the lips, knees and extremities. Although the effects are not usually serious, the symptoms in general outbreaks are both alarming and frightening. The *treatment* is supportive and symptomatic.

Nitrites, which prevent *Clostridium botulinum* growth, are also used to preserve the color of meat, fish, etc. in pickling or salting processes. The allowable residue in food is 0.01 per cent. However, occasionally, unscrupulous local markets often adulterate their fresh products with larger amounts of sodium nitrite than the law permits, which has resulted in several outbreaks of food poisoning with severe and fatal methemoglobinemia.

Current regulations permit up to 98 gm of sodium or potassium nitrate in 45 kg of meat when meat is dry cured, and 77 gm/45 kg when used in chopped meat. The nitrites, sodium and potassium, are permitted at a concentration of 28 gm/45 kg of meat dry cured and 7 gm/45 kg of chopped meat.

There is a special interest in nitrites consumed by infants because the normally low stomach acidity of infants facilitates the transformation of nitrate to nitrite by bacteria. Changes in the hemoglobin of infants who have been fed spinach puree high in nitrates have been reported. Nitrates are not added to baby foods but are sometimes present as natural constituents in green vegetables and in some water supplies.

Nitrites have been shown to convert in the stomachs of laboratory animals to nitrosa-

TABLE 157
FUNCTIONS OF SOME COMMONLY USED ADDITIVES

| *Function* | *Why These Additives Are Used* | *Examples of Additives Used* | *Foods in Which Such Additives are Used* |
|---|---|---|---|
| To improve nutritive value | The addition of certain nutrients to specific processed foods is heartily endorsed by medical and public health authorities as an important step in the elimination and prevention of certain types of disease. For example: where iodized salt is used, simple goiter has almost disappeared; vitamin D added to some dairy products and infant foods has practically eliminated rickets; the enrichment and restoration of bread, corn meal, and cereals have helped eliminate pellagra from the South and substantially increased the dietary intake of some essential B vitamins and iron. | vitamin A<br>thiamine<br>niacin<br>riboflavin<br>vitamin D<br>ascorbic acid<br>iron<br>potassium iodide | wheat flour<br>bread<br>breakfast cereals<br>corn meal<br>margarine<br>macaroni and noodle products<br>milk<br>iodized salt |
| To enhance the flavor of certain foods | A wide variety of spices and natural and synthetic flavors are used in processed foods to provide us with many of the flavorful foods we enjoy. Without them there would be no such foods as spice cake, gingerbread, or sausage. Nor is there enough natural flavoring in the whole world to flavor all the ice cream eaten in the United States in one year. | cloves<br>ginger<br>citrus oils<br>pepper<br>monosodium glutamate<br>amyl acetate<br>carvol<br>benzaldehyde | spice cake<br>gingerbread<br>ice cream<br>soft drinks<br>candy<br>sausage<br>fruit-flavored toppings<br>fruit-flavored gelatins |
| To maintain appearance, palatability, and wholesomeness of many foods | These additives are used to delay undesirable changes in food caused by microbial growth or oxidation. Food spoilage caused by such microorganisms as mold, bacteria, and yeast can be prevented or inhibited by the use of additives. Other additives—antioxidants—help prevent oxidation which might otherwise cause fats to turn rancid and certain fresh fruits (for processing) to darken when cut and exposed to air. | propionic acid<br>sodium and calcium salts of propionic acid<br>ascorbic acid<br>butylated hydroxyanisole<br>butylated hydroxytoluene | frozen fruit<br>dried fruit<br>bread<br>cheese<br>syrup<br>margarine<br>lard<br>nuts<br>dry soup mixes<br>candy<br>potato chips<br>crackers<br>shortening<br>pie fillings<br>fruit juices<br>cake mixes<br>sausage |
| To impart and maintain desired consistency in certain foods | Emulsifiers are additives which permit the distribution of tiny particles of one liquid in another liquid, thereby improving the texture, homogeneity, and keeping quality of many foods. Stabilizers and thickeners function in a similar way to give smooth uniform textures and flavors as well as desired consistency to certain foods. | lecithin<br>mono– and diglycerides<br>gum arabic<br>agar-agar<br>methyl cellulose<br>carrageenan* | baked goods<br>cake mixes<br>frozen desserts<br>ice cream<br>candy<br>evaporated milk<br>chocolate milk<br>beer<br>salad dressings<br>bread doughs<br>puddings<br>pie fillings |

*Carrageenan, an extract of red seaweed, has been removed from the "Generally Recognized as Safe" (GRAS) list by the FDA, because tests have shown it leads to birth defects in animals when administered in high doses.

| | | | |
|---|---|---|---|
| To control the acidity or alkalinity in many processed foods | One of the most important uses of these additives is as chemical leavening agents in the baking industry, to make cakes, biscuits, waffles, muffins, and other baked goods. These additives help make fruits and tubers easier to peel (for canning); neutralize sour cream when used to make butter; and help control the texture of candy. | potassium acid tartrate<br>tartaric acid<br>sodium bicarbonate<br>citric acid<br>lactic acid | cakes<br>cookies<br>quick breads<br>crackers<br>soft drinks<br>butter<br>process cheese<br>cheese spreads<br>chocolates |
| To give desired and characteristic color to certain foods | Both natural and synthetic food colors are used in processed foods, and play a major role in increasing the acceptability and attractiveness of these products. | F.D. & C. colors† cochineal<br>annatto chlorophyll<br>carotene<br>tartrazine (yellow no. 5)‡ | confections<br>bakery goods<br>soft drinks<br>frankfurters<br>cheese<br>ice cream<br>jams and jellies<br>dog food |
| To act as maturing and bleaching agent | Maturing and bleaching agents are used to change the yellow pigments in wheat flour to white and to modify the gluten characteristics to improve baking results. They are also used to improve the appearance of certain cheeses. | chlorine dioxide<br>nitrosyl chloride<br>chlorine<br>potassium bromate and iodate | wheat flour<br>certain cheeses |
| To perform other special functions | Humectants help retain moisture in certain foods. Anticaking agents help keep salts and powders free-flowing. Curing agents give flavor and color to certain meats. Nonnutritive sweeteners are used to take the place of sugar. | glycerine<br>magnesium carbonate<br>sodium nitrate and nitrite<br>calcium and sodium cyclamates<br>saccharin | coconut<br>table salt<br>frankfurters and other sausages<br>dietetic foods<br>marshmallows |

†A list of approved coal-tar colors formerly included Red 2, Red 4 and Carbon Black, which have now been banned. Red 40, the principal red food coloring in the United States since the ban of Red 2, is presently under investigation because of unexpected malignant lymphomas found in a long-term mouse-feeding study.

‡Tartrazine (yellow no. 5) is the food color additive formerly used in dry drink powders, carbonated beverages and colored candy. It was also used in margarine and butter and as a dye for drug solutions and drug capsules. Allergic urticaria and nonthrombocytopenic vascular purpura have been documented by this salicylate-related compound. Sensitized persons should limit their food to fresh red meats and green vegetables and medication to white tablets ("Roman diet," the red, white and green national colors of Italy).

mines, which are carcinogens. With bacon, nitrosamines are formed during the cooking process before reaching the gastrointestinal tract. Table 157, from Public Affairs Pamphlet No. 320, shows examples of additives used and why they are needed.

### *Sorbic Acid*

Sorbic acid is an unsaturated fatty acid which is used commercially in a synthetic form but may also be obtained from the berries of the mountain ash, *Sorbus aucuparia* (Lin) rosacaea. Sorbic acid and its sodium and potassium salts are recognized as safe for use in foods under regulations of the Food and Drug Administration. These food additives are effective preservatives at low concentration for the control of mold and yeast in cheese products, baked goods, fruit juices, fresh fruits and vegetables, wines, soft drinks, pickles, sauerkraut and certain meat and fish products.

# FOOD POISONING

The term "ptomaine poisoning," frequently used in newspaper accounts of outbreaks of food poisoning, is a misnomer. The term has been in use since 1870. The ptomaines are ammonia substitution compounds resulting from decomposition of the protein molecule and can be produced by any bacteria which bring about this degree of proteolysis. Only a few of the ptomaines are physiologically active; if injected parenterally, some are poisonous. When given by mouth, even in relatively large doses, the more poisonous ones do not produce gastrointestinal symptoms. The majority of so-called ptomaine food poisoning outbreaks are thought to be due to staphylococci.

In all cases of food poisoning, it is important to recognize the type so recurrences can be prevented. Often there is no really specific *treatment.* Vomiting and diarrhea serve the useful purpose of eliminating poisons not already absorbed. Symptomatic treatment should be given, and in those types of poisoning characterized by severe vomiting and diarrhea, parenteral fluids should be administered if dehydration and loss of electrolytes have been severe.

Inadequate reporting of incidence prevents a truly accurate figure, but it is estimated that more than 1 million cases of food poisoning occur annually in the United States. Many incidences of upset stomach, flu or indigestion may actually be mild cases of food poisoning. The frequency and type of food poisoning outbreaks vary with sanitary standards and eating and food preparation habits of countries and races. The bacterial types seem to be the most common and the most serious. In the United States, staphylococcal enterotoxin food poisoning is the most frequent type seen, with an average of 1700 cases reported annually over the past few years. (In England and throughout continental Europe, *Salmonella* food poisoning, or more properly, "infection," is the type most frequently seen.)

## Public Health Aspects

Control of food poisoning and infection depends mainly on proper methods of sanitation. Disease-producing bacteria in milk can be eliminated by sanitary processing, and most pathogens are destroyed in the pasteurization process. Water is subjected to a number of processes, such as chlorination, so that the real concern in controlling outbreaks today lies with food. Many of the foods which cause poisoning receive no terminal sterilization, although some germicidal heat treatment may be incidental to the cooking process. However, staphylococcal toxin is thermostable, so symptoms are produced even without live bacteria. In addition, food cooked in public institutions and restaurants is exposed to many different handlers who are often unaware of, or indifferent to, the most elementary sanitary techniques.

Most food poisonings, it is true, are relatively mild. Often affected persons receive no medical treatment, and deaths are rare. Therefore many outbreaks go unreported. This may be due to an understandable desire to avoid unfavorable publicity or even, in extreme cases, lawsuits for personal injury. This is unfortunate, because reporting of one outbreak may prevent others by making public institutions and restaurants more conscious of the dangers of inadequate sanitary conditions.

Health agencies must be concerned with fuller detection and reporting of individual cases and outbreaks. A stronger emphasis on the necessity of teaching sanitary techniques in secondary schools will also be helpful in further enlightening people to the perils of food poisoning.

## Differential Diagnosis

Outbreaks of food poisoning caused by toxins of staphylococci are typically explosive in nature. In gastrointestinal infections, e.g. those due to *Salmonella, Shigella,* pathogenic *Escherichia coli, Streptococcus,* etc., new cases continue to appear for many days as the result of person-to-person contact. Other conditions which may at times resemble food poisoning are chronic ulcerative colitis, bacillary dysentery, amebiasis, etc.

Trichinosis resembles food poisoning in that it can affect simultaneously many people who have eaten the same food. Since only about 70 per cent of the pork raised in this country is processed in plants which are under close sanitary inspection, a large part of our total supply of pork products may carry live parasites. The cysts do not calcify in pork and are almost invisible to the naked eye; they are not looked for in government inspection of meat.

If meat is heavily infested, invasion of the intestinal mucosa one to four days after ingestion may cause local irritation, producing symptoms of nausea, vomiting and diarrhea which resemble those of food poisoning. In other cases, these symptoms may be completely absent. By the seventh day, migration of the larvae usually produces muscular weakness and stiffness or pain accompanied by remittent fever, which may reach 104° F. Orbital edema is the next most common finding. Occasional skin rashes are transient. Central nervous system complaints (headache, delirium and psychic or visual disturbances) suggest encephalitis but are usually of short duration. The great variety of symptoms, the variation in their intensity and the irregularity in their course are characteristic of trichinosis.

If the parasite can be demonstrated in the suspected meat while the patient is still having gastrointestinal symptoms, administration of an anthelmintic may remove some of the adult worms. No drug, however, has been found effective against the larvae (which occasionally are also found in the spinal fluid).

Viral enteritis, so-called nonbacterial gastroenteritis, is characterized by watery diarrhea, abdominal cramps, nausea and vomiting, with or without fever. A number of viruses have been implicated. However, many respiratory viral illnesses begin with gastrointestinal symptoms.

Culture and microscopy of the feces are important in differentiation of nonbacterial gastroenteritis from shigellosis, salmonellosis or amebiasis, particularly in epidemics of the afebrile type. Food poisoning can often be excluded by the distribution and timing of new cases, which may continue to appear for over a week.

## Toxins

### *Staphylococcus Enterotoxin*

Staphylococcal food poisoning, the most common type of all food poisonings in the United States, involves almost everyone at one time or another. It is really food "poisoning" since an exotoxin is produced.

Although the bacteria are easily destroyed in cooking, they produce a heat-resistant toxin. Not all strains of staphylococci produce enterotoxins, and it is probable that only a few of the total strains in nature have this property. A wide variety of foods have been implicated in poisonings, including milk, cheese, ice cream, cream-filled bakery goods, tongue, rapid-cured hams, chicken or potato salad, dried beef, sausage and chicken gravy. Usually there is a history of food having been kept warm for several hours before being served. Foods may be contaminated from superficial infections in food handlers or by nasal droplets containing pathogenic staphylococci.

Symptoms usually appear within three hours after eating. This incubation period is influenced by the amount of enterotoxin consumed and the particular susceptibility of the person involved. The first symptom observed is salivation, followed by nausea, vomiting, retching, abdominal cramps, prostration and diarrhea. In severe poisoning, marked prostration accompanies vomiting and diarrhea. Symptoms of shock have also been observed. As a rule, acute symptoms are of short duration and generally subside after five to six hours. A few fatal cases have occurred, usually in the very young, the aged or the debilitated and immune compromised patients.

The best control of staphylococcal food poisoning consists of adequate refrigeration of perishable foods. It should be kept in mind that heat kills the staphylococci but usually does not destroy the enterotoxin.

DIAGNOSIS. Diagnosis is based on a brief interval between eating incriminated food and onset of symptoms. Bacteriologic examination establishes the presence of staphylococci. When individuals rather than large groups are stricken, it is essential to eliminate other possible causes such as gall bladder disease, appendicitis and functional bowel distress associated with emotional upsets. Enterotoxin may be produced by staphylococci in patients under treatment with large doses of broad-spectrum antibiotics.

*Treatment.* Symptoms of shock are due to loss of body fluids and electrolytes resulting in decreased circulating blood volume. This should be corrected by parenteral administration of the appropriate electrolyte solutions. The amount of fluid should be governed by the patient's age and the severity of vomiting and diarrhea.

### *Botulinus Exotoxin*

Botulinus exotoxin is produced by *Clostridium botulinum,* a large, gram-positive, rod-shaped organism which is an anaerobic spore former. Although the spores are not toxic, they are heat resistant and can germinate, in the absence of oxygen and acid, into cells that produce a deadly toxin. The organism is a natural saprophyte and is commonly found in the soil and some fresh waters. The term "botulism" is derived from a word meaning "sausage" and was coined by German physicians at the beginning of the nineteenth century, probably because the poisoning was sometimes seen in persons who had eaten contaminated sausage.

Six types of toxin have been distinguished, which have been designated A, B, C, D, E and F. The toxin of one type is not neutralized by the antitoxin of a heterologous type. Man is affected mainly by Types A and E, less frequently by Types B and F and rarely by C and D.

In the majority of cases there is a history of ingestion of home-canned foods, especially nonacid fruits and vegetables such as beets, corn or string beans. The food frequently has a rancid or slightly putrefactive odor or taste. In 1963, nine deaths were reported from botulism from commercially canned tuna and smoked whitefish. The deaths were among twenty-four cases of botulism linked to commercial foods, two more than the total caused by home-preserved foods. Type E botulism, one of five varieties, was responsible for twenty-two cases related to commercial fish products.

In March, 1963, three Detroit, Michigan, women were reported victims of botulism following a meal which included tuna fish sandwiches. The salad had been freshly prepared from canned tuna which allegedly had an abnormal odor when it was opened. This was the first outbreak of botulism from United States commercially canned products in forty years. Two of the women died; the third, who had eaten only a small portion of the tuna, recovered three to four days later.

In 1966, seven botulism deaths were caused by smoked Great Lakes whitefish not in the frozen state. The FDA now requires all Great Lakes fish smokers to freeze their product, since the botulism toxin is not known to develop at low temperatures. In five of the cases, the whitefish had been packed in vacuum-sealed plastic bags.

Prevention of botulism depends on careful examination of food, watching for abnormal taste, odor, gas, turbidity or softening. It should be kept in mind, however, that there may be no observable alteration in the food. When possible, home-canned products should be baked for fifteen minutes before using. Any food which appears to be spoiled should be destroyed without tasting. Contaminated food should not come in contact with cuts on the hands, because a dangerous quantity of toxin might conceivably be absorbed. A program for active human immunization with a pentavalent (ABCDE) aluminum phosphate absorbed botulinus toxoid on an investigational basis has been instituted. This vaccine is available from the Investigational Vaccines Program, Communicable Disease Center, Atlanta, Georgia, 30333.

DIAGNOSIS. Characteristic symptoms of botulism are preceded by an active digestive disturbance and vomiting. Typical symptoms appear in twelve to thirty-six hours. Incubation period can be as short as six hours and as long as eight days. Prognosis is poorest in patients with an incubation period of less than twenty-four hours. The earliest symptom is usually a peculiar lassitude or fatigue, sometimes associated with dizziness or headache attributable to constipation. Diplopia is an early occurrence. Photophobia, nystagmus and vertigo occasionally occur. The tongue is usually coated and swollen; there is an occasional sense of constriction of the throat. Difficulty in swallowing and in speech is observed.

It is not uncommon for fluids to be regurgitated through the nose and mouth. Neck muscles are often weakened and there may be muscular incoordination. There is no retention of urine, although the volume may be slight since the patient cannot swallow and proper fluid balance is not maintained. The pulse may be normal but often becomes rapid in the late stage. Temperature is usually normal or subnormal. Bronchopneumonia may develop because of aspiration of stomach contents.

In fatal cases, death usually occurs three to six days after ingestion of the poisonous food. Although paralysis of pharyngeal muscles is an early sign, death is the result of respiratory failure.

*Treatment.* Type E (responsible for recent cases and primarily associated with fish and marine mammal products) antitoxin has only recently been combined with types A and B in a trivalent form and is now available through the Communicable Disease Center, U.S. Public Health Service, Atlanta, Georgia. (The telephone number for day coverage is 404-633-3311, extension 3753, 4, 5, and 6, and 634-2561 for nights and weekends.) Because of the availability of antitoxin A, B and E combined, this should be given immediately until laboratory tests demonstrate which toxin is responsible, at which time the definitive antitoxin can be administered. The majority of cases are due to types A or B (associated mainly with the consumption of inadequately processed vegetables and meats). Poisoning is rarely caused by types C or D.

When the symptoms are already present, the antitoxin given is often too late, since it cannot reverse the damage already done by the toxin. Even though the disease is well advanced, antitoxin should be given in the hope of neutralizing any toxin not already fixed in tissues. The patient should first be tested for serum hypersensitivity and, if necessary, desensitized.

Antitoxin should prove of great value in patients who have eaten very small amounts of poisonous food. In the presence of pharyngeal paralysis, an airway should be maintained and fluids administered parenterally. Penicillin should be given because the toxin is released by spores in the germination phase.

Guanidine hydrochloride, an investigational drug, enhances the release of acetylcholine at the neuromuscular junction and improves the profound muscular weakness, ptosis and extraocular palsies that occur. The drug is given orally (by nasogastric tube, if necessary) 15 to 35 mg/kg/day in four to six doses. It should be discontinued as soon as the muscle weakness and paralysis improve. The patient should be kept quiet and inactive. One attack of botulism does not confer immunity; individuals have suffered repeat attacks.

To *prevent* botulism, the following measures are important.

1. Use only the pressure-canner method of canning vegetables, meats or poultry. High temperatures required to kill spores cannot be achieved by other home-canning methods. Tomatoes, pickled vegetables, and fruits, because of their acidity, may be canned in a boiling water bath.
2. Obtain reliable canning instructions, such as those available from the U.S. Department of Agriculture, and make certain that equipment is functioning properly.
3. Throw out foods with off-odors. (Remember, however, that an off-odor is not necessarily detectable in a food containing the toxin.)
4. Do not even taste food that is suspect. If doubtful about the canning procedure used, boil meats, poultry, corn, or spinach for twenty minutes and other vegetables for at least ten minutes.
5. Avoid food from cans (commercial or home-canned) that bulge or leak.
6. Keep frozen foods frozen until ready for use.

### *Clostridium perfringens*

Meat and meat products (gravy, creamed chicken, stew, soup) contaminated with *Clostridium perfringens,* type A, have been responsible for outbreaks of acute gastroenteritis. This anaerobic organism, which also produces gas gangrene, grows best at temperatures from 85° to 115°F, produces heat-resistant spores and is rapidly supplanting enterotoxin-producing staphylococci as the most common cause of food poisoning in this country. Typical symptoms of diarrhea with abdominal pain develop eight to twenty-four hours after ingestion of food stored at a warm temperature for several hours after cooking. *Clostridium* spores are ubiquitous on meat and gravies; when conditions are favorable they can germinate and have prolific growth within a few hours after cooking. Nausea is common but vomiting is rare. Systemic manifestations are usually mild or absent. Recovery is uneventful in twelve to twenty-four hours.

## Infections

### *Salmonella*

*Salmonella* strains *(S. enteritidis, S. cubana, S. aertrycke, S. choleraesuis)* have long been associated with food infection and are thought to have been causative agents when bacteriologic studies were negative or inconclusive. In 1963, 2300 cases of *Salmonella* poisoning were reported with a substantially increased incidence each year since then. Sources of the poisoning include meat from "cold slaughter" or sick animals, raw or improperly pasteurized milk, frozen eggs or egg powder products, foods contaminated by flies or sick rats, and last but not least, human carriers. By-products of the meat-packing industry (bone meal, fertilizer and pet foods) may constitute an important medium for the spread of salmonellosis. Carmine dye, which is used primarily to color foods, drugs and cosmetics, is derived from an insect which may harbor the bacterium *Salmonella cubana.* Twenty-six incidences of infection have been recently reported from the use of this product. It is more proper to speak of salmonellosis as "food infection," since it is the infection with and multiplication of bacteria that give rise to symptomatology.

Sanitation is the key to control of the infection. Meat and eggs should be adequately cooked; water and milk supplies controlled; fresh foods properly handled; and carriers treated and eliminated as food handlers.

DIAGNOSIS. The onset of symptoms varies from seven to seventy-two hours after contaminated food has been eaten. Headache and chills may be the initial symptoms. These are usually followed by abdominal cramps and persistent foul-smelling diarrheal stools, which may become watery and green. Nausea, vomiting, fever, prostration, muscle weakness, faintness and thirst are usually present. Also noted are restlessness, muscle twitching, drowsiness and herpes labialis.

Bateriologic diagnosis of *Salmonella* infection is made by isolation of the organisms from blood, feces, urine or local focus of infection.

*Treatment.* Symptomatic treatment should include restriction of food intake to liquids and bland soft solids, and if necessary, administration of parenteral fluids for dehydration. Specific antibiotic therapy (chloramphenicol, ampicillin or a tetracycline) should be used only if the infection is severe.

### *Streptococcus*

Food infection due to streptococcal strains is caused by cream-filled pastries, by dressings in meat and fowl and by canned foods or leftovers that have not been recooked. Colic, diarrhea, nausea and vomiting occur four hours after eating the poisoned food.

DIAGNOSIS. Bacteriologic diagnosis is based on streptococcal culture producing alpha hemolysis (viridans) on a blood agar plate.

*Treatment.* Treatment should follow that outlined previously for *Salmonella* infection.

### *Vibrio parahaemolyticus*

*V. parahaemolyticus,* a close relative of the cholera organism lives in seawater and is known to produce about half the food-borne diseases in Japan, probably because raw fish is very popular there. Shipboard outbreaks on cruise liners have occurred when food had been inadvertently contaminated by seawater. The organism's toxin is not known to be fatal, and *treatment* is symptomatic and supportive.

### *Anisakiasis*

A growing number of Americans have developed a taste for raw fish delicacies. Hundreds of cases of anisakiasis have been reported in Japan and confirmed cases of larvae from humans in North America have occurred since 1972.

Human anisakiasis can involve tissue penetration, with symptoms mimicking appendicitis or intestinal obstruction. Most human cases are attributed to *Anisakis* sp., although the two worms recovered in California belong to the *Phocanema* genus.

Many saltwater fish species harbor anisakian larvae. The parasite can survive refrigeration in shipping and marketing and smoking at low temperatures but is killed by normal cooking temperatures or by freezing.

### *Mycotoxicosis*

Since ancient times, an uncounted number of human beings have grown ill and died as a result of ingesting foods containing mycotoxins, the metabolites that develop on certain foodstuffs. For centuries in the Middle Ages, epidemics of ergot poisoning raged uncontrolled and must have killed hundreds of thousands, perhaps millions, of people.

But it took the unexpected and untimely death of thousands of young turkeys in England in 1960 (aflatoxin was the culprit) to spark what has developed into a major worldwide research effort directed toward identifying as many as possible of the apparently vast number of fungus-derived toxic compounds and determining their mechanisms of action. Mycotoxins may turn out to be responsible for more than one human ailment about which current textbooks say "pathogenesis unknown."

Most of the deaths from various forms of mycotoxicosis have been in animals rather than in man. Dogs, pigs, sheep, cattle, horses and donkeys have all figured at one time or another in outbreaks of fatal disease later traced to mycotoxins in their food.

## Chemicals

### *Arsenic*

Small doses of arsenic usually cause no acute gastrointestinal symptoms. Ten minutes after ingestion of large amounts, dryness of the throat; abdominal pain; vomiting; diarrhea with tenesmus, mucus and blood; hematuria; and cardiac and respiratory depression occur.

*Treatment* (*see* Arsenic page 138).

### *Lead*

Large doses are rarely ingested; however, contamination in the preparation of food, with the insecticide lead arsenate, occasionally occurs. Nausea, vomiting, diarrhea and cramps are early symptoms, followed later by more pathognomonic signs of lead intoxication.

*Treatment* (*see* Lead Arsenate).

### *Cadmium*

If acid foods (citrus fruit juices) are placed in cadmium-plated utensils, such as pitchers or refrigerator ice trays, a sufficient amount of cadmium is dissolved to cause abdominal cramping, severe diarrhea and vomiting within fifteen to thirty minutes after eating or drinking contaminated foods or beverages. Supportive and symptomatic *treatment* should be given.

### *Copper*

Copper utensils are not usually used in the preparation of food, due to the catalytic properties of this element, and therefore present no particular health hazard (*see* Copper page 179).

### *Tin*

Food poisoning has resulted from contamination of fruit punch with tin. Unusually high acidity of the punch (pH 3) caused a reaction with the lining of the container, resulting in gastrointestinal irritation.

Recovery occurs in five to six hours. *Treatment* is symptomatic and supportive.

### *Zinc*

Acid food or liquids prepared or stored in galvanized zinc containers may dissolve sufficient zinc salts to produce severe vomiting, diarrhea and prostration. *Treatment* is symptomatic.

### *Antimony*

Antimony was often used as a binder between enamel and metal in old cooking utensils. Citric acid in fruit beverages may dissolve the binding in the worn enamel coating of large pans or other containers, thus releasing sufficient antimony to cause symptoms of intoxication.

*Treatment* is the same as that for arsenic poisoning and includes BAL. Circulatory collapse, which occurs early, requires vigorous supportive treatment (*see* Antimony page 155).

### *Sodium Fluoride*

This insecticide is widely used to exterminate cockroaches from food establishments. Since it is a white powder, it can easily be mistaken for baking powder, soda or flour. Illness follows within a few minutes to two hours after ingestion and is characterized by vomiting, diffuse abdominal pain and diarrhea. Convulsions, tonic or clonic spasms (tetany), paresis of certain groups of muscles (eye and facial muscles, hand extensors and those of the lower extremities), hiccups and contraction of the pupils may occur.

Initial home *treatment* should include milk. For further treatment, *see* page 140.

### *Mercury*

In two to thirty minutes after bichloride of mercury is swallowed, an astringent metallic taste occurs, accompanied by salivation, thirst, vomiting, abdominal pain, and after two hours, a watery diarrhea. For *treatment, see* page 144.

### *Polynuclear Hydrocarbons*

Charcoal-broiled meat contains polynuclear hydrocarbons similar to those in pyrolyzed cigarettes and coal. Most notable is benzo (*a*) pyrene at a concentration of 8 μg/kg of meat. A large steak contains the same amount of this substance as 600 cigarettes. The most likely source of the hydrocarbons is melted fat, which drips on hot coals and is pyrolyzed at a high temperature and deposits on the meat as the smoke rises. Meat protein apparently is not pyrolyzed, and cooking methods such as oven broiling or roasting are unlikely to produce carcinogens. No nitrogen heterocyclic compounds such as carbazoles and acridines found in tobacco, coal and wood smoke are found in the charcoal-broiled meat.

Analysis was performed by broiling fifteen 1.1 kg steaks to "well done" on a standard charcoal broiler. Wood charcoal was ignited with purified iso-octane and allowed to reach a glowing red heat. Meat was placed six inches above the fire and cooked on both sides. The outer layers were removed and extracted. Polynuclear material was extracted from lipids, and the polynuclear aromatic hydrocarbons were separated by column and paper chromatography. Identification and measurement were made by ultraviolet absorption and by fluorescence spectrometry. Fifteen hydrocarbons were identified, and the mixture was similar qualitatively to those obtained from materials such as cigarettes and coal, except that no nitrogen-containing polynuclear compounds were detected (Lijinsky, W. and Shubik, P.: *Science, 145*:53-55, 1964).

## Plants and Seafood

### *Mushroom*

The most poisonous of the mushrooms is *Amanita phalloides;* two or three of these white or yellow toadstools are sufficient to cause illness and death. More than half of those severely poisoned die. Findings include hypoglycemia which may be accompanied by convulsions, severe abdominal pain, intense thirst, nausea, retching, vomiting and profuse watery stools. Illness occurs within six to fifteen hours after ingestion.

It should be noted that cooking does not destroy all the toxins in poisonous mushrooms and thus does not protect against the lethal effects of failure of proper identification. Nor is there any truth in the statements that a silver spoon or coin added to the pan in which mushrooms are cooked darkens if poisonous species are present, or that if the skin can be peeled from the cap of the mushroom and/or if they fail to turn color when broken, they are nonpoisonous. (For major discussion and *treatment, see* pages 547 through 558).

### *Ergotism*

Ergot poisoning occurs from eating rye meal or rye bread prepared from diseased rye containing the fungus *Claviceps purpurea.* Symptoms are drowsiness, headache, giddiness, painful cramps of the limbs and itching of the skin. In severe cases, gangrene may occur, involving the fingers and toes and occasionally the ears and nose.

Aside from elimination of ergot, *treatment* is symptomatic and supportive.

### *Acid Beverages*

Considerable clinical and experimental evidence indicates that erosion, etching or decalcification of calcified tooth structure may be produced not only by injudicious consumption of lemon juice but by other highly acidic carbonated beverages, liquids or medicaments if the acids, organic or inorganic, are of low enough pH.

People who habitually use lemons may exhibit acid erosion, usually on the labial surfaces of the anterior teeth if they suck on the fruit and on the lingual surfaces if they chew it. Dilution of the lemon juice with water does not reduce its acidity appreciably; it may have a pH below 3. In the interproximal areas and on lateral surfaces of the anterior maxillary teeth, the acidity may remain very low for several minutes unless the involved surfaces are actively bathed by the passage of saliva or mouth rinsing. In severe cases, the total enamel cap of the tooth may be lost as well as the underlying dentin.

### *Ciguatera*

Food fish poisoning is common in the tropics. (For symptoms and *treatment, see* page 581).

### *Shellfish*

Shellfish poisoning has been traced to eating shellfish which have fed on *Gonyaulax.* The symptoms resemble curare poisoning. It is characterized by paralysis of different groups of muscles, especially those of respiration. They vary from trembling about the lips to complete loss of power in the neck muscles. Nausea, vomiting and diarrhea also occur. The illness develops within five to thirty minutes or longer after eating the poisoned mussels, clams or crab. The neurotoxin (saxitoxin) is not destroyed by cooking.

*Treatment* should be carried out as with any curare-like poisoning: Prostigmin methylsulfate given in a dose of 1 ml of 1:2000 solution intravenously, with artificial respiration and oxygen until the patient can breathe normally.

### *Water Hemlock*

Poisoning occurs when the leaves and roots of the water hemlock, *Cicuta maculata,* are eaten. Nausea, vomiting and convulsions occur one to two hours after ingestion. Gastric lavage, purgation, enema and sedation for convulsions comprise *treatment.*

### *Rhubarb*

Rhubarb leaves and other plants containing large amounts of oxalic acid cause vomiting and diarrhea when eaten in large quantities. Gastric lavage is indicated (*see* Oxalic Acid).

### *Potato*

Potato poisoning follows ingestion of raw sprouted potatoes which contain an alkaloid that causes an acute gastroenteritis, oliguria, collapse and, rarely, neurological manifestations. *Treatment* should include lavage, emetics, cathartics and parenteral fluids as needed to correct electrolyte imbalance.

(For other plants, *see* Table 139.)

## Idiosyncrasies

### *Favism*

A type of poisoning which might be termed a food allergy is caused by the *Vicia faba* bean, widely cultivated in New York, New Jersey, Illinois and California, and an important item in the diet of many Americans of Italian descent. Sensitization to the bean seems to be hereditary, since in certain families every member for generations has been reported to be severely affected. Glucose-6-phosphate dehydrogenase deficiency in the erythrocytes has been demonstrated in most patients and families. Susceptibility varies; a person long accustomed to eating the beans without ill effect may suffer a single, severe attack and experience none thereafter. The illness may follow inhalation of the pollen or within an hour after eating the beans. Symptoms are acute febrile hemolytic anemia with jaundice, hematuria and hemoglobinuria. *Treatment* is supportive with transfusions as needed.

### *Food Allergies*

Because certain foods may not cause symptoms every time they are eaten, food allergies are often difficult to manage. Constipation is the most common symptom, but it may alternate with diarrhea. Belching, nausea and epigastric discomfort are usually present, and cramps are frequent. Pain is due to spasm of the colon, which can be demonstrated by x-ray examination with barium enema. Mucous diarrhea with large numbers of eosinophiles in the mucous may occur, with or without painful rectal spasm. Severe pruritus ani is often a complaint.

Diagnosis depends on a history of previous individual and familial allergic symptoms. A record of symptoms and foods eaten over a period of time may reveal the offending food or foods.

*Treatment* consists of either elimination of foods responsible for symptoms or desensitization. Parenteral administration of epinephrine or an antihistamine compound is recommended for control of acute symptoms.

## Antibiotic Residues

Antibiotic residues in foods pose a potential hazard to the health of man for several reasons. Persons sensitive to drugs such as penicillin and streptomycin may suffer adverse reactions from eating foods that carry residues of these antibiotics. Continued exposure to such drugs also can contribute to the development of sensitization, which means that subsequent use of the antibiotics to treat an illness could cause adverse reactions. It is well established that bacteria which are continually exposed to antibiotics tend to develop resistance to these drugs. More recently, it has been shown that this action can be transferred by bacteria, even between species, through contact or conjugation. This transfer factor can result in a more rapid build up of a drug-resistant bacterial population. There is concern that organisms in animals which have developed resistance as the result of continuous exposure to antibiotics may move to human beings and establish a resistant population. In addition, the population of resistant organisms in man may be maintained or expanded through a constant low-level exposure to antibiotics from residues in food. The persistence of antibiotic residues in treated animals varies widely between drugs. Streptomycin, when used in combination with penicillin, has been shown to persist at the site of the injection for forty-seven days. It has persisted even longer in the kidneys of treated animals.

More restrictive use of antibiotics in food-producing animals reduces the potential risk to man from residues in foods. The FDA policy on antibiotics outlines a number of steps the Agency has taken to prevent unauthorized and unsafe residues in foods: all exemptions from food additive regulations which were on sanctions or approvals granted prior to the Food Additive Amendment of 1958 were revoked. Uses which are concluded to be safe will be covered by new food additive regulations. Antibiotic preparations now marketed under exemptions will be subject to regulatory action 180 days after such exemptions are revoked. The Agency initiated action to revoke or amend antibiotic regulations or to withdraw approval of new drug applications on products for which there are inadequate residue data. All antibiotic products, including medicated premixes for feeds, intended for use in food-producing animals are now considered as new drugs or certifiable antibiotics, which means evidence of their safety and effectiveness is required.

These actions apply to products that are given orally, injected, or used in the udder or uterus of food-producing animals. Topical and ophthalmic preparations are not affected because they produce no residues in foods.

### Tips for Avoiding Food Poisoning

1. Wash your hands before preparing food, after handling raw meats and after blowing your nose or smoking. Keep fingernails clean.
2. Use only clean clothing, aprons, towels and equipment.
3. Avoid using hands to mix foods and keep hands away from mouth, nose and hair.
4. A person with a skin infection or infectious disease should not prepare food. Avoid coughing or sneezing over foods.
5. Refrigerate all perishables soon after purchase and refrigerate leftovers promptly. In preparation, refrigerate cooked foods immediately and use shallow pans—they cool faster.
6. Keep hot foods at 150°F or higher and cold foods at 40° to 45°F or lower. Bacteria grow rapidly at in-between temperatures.
7. Do not remove cold foods from refrigerator more than one-half hour before serving. Add dressings to salads just before serving.
8. When eating out, beware of buffets where food may be displayed for hours.
9. Many of the above rules are especially important when preparing foods for picnics or large group dinners.

## RECOMMENDATIONS TO THE PUBLIC ON FIRST AID MEASURES FOR POISONING

The aim of first aid measures is to help prevent absorption of the poison. *Speed* is essential. First aid measures must be started at once. If possible, one person should begin treatment while another calls a physician. When this is not possible, the nature of the poison determines whether to call a physician first or begin first aid measures and then notify a physician. Save the poison container and material itself, if any remains. If the poison is not known, save a sample of the vomitus.

*Emergency Telephone Numbers*

Physician..................................................
Fire Department.....................................
(Resuscitator)
Hospital..................................................
Pharmacist...............................................
Police......................................................
Rescue Squad..........................................
Poison Control Center...........................

### Measures To Be Taken Before Arrival of Physician

I. *Swallowed Poisons*

Many products used in and around the home, although not labeled "Poison," may be dangerous if taken internally. For example, some medications which are beneficial when used correctly may endanger life if used improperly or in excessive amounts.

In all cases except those indicated here, *remove poison from patient's stomach immediately* by inducing vomiting. The importance of this cannot be overemphasized, for it is the essence of the treatment and is often a lifesaving procedure. Prevent chilling by wrapping patient in blankets if necessary. Do not give alcohol in any form.

A. *Do not induce vomiting if*
   1. Patient is comatose or unconscious.
   2. Patient is convulsing.
   3. Patient has swallowed petroleum products (kerosene, gasoline, lighter fluid).
   4. Patient has swallowed a corrosive poison (symptoms: severe pain, burning sensation in mouth and throat, vomiting). *Call physician immediately.*
      a. Acid and acid-like corrosives: sodium acid sulfate (toilet bowl cleaners), acetic acid (glacial), sulfuric acid, nitric acid, oxalic acid, hydrofluoric acid (rust removers), iodine, silver nitrate (styptic pencil).

b. Alkali corrosives: sodium hydroxide—lye (drain cleaners), sodium carbonate (washing soda), ammonia water, sodium hypochlorite (household bleach).

If the patient can swallow after ingesting a *corrosive poison,* the following substances (and amounts) may be given.

FOR ACIDS: milk, water or milk of magnesia (1 tablespoon to 1 cup of water).*

FOR ALKALIS: milk, water, any fruit juice or diluted vinegar.*

FOR PATIENT ONE TO FIVE YEARS OLD: 1 to 2 cups.

FOR PATIENT FIVE YEARS OR OLDER: up to 1 quart.

B. Induce vomiting when noncorrosive substances have been swallowed
   1. Give milk or water; do not use carbonated fluid. For patient one to five years old, 1 to 2 cups; for patient over five years, up to 1 quart.
   2. Induce vomiting by placing the blunt end of a spoon or your finger at the back of the patient's throat or by use of syrup of ipecac (do not use table salt for inducing vomiting at any age).

When retching and vomiting begin, place patient face down with head lower than hips. This prevents vomitus from entering the lungs and causing further damage.

II. Inhaled Poisons
   A. Carry patient (do not let him walk) to fresh air immediately.
   B. Open all doors and windows.
   C. Loosen all tight clothing.
   D. Apply artificial respiration if breathing has stopped or is irregular.
   E. Prevent chilling (wrap patient in blankets).
   F. Keep patient as quiet as possible.
   G. If patient is convulsing, keep him in bed in a semi dark room; avoid jarring or noise.
   H. Do not give alcohol in any form.

III. Skin Contamination
   A. Drench skin with water (shower, hose, faucet).
   B. Apply stream of water on skin while removing clothing.
   C. Cleanse skin thoroughly with water; rapidity in washing is most important in reducing extent of injury from absorption.

IV. Eye Contamination
   A. Hold eyelids open, wash eyes with gentle stream of running water *immediately.* Delay of few seconds greatly increases extent of injury.
   B. Continue washing until physician arrives. *Do not use chemicals;* they may increase extent of injury.

V. Injected Poisons (scorpions and snakes)
   A. Make patient lie down as soon as possible.
   B. Do not give alcohol in any form.
   C. Apply tourniquet above injection site, e.g. between arm or leg and heart. The pulse in vessels below the tourniquet should not disappear, nor should the tourniquet produce a throbbing sensation. Tourniquet should be loosened for one minute out of every fifteen minutes.
   D. Incise and suction area of the bite.
   E. Apply cold pack to site of the bite.
   F. Carry patient to physician or hospital; *do not let him walk.*

VI. Chemical Burns
   A. Wash with large quantities of running water (except those caused by phosphorus).
   B. Immediately cover with loosely applied clean cloth.
   C. Avoid use of ointments, greases, powders and other drugs in first aid treatment of burns.
   D. Treat shock by keeping patient flat, keeping him warm and reassuring him until the arrival of the physician.

## Measures to Prevent Poisoning Accidents

I. Keep all drugs, poisonous substances and household chemicals out of the reach of children and away from food.

---

*Use of neutralizing (even well-diluted) solutions because of their potential exothermic effects are being questioned.

II. Do not store nonedible products on shelves used for storing food.

III. Keep all poisonous substances in their original containers; do not transfer to unlabeled containers.

IV. When medicines are discarded, destroy them. Do not throw them where they might be reached by children or pets.

V. When giving flavored and/or brightly colored medicine to children, *always* refer to it as medicine—*never* as candy.

VI. Do not take or give medicine in the dark.

VII. READ LABELS before using chemical products.

VIII. Use cleaning fluids with *adequate ventilation* only, and avoid breathing vapors.

IX. *Protect your skin and eyes* when using insect poisons, weed killers, solvents and cleaning agents. Be sure to wash thoroughly after their use and promptly remove contaminated clothing.

X. Always reseal safety closures and packages.

TABLE 158
SYMPTOMS WHICH MAY INDICATE THAT AN INDIVIDUAL IS TAKING DRUGS

| *Drugs* | *Symptoms* |
|---|---|
| Marihuana | Strong odor of burnt leaves on breath and clothes, dilation of pupils of the eyes, sleepiness, wandering mind, lack of coordination, craving for sweets, increased appetite |
| LSD<br>DMT<br>DOM or STP | Severe hallucinations, panic, feelings of detachment, incoherent speech, cold hands and feet, vomiting, laughing and crying jags, strong body odor, toxic psychosis and suicidal attempts |
| Amphetamines (pep or "up" pills) | Aggressive behavior, rapid speech, giggling and silliness, confused thinking, increased activity followed by fatigue, tremors, insomnia, no appetite |
| Heroin or morphine | Stupor, watery eyes, loss of appetite, needle marks on body, bloodstains on shirt, paraphernalia for injections |
| Glue sniffing | Drunk appearance, euphoric, incoordination, dreamy or blank expression |
| Barbiturates ("down" pills) | Stupor, dullness, blurred speech, drunk appearance, vomiting |

Screening by urinalysis usually employs thin-layer chromatographic techniques that will detect most drugs, although they cannot detect LSD and marihuana. Positive tests should be confirmed by another technique, such as gas-liquid chromatography.

## CARBON MONOXIDE POISONING

Approximately 1500 persons die in the United States from carbon monoxide gas, but this is only the "tip of the iceberg." Public health and medical authorities believe there are many more deaths and injuries from carbon monoxide that are not reported as such, because they are not suspected or correctly diagnosed and therefore not tabulated statistically (*see* pp. 239 through 243).

It takes a combination of two causes to bring about CO poisoning: improper burning of fuel and insufficient ventilation.

When one happens without the other, you may "get up." When both happen at the same time, you cannot escape poisoning. For instance, if the motor in your car is burning fuel properly and there is enough air intake, you can sit for some hours in a closed, parked car during a blizzard, with motor running, and still suffer no harm from CO. But if fuel is not burning properly (and how can you be sure?), and air cannot enter the car through the air-intake (this may be clogged by snow), CO poisoning may take your life.

CO poisoning may happen, and often does, when someone

1. Starts a car in a closed garage and lingers there while the motor warms.
2. Lights a heater, stove or furnace after a long period of disuse without checking to

see if it is in good operating condition and that the flue or chimney is unobstructed.

3. Uses a space heater in a small, unventilated room.
4. Overloads the fire in a coal furnace with fresh fuel, then closes the damper too soon.
5. Uses the kitchen oven of a gas stove for overnight heating purposes.

Just a few simple precautions that anyone may take remove most danger of CO poisoning.

### In the Home

1. Make sure all furnaces, stoves and heaters are connected by proper-sized flue pipes to chimneys or other approved outlets to the outside air (except in cases where the equipment meets approval of National Standards without such connections).
2. Use only approved, rigid-metal piping, or special types of semi-rigid piping (or flexible-metal tubing, if approved by local authorities), to connect room heaters, cookstoves, refrigerators, clothes dryers and similar gas-burning equipment to gas supply lines. *Never* use a rubber hose for such connections!
3. Keep all fuel-burning equipment, flue pipes and chimneys in good condition. Inspect all flues and chimneys regularly (at least annually). Replace or repair corroded sections or cracked linings. Clean out flues and chimneys and remove soot, tar, debris or any other obstructions which may be found after inspection. (There are cases on record where even a bird's nest in a chimney has caused CO deaths.) Have furnaces inspected for cracks in combustion chambers where gas might escape. Have burners of oil and gas furnaces, water heaters, gas refrigerators and similar equipment inspected regularly to make sure they are in proper adjustment and repair. (When this is done, fuel will be completely burned and there will be no dangerous amounts of CO in the flue gases.)
4. Do not substitute one type of gas for another in any gas-burning appliances unless a qualified serviceman has made the necessary changes in the parts affected and has tested the operation and made necessary adjustments.
5. Never try to change or interfere with the way an appliance was designed to be used. Keep all vents *open.* Do not block or cover vents of water heaters, range ovens or space heaters in any way. Do not try to patch gas pipes or tubing with tape, gum or other weak and temporary materials.
6. Never operate furnaces, fireplaces, space heaters or water heaters without providing some dependable means of supplying fresh air continuously to make up for the supply exhausted by burning.
7. Never tune up your lawn mower in an enclosed space, such as a closed garage; always start it out-of-doors.
8. Never use a hibachi or charcoal grill indoors for the purpose of cooking, heating or taking the chill off a particular room such as a basement or closed garage.

### In The Car

1. Check automobile exhaust systems regularly, especially for blown-out gaskets, loose manifolds, leaking exhaust pipe connections and holes in mufflers.
2. Be sure the doors are open in the garage or space where an automobile motor is running. Do not allow the engine to run more than a few minutes, even with the garage door open.
3. Shut the engine off when sitting in a parked car for more than a few minutes, unless the windows are open.
4. In slow-moving, closely spaced traffic, or while traveling through tunnels, keep air-intakes of car closed to be sure that CO from the exhaust pipes of the cars in front of you does not collect in large amounts in your own car.

### In Summer Homes, Camps and Motels

1. Give special and close attention to heating units in buildings which have been closed

for a season and are about to be occupied again. (Heating units may have broken down because of weather or other conditions; chimneys may have become blocked. They will probably need some adjustments before use during the new season.)

2. If you are a tourist camp operator who uses individual gas heaters in each cabin, keep a careful check on equipment. (Because of daily turnover of guests, many of whom are inexperienced in operating such appliances, heaters can easily be thrown out of adjustment.)
3. When stopping overnight at motels, auto courts, tourist homes and the like, where oil– or gas-burning heaters are located in bedrooms, ask how such appliances operate, and make sure that there are flue connections to such appliances before you use them. Open windows when heaters are in use, or make sure there is some other means of providing enough ventilation.

### First Aid for CO Poisoning

Prevention is always the best way to deal with accidents, but sometimes they happen despite our best efforts to foresee all possibilities. Be alert to signs of mild CO poisoning and investigate to determine the cause. Keep in mind that the first symptoms—headache, nausea and dizziness—resemble other illnesses. When they do occur, knowing what to do and acting quickly can save a life. This is especially true in cases of acute CO poisoning where time is of the essence. These are the steps to take.

1. Remove the victim to fresh air immediately. If he is not breathing, or is breathing irregularly, begin artificial respiration AT ONCE!
2. Call, or have someone else *Call a Doctor* immediately. Also send for an ambulance service, rescue squad, or fire or police department for special equipment to help revive the victim. However, do not wait for this help to arrive; start first aid without delay.
3. Continue artificial respiration when the emergency equipment arrives, providing both kinds of treatment at the same time until natural breathing returns, unless otherwise directed by a physician. Continue artificial respiration for two hours or more, if natural breathing is not restored.
4. Keep the victim warm, but not overly so, with blankets or other covering. If hot water bottles, bricks or metal are used to warm him, wrap them to make sure they do not come in contact with his body, since they may burn.
5. Meanwhile, if poisoning occurred in the house, have someone check the heating equipment, shut off the fuel supply and ventilate the premises.
6. Continue application of oxygen as provided through the emergency equipment for fifteen to thirty minutes after natural breathing returns. This assists in quickly ridding the blood of carbon monoxide.
7. After the victim begins to breathe again, keep him still, warm and quiet to help prevent any danger of shock.
8. Avoid the use of stimulants such as coffee or tea, since these may increase the heart rate unnecessarily.
9. Aid circulation by rubbing the arms and legs. The earlier proper circulation is restored, the sooner the patient recovers.
10. See that the patient has rest and time to recover slowly in order to avoid heart stress.
11. For persistent respiratory distress, perform chest x-rays to rule out diffuse pulmonary edema.

## HAZARDS OF SOLVENTS AT HOME AND ON THE JOB

Exposure to solvents in housekeeping, home maintenance, hobby activities or on the job may be the obscure cause of vague symptoms or serious disability.

Autoimmune glomerulonephritis apparently can be caused by the massive accumulation of inhaled toxic chemicals. Chemical interaction with lung or kidney basement membranes occurs in susceptible individuals, and these "autoantibodies" then mediate further kidney or lung injury.

Evidence of exposure to gasoline, degreasing and paint-removing solvents, fuel oils and other hydrocarbon solvents should be diligently sought in all patients who have rapidly progressing glomerulonephritis with or without associated pulmonary hemorrhage.

## General Principles Applying to Solvent Vapors

1. All solvents have toxic properties; some are more toxic than others.
2. All solvents can cause dermatitis by their action in removing normal skin oils, or by sensitizing.
3. All solvent vapors are heavier than air; vapor concentration is greater closer to the floor.

Use out-of-doors, if possible. If used inside, open windows and doors and let vapors flow out. Select a breezy day. Always ventilate DOWN and AWAY from the breathing zone. Use exhaust hoods whenever possible.

4. All solvents in very high concentrations have a rapid narcotic, anesthetic action. Systemic poisoning and fatal results are common.
5. Many solvents can cause cumulative systemic damage by repeated exposure to low, but unsafe, concentrations.

Systemic effects vary.

BENZENE (BENZOL): Principal effects are on the blood and blood-forming organs.

CARBON TETRACHLORIDE: Principal effects are on the liver and kidneys.

TRICHLOROETHYLENE: Principal effects are on the nervous system.

METHYL BUTYL AND ETHYL KETONE: Peripheral neuropathy.

There are great variations in individual susceptibility.

6. Nearly all solvents will *burn* and *explode* (except a few, such as carbon tetrachloride and trichloroethylene).
7. Watch pilot lights, sparking motors and cigarettes. Be careful of carbon tet vapors when used on fires in small, unventilated places. Volatile solvents evaporate readily; a small amount of liquid makes a large amount of vapor or gas. For example, 15.2 fl. oz. (about a pint) of carbon tetrachloride evaporates to form 4 cu. ft. of pure carbon tetrachloride vapor, producing a concentration of 4000 ppm, when dispersed in a room 10 ft. x 10 ft. x 10 ft. = 1000 cu. ft. This is 160 times the safe concentration for prolonged exposure.
8. The liquid volumes shown in connection with maximum allowable concentrations produce the indicated vapor concentrations when volatilized and thoroughly dispersed in a closed room of 1000 cu. ft. (10 ft. x 10 ft. x 10 ft.).
9. Maximum allowable concentrations (MAC)

TABLE 159
COMPARISON OF CARBON DISULFIDE AND ACETONE

| *Carbon Disulfide* | *Acetone* |
|---|---|
| Maximum Allowable Concentration (MAC) for prolonged exposure—20 ppm of air | Maximum Allowable Concentration (MAC) for prolonged exposure—*1000* ppm of air |
| Highly toxic—Strongly Narcotic | Weakly Narcotic—Weakly Toxic |
| *Acute Poisoning* | *Acute Poisoning* |
| Exposure to 4800 ppm—fatal in 1½ hr. | Exposure to 20,000 ppm—fatal on brief exposure |
| Exposure to 1150 ppm—serious after 1½ hr. | Exposure to 2,000 ppm—mild intoxication, nausea, headache, irritation of mucous membranes after 8 hrs. |
| *Chronic Poisoning* | *Chronic Poisoning* |
| A common occurrence from repeated exposure to lower concentration—effects are cumulative and serious | No evidence of cumulative effects from repeated exposures to lower concentrations |

or threshold limits are the recognized safe concentrations for prolonged and repeated exposure. A complete printed list of those which have been established is available from the Council on Industrial Health of the AMA (*also see* Tables 65 and 66.).

*Solvents have become an indispensable part of our life. Used properly, they are a boon; used improperly, they endanger safety, health and life itself.* For example, *carbon tetrachloride,* widely used in the home and in industry and commonly regarded as a safe solvent, however, is more dangerous than chloroform or ether.

## Carbon Tetrachloride

SYNONYMS.
Carbon tet
Tetrachlormethane
Perchloromethane
Many trade names

PROPERTIES.
Chemical formula $CCL_4$
Colorless liquid with sweet aromatic odor like chloroform
Vapor pressure, high; evaporates rapidly at ordinary temperatures
Vapor density, 5.32 (air = 1)
Nonflammable, nonexplosive
Breaks down at high temperatures or in presence of flame to form hydrochloric acid and phosgene, an extremely poisonous gas

USES.
Metal cleaning and degreasing
Dry cleaning
Solvents for oils, greases, waxes, paints, rubber, etc.
Fire extinguishing agent
Chemical processing, etc.

OTHER USES *(with occasional fatal results).*
"Dry" shampoo
Anthelmintic for hookworm
Removing adhesive tape
Anesthetic

### *Effects of Carbon Tetrachloride*

SIGNS AND SYMPTOMS.

INHALATION.

ACUTE POISONING, IMMEDIATE OR DELAYED.
Headache and dizziness
Visual disturbances
Nausea and backache
Confusion and stupor
Respiratory failure
Narcosis
Muscle cramps
Severe abdominal pain
Myocarditis
Ventricular fibrillation

OTHER SEQUELAE.
Suppression of urine
Uremia and jaundice
Hepatitis and nephrosis
Pulmonary and cerebral edema

TREATMENT.
Prompt removal from exposure
Artificial respiration
Restrict fluid intake
Digitalis for cardiac failure
High-carbohydrate diet
Contraindicated
- Adrenalin
- Alcohol

Watch for delayed effects six hours to several days later

### *Chronic Poisoning*

Irritation of eyes and respiratory tract
Mild narcosis
Headache and dizziness
Restricted visual fields
Backache and nausea
Gastric disturbances
Bleeding from mucous membranes
Nephritis and hepatitis
Removal from exposure important
Tissues being damaged faster than they can be repaired

### *Safe Exposure*

For continuous eight-hour daily exposures, the recognized safe maximum allowable concentration of $CCL_4$ is 25 ppm of air.

The odor perception threshold for carbon tetrachloride is about 80 ppm.

"If you can smell it, it's unsafe."

### *Skin Contact*

Systemic poisoning
Dermatitis
  Defatting action on skin
  Sensitization
Protective clothing
Protective creams before exposure
Superfatted creams after exposure
Removal from exposure

### *Ingestion*

Accidental ingestion of more than a teaspoonful (5 ml) may be fatal. Liver necrosis is the usual pathologic effect.

Induce vomiting
Treat for acute poisoning

### *Individual Susceptibility*

Especially
  The alcoholic
  The obese or undernourished
  The diabetic
  Liver or kidney disease
  Pulmonary or heart disease
  Peptic ulcers

## Other Common Solvents

### *Benzene (Benzol)*

MAC 35 ppm for prolonged exposures (0.12 fl. oz. or 3.6 ml evaporated in 1000 cu. ft. of air).

COAL TAR DERIVATIVE. Do not confuse with petroleum benzine.

SYNONYMS.
Phenyl hydride
Coal tar naphtha

PROPERTIES.
Clear, colorless liquid
Pleasant odor, very volatile
Highly flammable and explosive
Flash point 12° F

USES.
Solvent for rubber, fats, greases, paints, lacquers, etc.
Paint and varnish removers
Lacquer thinners, fast-drying ink
Plastic solvents, rubber cements
Chemical processing, insecticides
Automobile gasoline (Some may contain as much as 20% benzol)

TOXIC EFFECTS.
Strongly narcotic, highly toxic
Acute poisoning: Weakness, dizziness, tremor, rapid pulse, cyanosis, "benzol jag," confusion, hysteria, convulsions, acute mania, collapse, coma, respiratory failure hours or days later.
Chronic poisoning is more usual: Cumulative effects of repeated exposures; irritation of eyes, nose, throat; nausea; malaise; weakness; bleeding from mucous membranes; marked blood changes, decrease in white and red cells; dermatitis from solvent action, sensitization.

### *Methyl Alcohol (Methanol)*

MAC 200 ppm for prolonged exposures (0.32 fl. oz. or 9.4 ml evaporated in 1000 cu. ft. of air).

### *Wood Alcohol*

SYNONYMS.
Methyl hydrate, methyl hydroxide
Acetone alcohol, wood spirits
Wood naphtha, columbian spirits
Colonial spirits, carbinol, etc.

PROPERTIES.
Clear, colorless liquid
Volatile
Very flammable and explosive

USES.
Solvent and thinner for shellac

Paint and varnish removers
Paint and varnish manufacture
Dry cleaning, auto antifreeze
Solvent for rubber cement
Celluloid, gums, resins
Chemical processing

TOXIC EFFECTS.

May be acute or chronic
Powerful nerve poison affects central nervous system, especially optic nerve, and causes degenerative damage of kidneys, liver and heart.
Symptoms are sometimes delayed as long as thirty-six hours, sudden dimness of vision, coma and respiratory failure.
Blindness may occur after temporary improvement in vision
Dermatitis

### *Trichloroethylene*

MAC 200 ppm for prolonged exposures (0.70 fl. oz. or 20.8 ml evaporated in 1000 cu. ft. of air).

SYNONYMS.

Ethylene trichloride
Acetylene trichloride

PROPERTIES.

Clear, colorless liquid
Pleasant odor
Very volatile
Nonflammable

USES.

Metal degreasing
Solvent for oils, greases, etc.
Paint, varnish, perfume
Dye, leather manufacturing
Dry cleaning
Refrigerant
Anesthetic
Substitute for carbon tetrachloride

TOXIC EFFECTS.

A strong narcotic, readily absorbed
Acute poisoning: Irritation of eyes, nose, throat, confusion; nausea; severe circulatory failure; collapse; coma; death may follow apparent recovery. Sequelae may include paralysis of trigeminal nerve, sense of taste or smell, tremor, visual disturbance.
Chronic poisoning (authorities are not agreed on cumulative toxicity)
Reported effects include headache, drowsiness, fatigue, giddiness, excitability, tremor, indigestion, nausea, irritation of mucous membrane, corneal inflammation, disturbances of sensation in extremities, addiction.
Dermatitis

### *Oil of Turpentine*

MAC 100 ppm for prolonged exposure (0.61 fl. oz. or 18 ml evaporated in 1000 cu. ft. of air).

SYNONYMS.

"Turpentine"
"Turps"
Spirits of Turpentine
Composition variable according to sources and method

PROPERTIES.

Clear, colorless liquid
Slightly irritating odor
Low volatility
Flammable
Explosive hazard low
Flash point 95° F

USES.

Solvent and thinner for paint, varnish and lacquer
Solvent for resins, oils, fats, rubber, asphalt, etc.
In leather dressings, creams and waxes
Chemical processing

TOXIC EFFECTS.

Weak narcotic
Strong irritant
Systemic poisoning
Acute poisoning: Ingestion or inhalation of high concentration causes kidney damage; can be fatal.
Lesser exposure causes mild narcosis, headache, giddiness, coughing, nausea, gastric pain, irritation of eyes, nose and throat
Cumulative poisoning from chronic minor exposures is doubtful
Severe dermatitis from irritating properties and solvent action

TABLE 160
SOLVENT EFFECTS

| *Solvent* | *Estimated Oral Lethal Dose (ml/kg.)* | *Irritant Effect* | *Narcotic Effect* | *Convulsant Effect* | *Organ Damage** | *Other Effects* |
|---|---|---|---|---|---|---|
| Acetone | 0.7 | + + | + + + | | | inebriation, collapse, hypoglycemia (rare) |
| Allyl alcohol | 0.1 | + + + | + + | + | L,K+ | skin burns |
| Amyl acetate | 0.7 | + + | + + | | L,K (Chr) | |
| Amyl alcohol | 0.4 | + + + | + + + | + | | methemoglobinemia possible |
| Benzaldehyde | 0.7 | | + + | + | | |
| Benzene | 0.2 | + + | + + + | + + | L,K± | delirium, agitation, ventricular fibrillation, aplastic anemia (esp. Chr) |
| Butanone | 0.7 | + + + | + + | | | |
| Butyl acetate | 0.7 | + | + | | | |
| Butyl alcohol | 0.4 | + | + + | | L (rare) | |
| Butyl carbitol | 0.3 | + + | + | + | K+ + | |
| Butyl cellosolve | 0.2 | + | + | | K+ + | |
| Carbitol | 0.4 | + | + | | K+ + | |
| Carbon tetrachloride | 0.05 | + + + | + + + | | L,K+ + + | circulatory collapse, delirium |
| Cellosolves | ?1-2 | + | + | | K+ + | hemolysis |
| Chloroform | 0.3 | + + | + + + | | L,K+ | |
| Cumene | ?0.1 | + + | + + + | | L,K± | pulmonary edema |
| Cyclohexane | ?5† | + + | + + | | | |
| Cyclohexanone | >0.7 | + | + | | | |
| Cyclohexyl alcohols | 0.4 | + | + + | + | | persistent tremor |
| Diacetone alcohol | 0.4 | | + + | | L,K+ | anemia possible |
| Dichloroethane (*see* Ethylene dichloride) | | | | | | |
| Diethylene glycol | 0.3 | similar to ethylene glycol | | | | |
| Dimethyl sulfoxide | 5-10 | + | + + + | + | K+ +,L± | hemolysis |
| DMSO (*see* Dimethyl sulfoxide) | | | | | | |
| Ethyl acetate | 1.5 | + | + | | | |
| Ethylene chlorohydrin | 0.1 | + + + | + + | + | L,K+ + | pulmonary edema |
| Ethylene dichloride | 0.07 | + + + | + + + | | L,K+ + + | pulmonary edema, hypotension, anemia |
| Ethylene glycol | 1.5 | + + | + + + | + + | K+ + + | see EM, December 1972 |
| Ethylene glycol diacetate | 0.4 | + + | + | | K+ + | |
| Ethylene glycol dinitrate | | | | | | methemoglobinemia |
| Ethylene glycol ethers (*see* Cellosolves) | | | | | | |
| Isoamyl acetate (*see* Amyl acetate) | | | | | | |
| Isophorone | 3.5 | + + | + + | | K+ | |
| Mesitylene | | + | + | | | bone marrow damage pneumonia |
| Mesityl oxide | 0.6 | | + + + | | | |
| Methyl acetate | 0.4 | + + | + | | | optic atrophy reported |
| Methylchloroform (*see* Trichloroethane) | | | | | | |
| Methylene chloride | 0.5 | + + | + + + | + | L,K± | pulmonary irritation, collapse |
| Methyl ethyl ketone (*see* Butanone) | | | | | | |
| Methyl isobutyl ketone | <0.7 | + + + | + + | | | |
| β-Naphthol | 0.06 | + + + | | + | L,K+ + | hemolysis |

TABLE 160
SOLVENT EFFECTS

| *Solvent* | *Estimated Oral Lethal Dose (ml/kg.)* | *Irritant Effect* | *Narcotic Effect* | *Convulsant Effect* | *Organ Damage** | *Other Effects* |
|---|---|---|---|---|---|---|
| Octyl alcohol | 0.4 | + + | + + + | | | |
| Perchloroethylene (*see* Tetrachloroethylene) | | | | | | |
| Polyethylene glycols | >5.0 | | ± | | K(?) | |
| Polypropylene glycols | 0.4 | | ± | | | ?cardiac arrhythmias |
| Propyl acetate | 0.7 | + + | + + | | | |
| Propyl alcohol | 5.0 | + + | + + + | | L + | hypoglycemia possible |
| Propylene glycol (nontoxic) | | | | | | |
| Tetra (*see* Tetrachloroethylene) | | | | | | |
| Tetrachloroethane | <0.01 | + | + + + | | L,K + + + | similar to carbon tetrachloride |
| Tetrachloroethylene | 0.2 | ± | + + | | L + | ventricular fibrillation possible |
| Toluene† | 0.3 | + + | + + + | (rare) | K ± | mania, hallucinations, anemia (Chr) |
| Toluol (*see* Toluene) | | | | | | |
| Trichloroethane | 0.03 | + + | + + | | L + | ventricular fibrillation possible |
| Trichloroethylene | 0.07 | + + | + + | | L,K + + | ventricular fibrillation possible, trigeminal neuralgia |
| Trilene (*see* Trichloroethylene) | | | | | | |
| Turpentine | 0.2 | + + + | + + | + + | K + + | chemical pneumonia |
| Xylene | 0.3 | + + | + + | (rare) | | |
| Xylol (*see* Xylene) | | | | | | |

*L = *Liver;* K = *Kidney;* Chr = *with chronic poisoning*
†Commercial preparations may be contaminated with varing quantities of benzene.
From Alan K. Done, *Emergency Medicine, 8*:170-171, 1976. Courtesy of publisher.

## PESTS ABOUT THE HOME

### *Fleas*

Cat and dog owners often return from summer vacation to find their homes overrun with fleas. These fleas are very hungry because of the absence of animals to feed on and readily attack humans.

Dog and cat fleas are the most common fleas in homes. They are very similar in appearance, and each kind attacks either cats or dogs. Adult fleas feed by sucking blood from the host animal; the females require this blood before laying eggs on the host, but the eggs fall to the ground, floor or animal bedding where the larvae live.

Effective control of dog and cat fleas involves the simultaneous treatment of the pets and their habitats. In some areas, fleas have developed resistance to the chlorinated hydrocarbon insecticides like DDT; in these areas, the use of phosphates and botanical insecticides is advisable (*see* Repellents [Flea Collars] ).

### *Carpenter Bees*

These insects resemble bumblebees but usually have a shiny black abdomen. They use their mouthparts to tunnel into wood. Some areas that may be attacked are porch railings, porch and shed ceilings and trim, porch furniture and dead tree limbs. Carpenter bees prefer unpainted, poorly painted or badly weathered dry wood as a place to make tunnels (keeping all outside wood well painted may help reduce infestations). These tunnels are about one-half an inch in diameter and may be one foot deep. They serve as homes for the young.

Carpenter bees may be controlled by saturating a piece of cotton with methylchloroform or carbon tetrachloride, inserting it into the tunnel and sealing the entrance to the tunnel with putty. Treating the area frequented by the bees with insecticides containing DDT, chlordane, dieldrin or malathion kills the adults present at time of treatment and reduces damage.

### *Millipedes*

These worm-like animals with many short legs often leave their hiding place (mulch) and move into homes. Carbaryl (Sevin®) applied as a spray or dust in a band five to ten feet wide around the house, with heavy applications near foundations and around doors, gives satisfactory control.

### *Bagworms*

They are getting larger and harder to kill. If evergreens are infested, treat with insecticides containing malathion, naled (Dibrom®), lead arsenate, toxaphene or dieldrin.

### *Wireworm Control in Sweet Potatoes*

Diazinon® 14% granules should be broadcast over the top of foliage at 21 lb./acre for summer wireworm treatment on sweet potatoes.

### *Squash Vine Borers in Cucurbits*

Borer injury to squash and pumpkin plants is common. Treat around the bases of all vines with a 1% lindane dust. Repeat applications three or four times at five– to seven-day intervals. Do not use lindane within one day of harvest or on land that will be planted to root crops or peanuts within two years after treatment.

Carbaryl (Sevin), endosulfan (Thiodan®) and naled (Dibrom) all have label approval. Read the label and follow directions.

Vines that are wilted because of the attack of squash vine borers should have the earth piled up around the base of the plants so that more roots may develop, or in some cases a shovelful of earth on the vine may cause roots to develop.

### *Chemical Pesticides: How to Use Them*

Householders, apartment dwellers and home gardeners have been using more pesticide chemicals to keep homes free of ants, roaches, silverfish and other pests, to protect flowers and trees from insect damage and to clear lawns of unwanted weeds.

*Like any tool,* these pesticides must be handled with care. Always read the label on each container before each use and follow the directions. Store the sprays and dusts in original, labeled containers. Note warnings and cautions each time before opening containers.

Keep pesticides out of the reach of children, pets and irresponsible people. Store the material in locked cupboards. Avoid smoking while spraying or dusting—many of the chemicals used are flammable.

Avoid inhaling sprays or dusts, and wear protective clothing and masks. Keep your sleeves rolled down and your collar up. Wash immediately with soap and water if you spill pesticide materials on your skin.

Wash your hands thoroughly after spraying or dusting and before eating or smoking. Change your clothes, too.

Cover food and water containers when treating around livestock or pet areas. Always dispose of empty containers so they pose no hazard to humans or animals.

Observe label directions to keep residues on edible portions of plants within limits permitted by law.

If you should suddenly feel sick while using a pesticide, or shortly afterward, call your physician immediately. Physicians now have available information for the quick and effective treatment of accidental overexposure to pesticides.

How can the farmer be sure that crops he raises with the aid of pesticides are safe for consumers to eat? Here are some answers from the National Agricultural Chemical Association.

There are three ways to be sure, and one of them—the most important one—depends directly upon the farmer himself. Directions for the safe use of every pesticide used in agriculture are printed on the label. These directions are registered by the United States Department of Agriculture. They are approved by the Federal Food and Drug Administration. These directions tell when and when not to use the pesticide, how much to use and the crops to use it on. The Federal Food and Drug Administration says that when these directions are followed, the farmer can be sure that residues of chemicals, if any, left on crops are within safe tolerances set by the Food and Drug Administration and that his crops are safe for consumers to eat.

If one could see the research that goes into producing and testing one of these chemicals, he could see how safety is built into it. A single chemical must be screened in the laboratory, tested for effectiveness against pests in the laboratory and in the field and then tested on laboratory animals in various amounts for as long as three years before the chemical can even be presented for registration to the U.S. Department of Agriculture or for clearance by the Food and Drug Administration.

During the three to five years of testing, hundreds of trained scientists test the chemical—physicians, toxicologists, chemists, entomologists and many others. When they are through, the chemical has few secrets left. Scientists know what it does to agricultural pests, how much it takes to get control under field conditions, what it does if the user inhales it or gets it on his skin, and what, if anything, happens if people consume even tiny amounts of its residue.

Scientists in the U.S. Department of Agriculture and Federal Food and Drug Administration then examine the data and make some tests of their own. If the chemical passes their scrutiny, the U.S. Department of Agriculture registers it for use against certain pests on certain crops, and a safe tolerance of residue permitted to remain in or on a crop at harvest times is set. They also make sure that when directions are followed, residues come within the safe tolerances set.

The label, which states the directions, is backed by years of scientific testing by many qualified scientists and has the approval of both the U.S. Department of Agriculture and the Food and Drug Administration. Few materials anywhere in the world today are given such thorough testing.

Where does the farmer come in? Of course, when the pesticide is applied to protect crops from insects, disease, weed or rodent damage, it is the farmer's responsibility to apply the pesticide according to the directions.

In most cases of human death from pesticides, the cause has been accidental misuse of a chemical poison. Because almost all pesticides are poisons, they should always be used with respect and great care. Following these safety rules for using pesticides is essential in the prevention of morbidity and mortality.

1. READ THE LABEL each time you use a pesticide—no matter how often you have used it and no matter how well you think you know the instructions—and FOLLOW THE LABEL DIRECTIONS EXACTLY.
2. Use a pesticide only when you are sure it is needed. Use the one best suited to your needs. The label on the product explains the proper uses.
3. Keep the pesticide in a plainly labeled container, preferably the one in which it was bought. *Never* transfer pesticides to unlabeled or mislabeled containers.

4. Store pesticides under lock and key, away from food items and OUT OF THE REACH OF CHILDREN, pets and people who might not be able to understand their danger.
5. When handling, mixing or applying pesticides, avoid inhaling dust and fumes and avoid getting materials on the skin.
6. Check the label of the product *before using* so that you know what to do quickly if there is an accident. In case of an accident, call a doctor or get the patient to a hospital immediately.
7. The very few people who suspect they may have a special sensitivity to pesticides should consult an allergist, and, if necessary, take steps to avoid *any* exposure to the offending agent.
8. Wash hands thoroughly after using pesticides and before eating or smoking.
9. Get rid of used pesticide containers in a way that does not leave the package of leftover contents as a hazard to people, particularly children, or to animals or plants. Unused or empty containers can be mailed for discarding to

   National Agricultural Chemical Association
   1145 19th Street, N.W.
   Washington, D.C. 20006

   The fee for this service is modest.
10. Work in a well-ventilated area to avoid inhalation of fumes.
11. Do not spray into the wind.
12. When so directed by the label, wear protective clothing, such as goggles, gloves, aprons, respirators and masks.
13. Change clothing after each day's operations and bathe thoroughly. If clothing or skin becomes contaminated, wash the skin and change to clean clothing.
14. When mixing or using flammable chemicals, be especially careful to avoid the fire hazards caused by smoking, defective wiring and open flames.
15. In applying pesticides to food plants and crops, (a) use the proper dose recommended for the purpose and (b) allow the full recommended time between applying the pesticide and harvesting the crop, to avoid having a harmful amount of pesticides remaining on food to be eaten. Do not plant food crops near ornamental plants which are to be sprayed.
16. Check sprayers before each use to make certain that hose connections are tight and that valves do not leak.
17. Cover food and water containers when using pesticides around livestock or pet areas.
18. Do not spray or treat plants or animals or animal feeding areas with pesticides unless you are certain such treatment is safe for that use.

### *Rates of Application*

1 oz./sq. ft. = 2722.5 lb./acre
1 oz./sq. yd. = 302.5 lb./acre
1 oz./100 sq. ft. = 27.2 lb./acre
1 lb./100 sq. ft. = 435.6 lb./acre
1 lb./1000 sq.ft. = 43.6 lb./acre
1 gal./acre = ⅓ oz./1000 sq. ft.
5 gal./acre = 1 pt./1000 sq. ft.
100 gal./acre = 2.5 gal./1000 sq. ft.
(1 qt./100 sq. ft.)
100 lb./acre = 2.5 lb./1000 sq. ft.

### *Important Facts*

Vol of sphere = cu. dia × .5236
dia = circum × .31831
area of circle = sq. dia × .7854
area of elipse = prod of both dia × .7854
Vol of cone = area of base × ⅓ ht.
1 cu. ft. water = 7.5 gal. = 62.5 lb.
pressure in psi = ht. (ft.) × .434
1 acre = 209 sq. ft.
ppm = % × 10,000

$$\% = \frac{\text{ppm}}{10{,}000}$$

1% by Vol = 10,000 ppm

### *What is one part per million?*

Most lay people have no conception of what constitutes one part per million residue on

TABLE 161
POTENTIAL TOXICITY OF PESTICIDES

| | *Safe* | *Intermediate* | *Dangerous* |
|---|---|---|---|
| Fumigants | Ethylene dichloride<br>Formaldehyde | Carbon tetrachloride<br>Chloropicrin<br>Ethylene dibromide | Hydrocyanic acid gas<br>Methyl bromide |
| Rodenticides | ANTU (α-naphthyl thiourea)<br>Barium carbonate<br>Red squill<br>Warfarin | | Barium fluoride<br>Fluoroacetamide<br>Fluoroacetate<br>Hydrocyanic acid<br>Strychnine<br>Zinc phosphide |
| Herbicides | Borates<br>Carbamates (for example, IPC)<br>Chlorates<br>2,4-dichlorophenoxy-acetic acid (2,4-D) and all related plant-growth hormones, including TBA<br>Monochloroacetates<br>Monuron (CMU)<br>Simazine<br>Trichloroacetates | Pentachlorophenol (also used as a timber preservative) | Arsenites<br>Dinitrobutyl-phenol (dinoseb)<br>Dinitrocresol (DNC)<br>Sulfuric acid<br>Endothal |
| Insecticides | Benzene hexachloride<br>Chlorbenzide<br>Chlordane<br>DDD<br>DDT<br>Derris<br>Dipterex<br>Malathion<br>Methoxychlor<br>Mineral oils<br>Pyrethrin<br>Tar oils | Aldrin<br>Chlorthion<br>Demeton-methyl<br>Diazinon<br>Dieldrin<br>Heptachlor<br>Lead arsenate<br>Phenkaptone<br>Rogor<br>Toxaphene | Demeton<br>Dimefox<br>Dinitrobutyl-phenol<br>Dinitrocresol (DNC)<br>Endrin<br>Fluoroacetamide<br>Guthion<br>Methyl-parathion<br>Nicotine<br>Parathion<br>Phosdrin<br>Schradan<br>Sulphotepp<br>TEPP (HETP) |
| Fungicides | Antibiotics<br>Captan<br>Copper compounds<br>Dithiocarbamates<br>Lime-sulfur | Organic mercurials used as seed dressing (1–3% Hg) | Organic mercury compounds used as concentrates, or indoors |

| | |
|---|---|
| | Sulfur |
| | TMTD (tetramethyl thiuram disulfide) |
| Growth depressants | Maleic hydrazide (MH-30) |
| | Tetrachloronitrobenzene |
| | Chlorinated phenoxyacetic acid salts (2,4-D; 2,4,5-T and MCPA) |
| Repellents | Naphthalene |
| | Paradichlorobenzene |

From Deichmann and Gerarde, *Symptomatology and Therapy of Toxicological Emergencies,* 1964. Courtesy of Academic Press, Inc. Publisher, New York, N. Y.

*Safe*—of low mammalian toxicity and correspondingly slight hazards in use.

*Intermediate*—of moderate toxicity, safe if used with some care. Care especially needed in hot climates, indoors and when handling concentrates.

*Dangerous*—of dangerously high toxicity and appreciable hazards. Require careful handling under almost all conditions.

crops. The following examples may help make this interpretation for them.

1. One inch is 1 ppm in sixteen miles.
2. A postage stamp is 1 ppm of the weight of a person.
3. A one gram needle in a one ton haystack is 1 ppm.
4. One minute in two years is 1 ppm.
5. Lay your hand on the ground and it covers 5 ppm of an acre.
6. If one pound of a chemical lands on an acre of alfalfa the hay has 500 ppm. One ounce of a chemical imparts 31 ppm.
7. A teaspoon of material on an acre of alfalfa imparts 5 ppm.
8. One teaspoon of DDT drifting onto five acres of alfalfa puts 1 ppm in the hay, and the federal law says that the hay must contain none.

## MATCHES

Years ago, when the principal components of matches were white or yellow phosphorus, potassium chlorate and sulfur, instances of poisoning, especially among workers in match factories, were not uncommon. With the replacement of white phosphorus by the red variety or by phosphorus sesquisulfide, matches became a safe household commodity, and cases of serious poisoning due to accidental ingestion are now quite rare.

References to match poisoning in published literature relate principally to contact with matches of the now obsolete variety and absorption of toxic agents through the skin. However, inasmuch as frequent calls are made to the various poison control centers concerning accidental ingestion by children, the following information from the Diamond Gardner Corporation should prove useful.

I. Types of Matches in Current Use

A. The "strike-anywhere" or kitchen match in general use in this country is made of a nonpoisonous paste containing 6 per cent phosphorus sesquisulfide ($P_4S_3$), 24 per cent potassium chlorate, plus zinc oxide, red ochre or other pigment, powdered glass, glue and water.

B. The "safety" or strike-on-box match, first made in Bohemia in 1894, is a nonpoisonous match that ignites when struck on a prepared surface. In the head, the chief ingredient is potassium chlorate. Other compounds rich in oxygen have been used in the past and also in other countries. The striking surface on the box is made from a paste of glue and powdered glass or sand containing red phosphorus and, at times, antimony sulfide, $Sb_2S_3$.

C. Book matches are similar in composition to the safety or strike-on-box match insofar as the composition of the head and striking surface are concerned.

II. Toxicological Properties of Match Ingredients

From the standpoint of toxicological interest, the principal ingredients of matches are potassium chlorate, red phosphorus, phosphorus sesquisulfide, and antimony sulfide.

Other ingredients contained in matches, such as glue, cornstarch, coloring agents, rosin or paraffin, offer no significant problem in regard to acute toxicity.

A brief statement of the toxicity and antidotal treatment for each major ingredient, considered individually, follows.

A. Potassium chlorate

1. Toxicity

Potassium chlorate is less toxic than the bromate but produces similar effects. It is irritating to the gastrointestinal tract and to the kidneys. It can cause hemolysis of red blood cells and methemoglobinemia. The toxic dose is approximately 5 gm, although a dose of 1 gm has been reported to be lethal in a child. Larger doses (15 to 46 gm) may produce vomiting, diarrhea, abdominal pain, collapse and death from renal failure.

2. *Treatment*
Gastric lavage with water or 1% sodium thiosulfate. Administer a demulcent and an analgesic, but avoid morphine. Oxygen may be given for the mild methemoglobinemia but not methylene blue (unless above 40% concentration) since it may enhance the latter effect. Apply symptomatic and supportive treatment to correct dehydration and to combat renal failure.

B. Red phosphorus

1. Toxicity
In contrast to white or yellow phosphorus (no longer used in matches), red phosphorus is relatively nonabsorbable, nonvolatile and nontoxic. Such cases of poisoning as have been claimed to result from the ingestion of red phosphorus are believed to be due to the presence of a trace of the white variety. Since 3 mg of *white* phosphorus has proved lethal to a two-year-old child, it might be considered that if red phosphorus were to contain as much as 0.6 per cent of white as an impurity, a large dose of red phosphorus such as 0.5 gm or more could be acutely toxic. However, it should be noted that this form of phosphorus is present on the striking surface and not in the head of present-day matches.

2. *Treatment*
Because of its nontoxicity, antidotal treatment for red phosphorus *per se* is not necessary. However, if the circumstances suggest that impure red phosphorus has been ingested in sufficient quantity or over a long enough period to induce toxic symptoms due to the presence of white phosphorus (of which a garlicky odor of the breath or excreta would be a strong indication), therapeutic measures directed toward the latter should be employed.

C. Phosphorus sesquisulfide
This compound is relatively nonpoisonous. It is scarcely attacked by cold water, and the conditions under which it may decompose in water at high temperatures probably do not prevail *in vivo.*

D. Antimony sulfide ($Sb_2S_3$)

1. Toxicity
Whereas contact with or inhalation of antimony compounds have been reported to cause dermatitis, keratitis, conjunctivitis and mucous membrane ulceration, their oral toxicity is dependent upon solubility. Antimony trisulfide, being quite insoluble, is relatively inert. (The intraperitoneal lethal dose in rabbits has been reported as 1 gm/kg of body weight.)

2. *Treatment*
In the event of accidental ingestion, the first step to be applied is evacuation. Vomiting may be stimulated by an emetic, or the stomach may be lavaged directly. The best antidote is tannic acid in warm water; this forms the insoluble tannate of antimony, which should be removed from the stomach by repeated lavage. Symptomatic treatment should follow.

III. Incidence of Match Poisoning

Whereas accidental ingestion of matches particularly by children often occurs, they produce relatively infrequent serious effects as compared, for example, with poisoning by household drugs.

The heads of a book of twenty matches, or an equal number of strike-anywhere (kitchen) matches, contain approximately 0.2 to 0.3 gm of potassium chlorate, which is about 1/20 of the usual toxic dose. From the evidence available, the oral ingestion of matches is not believed to have caused lethal effects in recent years, although the incidence of ingestion or mouthing must remain high because of the widespread availability and use of this product. During 1976, there were 531 reports of accidental ingestion of matches from the National Clearinghouse for Poison Control Centers. In almost all cases, no symptoms were reported.

IV. Accidental Ingestion of Matches

Since cases of match poisoning result more frequently from the licking or swallowing of *match heads* by children than from other causes, the principal toxic components of the heads should be considered in treating such cases. Gastric lavage as described above for potassium chlorate should receive first consideration inasmuch as red phosphorus or the sulfides of phosphorus and arsenic are relatively nontoxic and occur only in the striking surfaces. Since these abrasive strips are insolubilized, a child would not be able to ingest the striking surface material by merely licking the strip; he would actually have to chew and swallow it.

## FIREWORKS HAZARDS*

### *Sparklers*

Gold sparklers may contain barium nitrate, plus gums, paste, chalk, dextrin, iron and aluminum. Green sparklers contain barium nitrate, potassium perchlorate, plus wheat pastes, gum, dextrin and aluminum powder. Red sparklers contain strontium carbonate and nitrate, potassium perchlorate, plus gums, wheat pastes, dextrin and aluminum powder.

Soluble barium salts are highly toxic, causing vomiting, severe abdominal pain, bloody stools, rapid, shallow respiration, convulsions, coma and death from respiratory or cardiac failure. Barium stimulates smooth and cardiac muscle.

Strontium, in the form of the bromide salt, has been used in medications and was officially listed in the National Formulary until 1960. The adult therapeutic dose is 1 gm, which is in excess of the quantity of strontium salt found in a single sparkler. The nitrate radical may cause vomiting, abdominal pain, bloody stools and methemoglobinemia.

Perchlorates may produce methemoglobinemia, vomiting and abdominal pain.

*Treatment.* In cases where a sparkler has been eaten, emesis should be induced or gastric lavage performed, Sodium sulfate should be used in the lavage fluid if green or gold sparklers are involved. Intravenous solution of 1% methylene blue is recommended in the case of nitrate-induced methemoglobinemia but is contraindicated in cases involving chlorates.

### *Roll Caps*

Roll caps contain ingredients similar to gunpowder. One cap formulation is potassium chlorate, antimony sulfide, amorphous (red) phosphorus and gum. A roll of fifty caps contains approximately 200 mg total weight of these ingredients. Antimony sulfide is an insoluble salt. Red phosphorus has a low toxicity. Chlorates may cause methemoglobinemia; however, with the very small quantity present it is doubtful that any toxic manifestations would develop following ingestion.

### *Serpents*

Some of these preparations contain mercury thiocyanate, while other formulations are free of this compound. Nevertheless, because of the inability to discern their composition, emesis or gastric lavage is recommended following ingestion of these items.

## CHECKLIST FOR FIREWORKS SAFETY

1. Always read the directions.
2. Always have an adult present for proper supervision.

* New regulations of the U.S. Consumer Product Safety Commission now mandate that firecrackers and fireworks sold or distributed for consumer use be limited to a maximum of 50 mg of powder instead of 130 mg as in the past (rockets exempted).

3. Never experiment, take fireworks apart, mix anything with fireworks contents or try to make fireworks yourself.
4. Always light fireworks outdoors in a clear area away from houses and away from flammable materials.
5. Light one device at a time.
6. Keep a bucket of water nearby for emergencies.
7. Keep at a safe distance after lighting devices.
8. Dispose of fireworks properly; soak malfunctioning devices with water.
9. Never allow small children to handle fireworks.
10. Always store fireworks in a dry, cool place and avoid rough handling that might damage the fuses or handles.
11. Always allow enough room for proper function; never ignite fireworks in metal or glass containers.

## TOXIC CHRISTMAS DECORATIONS

During the Christmas season a flurry of reports and requests for information on Christmas trimmings are received by many poison control centers. Those listed below have created the most disturbance.

### *Bubbling Lights*

The modern Christmas tree is much safer than the old candlelit tree, but the candle-shaped, bubbling lights which have been introduced in the last ten years attract and tempt curious children. If the child is not discouraged by an electric shock or cut while removing a "candle" from the tree, he may be tempted to break the bulb and then inhale or swallow the contents. Generally this liquid is methylene chloride, a chlorinated hydrocarbon of low toxicity. The estimated lethal dose is 0.5 to 5.0 ml/kg. Symptoms can occur from inhalation or ingestion. Since there are about 4 ml of fluid in each "candle," the symptoms may include a mild central nervous system depression which may be preceded or followed by central nervous system excitement. If large amounts are ingested there may be the danger, as with other more potent chlorinated hydrocarbons, of liver and kidney damage. In *treating* such an accident, gastric lavage and artificial respiration, if necessary, should be used and followed by symptomatic treatment of any central nervous system effects.

### *Fire Salts*

This product, which is used to produce multicolored flames on the yule log, can cause heavy metal poisoning if swallowed. The colors result from burning the salts of copper, barium, selenium, lead, thallium, arsenic and antimony. Gastric irritation usually is severe enough to produce vomiting. Subsequent *treatment* includes ingestion of such demulcents as milk, raw egg whites, flour or starch. Provided that the original container is saved, the attending physician or a poison control center can prescribe a particular antidote where one exists.

### *Snow Sprays*

These decorations simulate snow and are applied to the object to be decorated by aerosol spray. The "snow" particles are usually composed of an inert plastic material and a long-chain fatty acid; ingestion should lead to no toxic consequences. The propellent vehicles for these particles are halogenated hydrocarbon substances, e.g. methylene chloride and Freon. These propellents evaporate after the aerosol mixture is sprayed onto an object; thus they are not ingested when the dry "snow" particles are ingested. Inhalation of the mixture during the spraying process could conceivably produce toxic manifestations due to halogenated hydrocarbon inhalation. Nausea and vomiting occurring in an adult as he was using a "snow" spray has been reported.

Nausea and vomiting, headache and central nervous system depression are the acute manifestations of halogenated hydrocarbon intoxication. The *treatment* is symptomatic and supportive in nature after the exposure has been terminated.

### *Icicles (Tinsel), Angel Hair*

Even the icicle decoration for the Christmas tree may be a menace. Fortunately, the metal constituents (40% tin and 60% lead) are poorly absorbed in the gastrointestinal tract, so icicle mishaps occur from the stringy nature of the material; intestinal obstruction and choking may be encountered.

Christmas tree ornaments made of thin metal or plastic (mold or foam) are only of concern for their mechanical potential to cut or obstruct. Paint or coloring on these objects would not cause poisoning.

Another trimming, misty "angel hair" (spun glass), can produce some irritations inside and outside of the gastrointestinal tract when children become enchanted with its cotton-candy appearance.

### *Berries, Holly (Ilex)*

The berries of this plant, which is commonly used in Christmas decorations, are reported to be toxic. Nausea, vomiting and central nervous system depression may occur following ingestion of holly berries. Vomiting should be induced as soon as possible after the berries are ingested. Further *treatment* is nonspecific, being dependent upon the nature of manifestations which occur.

### *Candles*

Wax and synthetic candles are inert and do not cause symptoms. Neither coloring nor scent is present in large enough amounts to be significant.

### *Mistletoe*

The American mistletoe *(Phoradendron flavescens)* plays a well-known traditional role during the Christmas season. The pharmacology and toxicology of the plant are not as renowned. Studies of the aqueous and alcoholic extracts of *Phoradendron flavescens* have demonstrated a direct stimulating effect on smooth muscles in arteries, intestine, bladder and uterus. Also, it has been stated that the berries contain an alkaloid pharmacologically similar to digitalis. However, the basis for this statement has not been substantiated.

A fatality following ingestion of a tea brewed from American mistletoe berries, has been reported. Prior to death, which occurred approximately nine and one-half hours after ingestion of the tea, the victim manifested signs and symptoms of acute gastrointestinal irritation and cardiovascular collapse. The postmortem examination revealed no cause for death. However, mistletoe leaves have been used for some time as a tea or coffee substitute without any reported ill effects.

It seems wise to recommend the induction of emesis following ingestion of mistletoe berries. Further *treatment* is symptomatic and supportive in nature.

### *Mothballs*

Recently "dancing mothballs" have been described in advertisements as a novel way of adding color and entertainment to the holidays. The stunt consists of placing mothballs in a colored solution of vinegar and water and then adding baking soda, which releases carbon dioxide at the surface causing the mothballs to dance. Most mothballs contain paradichlorobenzene, but some still have naphthalene. Both of these substances are capable of producing toxic symptoms following ingestion, although naphthalene is more toxic.

### *Model Trains*

In recent years, manufacturers of toys have developed electric model trains that are capable of producing smoke. The cartridges used contain meta-terphenyl or kerosene and cedar wood oil. The quantities are not great enough to have harmful effects by inhaling the smoke or ingesting small amounts, but care should be taken that only a few cartridges are available at one time. Also, there is a cleaning fluid for train tracks which should be used under adult management because it contains deodorized kerosene.

### *Paints*

Homemade Christmas cards or trimmings usually involve painting surprises in a closed room with the possibility that toxic fumes may accumulate. Some poster paints have a toxic volatile base. The nearness of the work further enhances exposure; headache, nausea and vomiting may result. The inhalation of bronze powder used for gilding Christmas cards has produced necrotizing pneumonitis, pleuritis and pulmonary edema in a two-year-old child. The powder is in the form of thin flakes consisting of 70 per cent copper, 30 per cent zinc and a trace of stearate lubricants.

### *Poinsettia*

There have been numerous warnings in the lay media that poinsettia is poisonous. These apparently arise from a single report of a fatality in Hawaii in 1919 from an indigenous wild plant. Although a number of incidents are reported each year to poison control centers of ingestion of parts of the poinsettia plant (leaves), only an occasional local irritation or vomiting has been documented (332 reports in 1975, 7 of whom had symptoms). $LD_{50}$ is greater than 25 gm/kg for rats.

## INSECTS AND MAN

The role of insects as vectors of disease in man is well documented throughout the history of medicine. The *Anopheles* mosquito and malaria, *Aedes aegypti* and yellow fever, the flea from infected rodents and bubonic plague, the wood tick and Rocky Mountain spotted fever are but a few examples. Their role in the production of allergic reactions in certain individuals is recognized and is receiving increased attention from those scientists and physicians working in the fields of immunology and allergy. It has long been known that allergic disorders of the respiratory system can be associated with insect particles, debris and emanations present in the air. Sporadic news reports are testimonials to the serious and often fatal allergic response to insect stings.

Common offenders in the production of allergy are the Hexapoda, or six-legged insects, of which there are over 1 million varieties; these include moths, butterflies, flies, mosquitos, bees, wasps, hornets, yellow jackets and beetles. The insect population to which the human race is exposed is of staggering proportions. Swarms of grasshoppers, locusts and butterflies may partially block out the sky and cover hundreds of acres of land. During the moulting season, mayflies literally cover beaches and buildings. Street cleaning equipment is required at times to clear the highway of mayflies and caddis flies along the shores of Lake Huron and Lake Erie. Heavier and stronger insects are near the ground, while the smaller and weaker species densely populate the air up to 1000 feet.

The reproduction rate of insects is phenomenal. The queen bee produces 2000 eggs daily for two months of the year. Some termites produce 40,000 eggs in a day, while the parasitic wasp may produce several thousand progeny from a dozen eggs. With such fantastic rates of reproduction and with their dispersal from the tropics to the frozen north, on the ground and in the air, there is little opportunity, despite widespread use of insecticides and pesticides, to avoid contact with some form or another of insects.

Some insects are benefactors of man, while others are annoying, pestiferous and a constant threat to our comfort and well-being. The honeybee is commercially produced and used extensively to increase cross-pollination of crops, which is most vital to our economy. We obtain silk from the cocoon of the silkworm. The resin secreted by the scale insect, *Tachardia lacca,* of India, is converted into shellac. The ladybug feeds upon insects and their eggs, while the dragonfly feeds voraciously on flies, gnats and mosquitoes. On the other hand, man is constantly battling such crop destroyers and pests as weevils, potato bugs, Dutch elm beetles and cutworms.

There is reason to believe that allergy to insects—next to pollen, mold and fungus spores—is the most important cause of respiratory allergy in temperate and tropical regions. Disintegrated insect dust in the soil and on vegetation and insect particles in the air are all part of the atmospheric dust that we breathe in with air. Asthma and other allergic disorders have been proven by careful studies to be due to such insect allergens. Desensitization with inhalant insect allergens has proven effective in controlling symptoms.

Much time and attention has been devoted to the study of more dramatic and serious allergic episodes caused by the stinging insects. Although the nature of the complex venom of the wasp, hornet, yellow jacket, bumblebee and honeybee is not fully understood, numerous reports point to insect body proteins as the excitants, or antigenic fractions, in the venom as the mediators of the allergic response.

The stinging mechanism of the bee and wasp consists of an acid gland which secretes inflammatory and toxic substances, an alkaline gland which secretes a convulsant factor and enzymes, and a poison sac. The mixed glandular substances are injected into the sting victim through a double hollow shaft. Formic acid is present in the glandular mixture but in amounts insufficient to cause primary effects. The toxicity of the venom alone is thought not to be great enough to account for the severe local and general reactions which are encountered. A person once sensitized by sting exposure to the insect body proteins could react violently to reexposure to varying amounts of the insect body protein in the venom mixture.

Immunological studies on whole body extracts of wasps, hornets, bees and yellow jackets indicate that several antigenic protein fractions are shared in common, while other fractions are specific for each insect. Patients, therefore, may have reactions to the sting of bees but none to wasps and hornets, or vice versa. This indicates that a person may become sensitive to individual antigenic protein fractions to the complete or partial exclusion of others. This is of practical significance and suggests that for full protection against this group of stinging insects, all of the common Hymenoptera (wasp, hornet, honeybee and yellow jacket) should be included in a polyvalent whole body extract for desensitization therapy. Immunotherapy (or hyposensitization) may be effective in the case of sensitivity to stinging insects, even if whole body extracts are used. When pure venom extracts become available for routine use, the rate of success will be higher and immunologic protection of the patient easier to achieve. The incidence of systemic reactions to the infections also will increase, since pure venom extracts are more potent antigens than whole body extracts. For the time being, however, with the materials presently available, immunization therapy takes a long time. In fact, it is presently recommended that the injections be continued for life, with booster doses given as frequently as once every four to six weeks.

## Prevention of Insect Stings

The arrival of warm weather means that for several months the outdoors will abound with great numbers of insects which inflict painful stings on human beings. To most of the victims, the sting is a tiny wound which is painful for a while and is then forgotten; but to people who have become sensitized to any of the various antigens in the bodies of the insects, the reaction to a sting can be overwhelming and even swiftly fatal. Therefore any measures which may be employed to reduce the incidence of stings should be considered as important as, or even more important than, remedial treatment.

Experience has taught that repellents are not as effective as desired for warding off stinging insects. The chemicals and odors of repellents may discourage biting insects whose assaults are motivated solely by the need for food, but they do not deter or lessen the determination of insects intent on defense or attack.

Most stings are inflicted by bees simply because there are more bees than any other stinging insect. Furthermore, bees are widely cultivated both for pollination and the production of honey. Some beekeepers who do not react too violently may, as a result of being stung frequently, develop a certain degree of immunity; unfortunately, however, immunity to one species of insects is not always accompanied by immunity to other species.

As a rule, the bee one meets in the garden is not inclined to sting unless touched, stepped on or molested in some other way. Professional beekeepers who may handle up to several million bees in a day's work usually receive less than fifty stings a day, and it is an exceptionally irritated colony in which 1 per cent of the population is provoked to attack.

Most flying insects do not venture forth in cool weather, and honeybees and other stinging insects are unlikely to be found flying about when the temperature is below 55° F. Honeybees seldom go out on bee business on dull or damp days, although other stinging insects and many which bite are encountered provided the temperature is sufficiently high.

The type of clothing one wears is an important factor affecting one's chances of being stung, and it is generally agreed that white or light-colored clothing with a smooth hard finish is less likely to incite bees to traumatic action than gaily colored, dark, rough or wooly materials. Leather, possibly because of its odor, seems to be particularly irritating to bees. It has been recommended that women wear a head covering such as a silk scarf where bees are present in order to prevent a bee from accidentally becoming caught in the hair. The odor of perspiration also irritates bees, and those who must go among them should change clothing frequently. It is advisable to avoid wearing perfumes and pomades since their floral odors attract bees; and if they become entangled in the hair or clothing, they may be inclined to sting even if such was not their original intention.

A moving person is more likely to incur a sting than one who is motionless. Thus one should never wildly swing the arms at an approaching bee or other insect, nor should one resort to headlong flight unless a colony of bees or a nest of wasps has been disturbed, in which event anyone lingering in the area will almost certainly be stung. The best method of retreating unpunctured from an errant bee is a slow withdrawal, using the hands with the fingers extended as a shield before the face. Other recommended measures are lying prone on the ground with the arms covering the face or taking unhurried refuge in nearby vegetation.

When a person has been stung, he should quickly examine the site of the sting; if the stinger can be seen, it should be removed at once by a scraping motion of the fingernail. He can also draw some consolation from the fact that the bee, by the act of stinging, has brought about his own doom. He will not sting again.

# APPENDIX A

## PAMPHLETS AND OTHER MEDIA*

The busy physician is often confronted with requests from patients, lay groups or organizations for pamphlets on the various aspects of poisoning. The following is a comprehensive (though by no means complete) list of materials for this purpose, particularly appropriate for use during the annual National Poison Prevention Week held during the month of March.

### Booklets and Charts

*Your Child and Household Safety* (Arena)
Chemical Specialties Manufacturers Association, Inc.
Suite 1120
1001 Connecticut Avenue, N.W.
Washington, D.C., 20036
50¢ each; bulk rates.

*The ABC of First Aid*
Norwich Pharmacal Company
Norwich, New York

*Cockroaches—How to Control Them*
(Leaflet No. 430)
Superintendent of Documents
U.S. Government Printing Office

*Dangers In The Kitchen*
*Poisoning In The Kitchen*
*Poisons In Your Home*
American Visuals Corporation
460 Fourth Avenue
New York, New York, 10016

*Malathion Handbook for Insect Control*
American Cyanamid Company
Agricultural Division
30 Rockefeller Plaza
New York, New York, 10020

*Some of these publications and materials may not be available, and the cost as indicated may now be changed.

*Poison Proofing Your Home*
Published as a public health service by
Johnson and Johnson
New Brunswick, New Jersey, 08903

*Obedience Means Safety for Your Child*
American Academy of Pediatrics
Evanston, Illinois, 60204

*Read the Label—It's Your Protection*
U.S. Department of Health, Education and Welfare
Food and Drug Administration
Washington, D.C., 20025

*Children and Poison Don't Mix*
Development in Infant and Child Care No. 7
Ross Laboratories
Columbus, Ohio, 43126

*CO and You*
Carbon Monoxide Poisoning
Public Health Service Publication No. 611
U.S. Government Printing Office
Washington, D.C., 20025

*Facts and Fallacies of Plumbism and What To Do About Them*
Lead Industries Association
420 Lexington Avenue
New York, New York, 10017

*How to Prevent Lead Poisoning In The Home*
*The Recognition of Lead Poisoning In The Child*
U.S. Department of Health, Education and Welfare
Public Health Service
Washington, D.C., 20201

*Painting Toys and Children's Furniture*
National Paint, Varnish and Lacquer Association
498 Chancellor Avenue,
Irvington, New Jersey, 07111

*The ABC'S of Child Safety*
A Scriptographic Booklet

Channing L. Bete Co., Inc.
Greenfield, Massachusetts, 01301

*For Safety's Sake (CHART)*
Haack Laboratories, Inc.
Portland, Oregon, 97201

*First Aid Measures for Poisoning (Chart)*
American Medical Association
535 North Dearborn Street
Chicago, Illinois, 60610

*Hazards of Solvents at Home—On The Job*
Council on Industrial Health
American Medical Association
535 North Dearborn Street
Chicago, Illinois, 60610

*First Aid for Poisoning*
Birk & Co., Inc.
3 West 57th Street
New York, New York, 10019

*A Supplement on Artificial Respiration*
Red Cross Textbooks

*Open Door to Plenty*
National Agriculture Chemicals Association
1145 19th Street, N.W.
Washington, D.C., 20006

*Occupational Health Hazards*
U.S. Government Printing Office
Washington, D.C., 20025

*Directory of Poison Control Centers*
U.S. Department of Health, Education and Welfare
Accident Prevention Program
National Clearinghouse for Poison Control Centers
Washington, D.C., 20201

*Handbook for Phosdrin Insecticide Formulations*
*Safe Handling of Methyl Parathion*
*Safe Handling of Phosdrin Insecticides*
*Safe Handling of Dieldrin, Aldrin, and Endrin*
*Handbook of Aldrin, Dieldrin, and Endrin Formulations*
*Handbook of Methyl Parathion Formulations*
Shell Chemical Company
460 Park Avenue
New York, New York, 10022

*Cooperative Economic Insect Report*
U.S. Department of Agriculture
Washington, D.C., 20025

*Phosphate Ester Insecticides*
American Cyanamid Company
Agricultural Division
30 Rockefeller Plaza
New York, New York, 10020

*First Aid for the Family*
*Caution Babies Learning*
Metropolitan Life Insurance Company

*Poison Peril in Your Home*
Koster-Dana Corporation
76 Ninth Avenue
New York, New York, 10011

*Accidental Poisoning*
*Is Your Child Being Slowly Poisoned*
Philadelphia Department of Public Health
Room 632, City Hall Annex
Philadelphia, Pennsylvania, 19107

*Diagnosis and Treatment of Poisoning*
Jay M. Arena, M.D.
Duke University Medical Center
Durham, North Carolina, 27710

*Clinical Memoranda on Economic Poisons*
Department of Health, Education and Welfare
Public Health Service
Washington, D.C., 20201

## Brochures, Flyers and Pamphlets

*Counterdoses For The Home*
*(An 8½" x 11" chart of first aid instructions for poisoning and overdose emergencies)*
Black and white reproduction proof available from American Druggist, 1790 Broadway, New York, New York, 10019.

*Danger Lurks (HE–121)*
*(A card for the medicine cabinet door. Describes first aid for and preventive measures against poisoning. In English or Spanish.)*
10¢ each; $8/100; $40/1000. American Medical Association, 535 North Dearborn Street, Chicago, Illinois, 60610.

*Dennis the Menace Takes a Poke at Poison*
*(A 16-page, 4-color comic book.)*
Quantities available from the Division of Direct Health Services, U.S. Public Health Service, Washington, D.C., 20201, or the National Center for Urban and Industrial

Health, U.S. Public Health Service, Cincinnati, Ohio, 45202.

*Everyday Facts About Agricultural Chemicals*
*(A 12-page pamphlet which includes cautions against accidents involving pesticides.)*
Single copies free; $4/100. Manufacturing Chemists' Association, 1825 Connecticut Avenue, N.W., Washington, D.C., 20009.

*First Aid For Poisoning*
*(A revised 5" x 8" card of first aid instructions for poisoning emergencies.)*
Available through the courtesy of Plough, Inc. Limited quantities free on request. Those requiring a large supply may obtain free reproduction proof. American Association of Poison Control Centers, c/o Academy of Medicine of Cleveland, 10525 Carnegie Avenue, Cleveland, Ohio, 44106.

*First Aid Manual (OP–15)*
*(Pocket size, 46 pages.)*
15¢ each; $12/100; $80/1000. American Medical Association, 535 North Dearborn Street, Chicago, Illinois, 60610.

*How to Prevent Poisoning (599.05)*
*A 4-page, 2-color leaflet containing basic information on steps to take to prevent home poisonings.)*
Available in quantities of 50: 50 - 499, $.039 each; 500 - 999, $.027 each; 1000 - 4999, $.024 each. National Safety Council, 425 North Michigan Avenue, Chicago, Illinois, 60611.

*Locked Up Poisons Prevent Tragedy*
*(Brochure tells in words and pictures the methods of preventing accidental poisonings.)*
Quantities available from Secretary, National Planning Council for Poison Prevention Week, c/o U.S. Public Health Service, Washington, D.C., 20201. Black and white print on request for reproduction locally.

*Mainly for Mothers*
*(Health and safety folder with tips to protect youngsters against home hazards.)*
Limited quantities free on request. Council on Family Health, Department GS, 485 Madison Avenue, New York, N.Y., 10022.

*Medicines and How to Use Them (OP–63)*
*(A 4-page pamphlet describing safe procedures for use and storage of medicines with particular reference to the danger to children of inadequately protected medicine cabinets.)*
10¢ each; $8/100; $40/1000. American Medical Association, 535 North Dearborn Street, Chicago, Illinois, 60610.

*Mother, Key to Safety in the Home*
*(Resource kit for safety programs.)*
Single copy free to leaders of groups of 25 or more. Council on Family Health, Department GS, 485 Madison Avenue, New York, N.Y., 10022.

*Poison and You*
*(16-page, 2-color booklet, 5½" x 8". Story on type of poisons, how to keep them from children and what to do in case of poisoning. Presented in scriptographic style.)*
100- 499, $.15 each; 500 - 999, $.10 each; 1000 - 9999, $.09 each. Other quantity prices furnished on request. Channing L. Bete Co., 45 Federal Street, Greenfield, Massachusetts, 01301.

*Poison Prevention Program Kit (599.73)*
*(Basic materials for community wide poison prevention program. Includes publicity material, group project ideas, data sheets, reprints, posters, leaflets, etc.)*
1 - 9, $1.50 each; 10 - 99, $1.40 each; over 100, $1.30 each. National Safety Council, 425 North Michigan Avenue, Chicago, Illinois, 60611.

*Program Guide for National Poison Prevention Week*
*(Brochure, in flip-chart form, offers suggestions and ideas for a coordinated, local community wide poison prevention effort.)*
Single copies available from Secretary, National Planning Council for Poison Prevention Week, c/o U.S. Public Health Service, Washington, D.C., 20201.

*Protecting Your Home from Unlabeled Poisons (OP - 8)*
*(Three fold pamphlet describing hazards of careless storage.)*
10¢ each, $8/100, $40/1000. American Medical Association, 535 North Dearborn Street, Chicago, Illinois, 60610.

*Solid and Liquid Poisons (429.04 –21)*
*(A 6-page data sheet containing practical*

*information on poisons in and around the home, pointing out special dangers to children.)*

Available in quantities of 10: 10 - 99, $.068 each; 100 - 999, $.056 each; 1000 - 4999, $.05 each. National Safety Council, 425 North Michigan Avenue, Chicago, Illinois, 60611.

*Ten Little Tasters*

*(A 3" x 4", 12-panel pamphlet-foldout depicting, in cartoons and rhyme, the problems and precautions in accidental poisoning in children. Also available in small one fold envelope stuffer.)*

Sample copies, imprinting information, and quantity prices available from Imagination, Inc., 2651 University Avenue, Saint Paul, Minnesota, 55114.

## Films, Addresses and Slide Talks

*Accidental Poisoning in the Home*

*(Twenty-nine 35 mm color slides with script.)*

Available on loan from the American Pharmaceutical Association, 2215 Constitution Avenue, N.W., Washington, D.C., 20037.

*Children at Play—with Poison*

*(A 10-minute, 16 mm sound color filmograph.)*

Available on loan from National Medical Audio-Visual Center Annex, Attention: Film Distribution Unit, Chamblee, Georgia, 30005. Can be purchased from Creative Arts Studio, Inc., 814 H Street, N.W., Washington, D.C., 20001, at $60/print. Also available from many state and local health departments. Approved for commercial television.

*Go Seek and Hide*

*(37-frame filmstrip with illustrated script. Teaches elementary school pupils about chemical hazards in their homes and how they can prevent accidental poisonings.)*

Available for purchase for $6.50 from the American Association of Poison Control Centers, c/o Academy of Medicine of Cleveland, 10525 Carnegie Avenue, Cleveland, Ohio, 44106.

*One Day's Poison*

*(A 30-minute, 16 mm, black and white, sound motion picture film.)*

Available on loan from National Medical Audio-Visual Center Annex, Attention: Film Distribution Unit, Chamblee, Georgia, 30005. Also, many state health departments and libraries. Approved for commercial television.

*Good Drug Manufacturing Practices: No Margin For Error*

*(A 25-minute color film.)*

Produced by the Food and Drug Administration as a training tool for all drug industry personnel showing the steps involved in the manufacture and packaging of a new drug, how errors can occur in the process and how they can be prevented. A free short-term loan (up to 2 wk.) can be arranged by contacting: Bureau of Voluntary Compliance, Food and Drug Administration, 200 C Street, S.W., Washington, D.C., 20204.

*Poison: Handle with Care*

*(35-frame filmstrip with script. Suitable for upper elementary grade levels through adult audiences. Covers common household chemicals, preventive measures and first aid suggestions.)*

Price, $6.00 color; $4.50 black and white. Visual Education Consultants, Inc., Madison, Wisconsin, 53701.

*Poison in the House*

*(A 1-minute, 16 mm, sound color motion picture film.)*

A print can be purchased from Association Films, Inc., 600 Madison Avenue, New York, New York, 10022, at $65, or rented from the same organization at $4 per day. Also available from many state and local health departments. Approved for commercial television.

### *Pesticide Films*

*Perspective on Pesticides (M-1484 - MP)*

*16 mm, color, sound, 15 minutes, 1968, cleared for television.*

Stresses the importance of proper use and storage of pesticides. Through various visual enactments, points out the dangers of storage in places easily accessible to children, storage in containers designed for other uses and improper disposal of pesticide containers.

*Epidemiology of Pesticide Poisonings (M–1668 - MP)*

*16 mm, color, sound, 16 minutes, 1969, cleared for television.*

Discusses epidemiology as related to pesticide poisonings. The various factors contributing to the occurrence of pesticide poisoning are described step by step and further dramatized by the portrayal of two actual cases of poisoning by pesticides.

*Organophosphate Pesticide Poisoning (M–1747 - MP)*

*16 mm, color, sound, 19 minutes, 1969, cleared for television.*

Describes for medical and paramedical audiences the symptoms of an organophosphate poisoning. The film includes a discussion of laboratory methods available for diagnosis and describes appropriate treatment for poisoned patients.

Order pesticide films by title and number from these sources (free loan service).

1. The film library of your local state department of health
2. National Medical Audiovisual Center (Annex)
   Station K
   Atlanta, Georgia, 30324
3. Environmental Protection Agency
   Pesticides Office
   Division of Pesticide Community Studies
   4770 Buford Highway
   Chamblee, Georgia, 30341

Films should be requested at least 2 weeks before the preferred showing date; if possible, two alternate showing dates should be given.

Purchase of films; contact:

Sales Branch
National Audiovisual Center (GSA)
Washington, D.C., 20409

(Prices will be given upon request. Requests should include title of film and number.)

*Public Address on National Poison Prevention Week*

*(Two 10– to 15-minute prepared speeches for presentation to lay audiences.)*

Single copies of each are available on request from the Secretary, National Planning Council for Poison Prevention Week, c/o U.S. Public Health Service, Washington, D.C., 20201.

*Prepared Speech Directed Toward Menace of Poisonous Substances in the Home*

*(Approximately 15 minutes; also can be used as newspaper article.)*

National Association of Retail Druggists, 1 East Wacker Drive, Chicago, Illinois, 60601.

*Slide Series (I)*

*(35 mm, color, with annotated script. Covers incidence, hazards, preventive measures and first aid suggestions.)*

Purchase price, $12.50; rental fee for 3-week period, $3.00. Available from American Association of Poison Control Centers, c/o Academy of Medicine of Cleveland, 10525 Carnegie Avenue, Cleveland, Ohio, 44106.

*Slide Series (II)*

*(24) 35 mm captioned slides, suitable for use in an automatic projector with a self-contained screen.)*

Purchase price $6. American Association of Poison Control Centers, c/o Academy of Medicine of Cleveland, 10525 Carnegie Avenue, Cleveland, Ohio, 44106.

*Rescue Breathing*

The Metropolitan Life Insurance Company has produced a set of 26 black and white 2" x 2" slides on rescue breathing. The slides illustrate the important steps to follow in applying mouth-to-mouth artificial resuscitation. Accompanying the slides is a discussion leader's guide. Local groups interested in using these slides may obtain them without charge by writing directly to the Metropolitan Life Insurance Company, Health and Welfare Division, One Madison Avenue, New York, New York, 10010.

## Radio and Television

*Spot Announcements*

*(Television and radio announcements in lengths varying from 10 to 60 seconds.)*

Complete set sent directly to all radio and television stations. Single copies available from Secretary, National Planning Council for National Poison Prevention Week, c/o U.S. Public Health Service, Washington, D.C., 20201.

*Television Slide*

One slide designed for National Poison Prevention Week sent to all television stations.

## Newspapers

*Ad Mat for National Poison Prevention Week*

Free proof and order form available to individuals who wish to have their local newspapers order them. Address requests to the Secretary, National Planning Council for Poison Prevention Week, c/o U.S. Public Health Service, Washington, D.C., 20201.

*Editor's Fact Sheet*

Single copies available free on request from the Secretary, National Planning Council for Poison Prevention Week, c/o U.S. Public Health Service, Washington, D.C., 20201.

*Newspaper Article*

*(Suitable for publication in local newspapers.)*

National Association of Retail Druggists, 1 East Wacker Drive, Chicago, Illinois, 60601.

*Newspaper Mat*

*(Advertisement drawing attention to poison prevention.)*

National Association of Retail Druggists, 1 East Wacker Drive, Chicago, Illinois, 60601.

## Proclamations

*Suggested Proclamations*

Single copies of suggested proclamations for use by governors and local officials are available from the Secretary, National Planning Council for Poison Prevention Week, c/o U.S. Public Health Service, Washington, D.C., 20201.

*Presidential Proclamation*

Single copies of the presidential proclamation will be available after date of issue from the Secretary, National Planning Council for Poison Prevention Week, c/o U.S. Public Health Service, Washington, D.C., 20201.

## Posters and Miscellaneous

*Bus Card: Little Children Don't Read Labels*

*(11" x 28" card for display in buses.)*

Free copies of the art work suitable for reproduction are available from the American Association of Poison Control Centers, c/o Academy of Medicine of Cleveland, 10525 Carnegie Avenue, Cleveland, Ohio, 44106.

*Chemicals in Household Cleaning Products (Chart)*

National Association of Retail Druggists, 1 East Wacker Drive, Chicago, Illinois, 60601.

*Poison-Antidote Wheel (Chart)*

10¢ each; $10/100, postage prepaid. National Association of Retail Druggists, 1 East Wacker Drive, Chicago, Illinois, 60601.

*Exhibit (I)*

Diagram for construction of tabletop exhibit. Suggestions and ideas for simple, inexpensive display, which itemizes supplies and instructions necessary for "do-it-yourself" operation. Available from Secretary, National Planning Council for Poison Prevention Week, c/o U.S. Public Health Service, Washington, D.C., 20201.

*Exhibit (II)*

*(Three 23 " x 35 " posters in green, tan and violet, printed on heavy stock. Suitable as basic exhibit material with suggested ideas for use. Rolled and mailed in tube.)*

$3.50, postage prepaid. American Association of Poison Control Centers, c/o Academy of Medicine of Cleveland, 10525 Carnegie Avenue, Cleveland, Ohio, 44106.

*Guide for Teaching Poison Prevention in the Kindergartens and Primary Grades (PHS 1381)*

*(Manual for teachers who wish to introduce the subject into their classes. Includes ideas for games, songs, interviews, excursions and other activities.)*

55¢. Superintendent of Documents, U.S. Government Printing Office, Washington, D.C., 20402.

*Labels*

Sheet of ten various sizes of labels with "striking snake" design, reading "Warning—Keep Out of Reach of Children." Intended for use on containers of all potentially hazardous substances. Accompanying window or counter poster draws attention to the availability of the labels. Set of 100 with 1 poster, $5; set of 250 with 2 posters, $10; set of 500 with 3 posters, $18; set of 1000 with 4 posters, $35. American Pharmaceutical Association, 2215 Constitution Avenue, N.W., Washington, D.C., 20037.

*Poster*

*(23" x 29" in English or Spanish.)*

Courtesy of Ross Laboratories. Available from American Association of Poison Control Centers, c/o Academy of Medicine of Cleveland, 10525 Carnegie Avenue, Cleveland, Ohio, 44106.

*Is There a Killer in Your Medicine Chest?*

*(A multicolored poster, 18½" x 23", illustrating the potential poisoning hazards in the medicine cabinet.)*

Available through the courtesy of the American Medical Association. Limited quantities free on request from Secretary, National Planning Council for Poisoning Prevention Week, c/o U.S. Public Health Service, Washington, D.C., 20201.

*Medicines Can Cure or Kill (H–2524–A)*

*(An 8½" x 11" purple, black and white poster emphasizing the importance of keeping medicines out of the reach of children and knowing the bottle's contents for the safety of the elderly.)*

Available in quantities of 10: 10 - 99, $.146 each; 100 - 999, $.087 each. National Safety Council, 425 North Michigan Avenue, Chicago, Illinois, 60611.

*Poison Prevention (Poster)*

*(Multicolored, 18" x 24")*

National Association of Retail Druggists, 1 East Wacker Drive, Chicago, Illinois, 60601.

*Protect Your Family (H–2216–A)*

*(An 8½" x 11" colored poster depicting how to protect your family by keeping medicines and cleaning products properly labeled in safe containers, stored out of reach of children.)*

Available in quantities of 10: 10 - 99, $.146 each; 100 - 999, $.087 each. National Safety Council, 425 North Michigan Avenue, Chicago, Illinois, 60611.

*Safety With Chemicals, Off-the-Job Too (H–2884–A)*

*(An 8½" x 11½" two-color poster depicting the safe use and storage of pesticides around the home.)*

Available in quantities of 10: 10 - 99, $.146 each; 100 - 999, $.087 each. National Safety Council, 425 North Michigan Avenue, Chicago, Illinois, 60611.

*Syrup of Ipecac (Poster)*

*(An 8½" x 11" black and white reproduction proof, containing a picture of a bottle of syrup of ipecac and the legend "Parents Get Me and Keep Me Handy.")*

American Association of Poison Control Centers, c/o Academy of Medicine of Cleveland, 10525 Carnegie Avenue, Cleveland, Ohio, 44106.

*Stickers (I)*

Designed for National Poison Prevention Week; 1" x 2" for stationery and envelopes. Available from the Secretary, National Planning Council for Poison Prevention Week, c/o U.S. Public Health Service, Washington, D.C., 20201.

*Stickers (II)*

*(3 " x 5 " sticker with gummed back for pasting on inside cover of telephone book cover, door of medicine cabinet, etc. Carries poison prevention message and space for emergency telephone numbers.)*

$2/100; $3/300; $6/1000. Postage prepaid. National Association of Retail Druggists, 1 East Wacker Drive, Chicago, Illinois, 60601.

*National Poison Prevention Week*

*(8½" x 36 ", for windows, bulletin boards, etc.)*

Single streamers available free from the Secretary, National Planning Council for

Poison Prevention Week, c/o U.S. Public Health Service, Washington, D.C., 20201. Quantities can be purchased from the American Pharmaceutical Association, 2215 Constitution Avenue, N.W., Washington, D.C., 20037, at the following rates: 25, $2; 100, $7; 500, $30; 1000, $50.

*Window Placard*

*(Featuring skull and cross bones, 24" x 15 " fluorescent.)*

National Association of Retail Druggists, 1 East Wacker Drive, Chicago, Illinois, 60601.

## Source of Toxicology Information

### *National Library of Medicine (NLM)*

1. MEDLARS. Computer-based medical literature analysis and retrieval system, Computer-produced Index Medicus.
2. MEDLINE. Medlars on line, over 500,000 recent references.
3. TOXICOLOGY INFORMATION PROGRAM (TIP)

This program includes, on a computer-based system, several functional operations. Similar to Medline, it is a data bank of information from the toxicology literature and from the files of organizations, both governmental and nongovernmental.

TIRC. Toxicology Information Response Center gives information from Medline, Toxline, Chemline, Cancerline and ORNL (Oak Ridge National Laboratory). This center is located at ORNL, Oak Ridge, Tennessee.

TOXLINE. Toxicology information on line, computer based.

TOXICITY BIBLIOGRAPHY. A Quarterly publication covering the adverse effects of drugs and chemicals reported in the 2200 journals indexed for Index Medicus.

TOXICOLOGY DATA BANK. Chemical, physical, toxicological, pharmacological, use and manufacturing data on 4000 to 5000 chemicals and drugs.

LABORATORY ANIMAL DATA BANK. A new program to develop a computerized data bank of physiological baselines in laboratory control animals.

The NLM has fact sheets describing all of its services and programs. For these fact sheets and additional information write:

Toxicology Information Service
National Library of Medicine
8600 Rockville Pike
Bethesda, Maryland, 20014

TERATOLOGY LOOKOUT compiles references to articles found in Biological Abstracts, Medlars and Chemical Abstracts. For information write:

Biomedical Documentation Center
Karolinska Institutet FACK
S-10401 Stockholm 60, Sweden

### *The National Pesticide Telecommunications Network*

By utilizing toll-free telephone numbers, the network provides consultation for the management of pesticide poisonings for the 48 contiguous states with 24-hour physician coverage. Services offered include product active ingredient identification, toxicologic and symptom review, and specific treatment recommendations. This service is offered through the Medical University of South Carolina and is provided jointly by the South Carolina Pesticide Epidemiologic Studies Center and the Drug and Poison Information Center.

For pesticide poisoning information, call 1-800-922-0193 within South Carolina; from other states, 1-800-845-7633 *(Also see* pages 159 and 170).

# APPENDIX B

## NORMAL LABORATORY VALUES USED IN THE DIAGNOSIS AND TREATMENT OF POISONING

Drugs may alter laboratory test values through a variety of pharmacological, physical or chemical mechanisms. Through its pharmacological activity, a drug may affect the normal physiological levels in the blood or urine of the particular substance being measured. Some of these alterations are readily predictable even from a superficial knowledge of a drug's actions. Thiazide diuretics alter the serum levels of sodium, potassium and chloride ions; morphine produces an elevation in the catecholamine level; and probenecid decreases uric acid levels.

Through physical or chemical interference, a drug may not only alter the value of a test but actually prevent its determination by a particular method. Most contrast media used in radiography interfere with protein-bound iodine determinations because of their own iodine content. Edathamil, a chelating agent, ties up calcium ions to give a decreased or false negative value for serum calcium level. Phenazopyridine and dithiazanine impart their own characteristic colors to the urine, causing physical interference which negates many colorimetric or photometric determinations. Reducing agents excreted in the urine may enter into chemical reactions with test reagents to invalidate a particular procedure. Ascorbic acid, streptomycin and penicillin are but a few drugs which react with cupric sulfate to give invalid false positive Benedict's test results. Numerous drugs may alter the results of glucose determinations in blood and urine in two ways: by interfering with its measurement or by affecting its metabolism and excretion. The former effect gives rise to erroneous results and varies with the analytic method; the latter effect is the same for all methods.

Intermediate or end products of drug metabolism may also add to the complexity of the problem. Penicillin and tolbutamide metabolites give a false positive result for urine protein determination. The metabolite of quinine causes an elevation in urinary catecholamines. Aspidium, if absorbed, yields a metabolite which gives a false positive Benedict's test. Many more such examples could be cited.

The extended pharmacologic activity of a drug may often be responsible for unsuspected alterations in laboratory test values. Such altered values may thus more accurately reflect the side-effects or incipient toxicity of the drug than any true underlying pathology. The more that extremely potent or complex therapeutic agents are used, especially in multiple combinations, the more difficult and acute becomes the problem of evaluating the reported laboratory results. The tendency towards hepatotoxicity of such drugs as bismuth, gold salts, many of the phenothiazines and some of the monoamine oxidase inhibitors may make it difficult to evaluate results obtained from such laboratory tests as alkaline phosphatase, cholesterol, cephalin flocculation and others used to assess liver function. The administration of cortisone, with its normal side-effect of sodium retention, may complicate the assessment of renal tubular function by a determination of the serum sodium level.

CPK (creatine phosphokinase) is released from muscle when it is injured by direct trauma, as might be associated with intramuscular injections, but in addition, the administered medication may cause the release or activation of CPK. The mechanism of the release phenomenon may be related to histamine effects on muscle membranes. Margulies and Meltzer *(Univ Chgo Bull Med Alum Assoc, 25*:30-31, 1970) have reported that histamine and histamine liberators cause "very high serum CPK elevations," in the rat. One agent commonly given to patients with myocardial infarction by a variety of routes is morphine, a known histamine liberator. Other agents known to cause histamine liberation and also alter CPK activity which may be used in patients with myocardial infarction are chlorpromazine and tubocurarine chloride. Still other agents may augment CPK activity directly; one such is insulin (*Fed Proc, 25*:539, 1966). Clofibrate (Astromid-S®) can cause severe muscular cramping with a simultaneous increase in CPK. There are thus several agents—direct trauma, liberated histamine alteration of muscle membrane and direct enzyme activation—which may increase serum CPK activity following intramuscular or other forms of injection. There may be other mechanisms as well. It remains incumbent on the physician to properly interpret a CPK rise based upon the precise clinical context.

Many drugs interfere with the analysis of VMA (vanillylmandelic acid) and catecholamines in urine. For this reason, all drugs should be removed from patients undergoing these evaluations for a week prior to testing. When this is impractical, leave the patient on his medication, but be prepared to carefully reevaluate any positive results.

Chemical interference with laboratory tests by common anticonvulsant agents (diphenylhydantoin, phenobarbital, primidone, mephenytoin, ethosuximide, diazepam) though unusual, is not rare. All of them occasionally produce false positive results in programs that screen for drug abuse, though this should not be a serious problem if confirmatory tests are employed. Diphenylhydantoin often imparts a pink, red or red-brown color to urine that should not be mistaken for blood or bile. Both diazepam and phenobarbital produce falsely low responses when testing for urinary glucose with Clinistix® or Diastix® but have no effect on Tes-Tape®. Phenobarbital also falsely elevates measurements of urinary 5-hydroxyindoleacetic acid by interfering with the color reaction. When primidone is taken, phenobarbital will be detected in the bloodstream since phenobarbital is a major metabolite of this drug.

Another form of interference results from alterations in normal serum proteins. Diphenylhydantoin (through hepatic induction) increases serum ceruloplasmin. It also binds with great avidity to certain serum proteins, displacing other bound material in the process. For instance, methotrexate, cortisol and cardiac glycosides are displaced, and simply measuring serum levels underestimates their true activity since a larger portion of each is in the "free" or active form. Mephenytoin can decrease serum protein-bound iodine (PBI) and $T_4$ (thyroxine) by binding to thyroxine-binding globulin (TBG). Diazepam can decrease resin uptake of $T_3$ (triiodothyronine), but its effect on serum thyroxine is not known with certainty. Diphenylhydantoin decreases the PBI or thyroxine level by about 25 per cent; TBG binding and displacement are the generally accepted reason for this phenomenon. The reported effect on the $T_3$ resin uptake test is thought to be due to the acceleration of thyroxine metabolism, rather than displacing thyroid hormones from proteins.

The liver is the primary target through which anticonvulsants indirectly interfere with laboratory tests. The hepatic endoplasmic reticulum is the major site for the metabolism of a wide variety of exogenous and endogenous substances (drugs, bilirubin, thyroxine, steroids), and alteration of the activity of enzymes bound to this organelle directly affects the metabolism and therefore serum level of these materials. The anticonvulsants (particularly phenobarbital) stimulate the activity of mixed-function oxidases and both increase *de novo* synthesis and decrease degradation. Most of the changes in laboratory test results observed in patients taking anticonvulsant therapy chronically have been explained on the basis of this phenomenon.

Blood Clotting. The prothrombin time is decreased to less than expected as phenobarbital and primidone enhance the metabolism of administered coumarin anticoagulants. The prothrombin time may be prolonged when diphenylhydantoin is given since this drug inhibits coumarin degradation.

Function Tests. The well-known ability of phenobarbital to enhance conjugation and biliary excretion is the reason elevated bilirubin concentrations and increased BSP retention may be produced by this drug.

Corticosteroids. Steroid metabolism undergoes significant derangement when either phenobarbital or diphenylhydantoin is administered. In fact, concentrations of urinary steroids are virtually impossible to interpret when these drugs are given. Digitoxin is metabolized at a much faster rate than normal, and measured serum levels are much lower than expected.

Vitamin D. It is presumed that when the dietary intake of vitamin D is marginal, hepatic enzyme induction by diphenylhydantoin, phenobarbital and primidone may lead to vitamin D deficiency, hypocalcemia, hypophosphatemia, and, frequently, elevations of alkaline phosphatase.

Hepatic Enzymes. The elevation of hepatic enzymes (SGOT, SGPT, alkaline phosphatase, gamma glutamyltranspeptidase [GGT]) is often observed, but the reason for these changes is not always apparent. It is possible that enzyme induction may be a factor, but because hepatotoxicity is a recognized side-effect, it must always be considered as a possibility.

### *Hematopoiesis*

There are a number of hematologic side-effects of anticonvulsants which are manifested as altered laboratory values.

Megaloblastic anemia can be produced by primidone, phenobarbital and diphenylhydantoin, which interfere with folic acid absorption, producing increased renal loss of formiminoglutamic acid (FIGLU), decreased circulating folate and abnormal red cell formation.

Attacks of porphyria with increased urinary delta-amino levulinic acid (ALA) and porphyrins are well-recognized side-effects of diazepam and diphenylhydantoin therapy.

Mephenytoin is a known cause of hemolytic anemia, and all anticonvulsants have been implicated in the production of pancytopenia. Eosinophilia is a rare occurrence with ethosuximide, mephenytoin and diphenylhydantoin.

### *Immune phenomena*

A number of immunologic abnormalities can occur in some patients taking anticonvulsants.

The lupus erythematosus (LE) phenomenon has been reported in association with diphenylhydantoin, phenobarbital, mephenytoin, ethosuximide and primidone.

Direct and indirect positive Coombs' tests develop with diphenylhydantoin, mephenytoin and ethosuximide. The reason for this is quite obscure.

Antinuclear antibodies (ANA) have been noted in as many as 25 per cent of those receiving diphenylhydantoin. Ethosuximide is also known to induce ANA. In addition, diphenylhydantoin has been associated with decreases in lymphocytes as well as falls in the concentrations of IgA, IgG and C3 proteins.

### *Miscellaneous*

There are a number of other alterations in laboratory tests that can be grouped together only in a miscellaneous category. These include the following.

1. The formation of a characteristic crystal in urine with primidone overdosage.

2. A reversible nephropathy due to ethosuximide which is manifested by proteinuria and azotemia.
3. Diminished gastric acid and secretory volume caused by the central relaxant effect of diazepam.
4. The retardation of dopamine turnover by diazepam, resulting in reduced homovanillic acid secretion.
5. The inhibition of insulin secretion by diphenylhydantoin, causing, in turn, increased concentrations of glucose in serum and urine and decreased glucose tolerance.
6. The depletion of body pyridoxal phosphate by diphenylhydantoin.

"Drug Induced Modifications of Laboratory Test Values," by Sister Mary Paulette Elking and Hugh F. Kabat, *American Journal of Hospital Pharmacy, 25*:485-519 1968, is a comprehensive and useful review in tabular form of commonly ordered laboratory tests, their normal values and as altered by various drugs, of this poorly recognized phenomenon. This information is essential in the final evaluation of any laboratory procedure used in arriving at the diagnosis of poisoning. In addition, a computerized list of 17,000 drugs that interfere with medical tests has been recently developed at the Clinical Center, the research hospital of the National Institutes of Health. This registry, which is available in journal form to patient care and laboratory physicians, could be helpful in interpreting laboratory data, without undue delay, in the face of puzzling diagnoses.

## NORMAL LABORATORY VALUES USED IN THE DIAGNOSIS AND TREATMENT OF POISONING

**Blood, Plasma or Serum Values**

| *Determination* | *Normal Value* | *Material Analyzed* | *Minimal ml of Blood Required* | *Note* | *Method* |
|---|---|---|---|---|---|
| Acetoacetate plus acetone | 0.3–2.0 mg per 100 ml | Serum | 2 | | Behre: J Lab Clin Med 13:770, 1928 (modified) |
| Aldolase | 0.7–4.5 mU per ml | Serum | 4 | Use fresh, unhemolyzed serum | Beisenherz et al: Z Naturforsch 8b: 555, 1953 |
| Alpha amino nitrogen | 3.0–5.5 mg per 100 ml | Plasma | 5 | Collect with heparin | Szentirmai et al: Clin Chim Acta 7: 459, 1962 |
| Ammonia | 80–110 μg per 100 ml | Blood | 2 | Collect in heparinized tube; deliver *immediately* packed in ice. | Seligson, Hirahara: J Lab Clin Med 49: 962, 1957 |

**Blood, Plasma or Serum Values**

| *Determination* | *Normal Value* | *Material Analyzed* | *Minimal ml of Blood Required* | *Note* | *Method* |
|---|---|---|---|---|---|
| Amylase | 4–25 U per ml | Serum | 3 | | Huggins, Russell: Ann Surg 128:668, 1948 |
| Ascorbic acid | 0.4–1.5 mg per 100 ml | Blood | 7 | Collect in heparin tube before any food is given | Roe, Keuther: J Biol Chem 147:399, 1943 |
| Barbiturate | 0<br>Coma level; phenobarbital, approximately 11 mg per 100 ml; most other drugs, 2–4 mg per 100 ml | Serum | 5 | | Goldbaum: Anal Chem 24:1604, 1952 |
| Bilirubin (van den Bergh test) | One minute: 0.4 mg per 100 ml<br>Direct: 0.4 mg per 100 ml. Total: 0.7 mg per 100 ml. Indirect is total minus direct | Serum | 3 | | Malloy, Evelyn: J. Biol Chem 119:481, 1937 |
| Blood volume | 8.5–9.0 per cent of body weight in kg | | | | Isotope dilution technic with $^{131}$I albumin |
| Bromide | 0<br>Toxic level: 17 mEq per liter | Serum | 3 | | Adapted from Wuth: JAMA 82:2013, 1927 |
| Bromsulfalein (BSP) | Less than 5 per cent * retention | Serum | 3 | Inject intravenously 5 mg of dye per kg of body weight: draw blood 45 min later. | Goebler: Am J Clin Pathol 15:452, 1945 |
| Calcium | 8.5–10.5 mg per 100 ml (slightly higher in children) | Serum | 3 | BSP dye interferes | Bett, Fraser: Clin Chim Acta 4:346, 1959 Kessler, Wolfman: Clin Chim 10:686, 1964 (modified) |
| Carbon dioxide content | 24–30 mEq per liter. 20–26 mEq per liter in infants (as $HCO_3$) | Serum | 3 | Draw without stasis under oil or in heparinized syringe | Van Slyke; Neill; J. Biol Chem 61:523, 1924 Tech Auto Analyzer Meth |
| Carbon monoxide | Symptoms with over 20 per cent saturation | Blood | 5 | Fill tube to top; tightly stopper; use anticoagulant. | Bruchner, Desmond: Clin Chim Acta 3: 173, 1958 |
| Carotenoids | 0.08–0.40 $\mu$g per ml | Serum | 3 | Vitamin A may be done on same specimen | Natelson: Microtechniques of Clin Chem. 2nd ed. 1961 p. 454 |
| Ceruloplasmin | 27–37 mg per 100 ml | Serum | 2 | | Ravin: J. Lab Clin Med 58:161, 1961 |
| Chloride | 100–106 mEq per liter | Serum | 1 | | Modification of Schales. Schales: J. Biol Chem 140:879, 1941 Tech Auto-Analyzer Meth |

**Blood, Plasma or Serum Values**

| *Determination* | *Normal Value* | *Material Analyzed* | *Minimal ml of Blood Required* | *Note* | *Method* |
|---|---|---|---|---|---|
| Cholinesterase (pseudocholinesterase) | 0.5 pH U or more per hr<br>0.7 pH U or more per hr for packed cells | Serum<br>Packed cells | 1<br>1 | | Michel: J Lab Clin Med 34:1564, 1949 |
| Congo-red test | More than 60 per cent retention in serum | Serum | 5 | Inject 10 ml of 1 per cent Congo-red solution intravenously; draw blood from arm not injected 4 and 60 min later. | Unger, et al: J Clin Invest 27:111, 1948 |
| Copper | Total: 100–200 μg per 100 ml | Serum | 3 | | MGH Methodology |
| Creatine phosphokinase (CPK) | Female 2–25 mU per ml<br>Male 5–35 mU per ml | Serum | 3 | Immediately separate & freeze serum | Rosalki: J Lab Clin Med 69:696, 1967 (modified) |
| Creatinine | 0.7–1.5 mg per 100 ml | Serum | 3 | | Tech AutoAnalyzer Meth |
| Cryoglobulins | 0 | Serum | 8 | Collect and transport at 37° C | Barr, et al: Ann Intern Med 32:6, 1950 (modified) |
| Dilantin (Diphenylhydantoin) | Therapeutic level, 10–15 μg per ml | Serum | 5 | | Gas Liquid Chromatography |
| Doriden (Glutethimide) | 0 | Serum | 5 | | Rieder, Zervas: Am J Clin Pathol 44:520, 1965 |
| Ethanol | 0.3–0.4 per cent, marked intoxication; 4.5–0.5 per cent, alcoholic stupor; 0.5 per cent or over, alcoholic coma. | Blood | 2 | Collect in oxalate & refrigerate | Natelson: Microtechniques of Clin Chem. 2d ed, 1961, p. 208 |
| Gastrin | 0-200 pg per ml | Serum | | | Dent et al: Ann Surg 176:360, 1972 |
| Glucose | Fasting: 70–100 mg per 100 ml | Blood | 2 | Collect with oxalate-fluoride mixture. Micromethod: add 0.1 ml of blood to 1.9 ml of 0.01 per cent sodium fluoride solution | Tech AutoAnalyzer Meth<br>Huggett, Nixon: Lancet 2:368, 1957 (modified) |
| Iron | 50–150 μg per 100 ml (higher in males) | Serum | 5 | Shows diurnal variation higher in a.m. | Tech AutoAnalyzer Meth (modified) |
| Iron-binding capacity | 250–410 μg per 100 ml | Serum | 5 | | Scalata, Moore: Clin Chem 8:360, 1962 Tech AutoAnalyzer Meth |

**Blood, Plasma or Serum Values**

| *Determination* | *Normal Value* | *Material Analyzed* | *Minimal ml of Blood Required* | *Note* | *Method* |
|---|---|---|---|---|---|
| Lactic acid | 0.6–1.8 mEq per liter | Blood | 2 | Collect with oxalate fluoride mixture; deliver immediately packed in ice. | Hadjivassiliou, Rieder: Clin Chim Acta 19:357, 1968 |
| Lactic dehydrogenase | 60–120 U per ml | Serum | 2 | Unsuitable if hemolyzed | Wacker, et al: N Engl J Med 255:449, 1956 |
| Lead | 50 μg per 100 ml or less | Blood | 2 | Collect with oxalate fluoride mixture | Berman: Atom Absorp Newsl 3:9, 1964 (modified) |
| Lipase | 2 U per ml or less | Serum | 3 | | Comfort, Osterberg: J Lab Clin Med 20:271, 1934 |
| Lipids | | | | | |
| Cholesterol | 150–280 mg per 100 ml | Serum | 2 | Fasting | Tech AutoAnalyzer Meth |
| Cholesterol esters | 60–75 per cent of cholesterol | Serum | 2 | Fasting | Creech, Sewell: Anal Biochem 3:119, 1962<br>Tech AutoAnalyzer Meth |
| Phospholipids | 9–16 mg per 100 ml as lipid phosphorus | Serum | 5 | Fasting | Fiske, SubbaRow: J Biol Chem 66:2, 1925 |
| Total fatty acids | 190–420 mg per 100 ml | Serum | 10 | Fasting | Stoddard, Drury: J. Biol Chem 84:741, 1929 |
| Total lipids | 450–1000 mg per 100 ml | Serum | 5 | Fasting | Freedman: Clin Chim Acta 19:291, 1968 |
| Triglycerides | 40–150 mg per 100 ml | Serum | 2 | Fasting | Tech AutoAnalyzer Meth |
| Lipoprotein electrophoresis (LEP) | | Serum | 2 | Fasting; do not freeze serum. | Lees, Hatch: J Lab Clin Med 61:518, 1963 |
| Lithium | Toxic level 2 mEq per liter | Serum | 1 | | Flame photometry |
| Magnesium | 1.5–2.5 mEq per liter | Serum | 1 | | Willis: Clin Chem 11:251, 1965 (modified) |
| Methanol | 0 | Blood | 5 | May be fatal as low as 115 mg per 100 ml; collect in oxalate. | Natelson: Microtechniques of Clin Chem. 2d ed. 1961, p 298 |
| Mysoline (primidone) | Therapeutic level 4–12 μg per ml | Serum | | | Gas Liquid Chromatography |
| 5′Nucleotidase | 0.3–3.2 Bodansky U | Serum | 1 | | Rieder, Otero: Clin Chem 8:727, 1969 |
| Osmolality | 280–295 mOsm per kg water | Serum | 5 | | Crawford, Nicosia: J Lab Med 40:907, 1952 |

**Blood, Plasma or Serum Values**

| *Determination* | *Normal Value* | *Material Analyzed* | *Minimal ml of Blood Required* | *Note* | *Method* |
|---|---|---|---|---|---|
| Oxygen saturation (arterial) | 96–100 per cent | Arterial blood | 3 | Deliver in sealed heparinized syringe packed in ice | Gordy, Drabkin: J Biol Chem 227:285, 1957 |
| $Pco_2$ | 35–45 mm of mercury | Arterial blood | 2 | Collect and deliver in sealed heparinized syringe | By $CO_2$ electrode |
| pH | 7.35–7.45 | Arterial blood | 2 | Collect without stasis in sealed heparinized syringe; deliver packed in ice. | Glass electrode |
| $Po_2$ | 75–100 mm of mercury (dependent on age) while breathing room air<br>Above 500 mm of mercury while on 100% $O_2$ | Arterial blood | 2 | | Oxygen electrode |
| Phenylalanine | 0–2 mg per 100 ml | Serum | 0.4 | | Cullay, et al: Clin Chem 8:266, 1962 (modified) |
| Phosphatase (acid) | Male–Total: 0.13–0.63 Sigma U per ml<br>Female–Total: 0.01–0.56 Sigma U per ml<br>Prostatic: 0–0.7 Fishman-Lerner U per 100 ml | Serum | 1 | Must always be drawn just before analysis or stored as frozen serum; avoid hemolysis. | Bessey, et al: J Biol Chem 164:321, 1946<br>Babson, et al: Clin Chim Acta 13:264, 1966 |
| Phosphatase (alkaline) | 2.0–4.5 Bodansky U (infants to 14 U; adolescents to 5 U). | Serum | 1 | BSP dye interferes | Bessey, et al: J Biol Chem 164:321, 1945 |
| Phosphorus (inorganic) | 3.0–4.5 mg per 100 ml (infants in 1st year up to 6.0 mg per 100 ml) | Serum | 2 | Obtain blood in fasting state; serum must be separated promptly from cells. | Fiske, SubbaRow: J Biol Chem 66:375, 1925, Adapted for Tech AutoAnalyzer Meth |
| Potassium | 3.5–5.0 mEq per liter | Serum | 2 | Serum must be separated promptly from cells (within 1 hr) | Flame photometry |
| Protein: Total | 6.0–8.0 g per 100 ml | Serum | 1 | Patient should be fasting; avoid BSP dye. | Refractometry (American Optical Co) |
| Albumin | 4.0–5.0 g per 100 ml | Serum | 1 | | Doumas et al: Clin Chim Acta 31:87, 1971 |
| Globulin | 2.0–3.0 g per 100 ml | | | Globulin calculated | Gornall, et al: J Biol Chem 177:751, 1949 (modified) |

**Blood, Plasma or Serum Values**

| *Determination* | *Normal Value* | *Material Analyzed* | *Minimal ml of Blood Required* | *Note* | *Method* |
|---|---|---|---|---|---|
| Paper electrophoresis | Percent of total protein | Serum | 1 | Quantitation by densitometry | Kunkel, Tiselius: J Gen Physiol 35:89, 1951 |
| Albumin | 50–60 | | | | Durrum: J. Am Chem Soc 72:2943, 1950 |
| Globulin: | | | | | |
| $Alpha_1$ | 4.2–7.2 | | | | |
| $Alpha_2$ | 6.8–12 | | | | |
| Beta | 9.3–15 | | | | |
| Gamma | 13–23 | | | | |
| Pyruvic acid | 0–0.11 mEq per liter | Blood | 2 | Collect with oxalate fluoride. Deliver immediately packed in ice. | Hadjivassiliou, Rieder: Clin Chim Acta 19:357, 1968 |
| Quinidine | Therapeutic: 4-6 μg per 100 ml<br>Toxic: 10 μg per 100 ml | Serum | 1 | | Flourometry |
| Salicylate: | 0 | Plasma | 5 | Collect in heparin or oxalate | Keller: Am J Clin Pathol 17:415, 1947 |
| Therapeutic | 20–25 mg per 100 ml; 35–40 mg per 100 ml to age 10 yrs. | | | | |
| Toxic | Over 30 mg per 100 ml; over 20 mg per 100 ml after age 60. | | | | |
| Sodium | 135–145 mEq per liter | Serum | 2 | | Flame photometry |
| Sulfate | 0.5–1.5 mg per 100 ml | Serum | 3 | Avoid hemolysis | Letonoff, Reinhold: J Biol Chem 114:147, 1936 |
| Sulfonamide | 0 | Blood or Serum | 2 | Value given as unconjugated unless total is requested | Bratton, Marshall: J Biol Chem 128:537, 1939 |
| Thymol: | | | | | Maclagen: Nature 154:670, 1944 |
| Flocculation | Up to 1 + in 24 hr | Serum | 1 | Checked with phosphate buffer of higher molarity to rule out false-positive reaction | |
| Turbidity | 0–4 U | | | | |
| Thyroxine | | | | | Murphy: J. Lab Clin Med 66:161, 1965 (modified) |
| Total | 4–11 μg per 100 ml | Serum | 3 | | |
| Free | 0.8–2.4 ng per 100 ml | Serum | 6 | | Sterling, Brenner: J Clin Invest 45:153, 1966 (modified) |
| Transaminase (SGOT) | 10–40 U per ml | Serum | 1 | | Karmen, et al: J Clin Invest 34:126, 1955 |
| Urea nitrogen (BUN) | 8–25 mg per 100 ml | Blood or serum | 1 | Urea = BUN x 2.14. Use oxalate as anticoagulant. | Skeggs: Am J Clin Pathol 28:311, 1957 (modified) |

**Blood, Plasma or Serum Values**

| *Determination* | *Normal Value* | *Minimal ml Required* | | *Note* | *Method* |
|---|---|---|---|---|---|
| Uric acid | 3.0–7.0 mg per 100 ml | Serum | 2 | Serum must be separated from cells at once and refrigerated | Folin: J Biol Chem 101:111, 1933, Adapted for Tech AutoAnalyzer Meth |
| Vitamin A | 0.15–0.6 $\mu$g per ml | Serum | 3 | | Natelson, Microtechniques of Clin Chem. 2d ed, 1961, p 451 |
| Vitamin A tolerance test | Rise to twice fasting level in 3 to 5 hr | Serum | 3 | Samples taken fasting and at intervals up to 8 hr after test dose | Josephs: Bull Johns Hopkins Hosp 65: 112, 1939 |

**Urine Values**

| *Determination* | *Normal Value* | *Minimal Quantity Required* | *Note* | *Method* |
|---|---|---|---|---|
| Acetone plus acetoacetate (quantitative) | 0 | 2 ml | Keep cold | Behre: J Lab Clin Med 13:770, 1928 |
| Alpha amino nitrogen | 64–199 mg per day; not over 1.5 per cent of total nitrogen | 24-hr specimen | Preserve with thymol; refrigerate. | Hamilton, Van Slyke: J Biol Chem 150: 231, 1943 |
| Amylase | 24–76 U per ml | | | Huggins, Russell: Ann Surg 128:668, 1948 |
| Calcium | 150 mg per day or less | 24-hr specimen | Collect in special bottle with 10 ml of concentrated HCl | Atomic absorption |
| Catecholamines | Epinephrine: under 10 $\mu$g per day. Norepinephrine: under 100 $\mu$g per day | 24-hr specimen | Should be collected with 12 ml of concentrated HCl (pH should be between 2.0 and 3.0) | DuToit: WADC Tech Report no 59–175, 1959; MGH Methodology |
| Chorionic gonadotropin | 0 | 1st morning voiding | Specific gravity should be at least 1.015 | Immunologic technic |
| Copper | 0–100 $\mu$g per day | 24-hr specimen | | MGH Methodology Atomic absorption |
| Coproporphyrin | 50–250 $\mu$g per day | 24-hr specimen | Collect with 5 g of sodium carbonate | Schwartz: J Lab Clin Med 37:843, 1951 |
| | Children under 80 lb 0–75 $\mu$g per day | | | With: Scand J Clin Lab Invest 7:193, 1955 |

**Urine Values (Continued)**

| *Determination* | *Normal Value* | *Minimal Quantity Required* | *Note* | *Method* |
|---|---|---|---|---|
| Creatine | Under 100 mg per day or less than 6 per cent of creatinine. In pregnancy: up to 12 per cent. In children under 1 yr.: may equal creatinine. In older children: up to 30 per cent of creatinine | 24-hr specimen | Also order creatinine | Folin: Lab Manual Biol Chem. 5th ed. 1933, p.163 |
| Creatinine | 15–25 mg per kg of body weight per day | 24-hr specimen | | *Idem:* |
| Creatinine clearance | 150–180 liters per day per 1.73 m² of body surface | 24-hr specimen | Order serum creatinine also | Brod. Sirota: J Clin Invest 27:645, 1948 |
| Cystine or cysteine | 0 | 10 ml | Qualitative | Hawk, et al: Pract Physiol Chem. 13th ed, 1954, p 141 |
| Follicle-stimulating hormone | | 24-hr specimen | | Radioimmunoassay |
| Follicular phase | 5-20 IU per 24 hr | | | |
| Mid-cycle | 15-60 IU per 24 hr | | | |
| Luteal phase | 5-15 IU per 24 hr | | | |
| Menopausal | 50–100 IU per 24 hr | | | |
| Men | 5-25 IU per 24 hr | | | |
| Hemoglobin and myoglobin | 0 | Freshly voided sample | Chemical examination with benzidine | |
| Homogentisic acid | 0 | Freshly voided sample or 24-hr sample kept cold | Must be refrigerated if not determined at once; test also measures gentisic acid and may be positive in patients on high doses of salicylates | Neuberger: Biochem J 41:431, 1947 |
| 5-hydroxyindole acetic acid | 2–9 mg per 24 hr (women lower than men) | 24-hr urine | Collect in special bottle with 10 ml of concentrated HCl | Sjoerdsma, et al: JAMA 159:397, 1955 |
| Lead | 0.08 µg per ml or 120 µg or less per 24 hr | 24-hr specimen | | Willis: Anal Chem 34:614, 1962 (modified) |
| Phenolsulfonphthalein (PSP) | At least 25 per cent excreted by 15 min; 40 per cent by 30 min; 60 per cent by 120 min | Total output of urine collected 15, 30 and 120 min after injection | Inject 1 ml (6 mg) intravenously; BSP interferes. | Chapman: N Engl J Med 214:16, 1936 |
| Phenylpyruvic acid | 0 | Freshly voided sample unless quantitation needed | | Penrose, Quastel: Biochem J 31:266, 1937 |
| Phosphorus (inorganic) | Varies with intake; average 1 g per day | 24-hr specimen | Collect in special bottle with 10 ml of concentrated HCl | Tech AutoAnalyzer Meth |

**Urine Values (Continued)**

| *Determination* | *Normal Value* | *Minimal Quantity Required* | *Note* | *Method* |
|---|---|---|---|---|
| Porphobilinogen | 0 | 10 ml | Use freshly voided urine | Watson, Schwartz: Proc Soc Exp Biol Med 47:393, 1941 |
| Protein: | | 24-hr specimen | | |
| Quantitative | <150 mg per 24 hrs | | | Meulmans: Clin Chim Acta 5:757, 1951 |
| Electrophoresis | | | | See Blood Protein |
| Steroids: | | | | |
| 17-ketosteroids (per day) | Age / Males / Females<br>10 / 1–4 mg / 1–4 mg<br>20 / 6–21 / 4–16<br>30 / 8–26 / 4–14<br>50 / 5–18 / 3–9<br>70 / 2–10 / 1–7 | 24-hr specimen | Not valid if patient is receiving meprobamate | Vestergaard: Acta Endocrinol 8:193, 1951. Normal values taken from Hamburger: Acta Endocrinol 1:19, 1948 |
| 17-hydroxy-steroids | 3–8 mg per day (women lower than men) | 24-hr specimen | Keep cold; chlorpromazine and related drugs interfere with assay. | Epstein: Clin Chim Acta 7:735, 1962 |
| Sugar: | | | | |
| Quantitative glucose | 0 | 24-hr or other timed specimen | Collect with toluene; refrigerate. | Beach, Turner: Clin Chem 4:462, 1958 |
| Identification of reducing substances | | 50 ml | Use freshly voided urine; no preservatives. | |
| Fructose | 0 | 50 ml | Use freshly voided urine; also quantitate total reducing substances. | Roe, et al: J Biol Chem 178:839, 1948 |
| Pentose | 0 | 50 ml | Use freshly voided urine | Roe, Rice: J Biol Chem 173:507, 1948 |
| Titratable acidity | 20–40 mEq per day | 24-hr sample | Collect with toluene; refrigerate | Henderson, Palmer: J Biol Chem 17: 305, 1914 |
| Urobilinogen | Up to 1.0 Ehrlich U | 2-hr sample (1–3 p.m.) | | Watson, et al: Am J Clin Pathol 15:605, 1944 |
| Uroporphyrin | 0 | See Coproporphyrin | | Schwartz, et al: Proc Soc Exp Biol Med 79:463, 1952 |
| Vanilmandelic acid (VMA) | Up to 9 mg per 24 hr | 24-hr specimen | Collect as for catecholamine | Pisano, et al: Clin Chim Acta 7:285, 1962 |

**Special Endocrine Tests**

| *Determination* | *Normal Value* | *Minimal Quantity Required* | | *Note* | *Method* |
|---|---|---|---|---|---|
| Autoantibodies: | | | | | |
| Thyroid<br>Parietal cells<br>Skeletal muscle<br>Gonads<br>Kidney mitochondria | Absent. Occasionally positive in the elderly. | Serum | 2 | — | Ann NY Acad Sci 124:644, 1965; 124:730, 1965<br><br>Clin Exp Immunol 1:237, 1966 |
| Polypeptide hormones: | | | | | |
| Calcitonin | Undetectable in normals. > 100 pg per ml in medullary carcinoma | Plasma | 5 | Test done only on known or suspected cases of medullary carcinoma of the thyroid | Deftos, et al: Metabolism 20:1129, 1971<br><br>Deftos, et al: Metabolism 20:428, 1971 |
| Growth hormone | Below 5 ng per ml | Plasma | 1 | Fasting, at rest | Glick, et al: Nature 199:784,1963 |
| | Children: Over 10 ng per ml<br>Male: Below 5 ng per ml<br>Female: Up to 30 ng per ml | | | After exercise | |
| | Male: Below 5 ng per ml<br>Female: Below 10 ng per ml | | | After glucose load | |
| Insulin | 6–26 μU per ml | Serum or plasma | 1 | Fasting | Morgan, Lazarow: Proc Soc Exp Biol Med 110:29, 1962 |
| | Below 20 μU per ml | | | During hypoglycemia | |
| | Up to 150 μU per ml | | | After glucose load | |
| Luteinizing hormone | Male: 6–18 mU per ml | Serum or plasma | 2 | | Odell, et al: J Clin Invest 46:248, 1967 |
| | Female: 5–22 mU per ml | | | Pre- or postovulatory | |
| | 30–250 mU per ml | | | Midcycle peak | |
| Parathyroid hormone | <15 μl equiv per 150 μl | Plasma | 5 | Keep blood on ice, or plasma must be frozen if it is to be sent any distance. | Segre, et al: J Clin Invest 51:3163, 1972 |
| Renin activity | Supine: 1.1±0.8 ng per ml per hr<br>Upright: 1.9±1.7 ng per ml per hr | Plasma | 4 | EDTA tubes, on ice; normal diet | Haber, et al: J Clin Endocrinol Metab 29:1349, 1969 |
| | Supine: 2.7±1.8 ng per ml per hr | | | Low sodium diet | |
| | Upright: 6.6±2.5 ng per ml per hr | | | Low sodium diet | |
| | Diuretics: 10.0±3.7 ng per ml per hr | | | | |

**Special Endocrine Tests (Continued)**

| *Determination* | *Normal Value* | *Minimal Quantity Required* | | *Note* | *Method* |
|---|---|---|---|---|---|
| Steroid hormones: Aldosterone | 5–19 μg | 24-hr urine | 5 | Keep specimen cold. | Bayard, et al: J Clin Endocrinol Metab 31:507, 1970 |
| Cortisol | 8 a.m.: | Plasma | 1 | Fasting | Murphy: J Clin Endocrinol Metab 27:973, 1967 |
| | 5–25 μg/100 ml | | 1 | At rest | |
| | 8 p.m.: Below 10 μg/100 ml | | | | |
| | 4 hr. ACTH test: 30–45 μg/100 ml | | 1 | 20 U ACTH, IV/4 hr | |
| | Overnight suppression test: Below 5 μg/100 ml | | 1 | 8 a.m. sample after dexamethasone midnight. | |
| | Excretion: 20–70 μg/24 hr | Urine | 2 | Keep specimen cold. | |
| 11-Deoxycortisol | Responsive: Over 10 μg/100 ml Subnormal: 5–10 μg/100 ml Unresponsive: 0–5 μg/100 ml | Plasma | 2 | Preceded by 4.5 g of metyrapone P.O. per 24 hr. | Kliman: Adv Tracer Meth 4:227, 1968 |
| Testosterone | Adult male: Over 0.30 μg/100 ml Adolescent male: Over 0.10 μg/100 ml Female: Below 0.10 μg/100 ml | Plasma | 2 | a.m. sample | Chen, et al: Clin Chem 17:581, 1971 |
| Thyroid hormones: Thyroid stimulating hormone (TSH) | 1.6 ± 1.2 μU per ml | Serum | 2 | Fasting, a.m. | Patel, et al: J Clin Endocrinol Metab 33:768, 1971 |
| Thyroxine-binding globulin capacity (TBG) | 15–25 μg $T_4$ per 100 ml | Serum | 2 | Fasting, a.m. | Elzinga, et al: Am J Clin Pathol 36:125, 1961 |
| Total triiodothyronine by competitive binding ($TT_3$) | 150–250 ng per 100 ml | Serum | 3 | Fasting, a.m. | Benotti, et al: Further Adv Thyroid Res 1:1121, 1971 |
| Total triiodothyronine by radioimmunoassay ($TT_3$) | 70–190 ng per 100 ml | Serum | 2 | Fasting, a.m. | Larsen, et al: J Clin Invest 51:1939, 1972 |

**Hematologic Values**

| *Determination* | *Normal Value* | *Material Analyzed* | *Minimal ml of Blood Required* | *Note* | *Method* |
|---|---|---|---|---|---|
| Coagulation factors: | | | | | |
| Factor I (fibrinogen) | 0.15–0.35 g per 100 ml | Plasma | 4.5 | Collect in vacutainer containing sodium citrate | Ratnoff, Menzies: J Lab Clin Med 37: 316, 1951 |
| Factor II (prothrombin) | 70–130 per cent | Plasma | 4.5 | Collect in plastic tubes with 3.8 per cent sodium citrate | Owren, Aas: Scand J Clin Lab Invest 3:201, 1951 |
| Factor V (accelerator globulin) | 70–130 per cent | Plasma | 4.5 | Collect as in factor II determination | Lewis, Ware: Proc Soc Exp Biol Med 84:640, 1953 |
| Factor VII-X (proconvertin-Stuart) | 70–130 per cent | Plasma | 4.5 | Collect as in factor II determination | Same as factor II |
| Factor X (Stuart factor) | 70–130 per cent | Plasma | 4.5 | Collect as in factor II determination | Bachman, et al: Thromb Diath Haemorrh 2:29, 1958 |
| Factor VIII (antihemophilic globulin) | 50–200 per cent | Plasma | 4.5 | Collect as in factor II determination | Tocantins, Kazal: Blood Coag. Hemorrh Thrombosis, 2d ed. 1964 |
| Factor IX (plasma thromboplastic cofactor) | 70–130 per cent | Plasma | 4.5 | Collect as in factor II determination | *Idem:* |
| Factor XI (plasma thromboplastic antecedent) | 70–130 per cent | Plasma | 4.5 | Collect as in factor II determination | *Idem:* |
| Factor XII (Hageman factor) | 70–130 per cent | Plasma | 4.5 | Collect as in factor II determination | *Idem:* |
| Coagulation screening tests: | | | | | |
| Bleeding time | 3–8 min | | | | Mielke: Blood 34:204, 1969 |
| Clotting time | Below 15 min | Whole blood | 6 | Collect in 3 glass tubes (10 x 75 mm) | Lee, White: Todd-Sanford Clin Diag by Lab Methods. 11th ed. 1948, p.199 |
| Prothrombin time | Less than 2-sec deviation from control | Plasma | 4.5 | Collect in vacutainer containing 3.8 per-cent sodium citrate | Quick: Hemorrh Dis. 1957, p 379 |
| Partial thromboplastin time (activated) | 22–37 sec | Plasma | 4.5 | Collect in vacutainer containing 3.8 per-cent sodium citrate | Proctor, Rappaport: Am J Clin Pathol 36:212, 1961 (modified) |
| Whole-blood clot lysis | No clot lysis in 24 hr | Whole blood | 2.0 | Collect in sterile tube and incubate at 37° C | Page, Culver: Syllabus Lab Exam Clin Diag. 1960, p 207 |

**Hematologic Values (Continued)**

| *Determination* | *Normal Value* | *Material Analyzed* | *Minimal ml of Required Blood* | *Note* | *Method* |
|---|---|---|---|---|---|
| Fibrinolytic studies: | | | | | |
| Euglobulin lysis | No lysis in 2 hr | Plasma | 4.5 | Collect as in factor II determination | Sherry, et al: J Clin Invest 38:810, 1959 |
| Fibrinogen split products | | | | | |
| Method I latex agglutination with anti-D and -E antibody | Negative reaction at greater than 1:2 dilution | Serum | 4.5 | Collect in special tube containing thrombin and epsilon amino caproic acid | Garrey, Black: J Clin Pathol 25:680, 1972 |
| Method II (staphylococcal clumping) | Positive reaction at greater than 1:8 dilution | Serum | 4.5 | Collect as in Method I | Hawiger, et al: J Lab Clin Med 75:93, 1970 |
| Plasminogen | 3–5 casein U per ml | Plasma | 4.5 | Collect as in factor II determination | Alkjaersig, et al: J Biol Chem 234:832, 1959 |
| Thrombin time | Less than 5-sec deviation from control | Plasma | 4.5 | Collect as in factor II determination | Stefanini, Dameshek: Hemorrh Disord. 1962, p 492 |
| "Complete" blood count: | | Blood | 1 | Use EDTA as anticoagulant. The seven listed tests are performed automatically on the Coulter Counter Model S. The machine directly determines cell counts, hemoglobin (as the cyanmethemoglobin derivative) and MCV and computes hematocrit, MCH and MCHC. | |
| Hematocrit | Male: 42–50 per cent<br>Female: 40–48 per cent | | | | |
| Hemoglobin | Male: 13–16 g per 100 ml<br>Female: 12–15 g per 100 ml | | | | |
| Leukocyte count | 4,800–10,800 per mm$^3$ | | | | |
| Erythrocyte count | 4.2–5.9 million per mm$^3$ | | | | |
| Mean corpuscular volume (MCV) | 80–94 cu $\mu^3$ | | | | |
| Mean corpuscular hemoglobin (MCH) | 27–32 pg $\mu^3$ | | | | |
| Mean corpuscular hemoglobin concentration (MCHC) | 33–38 per cent | | | | |
| Erythrocyte sedimentation rate: | 1–13 mm per hr (men) | Blood | 5 | Use EDTA as anticoagulant | Westergren method as modified by Gambino et al: Am J Clin Pathol 35:173, 1965 |
| | 1–20 mm per hr (women) | Blood | 5 | | |

**Hematologic Values (Continued)**

| *Determination* | *Normal Value* | *Material Analyzed* | *Minimal ml of Blood Required* | *Note* | *Method* |
|---|---|---|---|---|---|
| Erythrocyte enzymes: | | | | | |
| Glucose-6-phosphate dehydrogenase | 5–15 U | Blood | 9 | Use special anticoagulant (3.8 per cent sodium citrate) | Beck: J Biol Chem 232:251, 1958 |
| 6-Phosphogluconate dehydrogenase | 2–5 U | Blood | 9 | Use special anticoagulant (3.8 per cent sodium citrate) | Brewer, Dern: Am J Hum Genet 16:472, 1964 |
| Glutathione reductase | 9–13 U | Blood | 9 | Use special anticoagulant (3.8 per cent sodium citrate) | Carson, et al: J Lab Clin Med 58:804, 1961 |
| Pyruvate kinase | 2–3 U | Blood | 8 | Use special anticoagulant (5 per cent polyvinylpyrrolidine and 3.8 per cent sodium citrate) | Tanaka, et al: Blood 19:267, 1962 |
| Folic acid | 6–15 ng per ml | Serum | 1 | | Baker, et al: Clin Chem 5:275, 1959; Goulian, Beck: Am J Clin Pathol 46: 390, 1966 |
| Haptoglobin | 100–300 mg per 100 ml | Serum | 1 | | Behring Diagnostic Reagent Kit |
| Hemoglobin studies: | | | | | |
| Electrophoresis for abnormal hemoglobin | | Blood | 5 | Collect with anticoagulant | Singer: Am J Med 18: 633, 1955 |
| Electrophoresis for $A_2$ hemoglobin | 2.0–3.0 per cent | Blood | 5 | Use oxalate as anticoagulant | Kunkel, et al: J Clin Invest 36:1615, 1957 |
| Fetal hemoglobin (alkali resistant) | Less than 2 per cent | Blood | 5 | Collect with anticoagulant | Miale: Lab Med-Hemat. 2d ed, 1962, p 845 |
| Hemoglobin, met- and sulf- | 0 | Blood | 5 | Use heparinized blood | Michel, Harris: J Lab Clin Med 25:445, 1940 |
| Serum hemoglobin | 2–3 mg per 100 ml | Serum | 2 | | Hunter, et al: Am J Clin Pathol 20:429, 1950 |
| Thermolabile hemoglobin | Negative | Blood | 1 | Any anticoagulant | Dacie, et al: Br J Haematol 10:388, 1964 |
| Lupus anticoagulant | Absent | Plasma | 4.5 | Collect as in factor II determination | Margolius et al: Medicine 40:145, 1961 |
| L. E.(lupus erythematosus) preparation: | | | | | |
| Method I | Negative | Blood | 5 | Use heparinized blood | Hargraves, et al: Proc Staff Meet Mayo Clin 24:234, 1949 |

**Hematologic Values (Continued)**

| *Determination* | *Normal Value* | *Material Analyzed* | *Minimal ml of Blood Required* | *Note* | *Method* |
|---|---|---|---|---|---|
| Method II | Negative | Blood | 5 | Use defibrinated blood | Barnes, et al: J Invest Dermatol 14:397, 1950 |
| Leukocyte alkaline phosphatase | 15–40 mg of phosphorus liberated per hr per $10^{10}$ cells | Isolated blood leukocytes | 20 | Special handling of blood necessary | Valentine, Beck: J Lab Clin Med 38:39, 1951 |
| Muramidase | Serum, 4–12 μg per ml<br>Urine, 0–2 μg per ml | Serum<br>Urine | 1<br>1 | | Osserman, Lawlor: J Exp Med 124:921, 1966 |
| Osmotic fragility of erythrocytes | Increased if hemolysis occurs in over 0.5 per cent NaCl: decreased if hemolysis is incomplete in 0.3 per cent NaCl. | Blood | 5 | Use heparin as anticoagulant | Beutler, in Williams et al: eds. Hematology, McGraw-Hill, 1972, p. 1375 |
| Peroxide hemolysis | <10 per cent | Blood | 5 | Use EDTA as anticoagulant | Gordon, et al: Am J Dis Child 90:669, 1955 |
| Platelet count | 200,000–350,000 per mm | Blood | 0.5 | Use EDTA as anticoagulant. Counts are performed on Coulter Counter Model B. When counts are low, results are confirmed by hand counting. | (Hand count): Brecher, et al: Am J Clin Pathol 23:15, 1955 |
| Platelet function tests | | | | | |
| Clot retraction | 50–100% at 2 hours | Plasma | 4.5 | Collect as in factor II determination | Benthaus: Thromb Diath Haemorrh 3:311, 1959 |
| Platelet aggregation | Full response to ADP, 1 epinephrine & collagen | Plasma | 18 | Collect as in factor II determination | Born: Nature 194:927, 1962 |
| Platelet factor 3 | 33–57 sec. | Plasma | 4.5<br>4.5] | Collect as in factor II determination | Rabiner, Hrodek: J Clin Invest 47:901, 1968 |
| Reticulocyte count | 0.5–1.5 per cent of red cells | Blood | 0.1 | | Brecher: Am J Clin Pathol 19:895, 1949 |
| Vitamin $B_{12}$ | 200–800 pg per ml | Serum | 12 | Special handling of blood necessary | Difco Manual, 9th ed. 1953, p 221 (modified) |

**Cerebrospinal-Fluid Values**

| *Determination* | *Normal Value* | *Minimal ml Required* | *Note* | *Method* |
|---|---|---|---|---|
| Bilirubin | 0 | 2 | | See Blood Bilirubin (adapted) |
| Cell count | 0–5 mononuclear cells | 0.5 | | |
| Chloride | 120–130 mEq per liter | 0.5 | 20 mEq per liter higher than serum; obtain serum for comparison. | See Blood Chloride |
| Colloidal gold | 0000000000–1111111111 | 0.1 | | Wuth, Faupel: Bull Johns Hopkins Hosp 40:297, 1927 |
| Electrophoresis | 80 per cent albumin | 5 | | See Blood Protein |
| Gamma globulin | 10 per cent of total protein | 5 | | |
| Glucose | 50–75 mg per 100 ml | 0.5 | 20 mg per 100 ml less than blood; compare with blood. | See Blood Glucose |
| Pressure (initial) | 70–180 mm of water | | | |
| Protein: | | | | |
| Lumbar | 15–45 mg per 100 ml | 1 | | Meulmans: Clin Chim Acta 5:757, 1960 |
| Cisternal | 15–25 mg per 100 ml | 1 | | |
| Ventricular | 5–15 mg per 100 ml | 1 | | |

**Miscellaneous Values**

| *Determination* | *Normal Value* | *Minimal Quantity Required* | *Note* | *Method* |
|---|---|---|---|---|
| Ascorbic acid load test | 0.2–2.0 mg per hr in control sample | Urine—approximate 1½-hr sample | Administer 500 mg of ascorbic acid orally | Harvard Fatigue Labs: Laboratory Manual, 1945 |
| | 24–49 mg per hr after loading | Urine—2 timed samples of about 2 hr each | | |
| Chylous fluid | | | Use fresh specimen | Todd, et al: Clin Diag 12th ed, 1953 p 624 |
| Duodenal drainage: | | | pH should be in proper range with minimal amount of gastric juice | |
| pH | 5.5–7.5 | 1 ml | | |
| Amylase | Over 1200 U per total sample | 1 ml | | Huggins, Russell: Ann Surg 128:668, 1948 |
| Trypsin | Values from 35 to 160 per cent "normal" | 1 ml | | Anderson, Early: Am J Dis Child 63:891, 1942 |
| Viscosity | 3 min or less | 4 ml | Run ice cold in 34-sec viscosimeter | |

**Miscellaneous Values (Continued)**

| *Determination* | *Normal Value* | *Minimal Quantity Required* | *Note* | *Method* |
|---|---|---|---|---|
| Gastric analysis | Basal: Females 2.0 ± 1.8 mEq per hr Males 3.0 ± 2.0 mEq per hr Maximal: (after histalog or gastrin) Females 16 ± 5 mEq per hr Males 23 ± 5 mEq per hr | | | Marks: Gastroenterology 41:599, 1961 |
| Immunologic tests: | | | | |
| Alpha-feto-globulin | Abnormal if present | 5 ml of clotted blood | | |
| Antinuclear antibodies | Positive if detected with serum diluted 1:10 | 10 ml clotted blood | Send to laboratory promptly | |
| Bence-Jones protein | Abnormal if present | 100 ml of urine | | |
| Complement, total hemolytic | 150–250 U per ml | 10 ml | Must be sent on ice | Hook, Muschel: Proc Soc Exp Biol |
| C3 | 145 mg per 100 ml (range 101–189) | 10 ml | | Med 117:292, 1964 |
| C4 | 45 mg per 100 ml (range 21–63) | 10 ml | | |
| Immunoglobins: | | 10 ml of blood | Mean values ± 1, standard deviation and range | Johnson, Bloch: Arch Ophthal 81:322, 1969 |
| IgG | 1180 (± 310) (720–1500) | | | |
| IgA | 218 (± 96) (90–325) | | | |
| IgM | 98 (± 41) (45–150) | | | |
| Viscosity | 1.4–1.8 | 5 ml of serum | Expressed as the relative viscosity of serum compared to water | Barth: Serum Proteins and Dysproteinemias. Editors, Sunderman, 1964, p 102 |
| Iontophoresis | Children: 0–40 mEq sodium per liter. Adults: 0–60 mEq sodium per liter | | Value given in terms of sodium | Gibson, Cooke: Pediatrics 23:545, 1959 |
| Stool fat | Less than 5 g in 24 hr or less than 4 per cent of measured fat intake in 3-day period | 24-hr or 3-day specimen, preferably with markers | | Van de Kramer, et al: J Biol Chem 177: 347, 1949 |

**Miscellaneous Values (Continued)**

| *Determination* | *Normal Value* | *Minimal Quantity Required* | *Note* | *Method* |
|---|---|---|---|---|
| Stool nitrogen | Less than 2 g per day or 10 per cent of urinary nitrogen | 24-hr or 3-day specimen | | Peters, Van Slyke: Quant Clin Chem Vol 2 (Methods), 1932, p. 353 |
| Synovial fluid: | | | | |
| Glucose | Not less than 20 mg per 100 ml lower than simultaneously drawn blood sugar | 1 ml of fresh fluid | Collect with oxalate-fluoride mixture | See Blood Glucose |
| Mucin | Type 1 or 2 | 1 ml of fresh fluid | Grades as: Type 1—tight clump Type 2—soft clump Type 3—soft clump that breaks up Type 4—cloudy, no clump | |
| D-Xylose absorption | 5–8 g per 5 hr in urine 40 mg per 100 ml in blood 2 hr after ingestion of 25 g of D-xylose | 5-hr collection of urine 5 ml of blood | For directions see Benson et al: New Eng J Med 256: 335, 1957 | Roe, Rice: J Biol Chem 173:507, 1948 |

* Normal Laboratory Values. New Eng J Med 234:24-28, 1946; 243:748-753, 1950; 254:29-35, 1956; 262:84-91, 1960; 268:1462-1469, 1963; 276:167-174, 1967; and 283:1276-1285, 1970.

† Prepared by: Mary Zervas, B.S., H. George Hamacher, M.S., and Olive Holmes, B.S., supervisors, and Sidney V. Rieder, Ph.D., chief of Chemistry Laboratory; Bernard Kliman, M.D., director of Endocrine-Steroid Laboratory; Gretchen Williams, chief technologist, Clinical Laboratories; William S. Beck, M.D., director of Clinical Laboratories, and Robert W. Colman, M.D., in charge of Special Clotting Laboratory.

# INDEX

Bold face—major discussion
t—table
f—figure
ft—footnote


**A**

AAS, (*see* Atomic absorption spectroscopy)
Abattoir, 519
Abietic anhydride (Rosin), 645
Abrasive cleaners, **525**
Abrin, 542, 543
*Abrus precatorius* (Jequirity bean), 541, 551t
ABS (Alkyl benzene sulfonate), 331, 518
Absinthe, 479, 481t, 546t
Acacia, 481t
*Acarina* (ticks), **580-581**
Acco Emulsifier #5, 526t
Acedicon (dihydrocodeinone enolacetate), 481t
Acenocoumarol (Sintrom), 481t
Acetaldehyde, 38, 144, 149, 202, 209, 211, 212, 220t, **221**, 274t, 648t
Acetaminophen (Amdil, Anelix, Apamide, Elixodyne, Febrolin, Fendon, Lestemp, Liquiprin, Lyteca syrup, Metalid, Nacetyl, Nebs, Tempra, Tylenol), 12t, 77, 81t, 90, 117t, **346-349,** 451, 461, 481t, 503t, 513t
Acetanilid, 7t, 12t, 17, 64, 97t, 274t, 339, 343t, 346t, **451-452**
  derivatives, 7t
Acetarsol (Acetarsone), 13t, 481t
Acetarsone (Acetarsol), 13t, 481t
Acetate, 209
  aluminum, 255, 350, 612
  ammonium, **31**, 51t, 612
  amyl, 87t, 94t, 202, 222, 247t, 636, 708t, 729t
  butyl, 94t, 247t, 729t
  cellulose, 95t
  cobalt ethylene diaminetetra, (*see* Kelocyanor)
  copper, 583
  Cortef, 69
  Cortogen, cortisone, Cortone, (*see* Cortisone)
  ethyl, 94t, 247t, 649, 729t
  mafenide, (*see* Mafenide acetate [Sulfamylon])
  methyl, 729t
  norethindrone, 143t
  oxyphenisatin, 346t
  propyl, 730t
  silver, 467, 649
  sodium, (*see* Sodium acetate)
  tetrahydrofurfuryl, 95t
  thallium, (*see* Thallium)
  vinyl, 314
Acetazolamide (Diamox), 13t, 16t, 81t, 248, 339, 347t, 360, 363t, 388, 466, 481t, 513t
Aceteen Stops Termites, 159t
Acetic acid, 20t, 38, 94t, 97t, 220t, 247t, 358, 481t, 533, 613, 614, 616, 635, 648t
  as treatment in poisoning, 31, 42, 83, 232
  glacial, 720
Acetoacetic acid, 209, 463
Acetoarsenite copper, 155t
Acetohexamide (Dymelor), 429, 481t, 513t
Acetomeroctol (Merbak), 481t
Acetone, 8t, 86, 87t, 94t, 97t, 184, 202, 216, 217, 220t, **221-222,** 247t, 271t, 274t, 482t, 513t, 580, 609, 621, 636, 725t
  alcohol, (*see* Wood alcohol)
  comparison with carbon disulfide, Table 159(725)
  cyanohydrin, 482t
  extraction, used for identification of poisons, 84
Acetonitrile extractions, used for identification of poisons, 84
Acetonitside, 482t
Acetonylbenzyl hydroxycoumarin (Warfarin), 179t
Acetophenetidin (Phenacetin), 12t, 13t, 65t, 191, 342, 343t, 425t, **451-452**
Acetrizoate (Urokon), 482t
Acetyl
  phenylhydrazine, 343
  strophanthin, 420
Acetylcholine, 93, 130, 131, 133, 156, 358, 452, 714
  effects of, 31, 98, 137
Acetylcholinesterase, 133
Acetyl-coenzyme A (Acetyl-Co A) 209
Acetylcysteine (Mucomyst), 349, 482t
N-acetylcysteine (NAC), 428
n-Acetyl-DL-penicillamine, 147, 148
Acetylene, 274t, 535
  trichloride, (*see* Trichloroethylene)
n-Acetyl-p-aminophenol (Acetaminophen), 204, 451
Acetylparaminophenol, 452
Acetylsalicylic acid, 65t, 93t, 97t, 341, 343t, 461, 516t, (*see* Salicylates)
Acetylurea(s), 359
  derivatives, 360
Achromycin, (*see* Tetracycline)
Acid(s), 4, 8t, 9t, 51t, 70, 85, 94t, **226-229,** 274t (*see also* individual acids)
  beverages, **718**
  caustic, 94t, 182
  corrosive, 7t, 51t, 82, 202, **226-229,** 720
  mineral, 36, 88
  neutralizing agents, **83**
  spot extractions, used for identification of poisons, 84
Acidol, 526t
Acidolate, 526t
Acidose, 526t
Acidosis, **49-58** (with tables)
Ackees *(Blighia sapida)*, 544, 548t
Acme All Round Insect Bomb, 159t
Acme Emo-Nik, 159t
Acme Flybait, 159t
Acme Garden Fungicide, 194t
Acme Weed Killer, 194t
Acne eruptions induced by drugs and chemicals, **312-313**
Aconite, 7t, 9t, 35t, 62t, 346t, **350,** 581
Aconitine, 6t, 7t, 97t, **350**
*Aconitum*
  *napellus* (monkshood), 541, 550t
  *uncinatum* (wild monkshood), 554t
ACP Brush Killer, 194t
ACP Grass Killer, 194t
Acridine, 274t, 455
Acriflavine, 346t, 609
Acrodynia, 53t, **608**
Acrolein (acrylaldehyde), 160t, 187t, 202, 221, 247t, 274t, 648t
Acro-osteolysis, 312
Acrylaldehyde (Acrolein), 202, **221**
Acrylonitrile, 87t, 153, 235
*Actaea alba, rubra, spicata* (baneberry, snakeberry), 548t
Acteen Stops Weeds, 194t
ACTH (Corticotropin), 19t, 253, 312, 320, 339, 568
Actinomycetes, thermophilic, (*see* Thermophilic actinomycetes)
Actinomycin D (Meractinomycin-Lyo), 347t, 398t
Activated charcoal, 20t, 30, **34-35** (with tables), 43, 45, 56t, 96t, 143, 152, 157, 158, 178, 186, 212, 217, 250,

349, 373, 385, 404, 416, 423, 427, 443, 445, 450, 454, 464, 475, 556
amount of substances absorbed by, Table 18(35)
and the artificial kidney, 66
ACTO, 526t
AD, 526t
Adamsite, 9t
Adanon (Methadone hydrochloride), 117t
Addiction, morphine (narcotic), **447-449**
Additives, food, **703-710** (with table)
functions of some commonly used, Table 157(708-709)
Adenosine
diphosphate (ADP), 467
triphosphate, 462
Adipate, dibutyl, (*see* Dibutyl adipate)
ADP (Adenosine diphosphate), (*see* Adenosine diphosphate)
Adrenal
corticosteroids, 71, 248, 571
steroids, 345t
Adrenalin (epinephrine), 19t, 21t, 351, 567
contraindications, 726
Adrenolutin, 98
Adriamycin (Doxorubicin), 399t
Advawet, 526t
*Aedes aegypti* (Mosquito), 741
Aerocyanate, 194t
Aerosect Ant Preventive, 159t
Aerosect Fly Spray, 159t
Aerosol(s), 325, **608-609**
Aerosol (AY, C-61, MA, OS, OT, SE, 18), 526t
Aerosporin, (*see* Polymyxin B sulfate)
*Aesculus* (buckeye), 549t
Afcophene, 159t
Aflatoxin, 604, 715
Agar-agar, 708t
*Agaricus campestris*, 556t
*Agave lecheguilla* (lechugilla), 548t
Agglutinins, 566, 574
Agicide Aerosol Bombs, 171t
Agicide Crab Grass Killer, 194t
Agicide Dog and Cat Flea Powder, 159t
Agicide Fly Spray, 159t
Agicide Houseplant Aerosol Bomb, 159t
Agicide Maggot Killer, 159t
Agicide Rat and Mouse Bait, 194t
Agicide Roach and Ant Powder, 159t
Agicide Rose Aerosol Bomb, 159t
Agicide Sabadust, 159t
Agicide Weed Wilt, 194t
Agicide Yellow Dot Fungicide, 194t
*Agkistrodon* (Moccasins, Copperheads), **562,** 564f
*mokeson* (venemous copperhead or highland moccasin) **562,** 564f
*piscivorus* (water moccasin or cotton-mouth), 562, 564f
Agranulocytosis, drugs and chemicals causing, 13-15t
Agrimul, 526t
Agritox Agrithion Dust, 159t
Agritox Cryolite Dust, 159t
Agro, 194t
*Agrostemma githago* (corn cockles), 549t
Ahcovel E, 526t
Ahcowet (ANS, N, RS), 526t, 527t
Air pollutants, Table 79 (329)
Air pollution, **322-330** (with figure and tables)
in the home, **327-329**
radioactive (fallout), **329-330**
Air Quality Act of 1967, 327
Air-Tox Household Aerosol Bomb, 159t
Ajax, 525, 527t
Akineton (Biperiden hydrochloride), 376
ALA (Delta-aminolevulinic acid), (*see* Delta-aminolevulinic acid)
Albamycin, (*see* Novobiocin)
Albasol BF, 527t
Albatex POK Paste, 527t
Albino Bleach Solution ("A", "B"), 527t
Albumin (Albumisol), 68t, 70, 144, 180, 389, 466, 544, 644t
Bilirubin binding, 124-125 (with table), 449
Albumisol, (*see* Albumin)
Alco Fly Cake, 159t
Alcohol(s), 6t, 7t, 8t, 9t, 35t, 86, 95t, 96t, 103, 110t, 115, 117t, 123, 181, 202, **209-219,** 274t, 334t, 366t, 437, 442, 443t, 456, 479, 518t, 523t, 524t, 533, 536, 538, 555, 628, 635
acetone, (*see* Wood alcohol)
allyl, **217,** 247t, 729t
amyl, 94t, 212, **217,** 729t
butyl, 94t, 95t, 212, 636, 729t
n-butyl, 87t
cetyl, 95t, **218,** 629
contraindications, 181, 454, 568
crisis, 64
cyclohexyl, 729t
dehydrogenase, 209, 213, 218
denatured, 94t, 95t, **216**
diacetone, 729t
ethyl, 6t, 20t, 36, 51t, 75, 77, 85, 87t, 89, 94t, 95t, 96t, 97t, 202, **209-212,** 213, 216, 217, 218, 220t, 247t, 271t, 454, 533, 536, 617, 649, 658
fetal syndrome, 103, 112t, 210
iso-amyl, (*see* Alcohol, amyl)
isopropyl, 4f, 94t, 95t, 97t, 89, **216-217,** 220t, 247t, 533, 636
methyl, 6t, 7t, 8t, 41, 51t, 58, 85, 87t, 89, 94t, 95t, 97t, 192, 193, 202, 212, **213-216,** 219, 220t, 533, 647, 727
octyl, 730t
propyl, 212, 730t
rubbing, (*see* Alcohol isopropyl)
tables:
approximate blood percentage, Table 59(211)
drug interactions with, Table 60 (214-215)
toxic substitutes, Table 61 (220)
terpene, 521, 636
tertiary amyl, 97t, 483t
tertiary butyl, 216
wood, 213, 649, **727-728**
Alcoholic liquors, **212-213**
beverages, % alcohol/volume, 212
Alcoholics Anonymous, 211
Alcopara (Hydroxynaphthoate), 354t
Aldactone, (*see* Spironolactone)
Aldarsone, (*see* Phenarsone sulfoxylate)
Aldehyde(s), 202, **219-222,** 274t, 324t, 327
gases, 647
Alder, striped or spotted (witch hazel) **657-658**
black *(Ilex opaca)*, 550t
Aldomet (Methyldopa), 15t, 16t, 81t, 494t
Aldrin, 126, 128, 130t, 137t, 159t, 161t, 169t, 734t
Ale, 212
*Aleurites fordii* (tung nut), 554t
Alexyl Disinfectant, 527t
Alfalfa *(Medicago sativa)*, 548t
Algae, producing photosensitization, 548t
Algaecides, 609, 610
Algin, **649**
Alginate, sodium (Algin), (*see* Sodium alginate)
Aliphatic
amines, 183, 313t
hydrocarbons, 87t, 224, 225, 609, 611, 636
thiocyanate (rhodanates), 170
Alkali(s), 8t, 9t, 45, 51t, 88, 94t, 97t, 148, **229-234,** 234t, 344, 454, 517
burns, 47
caustic, 51t, 94t, 182
dilute, 95t
chlorinated, 202, **232-233**
corrosive, 7t, 202, **229-234,** 721
neutralizing agents, **83**
therapy, 58
Alkaloids, 33, 39, 42, 45, 46, 55t, 84, 86, 366t, 538
ergot, **423-426**
rauwolfia, 371, 498t
Alkanolamines, 522t, 523t, 524t
Alkeran (Melphalan), 369t
Alkron, 159t
Alkylamines, 365t, 367t
Alkyl aryl sodium sulfates, 518t, 519
Alkyl aryl sulfonate, 94t, 233
Alkylating agents, polyfunctional, 369t
Alkyl-benzene sulfonate (ABS), 331, 518
Alkylphenyl polyethoxyethanol, (*see* Detergents [non-anionic])
Alkyl sodium isothionates, 519
Alkyl sulfates, sodium, 519, 522t
All detergent, 527t
Allen Tomato Dust, 194t
Allen Weed (Potato Vine) Killer, 194t
Allergens, 117t, 323
Allergies to food, **719**

Allethrin, 158t
pyrethrum, 157
Allopurinol (Zyloprim), 16t, 79t, 143t, 347t, 404, 481, 482t
Alloxans, 12t
All-Plan, 159t
Alltox 5 Bait, 159t
Allyl
alcohol, (*see* Alcohol, allyl)
bromide, 190
chloride, 190
cinerin, 158t
Allylisothiocyanate (oil of mustard), 495t, 659
N-allylnormorphine hydrochloride, (*see* Nalline)
Almond, 532
*Alocasia* (Arum family), 548t
Aloe, 122, 406t
Aloin, 117t
Alopecia, chemicals and drugs producing, 143t
Alpha-chloracetophenone, 654
Alpha-citral, 613
Alpha-lipoic acid, 556
Alpha-methyldopa, 40, 143t
Alphanaphthalene acetic acid, 182
Alpha-naphthol, 191
Alpha-naphthoquinone, 191
Alphanaphthylthiourea, (*see* ANTU)
Alphazurine 2 G, 609
Altafur, (*see* Furaltadone)
Althose syrup (Methadone hydrochloride), 117t
Alum (Aluminum ammonium sulfate) 350
ammonium, 653
chrome, 614t
Aluminum, 42, 269, 270t, 513t, 524t
acetate, 255, 350, 612
ammonium sulfate (Alum), 350
chloride, 350
hydroxide, 12t, 20t, 31, 83, 350, 438, 480
oxide, 311t
phosphate, 350, 644
pneumoconiosis, 323t
salts, 94t, 95t, 536
silicates, 315
sulfate, 615t
Alurate, (*see* Aprobarbital)
*Amanita* (mushrooms), 98, 547, 552t
*brunnescens,* 557f
*muscaria,* 358t, 547, 555, 556f
*phalloides,* 13t, 62t, 65t, 547, 555, 556(f)
*rubescens,* 557f
*verna,* 558
*verosa,* 558
Amanita toxins, 555
Amanitin, 555, 559t
Amantadine hydrochloride (Symmetrel), 119t, 482t
Amaze, 525
Ambenonium chloride (Mytelase), 117t, 482t
Amdil (Acetaminophen), 117t
A-Mean, 194t
Amebiasis, 592
American Academy of Pediatrics, Committee on Fetus and Newborn, 628
local branches working with poison control centers, 661
Subcommittee on Accidental Poisoning, 153
American Association of Poison Control Centers (AAPCC), 699ft, 700
American Conference on Governmental Industrial Hygientists, 221, 320, 657
American Hospital Association, 211
American laurel *(Kalmia)*, 551t
American Medical Association, 532
Committee on Toxicology, 532
Council on Industrial Health, 726
Department of Environmental Health, 327
American Standards Association, 261
Ames test, 273, 534
Amiben (Vegiben), 188t
Amicar (Aminocaproic acid), 482t
Amides, 352t
Amidoazotoluene (Toluazotoluidine), 482t
Amidopyrine, 97t
Amines,
aliphatic, 183, 313t
tricyclic, secondary, 65t
tricyclic, tertiary, 65t
9-Aminoacridine, 609
Amino-azotoluene (scarlet red), 499t
Aminobenzoate, sodium, methyl, ethyl-p-, 12t, 95t, 536
Aminobenzoic acid, 455
p- (PABA), 94t, 347t, 456
Amino benzol (Aniline), 203
4-Aminobiphenyl, 331t
Aminocaproic acid (Amicar), 482t
5-Amino-2,3-dihydro-1,4-phthalazinedione (Luminol), (*see* Luminol)
Amino-glutethimide (Elipten), 363t, 482t
p-Aminohippurate, 482t
p-Aminohippuric acid, 206, 482t
Aminometradine (Mictine), 482t
Aminophenol(s), 12t, 237
Aminophylline, 19t, 20t, 21t, 334t, **480-481,** 513t
as a treatment in poisoning, 31, 75, 251, 631
Aminopterin (4-Aminopteroylglutamic acid), (*see* Methotrexate)
Aminopteroylglutamate, sodium (Aminopterin) (*see* Methotrexate)
Aminopyrine, 10t, 13t, 339, 343t, 346t, 347t, **457**
Aminoquinoline(s)
4- , 460
8- , 338
Aminosalicylic acid (PAS), 11t, 15t, 77, 79t, 117t, 118t, 339, 343t, 347t, 355t, 437t, 482t
derivatives, 11t
Aminothiazole, 313t
Aminotriazole (Amizol), 182
Amiphenazole, 482t
Amisometradine (Rolicton), 483t
Amitriptyline (Elavil, Triavil), 10t, 11t, 358t, 359, 369t, 375t, 442, 443t, 472, 474, 513t
Amitrole (Aminotriazole, Weedazol), 188t
-T (Cytrol), 188t
Amizole, (*see* Aminotriazole)
Ammate X Herbicide, 194t
Ammonia, 8t, 65t, 85, 97t, 202, **234**(t), 245, 324t, 513t, 526, 534, 535, 621, 648t
aromatic spirits of, 20t, **31**
gas, 138, 247t, 526
water, 31, 94t, 721
concentrated, 28
Ammoniated mercury, 95t, 483t
Ammonium,
acetate, as a treatment in poisoning, **31,** 51t
alum, 653
bromide, 392
carbonate, 244
chloride, 101, 105t, 110t, 393, 459, 460, 461, 483t, 519, 523t, 611, 614t
ferric sulfate, 615t
ferrous sulfate, 615t
hydroxide, 20t, 31, 51t, 94t, 202, 233t, **234**(t), 523t, 524t, 533, 615t
nickel sulfate, 615t
nitrate, 94t, 621
phosphate, 621
picrate, **234**
quaternary compounds, 97t, 184, 470, 519, 525
salts, 183, 194t, 532, 656
sulfate, 621
sulfide, 95t, **237-239**
thioglycolate, 312
Amobarbital, 13t, 65t, 72t, 379t, 383t, 388, 503t
sodium (Amytal), 104t, 117t
Amodiaquin, 13t
hydrochloride (Camoquin hydrochloride), 460, 483t
*Amorphophallis* (Arum family), 548t
Amosite, 317
Amphenidone (Dornwal), 483t
Amphetamine(s), 7t, 9t, 31, 53t, 62t, 65t, 85f, 92t, 93t, 97t, 99, 101, 104t, 112t, 117t, 143t, 346t, 348t, 359, 360, 386, 416, 443t, 453, 470, 471, 513t, 722t (*see also* Sympathomimetic amines)
contraindications, 373
derivatives, 7t, 9t, 369t, 373
sulfate (Benzedrine), 117t
d-Amphetamine sulfate (Dexedrine), 19t, 35, 117t, 367
Amphotericin B (Fungizone), 79t, 355t

and tetracycline (Mysteclin-F), 357t
Ampicillin, 17t, 65t, 118t, 715
Amprotropine phosphate, 378
A.M.R. Insect Killer, 171t
AMS (Ammate), 188t
Amygdalin, 235, 236, 637
Amyl
acetate, (*see* Acetate, amyl)
alcohol, (*see* Alcohol, amyl)
nitrite, ( *see* Nitrite, amyl)
Amylene dichloride, 94t
Amylene hydrate (tertiary amyl alcohol), 97t, 483t
Amytal (Amobarbital), 117t, 379t, 383t
sodium (Amobarbital sodium), 19t, **41,** 71, 72t, 83
Anabolic agents, 359
*Anacardium occidentale* (cashew nut), 549t
Ana-Kit, 578ft
Analeptics, 204
Analgesics, 65t, 409
CNS, 12t
causing hemolysis in G-6-PD deficiency, 343t
narcotic, 117t
non-narcotic, 117t
public spending on, 332f
reactions in the aged, 345t
suicidal deaths, 334, 335t, 336t, 337f
urinary, 12t
Anap, 194t
Ancylostomiasis (dog hookworm), 592
Androgens, 80t, 110t, 347t, 348t, 359, 402t
Anectine, 338t
Anelix (Acetaminophen), 117t
Anemia(s)
drug-induced, Table 6 (13-15)
drug-induced hemolytic, **336-344** (with table)
Anesthesia, reactions in the aged, 345t
Anesthetics, 112t, 117t, 339, **426-427,** 443t
general, 7t, 9t, **351**
local, 7t, 112t, **351-353**
Table, 100
Angel hair (Christmas decoration), **740**
"Angel dust", 101
"Angel's trumpet", (*see Datura suaveolens*)
Anhydride,
carbonic acid gas, (*see* Carbon dioxide)
phthalic, 313t
Anhydron (Cyclothiazide), 469
Anhydro-o-sulfamine benzoic acid (Saccharin), 499t, 651
*Anicularíidae heteropodidae* (tarantula), **574**
Aniline, 7t, 13t, 65t, 82t, 95t, 97t, 202, **203-204**, 247t
derivatives, 7t, 12t, 17, 202, **203-204**
dyes, 10t, 37, 64, 224, 534, 632
Anilinoethanol, 12t
Animals (*see also* Zoonoses)
common poisons, Table 146 (605-606)
drug toxicity compared with man, Table 17(26)
Anionic detergents, (*see* Detergents)
Anisakiasis, **715**
Anise
Japanese star, 554t
oil, 453
Anisindione (Miradon), 11t, 17t
Anisotropine (Valpin), 358t
Annatto (food additive), 709t
Annelid
diseases (zoonoses), 598t
worms, 583, 585, 587t
*Anopheles* (mosquito), 741
Ansar, 187t
560-120, 187t
Ant(s), 579 (*see* individual listings)
Antabuse (Disulfiram), 81t, 181, 209, 211, 214t, 239, 429, 555
Antacid(s), 12t
Antazoline, 343t, 420
Ant-Foil, 159t
Anthelmintics, 12t, **353-354** (with table)
Anthophyllite, 317, 319
Anthozoa (elk horn coral), 584
Anthracene, 455
Anthralin, 346t, 483t
Anthraquinone(s), 10t, 122, 124
*Anthurium* (Araceae family), 543
Antiarrhythmic drugs,
adverse effects of, Table 20 (49)
dosages of, Table 19 (48)
Antibacterial agents, 11t, 12t, 536, 609
Antibactericidin, 566
Antibiotic(s), **82-83,** 116, 117t, 120, 122, 219, 225, 253, 267, 271, 355t, 370, 390, 431, 436, 447, 480, 503t, 567, 568, 584, 589, 645, 648, 712, 734t (*see also* individual drugs)
contraindications, 224
dosage in premature and newborn infants, Table 45 (121)
residues, **719-720**
Antichlorine compounds, 609, 610
Anticholinergics, 39
alkaloids, 358
compounds, **358-359,** 366t
syndrome produced by drugs and chemicals, 358t
Anticholinesterase, 134, 135, 358, 378, 566
Anticoagulants, 11t, 12t, 55t, 124, 143t, 214t, 566
and food interactions, 334t
drugs that diminish response of, 503t
drugs that increase response of, 503t
drugs whose effects are increased by, 503t
Anticonvulsants, 11t, 477
effects on fetus and newborn, 102, 112t
for epileptic therapy, **359-364** (with table)
untoward reactions, Table 104 (362-363)
Antidepressants, 11t
combinations, 369t
MAO inhibitors, 369t
miscellaneous, 369t
tricyclic drugs, 15t, 16t, 81t, **472-474**
Antidote(s), 11t, **47,** Table 21 (50-55)
universal, **45**
Anti-flea dog and cat collars, 136
Antifreeze, poisonous substances in, 95t
Antigens
causing hypersensitivity pneumonitis, Table 76 (322)
animal, 322t
bacterial, 322t
molds, 322t
plants, 322t
Antihistamines, 6t, 7t, 110t, 156, 214t, 339, 346t, **364-367,** 370, 372, 420, 428, 535, 573, 575, 578, 579, 582, 584, 719
common interactions, Table 106 (366)
contraindications, 349, 568
dosages, Table 105 (365-366)
duration of actions, Table 105 (365-366)
effects, Table 105 (365-366)
generic names, Table 105 (365-366)
lethal doses, 97t
trade names, Table 105 (365-366)
Antihistaminics, 117t
Antihypertensives, reactions to, 433t
Anti-infective agents, reactions in the aged, 345t
Antilirium (Physostigmine salicylate), 39, 54t, 376, 472
Antimalarials, 455
Antimetabolites, 124, 345t
Antimicrobials, 343t, 603, 628
in aquarium products, 609, 610
in breast milk, Table 44 (118-119)
interaction with alcohol, Table 60 (214)
Antimony, 32, 53t, 82t, 91, 97t, 127, **155,** 202, 269, 270t, 339, 346t, 633, **716**
chloride, 94t
compounds, 7t, 35t, 347t, 354t
hydride (Stibine), 155, 202
lactophenate, 168
potassium tartrate, 155t
salts, 739
sulfide, 155, 736, 737, 738
trichloride ("Butter of antimony"), 155, 373
trisulfide, 737
Antineoplastic agents, 16t
Antiparasitics, 609
Antiparkinson drugs, 443t
interaction with antihistamines, 366t
Antiprotozoal agents, 11t, 12t
Antipyretics, 182, 183, 336t, 338t, 409, 461
Antipyrine, 7t, 12t, 35t, 97t, 116, 339, 343t, 346t, 347t, **457**
Antirabies Prophylaxis, Table 144 (593)
Anti-riot gas (Mace), **250**
Antirot, 194t
Anti-rust products, poisonous substances in, 95t
Antithyroid drugs, 124

Antitoxin, 567, 603
botulinus (A,B,E), 20t, **713-714**
tetanus, 347t, 568, 589
Antituberculosis drugs, Table 123 (437)
Antivenin(s), 52t, 567 (*see* specific antivenins)
Antivenin Index Center, 568
Ant-Not Ant Trap, 159t
Antrenyl bromide, (*see* Oxphenonium bromide)
Ant-Roach Killer, 160t
Antrol, 194t
Antrol African Violet and House Plant Bomb, 159t
Antrol Ant Killer, 159t
Antrol Ant Powder, 171t
Antrol Ant Spray, 159t
Antrol Ant Syrup, 159t
Antrol Ant Trap, 159t
Antrol Lawntrol Granules, 160t
Antrol Push Button Ant and Roach Bomb, 171t
Antrol Rush Spray Flower Bomb, 171t
ANTU (Alphanaphthylthiourea), 97t, 173, **176-177,** 179t, 194t, 195t, 196t, 198t, 734t
Ant-X Ant Traps, 160t
Ant-X Jelly Bait, 160t
Apamide (Acetaminophen), 117t
Aphamite, 160t
Apiol, 8t, 479, 483t
*Apis mellifera* (honeybee), 575
Aplastic anemia
chemical causing, 13-15t
drug reactions causing, 339-340t
*Aplopappus heterophyllus* (rayless goldenrod), 539, 553t
*Apocynaceae* (dogbane), 540
Apomorphine, 35, 42, 43, 44, 373, 391, 444ft
contraindications, 43, 211, 445
hydrochloride, 19t, 44, 83, 420
hypodermic tablets, 31
Appendix
pamphlets and other media, 744-751
normal laboratory values used in the diagnosis and treatment of poisoning, 752-772
drugs that may alter normal laboratory values, 752-755
Apresoline (Hydralazine), 15t, 40, 345t, 490t
Aprobarbital (Alurate), 35t, 383t
Aqua fortis, 609
Aqualin Herbicide, 160t, 187t
AquaMEPHYTON (Phytonadione), 22t, 479
Aquarium
products, **609-610**
salts, 610
Aquathol, 187t
Arab Rat and Mouse Killer, 194t
Arab U Do-it Termite Control, 160t
Ara-C (Cytarabine, Cytosine arabinoside, Cytosar), 397t
Araceae, 543
Aralen (Chloroquine), (*see* Chloroquine)
Aramine bitartrate (Metaraminol), 22t, 133, 385
Aramite, 196t
Arasan, 194t
Arbor vitae (thuja), **655**
Arbutin, 10t, 656
*Areca catechu* (betel nut), 483t, 548t
Arecoline, 8t, 32, 483t
*Argemone mexicana* (Mexican poppy), 552t
Argo Gloss Laundry Starch, 650
Argon, 657
*Arisaema triphyllum* (jack-in-the-pulpit), 551t
Armazide (Algicide), 653
Arnica, 483t, 548t
*Arnica cordifolia, montana, sororia,* 548t
Arnofos detergent, 527t
Aromatic(s), **610**
hydrocarbons, 224, 225, 609, 610, 636
solvent, 184, 658
solvents, 187t, 610
spirits of ammonia, 31
Arrow grass, 606
Arsenate
calcium, 144, 160t, 161t, 164t, 165t, 166t, 167t, 168t, 187t, 194t, 197t
disodium methyl, 194t, 195t, 196t, 197t, 199t, 200t
lead, (*see* Lead arsenate)
sodium, 644t
Arsenic, 6t, 7t, 8t, 31, 32, 35t, 46, 53t, 56t, 65t, 69, 82t, 87, 91, 94t, 115, 117t, **138-140,** 143t, 164t, 165t, 167t, 168t, 194t, 195t, 198t, 201t, 202, 269, 270t, 271t, 272t, 311t, 314, 331t, 335t, 391, 496t, 513t, 604, 605t, 618, 620, 633, 646, 716
compounds, 45, 127, 173
salts, 739
sulfides, 738
trioxide, 13t, 62t, 85, 138, 155t, 159t, 194t, 196t, 199t, 200t, 488t
trisulfide, 647
Arsenicals, 7t, 82, 339, 346t, 347t, 455
Arsenious iodide, 619
Arsenite(s), 734t
lead, (*see* Lead arsenite)
potassium (Fowler's solution), 489t
sodium, 159t, 163t, 167t, 169t, 170t, 182, 187t, 194t, 195t, 196t, 197t, 198t, 199t, 201t
Arsenobenzene, 367
Arsine, 7t, 13t, 82t, 202, 247t, 324t
gas, 138
Arsonate, calcium propyl, 196t
disodium methyl, 201t
Arsphenamine, 62t, **367-370**
Arsthinol (Balarsen), 483t
Artane (Trihexyphenidyl), 104t, 143, 266, 373, 483t
Arthropods, **570-581**
diseases of animals (zoonoses), 599t
habits and effects, Figure 27 (576)
Artificial kidney, (*see* Extracorporeal dialyzer)
Artificial respiration, **59-61** (with figure)
Artox, 194t
Arum family, 548t
Arwell Fly Spray, 160t
Arwell Moth and Insect Spray, 171t
Arwell Rat and Mouse Bait, 194t
Arwell Roach Spray, 160t
Arwell Super Spray, 160t
Asbestos, 115, 311t, 316, 317
Asbestosis, 314, **316-318**, 323t, 331t
Ascorbate sodium (ascorbic acid), 19t, 31
Ascorbic acid, 18, 19t, 20t, 31, 37, 102, 152, 180, 343t, 344, 474, 659, 708t
Ash
as air pollutant, 324t
poison (*Rhus vernix*), 539, 553t
soda, 94t, 96t
ASL Spray Base, 160t
"Asp" (*Megalopyge opercularis*), 579
Asparaginase, (*see* L-asparaginase)
*Aspergillus*
*clavatus,* 322t
*flavus,* 322t, 558, 604, 606t
*fumigatus,* 322t
*Aspidium,* 97t, 483t
*oleoresin* (male fern), 353t
Aspirin, 4f, 9, 13t, 30, 36, 81t, 117t, 143t, 187t, 339, 343t, 345t, 347, 348, 452, 461, 463, 465, 477, (*see* Salicylates)
Assassin bugs, 579
Asterol (Diamethazole), 417
*Asthenosoma jimoni* (red sea urchin), 587t
Asthma
materials and industrial exposures associated with, Table 75 (313)
potters' (silicosis), 314
Asthmador, 93, 358t, 376
ATA (Aurintricarboxylic acid), (*see* Aurintricarboxylic acid)
Atabrine (Quinacrine), 7t, 11t, 79t, 214t, 354t, 459, 460
Ataractics, **370-376** (with table), 449
Atarax (Hydroxyzine), 15t, 118t, 366t
Atlacide Weed Killer, 188t, 194t
Atlas A, 194t
Triox, 187
Atomic absorption spectroscopy (AAS), 260
Atomic Bomb Casualty Commission, 329
Atox, 160t
Atrazine, 188t, 609
*Atropa belladonna* (deadly nightshade), 358t, 376, 544, 550t
Atropine, 6t, 7t, 8t, 9t, 21t, 32, 35t, 39, 45, 54t, 55t, 93, 97t, 101, 104t, 117t, 133, 134, 136, 157, 174, 238, 358t, **376-378,** 392, 408, 413, 415, 420, 421, 422, 423, 450, 452, 458, 473, 475, 480, 490t, 546t, 555, 579
contraindications, 122, 124, 135, 183
sulfate, 19t, 31, 52t, 421t, 424, 488t, 555
Auramine, 483t
Aurantia, 483t

Aureomycin, (*see* Chlortetracycline)
Aurintricarboxylic acid (ATA), 253
Aurothioglucose, (*see* Gold)
Aurothioglycanide, (*see* Gold)
Aurothionalate, (*see* Gold)
Authocyanin, 10ft
Autumn crocus, (*see* *Colchicum*)
Avadex, 187t
*Avena sativa* (oats), 548t
Aventyl (Nortriptyline), 358t, 472, 495t, 515t
Avertin (Tribromoethanol), 20t, 32, 72t, 471
Avlosulfon (Dapsone), (*see* Dapsone)
Avon Annalos Weed Killer, 194t
Axion, 525
Axurwhite Bleach, 527t
5-Azacytidine, 403t
Azak, 188t
Azapetine, 483t
Azathioprine (Imuran), 80t, 455, 483t
Azene, (*see* Clorazepate)
Azide-iodine, sodium, reaction, 239
Azine, 455
Azinphosethyl (Ethyl guthion), 137t
Azinphosmethyl (Methyl guthion), 137t
Azo dyes, 534
Azo Gantanol, 12t
Azo-Gantrisin, 11ft, 12t
Azolesterase, 378
Azolid (Phenylbutazone), 16t, 79t
Azotrex, 11ft
Azulfidine (Salicylazosulfapyridine), 11t, 338, 483t
Azure A, 203
Azurite, 615t

**B**

Bab-O-Ant and Roach Killer, 160t
Bab-O-Fly and Mosquito Killer, 160t
Bacikicide, 160t
Bacilicide Disinfectant, 527t
*Bacillus subtilis,* 322t, 450, 525
Bacitracin, 65t, 121t, 355(t), 702
Bacterial diseases epidemiology, animals (zoonoses), 594-595t
Bacteriostatic sulfonamides, 429
Bactocill (Oxacillin), 119t
Bactrim, 343t
Bagasse, 320
Bagassosis, 314, **320-321,** 323t
Bagworms, **731**
BAL (2,3-Dimercaptopropanol; dimercaprol; British anti-lewisite),
  contraindications, 254, 646
  in oil, 19t
  use in treatment of poisoning, 29, 32, 36, 41, 46, 139, 143, 147, 148, 155, 263, 264, 265, 266, 267, 338t, 341, 343t, 370, 392, 460, 608
Balantidiasis, 592
Balarsen, 483t
Bald-faced hornet, 577
Ball-point pen(s), poisonous substances in, 95t
Balsam of Peru, 496t, **610**
Banafly Bait, 160t
Banana
  oil (amyl acetate), **222**
  peel, dried, 108t
Banarat Bits, 194t
Banarat Premix, 194t
Bandane, 187t
Baneberry (*Actaea spicata*), 548t
Banthine bromide (Methantheline bromide), 493t
BAPN (Beta-aminopropionitrile), (*see* Beta-aminopropionitrile)
Barban (Carbyne), 188t
Barbital (Veronal), 35t, 65t, 379t, 383t, 513t
  sodium (Medinal), 35t, 83
Barbiturates, 6t, 7t, 8t, 9t, 35t, 71, 74t, 92t, 93t, 97t, 103, 112t, 116, 117t, 123, 129, 176, 178, 179t, 219, 249, 334, 335, 336, 338t, 339, 346t, 347t, 352, 359, 366, 367, 371, 373, 376, 377, **378-391,** 394, 404, 405, 411, 417, 437, 438, 442, 443t, 444, 446, 449, 452, 455, 456, 460, 468, 471, 472, 473, 480, 513t, 519, 568, 571, 589, 655, 722t
  blood levels at conscious return, Table 111 (383)
  contraindications, 341, 211
  interaction with alcohol, Table 60 (214)
  intoxication, 33, 36, 37, 38, 64, 66, 67, 73, 93, **378-391**
    treatment of, Table 112 (388)
  physicochemical properties of common, Table 110 (379)
  psychotic states with abuse of, 104t
  screening tests, 85f, 86, 92t, 390
  thio, 93t
Barbituric acid, (*see also* Barbiturates)
  derivatives, 86, 87, 336t, 360, 378
  chemical structure of, Figure 15 (379)
Barco Animal and Dairy Spray, 160t
Barekil, 160t
Baritosis, 323t
Barium, 6t, 7t, 8t, 9t, 37, 38, 54t, 62t, **173-174,** 269, 270t, 271, 315, 633, 739
  carbonate, 173, 179t, 734t
  chloride, 173
  fluoride, 734t
  fluosilicate, 173
  hydroxide, 173, 533
  nitrate, 173, 738
  soluble salts, 37, 97t, 738, 739
  sulfate, 173, 626, 653
  sulfide, 173, 535
    hydrate, 173
Barracuda (*Sphyraena*), 582, 583
  great, 586t
Base(s), (*see* individual listings)
Basicop, 194t
Bass, sea, 583
Batteries, **610-611**
Bauxite fume fibrosis (Shaver's disease), **318-319**
Baytex (Entex; Fenethion), 137t
BCNU (Carmustine), 400t
B-complex vitamins, (*see* Vitamins)
Beacon Ant Killer, 160t
Beacon Paste Wax, 527t
Beacon "Quick Gloss" Wax, 527t
Bead, Buddhist rosary, Indian, Seminole, (*see* Jequirity bean)
Bean, seed, 614t, (*see also* individual beans)
Beaver poison (*Cicuta virosa*), 554t
Bedbugs, 579
Bee(s), 741 (*see also* individual bees)
  sting, **575-580**
    prevention of, 743
  venom, 82t
Bee Brand Ant and Flea Killer, 160t
Beechnut (*Fagus sylvatica*), 548t
Beechwood creosote, 96t
Beer, 212, 443t, 444t
Beeswax, 95t
Beetles, 741
  blister (*Epicanta fabricii*), 578
Beets, causing urine color change, 10t
Beilstein test, 189
Belladonna, 6t, 7t, 8t, 9t, 93, 339, 346t, 358(t), **376-378,** 425t, 545 (*see also* Atropine)
Bellafoline, 424t, 425t
Bellergal, spacetabs, tablets, 424t
Bells Cleaning Fluid, 527t
Bemegride (Megimide), 8t, 37, 386, 427, 456, 494t
Benactyzine (Deprol), 358t, 369t
Benadryl (Diphenhydramine hydrochloride), 19t, 20t, 21t, 97t, 117t, 133, 358t, 373, 431, 455, 487t, 514t
Bendectin, 365t
Bendroflumethiazide (Naturetin), 469
Benedict's solution (Alkaline copper sulfate), 615t
Benefin (Balan), 188t
Benemid, (*see* Probenecid)
Benesan, 160t
Benexane (5,50), 160t
Bensulide (Betasan, Presan), 187t
Bentonite, 185, 186
Bentyl, (*see* Dicyclomine)
Benzahex, 160t
Benzaldehyde, 637, 708t, 729t
Benzalkonium chloride (Zephiran chloride), 484t, 519
Benzamide, chlorodiethyl, 193
Benzathine penicillin G (Bicillin, Permapen, Duapen), 357t
Benzedrex, (*see* Propylhexedrine)
Benzedrine (Amphetamine sulfate), 117t, 360, 362t
Benzene, 6t, 7t, 13t, 31, 82, 86, 87t, 94t, 97t, 127, 202, **225-226,** 247t, 513t, 609, 611, 636, **658-659,** 725, **727,** 729t
  alkyl derivatives, 225
  chlorinated, 95t

hexachloride (Lindane), 97t, 126, **129,** 130t, 162t, 331t, 339, 734t
Benzethonium chloride (Phemerol chloride), 484t, 519, 609, 632
Benzex, 160t
Benzidine, 203, 331t
Benzine, 97t, 216, 314
Benzo (a) pyrene, 717
Benzoate
benzyl, 581
caffeine sodium, 33, 468
methyl, (*see* Methyl benzoate)
salts, 611
sodium, (*see* Sodium benzoate)
Benzocaine, 12t, 649
Benzodiazepines, 81t, **364,** 411, 427, 455
Benzoic acid, 453, 484t, **611,** 624, 659
anhydro-o-sulfamine, (*see* Saccharin)
esters, 352t, 410, 610
Benzol, 13t, 62t, 225, 271t, **611,** 632
amino (Aniline), 203
Benzoylcholine chloride, 378
Benzoyl peroxide, 624
3,4-Benzpyrene hydrocarbons, 329t
Benzthiazide (Exna), 469
Benzyl benzoate, 484t, 581
Bephenium, 354t
Bergamot-Rul, 455
Berlou Instant Spray Moth Proofer, 160t
Berries, (*see* individual berries)
Beryllium, 82t, 97t, 202, 252-253, 269, 270t, 311t, 323, 513t
disease (pneumoconiosis), 323t
Beta-aminopropionitrile (BAPN), 231
Beta, beta-dimethyl-cysteine, (*see* Penicillamine)
Beta-butoxy-beta thiocyanodiethyl ether (Lethane 384), 170
Beta-chlor, (*see* Chloral betaine)
Beta-citral, 613
Betahistine hydrochloride (Serc), 484t
Beta-hydroxybutyrate, 209
Betamethasone, 69, 415t
Beta-naphthol, 94t, 191, 353t, 729t
Beta-naphthoquinone, 191
Beta-naphthylamine, 203, 331t
Beta-phenylethylamine tryptamine, 442
Beta-trichlorethane, 207
Betazole (Histalog), 393, 484t
Betel nut (*Areca catechu*), 483t, 548t
Beverages (*see also* individual listings)
acid, **718**
cola, 394
liquors, **212-213**
BHC (Benzene hexachloride), 130t, 160t, 161t, 162t, 163t, 168t
B-Hex, 160t
Bicarbonate, 178, 618
paste, 239
potassium, (*see* Potassium bicarbonate)
sodium, (*see* Sodium bicarbonate)
solution, 409
Bichloride of mercury, 4f, 95t, 717, (*see* Mercury)
Bichromates, 254
Bicillin, (*see* Penicillin)
Bidrin, 160t
Bif Ant and Roach Spray, 160t
Bif Insecticide Powder, 160t
Bif Stinky Control Fluid, 160t
Biguanide, 347t, 429
Bile pigments, causing urine color change, 10t
Bilirubin, 65t, 348
albumin binding, **124-125** (with table), 449
Binapacryl (Morocide), 137t
Bin-Fume, 160t
Bin-Treat, 160t
Biological pesticides, 127, **158-159**
Bionol Disinfectant, 527t
Biotin, 476t
Biperiden hydrochloride (Akineton), 376
Biphenyl, 82t
polychlorinated, 117t, 202, **208**
Bipyridylium methylsulfate or chloride (Paraquat), (*see* Paraquat)
Bird-of-paradise plant *(Strelitzia),* 543, 548t
Bis (chloromethyl [methyl] ) ether, 331t
Bisacodyl, 334t
Biscoumacetate, ethyl (Tromexan), 110t, 117t
Bishop's weed, 537
Bishydroxycoumarin (Dicumarol; Dicoumarin; Dicourmarol; Melitoxin), 110t, 117t, 484t
Bismuth, 10, 53t, 62t, 82t, 91, 94t, 95t, 97t, 269, 270t, 534
compounds, **391-392**
contraindications, 454
glycobiarsol, 391
glycolylarsanilate (Milibis), 12t
nitrate, 450
sodium thioglycolate, 391
sodium triglycollamate, 12t, 391
subcarbonate, 391
subgallate, 391, 392
subnitrate, 12t, 17, 391, 450
subsalicylate, 391
sulfide, 391
Bistrimate (Bismuth sodium triglycollamate), 12t
Bistrium bromide (Hexamethonium bromide), 110t
Bisulfate, sodium, 615t
Bisulfite, sodium, 614t
Bitartrate,
Aramine (Metaraminol), (*see* Aramine bitartrate)
Dihydrostreptomycin, (*see* Dihydrostreptomycin bitartrate)
Levarterenol, (*see* Levarterenol bitartrate)
Levophed, (*see* Levophed bitartrate)
Bites, (*see* Zoonoses)
Biting midges, 576f
Bitter almond, oil of, (*see* Cyanides)
Bitter principle, 657
Bittersweet (*Solanum dulcamara*), 358t, 539, 548t
Biz, 525
B-K Liquid Bleach, 527t
B-K Powder Disinfectant, 527t
Black alder (*Ilex opaca, verticillata*), 550t
Black cherry, (*see* Cherry, black)
Black elderberry (*Sambucus canadensis*), 550t
Black Flag Bug Killer, 160t, 171t
Black Flag Disinfectant, 527t
Black Flag Flea-Tick & Louse Powder, 160t
Black Flag Insecticide Powder, 171t
Black Flag Insect Spray, 171t
Black Flag Moth Ded, 160t
Black Flag Push Button Aerosol Insect Killer, 171t
Black Flag Push Button Flower Bomb, 171t
Black Flag Push Button Roach and Ant Killer, 171t
Black Flag Rat and Mouse Killer, 194t
Black Flag Special Roach Spray, 160t
Black fly, 576f
Black henbane (*Hyoscyamus niger*), 358t, 542f, 548t, 550t
Black laurel (Kalmia), 551t
Black Leaf, 160t, 171t
Black Leaf CPR Insect Killer, 160t
Black Leaf Crabgrass Killer, 194t
Black Leaf 11-36 Insect Killer, 160t
Black Leaf Mash-nic Powder, 160t
Black Leaf Mousekiller Bait, 194t
Black Leaf Pyrenone Insect Killer, 161t
Black Leaf Ready Mixed Bait, 194t
Black Leaf Slug and Snail Pellets, 160t
Black Leaf Spray, 171t
Black Leaf Weedkiller (Arsenical), 194t
Black locust (*Robinia pseudoacacia*), 544, 548t
Black nightshade (*Solanum nigrum*), 358t, 542f, 545, 548t
Black Panther Rat and Mouse Killer, 194t
Black widow spider (*Latrodectus mactans, curacaviensis*), **570-571,** 576f
bites of, 7t, 33, 570-571
venom, 52t, 570-571
Bladex, 160t
Blanket flower (*Gaillardia*), 539
Bleach(es),
chlorine, 4f, 525
common household, contents of, Table 62 (233)
composition of, 523-524t
effects of with household product mixtures, Table 63 (234)
first aid in poisoning by, 721
hair, 233t
optical, 233t
poisonous substances in, 94t
sodium hypochlorite, 233t, 526
sodium perborate, 233t
Bleachette Laundry Blue, 527t
Bleeding heart (*Dicentra pusilla*), 548t

Blenoxane (Bleomycin), 399t
Bleomycin (Blenoxane), 399t
*Blighia sapida* (Ackee, koenig tree), 544, 548t
Blind-X Cleaner, 527t
Blister beetles (*Epicanta fabricii*), 578
Blood,
  barbiturate levels at conscious return, Table 111 (383)
  causing urine color change, 10t
  chemistry values, factors for converting to milli-equivalents per liter, Table 26 (59)
  toxicologic analysis of, 10, **86**
  transfusions, **63-64**
Blood coagulants, as a component of venom, 566
Blood root (*Sanguinaria canadensis*), 549t
Blue Death Rat Killer, 194t
Blue, methylene, (*see* Methylene blue)
Blue nightshade (*Solanum dulcamara*), 542f, 545
Blue requiem shark (Carcharinidae family), 586t
Blue velvet, **611-612**
Bluing, laundry and gun, poisonous substances in, 96t
Blutene (Tolonium chloride; Toluidine blue), 11t, 203
Body fat, toxicologic analysis of, **87**
Body surface area (BSA), Figure 2(27)
  determination of children's doses on basis of, Table 12(23)
Body water needs, guide to maintaining, Table 24(57)
Bold, 525
Bonadoxin (Meclizine and Pyridoxine hydrochloride), 484t
Boncep, 160t
Bone, toxicologic analysis of, 10, **87**
Bonide Ant Dust, 160t
Bonide Lintox, 160t
Bonide Outdoor and Garden Spray, 160t
Bonide Roton Fly Spray, 171t
Bonide Ryatox, 160t
Bonkil Insecticide Powder, 160t
Bontano Liquid Spray, 160t
Bontox, 160t
Bontu Prep. Rat Baits, 194t
Bontu Rat Powder, 194t
Booklets on poisoning, (*see* Appendix A) 744-751
Borate(s), 89, 90, 188t, 615t, 623, 734t
  sodium, 127, **152-153,** 155t, 533
Borax, 96t, 155t, 188t, **612**
  Borassu, 188t
  composition of, 523t
Bordeaux mixture, **612**
Boric acid, 6t, 7t, 65t, 97t, **152-153,** 164t, 411, 477, 513t, 612, 644, 645
Bormeol, 449
Boroglycerin, **612**
  glycerite, 612
Boron, 269, 513t, 623
  hydride (rocket fuel), 270t, **644-645**
Botanical insecticides, 127, **156-158** (with table), 605t
  toxicity of, 158t
Botulinus toxin, 6t, 7t, 8t
  antitoxin (A,B,E), 20t, **713-714**
  exotoxin, **712-714**
Botulism, 97t, **712-714**
Bougienage, 231
Bouquet-Aire Hang-Up Cakes, 160t
Bowlclene, 527t
Bowlene, 527t
Box (*Buxus sempervirens*), 549t
Bracken fern, 606t
Brain, toxicologic analysis of, **86**
Brake fluids, poisonous substances in, 95t
Bramble Weedicide, 194t
Bramblicide Brushkiller, 194t
Brandy, 212
Brasiere disease, 268
Brass founder's ague, 268
*Brassica napus* (cultivated rape), 548t
Brayton Dairy Farm Spray, 161t
Brayton E-M Farm Insecticide, 161t
Brayton's Fly Killer, 161t
Brayton's KO Fly Killer, 161t
Brayton's P-B Insecticide, 161t
Brayton's Raticide Cereal Bait, 194t
Brayton's Residual Insecticide, 161t
Breast milk
  drugs and chemicals in, **115-125**
  hyperbilirubinemia from, 111t
Breath-O-Pine Disinfectant, 527t
Breck's Ant and Earwig Spray, 161t
Breck's Ant Spray, 161t
Breeding
  budgerigars, 322t
  parakeets, 322t
  pigeons, 322t
Breeze, 527t
Bretylium, 48t
Brevital (Methohexital), 117t
Brewer's yeast, 20t, 33
Bridgeport Aer-A-Sol Insecticide, 171t
Bridgeport No. 400 Aer-O-Sol Insecticide, 171t
Bridgeport No. 12 Bug Bomb, 171t
Bridgeport Moth Bomb, 161t
Bridgeport No. 137 Moth Bomb, 161t
Bridgeport No. 424 Mothproofer, 161t
Bright Sail Air Deodorant Purifier, 527t
Bright Sail Bleach, 527t
Bright Sail Insect Killer, 171t
Bright Spot Bleach, 527t
Brildane, 171t
Brilliantines, poisonous substances in, 95t
Broad bean, (*see* Fava bean)
Brochures on poisoning, (*see* Appendix A) 745-747
Bromaceton, 6t
Bromacil (Hyvar X), 188t
Bromat Disinfectant, 527t
Bromate(s), 64, 82, **182-183,** 533
  potassium, 94t, 709t
  sodium, 233t
Bromide(s), 6t, 7t, 55t, 64, 65t, 89, 90, 104t, 112t, 117t, 118t, 122, 124, 336t, 339, 359, 360, 362t, **392-393,** 513t
  allyl, 190
  ammonium, 392
  ethyl, 190
  hexamethonium (Bistrium bromide), 110t
  manifestations of chronic intoxication, 393t
  methantheline (Banthine bromide), 493t
  methyl, 87t, 95t, 186, 187t, **192-193,** 195t, 202, 247t, 500t, 734t
  neostigmine (Prostigmin), 19t, 495t
  oxyphenonium (Antrenyl), 496t
  potassium, 392
  propantheline, 39, 358t, 473
  sodium, 83, 392
  strontium, 738
  tetraethylammonium, 500t
Bromine, 7t, 9t, 10, 247t, 312, 653
  compounds, 326
Bromoacetone (tear gas), 617, 654
Bromobenzene, 33, 52t, 87t, 144, 646
Bromobenzylcyanide (tear gas), 617, 654
Bromochlorodimethyl-hydantoin, 653
Bromoform (Tribromomethane), 484t
Bromomercuri-2-hydroxypropane, 644t
Bromomethylethylketone (tear gas), 617, 654
Bromo-Seltzer, 392
Bromothymol blue, 610
Brompheniramine (Dimetane), 117t, 347t, 513t
Broom weed, 539
Brown mixture, **612**
Brown Rat Poison, 194t
Brown recluse spider (*Loxosceles reclusa*), 70, **571-574** (with figure)
Brown-tail moth, 579
Bruce Cleaning Wax, 527t
Bruce Floor Cleaner, 527t
Bruce Self Polishing Wax, 527t
Bruce Tuf Lustre Wax, 527t
Brucine (alkaloid), 216
  sulfate, 216, 536
*Brugmansia* (herbs), 545
Brulin's 4-X Concentrate, 161t
Brulin's Insecticide Aerosol, 161t
Brulin's Insect Spray, 161t
Brulin's Liquid No-Tox, 161t
Brulin's Moth Spray, 161t
Brulin's Roach & Ant Toxicant, 161t
Brush-Bane, 194t
Brush-Kil, 194t
Brushoff, 194t
Bruweed, 194t
Bubbling lights (Christmas decoration), 739
  poisonous substances in, 95t
Buccinidae (mollusks),
  related species:
    *Buccinum leucostoma*, 582

*Neptunea arthritica,* 582
*Neptunea intersculpta,* 582
*Neptunea antiqua,* 582
Buckeye (*Aesculus*), 544, 549t
Buck moth, 579
Buckwheat (*Fagopyrum sagittatum*), 548t
Buddhist rosary bead, (*see* Jequirity bean)
Budgerigar fanciers, 321, 322t
Bufotenine, 98, 99, 555
*Bufus marinus* (toad), 590
Bug-A-Boo Moth Crystals, 194t
Bug-Ant Doom, 161t
Bug-A-Way, 161t
Bug Blast Aerosol, 171t
Bug Bomb, 161t
Bug Butcher, 161t
Bug-Dust, 171t
Bug-Geta Snail Bait Meal, 161t
Bug-Getta, 194t
Bug-Kill Pellets, 161t
Bulk cathartics, 406t
Bull nettle (*Solanum carolinense*), 554t
Bull requiem shark (Carcharinidae family), 586t
Bumblebee, 576f, 577, 742
Bunamiodyl, 82t
sodium (Orabilex), 484t
Burning bush (*Euonymus atropurpureus*), 549t
Burns,
chemical, first aid, 721
chemical, of the eye, **46-47,** 721
lewisite, 46
Burow's solution (Aluminum acetate), **612,** 621
Burton Cesspool Cleaner, 527t
Burweed, 539
Busulfan (1,4-dimethanesulfonoxybutane), 396t
Butabarbital (Butisol), 65t, 379t, 383t, 503t
Butamben picrate (Butesin picrate), 484t
Butanol, 247t
Butanone, 729t
Butazolidin, (*see* Phenylbutazone)
Butcher's Boston Polish, 527t
Butesin picrate (Butamben picrate), 484t
Butethal (Neonal), 383t
Buti-Glow Silicone Polish, 527t
Butisol, see Butabarbital
Butopyronoxyl, 193, 581
Butoxide, piperonyl, 14t, 170
Butter,
as a demulcent, 83
cocoa, 95t
Buttercup (*Ranunculaceae*), 539, 549t
Butterflies, 741
Butyl
acetate, 94t, 247t, 729t
alcohol, 94t, 95t, 212, 636, 729t
cellosolve, **613,** 729t
methyl, 725
n-Butyl alcohol, 94t, 95t (*see also* Alcohol, butyl)
Butylated hydroxyanisole, 708t
Butylated hydroxytoluene, 708t
Butyl-3,4-dihydro-2,2-dimethyl-4-oxo-2H-pyran-6-carboxylate (Butopyronoxyl), (*see* Butopyronoxyl)
Butyl ethyl propanediol, 193
n-Butyl nitrite, 450
Butyraldoxime, 209
Butyric acid, 613
*Buxus sempervirens* (boxwood), 548t
Byssinosis, 314, **319-320**

**C**

Cabbage, skunk (*Symplocarpus foetidus*), 554t
Cacodylic acid (Ansar 500, 120), 188t
Cactus,
peyotl (*Lophophora williamsii*), 98, 102t, 552t
Caddis flies, 741
Caddy, 194t
Cadmium, 7t, 10t, 32, 53t, 62t, 82t, 97t, 113, 114, 194t, 202, 252t, **253-254,** 255, 262, 269, 270t, 271, 272t, 311t, 314, 331t, 513t, 533, 633, 716
Cafergot PB tablets, suppositories, 92t, 425t
Caffeine, 6t, 9t, 117t, 122, 211, 345t, 347t, 367, 373, **394,** 416, 425t, **480-481,** 484t, 513t, 632
sodium benzoate, 19t, 33, 124t, 468
contraindications, 351
"Caine" (Cocaine) phases, Table 116(411)
Calabar bean (*Physostigma venenosum*), 549t
Caladium (Arum family), 548t
Calamine USP, **612**
Calcium, 65t, 68t, 113, 117t, 120, 252(t), 269, 271, 315, 347t, **394-395,** 409, 410, 455, 519, 520, 626, 630
arsenate, 144, 160t, 161t, 164t, 165t, 166t, 167t, 168t, 187t, 194t, 197t
carbonate (chalk), 83, 229, **395,** 613, 614t, 626, 647, 648
chloride, 21t, 33, 141, 228, 229, **394,** 410, 438, 614t, 644t
cyanamide, 188t, 236, 621, 623
cyclamate (Sucaryl), 455, 486t, 651, 709t
disodium edetate, (*see* EDTA)
disodium versenate, (*see* EDTA)
edathamil, 180
edetate, 253, 254, 266, 268, 540
fluoride, 140, 141
gluconate, 19t, 33, 34, 52t, 62, 141, 144, 190, 218, 228, 229, 263, **394,** 408, 410, 424, 426, 438, 571, 574, 579, 584, 590
hydroxide, 20t, 36, 83, 141, 229, 629
hypochlorite, 524t, 615t, 652
lactate, 20t, 34, 53t, 229, **395**
leucovorin, 404
levulinate, **395**
monophosphate, 614t
nitrate, 615t
oxalate, 228, 229
crystals, 218
oxide, 615t, 629, 630
pantothenate (Modane), 11ft
phanodorn, 35t
phosphate, **395,** 621
polysulfide, **237-239,** 630
salts, 229
sulfate, anhydrous (Plaster of Paris), 636
sulfate, hydrous, 614t, 621
thioglycolate, 94t, 535
trisodium pentetate, (*see* DTPA)
Calgon, 527t
Calgonite, 527t
Calgreen, 194t
Calla lily (Arum family), 543, 548t
Calo-chlor, 194t
Calomel (Mercurous chloride), 117t, 144, 406t, 608
*Caltha palustris* (marsh marigold), 550t
Calvatia family (puffball), 556f
Camas lily (*Zygadenus, Camassia*), 540, 550t
*Camassia* (Camas lily), 540
Camoquin hydrochloride (Amodiaquin hydrochloride), 483t
Camphene, chlorinated (Toxaphene), 126, **129,** 130t
Camphor, 4f, 6t, 7t, 8t, 9t, 35t, 65t, 66, 94t, 97t, **404-405,** 453
in oil, 19t, **404-405,** 224
Camphorated tincture of opium (Paregoric), 422, **453,** 496t
Camp Instant Drain Pipe Cleaner, 527t
*Canavalia gladiata,* see *Vicia faba*
Cancer chemotherapeutic agents, 112t, **395-404** (with table)
some leading occupational agents, 331t
toxicity of, Table 114(396-403)
Candles, **740**
*Cannabis sativa,* (*see* Marihuana)
Cantharides, 7t, 8t, 35t
Cantharidic acid, 405
Cantharidin (Spanish fly, Cantharone), 94t, 97t, **405,** 484t, 578
Cantharone (Cantharidin), 484t
Cantil, (*see* Mepenzolate)
Capastat (Capreomycin), 15t
sulfate (Capreomycin sulfate), 437t, 484t
Capreomycin (Capastat), (*see* Capastat)
Caproate, hydroxyprogesterone (Delalutin), 402t, 490t
Capsicum, 484t
Captan, 194t, 198t, 734t
Carac Ant and Lawn Grub Killers, 161t
Carac Crabgrass Killer, 194t
Carac Kills All Insecticide, 161t
Carac Lawn Weed Killer, 194t
Caramel, 218

Caramiphen (Panparnit) hydrochloride, 157
Carbamate(s) (Carbaryl, Sevin), **136-138,** 196t, 198t, 734t
  chlorphenesin (Maolate), 485t
  dimethyl, 193, 581
  zinc ethylene bisdithio, 194t, 195t
Carbamazepine (Tegretol), 16t, 17t, 80t, **364,** 513t
Carbanilides, halogenated, 455
Carbaryl (Carbamates, Sevin), **136-138,** 731
Carbarsone, 339, 484t
Carbencillin (Geopen, Pyopen), 118t
Carbide, silicon, 331t
Carbimazole, 484t
Carbinol, (*see* Wood alcohol)
Carbitol, 729t
  butyl, 729t
Carbocaine (Mepivacaine), 110t, 352(t)
Carbohydrate, 57t
Carbolic acid, 485t (*see also* Phenol)
Carbon, **326**
  in dry cell batteries, 611
  oxides, **326**
Carbona Cleaning Fluid, 527t
Carbonate(s), 520, 521t, 618
  ammonium, (*see* Ammonium carbonate)
  barium, 37, 173, 179t, 734t
  calcium, (*see* Calcium carbonate)
  creosote, 618
  lead, **255-265,** 434
  lithium, 375t, 630, 631
  magnesium, (*see* Magnesium carbonate)
  potassium, 202, 230, 533, 621
  sodium, 94t, 95t, 139, 180, 202, 230, 233t, 234, 246, 520, 522t, 523t, 524t, 615t, 629, 721
  strontium, 738
Carbon dioxide, 6t, 7t, 9t, 87t, 202, **243,** 247t, 250, 324, 326
  as propellant, 95t
Carbon disulfide, 97t, 195t, 196t, 197t, 202, **237-239,** 247t, 725t
  comparison with acetone, Table 159(725)
Carbonic acid, 58, 326
Carbonic acid gas, anhydride, **243**
Carbonic anhydrase inhibitors, 359, 360, 468
Carbonic Met Metal Cleaner, 527t
Carbon monoxide, 6t, 7t, 9t, 13t, 62t, 65t, 73, 74t, 82t, 85, 86, 87t, 89, 97t, 112t, 202, **239-243,** 247t, 250, 267, 271t, 314, 321, 323, 324(t), 326, 328f, 329t, 334, 513t, 625, 637
  blood percentage producing symptoms, Table 65(242)
  first aid for poisoning, **724**
  poison prevention, **722-724**
Carbon tetrachloride, 6t, 13t, 62t, 65t, 77, 82(t), 86, 87t, 94t, 95t, 97t, 160t, 162t, 168t, 186, **189-190,** 192, 195t, 196t, 197t, 198t, 200t, 201t, 202, 205, 247t, 314, 353t, 471, 513t, 533, 636, 725, **726-727,** 729t, 731, 734t
Carbonyl
  chloride (phosgene), 202, **250-252,** 324t
  nickel, 203, **266-267**
Carboxyhemoglobin, 10, 73, 239, 240, 241
Carboxymethylcellulose, 233
Carbromal, 485t
Carburetor cleaners, poisonous substances in, 95t
Carbutamide, 77, 455
Carcharinidae family (sharks), 586t
Carcinogens, occupational, 331t, 642
Cardiac
  glycosides, 177, 417, 421, 540
  massage closed chest, **61-63** (with figure)
  therapy, **61-63**
Cardiotoxin, 566, 574
Cardiovascular drugs, reactions in the aged, 345t
Carisoprodol (Soma), 485t, 513t
Carmine dye, 534, 714
Carmustine (BCNU), 400t
Carnauba wax, 95t
Carogol, 527t
Carotene(s), 478, 709t
Carpenter bees, **730-731**
Carrageenan, 708t
Carvol (food additive), 708t
Cascara, 10t, 11t, 117t, 122, 406t
Cashew nut (*Anacardium occidentale*), 549t
  oil, 485t
Cassava (*Manihot utilissima*), 549t
Castor bean (*Ricinus communis*), 313t, 322t, 540, 542, 543, 549t
Castor oil, 56t, 95t, 532, 626, 656
  as a cathartic, 7t, 8t, 406t
  emulsion lavage, 30, 427, 449, 454, 480
  plant (*Ricinus communis*), 542
  sulfonated, 95t
Cat
  anti-flea collar, 136
  drug toxicity compared with man, 26t
  scratch disease, 591, 592
Cataria (Catmint, Catnep, Catnip), 546t, **613**
Catecholamines, 334t
Caterpillars (*Megalopyge opercularis*), 579
Catfish, 585
Cathartic(s), 7t, 8t, 11t, 12t, 117t, 347t, **405-408** (with table)
  bulk, 406t
Cathomycin, (*see* Novobiocin)
Cationic detergents, (*see* Detergents)
Catmint (Cataria), **613**
Catnep (Cataria), **613**
Catnip (Cataria), 546t, **613**
Caustic(s), 45
  acids, 182
  alkalis, 182
  soda, 94t
Caustic Poison Act, (*see* Federal Caustic Poison Act)
CDAA (Randox), 187t
CDEC (Vegadex), 187t
Cedarleaf, oil of, 224
Cedar oil, 82, 517
Cedarwood, oil of, 224, 741
Cedar, yellow (thuja), **655**
Cedilanid (Lanatoside C), 19t
Cee-Dee Disinfectant, 527t
Ceepryn chloride (Cetylpridinium chloride), 519
Celandine (*Chelidonium majus*), 549t
Cellosolve, 82t, 94t, 96t, **613,** 729t
  butyl, **613,** 729t
  diethyl, **613**
  ethyl, **613**
  methyl, **613**
Cellulose
  acetate, 95t
  methyl, 652, 708t
Celontin (Methsuximide), 8t, 345t, 361, 363t, 456, 515t
Cement(s), 314
  for jewelry, poisonous substances in, 95t
  plastic, **636**
*Cemophora coccinea* (scarlet snake), 564
Center for Disease Control, 593ft
Centipedes, **574-575**
Central nervous system, see CNS
*Centrurorides gertschii* and *sculpturatus* (scorpions), **574**
Cephaëline, 83
Cephalin, 65t
Cephalopods, 584
Cephaloridine (Loridine), 65t, 356t
Cephalosporins, 16t, 79t, 118t
  antibiotics, 15t
Cephalothin (Keflin), 356t
Ceresan, 194t
Ceresan-M, 194t
Certo-Kill, 161t
Cesium, 269, 270t
Cestode diseases (zoonoses), 597-598t
Cetol Disinfectant, 527t
Cetyl
  alcohol, (*see* Alcohol, cetyl)
  palmitate, 650
  pyridinium chloride (Ceepryn chloride), 519
Cetylon Disinfectant, 527t
Cevadine, 158
Chalk (Calcium carbonate), 83, **613**
Chaperone Insect Killer, 171t
Chapman Roach and Pest Killer, 161t
Charcoal, activated, (*see* Activated charcoal)
Check Pest Livestock Spray, 161t
Check Pest Outdoor Insecticide, 161t
Check Pest Systemic Insecticide, 161t
Cheer, 527t
Chelate, definition, 33
*Chelidonium majus* (Celandine), 549t
Chem-Chlor, 161t
Chem-Drin, 161t

Chem-Fog, 161t
Chemform Fly & Mosquito Aerosol Bomb, 171t
Chemform Home Termite Concoction, 161t
Chemform Turfacide, 161t
Chem-Hex, 161t
Chemical(s)
acne eruptions induced by, **312-313**
and food poisoning, **716-717**
classification of detergents, Table 132(518)
household, poisonous substances in, 95-96t
in breast milk, **115-125**
insecticides, inorganic, 127, **138-155**
pesticides, how to use them, **731-736** (with table)
pollutants to water, 330t
producing alopecia, 143t
producing anticholinergic syndrome, 358t
producing photosensitization, **455-456**
toxic hepatitis, **75-82** (with table)
Chemical burns,
first aid, 721
lewisite, 46
of the eye, **46-47**
Chemical Transportation Emergency Center (CHEMTREC), **159, 170**
Chemistry hobby sets, **613-616** (with table)
Chem-Klor, 161t
Chem-Lin, 161t
Chem-Mite, 161t
Chemotherapeutic(s), 117t, **354-357** (with tables)
for cancer, 112t, **395-404**
toxicity of cancer agents, Table 114(396-403)
Chemrat, 194t
Chem-San, 194t
Chem-Sect Brand Rat Powder, 194t
CHEMTREC (Chemical Transportation Emergency Center), **159, 170**
Chem-Weed P.I. & Brush Killer, 195t
Chenopodium, 485t
oil, 353t
Cherry,
black (*Prunus serotina, demissa, melanocarpa*), 549t, 606
finger (*Rhodomyrtus macrocarpa*), 550t
Jerusalem, 540, 551t
Cherry Coposil Fungicide, 195t
Chicken mushroom, 556f
Chickory, 539
Chiffon Liquid, 527t
Chigger mite, 576f, 580, 581
China berry (*Melia azedarach*), 549t
Chinese restaurant syndrome, (*see* Glutamic acid)
Chipman Fungicide Dust, 195t
Chipman Grain Fumigant, 195t
Chipman Top Killer, 195t
Chipman Toxaphene 8 L, 195t
Chloracetophenone, **616-617**
Chloracne (occupational acne), 311-312
Chloral, 312
betaine (Beta-Chlor), 409
Chloral hydrate, 6t, 7t, 8t, 9t, 33, 65t, 83, 85, 97t, 112t, 118t, 212, 214t, 346t, 377, 404, **408-409,** 448, 471, 485t, 492t, 503t, 513t
Chlorambucil (Leukeran), 77, 80t, 110t, 396t, 485t
Chloramine
fumes, 234t
-T, 313t, 485t
Chloramphenicol (Chloromycetin), 13t, 16t, 65t, 77, 79t, 102, 110t, 117t, 118t, 120, 121t, 214t, 334t, 339, 343t, 344, 347t, 355t, 485t, 503, 702, 715
Chloraniline(s), 12t
Chlorate(s), 7t, 12t, 13t, 17, 37, 64, 85, 97t, 197t, 200t, 734t, 738
potassium, 94t, 96t, 182, 346t, 736-737, 738
sodium, 65t, **182-183,** 188t, 194t, 195t, 198t, 200t, 201t
Chlorax-40, 195t
Chlorbenzide, 734t
Chlor-Clean, 527t
Chlordane (Octachloro-hexahydro-methanoindene), 13t, 97t, 126, 128, 130t, 137t, 159t, 160t, 161t, 162t, 163t, 164t, 165t, 166t, 167t, 168t, 169t, 170t, 311t, 731, 734t
Chlordecone (Kepone), 126
Chlordiazepoxide hydrochloride (Librium), 65t, 77, 104t, 138, 212, 214t, 339, **364,** 514t
Chlordust, 161t
Chlorfectant, 527t
Chlorgran, 161t
Chloride(s), 65t, 117t, 190, 392, 614t, 625
allyl, 190
aluminum, 105t, 350, 393
ambenonium (Mytelase), 117t, 482t
ammonium, 110t, 459, 460, 461, 483t, 519, 523t, 611, 614t
antimony, 94t
barium, 173
benzalkonium, 484t, 519
benzethonium, 484t, 519, 609, 632
benzoylcholine, 378
cadmium, 194t
calcium, (*see* Calcium chloride)
carbonyl (Phosgene), 202, 250-252 (with figure), 324t
Ceepryn, 519
cetylpyridinium, 519
cobalt, 410, 615t
copper, **179-180**
cyanogen, (*see* Cyanogen chloride)
Diaparene, 519
dimethyl tubocurarine (Curare), **415**
edrophonium (Tensilon), 415
ethyl, 190, 426, 471, 488t, 514t
cyclopropane, 351
ferric, 373, 454
test, 463
hydrogen, 247t, 648t
mercuric, 96t, 97t, 145, 155t, 611
mercurous (Calomel), 117t, 406t, 608
methacholine, 493t
methyl, 87t, 186, **192-193,** 202, 247t
methylbenzethonium, 519, 632
methylene, 87t, 94t, 95t, 247t, 515t, 729t, 739
methyl mercury, 149
methylrosaniline (Gentian Violet), 354t, 389t, 494t
nitrosyl, 709t
Phemerol, (*see* Benzethonium chloride)
polyvinyl, 312
potassium, 22t, 58t, 142, 143, 387, 420, 422, 497t, 615t, 621
pralidoxime (2-PAM chloride), (*see* Pralidoxime)
sodium, (*see* Sodium chloride)
Stannic, (*see* Tin)
strontium, 614t, 644t
succinylcholine, 500t
tetraethylammonium, 470, 500t
tolonium (Blutene Toluidine blue), 203
tubocurarine dimethyl, **415**
vinyl, 87t, 149, 312, 314, 331t
vinylidene, 87t
Zephiran, (*see* Benzalkonium chloride)
zinc, (*see* Zinc)
Chlorinated
alkalis, 202, 232-233
benzene, 95t
camphene (Toxaphene), 126, **129,** 130t
compounds, 7t
hydrocarbons, 33, 34, 53t, 71, 82t, 128, 311, 604, 605t, 657, 730, 739
lethal doses of, Table 47(130)
naphthalene, 202, **208,** 605t
phenoxyacetic acid ([2,4-D], [2,4-5-T], and [MCPA]), 182, 735t
Chlorine, 9t, 97t, 148, 233, 250, 312, 324t, 629, 648t, 652, 653, 709t
bleach, 4f
dioxide, 709t
free, 205
gas, 202, 234t, **245-246,** 247t, 327, 526, 625
Chloriodized oil, 485t
Chlorkil, 161t
Chlormerodrin, 644t
Chloroacetophenone (Mace), **250,** 631, 654
Chlorobenzene(s), 10t, 13t
derivatives, 126, **127-128**
oral, producing methemoglobin, 12t
Chlorobenzilate, 137t
Chlorocide, 161t
Chlorodiethyl benzamide, 193
Chlorodiphenyl(s), 311(t)
Chlorodiphenyloxides, 311

Chlorofluoromethanes, 326
Chloroform (Trichloromethane), 6t, 7t, 8t, 20t, 62t, 76, 77, 86, 87t, 97t, 117t, 189, 202, 206-207, 247t, 351, 426, 471, 514t, 636, 729t
  methyl, 87t, 190, 207
Chloroguanide hydrochloride (Paludrine), 485t
Chlorohydrin, ethylene, 202, **208**
Chloromethapyrilene, **617**
Chloromycetin (Chloramphenicol), 16t, 79t, 110t, 117t, 118t, 214t, 355t, 485t
Chloronaphthalene(s), 10t, 311(t)
Chloronitrobenzene, oral, producing methemoglobin, 12t
Chlorophenothane (DDT), 13t, 117t, 130t
Chlorophyll, 709t
Chloropicrin, 87t, 734t
Chloroprocaine (Nesacaine), 352t
Chloroquine (Aralen), 11t, 181, 338(t), 341, 343t, 344, 354t, 459, 461
  diphosphate, 460
  phosphate (Arlen phosphate), 110t, 346t, 456, 485t
Chlorosalicylamide, 455
Chlorosalicylic acid anilide, 485t
Chlorothen, **617**
Chlorothiazide (Diuril), 13t, 15ft, 339, 347t, 455, 485t
  diuretics, 124, 455, 469
Chlorothion, 126, 132t, 734t
Chlorotrianisene (TACE), 401t
Chloroxuron (Tenoran), 188t
Chlorphenesin carbamate (Maolate), 485t
Chlorpheniramine, 358t, **364-367,** 514t
  maleate, 13t
Chlorphentermine hydrochloride (Pre-Sate), 486t
Chlorpromazine (Thorazine; Chlor-PZ), 9(t), 13t, 36, 40, 53t, 76, 77, 92t, 100, 107t, 118t, 144, 214t, 347t, 366t, 371, 372, 433, 447, 448, 471, 486t, 514t
Chlorpropamide (Diabinese), 65t, 77, 112t, 209, 214t, 339, 344, 347t, 429, 455, 486t, 503t, 514t
Chlorprothixen (Taractan), 514t
Chlor-PZ, (*see* Chlorpromazine)
Chlorquinaldol (Sterosan), 486t
Chlortetracycline (Aureomycin), 13t, 82, 102, 121t, 334t, 355, 357t, 702
  hydrochloride, 486t
Chlorthalidone (Hygroten), 16t, 469
Chlorthion (p-Nitro-m-chlorophenyl dimethylthiophosphate), 130
Chlorzoxazone (Paraflex), 11t
Choledyl, (*see* Oxtriphylline)
Cholesterol esters, 629
Cholestrin, 95t
Cholestyramine (Cuemid), 347t, 422, 477, 486t
Choline, 77, 358, 632
  derivatives, 452
  esters, 424
  nitrates, 424
Cholinergic (parasympathomimetic) agents, **452**
  effects, 131t
Cholinesterase, 566
  inhibiting compounds, 6t, 7t, 8t, 52t, 75, 98, 112t, 130, 131, 132, 133, 136, 137, 358, 452, 582
  pseudo apnea, 338t
  reactivators, 138, 271t
Cholografin, (*see* Iodipamide)
Choloxin, (*see* Dextrothyroxine sodium)
Chondodendron tomentosum extract (Curare), **415**
Christmas
  decorations toxic, **739-741**
  tree, bubbling lights, 739
    poisonous substances in, 95t
Christmas rose (*Helleborus niger*), 549t
Chromate(s), 7t, 94t, 254, 311t
  lead, 618, 633
  sodium, 644t
  zinc, 331t
Chromatography
  gas used for identification of poisons, **84-85**
  paper, **84-85**
Chrome, alum (Chromium potassium sulfate), 614t
Chrome Kleen, 527t
Chromic
  acid, 65t, 311t, 331t
  salts, 254-255
Chromium, 94t, 202, **254-255,** 270t, 271t, 313t, 317t, 657
  potassium sulfate, 614t
  trioxide, 254
Chrysanthemum, 549t
Chrysarobin, 10t, 486t
Chrysolite, 317
*Cicuta maculata* (cowbane, water hemlock), 545, 554t
*Cicuta virosa* (beaver poison), 554t
Cicutoxin, 545
Cigarette smoking, (*see* Smoking, cigarettes)
Ciguatera (Fish poisoning), **718**
C-I-L Louse Powder, 161t
Cimetidine, 348t
Cinchona compounds, **457-461**
Cinchophen, 10t, 97t, 345t, 346t, **409,** 458
Cinerin(s), **157,** 158t
  allyl, 158t
Cinnamic acid
  esters, 610
Cinnamon, 546t
  oil, 486t
CIPC (Chloro-IPC), 188t
Citanest (Prilocaine), 352t
Citrate
  orphenadrine (Norflex), 52t, 496t
  potassium (K-Lyte), 466
  sodium, 479
Citric acid, 355, **409-410,** 486t, 533, 709t, 716
Citronellal, 613
Citronella oil (lemon grass oil), **617**
Citrovorum factor (Leucovorin), 404
Citrus oils (orange, lemon, lime), 455
Claire Insect Repellent, 195t
Clam, giant (tridacna), 583
Clarc I, II, 9t
Class B poison pesticide chemicals, 126
*Claviceps*
  *paspali* (paspalum staggers), 606t
  *purpurea* (ergotism), 606t, 717
Clay, 626
Cleaners, 525 (*see also* individual cleaners)
  composition of, 523t, 524t
  poisonous substances in, 94t
Cleanesco, 527t
Cleaning,
  equipment, poisonous substances in, 95t
  fluids, 106t
    poisonous substances in, 94t
Cleaning agents, Table 135(526-531)
Cleanser 400, 528t
Clearpine Disinfectant, 528t
Cleartox, 195t
Clemizole, 366t
Click (Para) Crystals, 195t
Climbing lily (*Gloriosa superba*), 550t
Climbing sumac, 539 (*see also* Poison ivy)
Clindamycin, 347t
Clinitest Tablets (Glycosuria testing tablets), 230
Clioquinol, 430
C-I-L Brush Killer, 195t
Clofibrate (Astromid-S), 143t, 503t
Clonidine, 348t
Clorazepate (Azene, Tranxene), 214t
Cloroben, 528t
Clor-O-Tol Bleach, 528t
Clorox Bleach, 234t, 528t (*see also* Chlorinated alkalis)
*Clostridium*
  *botulinum,* 707, 712
  *perfringens,* **714**
Clove oil USP, **617**
Clovers (Trifolium), 548t
  sweet, 606t
Cloxacillin monohydrate, sodium (Tegopen), 357t
CMA (Super-Dal-E-Rad), 187t
CMU, (*see* Monuron)
C-N Disinfectant, 528t
CNS (Central nervous system) (*see also* individual drugs)
  depressant drugs, 30
  effects on, in organic phosphate ester poisoning, 131t
  interaction with antihistamines, 366t
  stimulants, 104t
Coagulants, blood, as a component of venom, 566
Coal
  dust, 316

gas, 240
tar, 611, 618, 225, 331t, 455, 453
derivatives, 115, 661
naphtha, 247t, 727
Coal workers' pneumoconiosis, (*see* Pneumoconiosis)
Cobalt, 53t, 269, **410,** 533, 623
chloride, 410, 615t
ethylene diamine tetra-acetate (Kelocyanor), 237
preparations producing methemoglobin, 12t
salts, 8t, 257t, 270t
Cobaltamine test, 390
Cobalt-thiocyanate test, 92t
Cobra snake venom, 565, 568
Cocaine ("snow" or "speedball"), 6t, 7t, 9t, 35t, 92t, 97t, 108t, 352t, **410-411,** 457, 471
"caine" phases, Table 116(411)
hydrochloride, 46
*Cocculus indicus* (fish berries), 550t
*Coccus lactis,* 647
Cochineal, 614t, 709t
Cocillana, 486t, **617**
Cocklebur, 539
Cockles, corn (*Agrostemma githago*), 549t
Cocoa butter, 95t
Coco de mono (lecythis), 551t
Codeine, 13t, 54t, 97t, 122, 249, 346t, **412,** 422, 443t, 445, 448, 514t, 540, 579
hypodermic tablets, 34
phosphate, 19t, 20t
Cod liver oil, 312
Coelenterates, 583, 584
Coffee,
Kentucky tree, 551t
Colchicine (Colchicum), 7t, 13t, 97t, 150, 347t, **412-413**
Colchicum (*Colchicum autumnale*), **412-413,** 549t
*Colchicum autumnale* (meadow saffron, autumn crocus, naked ladies), 549t
Colestipol, 347t, 422
Colistimethate, sodium (Coly-Mycin), 121t, 356t
Colistin, 355
sulfate, 121t
Collars, anti-flea dog and cat, 136
College Brand Blight Dust, 195t
College Brand Household Spray, 161t
College Brand Powdered Insecticide, 171t
College Brand Rodenticide, 195t
Collodion USP, **617**
Colloidal sulfur, 651
*Colocasia* (Arum family), 548t
Colocynth, 406t, 486t
Colonial spirits, (*see* Wood alcohol)
Colophony (Rosin), **645**
Color,
feces, affected by drugs, Table 4(12)
pigments, 95t
television receivers, safety of, **641-642**
urine, affected by drugs, Tables 2 & 3(10-11)
Color Additive Amendment of 1960, 707
Colorings, hair, poisonous substances in, 94t
Columbian spirits, (*see* Wood alcohol)
Columbium, (*see* Niobium)
Coly-Mycin (Colistimethate, sodium), 356t
Coma, **71-73,** Table 31(74)
conditions causing, Table 32(75)
Combustion products,
pulmonary irritants, toxic gases, Table 154(648)
toxic, of common substances, Table 154(648)
Committee on Fetus and Newborn, (*see* American Academy of Pediatrics)
Common Sense Cockroach Preparation, 161t
Common Sense Insect Spray, 161t
Common Sense Insect Spray, Plain, 161t
Common Sense Rat Preparation, 195t
Communicable Disease Center, 713
Compazine, (*see* Prochlorperazine)
Composition of dialysis fluids, Table 29(68)
Compoze, (*see* Methapyrilene)
Congeners (in alcoholic liquors), 212
Coniine, 545
*Conium maculatum* (poison and deadly hemlock, poison parsley), 545, 553t
Conjugated estrogens USP, **426**
Consumer Product Safety Commission, 703
Consumer Protection Act of 1972, 703
Contax Weed Killer, 195t
Contraceptives, oral, 40, 80t, 143t, 334t, 345t, 347t, **413,** 455
effects on lactation, 116, 123, 124
steroids, 477
Contrast agents, as nephrotoxic compounds, 82t
*Conus* (gastropod), 584
*Convallaria majalis* (lily of the valley), 540, 552t
Convulsions, drugs and treatment, **71,** Table 30(72)
Conway dish, 89(f)
Cook-Kill Bug Killer, 171t
Cook's Push Button Real-Kill Insect Bomb, 171t
Cook's Real-Kill Mothproofer, 161t
Co-Op 70-30 Dust, 161t
Co-Op One Shot Dust, 161t
Copaiba, 346t
Coparaffinate, 486t
Cope, (*see* Methapyrilene)
Copper, 32, 33, 53t, 65t, 82t, 117, 252t, 269, 270t, 271, 514t, 533, **608,** 609, 623, 657, **716,** 741
acetate, 583
acetoarsenite, 155t, 194t
chloride, **179-180**
compounds, **179-180,** 195t, 196t, 197t, 198t, 200t, 201t, 734t
oxide, **179-180**
phosphate, **179-180**
phosphide, 152
salts, 7t, 8t, 148, 179, 201t, 739
silicate, **179-180**
sulfate, 37, 53t, 97t, 152, **179-180,** 187t, 196t, 197t, 198t, 199t, 610, 612, 615t
as an emetic, 44, 45, 83
wire, in chemistry sets, 614t
Copper-ADust, 195t
Copper Brite, 528t
Copper Coin Cleaner ("CCC"), 528t
Copper-Cure, 195t
Copperhead (*Agkistrodon*), **562**
venomous (*Agkistrodon modeson*), **562,** 564f
Copper Hydro-Bordo, 195t
Coppo-Clear, 195t
Coppo-Regular, 195t
Coprinus comatus, 556t
Coproporphyrin, 271t, 410
Coproporphyrinogen, 257
dicarboxylase, 257
Coral,
abrasions (cuts), 584
elkhorn (Anthozoa), 584
fire, 584
sumac (*Metopium toxiferum*), 553t
Co-Ral (Diethyl-0 3-chloro-4-methyl-7-coumarinyl] phosphorothioate), 132t, 137t
Coral snake (*Micrurus fulvius*), 561, **563-565** (with figure), 568
false (non-poisonous), 563
venom, 52t
Coramine (Nikethamide 25% solution), 19t, 38, 367
*Corchorus olitorius, capsularis* (jute), 551t
Corn cockles (*Agrostemma githago*), 539, 549t
Cornell Cattle Spray, 161t
Cornell Household Aerosol Spray Insecticide, 171t
Cornell Penta-Gard, 195t
Cornell Residual Household Spray, 161t
Cornell WO 5 Rodenticide, 195t
Corning extract, 12t
Corn King Dairyland Fly Spray, 162t
Corn King Dead-White, 162t
Corn King De-Louser Powder, 162t
Corn King Fly Mort, 162t
Corn King Fly Spray, 162t
Corn King Verm-O-Phen Granules, 162t
Cornstarch,
in dry cell batteries, 611
in matches, 736
Corothion, 162t
Corrosive(s), 82, 85, 202, **226-252**
acids, 202, **226-229,** 720
alkalis, 202, **229-234,** 721
gases, 202, **235-252**
sublimate, 155t
Cortef acetate, 69

Cortical compounds, adrenal, (*see* individual drugs)
Corticoids, in shock therapy, 69
Corticosteroids, 80t, 112t, 225, 231, 246, 250, 264, 271, 312, 334(t), 347t, 370, 395, **413-415,** 460, 466, 469, 535, 555, 573, 579, 617, 636, 645, 659
  adrenal, 71
  relative potencies, Table 119(415)
Corticotropin (ACTH), 13t, 19t, 253, 312, 320, 339, 345t, 415, 469
Cortisol (Hydrocortisone), 415t
Cortisone, 9t, 102, 117t, 123, 253, 320, 339, 347t, 366t, 404, 415t, 568, 589
  acetate (Cortogen acetate; Cortone acetate), 110t
Cortogen acetate (Cortisone acetate), 110t
Cortone acetate (Cortisone acetate), 110t
Corundum fume fibrosis (Shaver's disease), **318-319**
Cosmegen (Dactinomycin), 398t
Cosmetic(s), **532-537**
  laws, 701-702
  poisonous substances in, 94-95t
Cotoran, 188t
Cotton dust, 319
Cottonmouth (*Agkistrodon piscivorus*), **562,** 564f
Cottonseed, 532
  meal, 621
Cotton States Fly Spray & Repellent, 162t
Cough syrups, 104-105t
Coumadin (Warfarin), 502t
  sodium (Sodium warfarin), 110t
Coumaphos (Co-Ral), 137t
Coumarin, 6t, 55t
  anticoagulants, 477
  derivatives, 55t
Cowbane (*Cicuta maculata*), 554t
Cowley Spray, 162t
CPK (Creatinine phosphokinase), 241, 242
CPR-GP Plant Spray, 162t
CPR Liquid Base, 162t
Crab-Erad Crabtex, 195t
Crab Fruit Fungicide, 195t
Crab-Not Powder, 195t
Crab-Not Special, 195t
Crab's eye, 541
Crab-spiders (*Heteropodidae*), 574
Crane's Moth-Ex Junior, 162t
Cranial hypertension, caused by poisoning, **70-71**
Crayon(s), **618**
  industrial, 618
  wax, 12t
    poisonous substances in, 95t
Cream of tartar, 228
Creams, poisonous substances in, 95t
Creeper, poison, 553t
Creol Disinfectant, 528t
Creoletta, 528t
Creosol, 82t, 94t, 335t, 618
Creosote NF, 453, **618**
  beechwood, 96t
  carbonate, 618
  oil, 618
Creotex, 528t
Creozone, 528t
Cresanol, 528t
Cresol, 453
  dinitro-ortho, 65t, 97t
Cresolene, 528t
Cresophan, 528t
Cristy Cooling System Cleaner, 528t
Crocidolite, 317
Crocus, autumn (*Colchicum autumnale*), 549t
*Crocus sativus* (saffron), 645
Crosley Special Furniture Polish, 528t
Cross Country Crabgrass Killer, 195t
Cross Country Fire Ant Killer, 162t
Crotaline antivenin, polyvalent, 567, 568
*Crotalus* (true rattlesnake), **561-562,** 564f, 565
  *adamanteus* (Florida diamondback), **561**
  antivenin for, 20t
  *atrox* (Texas diamondback), **561**
  *horridus* (Timber rattlesnake), **561**
  *oreganus* (Pacific rattlesnake), **562**
  *viridis* (Prairie rattlesnake), **561-562**
Crotamiton (Eurax), 486t
Croton (*Croton tiglium*), 549t
  as a cathartic, 7t, 8t
  oil, 7t, 8t, 37, 406t, 486t, 494t
Croupette, 225
Crowfoot family (*Ranunculaceae*), 549t
Crude oil, 165t
*Cryptostroma corticale,* 322t
Crystal violet, 633
Crystamet, 528t
Cubeb, 486t
Cucurbits, squash vine borers in, 731
Cuemid (Cholestyramine), 486t
Cultivated rape (*Brassica napus*), 548t
Cumene (Xylene), **658-659,** 729t
Cuprimine (D-penicillamine), (*see* Penicillamine)
Cupro-K, 195t
Cuprous oxide, 199t
Curare, 7t, 97t, 112t, 415, 486t, 581
Cured Flea Duster, 162t
Cúscohygrine, 545
Cusso (Kousso), 353t
Cuticle removers, poisonous substances in, 95t
Cuttlefish, 584
Cutworms, 742
Cyanamide, 209, 235
  calcium, 188t, 236, 621, 623
Cyanate, potassium, 182, **184,** 194t, 195t, 196t, 197t, 198t
  allyl isothiocyanate, 495t
Cyanhemoglobin, 236
Cyanide (Hydrocyanic acid), 6t, 7t, 8t, 9t, 52t, 55t, 85, 89, 90, 127, **153-155,** 173, 186, 195t, 202, **235-237,** 331t, 514t, 605t, 637
  hydrogen, 97t, 115t, 153, 247, 266, 342t, 648t
  mercuric, 237
  oil of bitter almond, 495t
  poison kit (Eli Lilly stock #M76), 53t
  potassium, 18, 94t, 97t, 153
  salts, 517
  sodium, 97t, 153, 195t
  treatment for poisoning, 31, 37, 41
  zinc, (*see* Zinc)
Cyanmethemoglobin, 86, 154
Cyano Gas A Dust, 195t
Cyanogen chloride, 235
Cyanogenetic glycoside, (*see* Glycoside cyanogenetic)
Cyanohydrin, acetone, 482t
*Cycas circinalis,* 558
Cycasin, 558
Cyclamate(s), 115, 651
  calcium (Sucaryl), 455, 486t, 651, 709t
  sodium, 651, 709t
Cyclamycin, (*see* Oleandomycin)
Cyclandelate (Cyclospasmol), 486t
Cyclazocine, 448
Cyclizine(s), 365t, 366t, 425t
Cyclobarbital (Phanodorn), 65t, 383t
Cyclogel, (*see* Cyclopentolate)
Cyclohexane, 87t, 247t, 624, 729t
Cyclohexanol, 624
Cyclohexanone, 624, 729t
Cyclohexyl alcohols, 729t
Cyclohexylsulfamic acid, 463
Cyclonene, piperonyl, 170
Cycloparaffins (Naphthenes), 225
Cyclopentolate (Cyclogel), 358
Cyclophosphamide (Cytoxan; Endoxan), 65t, 117t, 143t, 396t
Cyclopropane, 117t, 426
  ethyl chloride, 351
Cycloserine (Seromycin), 65t, 117t, 356t, 437t
Cyclospasmol (Cyclandelate), 486t
Cyclothiazide (Anhydron), 469
Cycrimine hydrochloride (Pagitane hydrochloride), 486t
*Cydonia oblonga* (quince seed), 637
Cygon (Dimethoate), 137t
Cymag, 195t
Cymothoids, 590
*Cypripedium hirsutum* (lady's slipper), 551t
Cyproheptadine hydrochloride (Periactin), 486t
Cypromid (Clobber), 187t
Cysteamine, 349, 452
Cysteine, 148, 190, 349
  penicillamine disulfide, 147
Cystine, 35, 65t, 77, 143, 147
*Cystisus laburnum* (laburnum, golden chain), 551t
Cytarabine (Cytosine arabinoside; Ara-C), 397t
Cytochrome oxidase, 153, 237
Cytolysins, **565-566,** 575
Cytosar (Cytosine arabinoside; Ara-C), 397t

Cytosine arabinoside (Cytarabine; Ara-C; Cytosar), 397t
Cytoxan (Cyclophosphamide), 117t, 396t
Cytoxin, 211

**D**

2,4-D, (*see* 2,4-Dichlorophenoxyacetic acid)
Dacarbazine (DTIC-Dome), 400t
Dactin Bleach & Germicide, 528t
Dactinomycin (Actinomycin D; Cosmegen), 398t
Daffodil (*Narcissus pseudonarcissus*), 550t
Dairy-Mist Fly Spray Concentrate, 162t
Dalapon, sodium (2-2 Dichloropropionic acid), 182, 188t
DAM (Diacetyl monoxime), 133
Damiana *(Turnera diffusa)*, 546t
Dampo, 162t
Dan-Dee Floor Polish, 528t
Danilone, (*see* Phenindione)
Danthron (Dionone; Dorbane; Istizin), 117t, 122, 619
Dantrium (Dantrolene sodium), 487t
Dantrolene sodium (Dantrium), 487t
Daphne (*Daphne mezereum*), 550t
berries, 540
*Daphne mezereum* (Daphne), 550t
Dapsone (Avlosulfon), 12t, 79t, 341, 343t, 347t
Daraprim (Pyrimethamine), 16t, 117t
Darbid, (*see* Isoprapamide)
Daricon, (*see* Oxyphencyclimine hydrochloride)
Darnel (*Lolium temulentum*), 550t
Darvon (Dextropropoxphene hydrochloride), 81t, 117t, **416-417,** 514t
Dash, 528t
*Dasyatidae* (stingrays), **582**
*Datura* (Solanaceae family),
*stramonium* (jimson weed), 106t, 358t, 376, 544, 545, 551t
*suaveolens* ("angel's trumpet"), 106t, 544
Daunomycin (Daunorubicin), 402t
Daunorubicin (Daunomycin; Rubidomycin), 402t
Dawson #3 Insecticide, 162t
Dawson #4 Insecticide, 162t
Dazzle Bleach & Disinfectant, 528t
2,4-DB (Butrac; Butoxone), 187t
DBI (Phenformin hydrochloride), 110t, 214t
DCMA (Dicryl), 188t
DCPA (Dacthal), 188t
DCU (Crag), 188t
DDA (Bis p-chlorophenyl acetic acid), 127, 128
DDD (TDE), 734t
DDE (Toxic dehydrochloride), 124, 127
D-D Soil Fumigant,
exposure hazard, 162t
odor of, 162t
DDT (Dichlorodiphenyltrichloroethane), 7t, 13t, 71, 77, 87, 97t, 116, 117t, 123, 124, 126, 128, 129, 130t, 137t, 160t, 161t, 162t, 163t, 164t, 165t, 166t, 167t, 168t, 169t, 170t, 196t, 197t, 201t, 311t, 514t, 544, 580, 730, 731, 734t
DDVP (Dichlorvos), 137t, 168t
Deadly hemlock (*Conium maculatum*), 553t
Deadly nightshade (*Atropa belladonna*), 358t, 544, 550t
Death camas (*Zygadenus*), 540, 541f, 550t
Debrom, 162t
Decaborane, 644, 645
Decadron (Dexamethasone), 21t
Decamethonium, 338t, 341
iodide, 487t
Declomycin, (*see* Demethylchlortetracycline)
Ded-Tox Dust, 162t
Dee-Dex, 162t
Dee-Dex "25", 162t
Deer fly, 576f
Deet (DEET-Diethyltoluamide), 186, **193,** 581
Deferoxamine B (Desferal), 10t, 53t, 81t, 434, 435
dosage for iron poisoning, Table 122(436)
Dehydrochloride, toxic (DDE), (*see* DDE)
Dehydrocholic acid, 339
Dehydrogenase,
alcohol, (*see* Alcohol dehydrogenase)
glucose-6-phosphate, see G-6-PD
lactic, 115
malic, 115
succinic, 115
De-icer, spray, poisonous substances in, 95t
Delalutin, (*see* Hydroxyprogesterone caproate)
Delaney clause (FDC act), (*see* Cyclamates)
Delcro Shampoo for Dogs, 162t
Delnav (Dioxathion), 137t
*Delphinium* (larkspur), 35t, 549t
Delta-aminolevulinic acid (ALA), 257, 258, 260, 264
dehydratase, 257
ferrochelatase, 257
synthetase, 257
Delvex (Dithiazanine), 12t
Delvinal, (*see* Vinbarbital)
Demerol (Merperidine), 38, 54t, 97t, 392, 408, 422, 448, 468, 492t, 515t
Demethylchlortetracycline (Declomycin), 121t, 356t, 455
Demeton (Systox), 137t, 734t
Denatured alcohol, 94t, 95t
Denoxo, 162t
Deodorant(s) **536**
oils, 95t
poisonous substances in, 95t
Deodorizers, poisonous substances in, 96t
Deodorizing tablets, poisonous substances in, 96t
2,4-DEP (Falone), 187t
Department of Agriculture, (*see* U.S. Department of Agriculture)
Department of Environmental Health, (*see* American Medical Association)
Department of Health, Education and Welfare, (*see* U.S. Department of Health, Education and Welfare)
Depilatories, **535-536**
poisonous substances in, 94t
Depressants, 442
Deprol, (*see* Benactyzine)
*Dermacentor andersoni* (Rocky Mountain wood tick), 580
Dermal poisons, **46**
Dermatitis, occupational, **311-313**
materials and industrial exposures associated with, Table 75(313)
Deroxide, 162t
*Derris* (Rotenone), 157, 158(t), 734t
DES (Diethylstilbestrol), (*see* Diethylstilbestrol)
Desert ant (*Pogonomyrmex barbatus*), 579
Desferal (Deferoxamine B), 10t, 53t, 81t, 434, 435
Desipramine hydrochloride (Norpramin; Pertofrane), 90, 358t, 472, 487t, 495t, 514t
Desoxycorticosterone, 348t
Des-Tex Dry Cleaner, 528t
Destruol Antroach Dust, 162t
DET, (*see* Diethyltryptamine)
Detergent(s), **517-531** (with tables), 532
anionic, 518t, **519**
cationic, 518t, **519**
chemical classification of, Table 132(518)
dishwasher granules, **520**
household products, **519-525** (with tables)
liquid, **520-525**
non-anionic, 233, 518t, **519**
poisonous substances in, 94t
products, composition of, Table 134(522-524)
toxicity of, Table 133(521)
with bleaching and bactericidal properties, **525**
with enzymes, **525**
DEV, (*see* Duck embryo vaccine)
Dexamethasone, 21t, 69, 415t
Dexedrine (d-Amphetamine sulfate), 19t, 20t, 35, 117t, 360, 362t
Dexodine Metal Cleaner, 528t
Dextran, 385
iron, (Imferon), 431
Dextroamphetamine, 443t, 470
sulfate (Dexedrine), 13t, 117t
Dextromethorphan hydrobromide, **416**
Dextropropoxyphene, 37, 65t
hydrochloride (Darvon), 117t, **416-417,** 514t
Dextrose, 19t, 67, 70, 334t, 370, 384, 466

Dextrothyroxine, 503t
sodium (Choloxin), 487t
DFDT (Difluorodiphenyltrichloroethane), 126
DFP (Diisopropylfluorophosphate), 6t, 7t, 8t, 9t, 98, 127
DHE (Dihydroergotamine), 425t
Diabinese (Chlorpropamide), 209, 214t, 344, 455, 486t, 514t
Diacetate,
ethylene glycol, 729t
germine, 540
Diacetone alcohol, 729t
Diacetyl monoxime (DAM), 133
Diacetylmorphine (Heroin), 444
*Diadema setosum* (Black sea urchin), 587t
Diagnostic criteria for lead poisoning, 257
Dial (Diallybarbituric acid), 8t, 35t, 383t, 456
Diallate, 187t
Diallybarbituric acid (Dial), (*see* Dial)
Dialose Plus, 407t
Dial soap, 528t
Dialysis,
composition of fluids, Table 29(68)
extracorporeal, **64-66** (with table)
hemo-, **64-66**
in barbiturate poisoning, 388t
lipid, **66-67**
peritoneal, (*see* Peritoneal dialysis)
Dialyzable poisons, Table 28(65)
3,3' Diamino-4,4' dihydroxyarsenobenzene dihydrochloride (Arsphenamine), (*see* Arsphenamine)
Diaminodiphenyl sulfone, 12t
Diamondback rattlesnake,
Florida (*Crotalus adamanteus*), **561**
Texas (*Crotalus atrox*), **561**
Diamox (Acetazolamide), 16t, 81t, 248, 360, 363t, 388, 466, 481t, 513t
Diamethazole (Asterol), **417,** 487t
Dianeal, 67, 389
Dianol Insect Killing House Spray, 162t
Diaparene chloride (Methylbenzethonium chloride), 519, **632**
Diasone, 338t
Diatomaceous earth, 614t
Diatomite pneumoconiosis, 314, **318**
Diatrizoate, 487t
Diazepam (Valium), 20t, 71, 72t, 100, 101, 107t, 112t, 118t, 122, 124t, 178, 213, 214t, **364,** 367, 376, 405, 436, 447, 448, 449, 487t, 514t
Diazinon (Diethyl-0- [2-isopropyl-6-methyl-4-pyrimidyl] phosphorothioate), 127, 132t, 137t, 160t, 162t, 169t, 731, 734t
Diazoxide, 101, 347t
Dibasic calcium phosphate, **395**
Dibenamine, 6t, 487t
Dibenzyline (Phenoxybenzamine hydrochloride), 69, 157, 471, 487t
Diborane, 644, 645
Dibrom, (*see* Naled)
Dibromide, ethylene, 195t, 201t, 734t
Dibucaine, **457**
Dibutyl
adipate, 580
phthalate, 95t
DIC, (*see* Disseminated intravascular coagulation)
DIC, see Drug Information Centers
Dicalcium phosphate, 655
Dicamba (Banvel D), 188t
Dicarboximide (Raticate), 173, **178-179**
n-Octyl bicycloheptene, 170
*Dicentra cucullaria, pussilla* (Dutchman's breeches; bleeding heart), 548t
*Dichapetalum cymosum* (gifblaar), 176
Dichlobenil (Casoron), 188t
Dichlone (Phygon), 188t
Dichloramine-T, 524t
Dichloran Disinfectant, 528t
Dichloride
amylene, 94t
ethylene, 94t, 202, 207-208, 247t, 636, 729t, 734t
propylene, 247t
Dichlorobenzene, 247t
para- (Dichlorocide), 96t, 97t
Dichlorobenzyl Triphenyl Phosphonium CL, 195t
Dichlorocide (Para-dichlorobenzene), 186, **192**
Dichlorodifluoromethane (Freon), 87t, **624-625**
Dichlorodiphenylethanol (Dimite), 126
Dichlorodiphenyl methyl carbinol (DMC), 126
Dichlorodiphenyltrichloroethane (DDT), (*see* DDT)
Dichloroisocyanurate(s), 233t, **618**
potassium, 523t, 524t, **618**
sodium, 523t, 524t, **618**
Dichlorophene, 162t, 487t
2,4-Dichlorophenol (weed killer), 311
2,4-Dichlorophenoxyacetic acid (2,4-D), 182ft, 194t, 195t, 196t, 197t, 198t, 199t, 200t, 201t, 734t
Dichloropropane, 166t
2,2-Dichloropropionic acid (Dalapon sodium), 182
2,2-Dichlorovinyl dimethyl phosphate (Vapona), 136
Dichlorvos (DDVP), 136, 137t
Dichromate,
potassium, (*see* Potassium)
zinc, (*see* Zinc)
Dicloxacillin, sodium (Veracillin; Dynapen), 357t
Dicobalt tetracemate (Kelocyanor), 154
Dicodid, 487t
Dicofol (Kelthane), 137t
Dicoumarin (Bishydroxycoumarin), 117t
Dicourmarol (Bishydroxycoumarin), 117t, 484t
Dicumarol (Bishydroxycoumarin), 110t, 112t, 117t
Dicyclomine (Bentyl), 358t
Didimac, 162t
*Dieffenbachia* (Arum family), 543, 548t
*picta,* 543
*seguine,* 543
Die Fly, 162t
Dieldrec, 162t
Dieldrin (Hexachloro-epoxy-octahydrodimethano-naphthalene), 126, 127, 130t, 137t, 162t, 163t, 165t, 167t, 168t, 169t, 311t, 514t, 731, 734t
Diendrin, 126
Diesel
fuel additives, 12t
oil, (*see* Petroleum distillates)
Diethazine (Diparcol), 157
Diethylamide, d-lysergic acid, (*see* LSD)
Diethylcarbamazine (Hetrazan), 354t, 487t
Diethyl cellosolve, **613**
Diethyldithiocarbamate, 267
Diethylene glycol, 82t, 95t, 202, **218-219,** 729t
stearate, 95t
Diethylenetriamine penta-acetic acid (DTPA), (*see* DTPA)
N,N-Diethyl-m-toluamide (DEET), 186, **193**
Diethylstilbestrol, 13t, 16t, 339, 346t, 456
therapy, 103, 401t
Diethyltoluamide (DEET), (*see* DEET)
Diethyltryptamine (DET), 99, 106t
Difluorodiphenyltrichloroethane (DFDT), 126
Digitalis, 6t, 9t, 13t, 35t, 53t, 62t, 97t, 111t, 339, 346t, 348t, **417-422,** 604
adverse effects, 49t
glycosides, 15t, 16t, 334(t)
*lanata* (foxglove), 550t
*purpurea* (foxglove), 540, 550t
tolerance tests,, 420
toxicity, drug therapy for, 33, Table 120(421)
toxic manifestations of, 418-419
Digitoxin, 13t, 15ft, 19t, 97t, 339, 417, 514t
Diglycerides, 708t
Diglycolstearate, 615t
Digoxin, 13t, 20t, 65t, 122, 124t, 347t, 417, 514t
Dihydrocodeine, 412
Dihydrocodeinone, 412
bitartrate, 13t
enolacetate (Acedicon), 481t
Dihydroergotamine, 423, 425t
Dihydromycin, 355
Dihydrostreptomycin, 13t, 487t
Dihdrotachysterol, 124
1,8-Dihydroxyanthraquinone (Dorbane, Doxan), 11t, 12t, 407t
Diiodohydroxyquin (Diodoquin; Floraquin), 487t
Diisocyanate, toluene (TDI), (*see* Toluene diisocyanate)
Diisopropylfluorophosphate (DFP), 98, 127
Dilan, 126

Dilantin, (*see* Phenytoin)
Dilaudid, 37, 448, 514t
Dille-Koppanyi's test, 92t
Dimefox, 734t
Dimenhydrinate (Dramamine), 487t
Dimercaprol (2,3-Dimercaptopropanol; BAL), 19t, 53t, 139, 140, 155t, 343t, 370, 392, 428, (*see also* BAL)
2,3-Dimercaptopropanol (Dimercaprol; BAL), (*see* BAL & Dimercaprol)
Dimetane, (*see* Brompheniramine)
Dimethisoquin (Quotane), **457**
Dimethoate (Cygon, Rogor), 137t
2,5-Dimethoxy-4-methyl-amphetamine (DOM; MDA; STP), 102t
Dimethyl (*see* common names for most compounds)
  carbamate, 581
  phosphate, 137t
  phthalate, 96t, 196t, 200t
  sulfate, 202, **219**
  sulfoxide (DMSO), **618-619,** 729t
  urea, 197t, 200t
Dimethylamine(s), 368t
p-Dimethylaminobenzaldehyde, 373
  paper spot test, 92t
Dimethylaniline, 12t, 202, **203-204,** 624
Dimethyl carbamate, 193
Dimethyl dithiocarbamate, ferric, 621
Dimethyl-1 hydroxy-2,2,2-trichloro-ethyl-phosphonate (Dipterex), 162t
Dimethyl phosphate (Vapona), (*see* Vapona)
Dimethylphthalate, 186, **193,** 580, 581
Dimethyltryptamine (DMT), 99, 106t, **415,** 722t
Dimethyl tubocurarine chloride (Curare), (*see* Curare)
Dimethyl tubocurarine chloride (DMT), (*see* Dimethyltryptamine)
Dimite (Dichlorodiphenylethanol), 126
Dimocillin-RT (*see* Methicillin)
Dinitrate, ethylene glycol, 12t, 729t
Dinitrobenzene, 12t
Dinitrobutyl-phenol (Dinoseb), 734t
Dinitrocellulose (Pyroxylin), 617
Dinitrocresol (DNC), 7t, 311t, 734t
Dinitro-ortho-cresol, 65t, 97t, 514t
Dinitrophenol(s), 7t, 12t, 17, 97t, 205, 339
  derivatives, 182, **183-184,** 199t
Dinitrotoluene, 12t
Dinoseb (Dinitro-phenol), 734t
Dioctyl sodium sulfosuccinate, 11ft, 407t, 608, **619**
Diodoquin, (*see* Diiodohydroxyquin)
Diodrast, (*see* Iodopyracet)
Diolene (Phenylenediamine), 534
Diols substituted, 368t
Dionin, 54t
Dionone (Danthron), 117t
Dioxane, 87t, 202, **222**
Dioxathion (Delnav), 137t
Dioxide(s), **249-250**
  carbon, (*see* Carbon dioxide)
  chlorine, 709t
  manganese, (*see* Manganese)
  nitrogen, 247t, 325, 329t, 547
  silicone, 647
  sulfur, 15t, 87t, 202, **243,** 247t, 313t, 324(t), 325, 329t
  thorium (Thorotrast), 15t, 340t, 501t
  titanium, 95t, 331t, 536
Dioxin (Tetrachlorodibenzo-p-dioxin), 182
Dioxypurine, (*see* Xanthine)
Diparcol (Diethazine), 157
Dipaxin (Diphenadine), 17t
Dipentene, 94t, 613
Diphenadine (Dipaxin), 17t
Diphenamid (Dymid; Enide), 188t
Diphenhydramine, 8t, 65t, 339, 343t, **364-367,** 376, 431
  hydrochloride (Benadryl), 20t, 53t, 117t, 133, 358t, 373, 487t, 514t, 543, 582
Diphenidol (Vontrol), 487t
Diphenoxylate hydrochloride (Lomotil), **422-423**
  with atropine sulfate, 488t
Diphenylhydantoin (Dilantin), (*see* Phenytoin)
Diphenylthio-carbazone (Dithizon), 143
Diphosphate, chloroquine, 460
Diphosphopyridine nucleotide (DPN), (*see* DPN)
Dip-It-Stain Remover, 528t
Dipotassium, 540
  edetate, 33, 422
  phosphate, 479
  salt, 395, 479
Dippit solution, **635**
Dippo Silver Cleaner, 528t
Diprotrizoate, 488t
Dipterex (Dimethyl-1-hydroxy-2,2,2-trichloroethylphosphonate), 132t, 137t, 162t, 163t, 734t
Dipyrone (analgesic), 13t, 339, **457**
Diquat (1,1-Ethylene 2, 2-dipyridium dibromide), 182, **184-185,** 187t
Dirilyte Polish, 528t
Dishwasher detergents,
  granules, **520**
  poisonous substances in, 94t
Disinfectants, 4f
  laws, 701-702
  swimming pool, **652-653**
Disodium
  calcium, (*see* EDTA)
  glutamate, 489t
  phosphate, 395
    duohydrate, 434
  salt, 395, 479
Disolfton (Di-syston; Scope), 132t, 137t
Disseminated intravascular coagulation (DIC), **70**
Distannoxane, hexakis (Vensex), 581
Distillate(s)
  petroleum, 82, 94t, 160t, 161t, 162t, 165t, 168t, 182, 196t, 202, **222-224,** 225, 517
  solvent, 202, **222-224**
Disulfide,
  carbon, (*see* Carbon disulfide)
  penicillamine-cysteine, 147
  tetraethylthiuram, (*see* Disulfiram)
  tetramethylthiuram (Thiram), (*see* Tetramethylthiuram)
Disulfiram (Antabuse; Tetraethylthiuram disulfide), 81t, 181, 209, 211, 214t, 312, 346t, 429, 503t, 555, 735t
Di-syston (Disolfton; Scope), 132t, 137t
Dithiazanine (Delvex), 12t
Dithio, 162t
Dithiocarb (Sodium diethyldithiocarbamate trihydrate), 267
Dithiocarbamates (Thiocarbamates), 136, 179, **181,** 734t
  ferric dimethyl, 621
Dithiono, 162t
Dithizon (Diphenylthiocarbazone), 53t, 143
Ditiglytelodine, 545
Diuretics, 11t, 16t, 112t, 124
  chlorothiazide, 124
  mercurial, 16t, 393
  sulfonamide, **469-470**
  thiazide, 16t, 110t, 393, **469-470**
Diuril (Chlorothiazide), 77, 469, 485t
Diuron (Karmex), 188t
Divinyl
  ether (Vinethene), 426
  oxide, 514t
DLP-787 2% Bait, 174
DLP-787 10% House Mouse Tracking Powder, 174t
DL-penicillamine, (*see* Penicillamine)
DMC (Dichlorodiphenyl methyl carbinol), 126
DMPA (Zytron), 188t
DMSO, (*see* Dimethyl sulfoxide)
DMT, (*see* Dimethyltryptamine)
DMTT (Mylone), 187t
DNBP, amine, 187t
DNC (Dinitrocresol), 734t
Dock, 539
Doctor gum (*Metopium toxiferum*), 553t
Dodecylamine hydrochloride, 653
n-Dodecylguanide acetate (Dodine), (*see* Dodine)
Dodine (n-Dodecylguanide acetate), 179, **182**
Dog
  anti-flea collar, 136
  drug toxicity compared with man, 26t
  hookworm (Ancylostomiasis), 592
Dogbane (*Apocynaceae*), 540
Dogfish, 585
Dogwood, poison (*Rhus vernix*), 553t
Dolene (Propoxyphene), 81t
Dolomite, 319
Dolophine (Methadone hydrochloride), 117t, **440-442,** 493t
DOM (Methyl dimethoxy methyl phenylethylamine), 99, 102t, 722t
Done-Died Perfumed Moth Killer, 171t

Done's method for estimating degree of salicylate intoxication, 464
Donovan's solution, **619-620**
Doomsday, 171t
Dopa (α-Methyl), 143t, 347t
Dopamine (Intropin), 21t
Dopram (Doxapram hydrochloride), 445
Dorbane (1,8-Dihydroxyanthraquinone; Danthron), 10t, 12t, 117t, 122, 407t
Dorbantyl, 11ft
Doriden (Glutethimide), 8t, 14t, 30, 97t, **427-428,** 456, 514t
Dormison, (*see* Methylparafynol)
Dornwal (Amphenidone), 483t
Doses (*see also* drugs and individual drug listings)
  lethal, Table 38(97-98)
Dosage, drug **22-26** (with tables)
  of antiarrhythmic drugs, Table 19(48)
Dover's powder (Opium), 391
Dow Brush Killer, 195t
Dowclene Dry Cleaner, 528t
Dowfume MC-2, 195t
Dowfume (V,C,F,G,H,J,75,80-20), 195t
Dow Grain Bin Spray, 162t
Dowpon, 188t
Dow Seed Protectant, 195t
Doxan (1,8-Dihydroxyanthraquinone), 12t
Doxapram hydrochloride (Dopram), 445
Doxepin hydrochloride (Sinequan), 358t, 472, 514t
Doxidan, 11ft
Doxorubicin (Adriamycin), 399t
Doxycycline, 357t
D&P Bulb Saver, 171t
D&P Cinch-Tox, 162t
D&P Double O Crab Grass Killer, 195t
D-penicillamine (Cuprimine), (*see* Penicillamine)
D&P Fruit Spray, 171t
DPH (Diphenylhydantoin), (*see* Phenytoin)
D&P Liquid Fungicide, 195t
DPN (Diphosphopyridine nucleotide), 18, 209
DPNH, 209
D&P Slug Tox, 162t
D&P Tomato Dust, 195t
D&P Trispray, 162t
D&P Weedkiller, 195t
*Dracunculus* (Arum family), 548t
Dragonfish, 585
Dragonfly, 742
Drain cleaners,
  composition of, 524t
  poisonous substances in, 96t
Dramamine (Dimenhydrinate), 19t, 156, 447, 487t
Drano, disinfectant, 230, 528t
Dried banana peel, 108t
Drive (detergent), 525
Dromoran, (*see* Methorphinan hydrobromide)
Dro Rose and Ornamental Plant Spray, 162t
Dro Snosphra, 162t
Drug(s), **332-516** (*see also* individual drug listings and antibiotics, antihistamines, and chemotherapeutic agents)
  abuse and misuse, Table 40(104-109), 112t
  antiarrhythmics, effects of, Table 20(49)
  antituberculosis, 437t
  bilirubin-albumin binding, 124-125 (with table)
  capable of causing fixed eruptions, Table 93(346)
  causing discoloration of feces, Table 4(12)
  causing discoloration of urine, Table 3(11)
  dosages, **22-26** (with tables)
  emergency treatment, **19-26** (with tables)
  in breast milk, **115-124** (with tables)
  interactions with anticoagulants, Table 129(503)
  interactions with food, **333-334** (with table)
  laws, **701-710** (with table)
  lethal doses, Table 38(97-98)
  medication during pregnancy, **102-125** (with table)
  miscellaneous compounds, Table 128(481-502)
  producing acne eruptions, **312-313**
  producing alopecia, 143t
  producing anticholinergic syndrome, Table 103(358)
  producing epidermal necrolysis, Table 96(347)
  producing exfoliative dermatitis, Table 95(347)
  producing gynecomastia, Table 99(348)
  producing hemolysis, 338t, 343t
  producing hemolytic anemia, **336-344** (with table)
  producing hyperglycemia, Table 98 (347)
  producing malabsorption, Table 97(347)
  producing photosensitization, **455-456**
  producing porphyria, 456
  producing Stevens-Johnson syndrome, Table 94(347)
  producing systemic lupus erythematosus, Table 91(345)
  producing toxic hepatitis, **75-78,** Table 33(79-81)
  producing vitamin deficiencies, **477**
  public spending on, 332 (with figure)
  reactions, **339-340**
  reactions in the aged, Table 92(345)
  reactions of anticonvulsants, Table 104(362-363)
  retinotoxic, **344-346**
  risks to fetus and newborn, **109-115** (with table)
  role in gastroduodenal ulcers, Table 90(345)
  role in suicides, **334-336** (with figures and tables)
  symptoms indicating a person is taking drugs, Table 158(722)
  therapy for digitalis toxicity, Table 120(421)
  toxicity in experimental animals compared with man, Table 17(26)
  treatment, **31-47** (with tables)
Drug blood levels,
  lethal, Table 131(513-516)
  therapeutic or normal, Table 131(513-516)
  toxic, Table 131(513-516)
Drug Enforcement Administration (DEA), 448
Drug Information Centers (DIC), **504-513** (with table)
Drugs that may alter laboratory values, (*see* Appendix B), 752-755
Dry cell batteries, 610, 611
Dry cleaning fluids, poisonous substances in, 94t
Dryolene Dry Clean, 528t
DSMA, 187t
DTPA (Diethylenetriamine penta-acetic acid), 264, 434, 435, 642
Duapen, (*see* Benzathine penicillin G)
Dubonnet, 458
Duck embryo vaccine (DEV), 593ft, 603
Ducozone Bleach, 528t
Duke Poison Control Center, (*see* Poison Control Centers)
Du-Kill, 162t
Dulcin (Sucrol), 488t
Dumbcane (*Dieffenbachia*), 548t
DuPont Dry Clean, 528t
DuPont Lawn Weeder, 195t
DuPont Liquid, 195t, 241
DuPont Liquid Fungicide, 195t
Duricide DDT, 162t
Dust(s)
  cobalt, 313t
  inert, maximum allowable concentrations, Table 74(311)
  producing hypersensitivity pneumonitis, Table 76(322)
  toxic, maximum allowable concentrations, Table 73(311)
Dust-A-Way Crab Grass Dust, 195t
Dustox, 162t
Dutch elm beetles, 742
Dutchman's breeches (*Dicentra cucullaria*), 548t
Dwin Aerosol Insect Killer, 171t
Dyazide (Triamterene plus hydrochlorothiazide), 488t
Dye(s), 8t, 95t, 96t, 455
  aniline, (*see* Aniline dye)

eosin, 95t
hair, poisonous substances in, 94t
leather, poisonous substances in, 95t
metallic, 94t
nigrosine, 95t
vegetable, poisonous substances in, 96t
Dylox (Trichlorfon), 137t
Dymelor (Acetohexamide), 429, 481t, 513t
Dynapen, (*see* Dicloxacillin, sodium)
Dyochlor Powder, 162t
Dyocide 8, 162t
Dyohex Dust, 162t
Dyrenium, (*see* Triamterene)

**E**

Earth, diatomaceous, 614t
Eastern oakleaf poison ivy (poison oak), 539
Eastern States Aerosol Insecticide, 171t
Eastern States Duocide Mixed Bait, 195t
Easy Aid Silver Cleaner, 528t
Easy Bleach, 528t
Easy Monday Mothproofer, 195t
Easy Off Oven Cleaner, 528t
Echinococcosis (hydatid cyst), 592
Echinoderms, 583, 585
Echothiophate iodide (Phospholine iodide), 488t
Ecthyma contagiosum (orf), 591
Edathamil, calcium, 180
E-D Bee, 195t
EDDHA, 435
Edecrin, (*see* Ethacrynic acid)
Edetate, 255, 434
calcium, (*see* calcium edetate)
calcium disodium, (*see* EDTA)
dipotassium, 422
sodium, 422
trisodium, 253
Edrophonium (Tensilon), 21t
adverse effects, 49t
chloride, 415
EDTA (Ethylenediaminetetra-acetate, calcium disodium edetate or Versenate), 19t, 33, 53t, 253, 259, 260, 263, 264, 265, 395, 421t, 422, 428, 434, 435, 436, 474, 566
Education,
for poison prevention, **3-6**
public safety, **660-743**
Eel,
electric (*Electrophorus*), 587t
moray (*Gymnathorax mordax*), 582, 583, 586t
Egg(s),
raw, as an antidote, 46
whites, as a demulcent, 46, 83
Elaterin, 35t, 406t
Elavil, (*see* Amitriptyline)
Elco-Cide, 163t
Elco Roach and Ant Powder, 163t
Elder,
marsh, 539
poison (*Rhus vernix*), 539, 553t
scarlet (*Sambucus pubens*), 550t
Elderberry, black and scarlet elder (*Sambucus canadensis* and *pubens*), 550t
Electric dishwasher detergent granules, **520**
Electric fish,
eels, 587t
rays, 590
Electric Paste, 195t
Electric shock, **620**
Electrocution, 620
Electrolyte concentrations of several commonly used parenteral fluids, Table 25(58)
imbalance, 112t, 347t
*Electrophorus* (eels), 587t
Electroshock, 82t
Electro-Silicon Polishing Cream, 528t
Electro-Sol Dishwashing Compound, 528t
Elephantfish, 585
Elephant's ear (*Dieffenbachia*), 548t
"Elephant tranquilizer", 101
Elipten (Amino-glutethimide), 363t, 482t
Elixodyne (Acetaminophen), 117t
Elkay-s Klens-All, 528t
Elk horn coral, 584
El Rey Mouse Bait, 195t
Emergency,
drugs, **19-26** (with table)
equipment, **26-27**
management (general), 27-28
Emetic(s), **42-46**
apomorphine, **43-44**
hydrochloride, 83
hypodermic tablets, **31**
contraindications, 42-43
copper sulfate, 83
ipecac powder, 83
mustard water, contraindicated, 42
saline, contraindicated, 42-43
syrup of ipecac, 43, 83
tartar, (*see* Tartar emetic)
zinc sulfate, 83
Emetine, 62t, 83, 97t, 488t
hydrochloride, 346t
Emivan, *see* Ethamivan
Emodin, 10t, 11t, 406t
Emo-Nik, 163t
Emulphogene Detergent, 528t
Emulsa Chlor, 163t
Emulsin, 236
End-O-Pest Arc Ant & Lawn Insect Dust, 163t
End-O-Pest Arc for Ants & Lawn Insects, 163t
End-O-Pest Crabgrass Killer, 195t
End-O-Pest Evergreen & Ornamental Spray, 163t
End-O-Pest Mosquito Killer, 163t
End-O-Pest Rose Dust, 163t
Endosulfan (Thiodan), 731
Endothal, 187t, 734t
Endotoxin, 65t
End-O-Weed Weed Killer, 195t
Endrin, 126, 164t, 201t, 734t
Enduron (Methyclothiazide), 469
Enflurane (Ethrane), 79t
Energine Cleaning Fluid, 528t
Engo, 163t
Enterotoxin, staphylococcus, 710, **711-712**
Enterovioform (Iodochlorhydroxyquinoline), 430
Entex (Baytex), 137t
Entoquel, (*see* Thihexinol methylbromide)
Environmental hazards, **322-331**
air pollution, **322-327** (with figure and tables)
in the home, **327-329**
radioactive, **329-330**
water, **330-331** (with table)
Environmental Protection Agency, 128, 256
Enzymes, detergents with, (*see* Detergents)
Eosin, 346t
dyes, 95t
Eosinophilia, **10**
drugs associated with, Table 7(15-16)
Ephedrine, 8t, 9t, 13t, 32, 62t, 97t, 117t, 154, 346t, 443t, 446, 470, 471, 575
contraindications, 190, 226
sulfate, 19t, 20t, 36
*Epicanta fabricii* (blister beetles), 578
Epidemiological aspects of some zoonoses, Table 145(594-602)
Epileptic therapy, use of anticonvulsants for, **359-364**
reactions of anticonvulsant drugs, Table 104(362-363)
Epinephrine (Adrenalin), 7t, 9t, 19t, 21t, 32, 36, 62(t), 97t, 98, 154, 219, 239, 334t, 347t, 352, 370, 373, 431, 462, 470, 471, 543, 568, 571, 574, 575, 578, 589, 625, 719
adverse effects, 49t
contraindications, 128, 176, 177, 190, 205, 206, 207, 226, 333, 367, 373, 450, 473, 659
hydrochloride, 351, 579
in oil, 19t
Epival, (*see* Hexobarbital, sodium)
EPN (Ethyl-p-nitrophenyl thionobenzenephosphonate), 127, 132t, 136
EPN 300, 137t
Epoxy resin glues, **620-621**
toxicity of, Table 148(622)
Epsom salts (Magnesium sulfate), 37, 173, 228, 589
Eptam (EPTC), 188t
EPTC (Eptam), 188t
Equanil (Meprobamate), 110t
Equilin, 426
Equipment,
cleaning, poisonous substances in, 95t
emergency, **26-27**
for gastric lavage, **28-30**

Equivalents,
dosage for grains and grams, Table 13(23)
numerical, Table 15(24-25)
Erbon (Baron; Novon), 188t
Erco Brush Kill, 195t
Ercocide, 195t
Ergomar tablets, 425t
Ergonovine, 423
Ergot, 6t, 7t, 8t, 9t, 97t, 98, 112t 117t, 122, 346t, **423-426**
alkaloids, **423-426**
derivatives, maximum dosage in use for migraine, Table 121(424-425)
Ergotamine, 65t, 92t, 423
alkaloids, 92t
tartrate, 424t, 425t
Ergotism, 606t, 715, **717**
ERL, 163t
Erythrityl tetranitrate, 12t, 488t
Erythrocin (Erythromycin), 356t
Erythrocytic acid-phosphatase, 342
Erythromycin (Erythrocin; Ilosone; Ilotycin), 13t, 77, 110t, 117t, 118t, 334t, 356t
estolate, 16t, 79t, 121t, 339, 355ft
ethylsuccinate, 121t
*Erythroxylon coca* (Cocaine), 410
*Escherichia coli,* 711
Eserine (Physostigmine), 452
Esidrix (Hydrochlorothiazide) USP, 469
Essential oils, (*see* Volatile oils)
Esso Weed Killers, 195t
Ester(s), 95t, 157, 202, 212, **219-222,** 479
benzoic acid, 352t
cholesterol, 629
choline, 424
para-aminobenzoic, 94t, 352t
phosphate, 52t, 55t, 98, 126, **129-136** (with table), 160t
phthalate, 624
sulfate, 426
Estericide Weed Killers, 195t
Esteron Weed & Brush Killers, 195t
Estracyt (Estramustine phosphate), 403t
Estradiol, 339
Estramustine phosphate (Estracyt), 403t
Estrogen(s), 80t, 110t, 112t, 117t, 181, 312, 339, 347t, 348t, 401t, 413, 455, 488t, 503t
and lactation, 116, 119, 123
conjugated USP, **426**
Estrone, 426
Ethacrynic acid (Edecrin), 81t, 347t, 349, 386, 387, 438, 488t
Ethambutol hydrochloride (Myambutol), 356t, 437t
Ethamivan (Emivan), 386, 488t
Ethane, 625
Ethanol, 6t, 62t, 65t, 86, 116, 176, **209-212,** 216, 217, 220t, 366, 514t, (*see also* Alcohol, ethyl)
Ethanolamines, 365t, 366t
Ethchlorvynol (Placidyl), 17t, 65t, 66, 90, 427, 488t, 503t, 514t
Ether, 6t, 7t, 8t, 72t, 82t, 86, 97t, 117t, 202, 206, **219-222,** 247t, 351, **426-427,** 479, 521, 636
derivatives, 222
divinyl (Vinethene), 426
ethyl, 87t, 514t
petroleum, 95t
Ethinamate (Valmid), 65t, 118t, 514t
Ethion, 137t
Ethionamide (Trecator), 356t, 437t
Ethosuximide (Zarontin), 345t, 361, 363t, 364, 514t
Ethotoin (Peganone), 360, 363t
Ethoxazene (Serenium), 11t
Ethrane (Enflurane), 79t
Ethyl,
acetate, 94t, 247t, 649, 729t
alcohol, (*see* Alcohol, ethyl)
biscoumacetate (Tromexan ethyl acetate), 110t, 117t
bromide, 190
bromoacetate, 617, 654
cellosolve, **613**
chloride, 190, 426, 471, 488t, 514t
chloride cyclopropane, 351
ether, 87t, 514t
guthion, 137t
hexanediol, 96t, 193, 195t, 581
ketone, 725
mercaptan, 625
methyl ketone, 247t, 624
morphine hydrochloride, 54t, 488t
nitrite, 12t, 449, 450, 488t
spirit, 612
p-aminobenzoate, 12t, 536
silicate, 314
sulfones, **468**
Ethylene, 351, 426
chlorohydrin, 202, **208,** 729t
dibromide, 195t, 201t, 734t
dichloride, 82t, 95t, 202, **207-208,** 247t, 636, 729t, 734t
glycol, 51t, 65t, 82t, 94t, 95t, 97t, 202, **218-219,** 220t, 514t, 613, 729t
glycol diacetate, 729t
glycol dinitrate, 12t, 82t, 729t
oxide, 87t, 208
trichloride, (*see* Trichloroethylene)
Ethylenediamine(s), 312, 313, 365t, 366t
Ethylenediaminetetra-acetate, (*see* EDTA)
Eucaine, 488t
Eucalyptol, 489t
Eucalyptus, 479
oil, 65t
Eugenol, 449, 617
*Euonymus,*
*atropurpureus* (burning bush, wahoo), 549t
*europaeus* (spindle-tree), 554t
*Eupatorium rugosum, urticaefolium* (white snake-root), 539, 554t
*Euphorbia,*
*maculata* (milk purslane), 548t
*pulcherrima* (poinsettia), 553t
Eurax (Crotamiton), 486t
*Eurythoë* (Annelid worms), 587t
Eutonyl, (*see* Pargyline hydrochloride)
Eutrophication, 518
Evipal sodium, 35t
Exchange transfusions, **63-64,** 153
Ex-L Pellets, 195t
Exna (Benzthiazide), 469
Exotoxin, botulinus, **712-714**
Expello Moth Baglets, 195t
Expello Moth Proofer & Wool Wash, 195t
Expello Moth Vapors, 195t
Extracorporeal dialyzer, **64-66** (with table)
Eye
-brow pencil, poisonous substances in, 95t
chemical burns of the, **46-47**
contamination, first aid for, 721
cream, poisonous substances in, 95t
shadow, poisonous substances in, 95t

**F**

Fab, 528t
Fabric softener, composition of, 523t
*Fagopyrum sagittatum* (Buckwheat), 548t
*Fagus sylvatica* (Beechnut), 548t
Fair Packaging and Labeling Act, 5
Falcon Roach Powder, 163t
Fall out (radioactive air pollution), **329-330**
False coral snakes, 563
False hellebore (*Veratrum viride*), 540, 541f
False morel (*Gyromitra esculenta*), 555, 556f
Farmer's lung (hypersensitivity pneumonitis; "silofiller's disease"), 314, **321-322**
Farm & Garden Brand Aphid Dust or Spray, 163t
Farm & Garden Brand Chlordane Dust, 163t
Farmrite Crab Grass Killer, 196t
Farmrite 21-10 Dust, 196t
Farmrite Tomato Blight Dust, 196t
FAS, (*see* Fetal alcohol syndrome)
Fasco Ant Poison, 163t
Fasco Bur-Gam Dust, 163t
Fasco Cuminoil Emulsion, 196t
Fasco Fly Flakes, 163t
Fasco Fume, 196t
Fasco Master Lice Powder, 163t
Fasco Peach Dust, 196t
Fasco Wy-Hoe, 196t
Fast Kill Bug Killer, 171t
Fatal doses, (*see* Lethal doses)
Fatal Prepared Rat & Mouse Bait, 196t
Fatty acid alkanolamine amide, (*see* Nonionic detergent)
Fat wolf herb, 545
Fava bean (*Vicia faba*), 7t, 10t, 13t, 191, 343t, 540, 550t
Favism, 62t, 338t, 343t, **718-719**
F & B Weed Killer, 196t

FDA, (*see* Food and Drug Administration)
Febrolin (Acetaminophen), 117t
Feces, discoloration by drugs, Table 4(12)
Federal Aviation Administration, 326
Federal Caustic Poison Act, 701, 702
Federal Coal Mine Health and Safety Act of 1969, 273, 316
Federal Consumer Product Safety Commission, 620ft
Federal Food and Drug Administration, (*see* Food and Drug Administration)
Federal Food, Drug and Cosmetic Act, 652, 701, 702, 703, 707
Federal Hazardous Substances Labeling Act, **702-703**
Federal Insecticide, Fungicide and Rodenticide Act of 1947, 126, 702
Federal laws,
regarding household articles, 5, **701-710** (with table) (*see also* labeling regulations and individual laws)
Federal Uniform Hazardous Substances Act of 1960, 5, **702-703**
Fehling's test, 189
Feldspar, 314, 315, 524t
Fenac, 188t
Fendon (Acetaminophen), 117t
Fenethion (Baytex), 137t
Fenfluramine, 347t
Fenuron (Dybar), 188t
-TCA (Urab), 188t
FEP, (*see* Free erythrocyte prophyrin test)
Ferbam (Fermate), 181, 196t, 198t, 199t, **621**
Fermate, (*see* Ferbam)
Fern, bracken (*Pteridium aquilinum, Pteris aquilina*), 606t
male, (*see* Aspidium)
Ferradow, 196t
Ferric
ammonium sulfate, 615t
chloride, 373, 454
test, 463
tincture of, 139
dimethyl dithiocarbamate, 621
ferrocyanide (Prussian blue), 143
oxide, 612
salts, 463
sulfate, 632
Ferricyanide(s) 236
sodium, 614t
Ferrioxamine, 435
Ferrocyanide, 236
ferric (Prussian blue), 143
potassium, 45, 180
sodium, 614t
Ferrosilicon, 140
Ferrous,
ammonium sulfate, 615t
carbonate, 434
fumarate, 432
phosphate, 434
sulfate, 12t, 41, 45, 97t, 355, 431, 432
Fertilizers, **621-623**
Fescue, as an animal poison, 606t
Fetal alcohol syndrome (FAS), **103-108,** 112t, 210
Fetus,
antibiotics, effects on, 355
drug dangers, **102-125** (with table)
drugs affecting, Table 41(110-111), Table 42(112)
radiation, effects on, 640t
Fiberglass, 314, **623-624**
Fibrinogen, 436, 566
Fibrosis
bauxite fume, **318-319**
corundum fume, **318-319**
Field Rat Powder, 196t
Films on poisoning, (*see* Appendix A) 747-748
Finger cherry (*Rhodomyrtus macrocarpa*), 550t
Fire ant, 576t
Fire coral, 584
Fire-extinguishing fluids, poisonous substances in, 95t
Fire salts (Christmas decoration), **739**
Fire-starting tablets, poisonous substances in, 96t
Firethorn *(Pyracantha coccinea)*, 553t
Fireworks hazards, **738-739**
safety precautions, **738-739**
First aid,
chart, inner cover of book
measures for carbon monoxide poisoning, **724**
measures for poisoning, **720-722**
Fischer test, for iron detection, 434
Fish, (*see also* individual fish listings)
berries *(Cocculus indicus)*, 550t
dragon, 585
electric, 587t, 590
elephant, 585
jelly *(Physalia palagica)*, 584, 587t, 590
lion *(Pterois volitans)*, 588t, 590
poisoning (Ichthyosarcotoxism), 581
poisonous, **581-591** (with table)
scorpion *(Scorpaena guttata)*, 585, 587t
stinging, **585**
sting, treatment of, **585-589**
Fixit Scratch Cover Furniture Polish, 528t
*Flacourtiaceae* (Ryania), 157
Flag Cryolite Dust, 163t
Flagyl (Metronidazole), 10t, 11t, 79t, 117t, 118t, 122, 212, 214t, 494t
Flax, 539
dust, 319
Flaxseed oil, **630**
Flea(s), 579, 581, **730**
anti-dog and cat collars, 136
Flea-Foil Flea Powder, 163t
Flea-Go, 163t
Flea-Not Powder, 163t
Fleet enema, 434, 455
Flexin, (*see* Zoxazolamine)
Flight Brand Melon Dust, 196t
Flit, 171t
Flit Aerosol Fly Mosquito Killer, 163t
Flit Aerosol House and Garden Insect Killer, 163t
Flit Aerosol Insect Spray, 171t
Flit Bug Killer, 163t, 171t
Flit Bug Killer Pressurized, 163t
Flit Double Action Insect Spray Aerosol, 171t
Flit Fly and Mosquito Killer, 163t
Flit Moth Proofer, 163t, 196t
Flit Roach and Ant Killer, 163t
Flit Roach and Ant Killer Pressurized, 163t
Flit with 5% DDT, 171t
Flor-A-Bomb, 171t
Floral odor in perfumes, 95t
Floraquin, (*see* Diiodohydroxyquin)
Floratox Herbicide, 196t
Floratox Weed Killer, 196t
Florbait, 163t
Florida diamondback *(Crotalus adamanteus)*, **561**
Flour, 313t
as a demulcent, 46
Flower Guard, 163t
Floxuridine (FUDR), 397t
Fluid(s)
brake, poisonous substances in, 95t
cleaning, poisonous substances in, 94t
fire-extinguishing, poisonous substances in, 95t
intravenous, 110t
therapy, **47-49** (with table)
thermometer, poisonous substances in, 96t
Fluid-Cress Disinfectant, 528t
Fluoaluminate sodium, 159t, 161t, 163t, 165t, 167t
Fluoride(s), 8t, 33, 53t, 65t, 69, 86, 88, 89, 90, 97t, 123, 127, **140-141,** 198t, 271t, 331t, 335t, 514t, 605t, 657
barium, 734t
calcium, 140, 141
hydrogen, 228, 2235, 247t, 324t, 625
sodium, 140, 155t, 163t, 166t, 167t, 168t, 228, **716-717**
Fluorine, 202, **235,** 312, 625, 632
derivatives, 202, **235**
Fluoroacetamide "1080", **176,** 734t
Fluoroacetate, 62t, 734t
sodium ("1080"), 54t, 62t, 173, **176,** 179t
Fluoroscopy, **638-640**
Fluorotricarboxylic acid, 176
5-Fluorouracil (5-FU), 65t, 143t, 345t, 347t, 397t
Fluorocarbons, 624, 625
Fluorspar, 314
Fluosilicate,
barium, 173
sodium, 166t, 200t
Fluothane (Halothane), 15t, 79t, 426, 514t
Fluoxymesterone (Halotestin), 402t
Fluprednisolone, 415t
Fly, 579 (*see* individual listings)

Fly-B-Gon Insect Spray, 163t
Fly Dair, 163t
Fly-Ded, 171t
Flyded Aerosol Insect Killer, 171t
Flyded Insect Spray, 171t
Fly Doom Spray, 163t
Fly-Dy, 163t
Flyers on poisoning, (*see* Appendix A) 745-747
Fly Hot Foot, 163t
Fly Hot Lunch, 163t
Fly Jinx Insect Spray, 163t
Fly-Tox Aerosol Insect Bomb, 171t
Foliafume, 163t
Folic acid, 118t, 216, 339, 347t, 359, 360, 361, 475, 476t, 632
  deficiency, 477
Folinic acid, 404
Food,
  additives, 115, **703-710**
    functions of some commonly used, Table 157(708-709)
  allergies, **718-719**
  drug interactions, 333-334 (with chart)
  poisoning, 606, **710-720**
    prevention, 720
  with MAO inhibitors, adverse reactions, Table 124(443)
Food Additives Amendment of 1958, 707, 719
Food and Agriculture Organization, 124
Food and Drug Administration (FDA), 125, 128, 129, 150, 208, 264, 394, 422, 536, 558, 625, 651, 701, 702, 707, 710, 713, 719, 732
Food and Drug Directorate, 125
Food, Drug and Cosmetic Act, (*see* Federal Food, Drug and Cosmetic Act)
Formaldehyde, 31, 51t, 95t, 97t, 202, 213, 216, 220t, **243-244,** 247t, 313t, 346t, 533, 535, 536, 648t, 734t
  sodium sulfoxalate, 19t, 41, 55t, 147
Formalin, 31, 51t, 58, 97t, **243-244**
Formcolor Disinfectant, 528t
Formic acid, 58, 192, 193, 213, 216, 220t, 244, 648t, 742
Forrest rapid urine color tests, Figure 14(372)
Fort Dodge Flea and Louse Powder, 171t
Four o'clock *(Mirabilis jalapa)*, 550t
Four X-D, 196t
Fowler's solution (Potassium arsenite), 489t
Foxglove *(Digitalis purpurea, lanata)*, 540, 550t
Freckle removers, poisonous substances in, 95t
Free erythrocyte porphyrin test (FEP), 260
French delivery and suction tubes, use in gastric lavage, 29
French's Flea Powder for Dogs, 163t
Freon (Dichlorodifluoromethane), 189, 350, 609, **624-625,** 739
Freon-11 (Trichloromonofluoromethane), 87t
  propellants, 95t
Freon-12 (Dichlorodifluoromethane), 87t
Frog, Kokoi, **590-591**
Fröhde's test, 92t
5-FU (Fluorouracil), 397t
Fuadin (Stibophen), 155, 342, 354t, 499t
FUDR (Floxuridine), 397t
Fuedeth Roach Powder, 163t
Fuels, rocket (Boron hydride), **644-645**
Fulex Blue Label, 196t
Fulex Green Label, 196t
Fulex Red Label, 196t
Fuller's earth, 186
Fulvicin, (*see* Griseofulvin)
Fumarate, ferrous, 432
Fumes, toxic maximum allowable concentrations for, Table 73(311)
Fumigants, **186-201**
  potential toxicity of, 734t
Fumo-Gas, 196t
Fungal toxicoses, 606t
Fung Chex, 196t
Fungicides, **179-182,** Table 58(194-201)
  potential toxicity of, 734-735t
Fungi, producing photosensitization, 548t
Fungizone (Amphotericin B), 79t, 355t
Fungtrogen, 196t
Fungus diseases (zoonoses), 595-596t
Furacin, (*see* Nitrofurazone)
Furadantin (Nitrofurantoin), 16t, 79t, 110t, 117t, 118t, 338t, 341, 356t, 495t, 515t
Furaltadone (Altafur), 489t
Furazolidone (Furoxone), 11t, 214t, 334t, 343t
Furniture Doctor, 528t
Furniture polish, 4f, 224, 225
  poisonous substances in, 94t
Furocoumarin compounds (Psoralens), 455, 537
Furosemide (Lasix), 16t, 21t, 102, 124t, 386, 387, 438, 489t
Furoxone (Furazolidone), 11t, 214t
Fusel oil, 212, 217
Fyne-Tex Disinfectant, 528t


### G


Gaillardia (Blanket flower), 539
Gain detergent, 525
*Galerina* (mushroom)
  *autumnalis*, 557t
  *venenata*, 555
Gallamine triethiodide, 65t
Gallate, iron, 96t
Gallic acid, 656, 657
Gallium, 270t
Galltox, 196t
Galvo, (*see* Metal fume fever)
Gamboge, 406t
Gamene, 129
Gamma benzene hexachloride (Gamma BHC), 13t, 130t, 137t, 160t, 161t, 162t, 163t, 165t, 168t, 339
Gamma glutamyl transferase (GGT), 209
Gamtox Mosquito Cone, 163t
Ganges shark (Carcharinidae family), 586t
Gantanol, (*see* Sulfamethoxazole)
Gantrisin, (*see* Sulfisoxazole)
Gardsite Rust Remover, 528t
Garlic, 539
Gas(es) (*see also* individual gases)
  anti-riot (Mace), 6t, **250**
  chlorine, (*see* Chlorine gas)
  coal, (*see* Coal gas)
  identification of poison, 85
  infrared analysis of, Table 35 (87)
  manufactured, **625**
  maximum allowable concentration of, Table 66 (247)
  mustard, 6t, 9t
  natural, (*see* Natural gas)
  nerve, 7t, 9t
  propane, (*see* Propane gas)
  suicidal deaths, 335t, 337f
  tear, 6t, 9t, **654**
  toxic, 648t
  war, 6t, 9t
  water, (*see* Water gas)
Gas chromatography, used for identification of poisons, 84, 85
Gasoline, 4f, 87t, 106t, 202, **222-224,** 265
  vapor, 202, **244-245** (*see also* Petroleum distillates)
Gastric lavage, **28-30** (with figure), (*see also* specific poisons)
Gastroduodenal ulcers, role of drugs in, Table 90(345)
Gastropods (univalve mollusks), 584
Gator Roach Hive, 163t
G.C. Flykiller, 163t
Geigy LO-V Brush Killer, 196t
Geigy Potato Vine & Weed Killer, 196t
Geigy Rat & Mouse Bait, 196t
Geller's Cedarized Insecticide, 172t
Geller's Moth Proofer, 196t
Geller's Roach Fel, 163t
Gelsemine, 6t, 489t
*Gelsemium sempervirens* (yellow jessamine), 6t, 489t, 540, 551t
Gemonil (Metharbital), 362t
Genidust D-10 Dust, 163t
Geniphene, 163t
Genithion P-25 Dust Base, 163t
Genitol, 163t
Gentamycin (Geramycin), 124t, 143t
Gentian violet (Methylrosaniline chloride), 203, 354t, 489t
Gentran, 385
Geopen (Carbencillin), 118t
Geramycin (Gentamycin), 124t
Geraniol, 449, 613, 617
Germa-Pine Disinfectant, 528t
Germine diacetate, 540
Germ-I-Tol Deodorizer, 528t

Germonil (Metharbital), (*see* Metharbital)
GGT (Gamma glutamyl transferase), (*see* Gamma glutamyl transferase)
Giant clam (tridacna), 583
Gibberellic acid, **626**
Gifblaar *(Dichapetalum cymosum)*, 176
Gila monster *(Heloderma suspectrum)*, **570**
Glacial acetic acid, 94t
Glamorene Rug Cleaner, 528t
Glass, 311t
Glassware detergents, poisonous substances in, 94t
Glass Wax, 528t
Glauber's salt (Sodium sulfate), 173
G.L.F. Dust (#8A, #10, #30A, #33, #34, #61), 164t
Globe Flea Bomb and Deodorant, 164t
Globe Liquid Grub Killer, 164t
Globe Sud-N-Deth Fly Bait, 164t
*Gloriosa superba* (gloriosa or climbing lily), 550t
Glucagon, 209, 347t
Glucocorticoid compound tablets, 401t, 413
Gluconate,
calcium, (*see* Calcium gluconate)
quinidine, (*see* Quinidine gluconate)
Glucose, 68t, 190, 209, 211, 212, 213, 347t, 386, 408, 436, 452, 465, 466, 473, 479, 544, 637, 646
Glucose-6-phosphate dehydrogenase (G-6-PD) deficiency, 18, 32, 37, 113, 181, 191, 203, **337-344** (with tables), 718
Glucoside(s), 42, 45, 538, 656
stibamine (Neostam), 499t
Glucuronic acid, 404, 444
Glue(s)
epoxy resin, **620-621**
toxicity of, Table 148(622)
poisonous substances in, 95t
sniffing, 106t, **658-659,** 722t
Glutamate
monosodium (MSG), 115, 708t
sodium and disodium (Glutamic acid), 489t
Glutamic acid (Glutamate, sodium and disodium), 489t
Glutarimide, methyl-ethyl (Megimide), 37
Glutathione (GSH), 148, 338, 343, 348, 349
GSH stability test, 343
Glutethimide (Doriden), 8t, 14t, 30, 66, 67, 97t, 104t, 112t, 122, **427-428,** 453, 456, 503t, 514t
amino- (Elipten), see Amino-glutethimide
Gluthion, 52t
*Glycera* (Annelid worm), 587t
Glycerin(e) (Glycerol), 20t, 95t, 218, 235, 454, 522t, 612, **626,** 636, 709t
Glycerol, (*see* Glycerin)
Glyceryl,
esters, 522t
monoacetate (Monoacetin), 176
trinitrate, **449-450**
Glycine, 611, 647, 648
Glycobiarsol (Milibis), 489t
bismuth, 391
Glycol(s), 95t, 202, **218-219,** 518t, 523t, 524t
diethylene, 95t, **218-219,** 729t
diethylene stearate, 95t
ethylene, 51t, 94t, 95t, 97t, 220t, 514t, 613, 729t
ethylene diacetate, 729t
ethylene dinitrate, 12t, 729t
hexylene, **218-219**
polyalkaline, (*see* Non-ionic detergents)
polyethylene, 730t
polypropylene, 730t
propylene, 95t, 202, **218-219,** 454, 730t
Glycolaldehyde, 218
Glycolic acid, 218
Glycolylarsanilate, bismuth (Milibis), 12t
Glycoside(s),
cardiac, 177, 417, 421, 540
cardioactive, 7t, 9t
cyanogenetic, 235
digitalis, 15t, 16t, 344
Glycosuria-testing tablets (Clinitest tablets), (*see* Clinitest tablets)
Glycuronate, 226
Glycuronic acid, 451
Glycyrrhetinic acid, 626
Glycyrrhiza, 612
Glycyrrhizin (Licorice), **626**
Glyoxalidine derivative, 195t, 196t
Glyoxylic acid, 218
Go-Crab, 196t
Go-Fecto Disinfectant, 528t
Gold, 6t, 32, 53t, 82t, 269, 270t, **428**
radioactive colloidal, 78, 644t
salts, 16t, 143t, 339, 347t, 455, 514t
Golden chain *(Cytisus laburnum)*, 551t
Goldenrod, rayless *(Aplopappus heterophyllus)*, 539, 553t
Golden Seal *(Hydrastis canadensis)*, 549t
Gold Seal Snowy Bleach, 529t
Golf balls, contents of, **626**
Golf Brand Weed Killer, 196t
Golf Crabgrass Preventer, 196t
G & O Moth Deodorant Nuggets, 196t
Gonadotropins, 123, 348t
Go-Nex, 164t
*Gonyaulax,* in shellfish poisoning, 718
Gopher Death, 196t
Gopher Go, 196t
G & O Plant Spray, 172t
Gordolobos tea, 545, 547
Gorham Silver Polish, 529t
G-6-PD, (*see* Glucose-6-phosphate dehydrogenase)
Grain, 314
alcohol, (*see* Alcohol, ethyl)
Grainfume, 196t
*Granatum* (pomegranate), 636
Granite, 331t
Graphite, **626,** 633
Grasshopper, 741
Gray nurse shark (Carcharinidae family), 586t
Grease remover, poisonous substances in, 94t
Great barracuda *(Sphyraena barracuda)*, 586t
Green Cross Basi-Cop, 196t
Green Cross Brushkil, 196t
Green Cross Couchgrass Killer, 196t
Green Cross Fruit Fungicide, 196t
Green Cross Karbam Black Fungicide, 196t
Green Cross Potato Top Killer, 196t
Green Cross Rat & Mouse Bait, 196t
Green Cross Residual Household Spray, 172t
Green Cross San Seed Disinfectant, 196t
Green Cross Slug Bait, 164t
Green Cross Tantoo, 196t
Green Cross Tantoo Bomb, 196t
Green Cross Weed-No-More Dust, 196t
Green Light Fire Ant Killer, 164t
Green Light Fly & Mosquito Bomb, 164t
Green Light Oil for Scale, 164t
Green Light Roach and Ant Killer, 164t
Green Paris, (*see* Paris Green)
Green tobacco sickness, 156
"Grey" syndrome, 110t
Grifulvin, (*see* Griseofulvin)
Grinder's rot (Silicosis), **314-315**
Griseofulvin (Grifulvin; Fulvicin), 8t, 79t, 214t, 334t, 345t, 348t, 455, 456, 489t, 503t
Ground rattlesnakes *(Sistrurus)*, **562,** 564f
Groundsel, 545
Growth depressants, potential toxicity of, 735t
GSH (Glutathione), (*see* Glutathione)
GTA Ant Base, 164t
G.T.A. Bait for Rats, Mice, 196t
Guaiacol, 14t, **453,** 489t, 618
Guanethidine sulfate (Ismelin), 489t
Guanidine hydrochloride, 714
Guardsman Cleaning Polish, 529t
*Guarea rusbyi* (Bolivian tree), 617
Guide to organization of a poison control center, **696-699**
Gulf Roach & Ant Killer, 172t
Gulfspray, 172t
Gulfspray Aerosol Bomb, 164t
Gulfspray Cone Aerosol Insecticide, 164t
Gum, arabic, 614t, 708t
Gun bluing, poisonous substances in, 96t
Guthion (Dimethyl-S-[4-oxo-1,2,3,benzotriazinyl-3-methyl] phosphorodithioate), 132t, 734t
ethyl, 137t
methyl, 137t
Gutzeit's procedure, 139
Gy-Cop, 196t
*Gymnathorax mordax* (Moray eel), 586t

*Gymnocladus dioica* (Kentucky coffee tree), 551t
Gynecomastia, drugs producing, Table 99(348)
Gynergen tablets, ampules, 424t, 425t
Gy-Phene, 164t
Gypsum (Calcium sulfate hydrous), 314, 614t, **636**
*Gyromitra esculenta* (False morel), 555
Gy-Tet, 164t
Gy-Zip, 172t

**H**

Hair,
  bleaches, contents of, 233t
  colorings, poisonous substances in, 94t
  dyes, **533-535**
    poisonous substances in, 94t
  lotions, poisonous substances in, 95t
  neutralizers, contents of, 233t
  preparations, poisonous substances in, 95t
  rinse, composition of, 524t
  sprays, **535**
    poisonous substances in, 95t
  straightening solutions, **533**
  tints, **533-535**
    poisonous substances in, 94t
  toxicologic analysis of, 87
  waving preparations, **533**
    poisonous substances in, 94t
Hairy caterpillars, 579
Halazone, (*see* Para-sulfonedichloramidobenzoic acid)
Haldol, (*see* Haloperidol)
Hallucinogens, 124
  psychoactive effects from herbal preparations, Table 136(546)
  psychotic states associated with use of, Table 40(106-109), 112t
Halogen(s), 7t, 312
  salts, 192
Halogenated
  carbanilides, 455
  hydrocarbons, 62t, 91, 106t, 186, 190, 202, **205-208,** 609, 739, 740
  hydroxyquinolines, 430ft
  phenols, 455
  salicylanilides, 455
Haloperidol (Haldol), 372, 471, 472, 490t
Halotestin (Fluoxymesterone), 402t
Halothane (Fluothane), 15t, 79t, 351, 426, 514t
*Halvella esculenta* (mushroom), 555
*Hamamelis virginiana* (Witch hazel), **657-658**
Hammerhead shark(s) (Sphyrindae family), 583, 586t
Hammond Do-Di Lawn Weed Killer, 196t
Hammond Tomato Dust, 196t
Hammond Weed Killer, 196t
Handy Killer, 164t
"Hard metal" pneumoconiosis, 323t
Harlequin snake (coral [*Micrurus fulvius*]), 563-565 (with figure)
Harmine, 98, 99, 546t
Harmless snakes, identifying features, 563f
Harris Roach Tablets, 164t
Harvester ant, 576f
Hash, (*see* Marihuana)
Hashish (Marihuana), 99, 102t, 106t (*see also* Marihuana)
Haviland 3D Insecticide, 164t
Hazardous Substances Labeling Act, (*see* Federal Hazardous Substances Labeling Act
HCA (HCA Weed Killer), 188t
HDCV (Human diploid cell vaccine), 593ft
Health departments, local, state, working with poison control centers, **697**
Heat,
  as a water pollutant, 330t
  stroke, as nephrotoxic, 82t
Heavenly blue morning glory, 552t
  seeds *(Rivea corymbosa)*, 98
Hedeoma plant (Pennyroyal), 496t
Hedulin (Phenindione), 11t, 17t, 81t
Hellebore, false *(Veratrum viride)*, 540, 541f, 550t
*Helleborus niger* (Christmas rose), 549t
*Heloderma suspectum* (Gila monster), **570**
Helvellic acid, 555, 559t
Hematinic agents, 11t, 12t
Hemlock,
  deadly, 35t, 553t
  poison *(Conium maculatum)*, 545, 553t
  water *(Cicuta maculata)*, 544t, 545, **718**
Hemodialysis, 348t (*see also* Extracorporeal dialyzer)
  in children, 66, 67
Hemoglobin, 10t, 239, 240, 241
  met-, (*see* Methemoglobin)
  sulf-, (*see* Sulfhemoglobin)
Hemolysins, as nephrotoxic, 82t
Hemolytic anemia, 7t, 93
  chemicals causing, 13-15t
  drug-induced, **336-344** (with table)
  genetic polymorphisms producing, 338t
Hemostatic agents, 11t
Hemotoxins (Cytolysins), **565-566**
Hemp dust, 319
Henbane, black *(Hyoscyamus niger)*, 548t, 550t
Henna, 533
Hep Ant & Roach Killer, 164t
Heparin, 6t, 16t, 55t, 143t, 248, 339, 490t
  use in DIC, 568
Hepatitis,
  chemical-induced, **75-82** (with tables)
  drug-induced, **75-82** (with tables)
  radiation-induced, 78
  toxic, **75-82** (with tables)
Hepatogenic plants, producing photosensitization, 548t
Hep Bug Killer, 164t
Hep 5% Insect Killer, 164t
Hep Surface Spray, 172t
Heptabarbital, 503t
Heptachlor, 117t, 126, 128, 137t, 164t, 166t, 169t, 734t
Heptagran, 164t
Heptal, 164t
Heptane, 225
Heptenone, methyl, (*see* Methyl heptenone)
Herbal preparations with psychoactive effects, Table 136(546)
Herbicide(s), **182-186,** 605t
  potential toxicity of, 734t
  relative toxicity of, to mammals, Table 57(187-188)
  trade names and harmful ingredients in, Table 58(194-201)
Hermodice (Annelid worms), 587t
Heroin, 37, 54t, 65t, 108t, 110t, 117t, 348t, 444, 445, 448, 463, 471, 490t, 722t (*see also* Diacetylmorphine)
Hess, (Dr.) Anturat, 196t
Hess Bomb, 172t
Hess, (Dr.) Powdered Louse Killer, 164t
Hess, (Dr.) Rat & Mouse Killer, 196t
Hess, (Dr.) Warfarat, 196t
*Heteropodidae* (Giant crab-spiders), 574
HETP, 6t, 7t, 8t, 734t
Hetrazan (Diethylcarbamazine), 354t, 487t
Hexachloride, benzene (Lindane), 97t, 126, 129, 130t, 162t, 734t
Hexachlorobenzene, 8t, 117t, 120, 179, **181-182,** 455, 456
Hexachlorocyclohexane (Benzene hexachloride, BHC), 130t, 181
Hexachloro-epoxy-octahydro-dimethanonaphthalene (Dieldrin), 130t
Hexachloro-hexahydro-dimethanonaphthalene (Aldrin), 130t
Hexachlorophene, 455, 497t, 522t, **626-627**
  and skin care of newborn, **627-629**
Hexadecanol (Cetyl alcohol), (*see* Alcohol, cetyl)
Hexahydric alcohol (Mannitol), (*see* Mannitol)
Hexakis distannoxane (Vendex), 581
Hexametaphosphate, 520
  sodium, 94t
Hexamethonium, 112t, 470
  bromide (Bristrium bromide), 110t
  salts, 490t
Hexamethylenamine, 312, 313, 403t
Hexamethylenetetramine (HMT), 252
Hexanediol, ethyl, 96t, 193, 195t, 581
Hexapoda (six-legged insects), 741
Hexethal (Ortal), 383t
Hexobarbital sodium (Epival), 383t
Hexol, 226
Hexylene glycol, **218-219**
Hexylresorcinol, 354t, 490t
Highland moccasin *(Agkistrodon mokeson)*, **562**
Hil Flea Powder, 172t

*Hippomane mancinella* (Manchineel), 552t
Hippuran, (*see* Iodohippurate)
Hippuric acid, 271t, 610, 611, 659
Histadyl (Methapyrilene), 16t
Histalog (Betazole), 393, 484t
Histamine, 345t
HMT, (*see* Hexamethylenetetramine)
Holger-Nielsen method of artificial respiration, 59
Holly *(Ilex aquifolium opaca)*, 550t
  berries, **740**
Holly Pine Cleaner, 529t
Homatropine, 358t, 376, 378, 490t
Home,
  hazards of solvents in, **724-730**
  pests about the, **730-736**
  polluted air, **327-329**
  prevention of carbon monoxide poisoning in the, **723**
Honey, 490t, 626
Honeybee *(Apis mellifera)*, 575, 576f, 577, 742
Hops *(Humulus lupulus)*, 313t, 546t
Hormone(s), 95t, 112t, 312
  reactions in the aged, 345t
Hornet(s), 576f, 577, 741, 742
  bald-faced, 577
Horse bean, (*see* Fava bean)
Horsebrush *(Tetradymia)*, 548t
Horse chestnut tree, 544
Horse fly, 576f
Horse nettle *(Solanum carolinense)*, 554t
Hospitals, working with poison control centers, 696-697
Hot Spring Buttons, 196t
Household,
  antidotes, Table 22(56)
  articles, federal law regarding, 701-710 (with table)
  bleach, 721
    contents of, Table 62(233)
  detergent products, **519-525** (with tables)
  measures, approximate, Table 14(24)
Howard Insect Aerosol Bomb, 172t
Howard Rat Kill Cone, 196t
Howard Ready-To-Use Rat Kill, 196t
Howard Warficide Rat Kill, 196t
H-T-H Bleach, 529t
HTH (Calcium hypochlorite), 652
Hubbard Blight Control Dust, 196t
Hubklor Dust, 164t
Human diploid cell vaccine (HDCV), 593ft
Huntington Vaporizing Fluid and Roach Spray, 164t
Hyacinth *(Hycinthus orientalis)*, 550t
Hyaluronidase, 566
Hydantoin(s), 346t, 359
  derivatives, 339, 359, 360
  methylphenylethyl (Mesantoin), 14t, 360, 362t
Hydralazine (Apresoline), 15t, 40, 339, 345t, 346t, **428**, 475, 477
  hydrochloride, 345t, 490t
Hydrangea, wild hydrangea, 546t, 551t
Hydrastine, 42
*Hydrastis canadensis* (Golden seal), 549t
Hydrate,
  alcohols, 8t
  amylene, 97t, 483t
  chloral, (*see* Chloral hydrate)
  methyl, (*see* Wood alcohol)
Hydrazide
  isonicotinic acid, 477
  maleic (MH-30), 182, 735t
Hydrazine, 247t, 341
Hydrazol (Acetazolamide), 16t
Hydrea (Hydroxyurea), 401t
Hydride,
  antimony (Stibine), 155
  boron (rocket fuel), **644-645**
  lithium, 630
  phenyl, (*see* Benzene)
Hydrobromide,
  dextromethorphan, **416**
  methorphinan (Dromoran), 494t
  scopolamine, (*see* Scopolamine)
Hydrocarbons, 202, **222-226,** 323, 324, **326,** 328f, 479, 521, 618, 625, 636
  aliphatic, (*see* Aliphatic hydrocarbons)
  aromatic, (*see* Aromatic hydrocarbons)
  benzpyrene, 329t
  chlorinated, (*see* Chlorinated hydrocarbons)
  halogenated, (*see* Halogenated hydrocarbons)
  olefinic, 329t
  petroleum, 169t
  phosphorylated, 518t
  polycyclic, 329t
  polynuclear, **717**
  sulfonated, 518t
Hydrochloride,
  n-allylnormorphine (Nalline), 19t, 37, 38, 54t, 441
  amantadine (Symmetrel), 482t
  amodiaquin, 460, 483t
  apomorphine, 19t, 44, 83, 420
  benadryl, 20t
  betahistine (Serc), 484t
  biperiden (Akineton), 376
  camoquin, 483t
  caramiphen (Panparnit), 157
  chlordiazepoxide (Librium), 212
  chloroguanide, 485t
  chlorphentermine, 486t
  chlortetracycline, 486t
  cocaine, 46
  cycrimine (Pagitane), 486t
  cyproheptadine (Periactin), 487t
  desipramine (Pertofrane), 472, 495t
  dextropropoxyphene (Darvon), 117t, **416-417**
  diphenhydramine (Benadryl), 53t, 117t, 373, 487t, 543, 582
  diphenoxylate (Lomotil), **422-423,** 488t
  dodecylamine, 653
  doxapram (Dopram), 445
  doxepin, 472
  emetine, 346t
  epinephrine, 351, 579
  ethambutol (Myambutol), 356t
  ethylmorphine, 54t, 488t
  guanidine, 714
  hydralazine (Apresoline), 345t, 490t
  hydroxyzine (Vistaril), 449, 490t
  imipramine (Tofranil), 117t, 491t
  Inversine, 493t
  Isuprel, 492t
  ketamine (Ketaject; Ketalar), 351
  lidocaine, (*see* Lidocaine)
  lucanthone, 492t
  meperidine, 54t, 492t
  methadone (Dolophine), 117t, 493t
  methamphetamine, 493t
  methixene (Trest), 494t
  methylphenidate (Ritalin), 14t, 373
  morphine, 488t
  nalorphine, 54t, 416, 441
  naloxone (Narcan), 19t, 37, 43, 44, 54t, 416, 423, 441
  nortriptyline (Aventyl), 472, 495t
  oxophenarsine (Mapharsen), 367, 496t
  oxymorphone, 496t
  oxyphencyclimine (Daricon), 496t
  pagitane, 486t
  papaverine, 424
  pargyline (Eutonyl), 496t
  phenazopyridine (Pyridium), 496t
  phenformin (DBI), 110t
  phenoxybenzamine (Dibenzyline), 69, 471
  phentolamine (Regitine), 475
  priscoline, 501t
  procainamide (Pronestyl), 19t, 174, 345t
  procaine, (*see* Procaine)
  promazine, 498t
  propranolol (Inderal), 49t, 174, 498t
  protriptyline, 472, 498t
  pyribenzamine, 19t, 20t
  pyridoxine, 438, 484t
  quinacrine, 346t, 460, 498t
  quinidine, 19t, 40
  tetracycline, 120
  tetrahydrozoline, 500t
  thiamine (Vitamin $B_1$), 20t
  tolazoline (Priscoline), 501t
  tripelennamine, 15t
Hydrochloric acid, 8t, 83, 94t, 97t, 205, **226-228,** 245, 250, 268, 270, 467, 526, 633
Hydrochlorothiazide USP (HydroDIURIL; Esidrix; Oretic), 469, 490t
  plus triamterene (Dyazide), 488t
Hydrocodone (Codeine), 412
Hydrocortisone (Cortisol, Solu-Cortef), 14t, 19t, 69, 124t, 385, 415t
  sodium succinate, 21t, 69, 575
Hydrocupreine(s), 459
Hydrocyanic acid (Cyanide), 127, **153-155, 235-237,** 606, 637, 734t (*see also* Cyanide)
HydroDIURIL (Hydrochlorothiazide USP), 469, 490t

Hydroflumethiazide (Saluron), 469
Hydrofluoric acid, 95t, 202, **228,** 720
Hydrogen,
chloride, 247t, 648
cyanide, 97t, 153, 155t, 202, **235-237,** 247t, 266, 324t, 648t
fluoride, 228, 235, 247t, 324t, 625
peroxide, 54t, 152, 233t, 237, 490t, 532, 534, 537, 584, 634
sulfate, 656
sulfide, 85, 97t, 173, 237-239, 247t, 323, 324t, 326, 514t, 630, 648t
Hydroids, (*see* Coelenterates)
Hydrolysate, 555
Hydromix Crabgrass Killer, 196t
Hydromix Crabgrass & Weed Preventer, 197t
Hydromix Garden Insecticide, 172t
Hydromix Lawn and Termite Spray, 172t
Hydromorphone (Dilaudid), 514t
Hydromix (Quinethazone), 469
Hydroquinone, 10t, 656
oral, 12t
Hydroxide,
aluminum, (*see* Aluminum hydroxide)
ammonium, (*see* Ammonium hydroxide)
barium, (*see* Barium hydroxide)
calcium, (*see* Calcium hydroxide)
lithium, (*see* Lithium hydroxide)
magnesium, (*see* Magnesium hydroxide)
methyl, (*see* Wood alcohol)
potassium, (*see* Potassium hydroxide)
sodium, (*see* Sodium hydroxide)
triethanolamine, (*see* Triethanolamine hydroxide)
Hydroxyanisole, butylated, 708t
2-Hydroxybenzamide (Salicylamide), **461**
Hydroxychloroquine (Plaquenil), 338, 344, 459, 460, 555
Hydroxycoumarin, acetonylbenzyl, (*see* Warfarin)
Hydroxydione succinate sodium (Viadril), 490t
Hydroxylamine, 12t
2-Hydroxy-4-methoxy-benzophenone-5-sulfonic acid, (*see* Sulisobenzone)
Hydroxynaphthoate (Alcopara), 354t
Hydroxyprogesterone caproate (Delalutin), 402t, 490t
Hydroxyquinolines, halogenated, 430ft
Hydroxystilbamidine, 490t
Hydroxytoluene, butylated, 708t
Hydroxyurea (Hydrea), 401t
Hydroxyzine (Atarax; Vistaril), 15t, 118t, 366t
hydrochloride, 449, 490t
pamoate, 490t, 573
Hygroton (Chlorthalidone), 16t, 469
Hykinone, 112t
Hymenoptera group (honeybee, wasp, hornet, yellow jacket), 742
Hymenoptera stings, reaction types, Table 142(577)
Hyoscine (Scopolamine), 8t, 117t, 358t, 490t, 545
Hyoscyamine, 376, 545, 546t
sulfate, 14t
Hyoscyamus, (*see* Atropine)
*Hyoscyamus niger* (Black henbane), 358t, 548t, 550t
*Hypericum perforatum* (St. Johnswort, Klamath weed), 548t
Hyperosmolar state, 65t
Hypersensitivity pneumonitis (Farmer's lung), 314, **321-322**
antigens causing, Table 76(322)
Hypertension cranial, caused by poisoning, **70-71**
Hypertonic
saline, 58t
solutions, 70, 71
Hypervitaminosis,
A, 6t, **477-478**
D, 55t, 477, **478-479**
K, **479**
*Hypnos* (Rayfish), 587t
Hypnotics, 7t, 9t, 38
reactions in the aged, 345t
Hypochlorite, 97t, **232-233**
calcium, 524t, 615t, 652
potassium, 629
sodium, 51t, 94t, 95t, 96t, 230, 524t, 629, 652
bleaches, 233t, 234t, 526
Hypochlorous acid, 245
Hypoglycemic(s)
interaction with alcohol, 214t
oral agents, 110t, **429,** 503t
sulfonylurea, 455
Hypoglycine, 544
Hyposulfite, sodium, (*see* Sodium hyposulfite)
Hypotonic saline, 58t
Hy-Tox Fly Bait, 164t
Hy-Tox Insect Spray, 172t

**I**

Ibuprofen (Motrin), 490t
I.C. Degreaser, 529t
Ichthammol (Ichthyol), 490t
Ichthyoacanthotoxism, 581
Ichthyol, (*see* Ichthammol)
Ichthyosarcotoxism (fish poisoning), 581
Ichthyotoxism, 581
Icicles (tinsel), **740**
Ideal Brand Perk, 197t
Identification of poisons, isolation and separation techniques, **84-85**
Idoxuridine (IDU), 491t
IDU, (*see* Idoxuridine)
*Ilex,* 740
*aquifolium opaca, verticillata* (holly, black alder), 550t
*paraguayensis* (Mate), 631
*Illicium anisatum* (Japanese anise), 554t
Ilosone (Erythromycin), 16t, 79t, 110t
Ilotycine (Erythromycin), 356t
Imferon (Iron dextran), (*see* Iron)
Iminodibenzyl derivatives, 369t
Imipramine (Tofranil; Presamine), 14t, 90, 358t, 359, 364, 371, 442, 443t, 472, 474, 491t, 514t
hydrochloride, 117t
Impregno, 164t
Imuran (Azathioprine), 80t, 455, 483t
Indalone, 96t, 186, **193,** 580
Indane derivatives, 126, **128-129,** 166t
Indanedione,
anticoagulants, 16t, 17t
derivatives, 11t
Inderal (Propranolol hydrochloride), 17t, 174, 411, 421t, 498t, 515t
adverse effects, 49t
Indian balsam, **610**
Indian bead, (*see* Jequirity bean)
Indian hemp, (*see* Marihuana)
Indian tobacco (*Lobelia inflata*), 551t
Indigo, 533
Indocin, (*see* Indomethacin)
Indomethacin (Indocin), 7t, 10t, 12t, 17t, 79t, 344, 347t, 477, 491t
Industrial alcohols, 517
Industrial dermatitis, **311-313**
Industrial hazards, **202-272**
Industrial methylated spirit, 95t
Infant
adverse reactions and antibiotic dosage in the premature and newborn, Table 45 (121)
drug dangers, **102-125** (with tables)
skin care (hexachlorophene), **627-629**
Infections, 6
food poisoning, **714-716**
Infectious agents,
as water pollutants, 330t
from vertebrate animals and man (zoonoses), Table 145(594-602)
Influenza vaccination, 110t
Infrared analysis of gases and vapors in expired air, Table 35(87)
Infuco 80-20 Fumigant, 197t
INH (Isonicotinic acid hydrazide—Isoniazid [*Nydrazid*], 16t, 79t, 118t, 122, 338t, 341, 356t, 437t, 477
Inhalation of poisons, 46, 721
Injected poisons, 46, 721
Ink(s), eradicators, poisonous substances in 95t
laundry, poisonous substances in, 95t
laundry indelible, poisonous substances in, 95t
poisonous substances in, 95t, 96t
stamping, poisonous substances in, 95t
Inkberry (*Phytolacca americana*), 553t
Inorganic,
chemicals as pollutants to water, 330t
insecticides, (*see* Insecticides)
nonmetals, 85
Impersol, 67, 389
Insect(s), **570-581**
and man, **741-743**

and spiders (North American) harmful to man, Table 141(573)
bites, 33, 70
repellent, poisonous substances in, 96t
stings, prevention of, **742-743**
Insecticidal Freewax for Floors, 529t
Insecticide(s), **126-172**, 605t
biological pesticides, 127, **158-159**
botanical origin, 127, **156-158**
toxicity to man, Table 53(158)
chemical classification, **126-127**
chlorinated hydrocarbons, lethal doses of, 130t
combination sprays and powders, **170-172**
inorganic-chemical type, **138-155**
toxicity of, Table 52(155)
miscellaneous, **170-172**
organic, phosphorus containing, 71
acute toxicity of, 132t
potential toxicity of, 734t
synthetic organic, 126, **127-138** (with tables)
trade and common names, Table 50(137)
trade names and harmful ingredients, Table 54(159-170)
Insecticide, Fungicide and Rodenticide Act of 1947, (*see* Federal Insecticide, Fungicide and Rodenticide Act of 1947)
Insecto-Fog, 164t
Instant Dip Silver Cleaner, 529t
Insulin, 7t, 112t, 339, 443t, 491t, 702
Intravenous fluids, excess of, 110t
Intropin (Dopamine), 21t
Inversine hydrochloride (Mercamylamine), 493t
Invertebrates (stinging marine animals), **583-585**
Investigational Vaccines Program, 713
Iodate, potassium, 709t
Iodide(s), 65t, 97t, 117t, 122, 339, 345t, 347t , **415**
arsenious, 619
decamethonium, 487t
echothiophate, 488t
mercuric, 619
methyl, 186, **192-193**
phospholine, 488t
potassium, (*see* Potassium)
pralidoxime (2-PAM iodide), (*see* Pralidoxime)
sodium, 143, 614t, 644t
Iodine, 7t, 35t, 46, 53t, 97t, 102, 112t, 143t, 312, 346t, **429-431**, 720
antidote for, 41, 42, 55t, 56t,
radioactive, 122
radiologic contrast media, 16t
tincture of, 4f, 20t, 36, 430, 584
as an antidote, 54t, 178, 445
Iodipamide (Cholografin), 491t, 644t
Iodoalphionic acid (Priodax), 491t
Iodochlorhydroxyquin, 430
Iodochlorhyroxyquinoline (Enterovioform), 430
Iodoform, 430, 491t
Iodohippurate (Hippuran), 491t, 644t
Iodomethamate (Neo-Iopax), 491t
Iodopyracet (Diodrast), 491t
compound, 491t
concentrated, 491t
Iodopanoic acid (Iopanoic acid-Telepaque), 491t
Io moth, 579
Iopanoic acid (Telepaque), 117t, 491t
Iophendylate, 491t
Iophenoxic acid (Teridax), 110t
Iothiouracil (Itrumil), 491t
IPC (Propham), 188t, 734t
Ipecac, 35t, 62t, 346t
contraindications, 420, 445
fluidextract, 43, 83, 97t
powder, 83, 391
syrup of, 20t, 43, 44, 83, 525, 721
Ipecacuanha (Ipecac), 44, 83
*Ipomoea tricolor* (ololiugui seed), 98
*violacea* (morning glory), 552t
Iproniazid, phosphate-Marsilid (Isonicotinoyl-2-ispropylhydrazine), 76, **431**
Iris (*Iridaceae*), 551t
Irish potato, 544
Iron, 8t, 33, 53t, 65t, 82t, 90, 94t, 119, 252t, 262, 270t, 317, 347t, **431-436,** 514t, 533, 623, 708t
dextran (Imferon), 431
ferric, in methemoglobinemia, 17
gallate, 96t
metal, in chemistry sets, 614t
oxide, 95t, 331t, 652, 657
pigment, 536
preparations, 12t
salts, 10t, 77, 334t, 616
-sorbitol-citric acid complex (Jectofer), 11t, 431
Isethionate, stilbamidine, 499t
Ismelin, (*see* Guanethidine sulfate)
Iso-amyl alcohol, (*see* Alcohol, amyl)
Isobornyl thiocyanoacetate (Thanite), 170
Isobutane, 609
Isobutyl, methyl ketone, 216, 247t, 649, 729t
Isocarboxazid, 65t
ISOCIL (Hyvar), 188t
Isocyanates, 648t
Isoeugenol, 449
Isolation and separation techniques for identification of poisons, **84**
Isolette, 225
Isoniazid (INH; Nydrazid), 14t, 16t, 40, 65t, 79t, 117t, 118t, 122, 214t, 339, 343t, 345t, 347t, 348t, 356t, **437-438**, 455, 491t
Isonicotinic acid hydrazide (INH), 338t, 341, **437-438**, 477
Isonicotinoyl-2-isopropylhydrazine, **431**
Isonitrile test, 189
Isophorone, 729t
Isopoda (Sea lice), 590
Isopropamide (Darbid), 358t
Isopropanol, 65t, 89, 220t, 514t
Isopropyl alcohol (rubbing), 94t, 95t, 97t, 220t, 247t, 533, 636
Isoproterenol, 21t, 334t, 578
adverse effects, 49t
contraindications, 473
Isothionate(s), alkyl sodium, 522t
Isotonic saline, 58t, 184
Isotopes, radioactive, **642-644** (with table)
Isotox Dairy Spray, 164t
Isotox Garden Dust, 164t
Istizin (Danthron), 117t
Isto Insect Killer, 172t
Isuprel hydrochloride, 21t, 492t
Isuridae family (sharks), 586t
"Itai-itai" (ouch-ouch) disease, 114, 253
Itrumil, (*see* Iothiouracil)
Itso Insect Killer, 164t
Ivy,
oakleaf (poison oak), 539
poison (*Rhus toxicodendron*), 538, 539, 553t

## J

Jack-in-the-pulpit *(Arisaema triphyllum),* 543, 551t
Jake (fluidextract of ginger), 219
Jalap, 406t
*mirabilis* (four o'clock), 550t
Jamaica ginger (fluidextract of ginger), 219
Jamestown weed (jimson weed), 544
Japanese star anise *(Illicium anisatum),* 554t
Japanese puffer fish, 590
Jap Beetle Killer, 164t
*Jatropha* (physic nut), 553t
Javelle water, **629**
Jectofer (Iron-sorbitol-citric acid complex), 11t, 431
Jellyfish (Scyphozoa), 584, 587t, 590
Jelly, royal, **536**
Jequirity bean (*Abrus precatorius*), 540, 541, 542, 543, 551t
Jerusalem cherry (*Solanum pseudocapsicum*), 358t, 540, 544, 551t
Jessamine, yellow, *see Gelsemium sempervirens*
Jet berry bush (*Rhodotypos*), 551t
Jewelry cleaners, poisonous substances in, 95t
Jimson weed (*Datura stramonium*), 358t, 376, 539, 544, 545, 551t
Jitter Bug Insect Repellent, 164t
Johnsongrass, 606
Johnson's Carnu Gloss, 529t
Johnson's Carplate Auto Wax, 529t
Johnson's Cream Wax, 529t
Johnson's Glo-Coat, 529t
Johnson's Jubilee, 529t
Johnson's Liquid Wax, 529t
Johnson's Paste Wax, 529t
Johnson's Pride, 529t
Johnson's Super No-Roach Killer, 164t

Jonquil (*Narcissus jonquilla*), 550t
J-O Paste, 197t
Juniper (*Juniper macropoda*), 546t
See also Volatile oils
Jute (*Corchorus olitorius, capsularis*), 314, 551t

**K**

Kalite, 164t
*Kalmia* (American, black, mountain, sheep laurel), 551t
Kanamycin (Kantrex), 16t, 65t, 118t, 347t, 355, 356t, 437t
sulfate, 121t
Kan-Kil, 172t
Kantrex, (*see* Kanamycin)
Kaolin, 95t, 314, 315
contraindications, 454
poultices, 584
Kaolinosis, 323t
Karathane, 194t
Karaya gum,
causing dermatitis and/or asthma, 313t
causing fixed eruptions, 346t
Karith Cleaning Fluid, 529t
Karmex Herbicide DL, 197t
Karmex Herbicide W, 197t
Kavakava (*Piper methysticum*), 546t
Kayo Bug Killer, 164t
Kayo Killer, 197t
Keflin (Cephalothin), 356t
Kelade (Yarn), 543
Kel-F (Teflon), **654**
Kellogg's Ant Paste, 164t
Kelly's Red-Mix Rat & Mouse Killer, 197t
Kelocyanor (Dicobalt tetracemate), 154, 237
Kelthane (Dicofol), 137t
Kemtex Cleaner, 529t
Kentucky coffee tree (*Gymnocladus dioica*), 544, 551t
Kepone (Chlordecone), 117t, 126, 128
Kerosene, 4f, 37, 94t, 96t, 97t, 127, 157, 187t, 202, **222-224,** 225, 250, 741
deodorized, 94t, 95t
first aid for, 224
Ketaject (Ketamine hydrochloride), 351
Ketalar (Ketamine hydrochloride), 351
Ketamine, 101
hydrochloride (Ketaject; Ketalar), 351
Ketobemidone, 492t
Ketokil No. 2, 164t
Ketone(s), 95t, 96t, 202, **219-222,** 404, 464, 479
methyl ethyl, 247t, 725
methyl isobutyl, 216, 247t, 649, 729t
oxides, 115
Khellin, 492t
Kidney
artificial (extracorporeal dialyzer), **64-66** (with table)
toxicologic analysis of, **86**
Kilbrush Brush Killer (Bonide), 197t
Killer, 164t
Killer Blightex, 197t
Killer Dust D-10, 164t
Killer Dust Tox, 164t
Killer Kane Kartridges, 197t
Killer katz, 197t
Killer whales (*Orcinus orca*), 583, 586t
Kill-Ogen Instant Spray, 164t
Kill Wood Dust, 197t
Kilmice, 197t
Kilmite, 165t
Kil-Mor Moth Proofer, 197t
Kil-Mor Roach Ant Killer, 164t
Kilspray Aerosol Insecticide, 172t
Kilz-Moths, 197t
King snake, 564
scarlet kingsnake, 565
King Special Bug Killer, 165t
King Warble Fly Spray, 165t
Kissing bug, 576t
Kiszka, 12t
Klamath weed (*Hypericum perforatum*), 548t
Klane, 165t
Klean Spot Kit, 529t
Kleenal, 529t
Kleenize Disinfectant, 529t
Klenzade Fly Spray, 165t
Klenzade Roach Spray Ins-40,165t
Kling-Tite Dry, 197t
Klinzmoth Flakes, 197t
K-Lyte (Potassium citrate), 466
"Knockout drops" (Chloral hydrate), 492t
Knoxout Farm Insecticide, 165t
Knoxout Insect Spray and Powder, 165t
Knoxweed Contact Weed Killer, 197t
*Kochia scoparia* (Summer cypress), 548t
KOCN, 187t
Koenig tree (*Blighia sapida*), 544
Kokoi frog, **590-591**
Kolocide, 165t
Kola nut, 546t
Kolorsmear Screw-Worm Remedy, 165t
Kolotex, 165t
Konakion (Phytonadione), 479
Koneprox, 197t
Konex, 197t
Kopper Moth Balls, 197t
Korlan (Ronnel), 137t
12E, 25W, 24E, 165t
Korsakoff's syndrome, 210
See Alcohol
Kot-O-Fom Cleaner, 529t
Kousso (Cusso), 353t
Krab Crabgrass Killer (Bonide), 197t
Kritter Kote, 165t
Kritter Spray, 165t
K-R-O Powder, 197t
K-R-O Rat & Mouse Killer, 197t
K-R-O Ready Mixed Bis-Kit, 197t
Kryfax, 165t
Kryocide, 165t
Krytox, 165t
Kuron (Weedone-TP), 187t, 197t
Kwell, 129
Kwik-Kold (cold therapy), 36
Kynex (Sulfamethoxypyridazine), 338, 492t

**L**

Labarraque's solution, **629**
Labeling regulations, **701-710** (with table)
hazardous substances, **702-703**
Laboratory values, normal, used in the diagnosis and treatment of poisoning, **752-772**
altered by drugs, 752-755
Laburnum, golden chain, (*Cytisus laburnum*), 551t
Lacquer removers, poisonous substances in, 95t
*Lactarius* (mushrooms)
*deliciosus*, 557f
*helvus*, 557f
*vellereus*, 555
Lactase, 180
Lactate, 386
calcium, (*see* Calcium lactate)
molar sodium, 190
sodium, 19t, 41, 58, 387, 388, 461, 466, 631
Lactated Ringer's injection, 58t
Lactic acid, 65t, 450, 492t, 709t
Lactogen, 116, 119
Lactones, saturated, 421
Lactose USP, 355, 446
Ladybug, 742
Lady's slipper (*Cypripedium hirsutum*), 551t
Laetrile (Amygdalin), 235
Lake Nicaragua shark (Carcharinidae family), 586t
Lampblack, 95t
Lanatoside C (Cedilanid), 19t, 420
Lannate (Methomyl thioacetimidate), 137t, 138
Lanolin, 522t, 524t, **629**
Lanoxin (Digoxin), 21t
Lantana (*Lantana camara*), 548t, 551t
*Lantana camara* (Lantana; red and wild sage), 358t, 548t, 551t
Lanthanum, 270t
*Larkspur (Delphinium)*, 549t
seed, 540
Larvatox, 197t
Larvex, 197t
LAS (Linear alkylate sulfonate), (*see* Linear alkylate sulfonate)
Lasix (Furosemide), 16t, 21t, 102, 124t, 387, 489t
L-asparaginase, 80t, 402t, 414
Latex, 96t
Lathyrogens, 231
*Lathyrus odoratus* (sweet pea), 553t
*Latrodectus mactans, curacaviensis* (Black widow spider), **570-571**
antivenin, 52t, 571
Laudanum (tincture of opium), 492t (*see* Morphine)

Laundry,
detergents, poisonous substances in, 94t
indelible ink, poisonous substances in, 95t
Laurel, mountain, black, sheep, American (*Kalmia*), 551t
Lavage,
castor oil emulsion, (*see* Castor oil)
gastric, (*see* Gastric lavage)
Laws, state enforcement agencies and principal provisions, Table 156 (704-706)
Laxatives, 11t, 12t, 117t
L-dihydroxyphenylalanine (L-dopa), (*see* L-dopa)
L-dopa (L-dihydroxphenylalanine), 266, 334t, 477
Lead, 6t, 7t, 8t, 9t, 10, 14t, 31, 32, 33, 35t, 36, 37, 42, 53t, 54t, 65t, 82t, 87, 94t, 97t, 111, 112t, 113, 117t, 202, **255-266**, 269, 270t, 271, 272t, 314, 323, 328f, 391, 514t, 533, 605t, 609, 618, 740
alkyls, 113, 329t
arsenate (arsenite), 163t, 196t, **265**
carbonate, **255-265**
chromate, 331t, 618, 633
diagnostic criteria for poisoning, 257
in food poisoning, 113, **716**
oxide, **255-265**
soluble salts, 97t, 331t, 739
sulfide, 238, 256, 331t
tetraethyl, 97t, **265-266**, 271t, 331t
tolerable levels in young children, Table 68(256)
treatment, 263-265
Leather preservatives, polishes and dyes, poisonous substances in, 95t
Lebanon Arisod Grass & Weed Killer, 197t
Lebanon Bait Kills Rats and Mice, 197t
Lebanon Brush Killer, 197t
Lebanon Crab Grass Killer, 197t
Lebanon Japanese Beetle Spray, 165t
Lebanon Klor Dust, 165t
Lebanon Parafume Moth Crystals, 197t
Lebanon Tomato Blight Dust, 197t
Lechugilla (*Agave lecheguilla*), 548t
Lecithin, 95t, 708t
Lecythis (monkey pod; coco de mono), 551t
Leech, 581
Legumes, causing fixed eruptions, 346t
Lemcke's Dip-N-Rinse, 529t
Lemon
grass oil, 224, **617**
shark (Carcharinidae family), 586t
*Lepiota* (mushrooms)
*molybdites*, 557f
*morgani*, 555
*rhachodes*, 557f
Leptophos, 127, 136
Leptospirosis, 592
Lestemp (Acetaminophen), 117t
Lestox Fly Spray, 165t
Lethal doses, **91-93**, Table 38(97-98)
for chlorinated hydrocarbon insecticide, Table 47(130)
for inorganic insecticides, Table 52(155)
for organic phosphate insecticides, Table 49(132)
for rodenticides, Table 56(179)
Lethalaire G-57, 165t
Lethane(s), 168t
384 (beta-butoxy-beta thiocyano diethyl ether), 170
Leucovorin (Citrovorum factor), 404
calcium, 404
Leukeran (Chlorambucil), 80t, 110t, 369t, 485t
Leukopenia, drugs and chemicals causing, 13-15t
Levallorphan (Lorfan), 19t, 37, 38, 416, 447
tartrate, 54t, 416, 441
Levarterenol (Levophed), 21t, 367, 373, 385, 405, 411, 444, 458, 471, 473, 573
bitartrate, 333, 353
Levodopa, 143t, 472
Levohyoscyamine (Myceto-atropina), 555
Levophed bitartrate (Norepinephrine; Levarterenol), 19t, 21t, 36, 353, 385, 435, 473
Levoprome, (*see* Methotrimeprazine)
Levopropoxyphene (Novrad), 117t
Levorphanol, 416
Levothyroxine, 472, 492t
Levulinate, calcium, (*see* Calcium levulinate)
Lewisite burns (chemical), 46
Lexone Insecticide, 165t
Librium, (*see* Chlordiazepoxide)
Lice, 579
sea, (*see* Sea lice)
Licorice, 334t, **626**
Lidocaine (Xylocaine), 12t, 22t, 48t, 141, 352t, 421t, 459, 514t
adverse effects, 49t
hydrochloride, 619
Lights, bubbling (Christmas decoration), poisonous substances in, 95t
Lignasan, 197t
*Ligustrum vulgare* (common privet), 553t
Lily,
calla, 543, 548t
camas (*Zygadenus*), 540
climbing (*Gloriosa superba*), 550t
of the valley, (*Convallaria majalis*), 540, 552t
Lima bean (*Phaseolus limensis, lunatus*), 552t
Lime, **629-630**
quick (Calcium oxide), 612, 629
slaked ( Calcium polyhydroxide), 629
-sulfur (Calcium polysulfide), 605t, 630
water (Calcium hydroxide solution USP), 36
Limestone, 331t
Limonene, 613
Linco, 529t
Lincocin, (*see* Lincomycin)
Lincomycin (Lincocin), 118t, 334t
Lindane (Benzene hexachloride), 126, 127, **129**, 130t, 137t, 159t, 160t, 161t, 162t, 163t, 164t, 165t, 166t, 167t, 168t, 169t, 170t, 196t, 198t, 313t, 331t, 544, 731
Lindex Dust No. 10, 165t
Linear alkylate sulfonate (LAS), 519, 522t, 523t, 524t
Linoleic acid, 630
Linseed,
meal, 621
oil, **630**
Lintodd No. 102, 165t
Lintox, 165t
Linuron (Lorox), 188t
Lionfish (*Pterois volitans*), 588t, 590
Lipid dialysis, **66-67**
Lipoic acid, 558
Lipsticks, poisonous substances in, 95t
Liquid Plum'r, 230
Liquiprin, 451, 481t, 492t (*see also* Acetaminophen)
Liquor arseni et hydrargyri iodidi (Donovan's solution), **619-620**
Liquors, alcoholic, (*see* Alcoholic liquors)
Lithium, 65t, 112t, 269, 270t, 272t, 514t
carbonate, 375t, 630, 631
hydride, 630
hydroxide, 630
salts, **630-631**
side effects, Table 149(631)
Little David Insect Spray, 165t
Liver
extract, 339
toxicologic analysis of, 86
*Lobelia inflata*, (*see* Lobeline)
Lobeline (*Lobelia inflata*), 9t, 492t, 546t, 551t
sulfate, 649
Loco's disease, 143
Locust, 741
black (*Robinia pseudoacacia*), 548t
Logwood, 614t
extract, 533
*Lolium temulentum* (Darnel), 550t
Lomotil (Diphenoxylate hydrochloride), **422-423**, 488t
Lomustine (CCNU), 400t
*Loncho-carpus* (Rotenone), 157
*Lophophora williamsii* (Peyotl cactus), 98, 102t, 552t (*see also* Mescal, peyote)
Lophophorine, 99
Lorenz Activated Knockdown Concoction, 165t
Lorfan (Levallorphan), 19t, 37, 38
tartrate, 54t, 416, 441
Loridine (Cephaloridine), 356t
Lotion(s),
hair, poisonous substances in, 95t
skin, poisonous substances in, 94t
sun-tan, poisonous substances in, 94t

Love bean, (*see* Jequirity bean)
Lovester, 197t
Lo-Voi Brush Killer, 197t
Low-Dee, 197t
*Loxosceles*
*laeta* (South American brown spider), 572
*reclusa* (Brown recluse spider), 70, **571-574** (with figure)
L-penicillamine, (*see* Penicillamine)
LSD (d-Lysergic acid diethylamide), 92t, 98, 100, 347t, 514t, 722t
compared with other hallucinogens, 99, Table 39(102), 106t
Lucanthone hydrochloride, 492t
Lucide, 165t
Lucky bean, 541
Lugol's solution, 430
Lumber Last, 197t
Luminal, (*see* Phenobarbital sodium)
Luminol (Phthalazinedione), 519
Lung storage disease (thesaurosis), 95t
Lupin (*Lupinus*), 552t
Lupines, 539, 546t
*Lupinus* (Lupin), 552t
Lupus systemic erythematosus, drug-induced, Table 91(345)
Luteotrophic hormone (Prolactin), 119, 123
Lututrin, 492t
Lycons Cleaner, 529t
Lycopene, 478
Lycopenemia, 478
*Lycoperdon pyriformis*, 322t
Lye, 4f, 82, 234t, 335t, 526
first aid, 721
*Lyonia mariana* (Staggerbush), 554t
Lyovac (antivenin for *Latrodectus mactans*), 571
Lypressin, 492t
d-Lysergic acid diethylamide (LSD), (*see* LSD)
Lysodren (Mitotane), 401t
Lysol Disinfectant, 529t
Lyteca syrup (Acetaminophen), 117t

**M**

MAC (Maximum allowable concentration)
biological, Table 70(271)
for gases and vapors, Table 66(247)
for mineral and inert dust, Table 74(311)
for toxic fumes and dusts, Table 73(311)
Mace, 449
anti-riot gas, 108t, 202, **250**, **631**
"Machine oil" (Tri-ortho-cresyl phosphate), 202, **219-221**
Mackerel shark (Isuridae family), 583, 586t
Mackodiel, 165t
Mack-O-White, 165t
Macrodantin (Nitrofurantoin), 16t, 79t, 118t
Macroglobulin, 15ft
Macromolecules, in hair sprays, 95t
Mad-Hatter syndrome, in mercury poisoning, 98, 146
Madribon, (*see* Sulfadimethoxine)
Mafenide, 609
acetate (Sulfamylon), 232
Magclor Defoliant, 197t
Magikil Ant and Roach Duster, 165t
Magikil Jelly Ant Bait, 165t
Magik-Mist Insecticide, 165t
Magik-Mist Year Round Insecticide, 172t
Magik Rid, 172t
Magitrack Mouse Duster, 197t
Magnesia magma, (*see* Milk of magnesia)
Magnesium, 65t, 68t, 117t, 141, 252(t), 269, 271, 410, **438-439**, 515t, 519, 623, 631
carbonate, 229, 709t
hydroxide (milk of magnesia), 36, 45, 83, 233
oxalate, 229
oxide, 20t, 36, 51t, 141, 228, 235, 350
salts, 197t, 229, 408, 463
silicate, 316, 319
sulfate (Epsom salts), 19t, 20t, 37, 41, 54t, 112t, 147, 152, 173, 176, 179t, 186, 190, 228, 229, 263, 395, 420, 421t, 438, 458, 479, 544, 584, 589, 614t, 659
trisilicate, 347t, 350
Magnetite, 319
Maid Easy Stain Remover, 529t
Mainliner's lung (drug addicts), 314, **322**
Make-up, liquid, poisonous substances in, 95t
Mako shark (Isuridae family), 586t
Malachite green, 609
Malafog, 165t
Malanox Residual Bait Spray Concentrate, 165t
Malathion (Dimethyl-S-[1,2-bis-carboethoxy] ethyl phosphorodithioate), 52t, 127, 130, 132t, 137t, 159t, 160t, 161t, 162t, 163t, 164t, 165t, 166t, 167t, 169, 170t, 544, 731, 734t
Maleate
chlorpheniramine, 13t
methysergide (Sansert), 424, 425t
pheniramine, 14t
prophenpyridamine (Trimeton), 498t
Male fern, (*see* Aspidium)
Maleic hydrazide (MH-30), 182, 197t, 735t
Malic acid, 656
MAMA (Ansar; Methar), 187t
Mamba, 568
Manchineel (*Hippomane mancinella*), 544, 552t
Mandelamine, (*see* Methenamine)
Mandelic acid, 117t, 122, 492t
Mandelin's test, 92t
Mandrake (*Mandragora officinorium*), 546t
Man-eating shark, 583
Maneb (Dithiocarbamate), 181
Manganese, 6t, 14t, 33, 202, 252t, **266**, 269, 270t, 331t, 515t, 623
dioxide, 266, 611
oxides, 652
sulfate, 614t
Mango (*Mangifera indica*), 552t
*Mangifera indica* (Mango), 552t
*Manihot utilissima* (Cassava), 549t
Mannitol (Osmitrol), 22t, 65t, 70, 71, 82t, 143, 190, 218, 359, 373, 387, 438, 446, 474, 631
Man-of-war, Portuguese (*Physalia palagica*), 584, 587t, 590
Manta ray fish, 583
Manufacturers and other sources (hot lines), **693-696**
MAO inhibitors, (*see* Monoamine oxidase inhibitors)
Maolate (Chlorphenesin carbamate), 485t
Mapharsen (Oxophenarsine hydrochloride), 367, 496t
Marezine, 447
Marigold, marsh (*Caltha palustris*), 550t
Marihuana (Hashish—*Cannabis sativa*), 6t, 7t, 99, 102t, 106t, 123, 347t, 348t, **439-440**, 552t, 722t
psychotic states associated with use of, 106-109t
Marine animals, stinging, **583-585**
Markweed, 539
Marlate (Methoxychlor), 137t, 165t
Marplan, **442-444**
Marquis' test, 93t
Marsh,
elder, 539
marigold (*Caltha palustris*), 550t
Marsilid, iproniazid-phosphate, 76, **431**
Martin's Mar-Chlor, 165t
Martin's Mar-Fin Ready Bait, 197t
Martin's Mar Penta, l97t
Martin's Mar-Termino, 165t
Martin's Multi Kill, 172t
Martin's Rat Stop Liquid, 197t
Martin's Stock Tox, 165t
Martin's Wonderiex, 197t
Mascara, poisonous substances in, 95t
Mash-Nic Powder, 165t
Massasauga (*Sistrurus catenatus*), **562**
Matches, **736-738**
accidental ingestion, 737-738
incidence of poisoning, 737
toxic properties of, 736-737
types in current use, 736
Mate, 546t, **631-632**
Maternal medications,
drug dangers, **102-103**
effects on fetus and newborn, Table 42(112)
Matromycin, (*see* Oleandomycin)
Matulane (Procarbazine), 400t
Maximum allowable concentrations, (*see* MAC)
Mayapple (*Podophyllum peltatum*), 552t

May flies, 741
MCPA (2-Methyl-4-chlorophenoxyacetic acid), 182ft, 187t
MCPP (Mecoprop; Mecopex), 187t
MDA, *see* Methylenedioxyamphetamine)
Meadow saffron (*Colchicum*), 412-413, 549t
Measles vaccine, 347t
Mebaral, (*see* Mephobarbital)
Mebendazole (Vermox), 354t
Mechlorethamine (Nitrogen mustard; Mustargen), 396t, 492t
Mecholyl (Methacholine), 378, 424, 452, 458, 493t
M-E Cleaner, 529t
Meclizine (Bonadoxin), 156, 484t
Mecopex (MCPP), 187t
Mecoprop (MCPP), 187t
Media,
occupational hazards associated with, **313-314**
on poisoning, (*see* Appendix A) 744-751
*Medicago sativa* (Alfalfa), 548t
Medical colleges, working with poison control centers, 698
Medihaler-Ergotamine, 425t
Medinal (Barbital sodium), 35t, 83
Medroxy-progesterone acetate, 402t
Mefenamic (Ponstel), 117t
Megace (Megestrol acetate), 402t
*Megalopyge opercularis* (Stinging caterpillar), 579
Megestrol acetate (Megace), 402t
Megimide (Bemegride; Methetharimide), 8t, 37, 386, 427, 456, 494t
Melamine, triethylene (T.E.M.), 455, 502t
*Melia azedarach* (China berry), 549t
Melitoxin (Bishydroxycoumarin), 117t
Mellaril, (*see* Thioridazine)
Meloidae family (Blister beetles), 578
Melphalan (Alkeran), 396t
Melsan, 197t
Meltrol (Phenformin; DBI), 214t
Mema, 197t
Menadione (Vitamin K), 42
*Menispermum canadense* (Moonseed), 552t
Mental function and poisons, **93-102**
Menthol, 12t, 94t, **453**, 479, 492t
Mepacrine, 343t
Mepazine, 14t, 77
Mepenzolate (Cantil), 358t
Meperidine hydrochloride (Demerol), 6t, 37, 54t, 92t, 93t, 97t, 339, 393, 408, 422, 443t, 492t, 515t, 579
Mepesulfate, 143t
Mephenesin (Tolseram), 178, 492t
Mephenoxalone (Trepidone), 117t
Mephentermine (Wyamine), 22t, 93t, 104t, 443t
sulfate, 567
Mephenytoin (Mesantoin), 8t, 143t, 339, 345t, 456
Mephobarbital (Mebaral), 360, 383t
Mephyton (Vitamin $K_1$ emulsion), 19t, 42
Mepivacaine (Carbocaine), 110t, 352(t)
Meprobamate (Miltown; Equanil; Wyseals; Meprospan; Metrotabs), 8t, 14t, 30, 65t, 97t, 104t, 110t, 215t, 336(t), 339, 346t, 371, 373, 456, 493t, 503t, 515t (*see also* Ataractics)
Meprospan (Meporbamate), 110t
Meprotabs (Meprobamate), 110t
MER/29, (*see* Triparanol)
Meractinomycin-Lyo (Actinomycin D), 347t, 398t
Meralluride, sodium (Mercuhydrin), 124t
Meratran, (*see* Pipradrol)
Merbak (Acetomeroctol), 481t
Merbromin (Mercurochrome), 493t, 609
Mercamylamine (Inversine hydrochloride), 493t
Mercaptans, 202, **237-239**
ethyl, 625
6-Mercaptopurine (6-MP; Purinethol), 77, 80t, 398t, 404, 503t
Mercocresol, 493t
Mercuhydrin (Sodium meralluride), 105t, 124t
Mercupurin, 339
Mercurial(s), 339, 346t, 347t
diuretics, 16t, 393, 418
inorganic, 144, 146, 148
organic, **144-146**, 734t
Mercuric,
chloride, 7t, 35t, 41, 96t, 97t, 145, 147, 155t, 194t, 611
compounds, 45
iodide, 619
oxide, 611
phenyl propionate, 145, 608,
salts, 41, 194t, 195t, 196t, 197t, 199t, 200t
Mercurochrome (Merbromin), 8t, 145, 493t
Mercurous chloride (Calomel), 117t, 194t, 198t, 406t, 608
Mercury, 6t, 7t, 8t, 32, 36, 41, 46, 53t, 54t, 56t, 65t, 82(t), 87, 91, 95t, 96t, 98, 109, 112t, 117t, 127, **144-148**, 201t, 202, 269, 271t, 272t, 331t, 335t, 515t, 605t, **608**, 620, 633
ammoniated, 95t, 483t
bichloride of, 4f, 8t, 85, 95t, 198t
cell battery, 610, 611
compounds, 179
in food poisoning, **717**
metallic, 145, 148, 262, 611
methyl, 102, 109, 111(t), **148-151**
chloride, 149
protoiodide, 493t
salts, 55t, 194t, 195t, 196t, 197t
thiocyanate, 738
"Mercury", (*see* Poison ivy)
Mergamma, 197t
Merphenyl Disinfectant, 529t
Mersolite-8, 197t
Merthiolate, (*see* Thimerosal)
Mesantoin (Mephenytoin; Methylphenylethyl hydantoin), 8t, 14t, 345t, 347t, 360, 362t, 456
Mescal (*Lophophora williamsii*), 552t, **632**
Mescaline (3,4,5-Trimethoxyphenylethylamine), 98, 99, 102t, 106t, 632
Mesityl oxide, 729t
Mesitylene, **658-659**, 729t
Mestinon (Pyridostigmin), 376
Mestranol, 123, 343t
Metabolic acid, 58
Metabolic disorders (drug-induced hemolytic anemia), **336-344** (with tables)
Metachloroaniline, 12t
Metacide, 127, 165t
Metag Agricultural Bait, 165t
Metahydrin (Trichlormethiazide), 469
Metal(s), 7t, 45, 46, 82, 85, 86, 88, 93, 98, 117t, 345t (*see also* individual metals)
average levels of, Table 69(270)
blood, urine, tissue levels of, Table 71 (272)
cleaners, poisonous substances in, 94t
functions in man, Table 67(252)
"hard" in pneumoconiosis, 323t
identification of poison, 85
polishes, poisonous substances in, 94t
sulfide, 238
trace, 102, 203, **269-270**
Metaldehyde, 127, **144**, 202, **221**, 604
Metal fume fever, 253, 268, 314, 654
Metalid (Acetaminophen), 117t
Metallic
dyes, 94t
mercury, 145, 611
poisons, 202, **252-272**
Metaphen, (*see* Nitromersol)
Metaphosphate, sodium, (*see* Sodium phosphate)
Metaphydrin (Trichlormethiazide), 469
Metaraminol (Aramine bitartrate), 22t, 133, 385, 443t, 473
Metasilicate, sodium, 94t, 520
Meta-terphenyl, 741
Meteloidine, 545
Metformin, 477
Methacholine (Mecholyl), 31, 377, 378, 452
chloride, 493t
Methacycline (Rondomycin), 334t, 357t
Methadone, 37, 54t, 92t, **440-442**, 448, 463, 493t, 515t
hydrochloride (Dolophine; Adanon; Althose syrup), 117t
Methamphetamine hydrochloride, 65t, 92t, 104t, 333, 443t, 470, 471, 493t, 515t
Methandrostenolone, 503t
Methane, 7t, 625, 648t
bromine derivatives, 471
chlorine derivatives, 471
Methanol, 14t, 58, 62t, 65t, 82t, 89, 94t, 95t, 96t, **213-216**, 220t, 247t, 515t, 727

Methanox Residual Fly Spray Concentrate, 165t
Methantheline, 340, 358t
bromide (Banthine bromide), 493t
Methapyriline (Sominex; Compoz; Cope), 16t, 93t, 358t, **366**, 378, 392, 515t
Methaqualone (Quaalude), 65t, 66, 427, 493t, 515t
Methar, 187t, 197t
Metharbital (Gemonil), 360, 362t
Methate, 197t
Methdilazine (Tacaryl), 117t
Methemoglobin(s), 10, 18, 37, 41, 120, 154, 203, 204, 237, 348, 450, 451, 468
as nephrotoxins, 82t
known compounds producing, Table 5(12)
reduction test, 343
Methemoglobinemia, **17-18**, 31, 56t, 64, 73, 93, 154, 183, 192, 203, 204, 205, 217, 237, 352, 391, 392, 450, 452, 453, 457, 459, 468, 469, 534, 535, 618, 623, 707, 736, 737, 738
Methenamine (Mandelamine), 96t, 244, 346t, 493t
Methetharimide (Megimide), 494t
Methicillin (Staphcillin; Dimocillin-RT), 125, 357t
Methimazole (Tapazole), 14t, 81t, 110t, 117t, 143t, 340, 494t
Methionine (Pedameth), 77, 143, 190, 349
selenium, 644t
Methixene hydrochloride (Trest), 494t
Methocarbamol (Robaxin), 11t, 52t, 117t, 494t, 571, 645
Methohexital (Brevital), 117t
Methomyl thioacetimidate (Lannate), 137t, 138
Metho-Penn, 165t
Methorphinan hydrobromide (Dromoran), 494t
Methotrexate (Aminopterin; Amethopterin; Aminopteroylglutamate sodium), 65t, 80t, 102, 110t, 143t, 258, 347t, 397t, 404, 456, 477, 482t
Methotrimeprazine (Levoprome), 494t
Methoxamine (Vasoxyl), 333, 446
Methoxide, 165t
Methoxlin Insect Spray, 165t
Methoxychlor (Methoxy DDT; Trichloro-bis [p-methoxyphenyl] ethane), 126, 130t, 137t, 159t, 161t, 165t, 166t, 167t, 168t, 734t
Methoxyflurane (Penthrane), 79t, 351
Methsuximide (Celontin), 8t, 361, 363t, 456, 515t
Methyclothiazide (Enduron), 469
Methyl,
acetate, 729t
alcohol, (*see* Alcohol, methyl)
alkyl dipolyoxypropylene ammonium methyl sulfate, 653
p-aminobenzoate, 536
arsenate, (*see* Arsenate, methyl)
benzoate, 96t
bromide, 87t, 95t, 186, 187, **192-193**, 195t, 202, 247t, 500t, 734t
butyl, 725
cellosolves, **613**
cellulose, 652, 708t
chloride, 87t, 186, **192-193**, 202, 247t
2,4-chlorophenoxyacetic acid, (*see* MCPA)
-demeton, 734t
dimethoxy methyl phenylethylamine, (*see* DOM)
ethyl ketone, 247t
peroxide, 624
guthion, 137t
heptenone, 617
hydrate, (*see* Wood alcohol)
hydroxide, (*see* Wood alcohol)
iodide, 186, **192-193**
isobutyl ketone, 216, 247t, 649, 729t
mercury, 111t, **148-151**
chloride, 149
parathion (Dimethyl-p-nitrophenyl thiophosphate, 137t, 734t
perchloroformate, 9t
polysiloxane, 647
salicylate, 65t, 94t, 97t, 224, 461, 462, 466, 495t
violet, 633
Methylal, 247t
Methylated spirits, 94t
industrial, 95t
Methylazoxymethanol, 558
Methylbenzethonium chloride (Diaparene chloride), 519, **632**
Methylbromide thihexinol (Entoquel), 500
Methylchloride, 2-pyridine aldoxime, 133
Methylchloroform, 190, 731
Methyldopa (Aldomet), 15t, 16t, 81t, 143t, 343t, 443t, 494t
Methylene blue, 10t, 11t, 12t, 17-18, 19t, 35t, 56t, 203, 204, 338t, 341, 343t, 609, 645
basic fuchsin stain, Seller's in rabies, 603
contraindications, 183, 242
use in cyanide poisoning, 37, 154
use in treatment of methemoglobinemia, **18**, 31, 37, 217, 392, 450, 452, 457, 469, 535, 623, 738
Methylene chloride, 87t, 94t, 95t, 247t, 515t, 729t, 739
Methylenedioxyamphetamine (MDA), 99, 102t, 515t
Methylergonovine, 423
Methyl-ethyl glutarimide (Megimide), 37 (*see also* Bemegride)
Methyliodide, 2-pyridine aldoxime, 133
Methylparaben USP, 352, **632**
Methylparafynol (Dormison), 494t
Methyl parasept, **632**
Methylphenidate
hydrochloride (Ritalin), 14t, 373, 470, 494t, 503t
use in coma, 73
Methylphenylethyl hydantoin (Mesantoin), 14t, 360, 362t
Methyl-p-hydroxybenzoate (Methylparaben USP), **632**
Methylprednisolone, 69, 224, 415t
sodium succinate (Solu-Medrol), 22t, 69
Methylrosaniline chloride (Gentian violet), 354t, 489t, 494t
Methylsulfate
neostigmine, 495t
prostigmin, 718
Methyltestosterone, 76, 494t
Methylthiouracil, 494t
Methyprylon (Nodular), 8t, 65t, 427, 456, 494t, 515t
Methysergide maleate (Sansert), 424, 425t
Meticorten (Prednisone), 14t, 69, 401t, 413, 415t
*Metopium toxiferum* (Poisonwood tree), 553t, 544
Metrazol (Pentylenetetrazol), 19t, **38**, 97t, 351
Metronidazole (Flagyl), 10t, 11t, 79t, 118t, 122, 212, 214t, 494t
Mevinphos (Phosdrin), 137t
Mexican poppy (*Argemone mexicana*), 552t
M.G.K. Repellant, 11, 197t
MH (amine) (MH-30), 188t
MH-30 (Maleic hydrazide), 188t, 197t
Mica, 314, 315, 319, 331t
Mice Doom Pellets, 197t
Mice & Rat Doom, 197t
Mickey Finn drops (Croton oil or tartar emetic mixed with alcoholic beverage), 494t
Micro-Bu Cop, 197t
Microdiffusion test, **89-90**, 189
Microlin Disinfectant, 529t
*Micromonospora vulgaris* (thermophilic organism), 321, 322t
Micro Penta, 197t
*Micropolyspora faeni* (thermophilic organism), 321, 322t
*Micrurus fulvius* (coral, harlequin snakes), 563-565 (with figure)
antivenin for, 20t, 52t
Mictine (Aminometradine), 482t
Midges, biting, 576f
Midland Insecto-LOH 58, 165t
Midland Mill-O-Cide Formula B-9, 165t
Midland Ware-O-Cide Super Strength, 165t
Mienie-mienie, 541
Migral tablets, 425t
Migraine, maximum dose of ergot in treatment, Table 121(424-425)
Milibis (Glycobiarsol; Bismuth glycolyarsanilate), 12t, 489t
Milk,
as a demulcent, 37, 46, 82

breast, 110t
drugs and chemicals in, 115-124 (with tables)
contraindications, 43
evaporated, 37
Milk of magnesia (Magnesia magma; Magnesium hydroxide), 36, 45, 83, 233, 239
Milk purslane (*Euphorbia maculata*), 548t
Miller Pesticide Amendment to the Federal Food, Drug and Cosmetic Act, 126
Miller's Bordo, 197t
Miller's Chlorospra, 165t
Miller's DDT Household Spray, 166t
Miller's Fly-Ro-Cide, 166t
Miller's Malaspra, 166t
Miller's Methoxo, 166t
Miller's Microcop, 197t
Miller's Paraspra, 166t
Miller's Pestkil, 166t
Miller's Postreat, 198t
Miller's Rotefive, 166t
Miller's Rotefour, 166t
Miller's Spray-O-Cide, 166t
Miller's Texaspra, 166t
Millfume, 197t
Milliequivalents
definition of, 58
formula for, 58
per liter, factors for converting blood chemistry values to, Table 26(59)
Millipedes, **731**
Milontin (Phensuximide), 8t, 11t, 345t, 361, 362t, 456, 515t
Miltown, (*see* Meprobamate)
Minamata disease, 11, 150
Mineral(s), 117t
acid, 88
maximum allowable concentrations for, Table 74(311)
oil, 20t, 37, 56t, 152, 175, 449, 503t, 734t
contraindications, 177, 454
seal oil, 94t, **224-225**, 517
spirits, 94t, 184
Miners'
consumption (silicosis), **314-315**
phthisis (silicosis), **314-315**
Mintezol (Thiabendazole), 79t, 353t, 354t
Miosis, 6t
*Mirabilis jalapa* (four o'clock), 550t
Miracil D (Nilodin), 354t
Miracle Kill Roach Death, 166t
Miradon (Anisindione), 11t, 17t
Mirasect, 166t
Mirbane (Nitrobenzene), **632**
Mirex, 137t
Miscellaneous
compounds, **608-659**
drug compounds, Table 128(481-502)
insecticides, 170-172
Mission Brand Ant Powder, 166t
Mission Brand Ant Roach Killer, 166t
Mission Brand Gam-O-San, 198t
Mission Brand Pesticide Spray, 172t
Mission Brand Tix-Toc, 166t
Mission Brand Weedkiller, 198t
Mistletoe *(Phoradendron falvescens)*, 552t, **740**
Mites (Trombicula), **580-581**
rat, 580
Mithracin (Mithramycin), 80t, 398t
Mithramycin (Mithracin), 80t, 398t
Mitomycin C (Mutamycin), 399t
Mitotane (Lysodren), 401t
Moccasin (*Agkistrodon mokeson*), **562**
highland (*Agkistrodon mokeson*), **562**
water (*Agkistrodon piscivorus*), **562**, 564f
Modane (Calcium pantothenate), 11ft
Model trains, **740-741**
Mo-GO, 198t
Molar sodium lactate, 190, 218
Mole Nots, 198t
Mollusks, 583, 584
univalve, 584
Mologen, 198t
Molybdenum, 252t, 262, 269, 270t, 605t, 623
Monkey pod (*Lecythis*), 551t
Monkshood (*Aconitum napellus*), 350, 541(f), 550t
wild (*Aconitum uncinatum*), 554t
Monoacetate, glyceryl (Monoacetin), 176
Monoacetin (Glyceryl monoacetate), 54t, 176
Monoamine oxidase inhibitors, 65t, 81t, 215t, 334t, 340, 352, 366t, 369t, 376, 429, 437, **442-444**, 472, 473
adverse effects with concurrent administration of food, alcohol and drugs, Table 124(443)
Monochloroacetates, 734t
Monochlorobenzene, 247t
Monoethanolamine, 312, 533
Monoglycerides, 708t
Mono-Kay (Phytonadione), 479
Monopersulfate, **233-234**
potassium, 523t
Monophosphate, 614t
Monopotassium, phosphate, 395, 479
Monosodium glutamate (MSG), 115, 708t
Monothiols, 148
Monoxide, carbon (*see* Carbon monoxide)
Monsanto Niran, 166t
Monsanto Santobane, 166t
Monsanto Santochlor, 198t
Monsel's solution, **632**
*Monstera*, 543
Monuron (Telvar), 188t, 609
CMU, 734t
-TCA, 188t
Moonseed (*Menispermum canadense*), 552t
Mop-N-Mix, 166t
Moray eel (*Gymnathorax mordax*), 582, 583, 586t
Morel, false (*Gyromitra esculenta*), 555, 556f
Morning glory (*Ipomoea violacea*), 552t
pearly gates (*Rivea corymbosa*) seeds, 98, 106t
Morocide (Binapacryl), 137t
Morphine, 6t, 7t, 33, 35t, 45, 46, 54t, 85, 97t, 102, 110t, 117t, 122, 155, 219, 227, 229, 336t, 346t, 391, 411, 412, 413, 431, 443t, **444-449**, 453, 515t, 571, 574, 584, 722t
addiction, **447-449**
analogues, 7t, 8t, 9t
contraindications, 133, 178, 251, 390, 589, 737
derivatives, 7t, 8t, 9t, 102
hydrochloride, 488t
intoxication, 33, 36, 37
sulfate, 19t, 263, 468, 579
*Morus rubra* (Red mulberry), 552t
Mosquito, 579, 741
*anopheles*, 741
Moth, 579, 741
brown-tail, 579
buck, 579
io, 579
tussock, 579
white, 579
Moth balls, 97t, 338, **740** (*see also* Naphthalene)
Moth Chaser, 198t
Moth-Ded Button Moth Proofer, 172t
Moth-Ded Mothproofing Spray, 172t
Mothene, 166t
Moth-Ray,198t
Moth-Tox, 198t
Motrin, (*see* Ibuprofen)
Mountain laurel (*Kalmia*), 551t
Moura seed, 314
Mouse Lure, 198t
Mouse Nots, 198t
Mouse Seed, 198t
Mouth-to-mouth resuscitation, **59-60**, Figure 6(61)
Movellan, 495t
6-MP (6-Mercaptopurine), 80t, 398t
MSG (Monosodium glutamate), 115, 708t
MSMA (Weed-E-Rad; Ansar), 187t
MTT (Tetrazolium dye), 343
Mucomyst (Acetylcysteine), 349, 482t
*Mucor stolonifer*, 322t
Mud-dauber wasp, 576f
Mufti Spot Remover, 529t
Mulberry, red (*Morus rubra*), 552t
Mulch-Rite, 166t
Mullen, 545
Multi-Tox C,L, 166t
*Muraeva* (fish), 582
Muriatic acid (Hydrochloric acid), **633**
*Muscaria* (mushroom), 358t, 552t
Muscarine, 7t, 8t, 9t, 31, 35t, 97t, 452, 555, 559t, 581
effects, 131t
Muscle relaxants (Curare), 11t, 415
Mushroom(s), 7t, 31, 52t, **547-558** (with table), **717**
anticholinergic effects, 358t
as nephrotoxin, 82t

hallucinogenic properties, 98
Mussels (shellfish), 718
Mustard(s), 8t, 539
gas, 6t, 9t, 47
nitrogen (Mustargen), 396t, 492t
oil (Allylisothiocyanate), 659
phenylalinine, 404
uracil, 143
water, contraindicated as an emetic, 42
Mustargen (Nitrogen mustard), 396t, 492t
Mutamycin (Mitomycin C), 399t
Myambutol (Ethambutol hydrochloride), 356t
Myasthenia gravis, 65t
Mycetismus (mushroom poisoning), 547
Myceto-atropina (Levohyoscyamine), 555
Mycifradin, (*see* Neomycin sulfate)
Mycostatin, (*see* Nystatin)
Mycotoxicosis, **715-716**
Mydriasis, 6t
Myerkill, 198t
Myleran (1,4-Dimethanesulfonoxybutane), 396t
Myocardiopathy, Table 27(62)
Myristic acids, 630
*Myristica fragrans* (Nutmeg), 102t, 552t
Myristicin, **449**, 546t
Myro Range & Porcelain Cleaner, 529t
Mysoline (Primidone), 345t, 360, **361**, 362t, 498t, 515t
Mysteclin-F, 357t
Mysterious Roach Killer Outfit, 166t
Mystic Foam Cleaner for Fabrics, 529t
Mytelase (Ambenonium chloride), 117t, 482t

N

Nabam (Dithiocarbamate), 181
NAC, (*see* N-acetylcysteine)
Nacolene Dry Clean Detergent, 529t
Nacetyl (Acetaminophen), 117t
Nail(s),
preparations, poisonous substances in, 94t
toxicologic analysis of, 87
Naked ladies plant (*Colchicum*), 549t
Na-Klor Dust, 166t
Naled (*Dibrom*), 137t, 731
Nalidixic acid (NegGram), 118t, 343t, 347t, 455, 495t
Nalline (Nalorphine; N-Allylnormorphine hydrochloride), 19t, 37, 38, 54t, 441
Nalorphine (Nalline), **37-38**, 416, 447
hydrochloride, 54t, 416, 441
Naloxone hydrochloride (Narcan), 19t, 22t, 37, 38, 43, 44, 54t, 416, 423, **441**, 446, 447
Naphazoline, 470
Naphtha, 94t, 95t, 222, 524t
coal tar, 247t, 727
petroleum, 94t, 247t, 650
wood, 95t, 727
Naphthalene, 77, 82, 94t, 96t, 97t, 102, 136, 160t, 164t, 166t, 186, 189, **191-192**, 197t, 198t, 199t, 200t, 201t, 202, 216, 338(t), 340, 343t, 526, 735t, 740
chlorinated, 202, **208**, 605t
dimethano, 130t
Naphthenate compounds, 195t
Naphthenes (Cycloparaffins), 225
Naphthoate, pamaquine, 11t, 496t
Naphthol, 10t, 14t, **453**
alpha, 191
beta, 136, 191, 353t
Naphthoquinone,
alpha, 191
beta, 191
Naphthylamine(s), 12t
Naprosyn (Naproxen), 17t
Naproxen, (*see* Naprosyn)
Naqua (Trichlormethiazide), 469
Narcan (Naloxone hydrochloride), 19t, 22t, 37, 38, 43, 44, 54t, 416, 423, **441**, 446, 447
*Narcine* (rayfish), 587t
*Narcissus*
bulbs, 540
*jonquilla* (jonquil), 550t
*pseudonarcissus* (daffodil), 550t
Narcotic(s), 85f, 112t, 117t, 373
addiction, **447-449**
interaction with alcohol, Table 60(214)
Narcotic Addict Treatment Act of 1974, 448
Nardil, **442-444**
Natco Fabric Cleaner, 529t
National Academy of Sciences/National Research Council, 638
National Agricultural Association, 126
National Agricultural Chemical Association, 159, 732, 733
National Cancer Institute, 128, 207
National Clearinghouse for Poison Control Centers, 332, 517, 609ft, 613ft, 658, 662, 701, 737
National Council on Radiation Protection and Measurement (NCRP), 641
National Institute for Occupational Safety and Health, 535
National Institute of Health (NIH), 558
National Institute of Nutrition (Toyko), 271
National Office of Vital Statistics, 218, 334, 335t, 336t
National Poison Prevention Week, material for, (*see* Appendix A) 744-751
Natural gas, 240, **625**
Naturetin (Bendroflumethiazide), 469
Nautilus, 584
Navane (Thiothixene), 455
NCRP, (*see* National Council on Radiation Protection and Measurement)
Neatsfoot oil, **633**
Nebs (Acetaminophen), 117t
NegGram (Nalidixic acid), 118t, 455, 495t
Neguvon (Trichlorfon), 137t
Nemagon Soil Fumigant, 166t
Nematode diseases (zoonoses), 598t
Nembutal (Pentobarbital), 379t, 383t
sodium (Pentobarbital sodium), 71, 72t
Neo-A-Fil, 455
Neoarsphenamine (Neosalvarsan), **367-370**
Neobiotic (Neomycin sulfate), 117t
Neocinchophen (Cinchophen), **409**
Neo-Iopax, (*see* Iodomethamate)
Neomycin, 65t, 347t, 355, 356t
sulfate (Mycifradin; Neobiotic), 117t, 121t, 495t
Neonal, (*see* Butethal)
Neosalvarsan (Neoarsphenamine), **367-370**
Neostam, (*see* Stibamine glucoside)
Neostigmine (Prostigmin), 358, 376, 378, 415, 452
bromide, 19t, 495t
methylsulfate, 495t
Neo-Synephrine (Phenylephrine), 22t, 69, 446
Neotrane, 126
*Nepeta cataria* (Cataria), 613
Nephroallergens, as nephrotoxic, 82t
Nephrotoxic compounds, Table 34(82)
*Neptunea* (Mollusk)
*antiqua* (Red whelk), 582
*arthritica*, 582
*intersculpta*, 582
*Nerium oleander* (Oleander), 540, 552t
Nerol, 613
Nerve gas(es), 7t, 9t
Nesacaine (Chloroprocaine), 352t
Nettle
bull, horse *(Solanum carolinense)*, 554t
sea, 584
Neurotoxins, **565**, 566, 574
Neutralizers, poisonous substances in, 94t
Neutro Cop, 198t
New Larvex, 166t
Newspapers on poison prevention, (*see* Appendix A) 749
Niacin (Nicotinic acid), 118t, 495t, 708t
deficiency, 477
Niacinamide (Nicotinamide), 175, 179t
Niagara Brush Killer, 198t
Niagara Chlorkil Spray, 166t
Niagara Copodust, 198t
Niagara Copotex, 198t
Niagara Kalophoskil 1 Dust, 166t
Niagara Phoskil Spray, 166t
Niagara Quik-Kil Poison, 166t
Niagara Ro-Kil Spray, 166t
Niagara Thiodan 4 Dust, 166t
Niagara Thiodan Miscible, 166t
Niagara Toxakil Dust, 166t
Niamid, **442-444**
Nice Room Deodorant, 529t
Nichrome wire, in chemistry sets, 614t
Nickel, 32, 33, 53t, 114, 203, 262, **266**, 270t, 272t, 317, 533, 515t

ammonium sulfate, 615t
carbonyl, 203, **266-267**
salts, 8t
steel wire, in chemistry sets, 614t
NIC Odorless Fly Killer, 172t
Nico-Dust 10, 166t
Nico-Fume Liquid, 166t
Nico-Mulsion, 166t
Niconyl (Isoniazid; INH), **437-438**
*Nicotiana glauca* (Wild tobacco), 554t
Nicotinamide (Niacinamide), (*see* Niacinamide)
Nicotinate, sodium (food additive), **707-710**
Nicotine, 6t, 7t, 8t, 9t, 35t, 39, 55t, 62t, 97t, 117t, 127, **156-157**, 158t, 159t, 160t, 163t, 165t, 166t, 168t, 169t, 170t, 201t, 347t, 499, 515t, 633, 649, 734t, (*see also* Tobacco)
Nicotinic
acid (Niacin), 107t, 190, 347t, 476t, 495t
effects, 131t
Nicotrol, 166t
Nicotrox 10-X, 166t
Nightshade,
black (*Solanum nigrum*), 548t
blue (*Solanum dulcamara*), 542f, 545
deadly (*Atropa belladonna*), 550t
yellow (*Urechites suberecta*), 554t
Nigrosine dyes, 95t
ammonium derivatives, 583
NIH, (*see* National Institute of Health)
Nikethamide (Coramine), 9t, 19t, 38, 213, 367
Nilodin (Miracil D), 354t
Ninhydrin, 615t
Niobium, 114, 270t
Niocide 10 Dust, 166t
Nip-An-Tuck Roach Powder, 166t, 172t
Nipride (Nitroprusside sodium), 22t
Niran (Parathion), 137t
Nitrate(s), 7t, 9t, 12t, 17, 64, 97t, **449-450**, 605t, 623
ammonium, 94t, 621
barium, 173,
bismuth, 450
calcium, 615t
choline, 424
peroxyacetyl (PAN), **327**
pilocarpine, 377
potassium (Saltpeter), 499t, 707
silver, 7t, 55t, 96t, 97t, 451, 467, 720
sodium, 621, 707, 709t
strontium, 615t, 738
strychnine, 35t
Nitric acid, 7t, 8t, 97t, **226-228**, 609, 621, 632, 720
Nitric oxide, 325
Nitrilotriacetate (NTA), 115, 520
Nitrite(s), 7t, 9t, 10t, 12t, 14t, 17, 37, 62t, 64, 97t, 115, **449-450**, 605t, 616, 623, 707
amyl, 7t, 12t, 37, 154, 173, 237, 238, 449, 450, 458, 483t
pearls, 20t, 31, 53t, 154, 155
n-butyl, 450
ethyl, 12t, 449, 450, 488t
spirit, 499t, 612
sodium, 17t, 20t, 37, 41, 53t, 154, 155(t), 174, 237(t), 238, 449, 450, 471, 707, 709t
variation of child's dose with hemoglobin concentration, Table 64(237)
Nitroaniline, 202, **203-204**
para-, 12t, 203, 618
Nitrobenzene, 7t, 8t, 10t, 12t, 14t, 64, 94t, 95t, 98t, 202, **204**, 247t, 632
Nitrocellulose, 95t
in ketone, 96t
Nitrochlorobenzene, 12t
Nitrofurans, 12t
Nitrofurantoin(s) (Macrodantin; Furadantin), 10t, 14t, 16t, 65t, 79t, 110t, 117t, 118t, 122, 338t, 340, 341, 343t, 347t, 356t, 495t, 515t
Nitrofurazone (Furacin), 343t, 495t
Nitrogen, 621, 623
compounds, 202, **203-205**, 618
dioxide, 247t, 325, 329t, 547
mustard, 396t, 492t
oxides, 12t, 202, **249-250,** 322, 324(t), **325**, 328f, 625, 648t, 656
tetroxide, 250
Nitroglycerin(e), 17t, 62t, 449, 471
sublingual, 20t, 38
tablets, 38
Nitroglycerol, 12t
Nitromersol (Metaphen), 495t
Nitropropane, 247t
Nitroprusside(s), 235
sodium, (*see* Sodium nitroprusside)
Nitrosamines, 707, 710
Nitrosobenzene, 12t
Nitrosyl chloride, 709t
Nitrous oxide, 7t, 87t, 351, 426
N-K Seed Protectant, 166t
No-Bunt, 198t
Noctec, (*see* Chloral hydrate)
Nodar, 198t
Nolina texana (Sacahuiste), 548t
Noludar (Methyprylon), 8t, 456, 494t, 515t
Nomogram,
BSA (body surface area), Figure 2(27)
Done's, Figure 18(465)
No Moth, 198t
Non-ionic detergents, (*see* Detergents)
Nonmetals, inorganic, identification of, 85
Nonvolatile organics, identification of, 86
Nopocide-K Disinfectant, 529t
Norea (Herban), 188t
Norepinephrine (Levophed bitartrate), 19t, 36, 353, 373
l-, 473
Norethandrolone, 503t
Norethindrone acetate, 143t
Norethynodrel, 123
Norflex, (*see* Orphenadrine citrate)
Nor-hyoscyamine, 545
Norit A, 34
Normal laboratory values used in the diagnosis and treatment of poisoning, (*see* Appendix B) 752-772
altered by drugs, 752-755
No Ro, 166t
Norpramin, (*see* Desipramine hydrochloride)
Nortriptyline hydrochloride (Aventyl), 358t, 472, 495t, 515t
Norway Penetrating Oil, 529t
Nostyn, 77
Nott's Rat-TU, 198t
Nott's Roach Powder, 166t
Nott's 3-Way Bulb Saver, 166t
Novobiocin (Albamycin; Cathomycin), 14t, 120, 121t, 340, 356t
sodium (Albamycin sodium; Cathomycin sodium), 110t, 117t
Novocain (Procaine), 352t
Novrad (Levopropoxyphene), 117t
No Worry Household Bleach, 529t
Nox-Kwik High Test Insecticide, 166t
Noxon Metal Polish, 529t
NPA (Alanap), 188t
N.S.C. Detergent, 529t
NTA (Nitrilotriacetate), (*see* Nitrilotriacetate)
Nuchar C, 34
Nucleotide, diphosphopyridine, see DPN
Nu Leaf Dust, 198t
Numoquin, 459
Numorphan, (*see* Oxymorphone hydrochloride)
Nuplate Silver Cleaner, 529t
Nursing associations, working with poison control centers, 698
Nutmeg (*Myristica fragrans*), 102t, 108t, **449**, 479, 546t, 552t
Nux vomica, (*see* Strychnine)
Nydrazid, (*see* Isoniazid; INH
Nystatin (Mycostatin), 495t


**O**


Oak
poison *(Rhus toxicodendron)*, 538, 539, 553t,
western poison (yeara), 539
Oakleaf ivy (Poison oak), 539
Oats *(Avena sativa)*, 548t
Occupational
acne (chloracne), **311-312**
eruptions induced by drugs and chemicals, 312-313
asthma, materials and industrial exposures associated with, Table 75(313)
dermatitis, **311-313**
materials and industrial exposures associated with, Table 75(313)
hazards, **273-331** alphabetical listing of, Table 72(274-310) of painters and sculptors, **313-314**

some leading carcinogens, Table 81(331)
urticaria, materials and industrial exposures associated with, Table 75 (313)
Occupational Safety and Health Act of 1970, 273
Occupational Safety and Health Administration (OSHA), 273, 316
Occupations potentially associated with pneumoconioses, Table 77(323)
O-Cedar All Purpose Polish, 529t
O-Cedar Dri-Glo, 529t
O-Cedar Glass Polish, 529t
O-Cedar Paste Wax, 529t
O-Cedar Self Polishing Wax, 529t
O-Cedar Touch Up Furniture Polish, 529t
O-Cedar Upholstery & Rug Cleaner, 529t
Octachloro-hexahydro-methanoindene (Chlordane), 130t
Octadecanois acid (Stearic acid), **650**
Octafluoroisobutylene, 648t
Octamethyl pyrophosphoramide (OMPA), 127, 132t, 161t, 166t
Octane, 225
Octin, 495t
Octopus, 584, 588t
Octyl
alcohol, 730t
n-bicycloheptane dicarboximide, 170
Office of Vital Statistics, (*see* National Office of Vital Statistics)
Oil(s), 95t, 182, 312 (*see also* individual listings)
irritant, 406t
mineral, 83, 503t
of bitter almond, (*see* Cyanides)
of mustard, 495t, 659
of sassafras, (*see* Sassafras)
of turpentine, (*see* Turpentine)
of wintergreen, (*see* Methyl salicylate)
tar(s), 734t
volatile (essential), 95t
O.K. Plant Spray, 166t
Old English Red Oil Polish, 529t
Old English Scratch Cover Polish, 529t
Oleander (*Nerium oleander*), 540, 552t
Oleandomycin (Matromycin; Cyclamycin), 14t, 348t, 356t
Oleandrin, 540
Olefinic hydrocarbons, 329t
Oleic acid, 95t, 630, 633
Oligomeric resin, 621
Oligomers, 620
Olive oil, 532
as a demulcent, 83
topical application, 239
Ololiuqui seed (*Ipomoea tricolor*), 98
Omazene, 198t
Omnicide, 166t
"BB", 172
OMPA (Octamethyl pyrophosphoramide), 127, 132t
Ompa Aerosol, 166t
Oncovin (Vincristine sulfate), 400t
Onions, wild, 539
Onyx Disinfectant & Deodorant, 529t
Ophidism, **558-570**
therapy, Table 140(569)
Opiates, 449, 471, 568
drug reactions in the aged, 345t
poisoning, 38
Opipramol, 472
Opium, 6t, 8t, 35t, 38, 74t, 92t, 93t, 336t, 346t, 391, 453, 612
alkaloids, 54t, 92t, 340
camphorated tincture of (Paregoric), **453**
poppy (*Papaver somniferum*), 540
Optical bleaches, contents of, 233t
Optochin, 344, 459
Orabilex (Bunamiodyl sodium), 484t
Oral,
contraceptives, (*see* Contraceptives, oral)
hypoglycemic agents, **429**
poisons, 42
progestogens, 110t
Orchard Brand 400 Spray Powder, 166t
*Orcinus orca* (Killer whales), 586t
Oretic (Hydrochlorothiazide USP), 469
Orf, 591
Organic(s),
acids, 212
chemical pollutants to water, 330t
compounds, 17, 183
insecticides, synthetic, 126, **127-138**
mercurials, **144-146**, 734t
nonvolatile, 86
phosphate, 32, 75
ester poisoning, **129-136** (with table) insecticides, 71, Table 49(132), 604, 605t
solvents, 9t, 94t
Organomercurials, 386
Orinase (Tolbutamide), 15t, 122, 124t, 209, 214t, 455, 501t, 516t
Ornade, (*see* Chlorpheniramine)
*Ornithodorus coriaceus* (Pajaroello tick), 580
*Ornithogalum umbellatum* (Star of Bethlehem), 554t
Orphenadrine citrate (Norflex), 496t, 515t
Orpine Disinfectant, 529t
Orsin (Para-phenylenediamine), 534
Ortal, (*see* Hexethal)
Ortho Aquatic Weed Killer, 198t
Ortho Bush Killer, 198t
Ortho C-40 Dust, 166t
Ortho C-56 Dust, 187t
Orthochlorobenzylidene malononitrile, 617, 654
Orthocide Garden Fungicide, 198t
Ortho-Cop Fungicide, 198t
Ortho Crab Grass Killer, 198t
Ortho Defoliant Weed Killer, 198t
Orthodichlorobenzene, 192
Ortho Earwig Bait, 166t
Ortho Fly Killer Dry Bait, 167t
Ortho Fly Killer M., 167t
Ortho Fly Spray, 172t
Ortho Grass Killer, 198t
Orthophosphate, sodium, (*see* Sodium phosphate)
Orthophos 4 Spray, 167t
Orthosil Detergent, 529t
Osmitrol, (*see* Mannitol)
Osmolality (m Os/liter), 68t
Osteolathyrogen, 231
Ouabain, 420
"Ouch-ouch" disease (cadmium poisoning), 114, 253
Ovex (Ovotran), 137t
Ovotran (Ovex), 126, 137t
Ovulatory agents, effects on fetus and newborn, 112t
Oxacillin (Prostaphlin), 119t, 120
sodium, 124t, 125, 357t
Oxalate(s), 33, 34, 35t, 53t, 62t, 98t, **228-229,** 515t, 538
calcium, (*see* Calcium oxalate)
magnesium, (*see* Magnesium oxalate)
potassium hydrogen, (*see* Potassium hydrogen oxalates)
Oxalic acid, 8t, 36, 94t, 95t, 96t, 202, 218, 220t, **228-229**, 547, 613, 718, 720
Oxalid (Oxyphenbutazone), 16t, 79t
Oxamycin (Cycloserine), 356t
Oxanamide (Quiactin), 496t
Oxazepam (Serax), 215t, **364**, 496t
Oxazine, 455
Oxazolidine(s), 359
derivatives, 360
diones, **364**
Oxazone, 455
Oxidants, 85, 343t
Oxidase, 180
cytochrome, (*see* Cytochrome oxidase)
ferricytochrome, 237
monoamine inhibitors, (*see* Monoamine oxidase inhibitors)
Oxide(s), 230
aluminum, 311t
cadmium, 62t, 331t,
calcium, 615t, 629, 630
copper, **179-180**
ethylene, 87t, 208
iron, 331t, 652, 657
iron pigment, 95t, 536
lead, **255-265**
magnesium (*see* Magnesium oxide)
mercuric, 611
mesityl, 729t
nitric, 325
nitrogen, 202, **249-250**, 322, 324(t), **325**, 328f, 625, 648t, 656
nitrous, 87t, 351, 426
pigments, 95t
silver, (*see* Silver oxide)
sulfur, 328f, 625
titanium, (*see* Titanium oxide)
zinc, (*see* Zinc oxide)
zirconium, 536
Oxophenarsine hydrochloride (Mapharsen), 367, 496t

Oxtriphylline (Choledyl), 496t
Oxycodone (Codeine), 412
Oxydicolchicine, 412
Oxydol, 529t
Oxygen, 111t, 202, **246-249**, 344
Oxygenate Bleach, 529t
Oxyhemoglobin, 240
Oxylapine Disinfectant, 529t
Oxymorphone hydrochloride (Numorphan), 496t
Oxyphenbutazone (Tandearil; Oxalid), 12t, 16t, 79t, 429, 503t
Oxyphencyclimine hydrochloride (Daricon), 496t
Oxyphenisatin acetate, 346t, 407t, 619
Oxyphenonium bromide (Antrenyl bromide), 496t
Oxyquinoline sulfate, 95t, 536
Oxytetracycline (Terramycin), 14t, 82, 121t, 355, 357t
Oxytocin, 112t, 119
Ozone, 247t, **326-327**, 329t, 656, 657, pneumonitis, 314

**P**

PABA ((p-Aminobenzoic acid), 347t, 455, 456
Pacific rattlesnake *(Crotalus oreganus)*, **562**
Packaging and Labeling Act, (*see* Fair Packaging and Labeling Act)
Pagitane hydrochloride (Cycrimine hydrochloride), 486t
Paint(s), 4f, 14t, **741**
brush cleaners and preservatives, poisonous substances in, 94t
removers, poisonous substances in, 94t
solvents, poisonous substances in, 94t
thinners, 14t
Painters, occupational hazards to, **313-314**
Pajaroello tick (*Ornithodorus coriaceus*), 580
Palmitate, cetyl, 650
Palmitic acid, 268, 630, 633
Paludrine (Chloroguanide hydrochloride), 485t
2-PAM
chloride, (*see* Pralidoxime chloride)
iodide, (*see* Pralidoxime iodide)
Pamaquine naphthoate (Plasmochin), 11t, 338, 343, 496t
Pamoate
hydroxyzine (Vistaril), 490t, 573
pyrantel, 354t
pyrvinium (Povan), 12t, 354t
Pamphlets and other media on poisoning, (*see* Appendix A) 744-751
PAN, (*see* Peroxyacetyl nitrate)
Pancytopenia, drugs and chemicals causing, 13-15t
Panic grasses (Panicum), 548t
Panicum (Panic grasses), 548t
Panmycin, (*see* Tetracyn)
Panoram, 198t
Panparnit hydrochloride, 157
Pan-Thion Spray, 167t
Pantopon, 37, 54t, 496t
Pantothenate, calcium (Modane), 11ft
Pantothenic acid, 118t, 476t
Panwarfin (Sodium warfarin), 110t, 502t
*Papaver bracteatum*, 540
Papaverine, 6t, 81t, 117t, 515t
hydrochloride, 424
*Papaver somniferum* (Opium poppy), 540, 553t
Para-aminobenzoic acid esters, 94t, 352t
Para-aminophenol analgesic compounds, **451-452**
Para-aminosalicylic acid (PAS), 14t, 345t
salts, 117t, 338t
Para-bromoaniline, 12t
Paracetamol (Acetaminophen), 65t, **346-349**
Para-chloroaniline, 12t, 200t
Para-Denoxo, 167t
Para-dichlorobenzene, 96t, 97t, 160t, 186, 189, **192**, 194t, 195t, 196t, 197t, 198t, 199t, 200t, 526, 735t, 740
Paradione (Paramethadione), 360, 362t
Paradize Moth Balls, 198t
Paradize Nuggets, 198t
Paradow, 198t
Paradust, 166t
Paraffin(s), 95t, 225, 618
Paraflex (Chlorzoxazone), 11t
Paraflow, 167t
Paraformaldehyde, 96t, 244
Paraldehyde, 7t, 19t, 20t, 38, 65t, 71, 72t, 83, 98t, 112t, 202, 220t, **221**, 367, 377, 417, 436, 471, 473, 496t, 515t, 589
Paramethadione (Paradione), 360, 362t
Paramethasone, 415t
Paramethoxyamphetamine (PMA), 187t, 515t
Para-nitroaniline, 12t, 203, 618
Para-nitrophenol (PNP), 132
Para-oxon, 127, 130
Para-phenylenediamine, 94t, 313t
Paraquat (Bipyridylium methylsulfate or chloride), 91, 182, **185-186**, 187t, 440
Para red, 95t
Parasept, methyl (Methylparaben), **632**
Parasitic diseases (zoonoses), 597-598t
Para-Sul, 167t
Para-sulfonedichloramidobenzoic acid (Halazone), 500t
Parasympatholytics, 6t
Parasympathomimetics, 6t, 366t, **452**
Parathion (Diethyl-p-nitrophenyl monothiophosphate), 7t, 35t, 52t, 91, 98t, 127, 130, 132(t), 159t, 160t, 161t, 162t, 163t, 164t, 165t, 166t, 167t, 168t, 169t, 196t, 27lt, 331t, 734t
methyl (Dimethyl-p-nitrophenyl thiophosphate), 132t, 137t, 734t
Parathyroid extract, 229
Paratoluene, 609
Para-toluidine, 12t
Parawet, 167t
Paregoric, 20t, 612
camphorated tincture of opium, **453**, 496t
elixir, 449
Parenteral fluids, electrolyte concentrations of, Table 25(58)
Pargyline hydrochloride (Eutonyl), 65t, 496t
Paris green, 155t, 198t, 496t, **633** (*see also* Arsenic)
Parnate (Tranylcypromine), **442-444**, 501t
Parsley (*Umbelliferae*)
poison, 541f, 553t
Parson Moth Crystals, 198t
Parson's Cal-C-Nate, 167t
Parson's Insecticide Dust, 167t
Parson's Kal-Zoo Ant & Roach Dust, 167t
Parson's Kilkane Contact and Residual Spray, 172t
Parson's Louse Dust, 172t
Parson's Mosquito Yard Spray, 172t
Parson's Rat Killer, 198t
Parson's Tomato Dust, 167t
Parson's Weed Killer, 198t
Parson's Wood Preservative, 198t
PAS (Para-aminosalicylic acid), 15t, 77, 79t, 118t, 343t, 355t, 437t, 482t
Paspulum staggers, 606t
Passion flower (*Passiflora incarnata*), 546t
*Pasteurella multocida*, 591, 603
Pasture sage, 539
Patco Pestkill, 167t
Patoran, 188t
Patterson's Fly Bye, 167t
Patterson's Household Fly Spray, 167t
Patterson's Mole & Gopher Killer, 198t
Patterson's Rate & Mouse Killer, 198t
Patterson's Super Brushkiller, 198t
Patterson's Weed Killer, 198t
PBA (Benzac; Zobar), 187t
PCB (Polychlorinated biphenyl), 115, 117t, 202, **208**
PCP (Pentachlorophenol), (*see* Pentachlorophenol)
PCP (Phencyclidine), (*see* Phencyclidine)
PCP (Sodium salt, weedbeads), 187t
"Peace pills", 101
Pear (Amyl acetate), **222**
Pearl Range, Refrigerator and Metal Polish, 529t
Pearly gates morning glory (*Ipomoea violacea*) 552t
seeds (*Rivea corymbosa*), 98, 106t
Pearson's Kwik-Kill Bait, 167t
Peas, sweet (*Lathyrus odoratus*), 553t
Pebulate (Tillam), 188t
Pedameth (Methionine), (*see* Methionine)
Peganone (Ethotoin), 360, 363t
Pelletierine, 636
tannate, 353t, 496t

Pen(s), ball-point, poisonous substances in, 95t
Pencil, **633**
lead, graphite in, 633
styptic (Silver nitrate), 720
Penco Cryocide, 167t
Penco-D-Phos, 167t
Penco-Hi-Gam, 167t
Penco Pencal, 167t
Penco Penite 6X, 198t
Penco Pentrete, 198t
Penco Super Seventy, 167t
Penicillamine (Cuprimine; Beta, beta-dimethyl cysteine), 16, 54t, 180, 231, 264, 477, 608
D- , 139, 147, 148, 344, 372, 428
DL- , 147, 148
L-, 148
n-acetyl-DL- , 147, 148
Penicillin, 14t, 16t, 17t, 35t, 39, 62t, 65t, 67, 80t, 82, 119t, 120, 148, 231, 313t, 334t, 340, 342, 345t, 346t, 347t, 591, 603, 609, 702, 714, 719
benzathine, 357t
benzyl, 117t
G, 117t, 125, 357t
phenoxymethyl, 121t
potassium G, 121 t
*Penicillium*
*casei*, 322t
*islandicum*, 558
*rubrum*, 606t
Penick Roach Insecticide No. 2, 167t
Penn-Dane, 167t
Pennyroyal (Hedoma plant), 479, 496t
Penphos, 167t
Pentaborane, 644, 645
Pentachlorophenol (PCP), 179, **180-181**, 194t, 195t, 197t, 198t, 200t, 331t, 453, 734t
Penta-Core, 198t
Pentadecylcatechol (Urushiol resin), 538
Pentaerythritol tetranitrate, 12t, 346t
Penta-Five, 198t
Penta-Kill, 198t
Pentane, 96t
Penta Plus-40, 198t
Penta-Preservative, 198t
Pentaquine phosphate, 496t
Pentavalent (ABCDE) aluminum phosphate, botulinus toxoid, 713
Penta Weed Killer Concentrate, 198t
Pentazocine (Talwin), 441, 496t, 515t
Penthrane (Methoxyflurane), 79t, 351
Pentobarbital (Nembutal), 65t, 66, 67, 72t, 104t, 130t, 153, 157, 379t, 383t, 388, 389, 425t
sodium, (*see* Sodium pentobarbital)
Pentonucleotide, 370
Pentothal (Thiopental),
sodium, 71, 72t, 117t, 383t
Pentoxide dust, 474
Pentylenetetrazol (Metrazol), 7t, 38, 351, 367
Perborate(s), 533
sodium, 94t, 153, 233t, 534
monohydrate bleaches, 233t
Perchlorate
potassium, 340, 738
sodium, 82t
Perchloroethylene, (*see* Tetrachloroethylene)
Perchloroformate, methyl, 9t
Perchloromethane, (*see* Carbon tetrachloride)
Perfumes, poisonous substances in, 95t
Periactin (Cyproheptadine hydrochloride), 487t
Peridial, 6t, 389
Peritoneal dialysis, 64, **67-69**, 153, 186, 265, 349, 388, 393, 423, 436, 461, 466, 471, 474, 479, 556, 631, 646, 654
in hypothermia, 65t
Periwinkle (*Catharanthus rosens*), 546t
Permanent wave solutions, poisonous substances in, 94t
Permanganate, 98t
potassium, (*see* Potassium permanganate)
Permapen, (*see* Benzathene penicillin G)
Permatox-A, 198t
Per-Mo Mothproofing Spray, 198t
Peroxide(s), 230, 533, 624
benzoyl, 624
hydrogen, 54t, 152, 233t, 237, 490t, 532, 534, 537, 584, 634
methyl ethyl ketone, 624
Peroxyacetyl nitrate (PAN), **327**
Perphenazine (Trilafon), 14t, 359, 515t
Persulfate, sodium, 534
Pertofrane, (*see* Desipramine hydrochloride)
Peru balsam, 496t, **610**
Pescocide A, 167t
Pest-B-Gon Spray, 167t
Pestene Insecticide Powder, 172t
Pesticide(s), 604
chemical: how to use them, **731-736**
laws, 701-702
potential toxicity of, Table 161(734-735)
rates of application, 733
safe use of, **731-736**
Pesticide Safety Team Network (PSTN), **159, 170,** 751
Pestroy, 167t
Pests about the home, 730-736
Peterman Ant Food, 167t
Peterman Roach Food, 167t
Peterman Roach Powder & Paste, 167t
Petox, 167t
Petrolatum, 95t, 406t
liquid (mineral oil), 152, 204, 480 as a demulcent, 83
Petroleum
derivatives, 127
distillates, 14t, 82, 94t, 160t, 161t, 162t, 165t, 168t, 182, 196t, 202, **222-224,** 225, 517, 521
ether, 95t
hydrocarbons, 96t, 169t, 199t
naphtha, 247t, 650
oils, 164t, 194t, 198t, 201t, 224
products, 455
solvents, 96t, 187t
spirits, 96t, 222
Peyote (*Lophophora williamsii*), 99, 106t, 552t, **632**
buttons, 99, 102t
Peyotl cactus (*lophophora williamsii*), 98, 102t, 552t
P-51 Fast Kill Insect Spray, 172t
P Forty, 167t
Pfeuger Shoo Fly Insect Repellent, 198t
*Phalloides* (mushrooms), 547, 552t
Phalloidine, 555, 559t
Phalloin, 555
Phanodorn (Cyclobarbital), 383t
calcium, 35t
Pharmicists, working with poison control centers, 698
*Phaseolus limensis, lunatus* (Lima bean), 552t
Phemerol chloride (Benzethonium chloride), 484t, 519
Phenacemide (Phenurone), 77, 340, 347t, 360, 362t
Phenacetin (Acetophenetiden), 7t, 12, 64, 98t, 117t, 340, 342, 343t, 346t, 348, **451-452**
Phenaglycodol (Ultran), 118t, 496t
Phenanthrene, 455
Phenarsone sulfoxylate (Aldarsone), 496t
Phenazone, 343t
Phenazopyridine (Pyridium), 10t, 11t, 12t, 64
hydrochloride, 496t
Phencyclidine (Sernylan; PCP), 101, 515t
Phenelzine, 65t, 334t, 341
Phenergan (Promethazine), 455
Phenethicillin, (*see* Penicillin)
Phenetidin, 12t
Phenformin, 429
hydrochloride (DBI), 110t, 241t
Phenindione (Danilone; Hedulin), 10t, 11t, 17t, 81t, 340, 497t
Pheniramine maleate, 14t
Phenistix Reagent Strip, 9, 463
Phenkaptone, 734t
Phenmetrazine (Preludin), 104t, 515t
Phenprocoumon, 55t
Phenobarbital (Luminal), 14t, 20t, 35t, 38, 65t, 72t, 80t, 83, 110t, 117t, 120, 130t, 138, 207, 347t, 360, **361,** 379(t), 380, 381, 383(t), 386, 388, 389, 424t, 449, 503t, 513t
elixir, 20t
intoxication, 383, 387
sodium, 8t, 19t, 128, 129, 456
Phenobarbitone (Phenobarbital), 120
Phenol(s), 7t, 8t, 10t, 12t, 14t, 35t, 45, 58, 95t, 96t, 98t, 335t, 353t, **453-454,** 538, 618, 622t, 634
derivatives, 7t, 197t, 201t, **453-454**

dinitrobutyl (Dinoseb), 199t
halogenated, 455
Phenolphthalein, 10t, 11t, 14t, 35t, 122, 340, 346t, 347t, 406t, **454,** 614t
Phenosulfonate, zinc, 94t
Phenothiazine(s), 11t, 40, 53t, 66, 81t, 91, 102, 110t, 112t, 162t, 340, 344, 345t, 346(t), 347t, 348t, 365t, 366t, 371, 372, 373, 376, 411, 455, 472
adverse reactions to, 6t, Table 109(374-375)
contraindications, 135, 378
derivatives, 103, 366t, 368t, 371, 372, 442, 443t
dimethylamines, 368t
piperazines, 368t
piperidines, 368t
thioxanthenes, 368t
Forrest rapid urine color test for metabolites, 464
N.F., 354t
ocular effects, Table 108(371)
Phenoxyacetic acid, chlorinated, 182, 735t
Phenoxybenzamine hydrochloride (Dibenzyline), 69, 471
Phenoxymethyl penicillin, 121t
Phensuximide (Milontin), 8t, 10t, 11t, 347, 360, 362t, 456, 515t
Phentolamine (Regitine), 22t, 215t, 475, 497t, 573
hydrochloride, 475
methane sulfonate, 444
Phenurone (Phenacemide), 360, 362t
Phenyl,
mercuric propionate, 608
mercuric salts, 194t, 196t, 197t, 198t, 199t, 200t
Phenylalinine, 355t, 359
mustard, 404
Phenylazopyridine, 12t
Phenylbutazone (Butazolidin; Azolid), 12t, 14t, 16t, 62t, 79t, 117t, 340, 345t, 347t, 429, 455, **457,** 472, 497t, 503t, 515t
Phenylcinchoninic acid, 76
Phenylenediamine, 12t
ortho-isomer (Diolene), 534
para- (Orsin, Ursol D), 94t, 534
Phenylephrine (Neo-Synephrine), 9t, 22t, 69, 333, 443t, 446, 470, 473
hydrochloride, 14t
Phenylhydrazine, 497t
acetyl, 343
Phenylhydride, (*see* Benzene)
Phenylhydroxylamine, 12t
Phenylketones, 463
Phenylmercuric salts, 497t
Phenylpropanolamine, 443t
Phenylpyruvic acid, 9
Phenylsalicylate (Salol), 10t, **634**
Phenyramidol, 503t
Phenytoin (Diphenylhydantoin; Dilantin), 8t, 10t, 11t, 12t, 13t, 22t, 48t, 65t, 72t, 77, 80t, 117t, 120, 143t, 215t, 339, 345t, 347t, 359, 360, **361,** 362t, 366t, 420, 421t, 456, 503t, 514t
adverse effects, 49t
*Philodendron* (Arum family), 543, 548t, 606
pHisoHex (Hexachlorophene), 497t, 530t, 627
Phoenix Brand Delnar Cotton Spray, 167t
*Pholiota curvipes* (poisonous mushrooms), 557f
*Phoradendron flavescens* (Mistletoe), 552t, 740
Phorate (Thimet), 137t
Phosdrin (Mevinphos), 132t, 137t, 734t
Phosfume, 167t
Phosgene (Carbonyl chloride), 9t, 14t, 87t, 189, 202, 205, **250-252,** 324t, 625, 648t
Phoskil, 167t
Phosphamidon, 137t
Phosphatase (serum alkaline), 76
erythrocytic acid, (*see* Erythrocytic acid phosphatase)
Phosphate(s), 117t, 233t, 518, 605t, 621, 730
alkaline salts, 520
aluminum, 350
gel, 644
ammonium, 621
amprotropine, 378
as cathartics, 406t
calcium, **395,** 621
chloroquine (Aralen phosphate), 110t, 456, 485t
codeine, 19t, 20t, 34
copper, **179-180**
dicalcium, 655
2,2-dichlorovinyldimethyl (Vapona), 162t, 164t
dipotassium, 479
disodium, 395, 479
duohydrate, 434
esters, 52t, 55t, 98, 126, **129-136,** 137, 160t
ferrous, 434
iproniazid-Marsilid, **431**
monopotassium, 395, 479
organic poisoning symptoms, Table 48(131)
pentaquine, 496t
poly, 522t, 523t, 524t
polymeric, 58
potassium, 621
primaquine, 498t
sodium, 230, 405
glass, 94t, 524t
tripoly, 522t, 523t, 524t
tetracycline complex, 121t
tetrasodium, 94t
tricalcium, **655**
triethyl, 96t
tri-ortho-cresyl (machine oil), 202, **219-221**
trisodium, 96t, 522t, 523t, 524t, 616t
Phosphide(s), 203
copper, 152
zinc, 173, **174,** 734t
Phosphine, 140, **152,** 174, 203, 247t
Phospholine iodide, (*see* Echothiophate iodide)
Phosphordithioate, 169
Phosphoric acid, 94t, 98t, 517, 526, 621
Phosphorus, 7t, 8t, 35t, 53t, 57t, 62t, 69, 77, 82, 97t, 127, **151-152,** 161t, 173, 183, 194t, 195t, 197t, 199t, 200t, 269, 350, 515t, 621, 623
metallic, 203
organic insecticides, toxicity of, Table 49(132)
red, 736, 737, 738
sesquisulfide, 736, 737
sulfides, 738
trisulfide, 151
white, 736, 737
yellow, 8t, 736
4-Phosphoryltryptamine (Psilocybin), 102t
Phospho-soda, 406t, 455
Phosvex, 167t
Photographic material, **634-636**
Photophobia, 6t
Photosensitivity,
algae producing, 548t
compounds and drugs producing, **455-456**
fungi producing, 548t
plants producing, Table 138(548)
Phthalate
dibutyl, 95t
dimethyl, 96t
ester, 624
Phthalazine derivatives, 428
Phthalazinedione (Luminol), 519
Phthalic anhydride, 313t
Phthalmic acid
N-naphthyl, 194t
Phthisis, stone masons' and miners' (silicosis), **314-315**
*Physalia palagica* (Portuguese man-of-war), 584, 587t
Physicians, working with poison control centers, 698
Physic nut (*Jatropha*), 553t
Physicochemical properties of common barbiturates, Table 110(379)
Physiologic saline, 213
*Physostigma venenosum* (Calabar bean), 549t
Physostigmine (Eserine), 7t, 8t, 9t, 39, 55t, 97t, 98, 358, 359, 378, 438, 452, 497t, 633
salicylate (Antilirium), **39,** 54t, 367, 376, 378, 472
Phytocide, 198t
*Phytolacca americana* (Inkberry, pokeberry, pokeweed, scoke), 553t
Phytonadione, 22t, 55t, 479, 503t
Phytotoxins, 538
Pica, 113, 255, 262
Picloram (Tordon), 188t
Pi-Co, 172t

Picrate
ammonium, **234**
butamben, 484t
butesin, 484t
Picric acid, 7t, 8t, **456,** 497t
Picrotoxin, 6t, 7t, 8t, 9t, 19t, 38, 39, 97t, 497t
contraindications, 367
Picry, (*see* Poison ivy)
Pied Piper Brush Killer, 199t
Pied Piper Chlor-O-Cide, 167t
Pied Piper Dog Shampoo, 167t
Pied Piper for Rats & Mice, 198t
Pied Piper Household Insecticide Containing DDT, 172t
Pied Piper Kwik-Kill Mouse Seed, 198t
Pied Piper Moth Crystals, 198t
Pied Piper Roachicide, 167t
Pied Piper Rodenticide, 199t
Pigmy rattler *(Sistrurus miliarius),* **562**
Pills, suntan, (*see* Suntan pills)
Pilocarpine, 7t, 8t, 9t, 32, 39, 55t, 95t, 97t, 143, 377, 452, 497t
nitrate, 377
Pine, 479
oil, 4f, 94t, 96t, 521, 522, 523t, **636**
Pine Sol, 530t
Pinuseptol, 560t
Pipamazine, 497t
Pipenzolate (Piptal), 358t
Piperazine, 12t, 343t, 354t, 371, 497t
compounds, 366, 368t
Piperidine derivatives, 73, 368t
Piperocaine, **457**
Piperonyl
butoxide, 14t, 170
cyclonene, 170
Piperoxane, 497t
Pipradrol (Meratran), 497t
*Piptadenia peregrina* (DMT in), 99
Piptal, (*see* Pipenzolate)
Pitch, 455, 605t
Pitressin, (*see* Vasopressin)
Pittabs (Calcium hypochlorite), 652
Pittsburgh Weed Killer, 199t
Pituitary, anterior, extract, 348t
posterior pituitary units (Lypressin), 492t
snuff (Pigorox protein), 322t
Pit vipers (poisonous snakes), 568
identifying features, 563f
Pival (Warfarin), 173, **177,** 194t, 195t, 196t, 199t
Pivalyn Packets, 199t
Placidyl, (*see* Ethchlorvynol)
Plan-A-Diel, 167t
Plane Dane, 167t
Planeto, 167t
Plan-O-Lin, 167t
Plan-O-Weed, 199t
Plant(s)
and food poisoning, **717-718**
food, **621-623**
nutrients, as water pollutant, 330t
poisoning, **538-558** (with tables), **717-718**
poisonous, Table 139(548-554)
producing photosensitization, Table 138(548)
algae, 548t
fungi, 548t
hepatogenic, 548t
toxic chemicals in, 538
Planter's Blue Mold Dust, 199t
Planter's Rat & Mouse Bait, 199t
Planters Save-A-Root, 167t
Planters Special Insect Spray, 167t
Planters Special Jap Beetle Killer, 167t
Planters Termitox, 167t
Planters Truk-Dust, 167t
Planthion Aerosol, 167t
Plaquenil, (*see* Hydroxychloroquine)
Plasmanate, 385
Plasmapheresis, **63-64**
Plasmochin (Pamaquine naphthoate), 11t, 97t, 344, 459
Plasmoquine, 12t
Plaster
of Paris (Gypsum), **636**
wall, to neutralize acids, 83
Plastic(s)
cement, **636**
menders, poisonous substances in, 95t
poisonous substances in, 96t
resin, **623-624**
Plasticizers, poisonous substances in, 95t
Platinum, 313
Plizatropine, 560t
Plumbago (Graphite), **626**
Plumite Drain Opener, 530t
Pluraturf Crabgrass Killer, 199t
Plutonium, 331t, 642, 643
PMA, (*see* Paramethoxyamphetamine)
PMF, see Progressive massive fibrosis
Pneumoconioses, **314-322** (*see also* specific listings)
aluminum, 323t
coal workers', 314, **315-316,** 323t
diatomite, 314, **318**
hard metal, 323t
occupations potentially associated with, Table 77(323)
Pneumonitis
hypersensitivity (Farmer's lung), 314, **321-322**
antigens causing, Table 76(322)
ozone, 314
PNP (Para-nitrophenol), 132
Pod jelly, **634-635,** 636
Podophyllum, 406t, 497t
*Podophyllum peltatum* (Mayapple), 552t
*Pogonomyrmex barbatus* (Desert ant), 579
Poinsettia *(Euphorbia pulcherrima),* 553t, **741**
Poison
ash *(Rhus vernix),* 539, 553t
beaver *(Cicuta virosa),* 554t
creeper *(Rhus toxicodendron),* 539, 553t
dogwood *(Rhus vernix),* 539, 553t
elder *(Rhus vernix),* 539, 553t
hemlock *(Conium maculatum),* 545, 553t
herbal preparations, 546t
ivy *(Rhus toxicodendron),* 538, 539, 553t
oak *(Rhus toxicodendron),* 538, 539, 553t
western (yeara), 539
parsley *(Conium maculatum),* 541f, 553t
sumac *(Rhus vernix),* 538, 539, 553t
tree, *(Metopium toxiferum),* 553t
Poison Control Centers, **661-662**
directory of, Table 155(662-692)
guide to the organization of, **696-699**
activities of participants in, 696-699
objectives, 696
suggested duties for poison control officer, 699
recommendations by American Association of Poison Control Centers, **700-701**
roles of, 5
standards for, **699-700**
Poisoning, (*see also* specific diseases and poisons)
antibiotics, **82-83**
antidotes, **47,** Table 21(50-56)
artificial respiration, **59-60** (with figure)
blood transfusions, **63-64**
booklets available on, (*see* Appendix A) 744-745
brochures available on, (*see* Appendix A) 745-747
cardiac therapy, **61-63** (with figure)
causes, 3
charts available on, (*see* Appendix A) 744-745
chemical burns, **46-47,** 721
compounds capable of producing toxicity, **608-659**
contents of common household substances, Table 37(94-96)
convulsions, treatment of, 71, Table 30(72)
dangerous products, Figure 4(4)
demulcents used, 83
dermal, 6, **46,** 721
diagnostic considerations, **6-17**
disseminated intravascular coagulation (DIC), 70
drugs used in treatment of, **19-26** (with tables)
emergency drugs used for treatment of, Tables 9 & 10(19-22)
emetics used, **42-46,** 83
equipment used in emergencies, **26**
extracorporeal dialyzer used in treatment of, **64-66**
eye contamination, **46-47,** 721
fatalities, 3, 84
films available on, (*see* Appendix A) 747-748
first aid measures, **720-722**
flyers available on, (*see* Appendix A) 745-747
gastric lavage in treatment of, **28-30**
in fetus and infant, **102-125**
ingested, 6, **42-46,** 84, 720-721
inhaled, 6, 46, 84, 88, 721

injected, 46, 84, 721
lipid dialysis in treatment of, **66-67**
mental functions and, **93-102,** Table 40(104-109)
neutralizing acids in treatment of, **83**
neutralizing alkalis in treatment of, **83**
newspapers available on, (*see* Appendix A) 749
normal laboratory values used in the diagnosis and treatment of, (*see* Appendix B) 752-772
pamphlets and other media available on, (*see* Appendix A) 744-751
peritoneal dialysis in treatment of, **67-69**
posters available on, (*see* Appendix A) 749-751
prevention of, **3-6**
proclamations available on, (*see* Appendix A) 749
public safety education, **660-743**
radio spots available on, (*see* Appendix A) 749
sedatives used, 83
shock therapy, **69**
signs and symptoms of, Table 1(6-9)
slides available on, (*see* Appendix A) 747-748
source of toxicology information, (*see* Appendix A) 751
suicidal intent, 3, **334-336** (with table)
supportive measures in treatment of, **47-58**
television spots available on, (*see* Appendix A) 749
treatment, general principles of, **42-47, 720-721**

Poisonous
arthropods
fish, **581-591** (with table)
insects, **570-581**
plants, 538-558 (with table), **717-718**
snakes, **558-570**
substances found in the household, Table 37(94-96)

Poison Prevention Packaging Act of 1970, 703
Poisons and mental function, **93-102**
Poisons, common animal, Table 146(605-606) (*see also* Zoonoses)
Poisonwood tree *(Metopium toxiferum),* 544
Pokeberry *(Phytolacca americana),* 553t
Pokeweed *(Phytolacca americana),* 553t
Polar Moth Balls, 199t
Polar Moth Flakes, 199t
Polar Moth Rings, 199t
Polaroid (photographic material), **634-636**
prints, 635-636

Polish(es)
for furniture and floors, poisonous substances in, 94t
leather, poisonous substances in, 95t
shoe, poisonous substances in, 95t

Polishers and cleaners (metal), poisonous substances in, 94t
Polishing agents, **517-531** (with table)
Polistes wasp, 577
Pollen(s), 323
extracts, 340
Pollutants, Table 78(324)
air, 329t
water, 330t
Pollution
air, **322-327**
in the home **327-329**
radioactive, **329-330**
water, **330-331**
Polonium, 266
Polyalkaline glycol, (*see* Detergents, non-ionic)
Polychlorinated biphenyl (PCB), (*see* PCB)
Polycyclic hydrocarbons, 329t
Polycycline, (*see* Tetracyn)
Polyethoxyethanol, alkylphenyl, 522t, 523t, 524t
lauric, 522t, 523t, 524t
myristic, 522t, 523t, 524t
nonyl, 522t, 523t, 524t
Polyethylene glycols, 730t
*Polygonum* (Smartweeds), 548t
Polymer fume fever (Polytetrafluoroethylene; Teflon), **637,** 654
Polymeric phosphates, 58
Polymorphism, genetic, producing drug-induced hemolytic anemia or altered therapeutic response, Table 88(338)
Polymyxin, 65t, 355
B sulfate (Aerosporin), 121t, 357t
Polynuclear hydrocarbons, **717**
Polyphosphates, 233, 519
Polypropylene glycols, 730t
Polysiloxane, methyl (Silicones), 647
Polysulfide, calcium, **237-239,** 630
Polytetrafluoroethylene (Teflon), **637,** 654
Polythiazide (Renese), 469, 497t
Polyvinyl chloride, (*see* Chloride, polyvinyl)
Polyvinylpyrrolidone (PVP), 535
Pomegranate, **636**
Ponstel (Mefenamic), 117t
Pontocaine (Tetracaine), 352t
Poppy,
California *(Eschscholtzie california),* 546t
Mexican *(Argemore mexicana),* 552t
opium *(Pavaver somniferum),* 540, 541f, 553t
prickly, *see* Mexican
Porcelain, poisonous substances in, 94t
Porphobilinogen, 257
Porphyria, 65t, 338t, 341
drugs inducing, 8t, **456**
Porphyria cutanea tarda (PCT), 312
Porphyrins, 10t, 144, 259
Port Brand Kryolite Dust, 167t
Port Brand Tepp-Tone Emulsion, 167t

Port Brand Than-O-Dust, 199t
Portuguese man-of-war *(Physalia palagica),* 584, 587t, 590
Posters available on poisoning, (*see* Appendix A) 749-751
Pot, (*see* Marihuana)
Potash, 335t, 621
Potassium, 48t, 57t, 65t, 68t, 117t, 141, 174, 190, 252t, 269, 315, 411, 466, 473, 626, 631
acid tartrate, 709t
antimony tartrate, 155t
arsenite (Fowler's solution), 489t
bicarbonate, 533
bromate, 94t, 709t
bromide, 392
carbonate, 202, 230, 533, 621
chlorate, 65t, 94t, 182, 346t, 736-737, 738
chloride, 22t, 58t, 96t, 143, 387, 420, 422, 497t, 615t, 621
chromium sulfate, 614t
citrate (K-Lyte), 466
cyanate, (*see* Cyanate)
cyanide, 18, 35t, 94t, 97t
dichloroisocyanurates, 523t, 524t, **618**
dichromate, 65t
ferrocyanide, 45, 180
hydrogen oxalate, 228
hydroxide, 611
hypochlorite, 629
in digitalis therapy, 421t
iodate, 709t
iodide, 110t, 270, 430, 708t
magnesium sulfate, 621
monopersulfate, 523t
nitrate (Saltpeter), 499t
penicillin G, 121t
perchlorate, 340, 738
permanganate, 8t, 20t, 35t, 39, 54t, 55t, 85, 146, 152, 154, 157, 174, 178, 237, 445, 533, 555, 610, **633**
phosphate, 621
salts, 62t, 182, 422, 469, 532, 618
silicate, 230
sulfate, 621
sulfide, 238
thiocyanate, 184, 654
thiosulfate, **195t**
Potato *(Solanum tuberosum),* 358t, 553t, **718**
bugs, 742
Irish, 544
*Pothos,* 543
Potosan, 127
Potters' asthma (silicosis), **314-315**
Poulins Rat Doom, 199t
Povan (Pyrvinium pamoate), 12t, 354t
Powco Brush Killer, 199t
Powder
Dover's (opium), 391
ipecac, 83, 391
Prairie rattlesnake *(Crotalus viridis),* **561**
Pralidoxime
chloride (2-PAM chloride, Protopam), 55t, 133, 138, 582

iodide (2-PAM iodide), 55t, 133, 138
Pratt's D-X Insect Spray, 172t
Pratt's 622 Insect Repellent, 199t
Pratt's Surfispray, 172t
Pratt's Tomato Dust, 199t
Pratt's Weed Killer, 199t
Prayer bead, (*see* Jequirity bean)
Prednisolone, 69, 231, 415t
Prednisone (Meticorten), 14t, 69, 401t, 413, 415t
Preen, 560t
Preenet, 560t
Pregnanediol, inhibitor in breast milk, 111t
Prelim, 530t
Preludin (Phenmetrazine), 104t
Premerge, 187t, 199t
Prentox Roach Powder, 167t
Presamine, (*see* Imipramine)
Pre-Sate (Chlorphentermine hydrochloride), 486t
Presidon, (*see* Pyrethyldione)
Pretoxicosis test, 239
Prevention
of carbon monoxide poisoning, **722-724**
of food poisoning, **720**
of insect stings, **742-743**
of poisoning, **3-6**
Prilocaine (Citanest), 12t, 352(t)
Primaquine, 11t, 12t, 336, 337, 338(t), 343t
phosphate, 498t
Primidone (Mysoline), 14t, 65t, 345t, 360, **361,** 362t, 498t, 515t
Primrose *(Primula),* 553t
Print coater solution, **635**
Priodax, (*see* Iodoalphionic acid)
Priscoline hydrochloride, (*see* Tolazoline hydrochloride)
*Pristonia amazonica* (DMT in), 99
Privet, common *(Ligustrum vulgare),* 553t
berries, 540
Privine, 498t
Pro-Banthine (Propantheline bromide), 39, 358t, 473
Probenecid (Benemid), 79t, 343t, 429, 498t, 515t
Procainamide, 20t, 22t, 48t, 176, 340, 343t, 421(t), 422, 515t
adverse effects, 49t
hydrochloride (Pronestyl), 16t, 19t, 40, 81t, 174, 345t
Procaine (Novocain), 7t, 33, 92t, 97t, 264, 340, 351, 352t, **457,** 568, 574, 589, 590
hydrochloride, 619
local anesthetics of, 455
Procarbazine (Matulane), 334t, 400t
Prochlorperazine, 14t, 77, 371, 515t
Proclamations on poisoning, (*see* Appendix A) 749
Progesterone, 312, 348t, 455, 498t
and lactation, 116, 119, 123
Progestin, 112t, 413
Progestogens, 110t, 402t
effect on lactation, 116
oral, 110t
Proglycem (Oral diazoxide), 17t
Progressive massive fibrosis (PMF), 316
Prolactin (Luteotrophic hormone), 119, 123
Promazine hydrochloride (Sparine), 9, 14t, 77, 92t, 371, 498t, 515t
Promethazine (Phenergan), 9, 14t, 112t, 455
Prometone, 188t
Prometryne (Caparol), 188t
Promizole, (*see* Thiazosulfone)
Promoxolane, 498t
Pronestyl (Procainamide hydrochloride), 16t, 19t, 20t, 22t, 40, 81t, 174, 345t, 421t
adverse effects, 49t
Pronto (floorwax), 230
Pronton Detergent, 530t
Propane
gas, 609, **625**
liquid, **637**
Propanediol, butyl ethyl, 193
Propanil (Stam F-34; Rogue), 188t
n-Propanol, 95t
Propanolol HCL (Inderal), 498t
Propantheline bromide (Pro-Banthine), 39, 358t, 473
Propazine, 188t
Propellants, Freon, 95t
Propenol (Allyl alcohol), (*see* Alcohol, allyl)
Prophenpyridamine maleate (Trimeton), 498t
Propionate, phenyl mercuric, 145, 608
Propionic acid, 321, 708t
calcium salts of, 708t
sodium salts of, 708t
Propoxyphene (Darvon; Dolene), 81t, 112t, 416, 463, 515t
Propranolol hydrochloride (Inderal), 17t, 48t, 103, 174, 411, 421(t), 515t
adverse effects, 49t
Propyl
acetate, 730t
alcohol, 212, 216, 730t
n-Propyl isomer, 170
Propylene
dichloride, 247t
gylcol, 202, **218-219,** 454, 730t
Propylhexedrine (Benzedrex), 515t
Propylthiouracil (PTU), 80t, 110t, 117t, 143t, 498t
Prostaphlin (Oxacillin), 119t, 120, 124t, 357t
Prostigmin (Neostigmine), 19t, 376, 378, 415
methylsulfate, 718
Protamine sulfate, 55t
Proteolysins, 566
Pro-Tex Moth Balls, 199t
Prothromadin (Sodium warfarin), 110t
Prothrombin, 348
Protoiodide, mercury, 493t
Protopam (Pralidoxime chloride, 2 PAM chloride), 133
Protoporphyrin, 257, 259
Protoveratrine (Veratrum alkaloid), 474
Protozoan diseases (zoonoses), 596-597t
Protriptyline hydrochloride (Vivactil), 358t, 472, 498t
*Prunus demissa, melanocarpa, serotina* (Black cherry), 549t
Prussian blue (Ferric ferrocyanide), 96t, 143
Prussic acid (Hydrocyanic acid), 235, 606, **637**
PSC Co-Op Cuprocide Dust, 199t
PSC Co-Op Slug Pellets, 168t
PSC Co-Op Weed Killer, 199t
PSC Co-Op Weevil Bait, 168t
Pseudocholinesterase, 341
Pseudoephedrine (Sudafed), 117t
*Pseudomonas aeruginosa,* 236
*Psilocybe mexicana* (mushroom), 98
Psilocybin (4-Phosphoryltryptamine), 98, 99, 102t, 106t, 555, 560t
Psoralens ("suntan pills"), 455, **537**
PSTN (Pesticide Safety Team Network), **159, 170**
Psychic energizer, 431
Psychosis (hallucinogens), (*see* Poisons and mental function)
Psychotrine, 83
Psychotropic agents, **370-376,** 449
manufacturer, Table 107(368-369)
side effects of, 112t, Table 107(368-369)
trade and generic names, Table 107(368-369)
uses of, Table 107(368-369)
*Pteridium aquilinum* (Bracken fern), 606t
*Pteris aquilina* (Bracken fern), 606t
*Pterois volitans* (Lionfish), 588t, 590
Ptomaine poisoning, 710
Public Health Service, (*see* U.S. Public Health Service)
Public safety education, **660-743**
Puff adder, 568
Puffball (Calvatia family), 556f
Pulmonary
irritants, Table 154(648)
siderosis, 314, **319**
Pumice, 524t, 525, **637**
Punch Detergent, 525
Puncture vine *(Tribulus terrestris),* 548t
Puraturf Crabgrass Killer, 199t
Pure Para, 199t
Purex Dry Bleach, 530t
Purex Pipe and Drain Cleaner, 530t
Purex Toilet Bowl Detergent, 530t
Purified silicons, 95t
Purifiers (swimming pool disinfectants), **652-653**
Purines, 632
Purinethol (6-Mercaptopurine), 80t, 398t, 404
Puss caterpillar *(Megalopyge opercularis),* 579
Putty, poisonous substances in, 94t

PVP (Polyvinylpyrrolidone), 535
Pyfos, 168t
Pyopen (Carbencillin), 118t
Pyracantha, firethorn *(Pyracantha coccinea)*, 544, 553t
Pyrantel pamoate, 354t
Pyrazinamide (PZA), 16t, 80t, 437t, 455
Pyrazolon, 10t
analgesics, **457**
Pyrazon (Pyramin), 188t
Pyrenone Concentrate, 161t
Pyrethrin(s), 97t, 127, **157,** 158t, 159t, 160t, 161t, 162t, 163t, 164t, 165t, 166t, 167t, 168t, 169t, 170t, 313t, 647, 734t
Pyrethrum, 158t, 166t, 170
allethrin, **157**
Pyrethyldione (Sedulon; Presidon), 498t
Pyribenzamine, 97t, 611, 612, 617
hydrochloride, 19t, 20t
Pyridine, 455, 498t
bases, 216
test, 189
2-Pyridine aldoxime methylchloride, (*see* Pralidoxime chloride)
2-Pyridine aldoxime methyliodide (2-PAM iodide), (*see* Pralidoxime iodide)
Pyridium (Phenazopyridine), 10t, 11t, 12t, 17, 64, 496t, 598t
Pyridostigmin (Mestinon), 358, 376, 378
Pyridoxine (Vitamin $B_6$), 112t, 148, 476t
hydrochloride, 438, 484t
N-3 Pyridylmethyl-N-p-nitrophenol urea (Vacor), 173, 174-175, 179t
Pyrilamine, 358t
Pyrimethamine (Daraprim), 16t, 117t, 477, 498t
Pyrogallol, 10t, 14t, 94t
Pyro-Phos, 168t
Pyrophosphate, tetrasodium, 520, 522t, 523t, 524t
Pyrophosphoramide, octamethyl (OMPA), 132t, 161t, 166t
Pyrosect, 168t
Pyroxylin (Dinitrocellulose), 617
Pyrrolizidine alkaloids, 547, 558
Pyrvinium pamoate (Povan), 12t, 354t
PZA (Pyrazinamide), 16t, 80t

**Q**

Quaalude, (*see* Methaqualone)
Quaternary ammonium compounds (Cationic detergents), 97t, 184, 470, 519, 525
Queen's root, 606
Quiactin, (*see* Oxanamide)
Quick Action Gulfspray, 172t
Quick lime, 612, 629
Quick-N-Brite, 530t
Quinacrine (Atabrine), 79t, 143t, 214t, 338, 340, 341, 347t, 354t, 459, 460
hydrochloride, 346t, 460, 498t
Quince seed, **637**
Quinethazone (Hydromox), 469
Quinidine, 8t, 9t, 14t, 16t, 48t, 62t, 81t, 117t, 182, 340, 341, 342, 343t, 345t, 347t, 421t, 422, 455, 458, 461, 503t, 515t
adverse effects, 49t
gluconate, 22t, 40
hydrochloride, 19t, 40
sulfate, 20t, **40,** 177
Quinine, 8t, 9t, 10t, 11t, 15t, 16t, 35t, 36, 39, 54t, 55t, 62t, 65t, 85f, 97t, 110t, 112t, 117t, 119t, 122, 312, 340, 342, 343t, 346t, 455, **457-461,** 515t, 610, 633
derivatives, 7t, 457
Quinocide, 338
Quinoline, 344
Quinones, 12t
Quotane (Dimethisoquin), **457**

**R**

Rabies, 592, 603
preexposure rabies prophylaxis, **603**
Rad Cleaner, 530t
Radiant Lemon Oil Polish, 530t
Radiation, 78, 82t, 110t, 112t
effects at various doses, Table 150(640)
syndrome, **638-642**
Radioactive
air pollution, **329-330**
drugs affecting fetus and newborn, 110t, 112t, 124
iodine, 122
isotopes, 122
poisoning, 112t, **642-644**
preparations, 124
substances, as water pollutants, 330t
Radioimmunoassay test, 101
Radioiodine, 348t
Radioisotope(s)
and organs subject to scanning, Table 153(644)
important, list of (used in medicine and biology), Table 152(643)
poisoning, 112t
representative diagnostic procedures, Table 151(641)
Radio spots on poisoning, (*see* Appendix A) 749
Radium, 270t
Radon gas, 329
Ragweed (short, giant, western), 313t, 539
Ragwort, tansy, 545
Raid Bug Killer, 168t, 172t
Raid Insect Spray, 168t, 172t
Raid Roach and Ant Killer, 168t
*Ranunculaceae* (Crowfoot or buttercup), 549t
Rasmussen, F., experiments in drugs and breast milk, 116
Rat and Mouse Controller Paste, 199t
Rataway, 199t
Rat-B-Gon Rat & Mice Bait, 199t
Rat-Deth, 199t
Ratfish, 585
Raticate (Dicarboximide), **178-179**
Rat-Kill, 199t
Rat mite, 580
Rat-Nip, 199t
Rat-Nix, 199t
Rat-Nots, 199t
Rat-O-Cide No. 2, 199t
Rat-O-Cide Rat Bait, 199t
Rat-Ola, 199t
Ratorex, 199t
Rat-Pak, 199t
Rat-Seed, 199t
Rat's End, 199t
Rat-Snax, 199t
Rattlesnake,
ground *(Sistrurus)*, **562,** 564f
pacific *(Crotalus oreganus)*, **562**
prairie *(Crotalus viridis)*, **561-562**
timber *(Crotalus horridus)*, **561**
true *(Crotalus)*, **561-562,** 564f
Rat-Trol Bait, 199t
Rauloydin (Reserpine), 110t
Raurine (Reserpine), 110t
Rau-Sed (Reserpine), 110t
Rauwiloid, (*see* Rauwolfia alkaloids)
Rauwolfia alkaloids (Rauwiloid), 346t, 368t, 371, 498t
Rawleigh's Car Cleaner, 530t
Rawleigh's Car Polish, 530t
Rawleigh's Cleanser, 530t
Rax-Powder, 199t
Ray(s), 585, 587t
electric *(Torpedinidae)*, 590
sting- *(Dasyatidae)*, 587t
Rayless goldenrod *(Aplopappus heterophyllus)*, 539, 553t
R-Deth Grain Killer, 199t
Real-Kill Bug Killer, 168t
Real-Kill Mothkiller, 199t
Re-Clean for Fabrics, 530t
Recommendations to public on first-aid measures for poisoning, **720-722**
before arrival of physician, 720-721
prevention, 721-722
Red bug (Chigger), 580
Red Cap Refresh-R Germicide & Deodorant, 530t
Red Devil Dust, 168t
Red ochre, 736
Red phosphorus, 736, 737, 738
Red Seal Rodenticide, 199t
Red squill, 62t, 173, **177,** 194t, 197t, 199t, 200t, 201t, 734t
Red Star Crabgrass Killer, 199t
Red veterinary petrolatum (RVP), 456
Red whelk *(Neptunea antiqua)*, 582
Redwood extract, 533
Refrigeration, deodorizers, poisonous substances in, 96t
Regitine, (*see* Phentolamine)
Rela, (*see* Carisoprodol)
Reliable Moth Balls & Flakes, 199t
Removers
cuticle, poisonous substances in, 95t
freckles, poisonous substances in, 95t

grease spots, poisonous substances in, 94t
lacquers, poisonous substances in, 94t
paint, poisonous substances in, 94t
scratch, poisonous substances in, 96t
wax, poisonous substances in, 94t
Renal failure in poisoning, **82**
Renese, (*see* Polythiazide)
Renofab, 530t
Renuzit All Purpose Dry Clean, 530t
Renuzit Spot & Stain Remover, 530t
Repel-A-Mist, 199t
Repellent(s), **186-201**
poisonous substances in, 96t
potential toxicity of, 735t
Repel-X-Fly Spray Concentrate, 168t
Reptiles, poisonous, **558-570**
Requa's (charcoal), 34
Requiem sharks (Carcharinidae family), 583
Reserpine, 15t, 103, 110t, 112t, 117t, 118t, 122, 124, 135, 138, 334t, 345t, 346t, 348t, 366t, 371, 546t
Reserpoid, 110t
Residol, 168t
Resin(s), 538
as cathartics, 406t
epoxy glues, **620-621**
toxicity of, Table 148(622)
natural, 95t
oligomeric, 621
plastics, **623-624**
poisonous substances in, 95t
shellac, 94t
sulfonamide, 95t
synthetic, 95t
urushiol (Pentadecylcatechol), 538
yellow, **645**
Resistopen, (*see* Oxacillin, sodium)
Resorcinol, 10t, 12t, 15t, **453,** 498t, 622t
Respiration, artificial, **59-60**
Respiratory
insufficiency, **73-75**
symptoms, 6
Retinotoxic drugs, **344-346**
Reviva Spot Remover, 530t
RH-787 Technical Material, 174
*Rheum rhaponticum* (Rhubarb), 554t
*Rhiocissus cuneifolia* (Wild grape), 554t
Rhodamine B, 95t, 96t
Rhodanates, 170
Rhodanese, 236
Rhododendrom *(Rhododendron albiflorum, macrophyllum),* 553t
*Rhodomyrtus macrocarpa* (Finger cherry), 550t
*Rhodotypos* (Jet berry bush), 551t
Rhothane (TDE), 137t
Rhubarb *(Rheum rhaponticum),* 10t, 11t, 117t, 406t, 498t, 554t
leaves, 547, **718**
stalks, 547
*Rhus*
*radicans,* **539**
*toxicodendron* (Poison ivy), 539, 553t
*vernix* (Poison sumac), 539, 553t
Riboflavin, 11t, 118t, 334t, 476t, 477, 708t
Richfield Weedkiller A, 199t
Ricin, 542
*Ricinus communis* (Castor bean), 542, 549t
Rickettsial diseases (zoonoses), 599t
Rid-O-Moth Flakes & Balls, 199t
Rid-O-Moth Nuggets & Crystals, 199t
Rid-O-Spot, 530t
Rid-O-Weed, 199t
Rid Roach, 168t
Ridsect Aerosol, 172t
Ridsect Household Spray, 168t
Rifadin, (*see* Rifampin)
Rifampin (Rifadin; Rimactane), 10t, 11t, 12t, 17t, 80t, 117t, 122, 357t, 437t
Rimactane, (*see* Rifampin)
Ringer's
injection, 58t
solution, 67, 409
Ristocetin (Spontin), 15t, 340, 357t
Ritalin (Methylphenidate), 73, 373, 470, 494t
*Rivea corymbosa* (Pearly gates morning glory seeds) 98
Roach Doom, 168t
Roach Go Insect Spray, 168t
Roachkil Insect Spray, 168t, 172t
Roach powder, 140
Roach Salt, 168t
Robaxin (Methocarbamol), 11t, 52t, 117t
*Robinia pseudoacacia* (Black locust), 548t
Robinson's Bentonite USP, 186
Robinson's Fuller's Earth USP, 186
Roccal Detergent, 530t
Rocket fuels (Boron hydride), **644-645**
Rockland Brush Killer, 199t
Rockland Weed Killer, 199t
Rocky Mountain wood tick *(Dermacentor andersoni),* 580
Rodalon Disinfectant, 530t
Rodene, 199t
Rodenticides, **173-179,** 605t
fatal (lethal) doses, Table 56(179)
potential toxicity of, 734t
Rodent-Rid, 199t
Rodent-Vev, 199t
Rodine, 199t
Ro-Do, 199t
Rogor (Dimethoate), 137t, 734t
Rohm & Haas Mosquito Larvicide No. 30, 168t
Ro-Kil Spray, 168t
Ro-Ko Liquid Spray, 168t
Rolicton (Amisometradine), 483t
Rolitetracycline, 121t
Roll caps (fireworks), **738**
Rondomycin, (*see* Methacycline)
Ronnel (Korlan), 137t
Rosary bean, (*see* Jequirity bean)
Rosary pea, 541f (*see* Jequirity bean)
Rose, Christmas *(Helleborus niger),* 549t
Rosemary oil, 499t
Rose Rat Killer, 199t
Rose-X-Bleach, 530t
Rosin, 95t, **645,** 647
Rotenone, 97t, 127, 157-158, 159t, 160t, 161t, 162t, 163t, 164t, 165t, 166t, 167t, 168t, 169t, 170, 201t
Rotenox, 168t
Rot Not, 200t
Rotocide, 168t
Roto-Dust, 168t
Rotrate, 5, 168t
Rough on Rats, 200t
Rough & Ready Mouse Mix, 200t
Rough & Ready Rat Bait, 200t
Rough & Ready Rat Paste, 200t
Roux Fanciful Rinse, 534ft
Roxex, 199t
Royal jelly, **536**
Rubber, synthetic, 96t, 312
Rubbing alcohol, (*see* Alcohol, isopropyl)
Rubidium, 269, 270t
Rubidomycin (Daunorubicin), 402t
Rue, (*see* Volatile oils)
Rug
adhesives, poisonous substances in, 96t
cleaners, poisonous substances in, 96t
Run Roach, 168t
Rust removers (Hydrofluoric acid), 720
Rutgers, 200t, 612
Ruthenium, 270t
RVP (Red veterinary petrolatum), 456
Ryania, 127, **157,** 160t, 168t
Ryanicide, 168t
Ryanine, 157
Ryanodine, 157
Ryatox, 168t


**S**


Sabadilla, 127, **158,** 159t, 168t, 169t, 201t
Sacahuiste *(Nolina texana),* 548t
Saccharin (Anhydro-o-sulfamine benzoic acid), 115, 216, 346t, 499t, 651, 709t
Saddleback caterpillars, 579
Safeguard Soap, 530t
Safety
closures, 4, 5
container, 5
councils, working with poison control centers, 698
of color television receivers, **641-642**
packaging, 4, 5
public education, 3-6, **660-743**
Safety matches, 736
Saffron, 499t, **645**
meadow, 549t
Safite Rodenticides, 200t
Safranin, 95t
Safrene, 633
Safrol, 449, 633
Sage, 499t
pasture, 539
red, wild *(Lantana camara),* 358t, 551t
Sage Dry Bleach, 530t
Sage-O-Pine Disinfectant, 530t
Sage Savers, 200t

Salicylamide (2-Hydroxybenzamide), 125, **461,** 499t
Salicylanilides, halogenated, 200t, 455
Salicylate(s), 7t, 8t, 9t, 12t, 17t, 35t, 45, 58, 62t, 64, 67, 91, 97t, 110t, 112t, 117t, 122, 124, 249, 336t, 340, 345t, 346t, 347t, 429, 455, 458, 461-467, 503t, 516t, 616
  acid-base disturbances of intoxication in children, 463f
  Done's nomogram, 465f
  interaction with alcohol, Table 60(214)
  methyl (oil of wintergreen), 94t, 224, 461, 462, 466, 495t
  pathogenesis of intoxication, 463f
  phenyl (Salol), **634**
  physostigmine (Antilirium), 54t, 367, 376, 378, 472
  poisoning treatment scheme, 467
  sodium, 117t, 124t, 465, 615t
Salicylazosulfapyridine (Azulfidine), 11t, 15t, 340, 343t, 347t, 483t
Salicylic acid, 35t, 95t, 632, 634
Saline (solution), 102
  cathartics, 18, 406t
  emetic, contraindicated, 42
  hypertonic, 58t
  hypotonic, 58t
  isotonic, 58t, 184
  physiologic, 213
*Salmonella*
  *aertycke,* 714
  *choleraesuis,* 714
  *cubana*
    in carmine dye, 714
  *enteritidis,* 714
Salmonella food poisoning, 534, 710, 711, **714-715**
Salmonellosis, 592
Salol (Phenyl salicylate), **634**
Salp, 168t
Salsbury's (Dr.) Nic-Sal, 168t
Salsbury's (Dr.) Pest Spray, 168t
Salsbury's (Dr.) Vapor-Roost, 168t
Salt(s), 7t, 65t, 117t, 605t
  aluminum, 94t, 95t, 536
  ammonium, 183
  calcium, 229
  cobalt, 8t, 257t, 270t
  copper, 7t, 8t, 148, 201t, 179, 739
  Epsom, (*see* Epsom salts)
  Glauber's (*see* Glauber's salt)
  gold, (*see* Gold)
  halogen, 192
  hexamethonium, 490t
  iron, 9t, 334t
  lead, 97t
  lithium, **630-631**
  magnesium, 197t, 229, 408, 463
  mercuric, 41, 194t, 195t, 196t, 197t, 199t, 200t
  mercury, 55t, 194t, 195t, 196t, 197t
  nickel, 8t
  para-aminosalicylic, 117t, 338t
  phenylmercuric, 497t
  potassium, 62t, 182, 422, 469, 532, 618
  silver, 7t, 42, 455, **467-468,** 610
  sodium, 71, 182, 422, 426, 532
  table, 188t, **645-646**
  tetraethylammonium, 500t
  thioglycolate, 94t
  zirconium, 95t
Saltpeter (Potassium nitrate), 499t
Saluron (Hydroflumethiazide), 469
Salvarsan (Arsenobenzene), 367
*Sambucus*
  *canadensis* (Black elder), 550t
  *pubens* (Scarlet elder), 550t
Sanaseed Mouse Seed, 200t
Sand briar *(Solanum carolinense),* 554t
Sand fly, 576f
Sandril (Reserpine), 110t
Sand shark (Carcharinidae family), 586t
Sani-Chlor, 530t
Sani-Deth Multi-Purpose Spray, 168t
Sani-Deth Will-Kill Water Bug Death, 168t
Sani-Flush, 530t
Sani-Stod Dry Clean, 530t
Sanitizing agents, **517-531** (with table)
*Sanquinaria canadensis* (Blood root), 549t
Sansert (Methysergide maleate), 424, 425t
Santonin, 6t, 7t, 10t, 97t, 353t, 499t
Saphex Fly Spray, 168t
Sapho 25% C.P.R. Insecticide Dust, 168t
Sapho Crystals, 200t
Sapho Flower and Garden Aerosol, 172t
Sapho Insect Bombs, 172t
Sapho Insect Powder, 168t
Sapho 622 Repulseur Liquid and Cream, 200t
*Sarothamnus scoparius* (Scotch broom), 554t
Sassafras, oil of, **633**
Saurine, 582
Savin, (*see* Volatile oils)
Savol Purified Bleach, 530t
Saxitoxin, 581, 718
Scale insect *(Tachardia lacca),* 742
Scarlet
  elder *(Sambucus pubens),* 550t
  kingsnake, 565
  red (Amino-azotoluene), 499t
  snake *(Cemophora coccinea),* 564, 565
Schizophrenia, 65t
Schradan, 734t
Schweinfurth green (Paris green), **633**
Sclerotinia sclerotiorum (pink rot fungus of celery), 313t
Scoke, (*see* Pokeweed)
*Scolopendra morsitans* (Centipede), **574-575**
Scombroid fish poisoning, 582
Scope (Di-syston; Disolfton), 132t
Scopolamine (Hyoscine), 7t, 39, 54t, 93, 117t, 122, 358t, 376, 546t
  hydrobromide, 392
*Scorpaena*
  *guttata* (Scorpionfish), 587t
  *scropha,* 590
Scorpion *(Centrurorides gertschii, sculpturatus),* **574,** 576f
  bite of, 7t
Scorpionfish *(Scorpaena guttata),* 585, 587t
Scotch broom *(Sarothamnus scoparius),* 546t, 554t
Scrap-iron (Alcoholic beverage), 216
Scratch remover, poisonous substances in, 96t
Screening tests
  for general drug category, Table 36(92-93)
  toxicological, **89-91**
Sculptors, occupational hazards to, **313-314**
Scutl, 200t
Scyphozoa (Jellyfish), 584
Sea
  anemone, 584
  bass, 583
  blubber, 584
  cucumber, 585
  lice, 590
  lion, 583
  nettle, 584
  snake, 585, **589-590**
  urchin, 585, 587t
  wasp, 584
Seafood poisoning, **717-718**
Seal Treat Preservative, 200t
Secobarbital (Seconal), 65t, 66, 104t, 117t, 379(t), 380, 381, 383t, 386, 387, 388, 389, 453, 503t
  sodium, 15t
Seconal, (*see* Secobarbital)
Security Brand New 3-Way Tobacco Dust, 168t
Security Brand Powdered Cube, 168t
Security Poison, 168t
Sedative(s), 7t, 9t, 83, 117t, 433
  interaction with alcohol, Table 60(214)
Sedicin, 499t
Sediment, as a water pollutant, 330t
Sedormid, 499t
Sedulon, (*see* Pyrethyldione)
Selenate, sodium, 155t, 167t
Selenium, 33, 52t, 127, **143-144,** 151, 269, 331t, 455, 633
  animal poisoning (alkali, blind staggers types), 605t
  derivatives, **646**
  methionine, 644t
  salts, 739
  sulfide (Selsun), 143t, 499t, 646
Sel-Kaps, 168t
Seller's methylene blue-basic fuchsin stain (in rabies), 603
Selsun, (*see* Selenium sulfide)
Sel-Tox, 168t
Seminole bead, (*see* Jequirity bean)
Semustine (Methyl-CCNU), 403t
Senco Corn Mix, 200t
Senco Microfine Powder, 200t

Senco Paste, 200t
Senco Poison Oat Kernels, 200t
Senna, 10t, 12t, 122, 406t
Sepiolite, 314
Septrin, 343t
Serax (Oxazepam), 215t, **364,** 496t
Serc (Betahistine hydrochloride), 484t
Serenium (Ethoxazene), 11t
Serfin (Reserpine), 110t
Sernylan, (*see* Phencyclidine)
Seromycin (Cycloserine), 117t, 356t
Serpasil (Reserpine), 110t, 371
Serpate (Reserpine), 110t
Serpentine, 315, 319
Serpents (fireworks), **738**
Serum(s), 340
  alkaline phosphatase, 76
  sickness, mycardiopathy in, 62t
  transaminase, 76
Sesame oil, **647**
*Sesamum indicum L.*, 647
Sesone, 188t
Sesquicarbonate, sodium, 520
Sesquisulfide, phosphorus, 736, 737
Sesquiterpene, 613, 658
Setrete, 200t
Sevin (Carbaryl), **136-138,** 731
Sewage, as water pollutants, 330t
Shale, 315
Shampoos, **532-533**
  composition of, 524t
  poisonous substances in, 94t
Shaple Rat & Mouse Killer, 200t
Shark(s), 583
  bites, treatment of, 583
  Chaser, 583
  Ganges (Carcharinidae family), 586t
  Gray nurse, (Carcharinidae family), 586t
  Hammerhead (Sphyrnidae family), 583, 586t
  Lake Nicaragua (Carcharinidae family), 586t
  Mackerel (Isuridae family), 583, 586t
  Mako (Isuridae family), 586t
  Man-eaters (Mackerel), 583
  repellent, 583
  Requiem (Carcharinidae family), 583, 586t
  Sand (Carcharinidae family), 583, 586t
  White (Isuridae family), 586t
Shasta, 530t
Shaver's disease (Corundum fume fibrosis; Bauxite fume fibrosis), 314, **318-319,** 323t
Shed-A-Leaf, 200t
Sheep laurel (Kalmia), 551t
Shellac, 95t, **647**
  resin, 94t
  solvent, 649
Shellfish, food poisoning from, **718**
Shells, stinging, 588t
*Shigella,* 711
Shirlan, 200t
Shock
  electric, **620**
  therapy in poisoning, **69**
Shoe, cleaners and polishes, poisonous substances in, 95t
Ship-Rite Bleach, 530t
Siderosis, 323t
  pulmonary, 314, **319**
Siduron (Tupersan), 188t
Silica, 314, 315, 331t, 517, 524t, 525, **647**
  dust, 315
  mixtures, 331t
  quartz, 331t
Silicate(s), 315, 520
  aluminum, 315
  copper, **179-180**
  ethyl, (*see* Ethyl silicates)
  magnesium, (*see* Magnesium silicates)
  potassium, (*see* Potassium silicates)
  sodium, 233t, 520, 522t, 523t, 524t, 615t, 656
  iron, 317
Silicatosis, 315
Silicon(s)
  carbide, 331t
  dioxide, 314, 647
  purified, 95t
Silicon(s) (Methyl polysiloxane), **647**
Silicosis, **314-315,** 317, 319, 323t
Silkworm, 742
Silo-filler's disease, 249
Silver, 32, 35t, 36, 54t, 82t, 96t, 269, 270t, 534
  acetate, 649
  nitrate, 41, 55t, 97t, 451, 720
  oxides, 610
  salts, 42, 455, **467-468,** 610
Silver Dust, 530t
Silvex, 187t, 200t
Simazine, 188t, 609, 734t
Simoniz Hi-Lite Furniture Polish, 530t
Sinequan, (*see* Doxepin)
Singletary Pest Control, 200t
Sinox, 187t
Sintrom (Acenocoumarol), 481t
*Sistrurus* (Ground rattlers), **562,** 564f
  *catenatus* (Massasauga), **562**
  *miliarius* (Pigmy rattler), **562,** 564f
Skookon, 168t
Skin
  contamination, first aid for, 721
  cream, poisonous substances in, 95t
  dermal poisoning, **46**
  food, poisonous substances in, 95t
  masks, poisonous substances in, 95t
  tonics and lotions, poisonous substances in, 94t
Skunk cabbage *(Symplocarpus foetidus),* 554t
Sla Cedarized Spray, 172t
Slaked lime, 629
Sla-Rat Prepared, 200t
Slate, 315
SLE, (*see* Systemic lupus erythematosus)
Sleep-eze, 392
Slide talks on poisoning, (*see* Appendix A) 747-748
Slug-a-Bug, 168t
Slug-a-Bug Aerosol, 168t
Smallpox vaccination, 110t, 322t, 347t
Smartweeds *(Polygonum),* 548t
SMDC (Vapam), 187t
Smo-Cloud, 168t
Smo-Cloud Bug Killer, 168t
Smog, photochemical, (*see* Air pollution)
Smoke
  as air pollutant, 324t
  poisoning, **647-648**
Smoking
  affecting the fetus and newborn, 110t, 112t, 115, 116, 123
  cigarette, 112t, 266
  deterrents, **649**
Snake(s), (*see also* individual snakes)
  poisonous (Ophidism), **558-570**
  sea, **589-590**
  venom, 15t, 52t, 82t
Snakeberry *(Actaea spicata),* 548t
Snakebite
  symptoms, **565-566**
  treatment, **566-569**
Snakeroot, white *(Eupatorium rugosum* or *urticaefolium),* 554t
  *Rauwolfia serpentina* (Reserpine), 546t
Snapping hazel (Witch hazel), **657-658**
Snarol Meal, 168t
Sneezeweed, 539
Sno-Bol Liquid Bowl Cleaner, 530t
Snow, (*see* Cocaine)
Snowflake Moth Spray, 168t, 200t
Snow sprays (Christmas decoration), **739-740**
Snow White Flakes, 200t
Soap, **517-531**
  poisonous substances in, 96t
  products, composition of, Table 134(522-524)
  solution, to neutralize acids, 45, 83
  toilet bars, **525**
  toxicity of, Table 133(521)
Social Security Administration, 314
Society of Toxicology, 532
Soda
  ash, 94t, 96t, 234
  caustic, 94t
  washing, 4f, 85
Sodar, 187t, 200t
Sodisil Detergent, 530t
Sodite, 168t
Sodium, 57t, 65t, 68t, 117t, 190, 252t, 269, 271, 315, 422, 430, 631
  acetate, 176, 232
  acid sulfate, 96t, 524t, 526, 720
  alginate, 269, **649**
  alkyl aryl sulfates, 519
  alkyl isothionates, 519
  alkyl sulfate, 519, 522t
  alurate, 35t
  aminopterin, (*see* Methotrexate)
  aminopteroylglutamate, (*see* Methotrexate)
  Amytal (Amobarbital), 41, 71, 83, 104t
  arsenate, (*see* Arsenate, sodium)

arsenite, (*see* Arsenite, sodium)
ascorbate, 19t, 31
azide-iodine reaction, 239
barbital (Medinal), 83
benzoate, 33, 124t, 211, 367, 416, 448, 351
bicarbonate, 19t, 20t, 22t, 51t, 58(t), 62, 83, 133, 147, 155, 183, 192, 211, 213, 218, 223, 227, 233, 243, 386, 387, 388, 434, 436, 438, 444, 456, 465, 466, 469, 473, 520, 523t, 543, 582, 614t, 709t
contraindications, 465
bisulfate, 615t
bisulfite, 614t
borate, 7t, 127, **152-153,** 155t, 533
bromate, 233t
bromide, 83, 392
bunamiodyl (Orabilex), 484t
caffeine benzoate, 19t, 41, 468
carbonate, 94t, 95t, 139, 180, 202, 230, 233t, 234, 246, 520, 522t, 523t, 524t, 533, 615t, 629, 721
chlorate, (*see* Chlorate, sodium)
chloride, 41, 55t, 65t, 70, 95t, 105t, 118t, 192, 233, 263, 387, 393, 457, 459, 466, 468, 522t, 524t, 610, 614t, 629, 630, **645-646**
chromate, 94t, 644t
citrate, 65t, 67, 479
colistimethate (Colymycin), 121t
cyanide, 97t
cyclamate, 651, 709t
dalapon (2,2-Dichloropropionic acid), 182
dantrolene, 487t
dextrothyroxine (Choloxin), 487t
Dial, 35t
dichloroisocyanurates, 523t, 524t, **618**
diethyldithiocarbamate trihydrate (Dithiocarb), 267
diphenylhydantoin, 456, 473
edetate, 421t, 422
equilin sulfate, 426
estrone sulfate, 426
ethylenediaminetetracetic acid, (*see* EDTA)
Evipal, 35t, 383t
ferricyanide, 614t
ferrocyanide, 614t
fluoaluminate, 159t, 161t, 163t, 165t, 166t, 167t
fluoride, 140, 141, 155t, 159t, 163t, 166t, 167t, 168t, 228, **716-717**
fluoroacetate (1080), 7t, 54t, 97t, 173, 179t
fluosilicate, 200t
formaldehyde sulfoxalate, 19t, 41, 55t, 147
glutamate, 489t
hexametaphosphate, 94t, 520
hexobarbital (Epival), 35t, 383t
hydrocortisone succinate, 21t, 69, 575
hydroxide, 94t, 95t, 96t, 219, 230, 234t, 454, 517, 526, 533, 610, 626, 629, 721
hydroxydione succinate, 490t
hypochlorite, 51t, 94t, 95t, 96t, 230, 524t, 629, 652
bleaches, 233t, 234t, 526, 721
hyposulfite, 246
iodide, 143, 614t, 644t
iron silicates, 317
lactate, 19t, 40, **41,** 58(t), 387, 388, 461, 466, 631
meralluride (Mercuhydrin), 124t
metasilicate, 94t, 520
methylprednisolone succinate (Solu-Medrol), 22t, 69
molar-lactate, 190
Nembutal, (*see* Pentobarbital sodium)
nicotinate, **707-710**
nitrate, 621, 707, 709t
nitrite, 17, 20t, 41, 53t, 154, 155(t), 174, 237, 238, 449, 450, 471, 707, 709t
variation of child's dose with hemoglobin concentrate, Table 64(237)
nitroprusside, 22t, 235, 424
novobiocin, 110t
oxacillin (Prostaphlin), 124t, 357t
para-aminobenzoate, 536
pentobarbital (Nembutal sodium), 14t, 71, 83, 128, 129, 213, 404
pentothal, 71, 72t, 117t, 383t
perborate, 94t, 153, 233t, 522t, 523t, 524t, 534
perchlorate, 82t
persulfate, 534
phenobarbital, (*see* Phenobarbital, sodium)
phenytoin, 362t
phosphate, 230, 405
biphosphate, 405, 455
metaphosphate, 520
monophosphate, 455
orthophosphate, 520
phosphate glass, 94t
salicylate, 117t, 124t, 465, 615t
salt, 71, 182, 422, 426, 532
secobarbital, 15t
selenate, 155t, 167t, 168t
sesquicarbonate, 520, 522t
silicate, 233t, 520, 522t, 523t, 524t, 615t, 656
soaps, 522t, 523t
succinate, 107t, 406t
sulfate (Glauber's salt), 20t, 41, 55t, 101, 147, 173, 177, 233t, 263, 395, 479, 520, 522t, 523t, 738
sulfide, **237-239,** 313t, 535
sulfite, 94t
sulfobromophthalein, 500t
tetraborate (Borax), 522t, 523t, 612
thiamylal (Surital), 383t
thiocyanate. 654
thiomalate, 428
thiopental (Pentothal), 71, 411, 501t
thiosulfate, 20t, 41, 45, 53t, 55t, 154, 155t, 183, 236, 237(t), 428, 430, 610, 614t, 737
tripolyphosphate, 233t, 519, 520, 522t, 523t, 524t
warfarin, 110t, 143t
Solacen, (*see* Tybamate)
Solan, 188t
Solanaceae *(Datura),* 545
Solanine, 7t, 97t
*Solanum*
*carolinense* (Bull nettle, horse nettle, sand briar, wild tomato), 358t, 545, 554t
*dulcamara* (Blue nightshade, bittersweet), 358t, 545, 548t
*nigrum* (Black nightshade), 358t, 545, 548t
*pseudocapsicum* (Jerusalem cherry), 358t, 551t
*tuberosum* (Potato), 358t, 553t
Solox, **649**
Solozine Bleach, 530t
Solu-Cortef (Hydrocortisone), 19t, 21t, 385
Solu-Medrol (Methylprednisolone sodium succinate), 22t
Solution 45 Insect Killer, 168t
Solvent(s), 15t, 82t, 86
aromatic, 610
hydrocarbon, 184, 187t
benzene, 9t
distillate, 202, 222-224
effects (systemic), Table 160(729-730)
hazards of, at home and on the job, **724-730**
organic, 94t
paint, poisonous substances in, 94t
petroleum, 187t
Stoddard, 95t, 184, **225,** 523t, **650**
Solvoterge Metal Cleaner, 530t
Soma, (*see* Carisoprodol)
Sominex, (*see* Methapyrilene)
Somnifene, 499t
Soot, as air pollutant, 324t, 326
Soporifics, 334, 335t
Sorbic acid, **710**
Sorghum, 606
*Sorghum vulgare sudanense* (Sudan grass), 548t
Soybean, 532
meal, 621
oil, in lipid dialysis, 67
Spandy Disinfectant, 530t
Spanish broom *(Sparteus junceum),* 554t
Spanish fly (Cantharidin), **405**
Sparine, (*see* Promazine hydrochloride)
Sparklers (fireworks), **738**
*Sparteus junceum* (Spanish broom), 554t
Special Outdoor Fogging Concoction No. 11, 168t
Speckman Deth-Bait, 200t
Speckman Durotox, 200t
Speckman Naptox, 200t
Speckman Permite, 200t
Speedball (Cocaine with heroin), 108t
Speed Up Bleach, 530t
Speed Up Cleaner, Disinfectant, 530t
Spermaceti, **650**

*Sphyraena barracuda* (Great barracuda), 582, 586t
Sphyrnidae family (Hammerhead sharks), 586t
Spider(s)
  Black widow *(Latrodectus mactans, curariensis),* **570-571**
  Brown recluse *(Loxosceles reclusa),* 70
  Giant crab *(Heteropodidae),* 574
  South American brown *(Loxosceles laeta),* 572
  venom, 82t
Spiders and insects (North American) harmful to man, Table 141(573)
Spindle oil, 94t
Spindle tree *(Euonymus europaeus),* 554t
Spiny dogfish, 585
Spirit of niter, (*see* Nitrites)
Spirit of turpentine, (*see* Turpentine, oil of)
Spironolactone (Aldactone), 147, 348t, 499t
Spontin, (*see* Ristocetin)
Spot test, **90**
Spotrete, 200t
Spotted alder (Witch hazel), **657-658**
Spray(s),
  de-icer, poisonous substances in, 95t
  hair, **535**
    poisonous substances in, 95t
  snow (Christmas decoration), **739-740**
Spray-Trol Brand MelaOTrol, 169t
Spray-Trol Brand Para-Trol, 200t
Spray-Trol Brand Rodent-Trol, 200t
Spray-Trol Brand Super Trol, 169t
Sprayway Bug-Go Insect Spray, 172t
Sprayway Fast Kill Bug Killer, 172t
Sprayway Moth Proofer, 200t
Sprayway Tru-Nox Insect Spray, 169t
Spray X-M Insect Repellent, 200t
Squash vine borers in cucurbits, **731**
Squid, 584
Squill, red, (*see* Red squill)
Stabchlor, 169t
Stable fly, 576f
Stachybotrys, 606t
STAC Weed Killer, 200t
Staggerbush (Lyonia mariana), 554t
Sta-Kleen Toiletabs, 530t
Sta-Klor, 200t
Stamping inks, poisonous substances in, 95t
Stannic chloride, (*see* Tin)
Stanozolol (Winstrol), 499t
Stanson Laundry Detergent, 530t
Stantox, 200t
Staphcillin, (*see* Methicillin)
Staphene, 530t
Staphylococcus enterotoxin (food poisoning), 710, **711-712**
Star anise, Japanese *(Illicium anisatum),* 554t
Starch, 614t, **650**
  antidotal, 20t, 46, 55t
  as a demulcent, 46, 83
  water, 42, 83
Starfish, 585
Stargazers, 585
Star of Bethlehem *(Ornithogalum umbellatum),* 554t
Star Water Deodorant, 530t
State Drug laws (Enforcement agencies and principal provisions), Table 156(704-706)
State health departments, working with poison control centers, 661
Status of household articles under federal law, **701-702**
Stauffer's Brush Killer, 200t
Stauffer's Brush Killer-Ready to Use, 200t
Stauffer's Rodent Bait Cone, 200t
Stauffer's Weed Killer, 200t
Stay-Dee Dusting Powder, 169t
Steamship Vaposector, 169t
Stearate
  diethylene glycol, 95t
  zinc oxide, 95t
Stearic acid, 95t, 268, 618, 630, **650**
Stelazine (Trifluoperazine), 117t
Sterminate Aerosol, 169t
Sternutators, 9t
Steroid(s), 124, 228, 230, 231, 252, 267, 321, 349, 370, 648
  adrenal, 345t
  adrenocortical, 248, 418
  complications encountered in therapy with, Tables 117 and 118(414)
  contraceptive, 477
Sterosan (Chlorquinaldol), 486t
Stevens-Johnson Syndrome, 347t, 364
Stibamine glucoside (Neostam), 499t
Stibine (Antimony hydride), 155, 202
Stibophen (Fuadin), 342, 499t
Stilbamidine, 455
  isethionate, 499t
Stilbestrol, 119
Sting
  bee, yellow jacket, wasp, **575-580**
  fish, treatment of, **585-589**
Stinging
  caterpillar *(Megalopyge opercularis),* 579
  marine animals, **583-585**
  shells, 588t
  vertebrates, **585**
Stingrays *(Urobatis halleri,* Dasyatidae), 587t
  bite of, 7t, 582
Stinkweed, 544, 551t
St. Johnswort *(Hypericum perforatum),* 548t
Stoddard solvent (Varsol), 95t, 184, 225, 523t, **650**
Stomach, toxicologic analysis of contents, **88**
Stonefish, 585
Stonemasons' phthisis (silicosis), **314-315**
Stop-Rat, 200t
Stop Spot, 530t
Stove cleaners, poisonous substances in, 94t
STP (Methyl dimethoxymethyl phenylethylamine), 99, 102t, 722t
Stramonium, 35t, 93, 358t, **376-378,** 499t, 545, 551t
*Strelitzia* (Bird-of-paradise plant), 543, 548t
*Streptococcus,* 711, **715**
  *lactis,* 450
Streptokinase-streptodornase (Varidase), 499t
*Streptomyces pilosus,* 434
Streptomycin, 8t, 15t, 65t, 67, 82, 110t, 117t, 119t, 120, 340, 346t, 355, 357t, 437t, 609, 702, 719
  sulfate, 121t
Streptozotocin, 403t
Striped alder (Witch hazel), **657-658**
Strontium, 65t, 252, 269, 270t
  bromide, 738
  carbonate, 738
  chloride, 614t, 644t
  nitrate, 615t, 738
  radioactive, 33, 644
Strophanthin, 500t
  acetyl, 420
Strychnine, 7t, 9t, 35t, 36, 39, 42, 45, 54t, 55t, 71, 93, 97t, **177-178,** 195t, 196t, 199t, 335t, 445, 495t, 516t, 604, 605t, 633, 734t
  nitrate, 35t
  sulfate, 173, 179t, 197t, 198t, 200t
Sturgeonfish, 585
Styptic pencil (Silver nitrate), 720
Styrene monomer, 247t
Subcarbonate, bismuth, (*see* Bismuth)
Suberosis, 322t
Subgallate, bismuth, (*see* Bismuth)
Subnitrate, bismuth, (*see* Bismuth)
Sucaryl (Calcium cyclamate), 486t, 651
Succinamides, 359, **364**
  derivatives, 360
Succinate, sodium, 107t
  hydrocortisone, 21t, 69, 575
  hydroxydione, 490t
  methylprednisolone, 22t, 69
Succinylcholine, 338t, 341, 411
  chloride, 72t, 500t
Succinylsufathiazole (Sulfasuxidine), 357t
Sucrol (Dulcin), 488t
Sucrose, 70, 82t, 645, 651
  octaacetate, 216, 217
Sudafed (Pseudoephedrine), 117t
Sudan grass *(Sorghum vulgare sudanense),* 548t, 606
Sudia Deodorant, 530t
Suicide
  international classification E970, Table 86(336)
  international rates, Table 84(335)
  methods of, 337f
  number due to barbiturates, other analgesic and soporific substances and meprobamate during 1954-1963, Table 87(336)
  number of deaths by specific causes, Table 85(335)

role of drugs in, **334-336** (with tables)
United States rates, Table 85(335)
Sulfacetamide, 343
Sulfadiazine (Sulfonamide), 15t, 124t, 340, 345t, 357t, 468, 516t
Sulfadimethoxine (Madribon), 117t, 340, 357t, 516t
Sulfafurazole, 343t
Sulfaguanide, 516t
Sulfamerazine, 357t
Sulfamethazine, 15t, 341
Sulfamethoxazole (Gantanol), 117t, 357t
Sulfamethoxypyridazine (Kynex), 15t, 340, 343t, 492t
Sulfamic acid, 94t
Sulfamylon (Mafenide acetate), (*see* Mafenide acetate)
Sulfanilamide, 12t, 35t, 64, 95t, 110t, 122, 218, 334t, 343t, 468, 516t
antibacterials, 91
Sulfapyridine, 122, 341, 343t, 468
Sulfasuxidine, (*see* Succinylsulfathiazole)
Sulfate,
alkyl aryl polyether, 518t
aluminum, 615t
aluminum ammonium (Alum), 350
ammonium, 621
amphetamine, 35, 117t, 367
atropine, 19t, 31, 52t, 421t, 424, 488t, 555
barium, 37, 173, 626, 653
benzedrine, 362t
brucine, 216, 536
calcium, hydrous, 614t, 621, 636
capreomycin (Capastat), 484t
chromium potassium, 614t
colistin, 121t
conjugated, 271t
copper, see Copper sulfate
d-amphetamine, 35
dexedrine, 20t, 362t
dextroamphetamine, 13t, 117t
dimethyl, 202, **219**
ephedrine, 19t, 20t, 36
ferric, 632
ammonium, 615t
ferrous, 12t, 41, 45, 97t, 355, 431, 432
ammonium, 615t
guanethidine (Ismelin), 489t
hydrogen, 656
hyoscyamine, 14t
Kanamycin, 121t
lobeline, 649
magnesium, 19t, 20t, 37, 41, 54t, 112t, 147, 152, 173, 176, 179t, 186, 190, 228, 229, 263, 395, 420, 421t, 438, 458, 468, 479, 544, 584, 589, 614t, 659
manganese, 614t
mephentermine, 567
morphine, (see Morphine)
neomycin (Mycifradin; Neobiotic), 117t, 121t, 495t
nickel ammonium, 615t
oxyquinoline, 95t, 536
polymyxin B (Aerosporin), 121t
potassium, 621
protamine, 55t
quinidine, 20t, 40, 49t, 177
salt particles, 329t
sodium, 20t, 41, 55t, 101, 147, 173, 177, 233t, 263, 395, 479, 520, 659, 738
acid, 526, 720
alkyl, 519
alkyl aryl, 519
equilin, 426
estrone, 426
streptomycin, 121t
strychnine, 173, 179t
thallium, 142, 159t, 160t, 164t, 165t, 166t, 169t, 179t, 196t, 197t
vinblastine (Velban), 399t
vincristine (Oncovin), 399t
zinc, (*see* Zinc sulfate)
Sulfathiazole, 122, 468, 609
Sulfhemoglobin, 10, 18
Sulfhydryl
compounds, 190
enzymes, 138
penicillamine (Beta, beta-dimethyl-cysteine), 147
Sulfide(s), 7t, 183, 202, 234, **237-239,** 651
ammonium, **237-239**
antimony, 155, 736, 737, 738
arsenic, 738
barium, 173, 535
bismuth, 391
hydrogen, 85, 97t, 173, **237-239,** 247t, 323, 324t, 326, 514t, 630, 648t
lead, 238, 256, 331t
metal, 238
phosphorus, 738
potassium, 238
selenium (Selsun), 143t, 499t, 646
sodium, 95t, **237-239,** 313t, 535
soluble, 94t
zinc, 626
Sulfisoxazole (Gantrisin), 15t, 124t, 340, 357t, 516t
Sulfite(s), 85
sodium, 94t
Sulfmethemoglobin, 238
Sulfobromophthalein (BSP), 340
sodium, 500t
Sulfocyanates, 236, 340
Sulfonal (Sulfonmethane), 7t, 8t, 98t, 181, 456, **468,** 500t
Sulfonamide(s), 9, 11t, 12t, 15t, 16t, 17t, 35t, 40, 62t, 65t, 76, 77, 80t, 102, 112t, 116, 117t, 119t, 122, 191, 338(t), 340, 343t, 345t, 346t, 347t, 455, **468-469**
bacteriostatic, 429
diuretics, **469-470**
resin, 95t
Sulfonate
alkyl aryl, (*see* Alkyl aryl sulfonate)
alkyl-benzene (ABS), 331, 518
linear alkylate (LAS), 519
phentolamine methane, 444
Sulfonated
castor oil, 95t
fatty alcohols, salts of, 533
hydrocarbons, 518t
oils, salts of, 533
Sulfonchloramide, 609
Sulfone(s), 12t, 343t
diaminodiphenyl, 12t
ethyl, **468**
Sulfonethylmethane (Trional), 8t, 456
Sulfonmethane (Sulfonal), 8t, 181, 456, 500t
Sulfonylurea
compounds, 81t, 347t, 429
derivatives, 110t, 429
hypoglycemics, 102, 455
Sulfosalicylic acid, **650**
Sulfosuccinate, dioctyl sodium, 406t, 608, **619**
Sulfoxide, 170
dimethyl (DMSO), **618-619,** 729t
Sulfoxone, 338t
Sulfoxylate, phenarsone (Aldarsone), 496t
Sulfoxylate, sodium formaldehyde, 19t, 55t
Sulfur, 96t, 117t, 151, 183, 196t, 197t, 201t, 238, 269, 314, **325-326,** 500t, 615t, 651, 735t, 736
colloidal, 651
dioxide, 14t, 87t, 202, **243,** 247t, 313t, 324(t), 325, 329t
lime, 605t, 630, 734t
oxides, 328f, 625
trioxide, 324
Sulfuric acid, 8t, 36, 85, 94t, 97t, 219, **226-228,** 322, 324, 325, 329, 331t, 373, 451, 464, 517, 524t, 656, 720, 734t
ester, 656
Sulfurous acid, 325
Sulisobenzone (2-Hydroxy-4-methoxy-benzophenone-5-sulfonic acid), 456
Sulphotepp, 734t
Sumac
climbing, 539
coral *(Metopium toxiferum),* 553t
poison, *(Rhus vernix),* 538, 539, 553t
swamp, (*see* Poison sumac)
Summer black oil, 94t
Summer cypress *(Kochia scoparia),* 548t
Suntan
lotions, poisonous substances in, 94t
pills (psoralens), 455, **537**
preparations, 536
poisonous substances in, 94t
Super Alkali Detergent, 530t
Super-Five, 169t
Superlarvex Mothproofer, 200t
Superoxol Bleach, 530t
Supportive measures, **47**
Suprep Metal Cleaner, 530t
Sure Detergent, 525
Surfactants, (*see* Detergents)
Surital, (*see* Thiamylal, sodium)
Surmontil (Trimipramine), 472

Swallowed poisons, first aid for, **720-721**
Swamp sumac, (*see* Poison sumac)
Swan Brand Dry Insecticide, 200t
Sweeney's Ant-Go, 169t
Sweeny's Poison Wheat, 200t
Sweet clover, 606t
Sweetening agents, **651-652**
Sweet potatoes, wireworm control in, **731**
Swep, 187t
Swift Metal Cleaner, 530t
Swift's Gold Bear (A-2-E, B-1-E, D-2-E, D-B-E), 169t
Swift's Gold Bear Brand Brush Killer, 200t
Swift's Gold Bear Brand Fly Spray, 169t
Swimming pool disinfectants (purifiers), **652-653**
Sylpho-Nathol, 530t
Symmetrel (Amantadine hydrochloride), 119t, 482t
Sympatholytics, 6t
Sympathomimetics, 6t, 7t, 9t, 442, 472
  amines, **470-471**
*Symplocarpus foetidus* (Skunk cabbage), 554t
Synephrin, 470
Synkayvite (Vitamin $K_1$), 20t
Synklor, 169t
Synthetic
  organic chemicals, as water pollutants, 330t
  organic insecticides, 126, **127-138**
  resins, 95t
  rubber, 96t
  Vitamin K, 102
Syrup
  althose (Methadone hydrochloride), 117t
  lyteca (Acetaminophen), 117t
  of ipecac, (*see* Ipecac, syrup of)
Systemic lupus erythematosus (SLE), drug-induced, Table 91(345)
Systox (Demeton); Diethyl-O-ethylmercapto-ethyl phosphorothioate, 127, 132t

**T**

2,4,5-T (2,4,5-Trichlorophenoxyacetic acid), 182ft, 187t, 194t, 195t, 196t, 197t, 198t, 199t, 200t, 201t
Table salt, (*see* Salts)
Tabu-X-Spray, 169t
Tacaryl (Methdilazine), 117t
*Tachardia lacca* (Scale insect), 742
Tacobromine, 500t
Tag Fungicide, 200t
Take-Off, 530t
Talc (Talcum), 315, 331t, **653**
Talcosis, 314, 319, 323t
Talcum, (*see* Talc)
Talloil, 96t
Talwin (Pentazocine), 441, 496t, 515t
Tandearil (Oxyphenbutazone), 16t, 79t
Tannate, 42
  pelletierine, 353t, 496t
Tannic acid, 20t, 42, 45, 46, 56t, 78, 81t, 178, 377, 444ft, 555, 616t, **653,** 658, 737
Tannin(s), 613, 632, 656, 657, 658
Tansy, 539 (*see also* Volatile oils)
  ragwort, 545
Tao (Troleandomycin), 80t, 356t
Tap Ant Trap, 169t
Tapazole (Methimazole), 81t, 110t, 117t
Tar, 312
  oils, 734t
Taractan, (*see* Chlorprothixine)
Tarantulas *(Anicularidae)*, **574,** 576f
Tartar
  cream of, 228
  emetic, 115(t), 346t, 494t, 500t, 612
Tartaric acid, 500t, 616t, 709t
Tartrate(s)
  acid potassium, 709t
  antimony potassium, 115t
  ergotamine, 424t, 425t
  Fuadin, 354t
  levallorphan, 54t, 416, 441
  thenalidine, 15t
Tartrazine (food color additive), 709t
Tat-Chloro-40, 169t
Tat-C-Lect, 187t
Tat Insect Repellent, 200t
Tavern Spot Remover, 530t
*Taxus baccata* (Yew), 554t
2,3,6-TBA (Tryben; Benzac), 188t, 734t
TCA, 188t
TDE (Tetrachlorodiphenylethane; DDD), 126, 137t, 162t
TDI (Toluene diisocyanate), (*see* Toluene diisocyanate)
Tea, 334t
  Mormon, 546t
  to neutralize alkalis, 83
Tear gas(es), 617, 631, **654**
Technetium, 122
Technitate, 644t
Tedion (Tetradifon), 137t
Teflon (Polytetrafluoroethylene), 637, **654**
Tegretol, (*see* Carbamazepine)
Teldrin, (*see* Chlorpheniramine)
Telepaque (Iopanoic acid), 117t, 491t
Television
  safety of color receivers, **641-642**
  spot announcements on poisoning, (*see* Appendix A) 749
Tellurium, 8t, 269
Telodrin, 169t
Telvar Weed Killer, 200t
TEM (Triethylene melamine), 455, 502t
Tempra (Acetaminophen), 117t, 451, 481t, 500t
Tenn-Creo Disinfectant, 530t
Tensilon (Edrophonium), 21t, 415
  adverse effects, 49t
Ten-Twenty Brush Killer, 200t
TEPP (Tetraethylpyrophosphate), 6t, 7t, 8t, 9t, 52t, 127, 132t, 137t, 160t, 162t, 164t, 165t, 167t, 168t, 169t, 170t, 311t, 734t
Teppcide, 169t
Teridax (Iophenoxic acid), 110t
Terminix BTL, 169t
Terminix OG6 Concentrate, 169t
Termitine, 172t
Terpene(s), 196t, 197t, 500t, 617, 658
  alcohol, 521, 636
Terramycin, (*see* Oxytetracycline)
Terratox Weed Killer, 200t
Terro Ant Killer, 200t
Tertiary amyl alcohol, (*see* Alcohol, tertiary amyl)
Tertiary butyl alcohol, (*see* Alcohol, tertiary butyl)
Test(s)
  Beilstein, 189
  cobaltamine, 390
  eye, for serum sensitivity, 571
  Fehling's, 189
  ferric chloride, 463
  Fischer, for iron detection, 434
  for barbiturate presence in blood, 390
  Forrest rapid urine color, Table 14(372)
  free erythrocyte prophyrin (FEP), 260
  intradermal skin for serum sensitivity, 571
  isonitrile, 189
  microdiffusion, 189
  pretoxicosis, 239
  pyridine, 189
  screening, general drug category, Table 36(92-93)
  toxicologic, **85-86**
Testor's Polystyrene Plastic Cement, 658
Testosterone, 312, 340
  derivatives, 76
  propionate, 402t
Tetanus
  antitoxin, 347t, 568, 589
  toxoid, 567, 568, 589, 592
TETD (Antabuse), 239
Tetraborate, sodium (Borax), 523t, **612**
Tetracaine (Pontocaine), 352t, **457**
Tetracemate dicobalt (Kelocyanor), 154
Tetrachloride
  carbon, see Carbon tetrachloride
  titanium, 203, **270-271**
Tetrachlormethane, (*see* Carbon tetrachloride)
Tetrachlorodibenzo-p-dioxin (Dioxin), 182
Tetrachlorodiphenylethane (TDE), (*see* TDE)
Tetrachloroethane, 202, **207,** 247t, 730t
Tetrachloroethylene (Perchloroethylene), 82t, 87t, 190, 202, **205,** 247t, 353t, 730t
Tetrachloronitrobenzene, 735t
Tetracycline(s), 9, 15t, 65t, 77, 80t, 110t, 112t, 119t, 121t, 334t, 340, 345t, 346t, 347t, 348t, 355, 357t, 455, 609, 610, 702, 715
  and amphotericin B (Mysteclin F), 357t

hydrochloride, 120
phosphate complex, 121t
Tetracyn (Panmycin; Polycycline), 357t
Tetradifon (Tedion), 137t
*Tetradymia* (Horsebrush), 548t
Tetraethyl, lead, see Lead
pyrophosphate, (*see* TEPP)
Tetraethylammonium
bromide, 500t
chloride, 470, 500t
salts, 500t
Tetraethylpyrophosphate (TEPP), (*see* TEPP)
Tetraethylthiuram disulfide (Disulfiram), (*see* Disulfiram)
Tetrafume Grain Fumigant, 200t
Tetrahydrocannabinol (THC; Marihuana), 123, 439, 440
Tetrahydrofurfuryl acetate, 95t, 197t
Tetrahydronaphthalene, 10t
Tetrahydrozoline hydrochloride (Tyzine), 500t
Tetraiodofluorescein, 346t
Tetrakil Grain Fumigant, 200t
Tetrakote, 172t
Tetralin, 12t
Tetramethylthionine, 609
Tetramethylthiuram disulfide (Thiram), 179, **181,** 194t, 198t, 200t, 331t, 346t, 735t
Tetramines, 582
Tetranitrate
erythrityl, 12t, 488t
pentaerythritol, 12t, 346t
Tetranitromethane, 12t
Tetrapropylene, 518
Tetrasodium
phosphate, 94t
pyrophosphate, 520, 522t, 523t, 524t
Tetrathionate, 430
Tetrazolium dye (MTT), 343
Tetrodotoxin, 590
Tetron, 169t
Tetronal, 12t, **468**
Tetrox, 169t
Tetroxide, nitrogen, 250
Tetryl, 331t
Texas diamondback *(Crotalus atrox),* **561**
Texatone Bleach, 530t
Texize Laundry Starch, 531t
Texize Rug Cleaner, 531t
Textolit Bleach, 531t
6-TG (6-Thioguanine), 398t
Thalidomide, 102, 103, 110t, 112t, 342
Thallium, 6t, 33, 35, 53t, 62t, 82t, 97t, 127, **141-143,** 143t, 160t, 173t, 199t, 201t, 270t, 331t
acetate, 142
salts, 739
sulfate, 142, 159t, 160t, 164t, 165t, 166t, 169t, 179t, 196t, 197t
Tham (Tris-hydroxy-methyl-amino-methane), 81t, 390, 466
buffer, 387, 389
Thanite (Isobornyl thiocyanoacetate), 170
THC, (*see* Tetrahydrocannabinol)
Thebaine, 445, 540
Thenalidine tartrate (Sandostene), 15t
Thenylethylenediamines, 365t
Theobromine, (*see* Xanthines)
Theophylline, **480-481,** 513t, 516t
Therapeutic agents, **82-83**
Thermometer fluids, poisonous substances in, 96t
Thermophilic actinomycetes, 321, 322t
*Thermopolyspora polyspora,* 321
Thesaurosis (Lung-storage disease), 95t
Thiabendazole (Mintezol), 79t, 353t, 354t
Thiamin, 118t, 152, 212, 340, 476t, 708t
hydrochloride (Vitamin $B_1$), 20t
Thiamylal, sodium (Surital), 383
Thiazide(s), 386
diuretics, 16t, 110t, 118t, 334t, 340, 345t, 347t, 393, 443t, **469-470**
Thiazosulfone (Promizole), 343t, 357t
Thihexinol methylbromide (Entoquel), 500t
Thimerosal (Merthiolate), 500t
Thimet (Phorate), 137t
Thioacetamide, 238
Thioacetazone, 437t
Thioacetimidate, methomyl (Lannate), 138
Thiocarbamates (Dithiocarbamates), **181,** 621
Thioctic acid, 556, 558
Thiocyanate(s), 6t, 65t, 91, 98t, 154, 236, 237, 500t, **654**
aliphatic, 170
mercury, 738
potassium, 184, 654
sodium, 654
Thiocyanoacetate, isobornyl (Thanite), 170
Thiodan, (*see* Endosulfan)
Thioglycerol, 501t
Thioglycolic acid, 37, 533
Thioglycolate(s), 533
ammonium, 312
bismuth sodium, 391
calcium, 94t, 535
salts, 94t, **655**
6-Thioguanine (6-TG), 398t
Thiol, 115
Thiomalate, sodium, 428
Thiomersol, 145
Thiopental (Pentothal), 15t
sodium (Pentothal sodium), 72t, 117t, 383t, 411, 501t
Thiophos (Parathion), 137t, 169t
Thiophosphates, 130, 162t
Thioridazine (Mellaril), 371, 516t
Thiosemicarbazide, 477
Thiosemicarbazone, 340, 501t
Thiosinamine, 501t
Thiosulfate, 154, 155, 195t, 237t
sodium, (*see* Sodium thiosulfate)
Thiotep, 169t
Thio-TEPA (Triethylenethiophosphoramide), 397t
Thio-TEPP, 127
Thiothixene (Navane), 455
Thiouracil, 15t, 40, 102, 118t, 122, 312, 340, 501t
Thiourea, 94t, 98t, 112t, 194t, 312, 501t, 517
derivatives, 345t
Thioxanthenes, 368t, 375t
Thiram, (*see* Tetramethylthiuram disulfide)
Thorazine, (*see* Chlorpromazine)
Thoriated tungsten, 657
Thorium, 269
dioxide (Thorotrast), 15t, 78, 340, 501t
Thornapple *(Datura stramonium),* 542f, 544, 546t, 551t
Thorotrast (Thorium dioxide), 15t, 78, 340, 501t
Three-leaved ivy, (*see* Poison ivy)
Thrombocytopenia, **10-11**
drugs and chemicals causing, 13-15t
drugs associated with, Table 8(16-17)
T-H Spot Fumigant, 200t
Thuja (Yellow cedar), **655**
Thunderwood, (*see* Sumac, poison)
Thymol, 10(t), 353t, 453, 501t (*see also* Phenol)
Thyroglobulin, 119
Thyroid, 118t, 501t
drug effects, 347t
Thyrotrophic hormone, 119
Thyroxin, 119
Tick(s), 576f, **580-581**
pajaroello *(Ornithodoros cariaceus),* 580
protection, 580-581
wood, 580
Tide, 531t
Tide XK, 525
Tigan, (*see* Trimethobenzamide)
Tiger shark (Carcharinidae family), 586t
Timber rattlesnake *(Crotalus horridus),* **561**
Timbertox, 200t
Timothy weed, 539
Tin (Stannic chloride), 35t, 114, 203, 269, **270,** 270t, 272t, 516t, 534, **716,** 740
oxide, 270
Tincture
of ferric chloride, (*see* Ferric chloride)
of iodine, (*see* Iodine, tincture of)
of opium, (*see* Morphine)
Tinsel (Christmas decoration), **740**
Tints, hair, poisonous substances in, 94t
Titanium, 35t, 94t, 114t, 255, 269, 270t
dioxide, 95t, 331t, 536
oxide, 271
tetrachloride, 203, **270-271**
Titan Oil Disinfectant, 531t
TMTD (Tetramethyl thiuram disulfide), 735t
TNT (Trinitrotoluene), 202, **204-205**
Toad *(Bufus marinus),* 590-591
Toxicologic
analysis, **86-88**

tests, "general unknown", **85-86**
Toadfish, 585
Tobacco, 8t, 158t, 313t, 546t, **655**
Indian, (*see* Indian tobacco)
nicotine content (cigarettes), 655
wild *(Nicotiana glauca),* 544(t)
wood (Witch hazel), **657-658**
Tocopherol, 77
Tofranil (Imipramine), 14t, 117t, 358t, 359, 371, 443, 472, 491t, 514t
Toilet
articles, **532-537**
bowl cleaners, **525-526,** 720
composition of, 524t
poisonous substances in, 96t
soap bars, **525**
Tok-Tik, 169t
Tolazamide, 429
Tolazoline hydrochloride (Priscoline hydrochloride), 501t
Tolbutamide (Orinase), 15t, 112t, 118t, 122, 124t, 209, 214t, 340, 343t, 347t, 429, 455, 501t, 503t, 516t
Tolonium (Blutene), 11t, 203
chloride (Toluidine blue), 203
Tolseram (Mephenesin), 492t
Toluazotoluidine (Amidoazotoluene), 482t
Toluene, 15t, 87t, 94t, 96t, 202, **225-226,** 247t, 516t, 609, 636, **658-659,** 730t
diisocyanate (TDI), 226, 247t, 313t, 659
Toluenesulfonate, sodium, 522t, 523t
potassium, 523t
Toluidine, 12t, 202, **203-204**
blue (Blutene), 203
Toluol, 94t, 271t
Tomato, wild *(Solanum carolinense),* 358t, 544(t)
Tonics, 610
skin, poisonous substances in, 94t
Top, 169t
Topzol Rat Baits, 200t
Topzol Rat Killing Syrup, 201t
Tornado Roach & Pest Killer, 169t
Torpedinidae (Rayfish), 590
Torpedo (Rayfish), 587t
Toxane, 169t
Toxaphene (Chlorinated camphene), 98t, 126, 129, 130t, 159t, 161t, 163t, 164t, 165t, 166t, 169t, 195t, 731, 734t
Toxic
Christmas decorations, **739-741**
combustion products of common substances, pulmonary irritants, toxic gases, Table 154(648)
episodes in the fetus and infant, **102-103**
hepatitis, **75-82** (with tables)
Toxicological screening tests, **89-91**
Toxicology, **84-88**
veterinary, **604-607**
Toxic Substances Control Act (1976), 273
Toxins (food poisoning), **711-714**
Toxocariasis (Visceral larva migrans), 592
Toxoid, tetanus, 567, 568, 589, 592
Tox-plan, 169t
*Toxpneustes elegans* (Red sea urchin), 587t
Tox-Sol, 169t
TPN (Triphosphopyridine nucleotide), (*see* Triphosphopyridine nucleotide)
Trace metals, 203, **269-270**
average levels of, Table 69(270)
*Trachnius draco* (poisonous fish), 590
Trains, model, **740-741**
Tramine, 470
Tranquilizer(s), 11t, 85f, 118t, 366 (*see also* Psychtropic agents, Table 107[368-369])
miscellaneous, 369t
reactions in the aged, 345t
Tranquilizing drugs, **370-376**
interaction with alcohol, Table 60(214)
tricyclic antidepressants, **472-474**
Transaminase, serum, 241
Transferrin, 432
Transfusions,
blood, **63-64**
exchange, **63-64,** 153
Tranxene, (*see* Clorazepate)
Tranylcypromine (Parnate), 65t, 334t, 501t
Travert, 385
Treatment, (*see also* specific poisons)
general principles of, **42-47, 720-721**
of convulsions, Table 30(72)
of fish stings, **585-589**
of poisoning, **31-47** (with tables)
Treburon, 501t
Trecator (Ethionamide), 356t
Tree-Mist, 169t
Treflan (Trifluralin), 182, **184,** 188t
Trematode diseases (zoonoses), 597t
Trematol, 540
Tremolite, 319
Trepidone (Mephenoxalone), 117t
Trest, (*see* Methixene hydrochloride)
Triacetyloleandomycin, 430
Triad Metal Cleaner, 531t
Triad Metal Polish, 531t
Triamcinolone, 15t, 69, 415t
Triamterene (Dyrenium), 10t, 11t, 15t, 418, 502t
Triavil, (*see* Amitriptyline)
Tribasic calcium phosphate, **395**
Tribromoethane (Bromoform), 484t
Tribromoethanol (Avertin), 20t, 32, 72t, 471, 516t
Tribromosalicylanilide, 522t
*Tribulus terrestris* (Puncture vine), 548t
Tricalcium phosphate, **655**
Trichinosis, 711
Trichlorfon (Dipterex; Dylox; Neguvon), 137t
Trichloride,
acetylene, (*see* Trichloroethylene)
antimony, 155, 373
ethylene, (*see* Trichloroethylene)
Trichlormethiazide (Naqua; Metaphydrin), 469
Trichloroacetates, 734t
Trichloroacetic acid, 200t, 206, 271t, 408, 655
salts of, 196t
Trichloro-bis-(p-chlorophenyl) ethane (Chlorophenothane; DDT), 130t
Trichloro-bis (p-methoxyphenyl) ethane (Methoxychlor), 130t
Trichlorocarbanilide (TCC degradation), 12t, 522t
Trichloroethane (Methyl chloroform), 87t, 96t, 202, **207,** 247t, 250, 516t, 524t, 609, 730t
Trichloroethanol, 408
Trichloroethylene, 65t, 86, 87t, 94t, 96t, 190, 202, **205-206,** 208, 247t, 271t, 426, 605t, 725, **728,** 730t
Trichloroisocyanurate(s), 233t
Trichloromethane (Chloroform), 202, **206-207**
Trichloromonofluoromethane (Freon-11), 87t
Trichlorophenol, 182
2,4,5-Trichlorophenol (weed killer), 311
2,4,5-Trichlorophenoxyacetic acid (2,4,-5-T), 115, 182ft
Trichlorophenyl, 165t
Triclane Household Spray, 172t
Tri-Clene Dry Clean, 531t
Tri-Cop, 201t
Tricyclic(s), 359, 427, 449, 455
antidepressant drugs, 15t, 16t, 81t, **472-474**
secondary amines, 65t
tertiary amines, 65t
Tridacna (Giant clam), 583
Tridione (Trimethadione), 72t, 80t, 98t, 345t, 360, 362t, 455
Triethanolamine, 95t, 96t, 197t, 533
hydroxide, 183
soaps, 524t
Triethylene,
glycol, 95t
melamine (TEM), 455, 502t
Triethyl phosphate, 96t
Triethylenethiophosphoramide (TSPA; Thio-TEPA), 397t
Tri-Excel Dust Concoction, 169t
Trifluoperazine (Stelazine), 77, 118t
Triflupromazine (Vesperin), 15t
Trifluralin (Treflan), 182, **184,** 188t
*Trifolium* (clovers), 548t
Triglycerides, 347t
Triglycollamate, bismuth sodium (Bistrimate), 12t, 391
Trihexyphenidyl (Artane), 104t, 143
Trihydrate, sodium diethyldithiocarbamate (Dithiocarb, (*see* Dithiocarb)
Trikop, 201t
Trilafon (Perphenazine), (*see* Perphenazine)
Trimaterene plus hydrochlorothiazide, 488t

Trimethadione (Tridione), 15t, 72t, 80t, 143t, 312, 345t, 347t, 360, 362t, 455
Trimethobenzamide (Tigan), 516t
3,4,5-Trimethoxyphenylethylamine (Mescaline), 102t
Trimethyl alkyl ammonium chloride, 653
Trimeton, (*see* Prophenpyridamine maleate)
Trimipramine (Surmontil), 472
Trinitrate, glyceryl, **449-450**
Trinitrophenol (Picric acid), **456**
Trinitrotoluene (TNT), 10t, 12t, 15t, 202, **204-205,** 331t
Tri-Ogen Rose Bomb, 169t
Trional (Sulfonethylmethane), 7t, 8t, 12t, 456, **468**
Tri-ortho-cresyl-phosphate (Machine oil), 202, **219-221**
Triox, 201t
Trioxide
  arsenic, (*see* Arsenic trioxide)
  chromium, (*see* Chromium trioxide)
  sulfur, (*see* Sulfur trioxide)
Trioxone, 201t
Triparanol (MER/29), 143t, 502t
Tripelennamine (Pyribenzamine), 103, 340, **364-367,** 453, 611
  hydrochloride, 15t
Triphenylmethane dye, 609
Triphosphopyridine nucleotide (TPN), 337, 338, 344
Triple D-Dust, 201t
Triple dye, 628ft, 629
Triple-X Rat Poison, 201t
Tripolyphosphate, sodium, 233t, 519, 520, 522t, 523t, 524t
Tris-BP (tris [2-3 dibromopropyl] phosphate), 656
  as flame retardant, 656
Tris-hydroxymethyl aminomethane (Tris; Tromethamine; Tham), 58
Tris (Tromethamine; Tris-hydroxymethyl aminomethane), 58
Trisodium
  edetate, 253
  phosphate, 96t, 522t, 523t, 524t, 616t
Tri-Spray, 169t
Trisulfide
  antimony, 737
  phosphorus, 151
Trithion (S- [p-chorophenylthio] -methyl-O, O-diethyl phosphoro-dithioate), 52t, 132t
Tritium, 65t
Troleandomycin (Tao), 80t
Trolene, 169t
*Trombicula* (mites), **580-581**
Tromethamine (Tris; Tris-hydroxymethyl aminomethane), 58, 81t, 389
Tromexan ethyyl acetate (Ethyl biscoumacetate), 110t, 117t
Tropines, 365t, 366t
Trox, 201t
True rattlesnake *(Crotalus),* **561-562,** 564f
Trypsin, 543
Tryptamine, beta-phenylethylamine, 442
Tryptophan, 190
Tubocurarine chloride, dimethyl, **415**
Tumbleweed, 201t
Tung nut *(Aleurites fordii),* 544, 554t
  oil, 544
Tungsten, thoriated, 269, 657
Turkey red oil, **656**
Turpentine, 4f, 8t, 82, 87t, 94t, 95t, 98t, 202, **226,** 247t, 479, 730t
  oil of, 224, 645, **728**
Turps, (*see* Turpentine, oil of)
Tussock moth, 579
Twenty X-N, 169t
Twin Light Dieldrin-Thane Dust, 169t
Twin Light Gam Dust No.1, 169t
Twin Light Granular Chloro Dust, 169t
Twin Light Malathion-Perthane Dust, 169t
Twin Light Nu Spray, 169t
Twin Light Para Dust No.1, 169t
Twin Light Rat-Away, 201t
Twin Light Sabadust, 169t
Tybamate (Solacen; Tybatran), 502t
Tybatran, (*see* Tybamate)
Tylenol, (*see* Acetaminophen)
Typewriter cleaner, poisonous substances in, 96t
Tyramine, 215t, 442, 443
  in foods and beverages, 333, Table 125(444)
Tyrosinase, 180, 372
Tyzine, (*see* Tetrahydrozoline hydrochloride)

**U**

Ulcers, gastroduodenal, role of drugs in, Table 90(345)
Ultran, (*see* Phenaglycodol)
Ultra-Violet Absorbing Lotion (UVAL), 456
Umbelliferae (parsley family), 545
Undecyclenic acid, 502t
Uniform Hazardous Substances Act, (*see* Federal Uniform Hazardous Substances Act of 1960)
United Chemical Clorblor Weed Killer, 201t
United Chemical Ester Weed Killer, 201t
United Chemical Garden Unifume, 201t
United Chemical General Weed Killer, 201t
United States . . . (*see* U.S.)
Univalve mollusks (Gastropods) 584
Universal antidote, **45**
University Brand Grain Fumigant, 201t
Unopette #5820, 132
Uracil mustard, 143t
Uranium, 82t, 270t
Urates, 10t
Urchins, sea, 585, 587t
Urea, 70, 71, 116, 194t, 387, 438, 621, 631
*Urechites suberecta* (Yellow nightshade), 554t
Uremic toxins, 65t
Urethane, 77, 502t
Uric acid, 65t, 404, 480, 481, 516t
Uricosuric agents, 409
Urine
  colored by drugs, Table 2(10)
  discolored by drugs, Table 3(11)
  Forrest rapid color tests, Figure 14(372)
  toxicologic analysis of, 9, 10
*Urobatis halleri* (Stingray), 587t
Urobilin, 144
Urobilinogen, 144
Urokon (Acetrizoate), 482t
Urox, 188t
Ursol D (Para-phenylenediamine), 534
Urticaria, materials and industrial exposures associated with, Table 75(313)
Urushiol resin, 538
U.S. Consumer Product Safety Commission, 656, 738ft
U.S. Department of Agriculture (USDA), 142, 702, 714, 732
U.S. Department of Labor, 316
U.S. Naval Research Laboratory, 583
U.S. Public Health Service, 256, 312, 316, 335t
  aspects of food poisoning, 713
  drinking water standards, 450
U.S. Sanitary Specialties Moth Flakes, 201t
U.S. Sulfur Fumigating Candles, 201t
UVAL, (*see* Ultra-Violet Absorbing Lotion)
Uva ursi, **656**

**V**

Vaccination(s)
  influenza, 110t
  smallpox, 110t
Vaccine(s), 17t, 340, 347t
  duck embryo, 593ft
  human diploid cell, 593ft
Vacor (N-3 pyridylmethyl N-p-nitrophenol urea), 173, **174-175,** 179t
VACOR Ratkiller, 174
Valerian *(Valeriana officinalis),* 546t
Valeric acid, 613
Valium, (*see* Diazepam)
Valmid, (*see* Ethinamate)
Valone (Warfarin), 173, **177**
Valpin, (*see* Anisotropine)
Vanadium, 9t, 114, 269, 270t, **474**
Vancocin, (*see* Vancomycin)
Vancomycin (Vancocin), 16t, 65t, 357t
Vanish Detergent, 531t
Vapam, 187t
Vapomite 1-3 Dust, 169t
Vapona (2,2-Dichlorovinyl dimethyl phosphate), 136, 137t, 169t
Vapophos Citrus Spray, 169t

Vapophos Dust, 169t
Vapophos Liquid Spray, 169t
Vapor(s)
  gasoline, 202, **244-245**
  infrared analysis of, Table 35(87)
  maximum concentration of, Table 66(247)
Vaposector, 169t
Vapotone, 170t
Varidase, (*see* Streptokinase-streptodornase)
Varnishes, poisonous substances in, 94t
Varsol (Stoddard solvent), (*see* Stoddard Solvent)
Vasopressin (Pitressin), 502t
Vasoxyl (Methoxamine), 446
Vegetable
  dye, poisonous substances in, 96t
  oil, as a demulcent, 83
Vel, 531t
Velban (Vinblastine sulfate), 399t
Velvet, blue, **611-612**
Vendex (Hexakis distannoxane), 581
Venom(s)
  bee, 82t, 578
  black widow spider, 52t
  caterpillar, 579
  cobra, 565, 568
  coral snake, 52t
  scorpion, 574
  sea snake, 589
  snake, 8t, 15t, 52t, 82t
  spider, 82t, 573
Venomous copperhead *(Agkistrodon mokeson),* **562**
Veratramine (Veratrum), **474-475**
Veratrine, 7t, 9t, 42, **474-475,** 540
Veratrum, 9t, 35t, 62t, **474-475**
*Veratrum viride* (False hellebore), 540, 541f, 550t
Verdasan, 201t
Vermouth, causing fixed eruptions, 346t
Vermox (Mebendazole), 354t
Vernax Beauty Cream for Furniture, 531t
Veronal, (*see* Barbital)
Vernolate (Vernam), 188t
Versenate, calcium disodium, (*see* EDTA)
Versene (Ethylenediamine tetraacetate), (*see* EDTA)
Vesprin (Triflupromazine), 15t
Vetches *(Vicia),* 548t
Veterinary
  association, working with poison control centers, 698
  toxicology, **604-607**
Viadril, (*see* Hydroxydione succinate sodium)
*Vibrio parahaemolyticus,* **715**
*Vicia* (vetches), 548t
*Vicia faba* (Fava bean), 7t, 550t, 718
Vinbarbital (Delvinal), 383t
Vinblastine sulfate (Velban), 143t, 399t
Vincristine, 143t, 348t
  sulfate (Oncovin), 400t
Vinegar, 526
  diluted, 83, 233t, 234t
Vines, borer control, **731**
Vinethene (Divinyl ether), 426
Vintox, 170t, 201t
Vinyl acetate, 314
Vinyl chloride, 87t, 149, 312, 314, 331t
Vinylidene chloride, 87t
Viocin, (*see* Viomycin)
Viomycin (Viocin), 340, 357t, 437t
Vio-Serpine (Reserpine), 110t
Vipers, (*see* Pit vipers)
Virus diseases (zoonoses), 599-602t
  arthropod-borne, 599-601t
  not arthropod-borne, 602t
Vistaril (Hydroxyzine), 15t, 118t, 490t, 573
Vitamin(s), 11t, 118t, 143t, **475-479**
  A, 17t, 327, 334t, 347t, 475, 476t, 477t, 478, 502t, 536, 708t
  $B_1$ (Thiamine hydrochloride), 20t, 502t complex, 152, 334t, 436, 476t, 536
  $B_6$, 476t, 477
  $B_{12}$, 347t, 476t, 477, 478
  C, 180, 334t, 475, 476t, 477(t), 536, 632
  D, 255, 475, 476t, 477(t), 479, 502, 708t
  daily requirements, Table 127(477)
  drugs capable of producing deficiencies, **477**
  E, 327, 334t, 422, 476t
  electron transport (riboflavin, nicotinic acid), 476t
  fat soluble (A,D,K,E), 347t, 476t
  K, 20t, 22t, 55t, 475, 477, 502t
    analogues, 110t, 334t, 338t, 341, 343t, 476t
  $K_1$
    emulsion (Mephyton), 19t
    (Menadione), 152
    oxide, 361
    (Synkayvite), 42, 179t
    Synthetic water soluble, 191
  nucleogenic ($B_{12}$, $B_6$-pyridoxine, folic acid) 476t
  physiologic requirements, Table 126(476)
  used in aquariums, 610
Vitriolic acid, **656**
Vivactil, (*see* Protriptyline hydrochloride)
Vodka, 212
Volatile(s), **85-86**
  oils, 9t, **479-480,** 610, 613, 657
Volk Isotox Spray, 170t
Vomiting, drugs used to induce (emetics), **42-46**
Vontrol, (*see* Diphenidol)
Voo-Doo, 42, 201t
Voo-Doo White Magic Mouse Killer, 201t


**W**


Wahoo *(Euonymus atropurpureus),* 549t
Wallpaper cleaner, poisonous substances in, 96t
Warfarin (Panwarfin; Pival; Valone; Acetonylbenzyl hydroxycoumarin), 55t, 173, 177, 604, 734t
  sodium (Coumadin sodium; Prothromadin), 110t, 143t, 179t, 194t, 195t, 196t, 197t, 198t, 199t, 200t, 201t, 502t, 516t
Warficide Rat Killer, 201t
War gas(es), (*see* Gases, war)
Washing soda, 4f, 85, 721
Wasp, **575-580,** 741, 742
  polistes, 577
Waspfish, 585
Watch cleaners, poisonous substances in, 95t
Water
  ammonia, 31, 94t, 721
    concentrated, 28
  contamination of, 17
  drug-induced malabsorption, 347t
  effects with certain solutes, Table 23(57)
  gas, 240
  glass, **656**
  guide to maintaining body needs and correcting fluid deficits, Table 24(57)
  intoxication, 65t
  lime, **36,** 83 (*see also* Calcium hydroxide)
  starch, as a demulcent, 83
Water hemlock *(Cicuta maculata),* 545, 554t, **718**
Water moccasin *(Agkistrodon piscivorus),* **562,** 564f
Water pollutants, Table 80(330)
Water pollution, **330-331**
Wax(es)
  carnauba, 95t
  crayons, 12t
    poisonous substances in, 95t
  for furniture and floors, poisonous substances in, 94t
  removers, poisonous substances in, 94t
Weather plant, 541
Weaverfish, 585
Weed(s)
  bishop's, 537
  broom, 539
  Jamestown, 544
  jimson, 358t, 376, 539, 544, 545, 551t
Weed A Bomb, 201t
Weedane Aero-Concoction, 201t
Weed-Bane, 201t
Weed-B-Gon, 201t
Weeded, 201t
Weeder, 64, 201t
Weedeth, 201t
Weedicide, 201t
Weed killer(s), 98, 311

Weed-No-More, 201t
Weednox, 201t
Weedone Sodar, 201t
Weedster, 201t
Weevils, 742
Wekill, 201t
Welding hazards, **656-657**
Western poison oak (yeara), 539
Westicide, 170t
West Pine Deodorant, 531t
West Rid-All, 170t
Whale(s), killer *(Orcinus orca),* 586t
Wheel bug, 576f
Whelk, red *(Neptunea antique),* 582
Whiskey, 212, 216
White
  moth, 579
  of egg, *see* Egg white
  phosphorus, 736, 737
  shark (Isuridae family), 586t
  snakeroot *(Eupatorium rugosum, urticaefolium),* 539
  -tipped shark (Carcharinidae family), 586t
Whitepine Disinfectant, 531t
Wick, poisonous substances in, 95t
Wigraine tablets and suppositories, 425t
Wilbert's Fresh Pine Deodorant, 531t
Wild
  grape *(Rhiocissus cuneifolia),* 554t
  hydrangea, 551t
  monkshood *(Aconitum uncinatum),* 554t
  onions, 539
  sage *(Lantana camara),* 358t
  tobacco *(Nicotiana glauca),* 554t
  tomato *(Solanum carolinense),* 358t, 544, 545, 554t
Will-Kill Bug Killer, 170t
Wilson Cleaner, 531t
Wilson Elect-O-Weed, 201t
Wilsonol, 170t
Wilson's disease, 109, 147
Wilson's Tri Rose, 201t
Windex, 531t
Windsor bean, (*see* Fava bean)
Wine, 212, 443t, 444t
Winru Pyrenone Fly Spray, 170t
Winstrol, (*see* Stanozolol)
Winter bloom (Witch hazel), **657-658**
Wintergreen, oil of, 4f, 224
Wireworm control in sweet potatoes, **731**
Wisteria *(Wisteria sinensis),* 554t
Witch hazel *(Hamamelis virginiana),* **657-658**
Wolfsbane, 350
Wonder Rodenticide, 201t
Wood
  alcohol, 213, 649, **727-728**
  dust, 313t
  naphtha, 95t, 727
  spirits, (*see* Wood alcohol)
  tar, 453, 455, 618
  tick, 580
Woodbrite Furniture Polish, 531t
Wooly worm *(Megalopge opercularis),* 579
Workmen's Compensation Act, 273
World Health Organization, 124, 335t, 558
  Expert Committee on Rabies, 603
Worms, annelid, 583, 585, 587t
Wormseed, causing fixed eruptions, 346t
Wormwood *(Artemisia absinthium),* 546t
Worm, wooly, (*see* Wooly worm)
Wrasse family (fish poisoning), 582
Wright's Silver Cream, 531t
WW 42, 201t
Wyamine (Mephentermine), 22t, 104t, 567
Wyseals (Meprobamate), 110t

**X**

Xanthines, **480-481,** 632
  derivatives, 394
  oxidase inhibitor, 404
X-It Rat and Mouse Poison, 201t
X-O Deodorant, 531t
XXX (Triple) Alcufe Fungicide, 201t
XXX (Triple) DDT Spray, 201t
XXX (Triple) Endrin Spray, 201t
XXX (Triple) Flowable 75, 201t
XXX (Triple) Liquid Thrip-Tox, 201t
XXX (Triple) Tox-R, 201t
XXX (Triple) Unicide, 201t
XXX (Triple) Vigrocide, 201t
XXX (Triple) Zinc Nutraspray 20, 201t
Xylene, 7t, 87t, 95t, 96t, 184, 247t, 502t, 523t, 609, 636, **658-659,** 730t
o-Xylene, 87t
m-Xylene, 87t
p-Xylene, 87t
Xylocaine, ( **see** Lidocaine)
Xylols, (*see* Xylene)
Xylose, 347t

**Y**

Yage, 99
Yarrow, 539
Yeara (Western poison oak), 539
Yeast, brewer's, 20t, **33**
Yellow
  cedar (thuja), 655
  jacket, **575-580,** 741, 742
  jessamine *(Gelsemium sempervirens),* 6t, 489t, 551t
  nightshade *(Urechites suberecta),* 554t
  phosphorus, 736
  resin, **645**
Yew *(Taxus baccata),* 544, 554t
Yohimbine, 98, 546t

**Z**

Zarontin (Ethosuximide), 345t, 361, 363t, 514t
Zebrafish, 585
Zelio, 201t
Zephiran chloride (Benzalkonium chloride), 484t, 502t, 519, 584,
Zest soap, 531t
Zinc, 65t, 94t, 114, 119, 197t, 203, 252t, **268-269,** 270t, 516t, 524t, 608, 611, 614t, 623, **716,** 741
  chloride, 268, 611
  chromate, 331t
  cyanide, **268**
  dichromate, **268**
  ethylene bisdithio carbamate, 195t
  oxide, 96t, **268,** 331t, 611, 612, 736
    fume, 331t
  phenosulfonate, 94t
  phosphide, 173, **174,** 734t
  salts, 201t, 268, 269
  stearate, **268**
    oxide, 95t
  sulfate, 44, 45, 49t, 83, 98t, **268-269,** 616t
  sulfide, 626
  trichlorophenate, 195t
Zineb (Dithiocarbamate), 181, 196t, 199t
Ziram (Dithiocarbamate), 181
Zirconium, 270t
  oxide, 536
  salt, 95t, 536
Zoonoses, **591-603**
  epidemiological aspects of some, Table 145(594-602)
Zotox Crab Grass Killer, 201t
Zoxazolamine (Flexin), 502t, 516t
Zurd Rodenticide, 201t
Zwikker's test, 93t
Zygadenine, 540
*Zygadenus* (Camas lily, death camas), 540, 550t
Zyloprim (Allopurinol), 16t, 79t, 404, 481, 482t

## PUBLIC INSTRUCTION

## FIRST AID TREATMENT FOR INJURY

A PHYSICIAN SHOULD BE CALLED IMMEDIATELY FOR ALL SERIOUS INJURIES OR SUSPECTED POISONING.

BRUISES—Rest injured part. Apply cold compresses for half hour (no ice next to skin). If skin is broken, treat as a cut. For wringer injuries always consult physician without delay (signs of hemorrhage, swelling, soft-tissue and muscle injury may not appear immediately).

SCRAPES—Use wet gauze or cotton to sponge off gently with clean water and soap.

CUTS—Minor—Wash with clean water and soap. Hold under running water. Apply sterile gauze dressing. Major—Apply dressing. Press firmly to stop bleeding—use tourniquet only if necessary. Bandage. Secure medical care. Do not use iodine or other antiseptics before the physician arrives.

PUNCTURE WOUNDS—Consult physician immediately.

SLIVERS—Wash with clean water and soap. Remove with tweezers or forceps. Wash again. If large or deep, consult physician.

NOSEBLEEDS—In sitting position blow out from the nose all clot and blood. Insert into the bleeding nostril a wedge of cotton moistened with any of the common nose drops. With the finger against the outside of that nostril apply firm pressure for five minutes. If bleeding stops remove packing (no rush, here). Check with your doctor if bleeding persists.

FAINTING AND UNCONSCIOUSNESS—Keep in flat position. Loosen clothing around neck. Summon physician. Keep patient warm. Keep mouth clear. Give nothing to swallow.

CONVULSIONS—Contact physician. If caused by fever, sponge body with cool water, apply cold cloths to head. Lay on side with hips elevated. Prevent biting of tongue with folded handkerchief between teeth.

HEAD INJURIES—Do not move unless additional danger would occur to injured persons. Consult physician immediately.

POISONING—See First Aid for Poisoning Chart.

BITES OR STINGS—A) INSECT—Remove stinger at base if present. Do not squeeze stinger as it is removed. Cold compresses. Consult physician promptly if there is any reaction. B) ANIMAL—Wash with clean water and soap. Hold under running water for two or three minutes if not bleeding profusely. Apply sterile dressing. Consult physician. If possible, catch or retain the animal and maintain alive for observation regarding rabies. Notify police or health officer. C) SNAKE—Non-Poisonous—No treatment necessary. If there is a question, treat as "Poisonous." Poisonous—(Keep calm & work fast.) Complete rest. Suction and apply constricting band above the bite (not too tight). Get victim to physician or hospital immediately. D) HUMAN—Wash thoroughly with soap and water. Notify or see physician.